CONSUMER HEALTH

A Guide to Intelligent Decisions

Seventh Edition

CONSUMER HEALTH

A Guide to Intelligent Decisions

STEPHEN BARRETT, M.D.
Author, Editor, Consumer Advocate
Board Chairman, Quackwatch, Inc.
Allentown, Pennsylvania

WILLIAM T. JARVIS, PH.D.
Professor of Public Health and Preventive Medicine (Retired)
Schools of Medicine and Public Health
Loma Linda University
Loma Linda, California

MANFRED KROGER, PH.D.
Professor Emeritus of Food Science
Professor Emeritus of Science, Technology and Society
The Pennsylvania State University
University Park, Pennsylvania

WILLIAM M. LONDON, ED.D, M.P.H.
Associate Professor of Health Care Management
Director, Graduate Program in Health Care Management
College of St. Elizabeth
Morristown, New Jersey

McGraw-Hill
A Division of The McGraw·Hill Companies

CONSUMER HEALTH: A GUIDE TO INTELLIGENT DECISIONS
SEVENTH EDITION

Published by McGraw-Hill, a business unit of The McGraw-Hill Companies, Inc., 1221
Avenue of the Americas, New York, NY 10020. Copyright " 2002, 1997, 1993, 1989,
1985, 1980, 1976 by The McGraw-Hill Companies, Inc. All rights reserved. No part of
this publication may be reproduced or distributed in any form or by any means, or stored
in a database or retrieval system, without the prior written consent of The McGraw-Hill
Companies, Inc., including, but not limited to, in any network or other electronic storage
or transmission, or broadcast for distance learning.

Some ancillaries, including electronic and print components, may not be available to
customers outside the United States.

 This book is printed on recycled, acid-free paper containing 10% postconsumer waste.

1 2 3 4 5 6 7 8 9 0 QPD/QPD 0 9 8 7 6 5 4 3 2 1

ISBN 0–07–232366–3

Vice president and editor-in-chief: *Thalia Dorwick*
Executive editor: *Vicki Malinee*
Senior developmental editor: *Melissa Martin*
Senior marketing manager: *Pamela S. Cooper*
Project manager: *Richard H. Hecker*
Production supervisor: *Enboge Chong*
Coordinator of freelance design: *David W. Hash*
Cover designer: *Lisa Gravunder*
Cover illustration: *Linda Frichtel*
Senior photo research coordinator: *Lori Hancock*
Supplement producer: *Jodi K. Banowetz*
Compositor: *Shepherd, Inc.*
Typeface: *11/13.2 Times*
Printer: *Quebecor World Dubuque, IA*

Library of Congress Cataloging-in-Publication Data

Consumer health : a guide to intelligent decisions / Stephen Barrett . . . [et al.]. æ 7th ed.
     p.   cm.
   Includes index.
   ISBN 0- 07- 232366- 3
     1. Medical care. 2. Health products. 3. Quacks and quackery. 4. Consumer education.
   I. Barrett, Stephen, 1933-   . II. Cornacchia, Harold J. Consumer health.

 RA410.5 .C645   2002
   362.1ædc21   2001030923
                                                                  CIP

www.mhhe.com

Stephen Barrett, M.D., a retired psychiatrist who resides in Allentown, Pennsylvania, has achieved national renown as an author, editor, and consumer advocate. In addition to heading Quackwatch, Inc., he is Vice-President and Director of Internet operations of the National Council Against Health Fraud (NCAHF); a scientific adviser to the American Council on Science and Health (ACSH); and a Fellow of the Committee for the Scientific Investigation of Claims of the Paranormal (CSICOP). In 1984, he received an FDA Commissioner's Special Citation Award for Public Service in fighting nutrition quackery. In 1986, he was awarded honorary mem-bership in the American Dietetic Association. From 1987 through 1989, he taught health education at The Pennsylvania State University. Since 2000 he has been listed in *Marquis Who's Who in America*. In 2001 he received the Distinguished Service to Health Education Award from the American Association for Health Education.

An expert in medical communications, Dr. Barrett operates five Web sites; edits *Consumer Health Digest* (a free weekly electronic newsletter); writes a weekly column for Canoe.ca; is medical editor of Prometheus Books; and is a peer-review panelist for several top medical journals. His 48 books include *The Health Robbers: A Close Look at Quackery in America* and six editions of this book. His other major works include *Dubious Cancer Treatment*, published by the Florida Division of the American Cancer Society; *Health Schemes, Scams, and Frauds*, published by Consumer Reports Books; *The Vitamin Pushers: How the "Health Food" Industry Is Selling America a Bill of Goods*, published by Prometheus Books; and *Reader's Guide to "Alternative" Health Methods*, published by the American Medical Association. His Quackwatch Web site, which serves as a clearinghouse for information on health frauds and quackery, has won more than 50 honors and awards.

William T. Jarvis, Ph.D., is an expert on the psychology, sociology, and epidemiology of quackery. He recently retired as Professor of Public Health and Preventive Medicine at Loma Linda University, where he taught courses dealing with controversial health practices. He founded and served for many years as president of NCAHF. He is a scientific adviser to ACSH and co-chairman (with Dr. Barrett) of CSICOP's paranormal health claims subcommittee. He has been a featured speaker at many health-fraud conferences and testifies in court and at government hearings on controversial health matters. He has served on the American Cancer Society's committee on questionable methods and wrote the society's booklets, "Questionable Methods of Cancer Management" and "Helping Your Patients Deal with Questionable Cancer Treatments." He also co-authored the American Dietetic Association's 1995 position paper on nutrition misinformation.

Manfred Kroger, Ph.D., is Professor Emeritus of Food Science and Professor Emeritus of Science, Technology and Society at The Pennsylvania State University, where he has won several teaching awards. He also serves as associate editor of the *Journal of Food Science*, a scientific adviser to ACSH, a technical editor for Prometheus Books, and a science communicator for the Institute of Food Technologists. He has conducted research in analytical chemistry (pesticide residues), food composition, fermented milk products, and dairy processing technology. Even though retired, he remains professionally active at Penn State, nationally, and internationally. His university courses included food laws and regulations, toxicology, introductory food science, dairy technology, and a very popular university-wide general education course entitled "Food Facts and Fads." His other professional activities include lecturing at public and professional meetings, expert testimony in court and at government hearings, and translation of German writings. In 1999 he was elected a Fellow of the Institute of Food Technologists.

William M. London, Ed.D., M.P.H., is Associate Professor of Health Care Management and Director of the Graduate Program in Health Care Management, College of St. Elizabeth, Morristown, New Jersey; a specialized faculty mentor in the Master of Science in Public Health program of Walden University; and President of NCAHF. He is also a scientific consultant to CSICOP. He has been an associate professor at Kent State University where, for 10 years, he taught health-education courses, including consumer health. During this period he co-founded and served as the first President of the Ohio Council Against Health Fraud. He has also been Director of Public Health of ACSH; Director of Communications at Columbia University's Mailman School of Public Health; and Executive Director of RAP, Inc., a private nonprofit mental health and senior citizens service agency in Genesee County, New York. He is an accomplished writer and editor with extensive knowledge of public health, controversial health issues, health policy, risk communication, and public relations.

You can gain a great deal from this book if you're interested in:

- Nutrition
- Physical fitness
- Bodybuilding
- High-level wellness
- Choosing trustworthy health-care professionals
- Participating actively in your care
- Accessing high-quality information sources
- Avoiding health rip-offs
- Getting more for your health dollar

More is known about achieving and maintaining good health today than ever before. Life expectancy is at an all-time high; and, although there is still room for improvement, health-related accomplishments have exceeded the fondest dreams of past visionaries. In 1890, when life expectancy at birth was 37 years, the imaginative Jules Verne predicted that in 1000 years the life expectancy would reach 58 years! In fact, it doubled to more than 74 years in less than a century. This progress has been due, in part, to a biologically safer environment: cleaner water, food, and living space. But we hear plenty of bad news about these, and it worries us. Medical care, both preventive and therapeutic, has made important contributions, yet we worry about the risks associated with immunization, cancer therapies, prescription drugs, surgery, and many other treatment modalities. How can we resolve our concerns and reap the benefits of what modern science is discovering about health? The key is to be informed about what is happening in the health marketplace.

Unfortunately, the explosion in knowledge about health has been matched by enormous increases in health misinformation. Worse yet, health misinformation is much more readily available than the sound information people really want. In 1984 a congressional subcommittee reported that Americans wasted billions of dollars on worthless and unproven health remedies. Medical quackery was found to be the No. 1 consumer fraud problem among the nation's elderly population. The congressional report estimated that more was spent on cancer and arthritis quackery than on research into cures for those diseases.

The promotion of dubious health practices is not limited to the elderly or sick. Young, healthy people are the targets of supplements; devices; weight-control plans; and products aimed at fulfilling dreams of the body beautiful, superior athletic performance, exceptional mental ability, and more. Quackery has something for everyone because we all have wishes that exceed reality.

The entrepreneurs who market dubious health practices are clever and persistent. They exploit the public's enthusiasm for healthful living and self-help. Their promotions far outstrip school and public health education efforts aimed at consumer protection and encouraging positive health behavior. In fact, the spread of health misinformation has itself become an industry and is the foundation upon which the purveyors of dubious health products and services rely. Individuals who spread the misinformation are protected by the First Amendment, which guarantees freedom of speech. A cadre of writers produce books, magazine articles, newsletters, pamphlets, and Web sites that promote quackery—much of which they now call "alternative" or "complementary" medicine. Misinformation that would be illegal on product labels or in advertisements is spread by modern mass-media techniques. Health theories and claims are repeatedly extolled on radio and television talk shows whose celebrity hosts make such claims appear legitimate. The Internet has greatly expanded the ability of shady operators to promote their wares.

Another aspect of modern quackery's modus operandi is multilevel marketing. Its pyramid-type schemes capitalize on people's financial ambitions. Its participants encourage their friends and relatives to become "satisfied users" so they, too, can "believe in" their products—an essential factor for successful selling. Their judgment becomes clouded by self-interest and a general inability to separate real from imagined effects of health practices. Cable television is used to amplify testimonials into the siren call of quackery on a national scale. Average consumers are no match for such promotionalism.

Health hucksters are aided by those who claim that consumer protection laws constitute overregulation. "Freedom of choice" is their battle cry, but a careful examination reveals this argument to be a red herring. It is quacks who seek the freedom to sell worthless and unproven health products and services to unwary consumers. True freedom of choice cannot be exercised by people who have been deceived or driven by desperation. Yet many lawmakers think our laws should be weakened rather than strengthened.

Consumers exist in a crisis of confidence and wonder who can be trusted for reliable health information. Consumer advocacy calls for justice and fair play in the marketplace. But many self-appointed "consumer advocates" do not act in the public's interest. Although some are sincere and make a contribution, others use their role to simply engage in irrational business-bashing, advance political causes, or act from motives of personal aggrandizement. Occasionally, business trade associations and lobbies even pose as "consumer groups" and seek self-serving legislation. This is where academic consumer health education comes in. Con-

sumer protection laws are based on fundamental principles—inseparable from those of science—including the Consumer Bill of Rights. These provide standards that can unmask the pretenders to consumerism.

Consumer Health offers a kaleidoscopic view of today's complex and exciting health marketplace. It can help you to become a more intelligent consumer and equip you to be a better citizen. Its message is twofold: "You can do much for yourself through good decision-making," but "buyer beware!" It reveals the tremendous innovation of the purveyors of quackery at a time when more caution than ever is needed in making choices in the health marketplace. It also advises what to do when you encounter deceptive practices.

Stephen Barrett, M.D.
William T. Jarvis, Ph.D,
Manfed Kroger, Ph.D.
William M. London, Ed.D., M.P.H.

Preface for Instructors

Consumers regularly must confront the complicated and confusing health marketplace where *caveat emptor* (let the buyer beware) is the dominant philosophy. The rapid expansion of medical science has created innumerable new health products and services. Many of these receive considerable publicity before they have been adequately subjected to scientific study.

Consumers often have difficulty in making intelligent decisions about products and services that are useless, worthless, or hazardous. Quacks, pseudoscientists, many advertisers, many journalists, and a multitude of well-intentioned promoters spread vast amounts of misinformation. Fraud and deception are rampant. Consumers are bilked out of billions of dollars each year, and many suffer loss of health as well. Unfortunately, government and community agencies provide far less protection than most people realize. Navigating the legitimate avenues of the health marketplace can also be difficult and complex.

Consumers who wish to protect their health and their pocketbooks therefore must shop with great care. They must become accurately informed. They must learn how to identify and use reliable sources of information. They must accept responsibility and speak out when they are victims of fraud and deception. They must raise objections to dubious products and services and report them to the appropriate regulatory agencies.

Goal for This Revision

This seventh edition of *Consumer Health* continues to emphasize the economic aspects of health and the social and psychologic factors that influence consumer choices. As with previous editions, *the book's fundamental purpose is to provide science-based facts and guidelines to enable consumers to select health products and services intelligently.* Its data have been selected from thousands of reliable reports in books, scientific journals, and other periodicals, as well as original investigations done by the book's authors. Consumers will find the information useful in applying the *caveat vendor* (let the seller beware) concept to the health marketplace.

The underlying principles of consumer health were identified in the Consumer Bill of Rights promulgated by President John F. Kennedy and have guided the development of this textbook. President Kennedy declared that consumers have the right to purchase safe products and services, to be correctly informed, to freely choose products and services, and to be heard by the government and others when injustices occur. We strongly support consumer awareness and advocacy of these rights.

Intended Audience

Consumer Health will be helpful to teachers, health educators, health professionals, and to the general public. It can be used as a basic text or for supplementary reading in courses such as consumer health, health education, consumer education, sociology, psychology, home economics, social welfare, and business. School districts will find *Consumer Health* useful as a reference for teachers and students, as well as an aid in curriculum development. Professional health-care providers can use this text to prepare for public presentations and can make it available in their offices for perusal by clients.

Timeliness of References

Every topic in this book has been carefully researched. In most cases, the more than 1700 cited references represent the latest authoritative information we could locate. Some references may appear outdated because they are 5 to 10 years old. Unless otherwise stated, however, we believe these still reflect the current marketplace. References more than 10 years old are included either for historical reasons or because they provide insights that are still timely. Chapter 1 provides information on how to read citations and locate references. Those that may be especially useful for students seeking additional information are listed with boldface numbers.

Features

All features from the sixth edition have been retained. Many chapters contain vignettes ("Personal Glimpses") to stimulate reader interest and "Consumer Tip" boxes that emphasize key points. Many checklists and "It's Your Decision" boxes reflect "real-life" decisions that readers may face. The "Key Concepts" box at the beginning of each chapter states what we believe are the most important lessons to be learned from the chapter material. Extensive searching of the scientific literature and personal investigation by the authors have provided information to update the contents of this edition. New material on "alternative" health care, dietary supplements, fad diets, herbs, hormone-replacement therapy, magnetic products, dubious cancer treatments, and questionable mental help procedures reflects an explosion of media interest in these topics, plus new information made available by investigative reporters. The nutrition chapter has been revised to incorporate the latest dietary guidelines. Other new topics include disability insurance, prenatal care, delivery options, and other women's health concerns.

The most important feature of this edition is its integration with the Internet. The Internet section of Chapter 2 has been expanded. References that are available in full text on the Internet are underlined. A special Web site (http://www.chsourcebook.com) provides links to many full-text articles and to abstracts of most of the journal articles. Suggestions for course objectives, teaching/learning activities, a sample course outline, and links to hundreds of organizations that provide reliable information are also posted.

Students and instructors are welcome to subscribe to *Consumer Health Digest*, a free weekly e-mail newsletter edited by Dr. Stephen Barrett. (To subscribe, see http://www.ncahf.org/digest/chd.html.) Relevant new items will also be posted in a "Chapter Update" section.

Organization

As in the sixth edition, the text is broadly divided into six parts:

Dynamics of the Health Marketplace focuses on past and present problems. After defining the major consumer health issues, it discusses how the scientific method is used to determine medical truths, how consumers can separate fact from fiction, how frauds and quackery can be identified, and how advertising and other marketing activities influence consumer decisions.

Health-Care Approaches covers basic medical care, the services of many types of science-based and

"alternative" practitioners, self-care, and health-care facilities.

Nutrition and Fitness integrates what consumers need to know about the extremely important topics of nutrition, weight control, and exercise. Its chapters provide the necessary tools for distinguishing between science-based methods and fads, fallacies, and scams.

Major Health Problems covers four of the leading causes of death and disability in our society: cardiovascular disease, arthritis, cancer, and AIDS.

Other Products and Services covers a myriad of other subjects that affect most, if not all, consumers. These include drug products; skin care and beauty aids; contraceptive methods; vision and hearing aids; and other devices.

Protection of the Consumer focuses on legal and economic issues involved in protecting consumers. These include death-related issues, health insurance, other economic issues, consumer-protection laws and agencies, and strategies for intelligent consumers.

The *Appendix* provides comprehensive lists of agencies, organizations, and publications that offer reliable information. The Consumer Health Sourcebook Web site links to most of them.

The *Glossary* continues to include many useful items not discussed elsewhere in the book.

Acknowledgments

No book like this could have been written without help from many experts and other providers of information. The authors offer special thanks to Robert S. Baratz, M.D., D.D.S., Ph.D.; Judith N. Barrett, M.D.; John E. Dodes, D.D.S.; and Timothy N. Gorski, M.D., F.A.C.O.G., each of whom reviewed part of the text.

The photograph on page 169 is reproduced with permission from Aurora & Quanta Productions, Portland, Maine.

Two members of McGraw-Hill's staff guided the book's planning and production: Vicki Malinee, whose vision made publication possible and Melissa J. Martin, our steadfast project coordinator. Freelance editor Sarah E. Fike, of Belleville, Illinois, did a superb job of copy editing.

Contents

I. DYNAMICS OF THE HEALTH MARKETPLACE

1. Consumer Health Issues, 3
Misleading Information, 4
Quackery and Health Fraud, 7
Problems with Products, 8
Problems with Services, 9
Problems with Costs, 10
The Need for Consumer Protection, 11
Intelligent Consumer Behavior, 12

2. Separating Fact from Fiction, 15
How Facts Are Determined, 16
Problems with Health Information, 20
Prudent Use of the Internet, 28
Further Suggestions for Consumers, 30

3. Frauds and Quackery, 35
Definitions, 36
Frauds and Quackery Today, 37
Why People Are Vulnerable, 38
Hazards, 39
Common Misconceptions, 40
Recognizing Quackery, 42
Conspiracy Claims, 44
The Freedom-of-Choice Issue, 44

4. Advertising and Other Marketing Practices, 47
Psychologic Manipulation, 48
Puffery, Weasel Words, and Half-Truths, 50
Advertising Outlets, 50
Professional Advertising, 51
Marketing by Hospitals, 53
Prescription Drug Marketing, 53
Nonprescription Drug Advertising, 55
Food Advertising, 56
Dietary Supplement Promotion, 56
Tobacco Promotion, 59
Mail-Order Quackery, 60

Weight-Control Promotions, 63
Youth and Beauty Aids, 63
Exercise and Fitness Products, 63
Infomercials, 64
Multilevel Marketing (MLM), 64
Telemarketing Schemes, 66
Industry Self-Regulation, 66
Government Regulation, 67

II. HEALTH-CARE APPROACHES

5. Science-Based Health Care, 71
Health-Care Personnel, 72
Choosing a Physician, 76
Basic Medical Care, 80
Surgical Care, 87
Quality of Medical Care, 89
Disciplining of Physicians, 91
The Intelligent Patient, 94

6. Mental Health Care, 99
Who Should Seek Help?, 100
Mental Health Practitioners, 100
Psychotherapy, 102
Drug Therapy, 103
Electroconvulsive Therapy, 105
Psychosomatic Disorders, 105
Selecting a Therapist, 105
Hospital Care, 107
Questionable "Self-Help" Products, 107
Questionable Practices, 109

7. Dental Care, 119
Dentists, 120
Auxiliary Dental Personnel, 120
Tooth Decay, 121
Fluoridation, 122
Periodontal Disease, 123
Self-Care, 124
Dental Products, 124
Dental Restorations, 127

Endodontics (Root Canal) Therapy, 127
Orthodontics, 128
Dentures, 128
Dental X-Ray Procedures, 129
Questionable Procedures, 130
Dental Quackery, 130
Smokeless Products, 133
Choosing a Dentist, 134

8. "Alternative" Methods, 137
Definitional Problems, 138
Acupuncture, Qigong,
    and "Chinese Medicine," 141
Reflexology, 144
Chiropractic, 144
Naturopathy, 151
Natural Hygiene, 152
Iridology, 153
Homeopathy, 154
Psychic Healing, 158
Occult Practices, 162
Astrology, 164
Biorhythms, 164
Transcendental Meditation, 165
Yoga Therapy, 167
Visual Training, 167
Other "Alternative" Practices, 167
Unscientific Medical Practices, 168
"Holistic Medicine," 172
"Medical Freedom" Laws, 173
The NIH Center for Complementary and
    Alternative Medicine, 174

9. Self-Care, 179
Purposes of Self-Care, 180
Health Promotion, 181
Self-Diagnosis, 184
Home Medical Tests, 185
Self-Treatment of Chronic Diseases, 187
Self-Help Publications, 188
Self-Help Groups, 189

10. Health-Care Facilities, 195
The Joint Commission, 196
Outpatient Medical Facilities, 196
Hospitals, 199
Home Care Services, 201
Nursing Homes, 202

III. NUTRITION AND FITNESS

11. Basic Nutrition Concepts, 211
Major Food Components, 212
Human Nutrient Needs, 214
Food-Group Systems, 219
"Junk Food," 222
Dietary Guidelines for Infants, 222
Vegetarianism, 224
Nutrients of Special Concern, 225
Nutrition Labeling, 226
Reliable Information Sources, 230

12. Nutrition Fads, Fallacies, and Scams, 233
Food Faddism and Quackery, 234
Dietary Supplements, 235
Megavitamin Claims vs. Facts, 242
Appropriate Use of Supplements, 244
"Organic" Foods, 245
"Health Foods," 246
"Natural" Foods, 246
"Medicinal" Use of Herbal Products, 251
Macrobiotic Diets, 254
Promotion of Questionable Nutrition, 254
Promoters of Questionable Nutrition, 263

13. Weight Control, 271
Basic Concepts, 272
Eating Disorders, 278
The Diet and Weight-Loss
    Marketplace, 278
Questionable Diets, 278
Prescription Drugs, 283
Nonprescription Products, 284
Low-Calorie Products, 287
Questionable Products and Procedures, 289
Government Regulatory Actions, 291
Surgical Procedures, 292
Weight-Control Organizations, 292
Suggestions for Weight Control, 295

14. Exercise Concepts, Products, and
    Services, 301
Public Perceptions, 302
Benefits of Exercise, 303
Types of Exercise, 304
Components of Fitness, 304
Starting an Exercise Program, 306
Sports Medicine Specialists, 310

Exercise Equipment and Supplies, 311
Exercise Facilities, 319
Children's Exercise Centers, 322
Exercise While Traveling, 322
Corporate Fitness Programs, 323
Exercise and Weight Control, 323
Nutrition for Athletes, 323
Anabolic Steroids, 325
Other "Ergogenic Aids," 326

IV. MAJOR HEALTH PROBLEMS

15. Cardiovascular Diseases, 333
Significance of Cardiovascular
    Disease, 334
Risk Factors for Coronary Heart
    Disease, 334
Blood Lipid and Homocysteine Levels, 335
Cholesterol Guidelines, 336
Dietary Modification, 340
Lipid-Lowering Drugs, 346
Preventive Use of Aspirin, 347
Questionable Preventive Measures, 348
High Blood Pressure, 349
Heart Attacks, 351
Diagnostic Tests, 352
Surgery to Restore Blood Flow, 354
Rehabilitation Programs, 355

16. Arthritis and Related Disorders, 359
Types of Arthritis, 360
Scientific Treatment Methods, 361
Susceptibility to Quackery, 364
Questionable Treatment Methods, 365
Sources of Information, 370
Guidelines for People with Arthritis, 371

17. Cancer, 373
Risk Factors for Cancer, 374
Preventive Measures, 375
Diagnosis, 375
Prognosis, 375
Evidence-Based Treatment Methods, 376
Diet and Cancer, 376
Susceptibility to Cancer Quackery, 379
Questionable Methods, 381
Promotion of Questionable Methods, 390
Reliable Information, 392

Treatment Guidelines, 392
Consumer Protection Laws, 392

18. AIDS, 395
Course of the Disease, 396
Testing Procedures, 397
Prevention, 397
Treatment, 399
Treatment Costs, 399
AIDS-Related Quackery and Fraud, 400

V. OTHER PRODUCTS AND SERVICES

19. Drug Products, 407
Medication Types, 408
Pharmacists, 409
Prescription Drugs, 410
Generic vs. Brand-Name Drugs, 411
Drug Interactions, 412
Drug Recalls, 415
Internet Pharmacy Sales, 415
Innovations in Drug Delivery, 415
Over-the-Counter Drugs, 416
FDA's OTC Review, 417
Allergy Products, 418
External Analgesics, 420
Internal Analgesics, 421
Antacids and H_2 Blockers, 423
Antibiotics, 424
OTC First-Aid Antimicrobials, 426
"Aphrodisiacs" (Alleged Sex
    Enhancers), 426
Remedies for Common Foot Problems, 427
Cough and Cold Remedies, 427
Sore-Throat Products, 429
Diarrhea Remedies, 429
Ophthalmic Products, 429
Alleged Hangover Products, 430
Hemorrhoidals, 430
Iron-Containing Products, 431
Laxatives, 431
Motion Sickness Remedies, 433
Sleep Aids, 433
Smoking Deterrents, 434
Stimulants for Fatigue, 434
Home Medicine Cabinet, 436
Prudent Use of Medication, 436

20. Skin Care and Beauty Aids, 441
 Cosmetic Regulation, 442
 Soaps, 442
 Moisturizers, 443
 Questionable Claims, 444
 OTC Tretinoin, 445
 Fade Creams, 446
 Antiperspirants and Deodorants, 446
 Acne Care, 446
 Hair and Scalp Care, 447
 Hair Loss, 449
 Sun Protection, 451
 Cosmetic Surgery, 452
 Laser Phototherapy, 456
 Camouflage Cosmetics, 456

21. Especially for Women, 459
 Menstrual Products, 460
 Menstrual Problems, 460
 Vaginal Hygiene, 462
 Vaginitis, 462
 Contraception, 463
 Voluntary Abortions, 468
 Infertility, 469
 Genetic Testing and Prenatal
  Counseling, 469
 Pregnancy and Delivery, 470
 Infant Feeding, 471
 Osteoporosis, 471
 Hormone-Replacement Therapy, 472
 Mastectomy Prostheses, 473

22. Health Devices, 477
 Medical Device Regulation, 478
 Vision Products and Services, 480
 Hearing Aids, 486
 Dubious Water Purifier Promotions, 489
 Humidifiers, 489
 Personal Emergency Response Systems,
  490
 The Latex Allergy Epidemic, 490
 Quack Devices, 491

23. Coping with Death, 495
 Advance Directives, 496
 Donations of Organs and Tissues, 499

 Hospice Care, 501
 Euthanasia and Assisted Suicide, 502
 Reasons for an Autopsy, 503
 Body Disposition, 503
 Grief and Mourning, 506
 Life-Extension Quackery, 507

VI. PROTECTION OF THE CONSUMER

24. Health Insurance, 513
 Basic Health Insurance, 514
 Major Medical Coverage, 516
 Contract Provisions, 516
 Types of Plans, 517
 Medicare, 519
 Medicaid, 522
 Long-Term Care Insurance, 522
 Dental Insurance, 523
 Loss Ratios, 523
 Indemnity vs. Managed Care, 524
 Medical Savings Accounts, 525
 Choosing a Policy, 525
 Collection of Insurance Benefits, 527
 Disability Insurance, 529

25. Health-Care Economics, 531
 Health-Care Costs, 532
 Cost-Control Methods, 536
 Insurance Fraud and Abuse, 540
 National Health Insurance (NHI), 541

**26. Consumer Laws, Agencies, and
  Strategies, 547**
 U.S. Food and Drug Administration, 548
 Federal Trade Commission, 558
 U.S. Postal Service, 561
 Other Federal Agencies, 563
 State and Local Agencies, 563
 Nongovernmental Organizations, 563
 Consumer Action, 567

**Appendix: Reliable Sources of
  Information, 569**
 Federal Government Agencies, 570
 Nongovernmental Organizations, 570

Glossary, 573

Index, 585

PART I

DYNAMICS OF THE HEALTH MARKETPLACE

Chapter One

CONSUMER HEALTH ISSUES

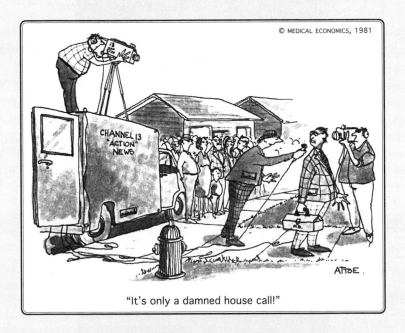

© MEDICAL ECONOMICS, 1981

"It's only a damned house call!"

Today everything that is wrong with the American health care system threatens everything that is right.

HILLARY RODHAM CLINTON[1]

A great deal of public confusion exists about who is a competent health authority.

JAMES HARVEY YOUNG, PH.D.[2]

Quackery—the promotion and sale of useless remedies promising relief from chronic and critical health conditions—exceeds $10 billion a year. The cost of quackery in human terms, measured in disillusion, pain, relief forsaken or postponed because of reliance on unproven methods, is more difficult to measure, but nonetheless real. All too often the purchaser has paid with his life.

CONGRESSMAN CLAUDE PEPPER[3]
QUACKERY—A $10 BILLION SCANDAL

Key Concepts

KEEP THESE POINTS IN MIND AS YOU STUDY THIS CHAPTER

- To get the most out of our health-care system, consumers must be knowledgeable and appropriately assertive.
- Virtually all legitimate health products and services have bogus counterparts.
- Intelligent consumers maintain an appropriate level of skepticism.
- Consumer protection agencies are unable to deal with many of the complaints they receive.
- Everyone in a free society has a stake in maintaining high standards in the health marketplace.

Consumer health encompasses all aspects of the marketplace related to the purchase of health products and services. It includes such things as buying a bottle of vitamins, a cold remedy, a dentifrice, or exercise equipment and selecting a physician, dentist, insurance policy, book, or other source of information. Consumer health has both positive and negative aspects. Positively, it involves the facts and understanding that enable people to make wise choices. Negatively, it means avoiding unwise decisions based on deception, misinformation, or other factors. Worksheet 1-1 provides an opportunity to test your knowledge of consumer health issues.

This chapter comments on misleading information; quackery; health frauds; and problems with products, services, and costs. It also outlines the strengths and weaknesses of consumer-protection forces and the characteristics of intelligent consumers.

MISLEADING INFORMATION

Health information has become increasingly voluminous and complex. Even well-trained health professionals can have difficulty sorting out what is accurate and significant from what is not. Table 1-1 lists questions faced by many of today's consumers.

The media have tremendous influence. Thousands of radio and television stations broadcast health-related news, commentary, and talk shows. Thousands of magazines and newspapers carry health-related items, and

Worksheet 1-1

TEST YOUR CONSUMER HEALTH I.Q.

1. Everyone should have a complete physical every year or two.   T F
2. Fluoride toothpaste works so well that water fluoridation is no longer important.   T F
3. It is difficult for busy people to eat a balanced diet.   T F
4. People intelligent enough to graduate from college are unlikely to be victimized by quackery.   T F
5. Accreditation of a school indicates that a regulatory agency considers its teachings sound.   T F
6. Cigarette smoking is the leading cause of preventable death in the United States.   T F
7. Sugar is a major cause of hyperactivity and other childhood behavioral problems.   T F
8. No special training is legally required to offer counseling to the public.   T F
9. Taking antioxidant vitamins has been proved to protect against heart disease, stroke, and cancer.   T F
10. Homeopathic remedies are a safe and effective alternative to many drugs that doctors prescribe.   T F
11. Taking large daily doses of vitamin C can cut the incidence of colds in half.   T F
12. People over age 21 should have their blood cholesterol level checked every year.   T F
13. The U.S. Postal Service screens many ads for mail-order health products before they are published.   T F
14. The American Medical Association can revoke the license of a doctor who is practicing improperly.   T F
15. Recent government reports indicate that the best person to consult for back pain is a chiropractor.   T F
16. Most health-food retailers are well informed about the products they sell.   T F
17. Protein or amino acid supplements help bodybuilders and other athletes improve their performance.   T F
18. The emergency department of a nonprofit hospital is a relatively inexpensive place to get medical care.   T F
19. Natural cancer cures are being suppressed because drug companies don't want competition.   T F
20. Most health-related books and magazine articles undergo expert prepublication review.   T F

Only #6 and #8 are true. Fifteen correct answers suggests that you are fairly well informed. Twenty correct suggests that you are very well informed.

Table 1-1

CONSUMER HEALTH QUESTIONS

How can the significance of research reports be judged?

How trustworthy are the media? How can reliable information sources be located?

What are the best ways to keep up-to-date on consumer health issues?

How can quacks and quackery be spotted?

What should be done after encountering quackery or health fraud?

Is it sensible to try just about anything for health problems?

How should advertisements for health products and services be analyzed?

How should physicians, dentists, and other health-care specialists be selected?

What should be done about excessive or unreasonable professional fees?

When is it appropriate to obtain a second opinion about recommended surgery?

What periodic health examinations are advisable? How much should they cost?

Where can competent mental help be obtained?

What kinds of toothbrushes and dentifrices are most effective?

Can mouthwashes and dentifrices control the development of plaque on teeth?

When are dental implants appropriate?

Do silver amalgam fillings pose any health hazard?

What rights should buyers and sellers have in the health marketplace?

How trustworthy are chiropractors, naturopaths, and acupuncturists?

Is it advisable for people with back pain to see a chiropractor?

Are over-the-counter pregnancy test kits reliable?

When are self-diagnosis and self-medication appropriate?

How should a hospital, nursing home, or convalescent facility be selected?

What are the pros and cons of using an ambulatory health-care center?

How can a balanced diet be selected?

Does vegetarian eating make sense?

When is it appropriate to use vitamin or mineral supplements?

Should extra vitamins be taken during pregnancy?

Should "organic foods" or "health foods" be purchased? Are they worth their extra cost?

Can taking vitamin C supplements prevent or cure colds?

Will taking calcium supplements help prevent osteoporosis?

Will taking antioxidants prevent future diseases?

Are any herbal products worth taking?

How trustworthy is the advice given in health-food stores?

Are food additives dangerous?

What is the safe way to lose and control weight? Are diet pills helpful or harmful?

Are electric vibrators and massage equipment useful for weight control or body shaping?

Which exercise equipment provides the greatest benefits? The fewest benefits?

Is it a good idea to join a health club or exercise center?

What principles should guide the use of blood cholesterol levels?

Can wearing a copper bracelet help arthritis?

Can any food or dietary measures prevent or influence the course of arthritis or cancer?

Are any AIDS remedies effective?

How do pain-relievers compare?

Should laxatives be used? By whom?

Is it a good idea to use generic drugs?

What products are appropriate for a home medicine cabinet?

What is the best strategy for protecting against sun exposure?

Can any product help to grow, restore, or remove hair?

Can wrinkles be removed with any product or with plastic surgery?

What forms of birth control are safest and most effective?

Are any over-the-counter drug products effective for menstrual cramps?

What can women do about premenstrual syndrome (PMS)?

Does the patenting of a health device ensure its safety and effectiveness?

How do the different types of contact lenses compare?

Who should determine the need for eyeglasses, contact lenses, or a hearing aid?

Are refractive surgery procedures safe and effective?

Does it make sense to prepay funeral expenses?

What can be done to limit extraordinary medical care if someone is terminally ill?

Which health coverage provides the best protection?

How can consumers reduce their health-care costs?

How much money should be budgeted for health care?

What agencies and organizations help protect consumers?

Are all consumer groups trustworthy?

How can one register a complaint about a health product or service?

thousands of health-related books and pamphlets are published each year. The *Star, Globe,* and other tabloids sell millions of copies weekly and influence many people's health behavior. Over 3000 books in print recommend unscientific health practices. The information available through the Internet and other computer channels is multiplying rapidly.

Gunther[4] has noted that the mass media have four main functions: to entertain, to inform, to carry advertisements, and to make money for their stockholders. In many cases what is transmitted depends on (a) how much it is expected to interest the target audience, and (b) how advertisers may feel about it. Larkin, for example, has noted that many women's magazines publish sensational claims and deliberately avoid information that might upset their advertisers.[5]

Fast-breaking news should be regarded cautiously. Many reports, though accurate, tell only part of the story. Unconfirmed research findings may turn out to be insignificant. The simplest strategy for keeping up-to-date is to subscribe to newsletters that place new information in proper perspective (see Chapter 2).

Advertising should also be regarded with caution (see Chapter 4). Many advertisers use puffery, "weasel words," half-truths, pictures, or celebrity endorsements to misrepresent their products. Some marketers use scare tactics to promote their wares. Some attempt to exploit common hopes, fears, and feelings of inadequacy.

◆ **Personal Glimpse** ◆

Doctors and Patients in Cyberspace

Physicians were once able to carry in their little black bags most of the tools needed to diagnose and treat patients. They could store in their own minds the information necessary for the majority of their work. Experience broadened one's ability to handle difficult or unusual cases, and patients relied upon their physicians as the primary source of information on both health and disease.

The logarithmic increase in biomedical knowledge over the last three decades has changed the doctor-patient relationship dramatically. The history and physical examination, once the basis for all medical practice, are now only the first exploratory steps in the process of making a diagnosis and planning a treatment regimen. The immense proliferation of laboratory tests, imaging techniques and diagnostic procedures is stunning. The specialties of medicine have further branched into subspecialties as basic research and clinical knowledge have greatly expanded. Medical journals and textbooks have multiplied in number, along with the arrival of new means of information delivery.

No individual physician, no matter how capable or experienced, is able to absorb and memorize more than a small portion of this database. This is true despite the fact that convenient access to the information is developing rapidly. One can search the literature rapidly with the National Library of Medicine's MEDLINE service to discover the latest in diagnosis, treatment and outcome for any disease, common or rare. Electronic textbooks are lavishly illustrated with high-quality images, and link the user (physician or layperson) directly to the references cited.

With the rapid growth and popularization of the Internet, access to the universe of medical information has been fundamentally altered. Physicians and the public may draw on the resources of medical discussion groups and reference databases with unprecedented ease.

But a new dilemma comes with this wonderful advance. For decades, inquisitive patients have turned to health letters and magazines to supplement the information gained from consultation with their physician. These publications filled a gap in doctor-patient communication. As demands on the physician's time have multiplied, the explanations offered patients are too often cursory and incomplete. As the concept of individual responsibility for health has grown, the computerized medical database has broadened the patient's horizons. Encyclopedias and other reference works on CD-ROM now put a "doctor on a disk." Interactive software has likewise placed diagnosis in the hands of patients, who can enter their symptoms into a formula and receive a digital assessment with suggestions for proper treatment. It is too early to analyze the virtues and problems of the information revolution. But some are obvious.

For example, a World Wide Web query for the keyword "health" found . . . documents, ranging from commercial health products and alternative therapies to issues of sexuality, obesity, aging, and environmental health. The *sci.med* Internet discussion forums, and others offered by the commercial online computer services, enable a patient to inquire electronically about an individual medical problem. The validity of the responses varies greatly and is often impossible to determine. Since even physicians can have difficulty sorting out the truth in cyberspace, imagine the problem for the average person browsing the Internet.

Michael Kashgarian, M.D.[6]

Cigarette ads use images of youth, health, vigor, and social acceptance to convey the opposite of what cigarette smoking will do to smokers. Alcohol ads stress fun and sociability and say little about the dangers of excessive drinking. Many ads for cosmetics exaggerate what they can do (see Chapter 20). Food advertising, though not usually deceptive, tends to promote dietary imbalance by emphasizing snack foods high in fat and calories.

Radio and television talk shows abound with promoters of health misinformation. Although many authoritative publications are available, greater numbers of books, magazines, and newsletters promote false ideas. Chapter 2 discusses this problem in detail and provides guidance on choosing reliable sources.

QUACKERY AND HEALTH FRAUD

Quackery is definable as the promotion of a false or unproven method for profit (see Chapter 3). Fraud involves deceit. Despite tremendous progress in medical science and health education, Americans waste billions of dollars each year on products and services that are unsubstantiated or bogus. Dr. William Jarvis[7] calls quackery "a national scandal." Barrett and Herbert have noted:

People generally like to feel that they are in control of their life. Quacks take advantage of this fact by giving their clients things to do—such as taking vitamin pills, preparing special foods, meditating, and the like. The activity may provide a temporary psychological lift, but believing in false things can have serious consequences. The loss may be financial, psychological (when disillusionment sets in), physical (when the method is harmful or the person abandons effective care), or social (diversion from more constructive activities). . . .

Quacks portray themselves as innovators and suggest that their critics are rigid, elitist, biased, and closed to new ideas. Actually, they have things backwards. The real issue is whether a method works. Science provides ways to judge and discard unfounded ideas. Medical science progresses as new methods replace less effective ones. Quack methods persist as long as they remain marketable.[8]

Quackery promoters are adept at using slogans and buzzwords. During the 1970s their magic sales word was "natural." During the 1980s the word "holistic" was popularized. Today's leading buzzword is "alternative." This term is misleading because methods that do not work are not reasonable alternatives to proven treatment. This textbook places the word "alternative" in quotation marks when referring to unsubstantiated methods that lack a scientifically plausible rationale. Chapter 8 discusses "alternative" methods in detail.

◆ Personal Glimpse ◆

Caveat Emptor

In 1990 in Duluth, Georgia, before getting ready for his high school prom, a teenager drank water mixed with two teaspoons of *Somatomax PM*, a powdery substance a friend had bought at a health-food store. He had heard it would give him a "high." It did not. Within 20 minutes he became comatose. Fortunately, his parents found him in time, but without prompt emergency treatment he might not have survived.

The substance was gamma-hydroxybutyrate (GHB), a product touted to build muscle, reduce fat, and induce sleep. It was sold under various names in health-food stores, bodybuilding and fitness centers, and through the mail. GHB is dangerous and was never approved for general distribution by the Food and Drug Administration (FDA). After the agency collected 57 cases of GHB-related illness, it initiated criminal charges against the local manufacturer. Poisonings were reported in at least nine states.[9] No deaths occurred, but most patients required emergency care.

Health-food stores sell hundreds of products claimed to build muscles and reduce fat. Most are harmless, except to one's budget, but none work.

Most people think of themselves as hard to fool. Yet the majority of Americans are victims of quackery. Contrary to popular beliefs, for example: (a) most people who take vitamin supplements don't need them; (b) vitamins do not make people more energetic, more muscular, or less stressed; (c) "organically grown" foods are neither safer nor more nutritious than conventionally produced foods; and (d) no nonprescription pill can produce rapid or permanent weight loss. Chapters 3, 12, and 13 cover these subjects thoroughly.

Victims of quackery usually have one or more of the following vulnerabilities:

LACK OF SUSPICION: Many people believe that if something is printed or broadcast, it must be true or somehow its publication would not be allowed. People also tend to believe what others tell them about personal experience.

DESPERATION: Many people faced with a serious health problem that doctors cannot solve become desperate enough to try almost anything that arouses hope. Many victims of cancer, arthritis, multiple sclerosis, and AIDS are vulnerable in this way.

ALIENATION: Some people feel deeply antagonistic toward scientific medicine but are attracted to methods that are "natural" or otherwise unconventional. They may also harbor extreme distrust of the medical profession, the food industry, drug companies, and government agencies.

BELIEF IN MAGIC: Some people are easily taken in by the promise of an easy solution to their problem. Those who buy one fad diet book after another fall into this category.

OVERCONFIDENCE: Despite P.T. Barnum's advice that one should "never try to beat a man at his own game," some strong-willed people believe they are better equipped than scientific researchers and other experts to tell whether a method works.

PROBLEMS WITH PRODUCTS

In light of scientific and technologic advances, it is not surprising that many people believe that health is purchasable. The health marketplace abounds with products of every description to accommodate people's desires. The problem areas include dietary supplements, herbs, homeopathic products, exercise devices, diet pills and potions, self-help tapes and gadgets, youth and beauty aids, magnets, and many types of over-the-counter drug products.

Thousands of "supplement" products are marketed with false claims that they can boost energy, relieve stress, enhance athletic performance, and prevent or treat numerous health problems (see Chapter 12). Ads for "ergogenic aids" feature champion bodybuilders or other athletes without indicating that the real reason for their success is vigorous training. Few supplement products have any usefulness against disease, and most that do—such as niacin for cholesterol control—should not be taken without competent medical supervision.

Although some herbs sold for medicinal purposes are useful, most are not, and some are dangerous (see Chapter 12). Because the U.S. Food and Drug Administration (FDA) does not require standards of identity or dosage for herbal products, consumers may be unable to tell what the products contain or how to use them. Moreover, many of the conditions for which herbs are recommended are not suitable for self-treatment.

The vast majority of mail-order health products are fakes (see Chapter 4). The common ones include weight-loss products (mostly diet pills), "hair restorers," "wrinkle removers," and alleged sex aids. Figure 1-1 illustrates the flamboyant claims found in ads for mail-order diet pills.

Many worthless devices are claimed to "synchronize" brain waves, relieve pain, remove unwanted fat deposits, improve eyesight, relieve stress, and ward off

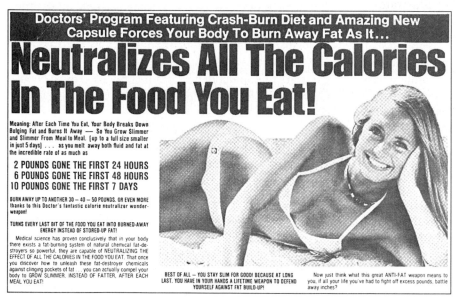

FIGURE 1-1. Ads for dubious mail-order products. The diet pill ad was published in many magazines during the late 1970s. Although no product can "neutralize calories" or fulfill the other promises in this ad, countless "weight-loss" products have been advertised in this way. The "nerve tonic" ad is from a 1996 flyer from a company that specializes in herbal products. Some of its statements about body physiology are true, but most are not related to each other, and the overall message is pseudoscientific gibberish. No ingredients are identified, and no product can remedy the long list of problems listed in the ad. Promotions like these persist in the marketplace because regulatory agencies lack the resources to control them; many people are unsuspecting enough to buy them; and many magazine and newspaper publishers value ad revenues more than ethics.

disease. Thousands of audiotapes and videotapes are marketed with false claims that they can help people lose weight, stop smoking, enhance athletic performance, quit drinking, think creatively, raise IQ, make friends, reduce pain, improve vision, restore hearing, cure acne, conquer fears, read faster, speak effectively, handle criticism, relieve depression, enlarge breasts, and do many other things (see Chapter 6). Magnets embedded in clothing, mattresses, or other products are falsely claimed to relieve pain, increase blood flow, boost immunity, and provide other health benefits (see Chapter 22).

Multilevel companies market a wide variety of health-related products, almost all of which are either inappropriate or overpriced (see Chapter 4). The products are sold by individual distributors who also attempt to recruit friends, neighbors, relatives, and others to do the same. More than a million people are involved in multilevel marketing.

Most over-the-counter drug products can be useful in self-care. However, many ads encourage pill-taking for insomnia, lack of energy, constipation, and other problems that may have better solutions. Homeopathic "remedies" are the only category of spurious products legally marketable as drugs. Figure 1-2 illustrates a product that contains no molecules of its alleged "active ingredient."

Exercise equipment varies greatly in quality, usefulness, and price. Before investing in equipment it is important to determine what it can do and whether it can meet one's needs or will be too monotonous for regular use (see Chapter 14). Some devices are gimmicks that have little or no effect on fitness.

PROBLEMS WITH SERVICES

Although health care in America is potentially the world's best, many practitioners fall short of the ideal, and some are completely unqualified.

Many physicians prescribe too many drugs, order too many tests, fail to keep up-to-date, or pay insufficient attention to preventive measures. Some do not spend sufficient time interviewing, examining, or advising their patients. Unnecessary surgery is also a significant problem. The percentage of physicians who furnish seriously deficient care is unknown. The Public Citizen Health Research Group (HRG)[10] has identified 13,012 medical and osteopathic physicians who were disciplined by state or federal agencies between 1985 and 1995. Some of these cases were not related to quality of patient care. Based on its analysis of the figures, HRG estimates that about 1% of physicians commit

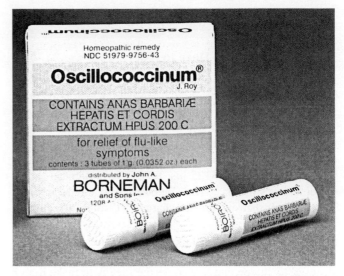

FIGURE 1-2. Homeopathic product "for the relief of colds and flu-like symptoms, such as fever, chills and shivering, body aches and pains." The box states that its active ingredient is "Anas barbariæ hepatis et cordis extractum HPUS 200C." This ingredient is prepared by incubating small amounts of a freshly killed duck's liver and heart for 40 days. The resultant solution is then filtered, freeze-dried, rehydrated, repeatedly diluted, and impregnated into sugar granules. The "200C" designation means that the dilution (1:100) is done 200 times. If a single molecule of the original substance were to survive the dilution, its concentration would be 1 in 100^{200}. The number 100^{200} is vastly greater than the estimated number of molecules in the universe. These numbers don't make sense, and neither does purchasing the product. Yet it is legal to market it as a nonprescription drug in the United States.

serious offenses each year, more than double the number actually disciplined.[11] These problems are addressed in Chapter 5.

Dodes and Schissel[12] warn that many dentists fail to get optimal results because they work too quickly (see Chapter 7).

Some optometrists fail to examine the eyes thoroughly when they prescribe glasses.

The mental health marketplace is replete with unqualified therapists, some of whom have no training whatsoever (see Chapter 6).

Many people who represent themselves as "nutritionists" lack adequate training and engage in unscientific and quack practices. A 1993 study sponsored by the National Council Against Health Fraud found that 58% of 618 Yellow-Page listings under the heading "Nutritionists" were either spurious or suspicious (see Chapter 12). Many commercial weight-loss clinics lack qualified personnel and promise too much in their advertising (see Chapter 13).

A wide variety of "alternative" practitioners engage in practices that are not science-based and have no proven value. This includes small percentages of medical and osteopathic physicians, large percentages of chiropractors and acupuncturists, and many others whose activities are described in Chapter 8.

The quality of care in hospitals and nursing homes varies considerably from one to another. The best ones have well-trained nurses who monitor their patients closely. In some facilities unlicensed personnel provide services for which they are not adequately trained. Patients confronted with a succession of tests and consultants may feel frustrated and bewildered if the reasons for them are not explained. Noise may interfere with getting adequate rest. In some nursing homes physical restraints or sedative drugs are used excessively, patients receive insufficient medical attention, and neglect by the nursing staff results in preventable

infections and bedsores. In 1995, following a lengthy investigation, *Consumer Reports* concluded that the quality of care at thousands of the nation's nursing homes was "poor or questionable at best" and that about 40% of the 16,000 facilities certified by the Health Care Financing Administration (HCFA) had repeatedly violated federal standards.[14] Hospitals and long-term care facilities are discussed in Chapter 10.

PROBLEMS WITH COSTS

Rising costs and lack of adequate insurance coverage have given rise to what many people call a health-care crisis. The cost of health care in the United States has risen about 11% a year from 1960 through 1990, about 8% from 1991 through 1993, and about 5% from 1994 through 1998. In 1998 it totaled $1.1 trillion ($4094 per person), which amounted to 13.5% of our gross domestic product (GDP).[15] In 1999 actuaries at the Health Care Financing Administration[16] estimated that the total would rise about 8% per year and would reach $2.2 trillion (16.2% of the GDP) by 2008.

In 1992 *Consumer Reports* estimated that overuse of medical services wasted at least $130 billion per year, and inefficient administration wasted about $70 billion more.[17]

In 1993, the White House Domestic Policy Council[1] concluded:

- The American health-care system was choked by paperwork and strangled by bureaucracy.
- Administrative costs were higher here than in any other country and were rising rapidly.
- Many consumers found insurance paperwork incomprehensible.
- In many cases, employers who chose insurance plans had the power to limit or determine the doctors and hospitals that their employees would use.
- Fraudulent claims were a serious problem.

About 44 million Americans have no health insurance and over 30 million more are underinsured.[18-20] The 1997 National Survey of Health Insurance Report found that 30% of uninsured persons said that cost had deterred them from getting needed medical care during the previous year, 55% had postponed care, and 24% did not fill a prescription.[21]

Attempts to control costs have included eliminating nonessential services. During the past few years, the number of people covered by managed-care programs has risen sharply. Although these programs tend to cut costs, they often restrict the freedom of patients to choose their treatment providers. Managed care can also result in decreased continuity of care. Suppose, for example, that an administrator decides that all patients with certain ailments (such as allergies or mental health problems) should see a specific physician who accepts a fixed annual fee from the program. Although this arrangement may save money for the program, it can force patients to abandon relationships with physicians who know them well.

Many wasted billions are attributable to "defensive medicine"—unnecessary procedures ordered in an effort to reduce the risk of a malpractice suit. Correction of this problem requires extensive changes in America's legal system that are staunchly opposed by the legal profession. The Clinton administration's health-reform proposals included many provisions for malpractice reform. Legislation embodying these proposals was introduced in 1993 but lobbying by business, hospital, and medical organizations quickly defeated it. Coverage of Medicare drug costs appears likely in the near future, but little attention to the other problems is expected.

The funeral industry has a disgraceful record of price-gouging. Many funeral directors fail to disclose costs, add dubious items to their bills, and/or pressure emotionally vulnerable survivors into spending more than necessary (see Chapter 23). Although comparison shopping or joining a memorial society can greatly lessen the cost of death care, many people are not in a position to do these things. Prepaid funeral plans that are badly managed or fraudulent are also a serious problem.[22]

THE NEED FOR CONSUMER PROTECTION

The *caveat emptor* doctrine ("let the buyer beware"), which originated in the Middle Ages, was based on the assumption that buyers and sellers had equal bargaining positions. This was reasonable because (a) goods (such as fresh vegetables and cloth) could be examined thoroughly for defects and (b) people bargained almost entirely with neighbors who risked severe social repercussions if they acted dishonestly. However, as trade expanded and technology advanced, it became apparent that individual caution is not enough. Even highly intelligent individuals may go astray in situations where they lack expert knowledge or are emotionally vulnerable.

Protective Forces
Today's consumers are protected, in part, by a myriad of forces that promote quality and fairness in the health marketplace.

The FDA is concerned about the safety, effectiveness, and marketing of foods, drugs, cosmetics, and medical devices. The FDA operates under powerful laws but lacks sufficient resources to handle the enormous number of violations it encounters. In addition, a recent campaign by the health-food industry and its allies has decreased the agency's ability to regulate claims for dietary supplements and herbs (see Chapters 12 and 26).

The Federal Trade Commission (FTC) has primary jurisdiction over most types of advertising. It administers a powerful law and has been enforcing it vigorously during the past few years.

The U.S. Postal Service (USPS) has jurisdiction over products sold through the mail. It administers a powerful law but has insufficient resources to deal with the vast number of frauds it encounters.

State attorneys general enforce several types of consumer-protection laws. In most states, however, few health-related cases are pursued.

Licensing laws set minimum requirements for training and knowledge but do not specify that practices must be science-based. Even physicians and dentists are not required by law to practice according to scientific principles, although they generally do so. The quality of state regulation varies from state to state and from board to board. Many licensing boards lack the resources to investigate all of the complaints they receive. Those that oversee chiropractors, naturopaths, and acupuncturists do almost nothing to protect consumers.

Accreditation agencies set standards for education and quality of care. Those serving schools for the science-based professions do an excellent job. Those that oversee chiropractic, naturopathy, and acupuncture schools make little or no effort to prevent unscientific teachings (see Chapter 8). Accreditation of hospitals, nursing homes, and other health-care facilities generally increases the quality of their care, but it also adds greatly to the cost of administering that care.

Hospitals oversee the activities of their staffs (see Chapter 10). Those that do so effectively provide a very valuable consumer-protection service to their communities.

Insurance companies and other third-party payers can refuse to cover services that are excessive or unsubstantiated. State legislatures and courts sometimes force them to pay for inappropriate treatment.

Professional societies set standards for their members. They lack the force of law and have little or no influence on nonmembers. Some societies can help consumers settle disputes over billing and ethical issues.

Table 1-2

ANALYSIS OF CONSUMER-PROTECTION FORCES

Agency/Organization	Potential Role	Limiting Factors
Accreditation of schools	Improve the quality of training	Teachings are not required to be science-based.
State licensing laws	Set standards for entry into profession	Licensure does not ensure that a profession practices scientifically
State licensing boards	Can act in cases of fraud, incompetence, or other unprofessional behavior	Resources are limited; courts may delay or overrule board actions; many dubious practitioners are unlicensed
Insurance companies	Gatekeeper function; can refuse to pay for unsubstantiated treatment	Laws or court actions may force companies to pay for unsubstantiated procedures
Medicare and Medicaid	Can eject errant practitioners	Fraud can be difficult to detect
Managed-care plans	Can exclude or eject practitioners who don't meet their criteria or who engage in unprofessional conduct	Selection criteria may be based on economic factors rather than quality of care; laws and court actions can force managed-care plans to accept practitioners they don't want
Professional societies	Set ethical standards for members	Have no legal power; cannot influence nonmembers
Specialty boards	Set high performance standards and ensure them by rigid examinations	Unrecognized boards may have low standards or be bogus
Advisory panels	Issue guidelines based on professional consensus	Have no legal power; some guidelines conflict with others
Hospitals	Credentialing and peer-review processes can restrict unqualified practitioners	Practitioners not on hospital staff are unaffected; some hospitals have lax standards
Food and Drug Administration (FDA)	Regulates food and drugs; can act against drugs and devices that are not proven safe and effective	Limited resources, especially if court action is required; current laws interfere with regulation of vitamins, herbs, and homeopathic products
Federal Trade Commission (FTC)	Can act against false advertising	Limited resources; tends to move slowly
U.S. Postal Service	Can stop frauds involving use of the mail	Can pursue only a small percentage of complaints
State attorneys general	Can stop fraudulent activities	Can pursue only a small percentage of complaints
Voluntary and consumer groups	Can educate public and campaign for stronger laws	Many groups are underfunded; some promote quackery

Recognized specialty boards set standards (through examinations) to identify practitioners who have achieved a high level of professional competence. Some "specialty boards" lack professional recognition, and some are bogus (see Chapter 8).

Many health-related agencies and organizations issue voluntary guidelines for science-based practices. The most comprehensive set was developed by the U.S. Preventive Services Task Force. Its 1996 report, discussed in Chapter 5, evaluates the cost-effectiveness of interventions for more than 80 potentially preventable diseases and conditions.[23]

Voluntary and consumer groups serve as watchdogs, information sources, and legislative advocates. Some deal with many health-related issues; others deal with few. Some advocate strengthening consumer-protection laws. Groups that represent the interests of "alternative" practitioners and the health-food industry want them weakened (see Chapters 8, 12, and 26).

Table 1-2 summarizes the functions and limitations of these protective forces.

INTELLIGENT CONSUMER BEHAVIOR

Intelligent health consumers have the following characteristics:

1. *They seek reliable sources of information.* They are appropriately skeptical about advertising claims, statements made by talk-show guests, and "breakthroughs" reported in the news media. New information, even when accurate, may be difficult to place in perspective without expert guidance. Most physicians, dentists, allied health professionals, health educators, government agencies, professional societies, and health-related voluntary organizations are reliable (for more information see Chapter 2 and the Appendix). Prominent organizations include the FDA, American Medical Association, American Cancer Society, American Dental Association, American Heart Association, National Council Against Health Fraud, and U.S. Public Health Service.

2. *They maintain a healthy lifestyle.* This reduces the odds of becoming seriously ill and lowers the cost

of health care. Prudent consumers avoid tobacco products, eat sensibly, exercise appropriately, maintain a reasonable weight, use alcohol moderately or not at all, and take appropriate safety precautions (such as wearing a seat belt when driving).

3. *They select practitioners with great care.* It has been said that primary-care physicians typically know a little about a lot and specialists typically know a lot about a little. The majority of people would do best to begin with a generalist and consult a specialist if a problem needs more complex management.

4. *They undergo appropriate screening tests and, when illness strikes, use self-care and professional care as needed.* Excellent guidebooks are available to help decide when professional care is needed (see Chapters 5 and 9).

5. *They communicate effectively.* They present their problems in an organized way, ask appropriate questions, and tactfully assert themselves when necessary.

6. *When a health problem arises, they take an active role in its management.* This entails understanding the nature of the problem and how to do their part in dealing with it. People with chronic illnesses, such as diabetes or high blood pressure, should strive to become

"experts" in their own care and use their physicians as "consultants."

7. *They understand the logic of science and why scientific testing is needed to test and to determine which theories and practices are valid.* Chapter 2 covers this in detail.

8. *They are wary of treatments that lack scientific support and a plausible rationale.* These are thoroughly discussed in Chapters 3 and 8.

9. *They are familiar with the economic aspects of health care.* They obtain appropriate insurance coverage, inquire in advance about professional fees, and shop comparatively for medications and other products.

10. *They report frauds, quackery, and other wrongdoing to appropriate agencies and law enforcement officials.* Consumer vigilance is an essential ingredient of a healthy society.

Worksheet 1-2 can help you evaluate your approach to the health marketplace.

SUMMARY

Consumer health encompasses all aspects of the marketplace related to the purchase of health products and

---

Worksheet 1-2

CONSUMER HEALTH PROFILE

This exercise can help you evaluate how you act when exposed to misinformation, fraud, and quackery.
Place an X in the column to the right that best represents your answer.
(VM = very much; M = much; S = some; L = little; N = none.)

	VM	M	S	L	N
Are you sufficiently informed to be able to make sound decisions?					
Do you maintain a healthy lifestyle?					
Where do you go for information when needed?					
Professional health organizations/individuals					
Health books, magazines, newsletters					
Government health agencies					
Advertisements					
Newspapers/magazines					
Radio/television					
Laypersons you know					
To what extent do you accept statements in news reports at face value?					
To what extent do you accept statements in ads at face value?					
How well can you identify quacks, quackery, fraudulent schemes, and hucksters?					
When selecting health practitioners, to what extent do you:					
Talk with or visit before the first regular appointment?					
Check/inquire regarding qualifications/credentials?					
Ask friend/neighbor about reputation?					
Inquire about fees and payment procedures?					
Do you undergo appropriate periodic medical examinations?					
Do you undergo appropriate periodic dental examinations?					
When you have been exposed to a fraudulent practice, quackery, or a substandard product or service, to what extent do you report your experience?					

services. Although health care in America is potentially the world's best, many problems exist.

Health information is voluminous and complex. Many practitioners fall short of the ideal, and some are completely unqualified. Quackery is widespread. The marketplace is overcrowded with products, many of which are questionable. Rising costs and lack of adequate insurance coverage have reached crisis levels. Consumer protection is limited.

Only well-informed individuals can master the complexity of the health marketplace. Intelligent consumers maintain a healthy lifestyle, seek reliable sources of information and care, and avoid products and practices that lack scientific substantiation.

REFERENCES

1. Clinton HR. Foreword to White House Domestic Policy Council. Health Security: The President's Report on the American People. Washington, D.C., 1993, US Government Printing Office.
2. Young JH. Why quackery persists. In Barrett S, Jarvis WT, editors. The Health Robbers: A Close Look at Quackery in America. Amherst, N.Y., 1994, Prometheus Books.
3. US House of Representatives, Select Committee on Aging, Subcommittee on Health and Long-term Care. Quackery: A $10 Billion Scandal (2 volumes). Washington, D.C., 1984, US Government Printing Office.
4. Gunther M. Quackery and the media. In Barrett S, editor. The Health Robbers: How to Protect Your Money and Your Life, ed 2. Philadelphia, 1980, George F Stickley Co.
5. Larkin M. Confessions of a former women's magazine writer. NutriWatch Web site, March 26, 2000.
6. Kashgarian M. Doctor and patient in cyberspace, or take two aspirins and e-mail me in the morning. Yale Medicine 30(2A):22–24, 1996.
7. Jarvis WT. Quackery: A national scandal. Clinical Chemistry 38:1574–1586, 1992.
8. Barrett S, Herbert V. The Vitamin Pushers: How the "Health Food" Industry Is Selling America a Bill of Goods. Amherst, N.Y., 1994, Prometheus Books.
9. Farley F. Prom night leads to GHB prosecutions. FDA Consumer 25(5):34-35, 1991.
10. Wolfe S and others. 13,012 Questionable Doctors. Washington D.C., 1996, Public Citizen Health Research Group.
11. Wolfe S. 13,012 questionable doctors. Public Citizen Health Research Group Health Letter 12(4):1–3, 1996.
12. Dodes JE, Schissel MJ. The Whole Tooth. New York, 1997, St. Martin's Press.
13. Markle GB. Dare to ask the cost. Public Citizen Health Research Group Health Letter 5(5):10-11, 1989.
14. Nursing homes: When a loved one needs care. Consumer Reports 60:518–528, 1995.
15. Highlights—National Health Expenditures, 1998. HCFA Web site, accessed Dec 10, 2000.
16. National Health Expenditures Projections: 1998-2008. HCFA Web site, accessed Dec 10, 2000.
17. Wasted health care dollars. Consumer Reports 57:435–448, 1992.
18. Second class medicine. Consumer Reports 65(9):42, 2000.
19. Shearer G. The Health Care Divide: Unfair Financial Burdens. Washington, D.C., 2000, Consumers Union.
20. Carrasquillo D and others. A reappraisal of private employers' role in providing health insurance. New England Journal of Medicine 340:109–114, 1999.
21. The Kaiser-Commonwealth 1997 National Survey of Health Insurance. New York, 1997, Commonwealth Fund.
22. Wasik JF. Fraud in the funeral industry. Consumers Digest 34(5):53–59, 1995.
23. U.S Preventive Services Task Force. Guide to Clinical Preventive Services, ed 2. Baltimore, 1996, Williams & Wilkins.

☑ Consumer Tip

How to Locate References

The format this textbook uses for references to magazine and journal articles is:

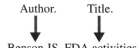

1. Benson JS. FDA activities protect public. FDA Consumer 25(1):7–9, 1991.

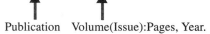

Publication   Volume(Issue):Pages, Year.

In this text, citations numbered in boldface type are recommended for further reading. Underlining of a reference number indicates that the document is available on the Internet and is easily accessed through the Consumer Health Sourcebook Web site (http://www.chsourcebook.com). Scientific journals are housed at medical school and hospital libraries, and some are available online. Librarians at most libraries can obtain books and article reprints through the interlibrary loan process.

Chapter Two

SEPARATING FACT FROM FICTION

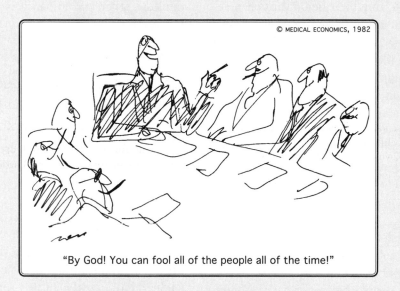

© MEDICAL ECONOMICS, 1982

"By God! You can fool all of the people all of the time!"

One of the factors that makes America great is our freedom of speech. To maintain this freedom, we must also run a risk. False prophets can get up on pedestals (such as radio and television talk shows) and tell you almost anything they please.

GABE MIRKIN, M.D.[1]

Finding the occasional straw of truth awash in a great ocean of confusion and bamboozle requires intelligence, vigilance, dedication and courage. But if we don't practice these tough habits of thought . . . we risk becoming a nation of suckers, up for grabs by the next charlatan who comes along.

CARL SAGAN[2]

An inability to comprehend even basic statistical concepts can transform modern youth into victims in search of an irrational belief system that will needlessly harm, panic, and abuse.

PASQUALE ACCARDO, M.D.
RONALD LINDSEY, M.D.[3]

Be careful about reading health books. You might die of a misprint.

MARK TWAIN

<table>
<tr><td align="center">Key Concepts</td></tr>
<tr><td align="center">KEEP THESE POINTS IN MIND AS YOU STUDY THIS CHAPTER</td></tr>
</table>

- The scientific process is essential for validating health claims and other information.
- Under the rules of science (and consumer protection), those who make a claim bear the burden of proof.
- Scientific research requires proper sampling techniques, the highest possible accuracy of measurement or observation, and appropriate statistical analysis of the findings.
- Don't assume that information is valid simply because it is broadcast or published. No magical superforce is protecting the marketplace against misinformation.
- The best way to avoid confusion is to use trustworthy sources of information.

The interest Americans have developed in maintaining and improving their health has been accompanied by a tremendous increase in the amount of information available. Several thousand health-related books, videotapes, and CD-ROMs are published each year. Radio and television stations conduct special programs on health issues, employ physicians as commentators, and provide talk shows on which health matters are discussed. Newspapers cover health issues in news articles and feature stories. Health products are advertised frequently. Ideas and experiences are also being shared through the Internet and other computer channels. Unfortunately, much of this information is inaccurate.

Consumers who wish to make intelligent decisions about health matters must address several questions: What are scientific facts? How can they be identified? To what extent should people believe what they read and hear about health matters? Where can valid information be found? This chapter explains how the scientific method is used to determine facts, how health information is disseminated, and how reliable information can be obtained.

HOW FACTS ARE DETERMINED

Reliable health information comes primarily through using the scientific method, a procedure for exposing hypotheses (assumptions) to critical examination and testing. The more we eliminate false information, the closer we get to what is true.[4] Hypotheses are scientific only if they are testable and can predict measurable events.[5]

The scientific method offers an objective way to evaluate information to determine what is false. It does not rely on testimonials as evidence of fact. Rather, it provides an objective way to collect and evaluate data.

Astronomer Carl Sagan said that "science is a way of thinking much more than it is a body of knowledge." He also noted:

At the heart of science is an essential tension between two seemingly contradictory attitudes—an openness to new ideas, no matter how bizarre and counterintuitive they may be, and the most ruthless skeptical scrutiny of all ideas, old and new. This is how deep truths are winnowed from deep nonsense. Of course, scientists make mistakes in trying to understand the world, but there is a built-in error-correcting mechanism: The collective enterprise of creative thinking and skeptical thinking together keeps the field on track.[2]

The scientific method has at least three noteworthy characteristics. First, it is self-correcting. Scientists do not assume that this method discovers absolute truth but rather that it produces conclusions that subsequent studies may modify. In this sense, science is cumulative. Second, the scientific method requires objectivity. Findings must not be contaminated by the personal beliefs, perceptions, biases, values, or emotions of the researcher. Only when the results speak for themselves should the conclusions be considered valid. Research results often lead to new questions that should be explored. Third, experiments must be reproducible. One study, taken alone, seldom proves anything. To be valid, one researcher's findings must be repeatable by others.

The long list of references cited in Chapter 15 of this text illustrates the enormous amount of effort that can be involved in developing important conclusions.

Research Design

Scientific research requires proper sampling techniques, the highest possible accuracy of measurement or observation, and appropriate statistical analysis of the findings. The conclusions are then used to develop new theories or modify old ones.

Science writer Rodger Doyle[6] has identified four types of studies used by medical scientists to investigate health and disease:

CASE STUDIES involve systematic observation of people who are ill.

LABORATORY EXPERIMENTS include studies of animals, living tissue, cells, and disease-causing agents.

EPIDEMIOLOGIC STUDIES analyze data from various population groups to identify factors related to the occurrence of diseases.

CONTROLLED CLINICAL TRIALS offer the most credible evidence.

Anecdotal reports are personal observations that have not been made under strict experimental conditions. Competent researchers may use anecdotes for suggesting new hypotheses, but never as supporting evidence. The fact that a person recovers after doing something is rarely sufficient to demonstrate that the recovery was caused by the action taken and is not simply coincidental. Moreover, reports of personal experiences can be biased, inaccurate, or even fraudulent. Well-designed experiments involving many people are needed to establish that a treatment method is effective. Without them, even honest, competent doctors can be misled by their clinical experiences.

Epidemiologists search for "risk markers" (predictors of a disease) by comparing people with different characteristics.[7] These markers can include personal characteristics (e.g., weight, blood cholesterol levels), personal activities (taking vitamins, exercising regularly, smoking cigarettes), and environmental factors (inhaling radon gas or tobacco smoke) that are statistically related to specific diseases. Before concluding that the relationship is causal rather than coincidental, however, epidemiologists must consider: (a) the strength of the association, (b) the consistency of the association in different studies, (c) whether it is clear that the risk marker preceded the disease, (d) whether the dose and not just the mere presence of the marker predicts disease risk, and (e) whether, in light of what else is known, it appears logical that the marker is responsible.

Controlled clinical trials compare an experimental group of people who receive the treatment being tested and a control group of people who receive a different treatment or no treatment. For example, members of the experimental group may receive a pill with active ingredients, whereas those in the control group receive another treatment, an inert substance (placebo), or no treatment. Studies may be conducted "blind" or "double-blind" to minimize or eliminate the effect of bias on data collection and interpretation. In blind studies the participants do not know which treatment they receive. In double-blind studies neither the people administering the treatment nor the experimental subjects know who gets what. In crossover studies participants in two or more groups are switched from one intervention to another after a specified period of time. Some studies do not use control groups. Ernst and others[8] have warned that experimental subjects who receive placebos should not be classified as "untreated" and that many people fail to distinguish between a placebo response and the improvement that results from the natural course of an illness. Chapter 3 discusses this subject further.

Large, randomized, well-controlled, double-blind studies in which several medical centers participate are considered the gold standard of research trials.[9] Because such studies are very expensive to conduct, they are reserved for questions of great importance. Long-term research ("outcomes research") is also needed to compare the effectiveness of proven alternatives.[10] Table 2-1 illustrates the typical steps in a clinical investigation.

It is important that research findings not be overgeneralized. Conclusions based on data from one population may not apply to another, and the results obtained from animal or test-tube studies may not be applicable to humans.

The importance of scientific testing was strikingly demonstrated by a study of mammary artery ligation, a surgical procedure used in the 1940s and 1950s for treating angina pectoris (chest pain resulting from coronary artery disease). Proponents believed that tying off the mammary arteries stimulated the growth of new blood vessels that would increase the supply of blood to the heart muscle. The procedure was considered effective until double-blind controlled tests demonstrated that pretending to operate (merely cutting the skin of the patient's chest wall) was as effective as tying off the mammary arteries.[11]

◆ **Personal Glimpse** ◆

The Scientific Method in Action[12]

In 1978 researchers at Mt. Sinai Hospital in Miami Beach, Florida, compared the effects of chicken soup, cold water, and hot water on the clearance rate of nasal mucus. Each liquid was consumed through a straw from a covered cup or open vessel. A videotaping system was used to record the advance of tiny radioactive discs as mucus carried them out the nose. Cold water slowed mucus flow, but chicken soup and hot water sipped from an open cup speeded it up. Since chicken soup outperformed hot water, the researchers concluded that it appeared to have a special ability to clear a stuffy nose. Mom and Grandma were right!

Table 2–1

TYPICAL STEPS IN CLINICAL INVESTIGATION

Step	Example
A question or problem is identified.	What is the effect of vitamin C on the common cold?
A hypothesis is formulated.	Supplementation with vitamin C can reduce the incidence of colds.
A limited aspect of the hypothesis is selected for testing.	Will daily administration of 1000 mg of vitamin C prevent colds?
A study is designed.	Sixty adults will be given 1000-mg tablets of vitamin C daily for 4 months, and 60 of comparable age, race, sex, and health status are given an inactive substance [placebo tablets]. The participants will not know which they receive [a blind study].
The study is conducted.	Volunteers are obtained and instructed on how to proceed.
Data are collected, recorded, and tabulated.	There were six colds in the vitamin C group and seven in the placebo group.
The data are analyzed to determine whether the results appear significant or were likely to occur by chance alone.	The small difference between the two groups could easily have occurred by chance alone and therefore is not "statistically significant."
A determination is made on whether hypotheses have been supported or refuted.	The hypothesis was not supported. The experiment found no evidence that vitamin C supplements reduce the incidence of colds.
The study may be repeated by the researchers or by others to verify their results or conclusions.	Many double-blind experiments have found that supplementation with vitamin C does not prevent colds (see Chapter 12).
Studies relevant to this area are reviewed.	Skilled reviewers agree that enough well-designed studies have been done to conclude that vitamin C megadoses do not prevent colds.

Misuse of Statistics

Many people tend to accept statistical data without question. To them, any information presented in quantitative form is correct. Advertisers, quacks, and pseudo-scientists often cite invalid data or misrepresent valid data to promote their wares. The following statistical errors can cause confusion:

BIAS: A factor that may cause people to make erroneous observations or draw erroneous conclusions. For example, in a study of vitamin C and the common cold, participants who knew they were taking vitamin C reported fewer colds than those who were taking it but did not know it.[13]

OMISSION OF AN IMPORTANT FACTOR: Many individuals who feel helped by an unorthodox remedy have taken it together with effective treatment but credited the unorthodox remedy.

NON SEQUITUR: Data may be interpreted illogically.

INSUFFICIENT DATA: Small amounts of data result in a high degree of uncertainty. Thus tests done on small numbers of individuals must usually be confirmed by larger studies.

NONCOMPARABLE DATA: Valid comparisons can be made only if data are logically comparable.

NONREPRESENTATIVE DATA: Improper sampling techniques (lack of random sampling) may yield data that do not accurately represent the population or universe. For example, to determine which car the average American likes best, it would not be appropriate to poll only owners of one make of car, or those living in one region, or even those listed in the telephone book (since many people have a non-published number or lack a phone). Similarly, the finding that vitamin supplementation reduces the incidence of cancer in a population of malnourished rural Chinese is not relevant to well-nourished urban Americans. Figure 12-1 provides another example.

CONFUSION OF ASSOCIATION AND CAUSATION: Things that occur together may not be causally related. Care must be taken to be sure that recovery after taking a remedy is not simply a result of the natural course of an illness.

In *How to Lie with Statistics*, Darrell Huff[14] describes how drug research data can be misrepresented by using biased samples, meaningless averages, purposeful omissions, apples-and-oranges comparisons, illogical conclusions, and deceptively drawn charts. He notes that a basic technique used by charlatans when they present testimonial evidence is the *post hoc, ergo propter hoc* fallacy: "This happened after that, therefore this was caused by that." The fact that someone who smokes 50 cigarettes and drinks heavily each day lives to age 95 does not mean that these habits are healthful. Huff says that to analyze a statement, one should ask, "Who says so? How does he know? How did he find out? Is anything missing? Does it all make sense?"

Manufacturers are quick to take advantage of preliminary research that may appear to support increased use of their products. In 1988 the Physicians' Health Study Group[15] reported that aspirin use every other day had reduced the incidence of heart attacks among 11,000 generally healthy physicians. The researchers concluded that although aspirin might help prevent heart attacks, the study's results should not be applied to the general population and that doctors should weigh potential risks as well as benefits when advising their patients. (Chapter 15 discusses this further.) Within days after the report was published, aspirin ads began referring to it and suggesting that consumers ask their doctors whether aspirin might help them. The FDA Commissioner, who believed that the ads were likely to encourage inappropriate self-medication, warned manufacturers that aspirin did not have FDA approval for preventing heart attacks in healthy people and that continuing the ads would trigger regulatory action. Fish oils, calcium supplements, antioxidant vitamins, and high-fiber products have also been marketed in ways that oversimplify or exaggerate the significance of research findings.

Peer Review

Peer review is a process in which work is reviewed by others who usually have equivalent or superior knowledge. It may be used during the development or execution of a study, as well as afterward. When studies are completed, researchers strive to publish their results in journals so that others can use or criticize the findings and science can advance. Detailed standards for reporting and evaluating studies have been published.[16] The best scientific journals are peer-reviewed by experts; papers submitted for publication are reviewed by two or more expert referees, then accepted, modified, or rejected by the editor. The peer review process is imperfect but can reliably screen out "obviously flawed and unreliable manuscripts."[17]

Reports from over 3500 peer-reviewed scientific journals are listed in the *Index Medicus* and its online counterpart Medline. (Such listing is a favorable sign but not a guarantee of quality.) The two most prestigious American medical journals are *JAMA* (*Journal of the American Medical Association*) and *The New England Journal of Medicine*. *JAMA* has more than 3000 names in its reviewer-referee file.

Expert review is also done by scientific organizations and government agencies. Several that have established formal review processes given great weight by the medical community are described here.

The American Medical Association (AMA)'s Council on Scientific Affairs studies many medical issues and reports to the AMA's House of Delegates. Once accepted, these reports help shape AMA public policies and may be published in *JAMA*.

The AMA Diagnostic and Therapeutic Technology Assessment (DATTA) project was established in 1982 to evaluate drugs, devices, procedures, and techniques, covering about 10 items per year. More than 1000 clinician-scientists from all areas of medicine have been selected by the AMA Council on Scientific Affairs to participate in the project. Evaluations typically take several months and represent a consensus of panelists considered experts in the technology under consideration; they judge whether it shall be considered safe and effective, investigational, indeterminate, or unacceptable. The topics selected are considered very important or controversial.

The National Institutes of Health Consensus Development Program, begun in 1977, has held about 100 consensus conferences in which experts meet for several days to discuss a topic and issue a report.

The National Academy of Sciences issues the Dietary Reference Intakes (see Chapter 11) and many other reports by expert committees.

The Office of Technology Assessment (OTA), which closed in 1995, was a nonpartisan support agency that provided congressional committees with analyses of emerging, difficult, and highly technical issues. In 1990

◆ Personal Glimpse ◆

Self-Persuasion

Charlatans are not the only people who engage in the *post hoc, ergo propter hoc* fallacy. As noted by Lisa Feldman Barrett, Ph.D., associate professor of psychology at Boston College:

People try to connect things that happen to them. In doing this, they lean toward ideas that fit their expectations and away from those that do not. Suppose somebody believes that vitamins provide energy. On a day when he feels energetic, he attributes that feeling to the vitamin, rather than to other factors, such as the quality of his sleep the night before. On a day when he feels fatigued, however, he doesn't register the experience as evidence against his belief. The scientific method safeguards against these tendencies by forcing people to look at disconfirmatory evidence and examine alternative explanations.

it prepared an excellent report on unconventional cancer treatments (see Chapter 17).

The American College of Physicians' Clinical Efficacy Assessment Project focuses primarily on relatively new procedures.

The U.S. Preventive Services Task Force publishes recommendations for preventive services that prudent health professionals should offer their patients in the course of routine clinical care. These recommendations, which represent the pooled judgment of many experts, are discussed in Chapter 5.

The Agency for Health Care Research and Quality (AHRQ), a component of the U.S. Public Health Service, was established in 1989 to enhance the quality, appropriateness, and effectiveness of health services. Formerly called the Agency for Health Care Policy and Research (AHCPR), it has published 18 clinical practice guidelines in separate versions for clinicians and consumers.

In 1990 the RAND Corporation, a private research organization in Santa Monica, California, teamed with the AMA and a 12-member medical school consortium to launch its Clinical Appropriateness Initiative. The project, which began publishing monographs in 1992, has prepared guidelines for many medical and surgical procedures. RAND has also done several studies related to spinal manipulation (see Chapter 8).

The *Cochrane Database of Systematic Reviews,* updated quarterly, is an electronic journal of systematic reviews produced by the Cochrane Collaboration, an international network of individuals and institutions committed to preparing systematic reviews of the effects of health care and disseminating them on CD-ROM and through the Internet. Established in 1993, it hopes to cover the entire spectrum of medical interventions.[18]

The National Guidelines Clearinghouse (NGC) is an Internet-based public resource sponsored by the AHRQ, in partnership with the AMA and the American Association of Health Plans. The Web site summarizes more than 900 evidence-based clinical practice guidelines that have met its criteria.

Scientific Fraud

Occasionally, individual scientists publish or attempt to publish bogus research data. The extent of this type of fraud is not known, but its existence presents one more argument for replicating studies. Peer review, high-quality journals, and the demand for replication make detection likely when fraud occurs. Physicist David Goodstein, who has worked with federal agencies to develop guidelines for defining misconduct in science,

reported that between 1980 and 1987 only 21 cases of misconduct involving doctors or biologists came to light—which was only three ten-thousandths of all scientists who received research grants.[19] Unconfirmed studies, particularly when inconsistent with other studies, seldom have major impact on what physicians do. Thus, although scientific fraud occurs, it seldom affects patient care.

PROBLEMS WITH HEALTH INFORMATION

Consumers obtain health information from individuals, educational institutions, and the media. The individual sources include nonprofessionals, pseudoscientists, and professionals. Nonprofessionals include friends, neighbors, relatives, and others who relate their experiences and ideas through informal talks and meetings. The pseudoscientists include charlatans and quacks. The professionals include practitioners, researchers, and others with specialized training who provide services and information. Educational institutions are schools at all levels that offer not only formal education provided by teachers, but also informal education through personal student contacts. The media include broadcasts, printed publications, and the Internet.

Reliability of Sources

It can be extremely difficult for consumers, and sometimes even for health professionals, to determine the reliability of health information. Separating fact from fiction can be a complex and time-consuming process. The reasons for this difficulty include:

- Advice from laypersons may be based on hearsay and personal experience rather than scientific data. Factual information, especially when several individuals are involved, is often distorted in transmission.
- Preliminary and limited scientific studies may be overemphasized by the media.
- Research data published by experts may conflict sufficiently to cause public confusion.
- Inaccurate health information may be disseminated purely for reasons of self-interest or profit.
- Claims that treatments are based on scientific evidence may not be true. Schick and Vaughn[5] have noted that unorthodox practitioners often cite or misconstrue "scientific findings" to support their views.
- Many false ideas "feel right" or seem commonsensical to people who lack the technical knowledge to evaluate them.

Nonprofessionals. Many consumers have misconceptions about the factors that influence health. People who share their experiences and knowledge may believe in unproven and unscientific methods. Such people often are highly motivated to spread their beliefs. Testimonials from movie stars, professional athletes, and other celebrities are commonly used to promote questionable health methods. National organizations exist to promote "alternative" cancer remedies (Chapter 17), the Feingold diet (Chapter 6), and other dubious methods. Millions of people have been involved in the sale of food supplements through multilevel companies such as Shaklee Corporation and Amway Corporation (see Chapter 4).[20]

Pseudoscientists. A pseudoscience is a set of ideas put forth as scientific when they are not. Pseudoscientists misuse and distort scientific evidence to support whatever products or services they promote. They may use scientific terminology and data to concoct theories that seem plausible to laypersons. They are often sophisticated in manipulating situations to gain notoriety and acceptance. They may write articles and books and may also reach consumers through television and radio programs. Some are "nutrition consultants" with "degrees" from diploma mills and nonaccredited schools.

Several observers have described characteristics that can help consumers distinguish pseudoscientists from true scientists. Hatfield,[21] for example, has noted:

Generally speaking, an establishment scientist has attended and graduated from an accredited university, belongs to one or more well-respected professional organizations, conducts carefully controlled and documented research, and reports these findings in professional journals that maintain high standards for accepting research papers.

By contrast, those claiming to be an alternative to establishment science have no common set of standards or practices from which measurements and comparisons can be made or quality of performance judged. Personal testimonies and

Consumer Tip

Any procedure proposed to treat human disease should be subject to the same standards of safety and effectiveness that apply to usual medical procedures. It is, however, unacceptable to require any scientific body to examine every proposed claim. There will never be enough facilities to consider the avalanche of proposals. Very simply, the burden of proof rests with the proponents. Ordinary claims require ordinary proof, and extraordinary claims require extraordinary proof. . . . Testimonials and anecdotal accounts, no matter how enthusiastic, do not constitute proof. Public enthusiasm and interest do not create validity.

Edward H. Davis, M.D.[22]

causal observations quite often serve as the basis of their research rather than act as the impetus to begin research.

Peterson[23] has likened improperly designed research to a man rowing a boat from only one side:

No matter how long or how hard he works, he never succeeds in doing anything except going in a circle, never realizing that it isn't his dedication or his strength but his method that is flawed. Until fringe research puts both oars in the water, it is doomed to remain where it has always been: spinning aimlessly near the shores of science.

True medical scientists have no philosophical commitment to particular treatment approaches, only a commitment to develop and use methods that are safe and effective for an intended purpose. Several observers have noted that pseudoscientists use hypotheses and data differently from scientists. Whereas scientists test hypotheses, abandon disproved ones, and welcome review of their findings and conclusions, pseudoscientists reject findings that contradict their beliefs and accuse critics of prejudice and conspiracy.[24,25]

In this regard, Criss[26] explains why we should not assume that people with strange ideas are modern Galileos:

To be a true analogy, these people would have to do experiments, make observations, and bring these results for all to see and question in an open forum. Further, they would have to be denied freedom of speech and press, or any expression all over the land—for that was the injunction against Galileo in 1616! It was as a result of this experience that the scientific method was adopted among scientists. . . . It has allowed the replacement of old ideas with new ones, and has provided a means of judging, and discarding, unfounded ideas.

Beyerstein[27] has noted that "alternative" practitioners rarely produce scientific data:

Unless an unconventional therapist keeps detailed records of a sufficiently large number of patients with the same complaint, we have no way of knowing whether the reported number of "cures" exceeds the normal unaided rate of recovery for the symptoms in question. Fringe practitioners rarely keep such data, preferring to publicize lists of satisfied customers rather than the percentage of the total cases that they represent. In addition, because alternative healers practically never carry out long-term follow-up studies, neither do we know how many of their clients receive temporary symptom relief rather than a genuine cure.

Professionals. Most health professionals give reliable advice, but scientific training does not guarantee reliability. For example, Adelle Davis promoted inaccurate and dangerous nutrition advice despite adequate training in nutrition. As noted in Chapter 13, many of the scientific studies she cited to back up her theories had no relevance to them. Dr. Andrew Ivy, a highly respected scientist, withdrew from the scientific community at the height of his career to promote the quack cancer remedy krebiozen (see Chapter 17). Chapters 3, 6, 7, 8, 12, and 27 of this book provide information on how to identify professionals who engage in unscientific practices.

During the past few years several lines of questionable nutrition products have been marketed with endorsements by scientists with respectable credentials. The most notable case occurred with United Sciences of America, Inc., a multilevel company that sold food supplements claimed to be effective in preventing cancer, heart disease, and many other diseases. Literature from the company said that its products had been designed and endorsed by a 15-person scientific advisory board that included two Nobel prize-winners. However, four members of the board told investigators that they had neither designed nor endorsed them. A few other multilevel companies claim to be guided by scientific boards, and a few supplement manufacturers have used endorsements by individual practitioners in advertisements. Barrett,[28] who believes that all such practitioners hold minority viewpoints, has warned that "vitamin product endorsements by doctors—no matter how prestigious they are—should be viewed with extreme caution. All I have seen so far have included claims that were unproved and also illegal."

Educational institutions. Educational standards are maintained through a system of accreditation by agencies approved by the U.S. Secretary of Education or the Council on Recognition of Postsecondary Accreditation. Accredited institutions tend to have well-trained faculty members and to provide reliable guidance to their students. Schools of chiropractic, naturopathy, and acupuncture are exceptions because much of what they teach is based on false beliefs (see Chapter 8). Nonaccredited schools that teach health subjects tend to be unreliable, and some are diploma mills that issue "degrees" and certificates whose only requirement is the payment of a fee. Chapter 12 discusses the problem of bogus nutrition credentials.

Many elementary and high school teachers of health subjects have had minimal formal training in these subjects and hold beliefs similar to those of the general public. Consequently, many misconceptions are passed from teacher to student. Dr. Roger Lederer, professor of biology, and Dr. Barry Singer, associate professor of psychology, California State University,[29] have noted that problems exist even at universities:

In recent years the teaching of pseudoscience and quackery in universities has become common and apparently accepted under the aegis of academic freedom. Typically the material is not formally presented as "Pseudoscience 101," but is offered as a component of a regular course.

Lederer and Singer, stating that pseudoscience is more evident in extension courses offered by institutions of higher learning, cited these examples:

- A community service course taught that manipulation of cranial bones can straighten teeth.
- Another course maintained that if infants were born using the Leboyer method, world peace would be achieved.
- A course approved for continuing education for nurses and pharmacists taught that high-frequency electronics can detect "the human aura, in all its various colors," that variations in auras may indicate the onset or presence of disease, and that "healing energy" can be transmitted by the laying on of hands.
- A course entitled "Spiritual Hypnosis" was claimed to help individuals probe multiple consciousness in numerous physical dimensions to make contact with spiritual guides for help with mental disorders.
- A conference sponsored by San Diego University offering relicensure credits for nurses and social workers advocated the use of mental imaging to cure cancer. It claimed that psyche and emotions are critical in the development of cancer and therefore hold the key to its treatment.

Many medical schools, hospitals, and professional organizations now offer courses related to "alternative" methods. Some are appropriately critical, but most provide a forum for promoters.

Print and Broadcast Media

Max Gunther[30] has succinctly described the role of the media in disseminating health information:

The media have four main functions: to entertain, to inform, to carry advertisements, and to make money for their stockholders. Because of the ways in which these functions are carried out, and the peculiar and intricate ways in which they are connected, an appalling amount of misinformation—ranging from the faintly biased to the downright wrong—is fed every day to an unfortunately gullible public. Hardly anywhere is this more evident than in the fields of medicine and its unwanted cousin, medical quackery.

Publicity is obviously a major factor in the success of quackery. Controversy often works to the advantage of quacks. During the mid-1970s Laetrile (amygdalin) promoters skillfully orchestrated publicity to increase their public following. Court cases of children whose parents wished to withhold conventional therapy became a rallying point. Laetrile supporters who sincerely believed it had saved their lives gained access to national television, where they appeared quite credible.[31] During the past several years chiropractic, homeopathy, and other "alternative" methods have received considerable publicity in mainstream publications with little or no attempt to examine their shortcomings.

When the media attempt to present health information, these problems are often evident: (a) coverage of a subject is inadequate because of the limited time allotment; (b) selection or screening of speakers or subject areas is poor; (c) pseudoscientific claims often are presented without rebuttal from qualified experts; (d) attempts are made to sensationalize and over-dramatize preliminary or new findings, especially about cancer, heart disease, arthritis, or alleged environmental dangers (see Figure 2-1); and (e) attempts are made to attract large audiences with claims that "alternative" methods are effective. Koren and Klein[32] have noted that the media have a natural tendency to report more on positive medical findings than on negative ones. This tendency contributes to the difficulty laypersons have in placing medical news in perspective.

Barrett and Herbert[33] note additional factors in the spread of misinformation by the media:

- Magical claims about health methods tend to be regarded as more newsworthy than established facts. Nationally televised talk shows provide enormous publicity for promoters of quackery.
- Time works to quackery's advantage. It is much easier to report a lie as a straight news event than it is to investigate it.
- Some journalists who have been misled by false ideas cannot write accurate papers.
- Most promoters of health misinformation are regarded as underdogs in a struggle against the establishment. As such, they tend to be treated with undeserved sympathy. Most editors insist that articles that attack false ideas be balanced so that the apparent "underdog" gets a fair hearing. Even science editors rarely feel a duty to issue effective public warnings against misinformation.
- Many more people are actively promoting misinformation than are actively opposing it. The sheer force of numbers works against the truth.
- Publications that accept ads for food supplements may be unwilling to risk offending their advertisers. For example, when *Self* magazine published an article by a freelance writer listing money-saving tips from the 1980 edition of this book, a tip about spending less money on vitamins was deleted from the writer's manuscript by the magazine's editors.
- Many editors fear that attacks on nutrition quackery will stir up controversy from readers who regard nutrition as their religion.
- Many editors fear that attacking the credibility of a quackery promoter will provide a libel suit.

Although libel suits related to health issues are extremely rare, other forms of economic reprisal are not. Some manufacturers cancel or threaten to cancel ads when magazines run articles that criticize their products, and "alternative" practitioners often initiate letter-writing campaigns or cancel their subscriptions when publications criticize their methods. After publication of the third and fourth editions of *Consumer Health*, chiropractors attempted to execute a boycott[34] and bring other pressure on the publisher to make the book's discussion of chiropractic more favorable.

Many publications use sensational claims to generate sales. Tabloids and women's magazines, for example, frequently carry articles on "quickie" reducing diets or "superfoods." Marilynn Larkin,[35] a freelance writer in New York City, has noted that topic selection is commonly based on sales appeal rather than scientific merit. Even a well-written article may be accompanied by a sensational headline that contradicts the article itself. Newspaper headlines are often composed by an editor who did not write the article and is not well-versed in the subject matter.

Lack of peer review. Scientists are generally eager to point out the deficiencies in each other's theories and experimental techniques. The comparable goal of most journalists is to report what happens. Journalists almost

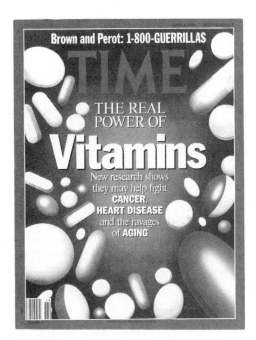

FIGURE 2-1. Magazine cover, 1992. Sales for this issue topped all others during the first half of the year. The six-page story, which speculated about antioxidant vitamins, was hailed by the health-food industry as a "watershed" event. In 1996, after studies refuting these speculations were published, *Time* covered the subject briefly.

never publicly criticize each other's coverage of the news. This is particularly true when health topics are involved. Stories about "alternative" methods rarely enable readers to judge whether proponents' claims are true. *Skeptical Inquirer*, *Priorities for Health* magazine, and *Probe* newsletter are among the very few that publish unrestrained criticisms of poor reporting.

The National News Council was founded in 1973 "to serve the public interest by . . . advancing accurate and fair reporting of news." It investigated complaints alleging unfairness, inaccuracy, or breaches of ethical standards by wire services, newspapers, news syndicates, news magazines, and television and radio networks and stations. The Council exerted some pressure on media outlets, but its findings were not widely publicized. It ceased operation in 1984, citing lack of media support as the primary reason.

Advertisements. Many periodicals contain ads encouraging their readers to buy vitamins and minerals, herbs, wrinkle removers, weight reducers, headache-relief drugs, pep pills, and various other health-related products. Advertising, however, is frequently misleading—often deliberately so. Advertising claims often have multiple meanings, one or more of which may be false. Many ads describe a product in terms of a mystical ingredient rather than specific contents or values.

Advertising dollars can also affect what gets published. Gunther[30] has observed: "Fear of losing good advertisers is one of the common reasons why worthless medicines and gadgets and treatment methods get free plugs and why you do not see honest medical rebuttals printed as often as could be wished." Chapter 4 discusses this subject further.

Table 2-2

NUTRITION ACCURACY OF POPULAR MAGAZINES (1995–1996)

Magazine	Score*	Comments
Consumer Reports	95	Objective, reliable, and scientifically sound
Better Homes & Gardens	92	Scientific recommendations are explained and demonstrated with food tips and recipes
Good Housekeeping	90	Smoothly translates complex information into lay language
Glamour	89	Concise, innovative educational articles and food ideas
Parents	88	Conscientious, expert advice, and thorough explanations
Health	87	Strives to present both sides of controversies
Reader's Digest	86	Despite come-on titles, information is sensible
Prevention	86	Objective reporting, but readers could be led to change dietary habits based on preliminary research data
Cooking Light	85	Seems to have the expertise to handle even the toughest topics, but brevity causes minor errors
Woman's Day	85	Innovative weight-control solutions; should consistently document scientific sources
McCall's	83	Sound advice mostly aimed at weight reduction; suffers from "studies show" syndrome where sources are missing
Redbook	83	Heavy reliance on renowned diet experts; should always document sources of preliminary nutrition findings
Runner's World	82	Recommendations to readers usually don't adhere to scientific consensus.
Shape	81	Articles vary widely in accuracy
Men's Health	81	Uses nutrition for cover-story appeal versus serious educational purposes
Fitness	79	Would benefit from scientific editorship to weed out subject matter that sounds too good to be true
Mademoiselle	79	Accuracy has dropped; fad diets and frivolous treatment of nutrition abound
Self	77	Inconsistent or downright inaccurate presentation style and recommendations
Cosmopolitan	74	Significantly better rating without "Dieter's Notebook" columns; up from "poor" rating for the first time in survey history, but still not trustworthy
Muscle & Fitness	70	Nutrition reporting at its worst; most advice completely unreliable
New Woman	69	Struggles to present anything on nutrition; needs a nutritional makeover from top to bottom

*Excellent: 90; Good: 80–89; Fair: 70–79; Poor: less than 70. Source: American Council on Science and Health.[36]

Newspapers. Many newspapers use overdramatization of incidents, inaccurate or exaggerated reports, quotations from unreliable sources, and misleading headlines to attract reader interest and attention. The weekly tabloids are notorious for this. Headlines like the following from tabloid newspapers have no credibility:

Breast-Feeding Can Prevent Pregnancies
Doctors Reveal Amazing Healing Powers of Water
Men Who Eat Slowly Make Better Lovers
Pizza Cuts Heart Attack Risk
Miracle of the Roses . . . Blooms From Shrine Are Curing Cancer, Arthritis and Even AIDS!
Researchers Claim Vasectomies May Lead to Heart Disease
Stars Use Crystals to Cure All Their Ills
Thousands Claim Cures From Radioactive Caves
Tomorrow's Drugs Will Make You Happier, Smarter, and More Creative
Vitamins—Guaranteed to Boost Energy and Slow Aging
World's Greatest Diet Pill—Eat What You Want and Still Lose 20 Pounds a Month

In 1987 Dr. Stephen Barrett[37] analyzed 322 articles on health, nutrition, and psychology appearing in five tabloid newspapers during a 3-month period and concluded that only 135 (42%) were reliable. A *National Examiner article*, for example, claimed that "a miraculous diet pill will flatten your tummy . . . and you can do it fast without a complicated diet program." The article discussed the Optifast system of weight control, a reputable medically supervised program. However, the program was not simple, the results were not instant, and the pills involved did not cause weight loss but simply added nutrients to the low-calorie program. Another article, "Bug Spray Makes Your Bosom Bigger," was accompanied by a photo captioned, "Flat-chested girls could look like Dolly Parton." The article stated that 30 men suing a federal detention center had claimed that exposure to a chemical intended to kill lice caused painful enlargement of their breasts. Nothing in the article indicated that the chemical is useful for women.

Dr. Barrett also examined 247 articles involving supernatural beliefs, faith healers, psychics, alleged kidnappings by space aliens, and similar topics. All but eight presented such occult events as factual.

Consumers should be wary of reports indicating that studies were completed on small numbers of subjects, done in foreign countries (evidence of accuracy is more difficult to ascertain), or based on animal studies alone. Preliminary findings can be important, but they do not become established as facts unless additional studies support them.

Even well-written articles about preliminary developments sometimes carry misleading headlines or begin with words that exaggerate their significance. For example, an article in the *San Francisco Examiner and Chronicle* had this headline: "New Hay Fever Drug May Replace Antihistamines." The article said the substance had to be inhaled, would require two-thirds fewer antihistamine tablets to control symptoms, and would not cause drowsiness. Later in the article, however, an allergy authority said it would work only for a small number of patients and would not replace antihistamines.[38]

Magazines and newsletters. Magazines and newsletters differ widely in the accuracy of the information they publish. Table 2-2 summarizes an evaluation by the American Council on Science and Health[36] of the nutrition information in 21 popular magazines in 1995 and 1996. Eight articles from each magazine were examined for accuracy, readability, substantiation of contents, and reliability of recommendations. *Consumer Reports, Good Housekeeping,* and *Better Homes & Gardens* were rated "excellent," and 12 other magazines were rated "good."

The major news magazines, *Time, Newsweek,* and *U.S. News & World Report*, are good sources of news on general health topics. Articles in these publications are usually timely, well-written, and based on interviews with recognized experts. However, all three of these magazines have publicized news about "alternative" health methods without appropriate critical analysis. *Newsweek* has also published several unduly alarmist articles about environmental factors and co-sponsored the 1996 Las Vegas Health Show, a large exposition at which many speakers and exhibitors promoted unscientific methods.

Two monthly magazines specializing in health topics deserve special comments: *Health* and *Prevention*. Both carry articles on a wide variety of topics. The articles on noncontroversial topics are generally well-written, but articles on controversial topics often give undeserved credibility to proponents of dubious methods. *Prevention* contains brief reports of preliminary research findings that can be difficult for readers to put into perspective. It also tends to exaggerate the ability of "positive thinking" to benefit health. Although the majority of their advertisers are reputable, neither magazine has maintained rigorous advertising standards for health products or services.

Many other periodicals specialize in health-related information. Dr. Barrett, who monitors more than 60 of them, has summarized his ratings in Table 2-3.

Books and other literature. Thousands of health-related books and pamphlets are published each year.

Table 2-3

HEALTH AND NUTRITION PERIODICALS ALIGNED WITH THE SCIENTIFIC COMMUNITY

Each of the newsletters and magazines in the chart below presents valuable information. Some deal with controversial topics much more than others, whereas some deal with them less accurately than others. Some cover many topics superficially, whereas others cover fewer topics deeply. Some balance this mix according to the importance of the topic. Generally the broader the scope, the less thorough, and vice versa.

R = How reliable?   4 = Excellent
D = How thorough?   3 = Good
P = How practical?   2 = Fair
S = How broad a scope?   1 = Inconsistent
T = How timely?   0 = Poor

General Health Newsletters	General Topics					Quackery			Comments
	R	D	P	S	T	R	S	T	
Consumer Reports on Health	4	4	4	4	4	3	3	4	Outstanding; packed with practical information
Executive Health's Good Health Report	3	3	2	2	2	1	2	2	Articles on controversial topics are often inconclusive
Harvard Health Letter	3	4	4	4	4	1	4	4	Excellent reports on research findings, but articles on "alternative" methods have been careless
Harvard Heart Letter	4	4	4	–	4	4	–	4	Outstanding but limited to cardiovascular topics
Harvard Women's Health Watch	3	4	4	4	4	1	3	4	Some articles on "alternative" methods have been promotional
HealthNews	3	4	4	4	4	2	4	4	In-depth interpretations of recent scientific findings, but inconsistent about "alternative" methods
Health Over 50 (Johns Hopkins Medical Letter)	4	4	4	3	4	4	3	4	Excellent and timely
Mayo Clinic Health Letter	4	3	4	4	4	4	3	4	Excellent and timely
Mirkin Report	4	2	4	4	4	4	4	4	Summarizes journal articles and provides practical tips
Public Citizen HRG Health Letter	2	3	1	1	4	2	2	2	Unduly negative about health marketplace; some conclusions based on inadequate data sampling
University of California at Berkeley Wellness Letter	3	4	4	4	4	3	4	4	Editors unwisely advise everyone to take antioxidant vitamins; a few articles on "alternative" methods have been inaccurate
University of Texas Health Letter	4	4	4	4	4	4	–	–	Seldom covers controversial topics
Women's Health Advocate	3	4	4	4	4	0	–	–	Consistently poor advice about "alternative" methods

The following *newsletters* provide reliable and useful information on specialized topics:
Cancer Smart; Georgia Tech Sports Medicine & Performance Newsletter; Harvard Mental Health Letter; Review of Natural Products (herbs and other substances); NCAHF News (from National Council Against Health Fraud); Probe (scientific controversies, misconduct, and quackery).

(In 1994, 3147 books categorized under "medicine" were registered with the Library of Congress.) The First Amendment of the Constitution protects free speech and thus, unfortunately, permits authors to embellish or distort facts and data and publish inaccurate and misleading health information. Writers and publishers, however, are subject to libel laws if they unfairly demean the character of any individual. In 1992, *Vegetarian Times* published a rebuttal[39] and paid $21,000 in an out-of-court settlement to the National Council Against Health Fraud and four of its board members who charged that they had been unfairly criticized in a 1991 article about "quackbusters."[40]

FTC laws protect consumers against false and misleading advertising. Federal laws and some state food and drug laws provide protection against improper labeling of products and advertising with false or unproved health claims. However, many independent publications extol the virtues of questionable products. Consumers should be alert to this situation and be aware that misinformation about food supplements is spread through many channels (see Chapter 12).

Bestseller lists often contain one or more books on diet, fitness, or "alternative medicine." These popular books are rarely reliable. The *Beverly Hills Diet,* by Judy Mazel, sold over 1 million copies and was on the bestseller list for many weeks. It is a bizarre diet primarily based on eating fruit and avoiding combinations of foods that supposedly cannot be digested at the same time. *Life Extension,* by Durk Pearson and Sandy Shaw, was based on the dubious premise that animal experiments suggest that taking various nutrients can prolong

Table 2-3

HEALTH AND NUTRITION PERIODICALS ALIGNED WITH THE SCIENTIFIC COMMUNITY - *CONT'D.*

Nutrition Newsletters	General Topics					Quackery			Comments
	R	D	P	S	T	R	S	T	
Environmental Nutrition	2	3	4	3	4	1	3	3	Best features are news and book reviews; some articles about vitamins have been inaccurate
Nutrition Action	3	3	3	1	3	1	1	3	Alarmist attitude toward nutrition and food safety
Healthy Weight Journal	4	4	4	–	4	4	4	4	Deals only with topics related to weight control
Tufts University Health & Nutrition Letter	4	4	4	4	4	4	4	4	Outstanding, informative, and practical
Magazines amd Journals									
FDA Consumer	4	4	4	3	4	4	3	4	Focuses on foods, drugs, devices, and FDA enforcement; full text available at http://www.fda.gov/fdac
Health	3	4	4	4	4	1	2	3	Advice often accurate but superficial; many articles on "alternative" methods are promotional
Men's Health	2	2	2	2	3	1	0	2	Breezy writing style sometimes obscures what is important
Prevention	3	3	1	2	4	–	–	–	Emphasizes lifestyle improvements; ome articles encourage inappropriate self-treatment; promotes worthless "alternative" methods
Priorities for Health	4	4	4	3	4	4	4	4	Emphasizes public health and environmental issues
Scientific Review of Alternative Medicine	4	4	4	4	4	4	4	4	Detailed, incisive analyses

The following are not recommended because they promote unscientific and/or unproven methods:

Newsletters: Allergy Hotline; Alternative Health Issues; Alternatives (written by David Williams, D.C.); Antha; Better Ways to Health; Bottom Line Health; Cancer Chronicles; Dr. Atkins' Health Revelations; Forefront; Health & Healing; Health Alert; Health & Longevity; Health Resource Newsletter; Health Wisdom for Women; HealthBeat; HealthFacts; Healthy Talk; The International DAMS Newsletter; The John R. Lee, M.D., Newsletter; The Lark Letter; The McDougall Newsletter; The Mindell Report; Naturally Well; New Century Nutrition; Nutrition & Healing; Nutrition Insight; Nutrition News (edited by Siri Khalsa); The Nutrition Reporter; Organic Food News; People's Medical Society Newsletter; Price-Pottenger Nutrition Foundation Health Journal; Prescriptions for Healthy Living; Pure Facts; Second Opinion; Self Healing; What Doctors Don't Tell You; Women's Health Advocate; Your Good Health.

Magazines: Alternative Medicine Digest; American Journal of Natural Medicine; Better Nutrition for Today's Living; Body, Mind & Spirit; The Choice; Choices; Counselor; Delicious!; Digest of Alternative Medicine; Energy Times; Explore More!; Flex; Forefront; Good Medicine; Health Consciousness; Health Counselor; Health Freedom News; Health Science; Health World; Healthier Times; Healthy & Natural; Herbs for Health; Holistic Medicine; The Human Ecologist; Innovation; Journal of Longevity Research; Let's Live; Life Extension; Massage & BodyWork; Muscle & Fitness; Muscular Development; Natural Health; The Natural Way; New Age Journal; New Body; Newlife; Nutrition & Fitness; Nutritional Perspectives; Prime Health & Fitness; Psychology Today; Search for Health; Senior Health; Total Health; Townsend Letter for Doctors and Patients; Vegetarian Times; Your Health. © 2000, Stephen Barrett, M.D.

human life to 150 years. The book stimulated sales of various substances it said have "anti-aging" properties. In recent years, Deepak Chopra, M.D., has charmed the public by declaring that health is a conscious choice; Andrew Weil, M.D., has promoted "integration" of standard and "alternative" medicine; and the Public Broadcasting System has promoted *Gary Null's Ultimate Anti-Aging Diet* for fundraising purposes. Amazon Books lists more than 1500 astrologic books written in English that are in print.

Many publishers are willing to publish books on unproven theories if they think that the books will be profitable. Only a few are unwilling to do so. The most noteworthy publishers of health-related books for the general public are Consumer Reports Books, which originates and reprints many books on health topics,

Healthwise, Inc., which publishes self-help materials, and Prometheus Books, which specializes in dissecting quackery and paranormal claims. Harvard Medical School and Johns Hopkins Medical School both publish excellent in-depth reports on timely subjects. Chapter 9 contains suggestions for a home health library.

Videotapes and CD-ROMs. Educational tapes and CDs are produced by many health organizations and commercial companies. Excellent videos have been issued by Time-Life Warner and Dartmouth Medical School. The Mayo Clinic has produced an outstanding series of CD-ROMs. Many public libraries have health-related tapes and CDs for public education.

The broadcast media. Thousands of radio and television stations provide a steady stream of health news and commentary. Many stations use physicians as commentators or consultants. Although news reports tend to be presented accurately, radio and television talk shows give frequent exposure to promoters of quackery,[41] and infomercials are almost always misleading (see Chapter 4). Talk-show guests are usually selected for their "entertainment" (audience-attracting) value rather than the soundness of their ideas. Some gain media access by hiring public relations firms to promote their media appearances. Critics of quackery are sometimes invited to debate, but are seldom permitted to appear unopposed. Stations rarely take corrective action when they receive complaints about their health programming.[41]

The quality of health information on CBS-TV's "60 Minutes" has been very inconsistent. The American Council on Science and Health used 65 experts to evaluate 97 transcripts of programs from 1978 through 1995 that addressed medical treatments or health scares. Each transcript underwent at least three reviews, during which they were assigned overall "report card" grades of A (4 points), B (3 points), C (2 points), D (1 point), or F (0 points). Fewer than 25% of the transcripts received a mean grade greater than 3.0; and more than 40% received a mean grade less than 2.0. The overall transcript grade was a "C."[42]

Heussner and Salmon[43] have noted three shortcomings of fallacious reporting: (1) large numbers of people may be led to doubt their doctors and acquire unrealistic hope in a risky procedure; (2) ensuing controversies can divert scientists' valuable time and attention or cause scarce research funds to be wasted on studies to formally disprove an obviously unworthy proposition; and (3) fallacious reporting wastes media resources that could be better used to provide useful information about health and disease issues.

PRUDENT USE OF THE INTERNET

The amount of health-related information accessible through computer channels is huge and expanding rapidly. These sources can be accessed through the Internet, the largest worldwide computer network. Anyone with access to a computer, a modem, and appropriate software can explore this wealth of information. Students often can do so, free of charge, through computers at their school. Free access is also available at public libraries.

Health information is available in several electronic formats.[44] Online databases can be searched by keyword. MEDLINE, the National Library of Medicine's

---

☑ **Consumer Tip**

American Telemedicine Association Advisory on the Use of Medical Web Sites (1999)

Since the use of the Internet for accessing health information and medical treatment is new, there exists little in the way of safeguards for consumers. These guidelines can help consumers who choose to use the Internet to obtain information about health care or to seek medical treatment:

1. Make sure that Web sites used to obtain information about health and medicine are provided by a reliable and credible source such as recognized and credentialed health care providers, and use sources that are based on qualified authorities. The source of the information should be clearly labeled and annotated.

2. In some cases commercial interests such as a drug manufacturer may sponsor or contribute information to a Web site. Consumers should look for assurances that the information provided in these cases is objective and does not favor the sponsor's products.

3. At this time consumers should exercise caution in using Web sites that offer online diagnosis of an individual's medical condition and prescribed treatment and medication for the diagnosed condition. There are currently no recognized accreditation or regulatory authorities overseeing the operation of these sites.

4. It is a widely recognized conflict of interest for health professionals that prescribe medicines to have any direct financial relationship with an entity that sells those medications. Therefore, consumers are cautioned against obtaining prescribed medicines from Web sites that offer both diagnosis of condition and direct sales of the prescribed medicine.

5. Consumers seeking medical treatment from health professionals over the Internet should receive clear assurances that they will be interacting with a qualified professional holding the appropriate credentials and that the professional is able to legally practice medicine in the consumer's location.

6. Clinical consultation over the Web by credentialed providers should include procedures that protect the patient including: informed consent; information security and privacy protection measures; and documentation of the clinical encounter.

database of references to the medical literature, can be accessed through various commercial and noncommercial channels. It is the world's largest such database, with more than 12 million references published since 1966 and about 10,000 new ones added per week.

The World Wide Web offers "pages" of text and graphics, similar to the pages of a magazine, on millions of topics. Pages can be accessed by clicking on a "link" (hyperlink) or entering their "URL" (unique resource locator) in a Web browser window. Newsgroups and bulletin boards enable individuals to hold discussions by posting and responding to messages. "Chat groups" permit discussions with all participants typing at once. Electronic mailing lists enable designated groups to hold discussions by electronic mail (unlike newsgroups and chat groups, which are available to all comers). Online sources provide peer communication, anonymity, convenience, and rapid responses. The information is voluminous but not necessarily accurate. Virtually anyone can create an online resource and make it generally available. This includes not only health professionals but also ordinary people who believe they have been helped by a product, companies with a financial stake in the information they provide, and even outright charlatans.

Locating Information
The Internet has no central index, but the World Wide Web offers special pages, called search engines, that index large portions of the Net. Examples are:

Altavista	http://www.altavista.com
Go	http://www.go.com
Yahoo	http://www.yahoo.com
Google	http://www.google.com

"Advanced search" options enable searches to be more focused. For most purposes, the most useful search engine is probably Google, which carries no advertising and can search more than 1.3 billion pages in about 1 second. Its advanced search page enables display of as many as 100 links at a time. The "Cached" links sometimes access pages archived on Google's servers that are no longer on the Web. The most efficient MEDLINE search engine is the National Center for Biology Information's "Clinical Queries" page located at http://www.ncbi.nlm.nih.gov:80/entrez/query/static/clinical.html.

Judging Credibility
The following questions can help evaluate the credibility of an online information source: (a) Who maintains the information? (b) Is it linked with other reputable

Table 2-4
WEB SITES RELATED TO CONSUMER HEALTH

Each of these sites contains extensive practical material. However, information about "alternative" methods on the sites marked with an asterisk (*) is not trustworthy and should be ignored.

American Academy of Family Physicians
http://www.aafp.org/family/patient.html

American Academy of Pediatrics
http://www.aap.org

American Cancer Society*
http://www.cancer.org

American Council on Science and Health
http://www.acsh.org

American Dietetic Association
http://www.eatright.org

American Heart Association (AHA)
http://www.americanheart.org

American Medical Association (AMA)
http://www.ama-assn.org

Chirobase
http://www.chirobase.org

Consumer Health Sourcebook
http://www.chsourcebook.com

Federal Trade Commission (FTC)
http://www.ftc.gov

Food and Drug Administration (FDA)
http://www.fda.gov
   Center for Food Safety & Applied Nutrition
   http://vm.cfsan.fda.gov

Health Care Reality Check
http://www.hcrc.org

InteliHealth*
http://www.intelihealth.com

Mayo Clinic Health Oasis
http://www.mayohealth.org

Museum of Questionable Medical Devices
http://www.mtn.org/quack/index.htm

National Cancer Institute (NCI)*
http://www.nci.nih.gov

National Council Against Health Fraud
http://www.ncahf.org

National Fraud Information Center
http://www.fraud.org

National Institutes of Health (NIH)*
http://www.nih.gov/

Oncolink (cancer database)
http://oncolink.upenn.edu

Quackwatch
http://www.quackwatch.com

sources of medical information? (c) When was it last updated? and (d) Is it selling a product? Larkin and Douglas[45] suggest that if you find something of interest, write it down (and the site's location) and ask your doctor about it. Quackwatch[46] recommends avoiding all sites that are marketing dietary supplements, herbs, or homeopathic products. Unsolicited commercial e-mail messages ("spam") for health-related products should also be ignored.

Many efforts are being made to develop quality standards and rating systems.[47] Two Canadian researchers examined 47 systems used to rate Web sites providing health information on the Internet and found that 14 of these described their rating criteria, only 5 provided instructions for their use, and none provided information on whether they had been validated. The researchers concluded: "Many incompletely developed instruments to evaluate health information exist on the Internet. It is unclear, however, whether they should exist in the first place, whether they measure what they claim to measure, or whether they lead to more good than harm."[48] Most of these systems excessively weighted appearance, ease of use, and other factors unrelated to information quality.[49] Reliable reviews of health-related Web sites suitable for laypersons are published regularly on Health Scout and MD net guide. Most guidebooks to health-related Web sites judge good sites accurately but fail to appropriately criticize bad ones.

The HONcode system encourages voluntary compliance with high standards, but it does not ensure that content is accurate. (See Consumer Health Insight box). Quackwatch's screening list enables rapid identification of "quacky sites" to avoid.[46] (See Consumer Tip box.) However, judging the accuracy of science-based sites requires expert knowledge. So even if a "perfect" yardstick were developed, no organization is likely to have sufficient resources to apply it to the huge number of sites available for laypersons. Table 2-4 on page 29 lists the URLs of several reliable sources.

FURTHER SUGGESTIONS FOR CONSUMERS

Individuals must act intelligently to protect themselves from misleading and fraudulent practices that abound in the health marketplace.

Johnson and Goldfinger[50] provide these tips for evaluating medical or health information:

- Proof that a new treatment is effective requires controlled studies that compare treatment under discussion to other treatments or to no treatment. Controls help to remove bias, and with large enough numbers the study can be statistically valid.

☑ Consumer Tip

Signs of a Quacky Web Site

The best way to avoid being quacked is to reject quackery's promoters. Each item listed below signifies that a Web site is not a trustworthy information source:

General Characteristics
- Any site used to market herbs or dietary supplements. Although some of these products are useful, it is impossible to sell them profitably without deception, which typically includes: (a) lack of full disclosure of relevant facts, (b) promotion or sale of products that lack a rational use, and/or (c) failure to state who should **not** use the products.
- Any site used to market or promote homeopathic products. No such products have been proven effective.
- Any site that **generally** promotes "alternative" methods. There are more than 1000 "alternative" methods. The vast majority are worthless.
- Any site that promotes "nontoxic," "natural," or "holistic" treatments.

False Statements about Nutrition
- Everyone should take vitamins.
- Vitamins are effective against stress.
- Taking vitamins makes people more energetic.
- Organic foods are safer and/or more nutritious than ordinary foods.
- Losing weight is easy.
- Special diets can cure cancer
- Diet is the principal cause of hyperactivity.

False Statements about "Alternative" Methods
- Acupuncture is effective against a long list of diseases.
- Chelation therapy is an effective substitute for bypass surgery
- Chiropractic treatment is efd ctive against a large number of diseases
- Herbs are generally superior to prescription drugs.
- Homeopathic products are effective remedies.
- Spines should be checked and adjusted regularly by a chiropractor.

False Statements about Other Issues
- Fluoridation is dangerous.
- Immunizations are dangerous.
- Mercury-amalgam ("silver") filings should be removed because they make people sick.
- All teeth that have had root-canal therapy should be removed because they make people sick.

- Reports should be based on studies published in peer-reviewed medical journals.
- Safety is not an absolute phenomenon but a relative one. All life activities, including medical treatment, involve some risk. The question is whether the risk is justified in comparison to other treatments and to the potential gain.
- Be wary of claims of unusual remedies for chronic or incurable diseases. The burden of proof rests with those who make the claims.

Fleiger[51] advises consumers to be skeptical of news of major drug "breakthroughs" because many such reports are exaggerated or inaccurate interpretations of scientific findings. Noting that truly significant advances in drugs and drug therapy are rare, he gives these tips:

- News stories about drugs producing complete cures, especially in patients with severe arthritis, AIDS, cancer, or other grave illnesses, are likely to be wrong. Except for

---

▶ Consumer Health Insight

Significance of the HONcode Seal

 The Internet's most widely recognized standard-setting organization is the Geneva-based Health on the Net (HON) Foundation (http://www.hon.ch). Sites that follow its code of conduct are welcome to display the HONcode seal. The HONcode principles evolved from discussions with Webmasters and medical professionals in several countries. These principles are sound, but compliance is voluntary and some sites displaying the seal contain unreliable information or link to other sites that contain unreliable information. To legitimately use the seal, a Web site must apply for registration. If accepted, it must subsequently comply with all the principles enumerated in the HONcode. When a noncompliant site is reported, HONcode officials ask that the seal be removed—and most sites comply. In January 2000, there were registered connections from about 5500 servers and 20,000 external Web pages. To check whether a site is actually registered, click on the HONcode seal, which should be linked to a registration status report on the HON site. The HON Foundation also reviews Web sites and posts the results. However, its reviews of sites providing unreliable information on "alternative" methods have been descriptive rather than critical—and thus offer little or no guidance to Web browsers. In addition, its search engine does not limit its searches to reliable sites. HON officials are aware of these problems and have indicated interest in correcting them.

1. Authority
Any medical or health advice provided and hosted on this site will only be given by medically trained and qualified professionals unless a clear statement is made that a piece of advice offered is from a non-medically qualified individual or organization.

2. Complementarity
The information provided on this site is designed to support, not replace, the relationship that exists between a patient/site visitor and his/her existing physician.

3. Confidentiality
Confidentiality of data relating to individual patients and visitors to a medical/health Web site, including their identity, is respected by this Web site. The Web site owners undertake to honor or exceed the legal requirements of medical/health information privacy that apply in the country and state where the Web site and mirror sites are located.

4. Attribution
Where appropriate, information contained on this site will be supported by clear references to source data and, where possible, have specific HTML links to that data. The date when a clinical page was last modified will be clearly displayed (e.g., at the bottom of the page).

5. Justifiability
Any claims relating to the benefits/performance of a specific treatment, commercial product or service will be supported by appropriate, balanced evidence in the manner outlined in Principle 4.

6. Transparency of authorship
The designers of this Web site will seek to provide information in the clearest possible manner and provide contact addresses for visitors that seek further information or support. The Webmaster will display his/her e-mail address clearly throughout the Web site.

7. Transparency of sponsorship
Support for this Web site will be clearly identified, including the identities of commercial and non-commercial organizations that have contributed funding, services or material for the site.

8. Honesty in advertising & editorial policy
If advertising is a source of funding, it will be clearly stated. A brief description of the advertising policy adopted by the Web site owners will be displayed on the site. Advertising and other promotional material will be presented to viewers in a manner and context that facilitates differentiation between it and the original material created by the institution operating the site.

—Version 1.5, July 1996

antibiotics, few drugs can make a disease disappear totally and permanently.

- The results of one study of a small number of patients are seldom, if ever, conclusive. News stories may place undue importance on these reports and jump to conclusions that the researchers themselves know are unjustified.
- Consider whether the report was made by a reporter or news service that regularly covers health and medical affairs and assigns reporters specializing in the subject. Be skeptical if the source emphasizes sensational stories on a regular basis.
- Ask your doctor. Although physicians cannot know everything, they are likely to be aware of truly important medical advances.

☑ Consumer Tip

How to Judge an Information Source

The following questions may be helpful in determining reliable sources of information:

- What is the purpose of the book, presentation, or statement? Is it to sell products or ideas and make money? Or is it to present data or to make a professional contribution?
- What is the procedure and style of presentation? Is it presented in an educational or scientific manner? Are propaganda devices used, such as testimonials, broad generalities, name-calling, and misleading statements? Does the information contain exaggerated claims or use gross superlatives?
- What are the qualifications of the author, speaker, organization, or agency? What is the educational background, professional experience, and training of the individual? If he has scientific credentials, are they in the field in which he is making claims?
- What is the standing of the individual in the professional community? Is the person listed in any recognized biographic sources such as *American Men and Women of Science* or in directories of health specialists?
- Are the data based on appropriate research by experts in the health field or on the testimony or opinions of one or a few individuals? Is the information based on scientific facts or on emotional appeal?
- Has the information been published in peer-reviewed professional journals and generally accepted as valid by the scientific community?
- Where there appear to be conflicting claims about a health matter, what is the extent of the evidence supporting or refuting the claims? Has the claimant generalized from a particular incident or from broad research?

To stay informed, consumers can do the following:

- Read reliable publications such as those recommended in Table 2-3. The most practical and reliable magazines are *Priorities for Health* and *FDA Consumer*. The best newsletters are *Consumer Reports on Health* and *Tufts University Health & Nutrition Letter*. The best source on "alternative medicine" is the journal *Scientific Review of Alternative Medicine*.
- Identify and use reliable sources of information on the Internet.
- Read the health and medical news in *Time, Newsweek,* and *U.S. News & World Report*, but be wary of their coverage of "alternative" health methods and alleged health threats.
- Take courses at accredited schools, colleges, and universities, but do not assume that all their courses are free of misinformation.
- Select health professionals and health educators carefully.
- Obtain information from federal, state, and local government agencies and reputable professional and voluntary organizations, such as the FDA, the AMA, the American Cancer Society, the American Dental Association, the U.S. Public Health Service, and others listed in Chapter 26 and the Appendix.

SUMMARY

Consumers obtain health information from nonprofessional, professional, and pseudoprofessional individuals as well as from educational institutions and from the media. Unfortunately, much of this information is misleading, inaccurate, or false.

The scientific method offers an objective way to evaluate information to determine what is false, but even scientists sometimes find it difficult to sort fact from fiction.

The intelligent health consumer should follow these practices:

- Maintain a healthy degree of skepticism toward health information received through the media.
- Select practitioners with great care.
- Become well-informed before making decisions to purchase and use health products and services; pay little or no attention to health advertising.
- Seek reliable sources of information.
- Be familiar with the fundamental concepts used in the scientific method, including statistical concepts.

REFERENCES

1. Mirkin G. Foreword to Barrett S, Herbert V. The Vitamin Pushers: How the "Health Food" Industry Is Selling America a Bill of Goods. Amherst, N.Y., 1994, Prometheus Books.
2. Sagan C. The fine art of baloney detection. Parade Magazine, p 12–13, Feb 1, 1987.

3. Accardo P, Lindsay R. Nutrition and behavior: The legend continues. Pediatrics 93:127–128, 1994.
4. Harper AE. Mythical thinking vs scientific thinking, ACSH News & Views 4(2):4–5, 1983.
5. Schick T Jr, Vaughn L. How to Think about Weird Things. Mountain View, Calif., 1994, Mayfield Publishing Co.
6. Doyle RP. The Medical Wars. New York, 1983, William Morrow & Co.
7. Savits DA and others. Methods in chronic disease epidemiology. In Brownson RC, Remington PL, Davis JR, editors. Chronic Disease Epidemiology and Control. Washington, D.C., 1993, American Public Health Association.
8. Ernst E and others. The importance of placebo effects. JAMA 273:283, 1995.
9. The gold standard of research trials. Harvard Heart Letter 2(2):6–7, 1991.
10. Wennberg JE and others, editors. Outcomes research, PORTs, and health care reform. In Warren KS, Mosteller F. Doing More Good than Harm: The Evaluation of Health Care Interventions. New York, 1993, The New York Academy of Sciences.
11. Beecher HK. Surgery as placebo: A quantitative study of bias. JAMA 176:1102–1107, 1961.
12. Sakethoo K and others. Effects of drinking hot water, cold water, and chicken soup on nasal mucus velocity and airflow resistance. Chest 74:408–410, 1978.
13. Karlowski TR and others. Ascorbic acid for the common cold: A prophylactic and therapeutic trial. JAMA 246:2235–2237, 1975.
14. Huff D. How to Lie with Statistics. New York, 1954, WW Norton & Co.
15. Physicians' Health Study Group. Preliminary report: Findings from the aspirin component of the ongoing Physicians' Health Study. New England Journal of Medicine 318:262–264, 1988.
16. Standards of Reporting Trials Group. A proposal for structured reporting of randomized clinical trials. JAMA 272:1926–1931, 1994.
17. Relman AS. Peer review in scientific journals: What good is it? Western Journal of Medicine 153:520–522; 1990.
18. Bero L, Rennie D. The Cochrane Collaboration: Preparing, maintaining, and disseminating systematic reviews of the effects of health care. JAMA 274:1935–1938, 1995.
19. Scientists deplore flight from reason. New York Times, June 6, 1995.
20. Barrett S. The mirage of multilevel marketing. Quackwatch Web site, Aug 26, 1999.
21. Hatfield D. In defense of the establishment. ACSH News & Views 6(2):6–7, 1985.

22. Davis EH. Complementary or alternative medicine. Journal of the American Board of Family Practice 9:70, 1996.
23. Peterson S. Spinning on science's shores. The Skeptical Inquirer 13(4):436, 1989.
24. Arseneau JC, Thigpen JT. The new quack: Pseudoscience, public relations and politics. Journal of the Mississippi State Medical Association, p 202–207, Aug 1981.
25. Radner D, Radner M. Science and Unreason. Belmont, Calif., 1982, Wadsworth Publishing Co.
26. Criss M. Science and nonscience. The Rocky Mountain Skeptic 5(2):5–8, 1987.
27. Beyerstein BL. Testing claims of therapeutic efficacy. Rational Enquirer 7(4):1–2, 8, 1995.
28. Barrett S. Be wary of medical endorsements. ACSH News & Views 8(3):3–4, 1987.
29. Lederer RJ, Singer B. Pseudoscience in the name of the university. The Skeptical Inquirer 7(3):57–62, 1983.
30. Gunther M. Quackery and the media. In Barrett S, editor. The Health Robbers, 2nd edition. Philadelphia, 1980, George F Stickley Co.
31. Wilson B. The rise and fall of Laetrile. Quackwatch Web site, Jan 22, 2000.
32. Koren G, Klein N. Bias against negative studies in newspaper reports of medical research. JAMA 266:1824–1826, 1991.
33. Barrett S, Herbert V. The Vitamin Pushers: How the "Health Food" Industry Is Selling America a Bill of Goods. Amherst, N.Y., 1994, Prometheus Books.
34. Kansas D.C. fights anti-chiropractic textbook—nationwide effort urged. ACA Journal of Chiropractic 25(12):19–20, 1988.
35. Larkin M. Confessions of a former women's magazine writer. NutriWatch Web site, March 26, 2000.
36. Woznicki D and others. Nutrition accuracy in popular magazines (January 1995—December 1996). New York, 1998, American Council on Science and Health.
37. Barrett S. Truth or trash? Health-related information in the tabloids. Priorities for Health, p 27–30, Summer 1989.
38. Saltus R. New hay fever drug may replace antihistamines. San Francisco Sunday Examiner and Chronicle, May 15, 1983.
39. Barrett S and others. "Quackbusters" respond. Vegetarian Times, p 10–14, March 1992.
40. Bloyd-Peshkin S. The health-fraud cops—are the quackbusters consumer advocates or medical McCarthyites? Vegetarian Times, p 49–59, Aug 1991.
41. Butler K. Lying for Fun and Profit: The Truth about the Media. Kula, Hawaii, 1999, Health Wise Productions.
42. London WM, Whelan EM, Kava R. Expert reviews of health reports on CBS Television's 60 Minutes, 1978–1995. Technology 7:539–552, 2000.
43. Heussner RC, Salmon ME. Warning: The Media May Be Harmful to Your Health: A Consumer's Guide to Medical News and Advertising. Kansas City, Mo., 1988, Andrews & McMeel.
44. Peters R, Sikorski R. Digital dialog: Sharing information and interests on the Internet. JAMA 277:1258–1260, 1997.
45. Larkin M, Douglas D. Health information in cyberspace: Steering a clear course through the clutter. Priorities for Health 7(4):15–18, 1995.
46. Barrett S. How to spot a "quacky" Web site. Quackwatch Web site, June 10, 2000.
47. Lundberg GM and others. Assessing, controlling, and assuring the quality of medical information on the Internet. *Caveat lector et viewor*—Let the reader and viewer beware. JAMA 277:1244–1245, 1997.

It's Your Decision

According to a local newspaper report, a researcher at a medical center claims to have discovered a substance that shows great promise for curing severe acne. How can consumers determine whether the report is valid? What questions should be raised about the research methodology, the use or misuse of statistics, the possibility of fraud, and whether the study has been peer-reviewed? How can the reliability of this information be checked?

48. Alejandro R and others. Rating health information on the Internet: Navigating to knowledge or babel? JAMA 279:611–614, 1998.

49. Internet rating systems: Knowledge or babel. (Letters to the editor.) JAMA 280:698–700, 1998.

50. Johnson GT, Goldfinger SE, editors. The Harvard Medical School Health Letter Book. Cambridge, Mass., 1981, Harvard University Press.

51. Fleiger K. A skeptic's guide to medical "breakthroughs." FDA Consumer 21(9):13, 1987.

Chapter Three

FRAUDS AND QUACKERY

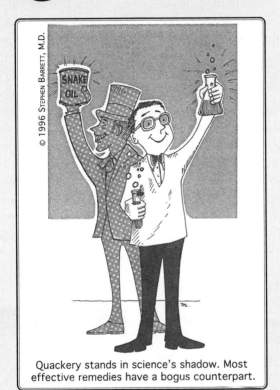

Quackery stands in science's shadow. Most
effective remedies have a bogus counterpart.

*There is nothing men will not do, there is nothing they have not done
to recover their health and save their lives. They have submitted to
being half-drowned in water, and half-choked with gases, to being
buried up to their chins in earth, to being scarred with hot irons like
galley slaves, to being crimped with knives like codfish, to having
needles thrust into their flesh, and bonfires kindled in their skins, to
swallowing all sorts of abominations, and to pay for all this, as if to
be singed and scalded were a costly privilege, as if blistering were a
blessing and leeches a luxury.*

OLIVER WENDELL HOLMES

There's a sucker born every minute.

OFTEN ATTRIBUTED TO P.T. BARNUM

There's also a crook born every hour who can take care of sixty suckers.

ANONYMOUS

Key Concepts
KEEP THESE POINTS IN MIND AS YOU STUDY THIS CHAPTER

- Anecdotes and testimonials are not reliable evidence that a product or service is effective.

- Spontaneous remissions and the placebo effect can make it difficult to determine whether treatments are effective.

- Quackery is far more widespread and pervasive than most people realize.

- The best way to avoid being tricked is to stay away from tricksters. Don't base your health-related decisions on the advice of people who exhibit the signs of quackery described in this book.

- Many quacks promote conspiracy theories and a "freedom of choice" concept to divert attention from the worthlessness of their methods.

Despite the tremendous advances in medical science, health frauds and quackery are still common. Newspapers, magazines, radio, television, and computer channels provide entrepreneurs with enormous opportunities to promote their wares to the public. Laws intended to control fraud and quackery have not been particularly successful. This chapter provides practical definitions of health fraud and quackery, explains why people are vulnerable, and tells how to identify and avoid quack practices. The remaining chapters in the text offer more detailed information about the practices listed, as well as many others that deserve attention.

DEFINITIONS

"Quackery" derives from the word *quacksalver* (someone who boasts about his salves). Dictionaries define *quack* as "a pretender to medical skill; a charlatan" and "one who talks pretentiously without sound knowledge of the subject discussed." These definitions suggest that the promotion of quackery involves deliberate deception, but many promoters sincerely believe in what they are doing. The FDA defines health fraud as "the promotion, for profit, of a medical remedy known to be false or unproven." This also can cause confusion because in ordinary usage—and in the courts—the word "fraud" connotes deliberate deception. Dr. William T. Jarvis,[1] former president of the National Council Against Health Fraud, stresses that quackery's paramount characteristic is promotion ("Quacks quack!") rather than fraud, greed, or misinformation.

Quack methods are sometimes referred to as "alternative" health care. However, the terms *unscientific*, *nonscientific*, or *dubious* are more appropriate. This book generally uses these terms and places the word "alternative" in quotation marks when using it to describe unscientific methods.

Most people think of quackery as promoted by charlatans who deliberately exploit their victims. Actually, most promoters are unwitting victims who share misinformation and personal experiences with others. Customers of multilevel companies that sell health-related products typically have been persuaded by friends, relatives, and neighbors who use the products because they believe them effective. Pharmacists also profit from the sale of nutrition supplements that few customers need. In most cases pharmacists do not champion the products but simply profit from the misleading promotions of others. Much quackery is involved in telling people something is bad for them (such as food additives) and selling a substitute (such as "organic" or "natural" food). Quackery is also involved in misleading advertising of dietary supplements, homeopathic products, and some

---

Historical Perspective
Quacks Quack

Why should a critter as cute and harmless-looking as a duck be used to symbolize the vicious social menace of quackery? A vulture would seem to be more appropriate. But vultures actually wait until death occurs before engaging their targets. Thus their conduct is too benign to symbolize quackery, which preys on the weak, the helpless, and the desperate.

Other birds of prey behave more like that of quacks, but the bald eagle, which is a national symbol, would not be suitable for derision. An ostrich might be appropriate, because of its reputation for hiding its head in the sand, thus symbolizing the denial so often seen in both quacks and their victims. The word *quack* is short for "quacksalver," which literally means to quack like a duck about one's salves. The duck personifies quackery because it makes a lot of noise about nothing.

William T. Jarvis, Ph.D.

nonprescription drugs. In many such instances no individual "quack" is involved—just deception by manufacturers and their advertising agencies.

Quackery is not an all-or-nothing phenomenon. A practitioner may be scientific in many respects and only minimally involved in unscientific practices. Also, products can be useful for some purposes but worthless for others. For example, vitamin B_{12} shots are lifesaving in cases of pernicious anemia, but giving them frequently to "pep you up" is quackery.

Quackery and malpractice overlap but are not identical. Quackery entails the use of methods that are not scientifically accepted. Malpractice involves failure by a health professional to meet accepted standards of diagnosis and treatment. It includes situations in which the practitioner was negligent while using standard methods of care. Leaving a surgical instrument in a patient's abdomen or operating on the wrong part of the body are examples of malpractice unrelated to quackery.

To avoid semantic problems, some experts suggest that quackery be broadly defined as "anything involving overpromotion in the field of health." This definition would include questionable ideas as well as questionable products and services, regardless of the sincerity of their promoters. In line with this definition, the word "fraud" would be reserved only for situations in which deliberate deception is involved.

Unproven methods are not necessarily quackery. Those that are consistent with established scientific concepts may be considered experimental. Legitimate researchers and practitioners do not promote unproven procedures in the marketplace but engage in responsible studies with proper protocols (see Chapter 2). Legitimate practitioners may try methods that have not been completely tested, but do not peddle them to build their practice. Methods not compatible with established scientific concepts should be classified as nonsensical or disproven rather than experimental. Homeopathy's claim that infinitesimally dilute solutions can exert powerful effects is the epitome of health nonsense (see Chapter 8).

FRAUDS AND QUACKERY TODAY

At least $15 billion is spent yearly on products and services that are falsely claimed to prevent or alleviate health problems. Some experts say this figure is too conservative, but no precise data are available. Many millions of dollars yearly are wasted on magnets and other health devices (see Chapter 22), exercise equipment (see Chapter 14), unnecessary and ineffective drug and beauty products (Chapters 19 and 20), and

worthless and possibly harmful cancer remedies (Chapter 17). The Arthritis Foundation states that $1 billion a year is spent on quack remedies (Chapter 16). It adds that 60% of patients continue to try questionable diets and nostrums such as alfalfa seed, sea brine, liniments, and iodine baths, even when under professional care. Billions are wasted annually for spurious food remedies, weight-reduction schemes and products, fad diets, "organic" and "natural" foods, and unnecessary vitamins and minerals (see Chapters 11 and 12).

The California Medical Association[3] has listed the following widely promoted practices as questionable: acupuncture, acupressure, applied kinesiology, bogus arthritis treatments, "cellular therapy," cellulite removal, chelation therapy, clinical ecology, colonic irrigation, cytotoxic testing, DMSO (dimethyl sulfoxide), enzymes and "glandular extracts," faith and psychic healing, figure enhancers, hair analysis, homeopathy, immune system protectors, iridology, Laetrile (amygdalin) treatment for cancer, live cell analysis, nutrition remedies for cancer, polarity therapy, reflexology, Touch for Health, vitamin megadoses, and youth prolongers.

A U.S. House of Representatives subcommittee report[4] detailed numerous fraudulent and quack endeavors including: (a) clinics inside and outside the United States that provide bogus treatments for chronic and terminally ill patients using diet, drugs, and enemas for arthritis, cancer, heart disease, and other ailments; (b) foundations that encourage the use of unproven remedies; and (c) phony healers who use a religious healing image or claim powers generated by Satan or witchcraft.

In 1989 the FDA[5] listed the following as the top 10 health frauds: (a) fraudulent arthritis products, (b) bogus AIDS cures, (c) instant weight-loss schemes, (d) fraudulent sexual aids, (e) spurious cancer clinics, (f) quack baldness remedies and other appearance modifiers, (g) false nutritional schemes, (h) unproven use of muscle stimulators, (i) chelation therapy (claimed to clean out clogged arteries), and (j) treatment for nonexistent yeast infections.

WHY PEOPLE ARE VULNERABLE

Despite the advanced state of medical science, many people with health problems turn to dubious methods. Faced with the prospect of chronic suffering, deformity, or death, many individuals are tempted to try anything that offers relief or hope. The terminally ill, the elderly, and various cultural minorities are especially vulnerable to health frauds and quackery. Many intelligent and well-educated individuals resort to unconventional medical procedures with the belief that anything is better than nothing. Former Arthritis Foundation official Jerry Walsh, who was stricken at age 18 with rheumatoid arthritis, admitted that during the early years of his illness he spent thousands of dollars on quack remedies—everything from radium gadgets to magic buckeyes.

Beyerstein[6] has noted:

Subtle forces can lead intelligent people (both patients and therapists) to think that a treatment has helped someone when it has not. This is true for new treatments in scientific medicine, as well as for nostrums in folk medicine, fringe practices in "alternative medicine," and the ministrations of faith healers.

Specific reasons why people turn to questionable methods include the following:

- Individuals may underestimate the degree of illness or may delay obtaining assistance because they believe they cannot afford such services.
- Religious and cultural beliefs can foster acceptance of faith healers, prayer, magic, sorcery, and the like. For example, some Chinese people consider acupuncture and herbal remedies as standard forms of treatment and regard the scientific medicine practiced in the United States as totally foreign.
- Physicians may be unable to communicate in language their patients understand. Patients may be unable to question their physicians; they may lack knowledge or fear that they will be criticized.
- Patients may distrust physicians or question the quality of their care. Doctors sometimes appear more concerned with treating illnesses than with helping the patient.
- Some people harbor extreme distrust of the medical profession, the food industry, drug companies, and government agencies. Some feel deeply antagonistic toward scientific medicine but are attracted to methods that are "natural" or otherwise unconventional.
- People fear social unacceptability, pain, death, and growing old (wrinkles, loss of hair and sensory acuity, decreased sexual potency, and incontinence). Elderly individuals are particularly vulnerable in this regard.
- Faced with a serious health problem that physicians cannot solve, many people become desperate enough to try almost anything that arouses hope. Many victims of cancer, arthritis, multiple sclerosis, and AIDS fall prey to unscrupulous entrepreneurs. Some squander their life's savings searching for a "cure."
- Many people suffer from chronic aches, pains, or other discomforts for which medicine cannot offer clear-cut diagnoses or effective treatment. The more persistent the condition, the more susceptible the sufferer may be to promises of a "cure." Many people in this category fall into the hands of doctors who make fad diagnoses such as hypoglycemia, "candidiasis hypersensitivity," or "multiple chemical sensitivity" (see Chapter 8).
- Many practitioners have difficulty in helping people whose symptoms are the result of emotional problems or are bodily responses to stress.
- Many people are gullible because of their ignorance of health matters. People also tend to believe what others tell them about personal experience. Many people believe that any health-related claim in print or in a broadcast must be true, and many are attracted by promises of quick, painless, or drugless solutions to problems.
- The mass media provide much false and misleading information in advertisements, news reports, feature articles, and books and on radio and television programs. News reports are often sensationalized, stimulating false hopes and arousing widespread fears. Many radio and television producers who promote unsubstantiated health claims say they are providing entertainment and have no ethical duty to check the claims.

- People fail to realize that some serious illnesses (even cancer and arthritis) have ups and downs. Temporary improvement may be mistakenly attributed to whatever product or service was used before it occurred.
- Many people do not understand the nature of the placebo effect (discussed later in this chapter).
- Self-confidence, which quacks tend to exude, is a powerful persuader. The "Self-Confidence Sells" Personal Glimpse box contains the condensed testimony of a defense witness in the 1990 trial of a Canadian couple whose infant daughter had died of malnutrition under the care of an unlicensed naturopath. The couple were charged with criminal negligence, but they were acquitted when a judge ruled that the problem was not neglect but misplaced trust.

Psychologist Anthony R. Pratkanis, Ph.D., has identified nine strategies used to sell pseudoscientific beliefs and practices. They include setting phantom goals (such as better health, peace of mind, or improved sex life), making statements that tend to inspire trust ("supported by over 100 studies"), and fostering granfalloons (proud and otherwise meaningless associations of people who share rituals, beliefs, jargon, goals, feelings, specialized information, and "enemies").[7] Multilevel sales groups, nutrition cultists, and crusaders for "alternative" treatments fit this description well.

HAZARDS

Consumers should be aware of quackery's dangers. Financial harm can range from minor expense to loss of one's life savings. Improper diagnosis can lead to a deterioration of health. Unsafe procedures can cause irreparable harm. Delay in getting proper treatment can have serious or fatal consequences. Psychologic harm can also occur.[8] The following well-publicized cases illustrate quackery's serious potential for harm.

In 1961, the parents of 8-year-old Linda Epping charged that a chiropractor had bilked them out of $739 by promising to cure her of cancer of the eye. Linda had been scheduled for surgery to remove her left eye and surrounding tissue. Her doctors thought cure was possible because it appeared that the tumor had not spread. But shortly before the operation was to be performed, Linda's parents met a couple who said that a chiropractor had cured their son's brain tumor without using surgery. After the chiropractor agreed to help by "balancing" Linda's body, her parents removed her from the hospital and took her for treatment with "spinal adjustments," vitamins, food supplements, and laxatives (up to 124 pills plus 150 drops of iodine solution daily). Despite the new "treatment," the tumor grew quickly. Within three weeks it was the size of a tennis ball and had pushed Linda's eye out of its socket. She died within

a few months. The chiropractor was subsequently convicted of second-degree murder and sentenced to prison.[9]

Ruth Conrad, an Idaho woman, consulted one of the state's many unlicensed naturopaths. While seeking treatment for a sore shoulder, she also complained of a bump on her nose. The naturopath stated that it was cancer and gave her a black herbal salve to apply directly. Within a few days, her face became very painful and she developed red streaks that ran down her cheeks. Her anxious phone call to the naturopath brought the explanation that the presence of the lines was a good sign because they "resemble a crab, and cancer is a crab." He also advised her to apply more of the black salve. Within 1 week, a large part of her face, including her nose, sloughed off. It took 3 years and 17 plastic surgery operations to reconstruct her face.

Caroline Copeland,[10] an Arizona journalist, consulted a leading "holistic" physician who seemed very attentive to her concerns. During most of the 16 years she remained under his care, his recommendations appeared logical and effective. Her initial diagnosis was hypoglycemia (low blood sugar). Later she was told she had hypothyroidism and was treated with thyroid hormone.

◆ Personal Glimpse ◆

Self-Confidence Sells

The herbalist was a very impressive man. He just glowed with health and was very charismatic, very jovial, charming, friendly, very nice, very knowledgeable. There was not a question that you could ask that he would not have an answer for. And he told a lot of stories about people who had come to see him and been cured by following his course of treatment. It's a very difficult thing to communicate just how mesmerizing this man was. He was so good, so positive. He just exuded this powerful aura about him. He told my father that his cancer was completely curable. He had to change his diet because this was the cause of the cancer. He would have to eat strictly fruits and vegetables, raw, or juices of those fruits and vegetables, and by doing this, the tumor would be dissolved. When my father lost weight, the herbalist said this was just the body ridding itself of toxins and poisons. During his final two weeks, my father developed a hole near his rectum and a lesion that grew bigger each day. The herbalist said it was just the radiation coming out, which was a good thing. I now know it was a gangrenous tumor. I look back now and can't believe that I fell under this man's spell.

Testimony of Magaly Bianchini[11]

A Traumatic Experience

In *The Faith Healers*, James Randi tells what happened to a youngster with twisted legs who attended televangelist Peter Popoff's "Miracle Crusade" with strong expectations that he would be made well :

> Following the . . . spectacle, I saw that little boy outside the Civic Center again, perched on his crutches and staring down at the pavement. At the service, the highly touted "healer" had not even come near the kid. . . .
>
> The boy looked up as I approached him. His smile was gone, and I saw tears running down his face. His eyes were red from weeping. I began to speak, intending to ask him what he now thought of Popoff and his promises. But I choked up and had to turn away. . . .
>
> I will never forget that terrible moment, as the child realized that he had witnessed a cruel callous hoax. Hundreds of people at that meeting had believed they would see miracles performed. . . . Some few had been touched by the preacher, but none had been healed. Most had given cash or checks, some in envelopes sent to them by mail before they attended. One way or another, they were all swindled.[12]

Then she developed a "stubborn case" of iron-deficiency anemia that was treated with very high oral doses of iron and several vitamins plus injections containing iron, liver extract, and vitamin B_{12}. She also developed persistent constipation with bouts of abdominal pain. When additional symptoms developed, she sought help elsewhere and learned that all of the previous diagnoses had been wrong and that her symptoms were caused by iron and vitamin poisoning, thyroid hormone overdose, a grapefruit-sized ovarian cyst, and endometriosis (which, undiagnosed, had prevented her from bearing children). When she complained, the state licensing board concluded that her care had been inadequate, but it permitted the doctor to remain in practice.

COMMON MISCONCEPTIONS

There are many misconceptions about quackery. The following are among those identified by Jarvis and Barrett:[13]

Quacks are frauds and crooks. Most promoters of quackery sincerely believe in what they do. Their deception of others may not be deliberate.

Most quackery is dangerous. Most victims of quackery are harmed economically rather than physically. Sometimes a bogus approach will relieve emotionally related symptoms by lowering a person's tension level. Although such an experience is likely to be perceived as beneficial, it can prove harmful in the long run if the individual decides to rely upon unproven approaches for future health problems.

The media are reliable. Most media are willing to publicize sensational viewpoints they believe are newsworthy and likely to increase their audience. Radio and television and talk shows abound with promoters of nutrition quackery. General magazines that carry vitamin ads almost never publish articles advising readers not to waste their money on vitamins.

Personal experience is the best way to tell whether a treatment works. When someone feels better after using a product or procedure, it is natural to credit whatever was done. However, this is unwise. Most ailments are self-limiting, and even incurable conditions can have sufficient day-to-day variation to enable quack methods to gain large followings. Taking action often produces temporary relief of symptoms (a placebo effect). In addition, many products and services exert physical or psychologic effects that users misinterpret as evidence that their problem is being cured. These "Dr. Feelgood" modalities include pharmacologically active herbal products, quack formulas adulterated with prescription drugs, colonic irrigations (which some people enjoy), bodywork, and meditation. Scientific experimentation is almost always necessary to establish whether health methods are really effective. Thus it is extremely important for consumers to understand the concepts of spontaneous remission and the placebo effect.

Spontaneous Remission

Recovery from illness, whether it follows self-medication, treatment by a scientific practitioner, or treatment by an unscientific practitioner, may lead individuals to conclude that the treatment received was the cause of the return to good health. Medical historian James Harvey Young, Ph.D.,[14] has noted:

John Doe does not usually realize that most ailments are self-limiting and improve with time *regardless of treatment*. When a symptom goes away after he doses himself with a remedy, he is likely to credit the remedy with curing him. He does not realize that he would have gotten better just as quickly if he had done nothing! Thousands of well-meaning John and Jane Does have boosted the fame of folk remedies and have signed sincere testimonials for patent medicines, crediting them instead of the body's recuperative power for a return to well-being. . . .

The unscientific healer does not need to observe the restraints of reputable medicine. Where true medical science is complex, the quack can oversimplify. . . . Where ailments are self-limiting, the quack makes nature his secret ally.

It is commonly said that if you treat a cold it will disappear in a week, but if you leave it alone it will last 7 days. Even many serious diseases have ups and downs. Rheumatoid arthritis and multiple sclerosis are prime examples. On rare occasions even cancer can inexplicably disappear (although most testimonials for quack cancer remedies are based on faulty original diagnosis or simultaneous administration of effective treatment).

Quackery's victims are not the only ones who can be fooled by the placebo effect, spontaneous remissions, and other coincidental events. The gratitude and adulation of people who think they have been helped can even persuade charlatans that their methods are effective!

Placebo Effect

You must know that the will is a powerful adjuvant of medicine — PARACELSUS

The power of suggestion has been demonstrated by many investigators in a variety of settings. In a classroom, for example, a professor sprayed plain water about the room and asked the students to raise their hands as soon as they detected an odor. Seventy-three percent managed to smell a nonexistent odor.

Persons with a dominant or persuasive personality often have considerable impact on others through their ability to create confidence, which enhances suggestibility. Many individuals who are taken in by a charlatan later tell their doctors, "But he talked to me; he explained things; he was so nice."

Individuals who are psychologically susceptible to suggestion often feel better under the influence of counseling or reassurance. One woman remarked, "I take a multivitamin pill that *Consumer Reports* says is useless. But I don't care. It makes me happy." Gullibility and wishful thinking are common human characteristics. People are willing to believe in untrue things in varying ways and to varying degrees. Even scientifically sophisticated people may respond to the power of suggestion.

In medicine the effect of suggestion is referred to as the "placebo effect." The Latin word *placebo* means "I shall please." A placebo effect is a beneficial response to a substance, device, or procedure that cannot be accounted for on the basis of pharmacologic or other direct physical action. Feeling better when the physician walks into the room is a common example.

A placebo may be used in medicine to satisfy a patient that something is being done. By lessening anxiety, placebo action may alleviate symptoms caused by the body's reaction to tension (psychosomatic symptoms). In certain circumstances a lactose tablet (sugar pill) may relieve not only anxiety but also pain, nausea, vomiting, palpitations, shortness of breath, and other symptoms. The patient expects the "medication" to cause improvement, and sometimes it does.

Many studies have shown that placebos may relieve a broad range of symptoms. In many disorders, one third

---

Table 3-1

PLACEBO MYTHS AND FACTS

Myths	Facts
1. Placebos work on the imagination, not the body.	1. Placebos affect people physiologically as well as psychologically. Emotions can trigger the release of hormones that can affect bodily functions in many ways.
2. Placebos may help, but they cannot hurt.	2. Adverse reactions can occur. Common complaints include dry mouth, nausea, headache, drowsiness, sleep disturbance, and rash.
3. Placebos work primarily on suggestible patients.	3. All kinds of people may respond. There does not appear to be a specific personality profile.
4. The patient must believe in the treatment for it to have a placebo effect.	4. Nonbelievers can experience placebo effects if they believe in the practitioner, are influenced by the setting, or are suggestible, even if they do not believe in the treatment.
5. Placebo response is not so important if the active drug really works.	5. Patients often respond to placebos as well as to active drugs; a placebo can make an active drug more effective.
6. Placebo response depends on the patient, not the practitioner.	6. How the placebo is given and by whom influences the outcome more than any characteristic of the patient.

or more of patients will get relief from a placebo. Temporary relief has been demonstrated, for example, in arthritis, hay fever, headache, cough, high blood pressure, premenstrual tension, peptic ulcer, and even cancer. The psychologic aspects of many disorders also work to the healer's advantage. A large percentage of symptoms either have a psychologic component or do not arise from organic disease. Hence, treatment offering some lessening of tension can often help. A sympathetic ear or reassurance that no serious disease is involved may prove therapeutic by itself. Beyerstein[15] has observed:

Pain is partly a sensation . . . and partly an emotion. . . . Anything that can allay anxiety, redirect attention, reduce arousal, foster a sense of control, or lead to . . . reinterpretation of symptoms can alleviate the agony component of pain. Modern pain clinics put these strategies to use every day. Successful quacks and faith healers typically have charismatic personalities that make them adept at influencing these psychological variables that can modulate pain. . . . But we must be careful that purely symptomatic relief does not divert people from proven remedies until it is too late for them to be effective.

Confidence in the treatment—on the part of the patient and the practitioner—makes it more likely that a placebo effect will occur. But the power of suggestion may cause even a nonbeliever to respond favorably. The only requirement for a placebo effect is the awareness that something has been done. It is not possible to predict accurately or easily a particular patient's reaction to a placebo at a particular moment. However, the psychologic predisposition to respond positively to placebos is present to some extent in most people. Some are very likely to obtain relief from placebos in a wide variety of situations, whereas others are very unlikely to do so. Most people's response lies somewhere in between.

Another factor that can mislead people is selective affirmation—a tendency to look for positive responses when improvement is expected. As Jarvis[16] has further noted:

A culturally significant setting can also produce a potent effect, as folk healers know well. Effective settings can be as divergent as the trappings of an oriental herb shop to Asians, a circle of witchcraft paraphernalia to a primitive tribesman, or the atmosphere of a modern clinic to a modern urban American. Social expectations can also play a role, as occurs in stoic cultures where people are taught to endure pain and suffering without complaining. . . .

Operant conditioning can occur . . . when behavior is rewarded. . . . Thus, people with a history of favorable responses to treatment are more apt to react well to the act of treatment.

Responses to the treatment setting can also be negative ("nocebo effects"). In one experiment, for example, some subjects who were warned of possible side effects of a drug were given injections of a placebo instead. Many of them reported dizziness, nausea, vomiting, and even mental depression. A recent review of 109 double-blind drug trials found that the overall incidence of adverse events in healthy volunteers during placebo administration was 19%.[17]

Placebo responses, such as feeling less pain or more energy, can occur without affecting the actual course of the disease. Thus placebo responses can obscure real disease, which can lead to delay in obtaining appropriate diagnosis or treatment.

The placebo effect is not limited to drugs but may also result from procedures.[18] Devices and physical techniques often have a tremendous psychologic impact. Chiropractors, naturopaths, and various other nonmedical practitioners use heat, light, diathermy, hydrotherapy, manipulation, massage, and a variety of gadgets. In addition to any physiologic effects, their use can exert a potent psychologic force that may be reinforced by the relationship between the patient and the practitioner. Of course, devices and procedures used by scientific practitioners can also have placebo effects.

Barrett[19] has expressed serious misgivings about over-reliance on the placebo effect in clinical practice:

Doctors are confronted by many people who complain of tiredness or a variety of vague symptoms that are reactions to nervous tension. Far too often, instead of finding out what is bothering them, doctors tell them to take a tonic, a vitamin, or some other type of placebo.

I am against people being misled. The quack who relies on a placebo effect is also pretending he knows what he is doing—that he can tell what is wrong with you and that he has effective treatment for just about everything. His customers are playing Russian roulette. The medical doctor who uses vitamins as placebos may not be as dangerous, but he is encouraging people to form lifelong habits of using things they don't need.

Most people who use placebos do not get relief from them. So we're talking about practices that are not only misleading. They are also a financial rip-off.

RECOGNIZING QUACKERY

Fraud and quackery are so pervasive that laws and enforcement agencies are unable to adequately police or resolve the problem by themselves. Consumers must be alert for the purveyors of quackery and be able to recognize how they operate in the health marketplace. Table 3-2 describes their characteristic behavior.

Table 3-2

CHARACTERISTIC BEHAVIOR OF PRACTITIONERS AND PROMOTERS OF QUACKERY

- They promise quick, dramatic, simple, painless, or drugless treatment or cures.
- They use anecdotes, case histories, or testimonials to support claims. Prominent people such as actors, writers, athletes, and even physicians may be involved.
- They use disclaimers couched in pseudomedical or pseudoscientific jargon. Instead of promising to treat or cure specific illnesses, they offer to "detoxify" the body, "strengthen the immune system," "balance body chemistry," or bring the body into "harmony with nature."
- They may display credentials or use titles that could be confused with those of reputable practitioners. Their use of the terms *professor*, *doctor*, or *nutritionist* may be spurious. Their credentials may be from a nonaccredited school or an organization that promotes nonscientific methods.
- The results they claim have not been verified or published in a reputable scientific journal.

- They claim that a single product or service can cure a wide range of unrelated illnesses.
- They claim to have a secret cure or one that is recognized in other parts of the world but not yet known or accepted in the United States.
- They claim to be persecuted by organized medi-cine and that their treatment is being suppressed because it is controversial or because the medical establish-ment does not want competition.
- They state that medical doctors should not be trusted because surgery, x-rays, and drugs cause more harm than good. They say most doctors are "butchers" and "poisoners."
- They claim that most Americans are poorly nourished and should take vitamins for "nutrition insurance."

Any of these behaviors should make you highly suspicious. Additional signs of nutrition quackery are listed in Table 12–2.

Quacks can be classified into three groups:

DUMB QUACKS: These people know not, and don't know that they know not. They may be uneducated, ignorant people who believe they have the secret formula or cure-all that no one else possesses. Generally they are small-time operators.

DELUDED QUACKS: These people know but have been misled into knowing not. They often have some educational background and may even have a medical degree. Their beliefs are based on faulty observations and equally faulty reasoning. They may command large audiences and thereby be dangerous.

DISHONEST QUACKS: These people know not, and know that they know not. Their primary goal is money. They have no scruples.

Jarvis and Barrett[13] warn that modern health quacks are supersalespeople:

Seldom do their victims realize how often or how skillfully they are cheated.

Do viewers of an ad for a weight-loss "breakthrough" stop to think that a *real* breakthrough would be headlined in the news? Does the mother who feels good as she hands her child a vitamin pill think to ask herself whether it is really needed? Do buyers of "extra-strength pain relievers" wonder what's in them or whether an unadvertised brand might cost less? Do users of "herbal energizers" realize that many herbs contain potent chemicals that may be harmful? Do subscribers to "health food" publications realize that articles are slanted to stimulate business for advertisers? Do people who

hear testimonials stop to think that for every success there may have been dozens of failures? Do chiropractic patients who sign up for "preventive maintenance" know there is no scientific justification for such care? Do patients understand that . . . "alternative medicine" refers to methods that have no proven value? . . . . Do people who lobby for "health free-dom" laws realize these are intended to excuse quacks from accountability rather than to improve consumer choice?

Not usually. Quackery confuses people with *double-speak*—language that makes bad things sound good.

Most people think that quackery and health frauds are easy to spot. Some are, but most are not. Today's promoters wear the cloak of science. They use scientific terms and quote (or misquote) scientific references. On talk shows, they may be introduced as "scientists ahead of their time." The very word "quack" helps their camouflage by making us think of an outlandish character selling snake oil from the back of a covered wagon—and, of course, no intelligent people would buy snake oil nowadays, would they?

Well, maybe snake oil isn't selling so well. But acupuncture? "Organic" foods? Mouthwash? Hair analysis? The latest diet book? Megavitamins? "Stress" formulas? Chelation therapy? Cholesterol-lowering teas? Homeopathic remedies? AIDS cures? Or vitamin shots to pep you up? Business is booming for health quacks. Their annual take is in the *billions!* Spot-reducers, "immune boosters," water purifiers, "ergogenic aids," bust creams, spinal adjustments for "preventive maintenance," devices to increase manhood, systems to "balance body chemistry," cults to give life new meaning, special diets for arthritis. The list is endless.

What sells is not the quality of their goods and services,

but their ability to influence their audience. To those in pain, they promise relief. To the incurable, they offer hope. To the nutrition-conscious, they say, "Make sure you have enough." To a public worried about pollution, they say, "Buy natural." To one and all, they promise better health and a longer life. Modern quacks can reach people emotionally, on the level that counts the most.

Many people lack knowledge of what should pass for proof that something works.[20] Because people tend to believe what they hear about the personal experience of others, testimonials can be powerful persuaders. Vissing and Petersen[21] stated that testimonials offer the most powerful type of persuasion to try an unconventional method. Many years ago, Smith[9] made this observation, which is still noteworthy:

Personal testimonials are not used in scientific medicine to prove or disprove the validity of therapies, and for good reason. There has never been a worthless or fraudulent treatment that could not produce a legion of persons who would swear that it helped or cured them.

CONSPIRACY CLAIMS

Quacks typically charge that the medical profession, drug companies, the food industry, government agencies, and/or other "vested interests" are conspiring against "alternative medicine," dietary supplements, and "natural" health cures and that these alleged conspirators put profits ahead of public safety. Some practitioners, for example, charge that the American Medical Association (AMA) and mainstream physicians are against them because their cures would cut into the incomes that doctors make by keeping people sick. Chelationists charge that doctors oppose chelation therapy because it would destroy the very profitable

bypass surgery industry, and cancer quacks claim that their methods pose an economic threat to the multi-billion-dollar "cancer industry." Many quacks charge that their critics have been "bought off" by drug manufacturers who view "natural" methods as a threat to their enormous profits. Antifluoridationists falsely claim that the driving force behind water fluoridation is a desire by the aluminum industry to sell waste products that are used to fluoridate public water supplies. Claims of "suppression" are used to market publications as well as treatments. Many authors and publishers purport to offer information that your doctor, the AMA, and/or government agencies "don't want you to know about."

The "conspiracy" charge is an attempt to gain sympathy by portraying the quack as an "underdog." Jarvis[22] has observed that, "Whereas individuals who complain about conspiracies directed toward themselves are likely to be regarded as mentally ill (paranoid), those who perceive them as directed against a nation, culture, or way of life may seem more rational." Novella[23] has noted:

Patients, especially those with a disease which is not curable by standard medicine, are eager to believe such conspiracy theories because they offer the hope they crave. It is far better to believe that there is a cure out there for you, with a small but dedicated band of rebels who will defy the establishment to bring it to you (for a fee of course), than to believe that no cure exists anywhere.

Although the accused parties profit from their current activities, the idea that great numbers of independent individuals, companies, and government agencies would—or could—conspire to suppress progress is complete fantasy. The elimination of serious diseases, for example, is not a threat to the medical profession. Doctors prosper by curing diseases, not by keeping people sick. Moreover, doctors and their families get sick themselves and would stand to lose if genuine treatments were suppressed.

It should also be apparent that modern medical technology has not altered the zeal of scientists to eliminate disease. When polio was conquered, iron lungs became virtually obsolete, but nobody resisted this advancement even though it meant that hospitals would have to change. Actually, the greatest threat to quacks would be for the medical profession to adopt their methods and compete with them for patients.

THE FREEDOM-OF-CHOICE ISSUE

Promoters of quackery tend to disparage accepted scientific methods as well as consumer-protection laws. They argue that personal experience determines what

It's Your Decision

One of your parents is seriously ill with cancer, with little hope of recovery. Treatment at a large medical center has not succeeded in curing or alleviating the condition. You have been told that your parent has only 6 months to live. A friend of your parents told them he was helped by a clinic in Mexico that uses a substance, unavailable in the United States, that cures a high percentage of cancer patients who receive it.

Despite its high cost, your parents are considering a trip to Mexico. What can you do to help your parents reach an intelligent decision? How sensible would it be for them to spend their life savings for the treatment?

FIGURE 3-1. "Healthcare Rights Amendment." A now-defunct "consumer group" gathered approximately 100,000 signatures supporting a constitutional amendment to establish "health freedom." If it were enacted, government agencies could no longer stop the marketing of unproven or dangerous remedies if even one consumer wanted them. Anyone, licensed or not, could engage in any practice labeled "health care" so long as a single consumer wished it to continue. Compulsory immunization would end, and courts could no longer protect children from parents who deny them access to effective treatment, even if such neglect will result in their death.

WE—THE PEOPLE of the United States, propose AMENDMENT XXVII to be known as the HEALTH-CARE RIGHTS AMENDMENT, which should read as follows:

HEALTHCARE RIGHTS AMENDMENT
SECTION 1.

The Congress shall make no law which restricts any individual's right to choose and to practice the type of healthcare they shall elect for themselves or their children for the prevention or treatment of any disease, injury, illness or ailment of the body or the mind.

works and that patients should be free to select any therapy they wish (Figure 3-1). They also argue that everyone should be free to market methods without the responsibility of ensuring that they are effective. The American Council on Science and Health[24] views this version of "health freedom" as "nothing more than a hunting license for quacks." Jarvis[1] describes it as a ploy:

The "health freedom" argument is a classic example of deception by misdirection. . . . The reality is that patients may freely choose to do a variety of things. Patients may refuse treatments, swallow vitamins, eat apricot pits or the whole tree if they wish. However, they may not sell their pet remedies in the marketplace if those remedies have not been proven safe and effective.

The reason that patients clamor for dubious treatments is that they have been deceived into believing that these therapies offer hope. By focusing attention on the patients, the deceivers direct attention away from themselves.

Several groups espousing unscientific methods are crusading to weaken consumer-protection laws. They include the National Health Federation (NHF), the National Council for Improved Health, the Foundation for the Advancement of Innovative Medicine (FAIM), Citizens for Health, the American Preventive Medical Association, People Against Cancer, and the Committee for Freedom of Choice in Medicine (CFCM).

To promote their legal strategies these groups lobby, stage news events, and generate letter-writing campaigns to legislators and government agencies. During the mid-1970s, for example, NHF and CFCM (then called the Committee for Freedom of Choice in Cancer Therapy) spearheaded passage of laws to permit the marketing of Laetrile (a bogus cancer remedy) within the borders of nearly half the states. In the 1990s several of these groups combined with health-food industry organizations to generate a massive letter-writing campaign that led to passage of the Dietary Supplement Health and Education Act of 1994, which greatly weakened the ability of the FDA to protect consumers against useless and dangerous dietary supplement and herbal products (see Chapter 13). In recent years a few states have passed laws preventing their medical licensing board from disciplining physicians solely because they engage in "alternative" practices. Efforts are also under way to obtain passage of laws that would prevent the FDA and state boards from interfering with "alternative" practitioners (see Chapter 8).

Consumers should have considerable right to choose the health products and services they wish to use. However, they will benefit from this only to the extent that the marketplace is trustworthy. The fundamental principle of consumer protection (and federal law) is that methods should not be marketed until they have been proven safe and effective by scientific study. Abolishing this safeguard would have disastrous consequences, especially for seriously ill people who must quickly decide what to do. Such people should not have to sort through a mix that includes cleverly worded but empty promises.

SUMMARY

Despite the tremendous advances in medical science and health education, health frauds and quackery are still common. Americans waste huge amounts of money on unproven and unscientific approaches to health care. Faced with the prospect of chronic suffering, deformity, or death, many individuals are tempted to try anything that offers relief or hope. Health frauds and quackery can cause financial, physical, and psychologic harm.

It is extremely important for consumers to understand the concepts of spontaneous remission and the placebo effect. The mere fact that someone feels better after trying a remedy does not prove that the remedy was effective. Most diseases are self-limiting, and placebos can relieve a broad range of symptoms.

Modern quacks can be difficult to recognize. However, certain behavior patterns should help consumers identify them. It also is important for consumers to complain to appropriate authorities when they encounter deception in the marketplace.

REFERENCES

1. Jarvis WT. How quackery is promoted. In Barrett S, Cassileth BR, editors. Dubious Cancer Treatment: A Report on "Alternative" Methods and the Practitioners and Patients Who Use Them. Tampa, 1991, Florida Division of the American Cancer Society.
2. Barrett S. Some notes on ImmuStim and the credentials of its proponent. Quackwatch Web site, Aug 21, 2000.
3. California Medical Association. The Professional's Guide to Health and Nutrition Fraud. San Francisco, 1987, The Association.
4. U. S. House of Representatives, Select Committee on Aging, Subcommittee on Health and Long-term Care. Quackery: A $10 Billion Scandal (2 volumes). Washington, D.C., 1984, US Government Printing Office.
5. Top 10 health frauds. FDA Consumer 23(8):29-31, Oct 1989 (updated April 5, 1999, on Quackwatch Web site).
6. Beyerstein BL. Why bogus therapies often seem to work. Quackwatch Web site, 1998.
7. Pratkanis AR. How to sell a pseudoscience. Skeptical Inquirer 19(4):19–25, 1995.
8. Jarvis WT. How quackery harms cancer patients. Quackwatch, Web site, 1997.
9. Smith RL. At Your Own Risk: The Case against Chiropractic. New York, 1969, Pocket Books.
10. Copeland C. Deception at a New Age clinic. Journal of Christian Nursing 6:5–7, Spring 1989.
11. Bianchini M. Testimony in Her Majesty the Queen v. Sonia Atikian and Khachadour Atikian. Toronto, June 28, 1991.
12. Randi J. The Faith Healers. Amherst, N.Y., 1989, Prometheus Books.
13. Jarvis WT, Barrett S. How quackery sells. In Barrett S, Jarvis WT, editors. The Health Robbers: A Close Look at Quackery in America. Amherst, N.Y., 1993, Prometheus Books.
14. Young JH. Why quackery persists. In Barrett S, Jarvis WT, editors. The Health Robbers: A Close Look at Quackery in America. Amherst, N.Y., 1993, Prometheus Books.
15. Beyerstein BL. Testing claims of therapeutic efficacy. Rational Enquirer 7(4):1–2, 8, 1995.
16. Jarvis WT. Arthritis: Folk remedies and quackery. Nutrition Forum 7:1–3, 1990.
17. Rosensweig P and others. The placebo effect in healthy volunteers: Influence of experimental conditions on the adverse events profile during phase I studies. Clinical Pharmacology and Therapeutics 54:578–573, 1993.
18. Turner JA and others. The importance of placebo effects in pain treatment and research. JAMA 271:1609–1614, 1994.
19. Barrett S. Health frauds and quackery. FDA Consumer 11(9):12-17, 1977.
20. Jarvis WT. Quackery: A national scandal. Clinical Chemistry 38:1574–1586, 1992.
21. Vissing MV, Petersen JC. Taking Laetrile: Conversion to medical deviance. CA—A Cancer Journal for Clinicians 31:365-369, 1981.
22. Jarvis WT. Why health professionals become quacks. Quackwatch Web site, 1998.
23. Novella S. Medical conspiracies and the myth of the "hidden cure." In Sampson WI, Vaughn L, editors. Science Meets Alternative Medicine: What the Evidence Says about Unconventional Treatments. Amherst, N.Y., 2000, Prometheus Books.
24. Barrett S. The unhealthy alliance: Crusaders for "health freedom." New York, 1988, American Council on Science and Health.

Chapter Four

ADVERTISING AND OTHER MARKETING PRACTICES

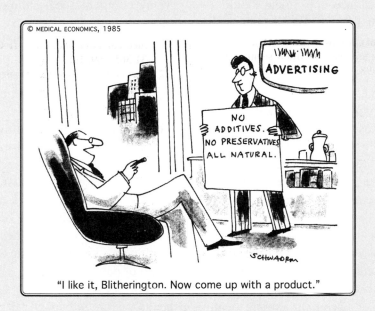

© MEDICAL ECONOMICS, 1985

ADVERTISING

NO ADDITIVES. NO PRESERVATIVES ALL NATURAL.

"I like it, Blitherington. Now come up with a product."

The public is constantly being bombarded by those who wish to promote their own views, sell a bill of goods, convert others to a cause or convince us that they have discovered a special truth or have found a unique road to salvation [to health].

PAUL KURTZ, PH.D.[1]

All things should be laid bare so that the buyer may not be in any way ignorant of anything the seller knows.

CICERO

Freedom of speech doesn't give a person the right to shout "fire" in a crowded theater (Oliver Wendell Holmes, Jr.). Nor should it give con artists the right to promote health frauds through ads in print or on the air. Yet, health fraud lives and thrives . . . because of successful advertising.

ROGER MILLER[2]
FDA CONSUMER, 1985

Key Concepts
KEEP THESE POINTS IN MIND AS YOU STUDY THIS CHAPTER

- The main purpose of advertising is to sell rather than to inform. Many ads that are not blatantly false do not tell the whole truth.

- Ads for alcohol and tobacco products are intended to distract attention from the risks involved in using them.

- Many health professionals who advertise do not represent their services accurately.

- The vast majority of health-related products that are advertised with health claims and marketed primarily by mail, by telephone, through infomercials, and from person to person are worthless, overpriced, or both.

- Misleading advertising is so widespread that government agencies cannot stop most law violators they detect.

The prevailing philosophy of the free-enterprise system is based on the profit motive. It permits sellers to supply what consumers want and buyers to select the products they believe will be advantageous. In the health marketplace, consumers should regard advertising cautiously and should follow the principle of *caveat emptor* (let the buyer beware).

Business leaders view marketing in different ways. One has said that "the solution to marketing problems is not one of giving consumers what they want, but rather to make consumers want what we, the marketers, want them to want." Another has stated that advertisers are "concerned not with finding an audience to hear their message, but rather with finding a message to hold their audience." Another has said that advertising has the obligation to communicate messages clearly, accurately, honestly, and with interest and impact.[3]

William Lutz,[4] author of *Doublespeak,* states that "the job of advertising is to make something out of nothing." The medical community tends to market its services far more cautiously and conservatively than the business community, but abuses exist among health professionals also.

Advertisements are not the only form of marketing. Many sellers beam their messages indirectly through the news and entertainment media. Some entrepreneurs host their own talk shows. Multilevel marketers spread their ideas from person to person. Many people are hawking their wares through computer channels, telephone lines, and direct mail.

This chapter describes how advertising and other marketing activities can mislead consumers. It also examines problems with the advertising of mail-order health products, professional services, drug products, foods, dietary supplements, homeopathic products, exercise and fitness products, weight-control products and services, and tobacco products.

PSYCHOLOGIC MANIPULATION

The business world uses insights from psychology and the social sciences to manipulate consumer behavior. Many companies base their marketing strategies on research that determines what governs people's choices. Armed with such knowledge, advertisers can often persuade people to buy things in a predictable manner.

Cosmetics manufacturers, for example, are not selling merely lanolin, but fantasies involving attractiveness. Women who normally would pay less than $1 for a bar of soap might be willing to pay $10 or more for a skin cream they hope will make them more attractive (see Chapter 20). What they are buying is a promise or hope. Purchasers of a cosmetic alleged to remove wrinkles are seeking everlasting attractiveness and social acceptance. Shampoo buyers may be seeking romance. Television ads for headache remedies often use soothing background music to promote their particular brand of pain reliever.

For decades, cigarette ads used images of youth, health, vigor, and social acceptance to convey the opposite of what cigarette smoking will do to smokers. A widely aired series of television ads has portrayed coffee as a valuable aid to friendship and romance.

Many ads attempt to convey simple answers to people's needs, ambitions, fears, hopes, and feelings of inadequacy. Ads suggest products to enhance sexual performance or provide relief from a boring or lonely life. Many offer quick, simple, painless methods of treatment. They encourage pill-taking for insomnia, tension, and lack of energy. Ads for baldness remedies, weight-control products, deodorants, impotence cures, bust enhancers, and penis enlargers exploit feelings of inferiority and suggest that using these products will lead to social success. Vitamin ads picture energetic people. Ads for alcoholic beverages show people relaxing with

Table 4-1

TECHNIQUES USED IN ADVERTISING

Technique	Questions to Raise
Power words to gain attention	
"Strengthens immune system"	Is this possible? Will it help treat AIDS?
"Fights . . ."	How? Is it effective?
"Provides relief three times longer"	Longer than what? Why not four times?
"Free," "Money back guarantee"	What is free? Is this a come-on? What do you pay for?
"It's natural"	What is "natural?" Is it better? More expensive?
"Amazing breakthrough"	Who says? What evidence? How effective?
"Less salt, fat, calories"	Than what? Is it still high?
"Ask your doctor"	Do doctors generally recommend this product?
"FDA-approved"	Did the FDA actually approve the product?
"Used by millions"	Is it really? Is popularity a good measure of effectiveness?
"Scientifically tested"	How? By whom? Were studies well-designed?
Misleading comparisons to encourage consumers to jump to conclusions	
"Contains twice as much . . ."	As what? Is it better? More economical?
"Wrinkle eraser"	Does it really erase? Or cover temporarily?
"Isn't it time you tried . . ."	Why? Because everybody does?
"Contains X"	What is X? What does it do? Is it better than the ingredient(s) of competing products?
"Up to 8-hour relief"	What is "up to"?
"Fast-acting," "Inexpensive"	How does it compare to other products?
"Guaranteed purity, potency, and quality"	Does the product work?
"Clinically proven safe and effective"	What's the evidence?
Imagery to appeal to emotion	
"Quiet world is like taking a vacation from tension"	Will it help you escape from problems? The real world?
"Beautiful people, places, things"	Will the product help you achieve this?
"The Marlboro man"	Is smoking macho or stupid?
"Look younger instantly"	How quickly? Possible? Temporary?
"Created by research scientist (or specialist) "	Aren't most products? Qualifications?
"Miracle beauty secret, no surgery"	What is? Why secret? Does it work?
"Used extensively in Europe"	Why not in the United States? Not FDA-approved?
"Before-and-after pictures	Do they depict typical results? Were they faked?
Weasel words	
"Helps . . ."	Does it? In what way? How much?
"Virtually . . ."	Does it or doesn't it do what surrounding words imply?
"New and improved"	How was it changed? Is it more effective?

friends and having fun. Ads for "ergogenic aids" feature bodybuilding champions without indicating that the real reason for their success was hard work. Table 4-1 illustrates common persuasive techniques.

Visual imagery is sometimes used to exaggerate the truth. For example, Crest toothpaste has shown a "fluoride eraser" rubbing out a substantial black carious area on a tooth. Fluoridated toothpaste is valuable because it helps prevent decay in its early stages, but it does not cure cavities.[5] Pratkanis and Aronson[6] have noted that appeals to fear are most effective when they terrify the recipient and offer a specific recommendation for overcoming the fear-arousing threat.

Many ads encourage self-diagnosis and self-treatment. Consumer interest in self-care (Chapter 9) increases vulnerability to advertising.

Consumer Reports has noted that some companies have found ways to plug health-related products by issuing press releases or canned video news reports.[7] The resultant press coverage may have greater impact and cost the manufacturer less than regular ads. Prescription drug manufacturers and supplement companies often use this way to call public attention to new products or preliminary scientific reports.

PUFFERY, WEASEL WORDS, AND HALF-TRUTHS

In many ads the primary technique is *puffery*, which Preston defines as praise that includes opinions, superlatives, exaggerations, or generalities, but no specific facts. Preston[8] states: "Puffery lies to you and it deceives you, but the law says it doesn't." In *The Great American Blow-Up*, he provides this illustration:

The book you are about to read is a superior piece of work. It demonstrates the sheerest true excellence in its treatment of one of the outstanding important topics of our time. You will find every moment informative and entertaining to a degree you have never before encountered in the world of fine literature. This much-applauded volume has earned for its author a rightful place as one of the top writers on the contemporary scene.

He then states:

The paragraph you have just read is the purest baloney. . . . It is puffery. It is the pretentious opinion of salesmen and advertisers exaggerating their wares, magnifying value, quality and attractiveness to the limits of plausibility and beyond. It is false, and I know it is false. I do not believe it. If you had believed it, and had bought this book because you relied upon the belief, you would have gotten less than you had bargained for in the marketplace. You would have been cheated.

Puffery is often used to promote nonprescription drugs. For example, Bayer aspirin has been said to "work wonders," and Pepto-Bismol has been touted as having "the famous coating action." Many pain-relievers, vitamins, and other products are identified as "advanced formulas." The most egregious puffs, however, appear on the jackets of books said to offer a "revolutionary" diet, "amazing health secrets," or the like.

Another selling trick is the use of "weasel words." These create the illusion of a promise but permit the advertiser to "weasel" out of the deal later. Here is an example from the catalog of a laboratory that supplies "glandular" products to chiropractors. These products are composed of dehydrated animal organs but contain no hormone or other pharmacologically active ingredient. They are mainly ordinary proteins made into pills or capsules. But according to the catalog:

These glandular concentrates *reportedly* go directly to the aid of the gland of the same name . . . liver to liver, eye to eye, prostate to prostate, and so forth. *Theoretically*, the nutrients found in glands *may* contain essential factors and when taken as a supplement, will *help* the body's glands reach and maintain proper functioning levels.

(The weasel words are italicized for the purposes of this text book.) Despite the illusion that the products are useful, the ad actually promises nothing. Another example would be a promised weight loss of "*up to* 20 pounds in 30 days."

Many statements in advertising, although literally true, could be misunderstood by consumers to mean things that are not true. For example, a claim that one food product has more "food energy" than its competitors may be literally true, because "food energy" is simply a synonym for calories. Yet the consuming public may relate "food energy" to feeling energetic and interpret the claim to mean something that is untrue. Many ad claims have multiple meanings, one of which may be false or unsubstantiated. To some consumers a "better" product should be better than competing products. To others, "better" may mean superior to previous versions of the product itself. If a product is claimed to be better, consumers should ask, "Better than what?"

Many advertisers believe they have license to mislead people as long as nothing explicitly false is said. Years ago, a *Harvard Business Review* poll of 2700 executives found that two out of three believed that advertising failed to present a true picture of the product advertised. They were uneasy about the truthfulness and the social impact of ads.[9] A similar poll of business school deans rated honesty in advertising to be 13%.[10]

ADVERTISING OUTLETS

The number of advertising outlets is enormous. There are tens of thousands of daily and weekly newspapers, magazines, and radio and television stations. Products also are marketed through direct mail, by telephone, by word of mouth, and through the Internet. Some sellers use less obvious marketing strategies in which free publicity is obtained through the use of public relations agencies and public appearances that generate news reports. It has been estimated that the average American is exposed to 1500 advertising messages a day.

The cost of advertising depends mainly on the size of the audience it can reach. Ads can cost anywhere from a few dollars for a 30-second radio spot on a small station to tens of thousands of dollars for ads in popular magazines to more than $2 million for a 30-second nationwide television ad aired during the Super Bowl.

Many people believe that advertising must be reasonably truthful or it would somehow not be permitted. However, standards for advertising acceptability vary greatly from outlet to outlet. Some do their best not to carry misleading ads, whereas others care very little about truth in advertising. Government regulation curbs many deceptive promotions, but it cannot stop them all.

The impact of advertising extends beyond the ads themselves. Many advertising outlets will not convey information that would place their advertisers in an unfavorable light. Some outlets deliberately promote their advertisers' wares. Radio talk shows sponsored by health-food stores, for example, interview a steady stream of guests who promote the types of products sold in the stores. Health-food industry and bodybuilding publications invariably boost the types of products marketed by their advertisers.[11]

The nature and extent of health-related advertising raise serious questions about its effect on people's health. What kind of society is being produced by the information transmitted? Is the selling of more health products and services a good thing for consumers? Does a belief in *caveat emptor* absolve the seller who encourages behavior detrimental to health? Is it right to profit by playing on people's hopes, fears, and anxieties? Regardless, consumers should still protect themselves by invoking the *caveat vendor* (let the seller beware) principle and intelligently analyzing the ads they encounter.

PROFESSIONAL ADVERTISING

Medical and dental societies traditionally have frowned on the use of advertising to solicit patients. Years ago, members who advertised might be expelled, and many state laws banned or severely restricted advertising by health professionals. However, court decisions and pressure by the Federal Trade Commission (FTC) have forced professional societies to abolish their ethical restraints on advertising.

The FTC is legally responsible for helping to foster competition and prevent price-fixing. In 1978 an FTC judge ruled that the American Medical Association (AMA) could no longer forbid advertising by its members. When the U.S. Supreme Court upheld the order, the AMA and the American Dental Association changed their guidelines. The AMA Council on Ethical and Judicial Affairs now places no restrictions on advertising "except those that can be specifically justified to protect the public from deceptive practices. . . . . The key issue is whether advertising or publicity, regardless of format or content, is true and not materially misleading." However, the Council has cautioned that

statements relating to the quality of medical services may be a problem because they may be difficult or impossible to measure by objective standards.[12]

The FTC believes that advertising lowers prices (by increasing competition) and provides consumers with additional information that will help them make appropriate decisions. Critics of this policy respond: (a) deceptive advertising can be difficult to stop; (b) advertising enables the least qualified practitioners to try to lure patients through salesmanship rather than demonstrations of competence; and (c) advertising does not lower medical fees because it tends to increase both the demand for services and the cost of delivering them. Yarborough,[13] for example, expressed doubt that ads by individual physicians would better inform patients. He said that the primary reasons for advertising by most physicians were to persuade rather than inform, to increase their practice, and to make money. Therefore they focus on convenience, friendliness, and personal attention rather than quality of care. He urged physicians to resist advertising unless their objective is to benefit patients rather than to boost their personal income and prestige.

The most appropriate approach in advertising is one that accurately informs the public of facilities and useful services offered. Figure 4-1 shows a responsible ad that attempts to attract patients by offering a discount coupon for a dental examination.

The amount of professional advertising has increased sharply since the 1982 Supreme Court decision. The leading medical advertisers include plastic surgeons, ophthalmologists (radial keratotomy, lens implants), dermatologists (wrinkle reduction, hair transplants), urologists (sexual dysfunction), obstetrics and gynecology specialists (free pregnancy tests), and orthopedists (sport injuries). Margo[14] noted that advertisements for ophthalmology services were almost exclusively designed to promote surgery. He stated that ads may mislead the public about the risks and indications for surgery. In cataract surgery the risk of complications is small, but it is unfair to claim that it is

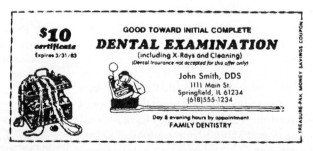

FIGURE 4-1. Straightforward ad with discount for first visit.

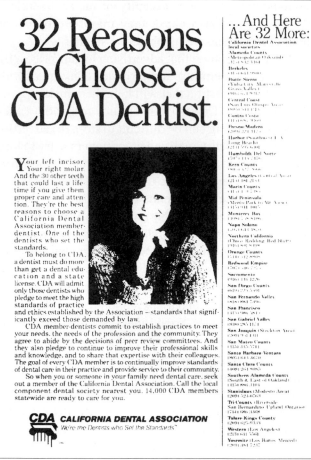

FIGURE 4–2. Dental association ad promoting dental care.

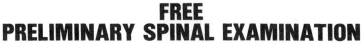

FIGURE 4-3. Innovative ad alluding to auto maintenance.

quick, simple, and without risks, or that there is no alternative. Flamboyant advertising is probably a sign of low-quality, mass-production service.

Gray[15] has documented how advertising can draw very large responses. For example, a Southern California ophthalmologist who advertised radial keratotomy received 900 phone calls in 3 days. A Virginia plastic surgeon who spent $20,000 monthly attracted enough patients to perform 40 cosmetic operations per week. On the other hand, ads placed by a West Coast radiologist antagonized colleagues on whom he depended for

referrals, and consequently his business suffered. And a large clinic that spent $280,000 advertising its services attracted many new patients, but it lost most of them because the patients did not want to wait 1 1/2 hours for service.

Telephone companies have shown little or no interest in preventing unqualified individuals from misrepresenting their credentials. In Allentown, Pennsylvania, for example, an anesthesiologist with an interest in hypnosis for pain relief was permitted to advertise himself as a psychiatrist despite protests made to both the telephone company and the state medical board. To counter this type of problem, the American Board of Medical Specialties[16] has been placing lists of board-certified physicians in many of the Yellow Pages. However, most board-certified physicians are not participating in the program because they do not wish to pay the required fee (over $200 per year). Many people advertising under the heading "Nutritionists" are unqualified (see Chapter 12).

Ads by medical and dental societies tend to be useful and informative. Figure 4-2 shows an informative ad used by the California Dental Association. Figure 4-3 shows one for an individual dentist. Chiropractic ads tend to be misleading. Many chiropractors offer "free" spinal examinations or postural screening that almost always results in a recommendation for lengthy treatment.[17] Figure 4-4 illustrates one such solicitation.

FIGURE 4-4. "Danger signal" ad from the Yellow Pages. The solicitation is misleading because: (a) the listed symptoms are not usually caused by "pinched nerves," (b) most cases involving such symptoms are not serious, and (c) some of the symptoms are likely to be appropriate for medical rather than chiropractic evaluation. Respondents to such ads are almost always told they have a spinal problem and should have prolonged chiropractic care.

ANXIETY . . . in the ELDERLY

Doctors at the Medical College of Pennsylvania are offering free screening evaluations for people 60 or older, who experience the following symptoms:

- Anxiety
- Worries
- Irritability
- Insomnia
- Shakiness
- Upset Stomach
- Difficulty Concentrating
- Fatigue
- Lump in the Throat
- Sweating

These evaluations will be offered as part of a new program designed to find out more about how anxiety affects your daily lives, and to offer opportunities for relief.
Call Natalie Carter, RN, at 555-5683 for more information.

MCP Hospital
The Medical College of Pennsylvania
3300 Henry Avenue, Philadelphia, Pennsylvania 19129

FIGURE 4-5. Straightforward ad for a hospital program that includes a free evaluation of anxiety-related symptoms.

MARKETING BY HOSPITALS

Rising overhead costs and decreased occupancy rates have placed many hospitals in a precarious financial position. In many communities, hospitals are engaged in extensive marketing plans intended to ensure that they fill their beds. These may include ads for emergency services; outpatient clinics; programs for alcoholism, drug addiction, and chronic pain; fitness programs; smoking-cessation courses; medical referral services; community lectures; and other activities designed to boost community awareness of the hospital and its facilities. Hospitals have also offered new services such as Saturday surgery (for convenience), gourmet food, newsletters to former patients, and free transportation. A few have used such gimmicks as a "$10 off" coupon for emergency room services. Many hospitals spend hundreds of thousands of dollars to market themselves. In many instances, these campaigns anticipate consumer needs and offer useful services. Figure 4-5 shows a straightforward ad for people experiencing symptoms related to anxiety.

PRESCRIPTION DRUG MARKETING

Prescription drug marketing traditionally has been directed toward physicians, dentists, and other health-care personnel in professional and technical magazines. The FDA regulates this and requires ads and package inserts to include full information about dosage, effectiveness, side effects, adverse reactions, precautions, and contraindications. Pharmaceutical companies spend several billions of dollars a year promoting prescription drugs to physicians. This promotion includes not only advertising but also individual visits by sales representatives, free samples, continuing education courses, dinner presentations, and other perks.

For many years the FDA opposed the advertising of prescription drugs to the public because the information needed to make intelligent decisions about them is generally too complex to place in a brief advertisement. But in 1983 the agency concluded that its regulations provided sufficient safeguards to protect consumers.

Manufacturers are now spending more than $1 billion per year to advertise prescription products in magazines and newspapers and on television.[18] A few companies have placed Web pages on the Internet for that purpose.[19] Some ads mention a product by name, whereas others encourage people with certain health problems to seek further medical advice. Most drugs in the latter category are either the only drug or the market leader in a category of drugs for the advertised problem. The products have included: *Seldane* (terfenadine), an antihistamine that did not cause drowsiness; *Rogaine* (minoxidil), an antibaldness drug that is somewhat effective for some people; and *Nicorette* (nicotine polacrilex gum), which that can help people stop smoking. *Rogaine* and *Nicorette* are now available without a prescription. Figures 4-6 and 4-7 show ads that provide helpful, informative messages.

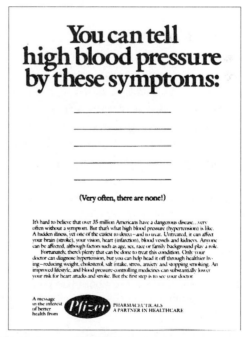

FIGURE 4-6. Informative ad advising people that it is possible to have high blood pressure without knowing about it. The ad mentions no product, but the manufacturer knows that some people who are discovered to have "silent" hypertension will be appropriately treated with one of its products.

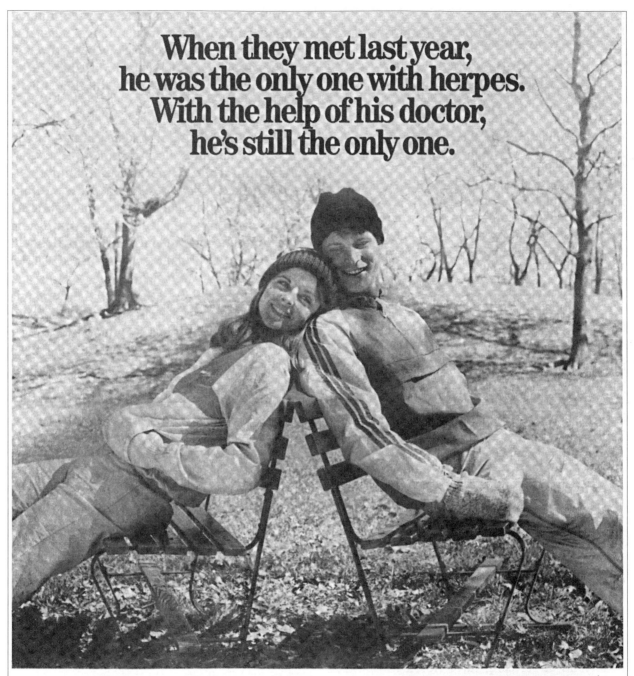

When they met last year, he was the only one with herpes. With the help of his doctor, he's still the only one.

Whether you have a mild, intermediate or severe case of genital herpes, you should see your doctor to help gain new control over your outbreaks— especially if you haven't seen your doctor within the past year.

The medical profession now has more information than ever before about the treatment of herpes, as well as effective counselling and treatment programs that can help you reduce the frequency, duration and severity of your outbreaks.

If in the past you were told that nothing could be done for herpes, it's no longer true. Herpes *is* controllable.

Ask your doctor about these treatment programs, and whether one of them would be suitable for you.

See your doctor...there is help for herpes

Burroughs Wellcome Co.
Research Triangle Park
Wellcome | North Carolina 27709

© 1986 BURROUGHS WELLCOME   RH 86 BW 6

FIGURE 4-7. A useful message from the manufacturer of a prescription drug that can help control the symptoms and reduce the transmission of genital herpes.

Consumer Tip

Prescription Drug Ads

- Remember that the primary purpose of the ad is to sell the product.

- Do not assume that the ad gives you the full story.

- Seek additional information from the company (a toll-free number may be given), a reliable drug reference book (see Chapter 19), and your physician.

Ads that mention a prescription drug by name must include "adequate directions for use." This includes full product information of the type found in package inserts and the *Physicians' Desk Reference*. This amount of information is often too technical for laypersons to understand. Less information is required in ads that do not name a specific product.[20]

Although prescription drug ads call attention to useful products, their primary purpose is to sell them. Some observers believe that direct advertising educates patients, alerts consumers to new treatments, encourages people to seek medical advice for conditions that would otherwise go untreated, increases consumer confidence in products already prescribed, and generally results in a more informed public.[18,21] Others argue that advertising prescription drugs interferes with the physician-patient relationship, confuses patients, increases the cost of drugs, puts undue emphasis on drug treatment alternatives, pressures doctors to prescribe products, and results in unnecessary use.[22] Nearly 90% of AMA members responding to a recent poll stated that direct-to-consumer advertising had resulted in increased patient demand for specified brand-name drugs, and 73% said that it caused physicians to spend more time supplying accurate information.

Consumer Reports on Health[23] has noted that consumer drug ads can call attention to symptoms that require medical attention; can publicize a vaccine; and can alert consumers to products that are safer, cheaper, or more convenient than those a person is using. But it warns:

Drug pitches are not public service messages—they're commercial advertisements . . . designed with the drug manufacturer's health in mind. Even when the ad seems to be merely alerting you to symptoms that may require drug treatment, the message is usually overstated. . . . You should regard consumer drug ads with the same type of skepticism as you would any other type of salesmanship.

It notes, for example, that *Rogaine*'s manufacturer has tried to hook worried men by asking whether "an emerging bald spot" can "damage your ability to get along with others" or "influence your chances of obtaining a job or a date." A similar pitch for *Estraderm*, a hormonal product, called attention to what it called "myth number one: No man in his right mind would be interested in a menopausal woman." The *Rogaine* ad failed to mention that only a small percentage of men can benefit and that the product is quite expensive. The *Estraderm* ad failed to consider risks, side effects, or whether a drug actually is needed to counter menopausal symptoms. A recent study of 28 ads concluded that two-thirds were factually accurate, but some of these left out important information or carried it in small print.[24]

NONPRESCRIPTION DRUG ADVERTISING

In 1972 the FDA began a lengthy review process that has led to the removal of many ineffective ingredients from nonprescription drugs (see Chapter 19). During this period, regulatory actions by the FTC have persuaded many major manufacturers to stop making blatantly misleading claims. As a result, except for homeopathic products (see Chapter 8), most nonprescription drugs sold today contain at least one effective ingredient, and ads for such products tend to be truthful. However, at least three problems remain:

1. Ads often fail to disclose the ingredients of the product. This makes it more difficult for consumers to choose the most suitable product or compare one product to another. Multi-ingredient products promoted for the relief of colds, for example, may not be better than products that contain fewer ingredients or a single ingredient.

Consumer Tip

Rational Choice of Nonprescription Drugs

- Ignore advertising hype. Be wary of ads that claim "special," "secret," or "foreign" formulas, use testimonials from satisfied customers, or promote a "miracle" or "wonder" cure that medicine has not yet discovered.

- Become informed with the help of a reference book plus guidance, as needed, from a physician.

- Select products according to their ingredients rather than advertising claims.

- Buy mostly single-ingredient products rather than combination products.

2. Many ads use imagery, puffery, or testimonials to suggest that a product is more effective than it actually is. Pain relievers, for example, may be described as "advanced," "new," and "extra-strength" even though they are identical or very similar to competing products.

3. Commercial television viewers, bombarded by ads, may incorrectly conclude that many of life's problems can be solved by drugs. Ads for "Excedrin headaches" are a classic example in which viewers were encouraged to use medication to relieve tension headaches with no mention that trying to resolve the underlying problem would be prudent.

FOOD ADVERTISING

The main problem with food advertising is that it tends to promote dietary imbalance. A study of television messages related to food and eating behavior, for example, found that between 8 and 11 PM food references occurred 4.8 times per 30 minutes of programming time.[25] About 60% were for low-nutrient beverages and sweets. Foods were also typically consumed as snacks. The most frequently expressed messages were claims of good taste and of food being "fresh and natural." Ads for fast-food restaurants, which were more frequent than those of any other category, did not mention salad bars. Of 261 commercials aired, only three mentioned fruit and none mentioned vegetables, although fruits and vegetables were pictured in 36% of the ads. The authors concluded that the "prime-time diet" is inconsistent with the U.S. dietary guidelines (see Chapter 11).

The American Academy of Pediatrics wants to stop television food advertising aimed at children. In a policy statement, the Academy charged that the primary goal of children's television is to sell products to children. According to the Academy, young children cannot distinguish between programs and commercials and do not understand that commercials are designed to sell products. The policy statement also noted, "Television shows promote toys. The same toys are used to promote cereals and other foods. Commercials for the cereals, named after the toys, indirectly promote the toy and the toy-based program as well as the cereal and other related products."

Public focus on the relationships between diet and various diseases, particularly heart disease and cancer, has spawned an enormous number of related advertising claims. In the mid-1980s many food manufacturers began suggesting that their products might protect, or help protect, against certain diseases. Many of these claims were misleading because they stressed individual foods rather than overall diet. In addition, ads for certain foods emphasized a potentially helpful quality (such as being low in cholesterol) when another characteristic (such as a high fat content) would negate any benefit. These problems have been largely solved by FDA labeling regulations that took effect in 1994 (see Chapter 11).

DIETARY SUPPLEMENT PROMOTION

Much of the advertising for vitamin products and other types of dietary supplements is misleading. Many companies falsely suggest that supplements be taken because it is difficult or impossible to meet nutrient needs with ordinary foods or in times of stress. Ads for supplements never inform people how to accurately judge whether they need them. Many products are marketed with false and illegal claims that they can prevent or treat various diseases. Supplements also are promoted through books, radio and television broadcasts, oral claims from person to person, and many other channels. Unwarranted claims made through these channels are protected by the doctrines of free speech and freedom of the press as long as they are not directly tied to the sale of specific products. These problems are described in Chapter 12.

Many supplement manufacturers suggest that their products have characteristics that make them unique or better than those of their competitors. Barrett and Herbert[11] have warned that products described as "sustained-release," "chelated," "targeted," "biologically activated," "protein-bonded," and "food-grown" are not significantly different from other products containing similar levels of ingredients. Some companies state that their supplement products are patented. The U.S. Patent Office does not require proof that a product actually works; the main requirement is that it be different from previously registered products.

The 1994 Dietary Supplement Health and Education Act (DSHEA) permits product labels to carry "structure/function" claims as long as the products are not falsely promoted for cure, mitigation, treatment, or prevention of disease. Manufacturers have responded by making hundreds of questionable claims that they previously were afraid to make. In December 1998, the FTC issued "Dietary Supplements: An Advertising Guide for Industry," a detailed document to clarify the need for substantiation.[26] The guide describes the steps the FTC uses to make its analyses and provides a roadmap for others who wish to do the same.

To determine whether an ad complies with FTC law, the first step is to identify all express and implied claims that the ad conveys to consumers. Once the claims are identified, the scientific evidence can be assessed to determine whether they are adequately supported. Ad-

---

Historical Perspective

"Tired Blood"

One of the catchiest advertising campaigns of all time was the promotion of *Geritol* for people with "tired blood." The admakers reasoned that since iron deficiency causes anemia, and anemia causes fatigue, people who are tired should take an iron tonic. This play on words was invalid because iron-deficiency anemia is not the usual cause of fatigue, and people who actually are iron-deficient need medical attention to ascertain why. (If, for example, the cause is intestinal bleeding from a curable cancer, delaying medical care could prove fatal.)

In 1968 the FTC charged that TV commercials had misrepresented the likelihood that *Geritol* would relieve tiredness, loss of strength, rundown feelings, nervousness, and irritability. In 1975 the J.B. Williams Company of New York City settled the matter by agreeing to pay $125,000 in penalties to the government. The ad, to the right, which was published at about that time in *Parade* magazine, does not refer to fatigue or "tired blood" but was still misleading. Although iron-deficiency anemia is not rare, few people should take an iron supplement (see Chapter 19).

IF YOU HAVE IRON POOR BLOOD ALL THE VITAMINS IN THE WORLD WON'T HELP

Iron poor blood is the most widespread nutritional ailment in America today. And taking vitamins can't help, because vitamins don't contain iron.

What you need is Geritol, every day. Geritol is so rich in iron, just one tablet contains more iron than even a pound of calf's liver. Plus vitamins important to your health.

Geritol's iron can actually build your blood day by day. That's what makes it different from vitamin pills—and so important to you.

---

vertisers must make sure that whatever they say expressly is accurate. Often, however, an ad conveys other claims beyond those expressly stated. Advertisers cannot suggest claims that they could not make directly. When identifying claims, advertisers should consider the ad as a whole, assessing the "net impression" conveyed by all elements of the ad, including the text, product name, and depictions.

For example, if an ad claims that "university studies prove" that a mineral supplement can improve athletic performance, the advertiser should have "university studies" that document the benefit as well as evidence that the studies are methodologically sound. And if advertisement for a vitamin supplement claims that 90% of cardiologists regularly take the product, the advertiser should have adequate support for both the percentage and the implied representation that taking the product is beneficial for the heart.

A statement about a product's effect on a normal "structure or function" of the body may also imply that the product is beneficial for treatment. If elements of the ad imply that the product is useful against a disease, the advertiser must be able to substantiate the implied claim even if the ad contains no express reference to the disease. Thus if an ad for "Arthricure" shows an arthritic woman using a walker before taking the products and dancing afterward, the manufacturers should be able to substantiate the implied claims that the product can cure or mitigate arthritis.

The FTC typically requires claims about the efficacy or safety of dietary supplements to be supported with "competent and reliable scientific evidence." Anecdotal evidence about the individual experience of consumers is not sufficient to substantiate claims. Even if those experiences are genuine, they may be attributable to a placebo effect or factors unrelated to the supplement. Individual experiences are not a substitute for scientific research. Ads that include testimonials should be backed by adequate substantiation that the testimonial experience represents what consumers will generally achieve when using the product. Vague disclaimers like "results may vary" are likely to be insufficient. Whenever an expert or consumer endorser is used, the advertiser should disclose any material connection between the endorser and the advertiser of the product that the consumers would not reasonably expect.

Claims based solely on traditional use should avoid implying that the product has been scientifically evaluated for efficacy.

When a claim, if unfounded, could present a substantial risk of injury to consumer health or safety, it can be held to a higher level of scientific proof. For example, a claim that a mineral supplement has been a popular American folk remedy for shrinking tumors should not be made without scientific evidence that the product is effective.

An advertisement can also be deceptive because of what it fails to say. For example, if an herbal weight loss product contains an ingredient that when regularly consumed can result in a significant increase in blood pressure, the advertiser should disclose this potentially serious risk.

When the disclosure of qualifying information is necessary, that information should be presented so that it is actually noticed and understood by consumers. A fine-print disclosure at the bottom of a print ad, a dis- claimer buried in a body of text, a brief video super- script in a television ad, or a disclaimer that is easily missed on an Internet Web site are not likely to be ad- equate. Table 4-2 analyzes several ads.

Table 4-2

ANALYSES OF FIVE RECENT AD SCRIPTS

NATURALIFE HERBAL PRODUCTS

If nature can heal itself, just think what it can do for you. . . . Just look at your body. Millions of little cells doing exactly what they're supposed to do. Most of the time. Unfortunately, sometimes your body isn't in perfect order. And that's why people reach for synthetic drugs. The question is why? Doesn't nature know your body better than anyone? That's why there's a Natural Pharmacy in food and drug stores near you. There you'll find a new line of all-natural herbal supplements that have been considered healthful to the body for centuries. . . . What would your body rather have: something from a laboratory, or something from nature?

Analysis: The key question should not be whether products are "natural," where they are made, or whether they have been used for centuries as folk remedies. The important issue is whether they have been proven safe and effective for their intended purpose. Most herbal prod- ucts have not (see Chapter 12).

CANCER TREATMENT CENTERS OF AMERICA

We specialize in treating cases others call "hopeless," cases in which previous treatments have often failed. . . . People fighting for a chance to live. We've given them the chance, time and again. . . . And we've done it without the side effects that can make other cancer treatments unbearable. One reason, we're certain, is our love-filled environment. Another is the quality and the scope of our cancer treatments.

Analysis: Is there a way to determine whether this hospital offers superior treatment? Have its results been published in a peer-reviewed scientific journal or any- where else? Is it possible to administer effective chemo- therapy that has no side effects? If so, why wouldn't ev- ery facility use it?

PURE FLORIDA ORANGE JUICE

After reading how research has found that certain nutri- ents like those in 100% pure Florida orange juice may help prevent some types of cancer (when part of low-fat, high-fiber diets rich in fruits and vegetables), Mr. Johnson, known for his frugality, finally relented to his employees' demands and improved the company's health plan.

Analysis: The ad, from the Florida Department of Citrus, pictures "Mr. Johnson" standing next to a water cooler filled with orange juice. Diets rich in fruits and vegetables are associated with a lower incidence of cancer, but no one knows what dietary components produce this effect. Orange juice is high in vitamin C—as are potatoes, tomatoes, and broccoli—but any diet rich in fruits and vegetables is likely to provide more vitamin C than people need. Drinking orange juice instead of water is unlikely to lower the incidence of cancer for anyone whose diet is otherwise balanced.

MEDICINES FROM NATURE

Unlike most over-the-counter medicines, Medicine from Nature works in harmony with your own body defenses and gets to the cause of your illness or discomfort. So rather than masking the symptoms of a cold . . . your body gets the support to work through the problem on its own. The result is no side effects, only relief.

Analysis: This message was used to promote a large line of homeopathic remedies, which, according to the ad, enhance the body's self-healing ability. Is this a testable claim? Has it been tested? Do you think that any medication potent enough to benefit people can have a zero incidence of side effects? Actually, most homeopathic "remedies" are so dilute that they exert no detectable effect on the body (see Chapter 8).

ENSURE AND ENSURE HIGH PROTEIN

Even if you've improved your diet by eating more lean meats, fruits and vegetables, you still may not be getting the balanced nutrition you need. So how can you help guarantee that you and the ones you love get the right nutrition? With Ensure and Ensure High Protein. Ensure is more than a vitamin supplement. It's complete, balanced nutrition in a delicious ready-to-serve drink that provides an excellent balance of protein, carbohydrate, vitamins and minerals. . . . Ensure is even recommended #1 by doctors as a complete source of nutrition.

Analysis: Doctors recommend these products for people whose appetite is impaired, usually as a result of severe illness or major surgery. They are not recom- mended for the general population. They contain significant amounts of vitamins and minerals but lack fiber, certain trace minerals, and many of the phyto- chemicals found in fruits and vegetables. There is no reason why young, healthy individuals (pictured in the ad) should waste their money on these products.

TOBACCO PROMOTION

Although cigarette consumption in the United States has declined in the last 25 years, over 430,000 deaths each year are attributable to smoking, and additional deaths are related to secondhand smoke.[27] Yet cigarettes are America's most heavily marketed consumer product.

Tobacco-product advertising has been banned on television and radio, and warnings about health risks are required on the labels of cigarettes and smokeless tobacco products. However, these products have been extensively promoted through print advertising and sporting and cultural events. In 1998 the FTC reported that the costs of cigarette advertising and promotion in the United States had totaled $5.1 billion in 1996 and that since 1987 the amount spent increased every year except for 1994. Tobacco ads associate smoking with affluence, glamour, slimness, visceral satisfaction, romance, popularity, escape from worry, winning friends, gaining independence, relaxation, fitness, and upward mobility.

Former U.S. Surgeon General C. Everett Koop[28] has criticized several ads that sent contrary and dangerous signals about the use of tobacco to readers. He said one that uses the slogan "Alive With Pleasure" perhaps should be changed to "Dying in Agony" in view of the deaths and other problems caused by smoking cigarettes. In a 1990 study of 20 leading magazines, the American Council on Science and Health (ACSH)[29] found that those carrying the most cigarette ads tended to publish the least about smoking and its dangers. Anti-tobacco activists suggest using the postage-paid subscription cards to send protest messages to the publishers of these magazines.

In 1985 R.J. Reynolds used the denial-of-death theme in an editorial-type ad suggesting that a major federal study (MRFIT) had cast doubt that cigarette smoking was a factor in causing heart disease. The FTC charged that the ad was deceptive because it misrepresented the study and omitted important findings. The company signed a consent agreement barring it from misrepresenting scientific studies in the future.[30]

Although tobacco companies claim that cigarette promotions are not aimed at people who are most at risk, ads do appear to be focused on youth, minorities, women, and the poor.[31] Kilbourne has noted that cigarettes have been directly marketed to women and girls as a way to control their weight. (For example, Virginia Slims have been promised to provide "more than just a sleek shape," while Capri cigarettes have offered "the slimmest slim in town.")[32]

Camel cigarettes were widely promoted by "Joe Camel," a cigarette-smoking cartoon figure described as a "smooth character." In one ad, Joe offered "foolproof dating advice" that included, "Always break the ice by offering her a Camel" on its list of "smooth moves." The Public Citizen Health Research Group charged that one of the moves listed for males in the Camel ad promoted violence against women.[33] A study of logo recognition found that 30% of 3-year-old children and 91% of 6-year-old children were able to match Camel's cartoon figure with a picture of a cigarette and that the 6-year-olds were as familiar with "Old Joe" as they were with Mickey Mouse.[33]

Joe B. Tye, founder of STAT (Stop Teenage Addiction to Tobacco), identified 43 movies involved in covert advertising that encourages cigarette smoking. For example, in "Beverly Hills Cop II," Eddie Murphy holds up a pack of Lucky Strikes and says, "These are very popular cigarettes with the children." "Superman II" has scenes that call attention to Marlboro cigarettes more than two dozen times.[34] Wolinsky[35] has described how the tobacco industry gained publicity, targeted mainly to youngsters, by subsidizing athletes and sponsoring sports events. For example, despite the ban on television advertising, tobacco companies still get their

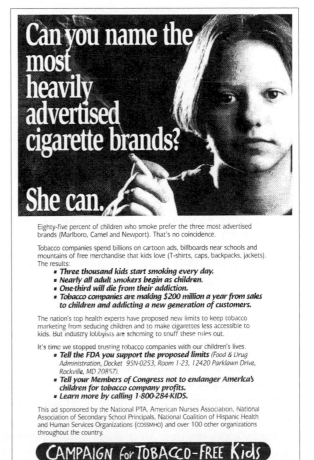

FIGURE 4-8. Ad supporting FDA proposal to curb tobacco marketing to children.

message across when television cameras show tobacco messages placed near scoreboards and shots of athletes chewing tobacco.

Cigarette companies encourage their customers to speak out for "smokers' rights."[37] R.J. Reynolds published a *Smokers' Rights Action Guide*, which advised how to overcome "discrimination" against smokers. Philip Morris sponsored an "accommodation" program to "revive public smoking," mainly in restaurants.

The AMA has called for a complete ban on cigarette advertising. In 1995 the *Journal of the American Medical Association* revealed the contents of secret Brown and Williamson Tobacco Corporation documents related to the dangers of smoking. The documents described how the company's public relations strategy had maintained that cigarettes were neither dangerous nor addictive even though the company's own research had found otherwise.[38] The FDA issued regulations that would limit tobacco promotions directed at children. The courts overturned them, but lawsuits by state attorneys general have led to a settlement in which tobacco companies agreed to stop billboard advertising, restrict brand-name sponsorships, stop using cartoon characters, and discontinue various other marketing methods.[39] Figure 4-8 shows an ad sponsored by more than 100 groups that supported the FDA proposal.

MAIL-ORDER QUACKERY

Many people believe that advertising claims for health products must be true or somehow they would not be "allowed." Many assume that media outlets screen such ads carefully, and some even think that the Postal Service licenses mail-order advertisers. Each of these beliefs is erroneous. Several large studies have shown that the vast majority of advertisements for mail-order health products are misleading. The names of people who respond to mail-order scams may be added to "sucker lists" that are sold to other scammers.

In 1985 the FDA conducted a 1-month survey of advertisements for health products in American newspapers and magazines. The survey found 435 questionable ads, 249 of them for weight-loss products (mostly diet pills). Gross deceptions appeared in ads for waist wraps, vibrating belts, and sauna suits advertised to help lose weight. There were 89 ads for hair restoration schemes, 42 of them for products and 47 for "clinics." Wrinkle removers were also common. Other ads found

---

Table 4-3

THE MAIL-ORDER HEALTH MARKETPLACE

Communication Channel	Typical Products
Magazines, astrology	Psychic help with health problems
Magazines, fitness/bodybuilding	"Ergogenic aids"
Magazines, general audience	Youth and beauty aids
Magazines, health	Nonprescription drugs sold through drugstores and supermarkets
Magazines, health food	Herbs, homeopathic, and supplement products sold through health-food stores Misleading claims tend to be made through articles rather than ads
Magazines, pornographic	Sex aids
Newspapers, general	Weight-reduction schemes
Newspapers, tabloid	Weight-reduction schemes, psychic healing
Classified ads	Mostly information and product catalogs rather than specific products
Direct mail	Weight-reduction schemes, anti-aging products, sex aids
"Post-it" ads	Weight-reduction schemes, anti-aging products, pinhole eyeglasses
Prizes (mail or phone)	Vitamins, water purifiers
Catalogs from mail-order supplement distributors	A multitude of herbal and "dietary supplement" products with misleading therapeutic claims
Multilevel companies	A multitude of supplement products with illegal claims made through brochures, videotapes, and word-of-mouth
Infomercials	Weight-loss schemes, beauty aids, hair-loss remedies, books, audiotapes, videotapes, and exercise devices
Internet	All of the above—and much more

---

in the survey included products for hemorrhoids, varicose veins, and indigestion; "rear end" kits for shaping; pills for the "ultimate orgasm"; and cheap, quick ways to treat arthritis, heart disease, alcoholism, depression, and high blood pressure.[2]

Some direct-mail solicitations look like reproductions of newspaper articles or ads, although they probably have not been published. They are accompanied by a handwritten endorsement in the margin or on a *Post-it* or other note addressed to the recipient by name or first initial. "Dear Bill," the note might read, "This really works! Try it. S."

In 1991 ACSH[41] published a study of magazines, tabloid newspapers, direct-mail catalogs, television infomercials, multilevel companies, and other channels through which health-related mail-order products are marketed. Table 4-3 lists products typically sold through these channels. The study examined one issue each of 463 magazines in national circulation during the summer of 1990. Dubious ads appeared in 56 out of 423 (13%) general audience magazines and 23 out of 40 (58%) health and fitness magazines. In the general audience magazines about 50 companies advertised about 70 dubious products. In health-food publications 15 companies advertised 24 dubious products. In fitness and bodybuilding magazines 26 companies advertised more than 60 products. All but one product (a device

for reducing sweat) were misrepresented. Tabloid newspapers (*Globe, National Examiner, Sun, National Enquirer,* and *Weekly World News*), which were surveyed for several months, contained several misleading ads per issue.

ACSH's report advises that no mail-order product can (a) cause effortless weight loss; (b) erase scars, wrinkles, or "cellulite;" (c) selectively reduce one part of the body; (d) increase bust or penis size; (e) prevent or cure hair loss; (f) increase stamina, endurance, strength, or muscle mass; prevent aging; (6) prolong life; (h) prevent senility; (i) increase memory; or (j) increase sexual stimulation or pleasure. Figure 4-9 illustrates ads from the FDA and ACSH surveys.

In 1992 Jack Raso, M.S., R.D., surveyed 94 periodicals and found more than 600 ads for nutrition-related products available by mail. He concluded that most of the products were safe but useless, but a few were dangerous for long-term use.[42]

The most agressive promoter of youth and beauty aids is probably A. Glenn Braswell, whose Gero Vita International distributes about 20 million mail-order brochures per month. Some of his products may have some effectiveness (though overpriced), but most have been promoted with misleading claims. Purchase of any product entitles the buyer to a free 1-year subscription (available separately for $39.95) to a monthly "journal"

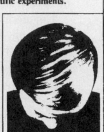
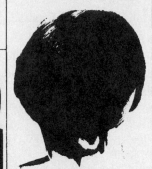

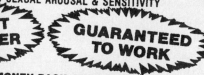
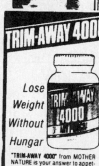

FIGURE 4-9. Ads for mail-order health products.

(Figure 4-10). Braswell was the object of 140 federal enforcement actions in the late 1970s and early 1980s and served a brief prison sentence for federal income tax evasion and perjury charges developed during a mail-fraud investigation. But after his release he bounced back, grossed over $1 billion, and was even pardoned by President Clinton for his earlier crime.[42]

The U.S. Postal Service has primary responsibility for combating mail-order fraud. Chapter 26 describes how the agency works.

WEIGHT-CONTROL PROMOTIONS

The $32 billion weight-control marketplace is rife with misleading ads for mail-order "diet" products, weight-loss clinics, spot reducers, cellulite removers, and similar products. The FDA has stated that there is no scientific or clinical evidence to support the use of body wraps or sauna suits for controlling weight. Nor are there any data to back up promoters' claims that these products eliminate cellulite and bulging fat, make spot reductions possible, control appetite, or increase the rate at which the body burns calories.[2] Commercial weight-loss clinics have come under heavy fire during recent years. Weight-control facts and frauds are covered in Chapter 13.

YOUTH AND BEAUTY AIDS

Many products and services are falsely claimed to make people appear more youthful and attractive. In 1993, for example, Revlon, Inc. and its subsidiary, Charles Revson, Inc., signed a consent agreement not to make unsubstantiated claims that their *Ultima II ProCollagen* anti-cellulite body complex would: (a) significantly reduce cellulite; (b) help disperse toxins and excess water from areas where cellulite appears; (c) reduce skin's bumpy texture, ripples or slackness caused by cellulite; and (d) increase sub-skin tissue strength and tone.[43]

Chapter 20 provides additional information about bogus youth and beauty aids.

Many creams, protein powders, and gadgets have been sold by mail with claims that they can enlarge the female breasts. All such products are fakes. In 1977 the Good Housekeeping Institute tested four bust developers advertised in leading magazines: a water-massage type and three "tension" devices (one clam-shaped, one rod-shaped, and one that used an oversized rubber band). The tests showed that none affected breast size.[44]

The breast itself is a gland and has no muscles. Since bust size is measured around the torso, resistance exercises that increase the size of chest and back muscles will slightly increase the bust measurement, but the actual breast and cup size are not affected. The growth of the breasts is influenced only by hormones—released during puberty and pregnancy—and by general weight gain. Estrogen prescribed for menstrual difficulty or birth control may produce some temporary breast enlargement, but the breasts return to their original size when the drug is stopped. Plastic surgery (discussed in Chapter 20) is the only procedure that can be used to permanently augment breast size.

EXERCISE AND FITNESS PRODUCTS

Regulatory agencies have paid much less attention to exercise and fitness products than they have to foods and drugs. The agencies appear to believe that misleading advertisements for these products generally have less potential to cause harm.

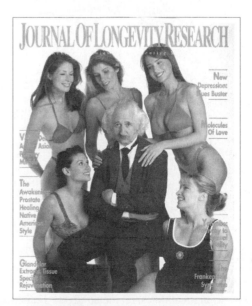

Figure 4-10. This magazine, given free to buyers of mail-order health products, consists of articles promoting the products' ingredients.

"Ergogenic aids" that are concoctions of vitamins, minerals, and amino acids have been promoted through fitness and bodybuilding magazines. In 1985 the market leader, Weider Health and Fitness, agreed not to falsely claim that two of its products could help build muscles or were effective substitutes for anabolic steroids (see Chapters 14 and 26). Weider still markets these and similar products with testimonial ads featuring bodybuilding champions and other athletes. Many other companies use similar ads, and some advertise with blatantly false claims. Figure 4-11 illustrates how one company used imagery to deliver a powerful message that might be illegal if made explicit with words.

In 1999, in response to an FTC complaint, Fitness Quest agreed not to make unsubstantiated weight-control or body-shaping claims. The company had falsely claimed that several of its devices could cause the user to burn 1000 calories per hour and that using its "Ab Isolator" 3 minutes a day would result in a significantly reduced waistline in 30 days.[45]

The FTC has also acted against misleading representations by health and fitness facilities. In 1989 the agency stopped two individuals from falsely claiming that their electric muscle stimulation treatments produced the same effect as exercise.[46] Other problems with health and fitness facilities are discussed in Chapter 14.

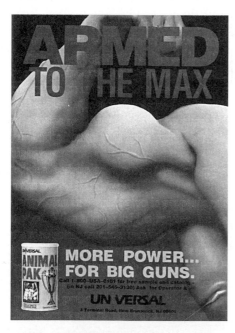

FIGURE 4-11. Ad from a bodybuilding magazine. The ad makes no claims, but a company catalog states that the product contains "mega doses of the vitamins and minerals normally required by strength athletes, fat metabolizers, branched-chain amino acids, complex carbohydrates, enzymes, and over 2000 milligrams of growth factors that can build a physique almost better than nature intended."

INFOMERCIALS

The FTC has warned consumers to be aware that some television programs that resemble talk shows are actually program-length commercials. Many such programs have promoted bogus weight-loss plans, hair-growth products, vitamin products, herbs, "skin rejuvenation" products, "body contouring" programs, cosmetics, exercise aids, books, tapes, and other health-related products. Some of these programs use a movie star, athlete, or other celebrity as a host or guest, plus one or more "experts" who are referred to as "doctor." Testimonials from "satisfied users" (some of whom are paid actors) also are a common feature.

One way to recognize an infomercial, says the FTC, is that the product promoted during "commercial breaks" is related to the program's content. During the past decade the agency has filed many complaints against companies marketing infomercials. When necessary, the settlement agreements require that future program-length ads be clearly identified as ads throughout the program. Some infomercial producers have voluntarily inserted such notices in their ads. But many do not, and most of the health-related products sold through infomercials are bogus.

MULTILEVEL MARKETING (MLM)

Many companies market dietary supplements, diet plans, homeopathic products, herbs, and other health-related products through person-to-person sales. Almost anyone can become an "independent distributor" by completing an application and paying a small fee (usually between $35 and $100) for a kit containing product literature and other sales aids. No knowledge of nutrition or health care is required. Distributors are urged to use the products themselves and to persuade others to become distributors who, in turn, use the products and recruit more distributors. With sufficient sales volume, distributors get a percentage of the sales in their "downline." Companies suggest that this process provides a great money-making opportunity. The sales of health-related MLM products total several billion dollars per year. However, people who do not join during the first few months of operation or become one of the early distributors in their community are very unlikely to prosper.

An Amway Corporation report indicates that the vast majority of its distributors make very little money. Amway's 1998 "Business Review" tabulates figures gathered from April 1994 through March 1995 from distributors who attempted to make a retail sale, presented the Sales and Marketing Plan, received bonus money, or attended a company or distributor meeting in the month surveyed. The average "gross income" for these "active distributors"—approximately 41% of all distributors of record—was $88 per month. The report defines "gross income" as the amount received from retail sales minus cost of products, plus any bonus. It does not take any business expenses into account. If this figure includes purchases for personal use, the potential profit would be less.[47]

Most MLM health products are marketed with claims that they can prevent or cure disease. Companies whose sales aids contain clear-cut health claims are easy targets for government enforcement actions. Some companies run this risk, hoping that the government will not act until their customer base is well established. Others make no claims in their "official" literature but rely on distributors to supply anecdotes, testimonials, and independent literature. Distributors typically encourage people to try their products and credit them for any improvement that occurs.

Many companies hold sales meetings at which people tell how products have supposedly helped them. Some sponsor telephone conference calls during which distributors describe their financial success, give sales tips, and describe their own experiences with the products. Testimonials may also be published in company magazines, audiotapes, and videotapes. Many distributors use testimonials—typically their own—to market their products through computer bulletin boards and other Internet outlets.[48]

During the past 20 years Dr. Stephen Barrett has examined promotional materials from more than 100 multilevel companies selling health-related products. Every single one has made false or deceptive claims. The products that have nutritional value (such as multivitamins and low-cholesterol foods) are invariably overpriced and usually not needed. Those promoted as remedies are either bogus, unproven, or intended for conditions that are unsuitable for self-medication. Today's most noteworthy companies include the following.

Mary Kay, well known for its cosmetic products, is now marketing a $29.50-per-month daily supplement packet alleged "to help bridge the gap between what a healthy diet provides and what a woman needs for optimum health and beauty." *Tufts University Diet & Nutrition Letter*[49] has observed that more rationally formulated multivitamin/mineral preparations are available elsewhere for one tenth the cost.

Matol Botanical International, a Canadian firm, markets *Km*, a foul-tasting extract of 14 common herbs.

Consumer Tip

Cyberwarning

Cyberspace has become the new frontier for scam artists. The scams aren't new, just the medium. . . .

Treat all ads or would-be ads with skepticism and *never* make an investment or health-related purchase decision based solely on information obtained from a single source in any medium—print, broadcast, or online.

Bureau of Consumer Protection
Federal Trade Commission[51]

Km was originally marketed as *Matol*, which was claimed to be effective for ailments ranging from arthritis to cancer, as well as for rejuvenation. Canada's Health Protection Branch took action that resulted in an order for the company to advertise only the product name, price, and contents. In 1988 the FDA attempted to block importation of *Matol* into the United States. However, the company evaded the ban by adding an ingredient and changing the product's name. The product literature acknowledges that *Km* has never been tested for effectiveness against any disease and states that distributors should not diagnose or recommend its products for any specific disease. However, many distributors do so.[51]

National Safety Associates markets Juice Plus+® products, which are made by extracting the vitamins and other phytochemicals from 17 fruits and vegetables. The products are claimed to be useful because diets high in fruits and vegetables are associated with lower rates of various diseases and many Americans fail to consume the recommended amounts. However, much of the protective effect of fruits and vegetables is due to their fiber content. Juice Plus+ pills have nearly all the fiber removed.[52]

Nature's Sunshine Products, of Spanish Fork, Utah, markets herbs, vitamins, other nutritional supplements, homeopathic remedies, skin- and hair-care products, water treatment systems, cooking utensils, and a weight-loss plan. Its more than 400 products include many that are claimed to "nourish" or "support" various body organs. Its salespeople, dubbed "Natural Health Counselors," are taught to use iridology (a bogus diagnostic procedure in which the eyes are examined), applied kinesiology (a bogus muscle-testing procedure), and other dubious methods to convince people that they need the products.[52]

Nu Skin International, Inc., of Provo, Utah, sells body-care products and dietary supplements. In 1993 the company and three of its distributors agreed to pay a total of $1,225,000 to settle FTC charges that they made unsubstantiated claims for *Nutriol Hair Fitness Preparation* and two skin-care products. Nu Skin's Interior Design division markets expensive antioxidant, phytochemical, and "active enzyme" products. The enzyme products are said to be important because "the majority of cooked or processed foods we eat lack an ideal level of enzyme activity" needed for digestion. This statement is nonsense because the enzymes needed for digestion are made by the body's digestive organs. In 1997, the company agreed to pay $1.5 million to settle charges that it had made unsubstantiated claims for five more of its products. The products, which contained chromium picolinate and L-carnitine, were falsely claimed to reduce fat, increase metabolism, and preserve or build muscle.[55]

Sunrider Corporation, of Torrance, California, claims that its herbal concoctions can help "regenerate" the body. Although some ingredients can exert pharmacologic effects on the body, there is little evidence they can cure major diseases or that Sunrider distributors are qualified to advise people about how to use them properly. During the mid-1980s the FDA ordered Sunrider to stop making health claims for several of its products. In 1989 the company signed a consent agreement to pay $175,000 to the state of California and to stop representing that its products have any effect on disease or medical conditions. The company toned down its literature but continued to make therapeutic claims in testimonial tapes included in its distributor kits.[55] In 1992 a jury in Phoenix, Arizona, concluded that Sunrider had violated Arizona's racketeering laws and awarded $650,000 to a woman who claimed she had been misled by company representations and had become ill after using some of its products.

TELEMARKETING SCHEMES

Fred Schulte,[56] a newspaper editor who spent more than 1 year investigating telemarketing schemes, concluded that millions of people had been robbed at an annual rate of more than $40 billion. The health-related schemes typically involve notification by mail or phone that the recipient has won a "valuable" prize. To collect, the recipient must order a large supply of vitamins, a water purifier, or something else that costs hundreds of dollars. If delivery is made, the prize almost always is worthless, the product overpriced, and the "money-back guarantee" not honored.

When the product has been ordered by credit card, the buyer can usually prevent loss by asking the credit card company to reverse the payment. But many buyers don't realize this or waste so much time trying to get a refund that the deadline for action through the credit card issuer expires.

In the early 1990s, the National Alliance for Fraud in Telemarketing predicted that telephone scams involving arthritis remedies, weight-loss plans, sexual aids, baldness cures, and other health and nutrition products would increase during the following decade.

In response to this burgeoning problem, state and federal agencies took action against hundreds of individuals and companies. A 1992 nationwide undercover investigation called Operation Disconnect resulted in 296 convictions and the seizure of $7.6 million in fraudulently obtained assets. Another major effort was Operation Sentinel, in which volunteers trained at seminars run by the American Association of Retired Persons helped the FBI and the Justice Department gather evidence used in 1996 to arrest more than 400 fraudulent telemarketers in 15 states.

The FTC, which has issued new telemarketing rules, advises consumers to report suspect telemarketing activities to their state attorney general and the National Fraud Information Center (1-800-876-7060). The rules, issued pursuant to the 1993 Telemarketing and Consumer Fraud and Abuse Prevention Act, enable state attorneys general to use federal courts to stop scams nationwide.

INDUSTRY SELF-REGULATION

In 1971, when the FTC was initiating an advertising substantiation program, the National Advertising Review Board (NARB) was formed "to promote higher standards of truth and accuracy in national and regional advertising." Its sponsors were the American Advertising Federation, American Association of Advertising Agencies, Association of National Advertisers, and Council of Better Business Bureaus. The review process is done primarily by the Council's National Advertising Division (NAD), which investigates questionable ads, draws conclusions, and sometimes negotiates settlements. Parties that disagree with NAD's findings can appeal to the NARB. Few cases go to the NARB.

NAD may initiate action as a result of its own monitoring of the advertising media. Complaints are also made by competing companies, local Better Business Bureaus, individual consumers, consumer groups, professional and trade associations, and government agencies.

When NAD decides to investigate a complaint, it asks the advertiser for substantiation, which may then be shown to the complainant for rebuttal. Closed cases are classified in the monthly *NAD Case Reports* as "substantiated" or "modified or discontinued." NAD closes about 100 cases a year. Anyone can initiate a complaint by sending a letter to NAD with a description of the ad (including a copy if it has been printed) and the reasons why it appears to be invalid.

NAD's impact on the health marketplace is very small. Barrett, who has complained about more than 20 health-related ads, found that NAD refused to open cases involving: (a) products or companies it did not consider basically legitimate; (b) dietary supplements whose manufacturers made illegal therapeutic claims; (c) services by licensed health professionals; and (d) ads that were not distributed nationally. NAD's investigations tend to be slow, and even ads that are discontinued as a result of an NAD inquiry usually have run long enough to achieve their purposes. NAD's findings are available on its Web site but are rarely reported by other news outlets.

GOVERNMENT REGULATION

The FDA has jurisdiction over the labeling of foods, dietary supplements, drugs, and devices. The FDA has been severely criticized for failing to stop many misleading promotions for foods and nutrition-related products.[56] Recently enacted regulations should keep misleading claims off the labels of food products. But the Dietary Supplement Health and Education Act of 1994 has greatly increased the number of false claims made for supplement products and made it more difficult for the FDA to stop them (see Chapters 12 and 26). Since passage of this act, the FDA has turned down citizen petitions asking it to ban "stress vitamins" and "ergogenic aids" and issue public warnings that they are ineffective.

The FTC has jurisdiction over the advertising of products and services except for prescription drugs. In recent years it has handled many health-related cases.

The U.S. Postal Service has jurisdiction over products marketed through the mail. However, in recent years, it has handled very few cases related to mail-order health products.

State and local agencies have jurisdiction over advertising within their own state, but they vary considerably in their attitude toward health frauds. Some states handle many cases, whereas others handle few or none. When a promotion is stopped in one state, it may be able to continue in others.

In many cases more than one agency may have authority to act against a particular ad.

Chapter 26 discusses the role of each of these agencies in detail. Consumers should keep in mind that the problem of health fraud is so vast that government agencies cannot stop most violations they detect.[57]

SUMMARY

Consumers should be aware that the health marketplace is flooded with misleading messages. Some marketers use scare tactics to promote their wares. Some attempt to exploit people's common hopes and fears. Many advertisers use puffery, weasel words, half-truths, or visual imagery to misrepresent their products. Except for chiropractors, most health professionals who advertise tend to represent their services accurately. Ads by professional societies, hospitals, and prescription drug manufacturers also tend to be useful and informative. Food advertising tends to promote dietary imbalance. Dietary supplements and alleged weight-control products are promoted in a wide variety of misleading ways. Ads for tobacco products appear intended to distract attention from their dangers. Health-related products promoted by mail, by telephone, by television infomercials, through the Internet, or through multilevel distributors rarely live up to the claims made for them. Although government agencies can stop many misleading promotions, regulatory action provides only limited protection and cannot substitute for intelligent consumer behavior.

It's Your Decision

A friend tells you he has been feeling extremely energetic since using product X. He thinks that everyone should use it. In fact, he is thinking about becoming a distributor for the company that makes the product. He invites you to try the product and to consider becoming a distributor. What things should you consider in making an intelligent decision?

68   Part One   Dynamics of the Health Marketplace

REFERENCES

1. Kurtz P. The responsibilities of the media and paranormal claims. Skeptical Inquirer 9(4):362, 1985.
2. Miller R. Critiquing quack ads. FDA Consumer 19(2):10–13, 1985.
3. Howard JA, Hulbert J. A staff report to the Federal Trade Commission: Advertising and public interest. From FTC hearings on modern advertising practices. New York, 1973, The Commission.
4. Lutz W. Doublespeak. New York, 1989, HarperCollins.
5. Oler C. "Low blows" in television advertising. Canadian Dental Association Journal 7:482, 1985.
6. Pratkanis AR, Aronson E. Age of Propaganda: The Everyday Use and Abuse of Persuasion. W.H. Freeman and Company, New York, 1992.
7. Advertising in disguise. Consumer Reports 51:179–181, 1986.
8. Preston IL. The Great American Blow-Up: Puffery in Advertising and Selling. Madison, Wis., 1975, University of Wisconsin Press.
9. DeBaggio T. Advertising image: Puffery or effrontery. The Nation 214:79–83, 1982.
10. Advertising Age, Dec. 7, 1981.
11. Barrett S, Herbert V. The Vitamin Pushers: How the "Health Food" Industry Is Selling America a Bill of Goods. Amherst, N.Y., 1994, Prometheus Books.
12. AMA Council on Ethical and Judicial Affairs. Code of Medical Ethics: Current Opinions with Annotations. Chicago, 1994, American Medical Association.
13. Yarborough M. Physician advertising: Some reasons for caution. Southern Medical Journal 82:1538–1544, 1989.
14. Margo CE. Sounding board: Selling surgery. New England Journal of Medicine 314:1575–1576, 1986.
15. Gray J. The selling of medicine. Medical Economics p 180–194, Jan. 20, 1986.
16. Edwards KS. The new ABMS listings. Ohio Medicine 86:653, 1990.
17. Magner GW. Chiropractic: The Victim's Perspective. Amherst, N.Y., 1995, Prometheus Books.
18. Year Two: A National Survey of Consumer Reactions to Direct-to-Consumer Advertising. Emmaus, Pa.,1999, Prevention Magazine.
19. Borzo B. Drug ads casting a wider net, finding a home on the Web. American Medical News 38(47):3,25, 1995
20. Kessler DA, Pines WL. The federal regulation of prescription drug advertising and promotion. JAMA 264:2409–2415, 1990.
21. Masson A, Rubin PH. Matching prescription drugs and consumers. New England Journal of Medicine 313:513–515, 1985.
22. Cohen EP. Direct-to-the-public advertisement of prescription drugs. New England Journal of Medicine 318:373–375, 1988.
23. Lipman MM. Office visit: Pitching prescription drugs to consumers. Consumer Reports on Health 3:22, 1991.
24. Drug advertising. Is this good medicine? Consumer Reports 61:62–63, 1996.
25. Story M, Faulkner P. The prime time diet: A content analysis of eating behavior and food messages in television program content and commercials. American Journal of Public Health 80:738–740, 1990.
26. Bureau of Consumer Protection. Dietary Supplements: An Advertising Guide for Industry. Washington, DC, 1998, Federal Trade Commission.
27. Tobacco advertising and the First Amendment. JAMA 264:1593–1594, 1990.
28. Koop CE. A parting shot at tobacco. JAMA 262:2894–2895, 1989.
29. Beck B. 1990 ACSH survey: An evaluation of reporting on the health hazards of smoking in American magazines. New York 1991, American Council on Science and Health.
30. R.J. Reynolds abuses MR FIT. Consumer Reports on Health 2:44, 1990.
31. Tobacco foes attack ads that target women, minorities, teens and the poor, JAMA 264:1505–1506, 1990.
32. Camel ad. Is male violence a "smooth move?" The Public Citizen Health Research Group Health Letter 5(9):11–12, 1989.
33. Fischer M and others. Brand logo recognition by children aged 3 to 6 years. JAMA 266:3145–3148, 1991.
34. Tye JB. The silver smoke screen: Covert cigarette ads in movies. Priorities, Summer 1991.
35. Wolinsky H. Tobacco and sports: An unhealthy alliance. Priorities, pp 8–11, Spring 1991.
36. Kilbourne J. Still killing us softly: Advertising and the obsession with thinness. In Fallon P, Katz MA, Wooley SC, editors. Feminist Perspectives on Eating Disorders. New York, 1994, Guilford Press, pp 395–418.
37. Tobacco companies "guide" smokers to action against nonsmokers. The Public Citizen Health Research Group Health Letter 5(9):4, 1989.
38. Glantz SA and others. Looking through a keyhole at the tobacco industry. JAMA 274:219–224, 1995.
39. Wilson JJ. Summary of the attorneys general master tobacco settlement agreement, March 1999.
40. Wellness Today, a speecial supplement to Health and Healing. Potomac, Md., 1991, Phillips Publishing, Inc.
41. Barrett S. Quackery by mail. New York, 1991, American Council on Science and Health.
42. Raso J. Mystical Diets. Amherst, N.Y., 1993, Prometheus Books.
43. Barrett S. Be wary of Gero Vita, A. Glenn Braswell, and Braswell's "Journal" of Longevity. Quackwatch, Sept 30, 2000.
44. Revlon, Inc. to settle charges of unsubstantiated ad claims for "anti-cellulite" and sunscreen products. FTC news release, Aug 24, 1993.
45. Do the bust developers really work? Good Housekeeping 185:153-154, Aug 1977.
46. Claims of weight loss for exercise gliders and abdominal devices not substantiated; FTC alleges. FTC news release, May 12, 1999.
47. FTC News Notes, Jan 8, 1990.
48. The Amway Business Review. Ada, Mich., 1998, Amway Corporation.
49. Barrett D. Bandits on the Information Superhighway. Boston, 1996, O'Reilley & Associates.
50. In the pink with Mary Kay? Tufts University Diet & Nutrition Letter 13:(11):1, 1996.
51. Online scams: Road hazards on the information superhighway. Washington, D.C., 1995, Federal Trade Commission.
52. Raso J. Bottled hype: The story of Km. Nutrition Forum 8:33–37, 1991.
53. Barrett S. Juice Plus+: Want a "carotenoid gloss"? Quackwatch Web site, April 22, 2000.
54. Raso J. The shady business of Nature's Sunshine. Nutrition Forum 9:17–23, 1992.
55. Barrett S. The multilevel mirage. Quackwatch Web site, Aug 26, 1999.
56. Schulte F. Fleeced! Telemarketing Ripoffs and How to Spot Them. Amherst, N.Y., 1995, Prometheus Books.
57. Barrett S. Quackery and the FDA: A complicated story. Nutrition Forum 8:42–45, 1991.
58. Barrett S. Strength and weaknesses of our laws. Quackwatch Web site, Aug 10, 2000.

PART II

HEALTH-CARE APPROACHES

Chapter Five

SCIENCE-BASED HEALTH CARE

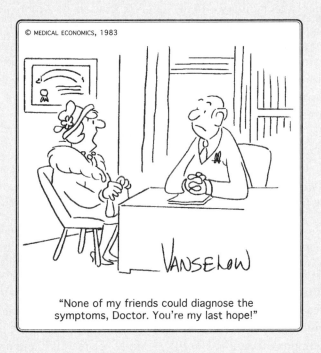

© MEDICAL ECONOMICS, 1983

VANSELOW

"None of my friends could diagnose the symptoms, Doctor. You're my last hope!"

The good physician treats the disease; the great physician treats the patient who has the disease.

SIR WILLIAM OSLER

Knowing about your problem will help you assert yourself in the doctor's office. And the more you know, the more intelligently you're apt to follow—or question—your doctor's advice.

MARVIN LIPMAN, M.D.[1]

Science-based health care is the prevention, diagnosis, and treatment of disease based on modern scientific principles. Most people in the United States accept physicians as the primary health authorities and healers of the sick. Aligned with physicians are other scientifically trained practitioners and ancillary (allied) providers who espouse scientific concepts of disease, such as the germ theory. These professionals advocate research based on scientific principles and prevention and treatment based on proven methods. They also advocate strict codes of professional ethics and rigorous procedures for education, licensure, and accountability.

This chapter discusses the training and work of medical and osteopathic physicians, podiatrists, nurses, and various allied personnel. Mental-health, dental, nutrition, sports medicine, pharmacy, and optometry professionals are discussed in Chapters 6, 7, 11, 14, 19, and 22, respectively.

HEALTH-CARE PERSONNEL

Most science-based practitioners are regulated by state licensing laws. To obtain a license one must first complete a specified amount of training at an accredited institution and then pass a licensing examination. Based on laws that define their scope of practice, practitioners may be divided into three groups:

1. Independent practitioners whose scope is theoretically unlimited: medical and osteopathic physicians.
2. Independent practitioners whose scope is limited: dentists, podiatrists, optometrists, psychologists (in some states), and dietitians (in some states),
3. Ancillary providers, most of whom practice under some degree of medical supervision or control: nurses, physicians' assistants, physical and occupational therapists, pharmacists, and many types of technicians

In many states practitioners must participate in continuing education to maintain their license or membership in their professional association.

Medical Doctors

The doctor of medicine (M.D.) degree requires 4 years of training at a medical school accredited by the Liaison Committee on Medical Education, a joint committee of the AMA Council on Medical Education and the Association of American Medical Colleges. The first 2 years of medical training cover basic and preclinical science courses, including anatomy, physiology, biochemistry, histology, pathology, epidemiology, and pharmacology. The last 2 years stress clinical work in hospital and clinic settings. A minimum of three years of premedical college work is required for admission to medical school, but 97% of matriculants have at least a baccalaureate degree. The grade-point average of students admitted in 1999 was 3.59 (on a 4.0-point scale). About 44% were women, and about 34% were members of racial or ethnic minorities.[2]

There are 125 accredited medical schools in the United States. Graduates of these schools must take state or national board examinations to become licensed. Some states require additional postgraduate training at a hospital. Graduates of foreign medical schools must take postgraduate education in the United States before they are eligible to take licensing examinations in most states. Currently there are about 690,000 medical doctors in the United States, about 250,000 of whom are AMA members.

Because modern medical knowledge is so vast, most medical school graduates take additional training before entering clinical practice. Those choosing to become specialists take at least 3 years of residency training during which they are designated as PGY 1 (postgraduate-year-one resident), PGY 2 (postgraduate-year-two resident), and so on. The recognized standard-setting organization is the American Board of Medical Specialties (ABMS), which is composed of 24 primary medical specialty boards and six associate members: the American Hospital Association, American Medical Association, Association of American Medical Colleges,

Council of Medical Specialty Societies, Federation of State Medical Boards of the United States, and National Board of Medical Examiners.

Medical specialty boards require high standards of training and performance and ensure them by rigid examinations. Successful applicants receive diplomas and are considered "board-certified." They are also referred to as "diplomates" in their particular specialties. Physicians who complete all requirements for certification except the examination may be identified as "board-eligible." Certificates are now available for about 100 specialties and subspecialties. Most expire within 7 or 10 years and require re-examination for renewal. Table 5-1 describes the scope of many of the recognized medical specialties and subspecialties.

Osteopathic Physicians

The principles of osteopathy originally were expressed by Andrew Taylor Still, M.D., in 1874, when medical science was in its infancy. A medical doctor, Still believed that diseases were caused by mechanical interference with nerve and blood supply and were curable by manipulation of "deranged, displaced bones, nerves, muscles—removing all obstructions—thereby setting the machinery of life moving." His autobiography states that he could "shake a child and stop scarlet fever, croup, diphtheria, and cure whooping cough in three days by a wring of its neck."

Still was antagonistic toward the drug practices of his day and regarded surgery as a last resort. Rejected as a cultist by organized medicine, he founded the first

---

Historical Perspective

The Rise of Medical Standards

In colonial America there were few trained physicians, no medical schools, and no standards of medical practice. Virtually anyone could practice medicine, but learning through apprenticeship was common. Much of the surgery was performed by barbers. In prerevolutionary America there were about 3500 practitioners, 400 of whom had obtained medical degrees from foreign schools. Many were immigrants. The first American medical school opened in 1765.

Death rates were high during the eighteenth century. The major killers were infectious diseases, the causes of which were unknown. Cathartics and herbal concoctions were used for treatment. When purging was combined with bloodletting, many patients became so weak they died.

During the nineteenth century, American medicine went from bad to worse. Many medical schools opened, but most had few if any standards of competence.[3] Programs generally were 2 years long, with little scientific training, clinical instruction in hospitals, or laboratory work. In 1870 the head of the Harvard Medical School said that written examinations could not be given because most of the students could not write well enough.[4] Dozens of schools sold diplomas, some for as little as $5. Many of the so-called healers were illiterates who peddled narcotic "cure-alls."

In the 1800s self-diagnosis and self-medication were practiced extensively. Most families had a supply of medical books, herbs, and nostrums. People who could nurse the sick were generally available, but doctors were seldom called when illness occurred. Few doctors were competent, patients lived considerable distances from physicians, and treatment was often too severe. Many

diseases that are now curable were simply accepted as "acts of God."

Few medicines used before 1900 were effective. Surgery often was successful, but postoperative infections exacted a heavy toll. For most ailments the best that could be done for the patient was to provide relief. Worthless nostrums were abundant, and charlatans flourished without interference from the law.

Until the work of Louis Pasteur, Joseph Lister, and Robert Koch established the bacterial theory of disease in the 1870s, the cause of infections was unclear. Pasteur was a chemist who studied contagious disease in animals and discovered the anthrax bacillus. He also developed diphtheria antitoxin, rabies vaccine, and the theoretical basis for pasteurization. Lister used carbolic acid for antiseptic surgery. Koch discovered the bacillus that causes tuberculosis.

By the 1880s infection-control measures were incorporated into medical practice, and scientific methods for seeking medical facts were known. The groundwork had also been laid for consumer-protection laws based on the ability to determine whether claims are valid.

In 1904 the American Medical Association and the Carnegie Foundation commissioned Dr. Abraham Flexner to investigate medical schools in the United States. His report, published in 1910, recommended standards for curricula, admissions, and clinical teachings. The report, plus tightening of the requirements for medical licensure, led to the closing of half these schools. By the 1930s, substandard medical schools were eliminated, accreditation procedures were established, and science-based health care was poised for explosive technologic growth.

Table 5-1

Selected Medical Specialties and Subspecialties

ALLERGY AND IMMUNOLOGY: Management of asthmatic, allergic, immunologic, and related disorders

ANESTHESIOLOGY: Administration of drugs to prevent pain or to induce unconsciousness during surgical operations or diagnostic procedures

CARDIOVASCULAR DISEASE (CARDIOLOGY): Subspecialty of internal medicine that deals with the heart and blood vessels

COLON AND RECTAL SURGERY (PROCTOLOGY): Diagnosis and treatment of disorders of the lower digestive tract

DERMATOLOGY: Diagnosis and treatment of skin problems

EMERGENCY MEDICINE: Evaluation and treatment of emergencies

ENDOCRINOLOGY: Subspecialty of internal medicine that deals with glandular and metabolic disorders

FAMILY PRACTICE: General medical services for patients and their families

FORENSIC PATHOLOGY: Subspecialty of pathology that deals with medicine and the law

GASTROENTEROLOGY: Subspecialty of internal medicine that deals with disorders of the digestive tract

GENERAL SURGERY: Surgery that deals with parts of the body that are not in the domain of specific surgical specialties (some areas overlap)

GERIATRICS: Care of problems of the elderly; family practitioners and internists can become certified with added qualifications in geriatric medicine; psychiatrists can become certified with added qualifications in geriatric psychiatry

HEMATOLOGY: Subspecialty of internal medicine that deals with disorders of the blood

INFECTIOUS DISEASE: Subspecialty of internal medicine

INTERNAL MEDICINE: Diagnosis and nonsurgical treatment of internal organs of the body of adults

NEONATAL-PERINATAL MEDICINE: Subspecialty of pediatrics that deals with disorders of newborn infants, including premature infants

NEPHROLOGY: Subspecialty of internal medicine that deals with kidney disorders

NEUROLOGIC SURGERY (NEUROSURGERY): Diagnosis and surgical treatment of diseases of the brain, spinal cord, and nerves

NEUROLOGY: Diagnosis and nonsurgical treatment of diseases of the brain, spinal cord, and nerves

NUCLEAR MEDICINE: Use of radioactive substances for diagnosis and treatment

OBSTETRICS AND GYNECOLOGY (OB/GYN): Care of pregnant women and treatment of disorders of the female reproductive system

OCCUPATIONAL MEDICINE: Preventive medicine subspecialty that deals with work-related illnesses and injuries

OPHTHALMOLOGY: Medical and surgical care of the eye, including the prescription of visual aids

ORTHOPEDIC SURGERY (ORTHOPEDICS): Care of injuries and disorders of the muscles, bones, and joints

OTOLARYNGOLOGY: Care of diseases of the head and neck, except for those of the eyes or brain

PATHOLOGY: Examination and diagnosis of organs, tissues, body fluids, and excrement

PEDIATRICS: Care of children from birth through adolescence

PHYSICAL MEDICINE AND REHABILITATION (PHYSIATRY): Treatment of convalescent and physically handicapped patients

PLASTIC SURGERY: Surgery to correct or repair deformed or mutilated parts of the body, or to improve the appearance of facial or body features

PREVENTIVE MEDICINE (PUBLIC HEALTH): Prevention of disease through immunization, good health practice, and concern with environmental factors

PSYCHIATRY: Treatment of mental and emotional problems

PULMONARY DISEASE: Subspecialty of internal medicine that deals with diseases of the lungs

RADIOLOGY: Use of radiation for the diagnosis and treatment of disease

RHEUMATOLOGY: Subspecialty of internal medicine that deals with arthritis and related disorders

SPORTS MEDICINE: Subspecialty available to practitioners of internal medicine, pediatrics, family practice, and emergency medicine

THORACIC SURGERY: Surgical treatment of the lungs, heart, and large blood vessels within the chest cavity

UROLOGY: Treatment of problems involving the male sex organs, male urinary tract, and female urinary tract

---

osteopathic medical school in Kirksville, Missouri, in 1892.

As medical science developed, osteopathy gradually incorporated all its theories and practices and abandoned Still's teachings.[5] Today, except for slight additional emphasis on musculoskeletal diagnosis and treatment, the scope of osteopathy is identical to that of medicine.

Currently there are about 44,000 practitioners of osteopathy and 19 accredited osteopathic colleges in the United States.[6] Admission to osteopathic school requires 3 years of preprofessional college work, but almost all of those enrolled have a baccalaureate or higher degree. The doctor of osteopathy (D.O.) degree requires more than 5000 hours of training over 4 academic years. The faculties of osteopathic colleges are about evenly divided between doctors of osteopathy and holders of Ph.D. degrees, with a few medical doctors at some colleges. Graduation is followed by a 1-year rotating internship at an approved teaching hospital. Specialization requires 2 to 6 additional years of residency training, depending on the specialty. A majority of osteopaths enter family practice. The American Osteopathic Association (AOA) recognizes more than 60 specialties and subspecialties. Many osteopathic physicians obtain their residency training at medical hospitals.

Osteopathic physicians are licensed to practice in all states and are legally equivalent to medical doctors. The licensing boards vary in makeup: some are composed entirely of osteopaths, some are composed entirely of medical doctors, and some have both.

Many observers believe that osteopathy and medicine should merge.[7] But osteopathic organizations prefer to retain a separate identity and have exaggerated the minor differences between osteopathy and medicine. According to a 1987 AOA brochure, for example: (a) osteopathy is "the only branch of mainstream medicine that follows the Hippocratic approach," (b) the body's musculoskeletal system is central to the patient's well-being, and (c) osteopathic manipulative treatment (OMT) is a proven technique for many hands-on diagnoses and often can provide an alternative to drugs and surgery. The AOA's Web site claims (falsely) that OMT "supports the body's natural tendency toward healing" and that combining it with all other medical procedures enables D.O.s to provide "the most comprehensive treatment available."[8]

Podiatrists

Doctors of podiatric medicine (D.P.M.) are independent practitioners who deal with problems of the foot and its governing structures. Podiatrists are licensed in all states to provide surgical and medical treatment of the feet, including corrective devices, drugs, and physical therapy. Most podiatrists have staff privileges at a hospital, and many belong to a medical group practice, health maintenance organization, or preferred provider organization.

Podiatry has its roots in the practice of chiropodists, practitioners who treated corns, warts, bunions, and other ailments of the foot and hand. The terms "chiropodist" and "chiropody" became obsolete during the mid-1960s.

Podiatric licensure requires a minimum of 90 semester hours of undergraduate course work plus 4 additional years of study at one of the seven accredited colleges of podiatric medicine in the United States. About two thirds of the states require an additional year of postgraduate work. Residency programs for 1 to 3 years of additional training are available to graduates. There are about 11,000 podiatrists in the United States, about 80% of whom belong to the American Podiatric Medical Association. About 90% of podiatrists are general practitioners, and the rest specialize in such areas as geriatrics, pediatrics, dermatology, surgery, orthopedics, public health, and sports medicine. Board certification is available in podiatric surgery and podiatric orthopedics and primary medicine.

Nurses

Registered nurses (R.N.s) are graduates of accredited nursing schools and have passed a state board examination for licensure. Their education may be acquired in several ways. Two-year programs leading to an associate degree are offered at community colleges or vocational technical schools. Three-year programs leading to a diploma are offered at hospital-based schools of nursing. Four-year programs leading to a baccalaureate degree (B.S.N.) are offered by colleges and universities. About 2 million registered nurses are licensed to practice in the United States.

The primary certifying body for nurses is the American Nurses Credentialing Center (ANCC), a subsidiary of the American Nurses Association (ANA). Certification in more than 30 specialty and advanced practice areas is available to registered nurses who meet educational and practice requirements and pass an examination. The ANCC's certification system was recently revised. As of 2000, nurses with an associate or higher degree are eligible to acquire the credential "Registered Nurse, Certified" (RN,C); and those with a baccalaureate or higher degree may be eligible for the credential "Registered Nurse, Board Certified" (RN,BC).

Nurse practitioners are registered nurses who undergo additional nursing education, usually at the master's level, to enable them to function in some states as primary care providers. Nurse practitioners and clinical specialists can achieve certification as a clinical nurse specialist. They must have a master's or higher degree in nursing, meet practice requirements, and pass an examination. Certification as an Advanced Practice Nurse entitles them to use the designation "APRN" or "APRN,BC." Certification is also available in nursing administration.

Registered nurses can work in hospitals, clinics, physicians' offices, public and voluntary health agencies, schools, industries, or independent practice. Some states require additional training for those who wish to work as school nurses.

Work as a public health nurse usually requires at least a baccalaureate degree. Specialization in public health may be acquired through nursing schools that offer a master of science (M.S.N.) degree. Schools of public health offer programs leading to a master of public health (M.P.H.) degree.

Nurse anesthetists are R.N.s who complete a 2-year program in anesthesia, usually at the master's level. Certified registered nurse anesthetists (C.R.N.A.s) must pass an examination administered by the American Association of Nurse Anesthetists.

Nurse-midwives are registered nurses who have completed an additional 1 to 2 years of training from an approved school of midwifery. By passing an examination given by the American College of Nurse-Midwives, they can earn a certified nurse-midwife (C.N.M.) certificate that allows them to practice midwifery in most states. Nurse-midwives care for mothers during pregnancy, manage labor and delivery, and watch for signs that require a physician's attention. They also help the mother care for herself and the baby and may serve as members of obstetric teams in medical centers and other community institutions.

Practical and vocational nurses (L.P.N.s and L.V.N.s) are graduates of state-approved schools of nursing who must pass a state board examination for licensing. Their training involves 12–18 months of work following a minimum of 2 years of high school. They usually work under the direction of a registered nurse.

Table 5-2 describes the work of several types of allied health-care personnel. Allied dental, mental health, nutrition, and optometric personnel are discussed in other chapters.

Choosing a Physician

In the past, basic medical care of individuals and families was provided by family physicians. Typically they were general practitioners who did not limit themselves to one area of medicine. Many delivered babies, and some even performed major surgery. When a specialist was needed, the family physician remained as the primary contact and medical advisor, with the specialist serving as a consultant.

As medicine became more complex, the percentage of physicians becoming specialists increased. As our society became more mobile, the number of group practices and walk-in facilities increased, and more people consulted specialists without coordination and referral by a family physician. Lack of coordination raises the cost of care and may lower its quality.

Managed care plans attempt to counter this problem by requiring authorization from a primary-care physician in order to consult a specialist (see Chapter 24).

The Good Physician

Because of the complexity of medical practice, it is difficult to construct yardsticks by which consumers can judge the quality of their medical care. In addition, what is good for one patient may not be what another needs or prefers. The "Consumer Tip" box on page 78 lists qualities of a good physician.

Alper[10] suggests that marginal physicians can often be identified by overuse of antibiotics for common infections, overuse of tranquilizers and injections, and use of "fad diagnoses" (discussed in Chapter 8 of this book). He states that antibiotic treatment is important for strep throats, but routine use for viral sore throats or ordinary colds is a sign of fuzzy thinking. Monthly B_{12} shots are lifesaving in cases of pernicious anemia, but giving shots to people who simply feel "rundown" is poor medical practice.

Locating Prospective Physicians

Medical authorities are unanimous in recommending affiliation with a primary care provider—a personal physician who becomes familiar with a patient's medical needs and can coordinate care with other physicians should consultations become necessary. Ideally, primary care doctors generally offer "one-stop shopping" and lower cost and convenience.[11] For many people the choice of physician is limited by the nature and scope of their insurance coverage. Student health services, for example, offer relatively few options. The following guidelines apply to the extent that a choice is possible.

A board-certified family practitioner (for adults and children), internist (for adults only), geriatrician (for elderly adults), or pediatrician (for young children or adolescents) is likely to be a good choice, because all of them have taken advanced training in the diagnosis and treatment of general medical problems. Staff affiliation with a hospital connected with a medical school indicates that a physician is working with up-to-date colleagues and is therefore likely to keep abreast of current medical developments and techniques. A teaching appointment at a medical school and affiliation with a hospital that trains residents are favorable signs. Lack of hospital affiliation is suspect because it may mean that the physician is isolated from the community's scientific mainstream. Even worse, it could mean that the physician's standard of practice is not high enough to merit membership on a hospital staff.

Table 5-2

ALLIED HEALTH-CARE PERSONNEL

More than 100 types of allied health-care personnel offer clinical services to the public.[9] The AMA Committee on Allied Health Education and Accreditation accredits training programs for 26 occupations. Some types of allied health-care personnel are licensed; others are not.

AUDIOLOGISTS test patients and recommend hearing aids. Work in this field requires a master's degree in audiology.

EMERGENCY MEDICAL TECHNICIANS (EMTs) respond to medical emergencies and provide immediate care to the critically ill or injured. Rating as an EMT requires completion of an 81-hour course approved by the U.S. Department of Transportation. An EMT-dispatcher rating requires an additional 2-day communication course. An EMT-paramedic rating requires a minimum 500-hour approved course with 6 to 12 months of prior EMT experience. EMT-paramedics can work in mobile intensive care vehicles under a physician's direction through voice contact relayed from a medical center. They may administer drugs intravenously or use a defibrillator to shock a stopped heart into action. The basic courses are given by hospitals; community colleges; and health, police, and fire departments. Advanced training is given by hospitals. Some 2-year associate degree programs exist.

MEDICAL ASSISTANTS work mainly in medical offices helping physicians to examine patients. They may also obtain laboratory specimens, function as receptionists, complete insurance forms, and order supplies. Their training may be a 2-year community college program, after which certification may be obtained from the American Association of Medical Assistants or on-the-job training by physician-employers.

MEDICAL TECHNOLOGISTS are college graduates whose education includes at least 1 year of clinical training in the performance of various laboratory tests and procedures. They may be assisted in their work by laboratory technicians. Certification is available from the American Society of Clinical Pathologists and several other professional organizations.

NURSE'S AIDES AND ORDERLIES, also referred to as nursing assistants or hospital attendants, provide basic patient care under direct nursing supervision. They may bathe and feed patients, change linens, and make beds. No formal training is required; most hospitals and nursing homes provide 6 to 8 weeks of on-the-job training. Programs are also available at vocational schools, community colleges, and elsewhere.

OCCUPATIONAL THERAPISTS help physically and emotionally handicapped persons with vocational or recreational activities. They are college graduates whose education includes at least 2 years of specialized training.

PHYSICAL THERAPISTS help to rehabilitate individuals who have temporary or permanent physical handicaps or other ailments. Their treatment methods include exercises to improve muscle strength, flexibility, and coordination, and the application of heat, cold, or electricity to relieve pain or to change the patient's condition. Physical therapists are college graduates whose education includes 1 or more years of specialized training. Traditionally they work under physician supervision, but some states permit direct access to patients.

PATIENT REPRESENTATIVES work mainly in hospitals, where they help patients interpret policies and procedures, respond to patient complaints, and help staff members understand how patients perceive the hospital experience. Academic training is not required, although most are college graduates and a few have master's degrees in health advocacy.

PHYSICIAN ASSISTANTS (PAs), under physician supervision, perform many tasks traditionally done by physicians. PAs perform physical examinations, treat certain ailments, prescribe certain drugs, and counsel patients on health problems. Training at community colleges, universities, medical schools, or in the military usually takes 2 years. Some training programs require prior college or patient-care experience. Most PAs work in physicians' offices, but some work in hospitals, health maintenance organizations (HMOs), prisons, and community clinics. Training is available at more than 60 programs accredited by the Commission on Accreditation of Allied Health Education Programs. All states except Mississippi regulate or license PAs. For licensure most require passage of an examination administered by the National Commission on Certification of Physician Assistants, which enables use of the title "Physician Assistant — Certified" (PA-C). To maintain national certification, PAs must complete 100 hours of continuing education every 2 years and pass a recertification examination every 6 years.

RESPIRATORY THERAPISTS, on physician's orders, treat patients with heart or lung problems, administering oxygen and various types of gases or aerosol drugs. They may also test respiratory function. Therapists complete a minimum of 2 years' training in a college or hospital.

SOCIAL WORKERS help people with their jobs, families, financial problems, and daily living tasks, particularly when their needs are related to illness or disability. They are usually college graduates.

SPEECH PATHOLOGISTS test patients and provide corrective therapy. Work in this field requires a master's degree in speech pathology.

A good physician:

- Is intelligent and knowledgeable
- Is sympathetic and interested in the patient
- Advocates preventive measures
- Is sufficiently organized to maintain a reasonably smooth appointment schedule
- Takes a detailed history and gives the patient enough time to discuss problems
- After examination, gives the patient a clear explanation of the diagnosis and treatment
- May indicate that knowledge or diagnosis is lacking
- Knows his or her limitations and refers patients to specialists when needed
- Is conservative about recommending surgery
- Will not abandon a patient once treatment has begun
- Is available for appropriate telephone consultations
- Is available for emergencies or provides a competent backup physician
- Charges reasonable fees and is willing to discuss them
- Is on the staff of an accredited hospital
- Keeps up-to-date by reading journals and attending educational meetings

McCall[12] has pointed out that older doctors are more likely to fall behind, but those who make the effort to stay current combine their broad knowledge with a wealth of clinical experience. He also states that the best way to discover whether a doctor is up-to-date is to become well informed about subjects that concern you.

Because a personal physician can significantly affect a person's health (and even life), considerable care should be exercised in looking for one. The best time to look is before becoming ill. Names can be obtained from many sources:

- The department of family practice or department of medicine at a nearby medical school
- A local accredited hospital
- A local health-care professional such as a dentist, nurse, or pharmacist
- The county medical society (names are usually given out on a rotating basis from a list of available members)
- Friends, neighbors, co-workers
- One's physician from a previous community
- A list of physicians participating in a managed-care program provided through one's employer or otherwise available; some managed-care organizations hold meetings to introduce primary care physicians to new or prospective members

Several years ago the Medical Association of Alabama asked people what counted most in choosing a family doctor. The following percentages indicate which characteristics the respondents thought were "important" or "very important":

Willingness to talk about your illness	100%
Access to a hospital you want	89%
Length of time to get an appointment	88%
Personality or appearance	84%
Fees	75%
Years of experience	73%
Office location	66%
Weekend and evening office hours	66%
Involvement in civic organizations	37%
Listing in Yellow Pages or other directories	30%

The *Washington Consumers' CHECKBOOK* has suggested asking friends the following questions:

- Does your physician seem to understand your symptoms when you describe them?
- Does your physician take time to explain your medical problems and their treatment?
- Is it easy to talk with your physician about concerns, however silly they may seem?
- How long do you usually have to wait for an appointment for a nonemergency medical problem?
- How long must you usually wait for an appointment for a full physical examination?
- How long do you usually wait in the physician's office?
- Is it usually easy to reach the physician by phone?
- Will the physician advise you on the phone?
- Do the physician's fees seem reasonable?

Another consideration that will become increasingly important is the use of electronic communication. Many medical offices will use the Internet to provide educational information and test results and to answer questions by e-mail.

Credentials may be ascertained by contacting the physician's office and may be verified by consulting a medical society, hospital, or managed-care program with which the physician is affiliated. They are also listed in the *Directory of Medical Specialists,* the ABMS *Compendium of Certified Medical Specialists,* and the *American Medical Directory*, which are commonly available at hospitals and public libraries. Most physicians identified as specialists in the Yellow Pages have completed accredited specialty training. However, telephone directory publishers rarely attempt to verify credentials, so self-proclaimed specialists may be listed also. Board certification is easily checked on the American Board of Medical Specialties Web site at http://www.abms.org. The Board has also been placing lists of board-certified physicians in many telephone directories, but many board-certified physicians are not included because they do not wish to pay the required fee (over $200 per year). Additional information about credentials and disciplinary action is available on Web sites operated by the AMA, state medical boards, and several commercial sites.[13]

Meeting the Physician

An excellent way to begin a relationship with a new physician is to have an evaluation that includes a thorough physical examination. Such an examination will provide a baseline against which future changes can be compared. Those who do not wish to have a complete physical examination might still wish to schedule a brief "get-acquainted" visit with the prospective physician. This will provide an opportunity to observe the physical characteristics of the office, to bring up troubling health questions, and to judge the physician's personality. If satisfied, one can also sign a release form to enable the new physician to obtain past medical records.

Advance registration has another advantage. Some physicians will not accept new patients under emergency conditions, particularly outside of regular office hours. Once a patient is accepted, however, the doctor has a legal obligation either to treat the patient or to provide a substitute.

Having chosen a primary physician, it is a good idea to try to learn about the doctor's routine. Most well-organized offices have printed information sheets for this purpose. If these are not available, ask questions. What are the office hours? Which are the days off? Who will cover in the doctor's absence? Does the doctor make house calls? Which hospital does the doctor use? Knowing the hospital affiliation is important. In an emergency, unless instructed differently, ambulance drivers usually take patients to the nearest hospital. The doctor may not be able to take care of a person who goes to the wrong hospital.

Emergency Care

In an emergency, try to phone the doctor immediately rather than just showing up at the hospital emergency room. Advance notice may enable one's doctor to provide the necessary service. It also will enable the

---

FUNDAMENTAL ELEMENTS OF THE PATIENT-PHYSICIAN RELATIONSHIP

From ancient times, physicians have recognized that the health and well-being of patients depends on a collaborative effort between physician and patient. Patients share with physicians the responsibility for their own health care. The patient-physician relationship is of greatest benefit to patients when they bring medical problems to the attention of their physicians in a timely fashion, provide information about their medical condition to the best of their ability, and work with their physicians in a mutually respectful alliance. Physicians can best contribute to this alliance by serving as their patient's advocate and by fostering the following rights:

1. The patient has the right to receive information from physicians, and to discuss the benefits, risks, and costs of appropriate treatment alternatives. Patients should receive guidance from their physicians as to the optimal course of action. Patients are also entitled to obtain copies or summaries of their medical records, to have their questions answered, to be advised of potential conflicts of interest that their physicians might have, and to receive independent professional opinions.
2. The patient has the right to make decisions regarding the health care that is recommended by his or her physician. Accordingly, patients may accept or refuse any recommended medical treatment.
3. The patient has the right to courtesy, respect, dignity, responsiveness, and timely attention to his or her needs.
4. The patient has the right to confidentiality. The physician should not reveal confidential communications or information without the consent of the patient, unless provided for by law or by the need to protect the welfare of the individual or the public interest.
5. The patient has the right to continuity of health care. The physician has an obligation to cooperate in the coordination of medically indicated care with other health care providers treating the patient. The physician may not discontinue treatment of a patient as long as further treatment is medically indicated without giving the patient sufficient opportunity to make alternative arrangements for care.
6. The patient has a basic right to have available adequate health care. Physicians, along with the rest of society, should continue to work toward this goal. Fulfillment of this right is dependent on society providing resources so that no patient is deprived of necessary care because of an inability to pay for the care. Physicians should continue their traditional assumption of part of the responsibility for the medical care of those who cannot afford essential health care. Physicians should advocate for patients in dealing with third parties when appropriate.

AMA Council on Ethical and Judicial Affairs (1993)[14]

doctor to alert the emergency room personnel so that they may begin treatment or arrange for necessary tests.

Should an emergency arise before a doctor has been selected, the best bet is to go to the emergency room of the nearest accredited hospital. If a private practitioner is preferred, some emergency rooms and medical societies maintain a roster of doctors who are on call 24 hours a day. If an ambulance is needed, one can be obtained by dialing 911 (or other community emergency number), contacting the police, or calling a company listed in the Yellow Pages of the telephone directory.

Many cities have freestanding emergency centers, where fees are in between those of office practitioners and emergency rooms. The advantages and disadvantages of using such facilities are discussed in Chapter 10. Elderly or ailing individuals who live alone can wear or install special devices for emergencies; by pressing a button they can signal that help is urgently needed.

Finding a Doctor Abroad

Americans traveling in foreign countries can locate suitable treatment facilities through the International Association for Medical Assistance to Travelers (IAMAT). Established in 1960, IAMAT is a voluntary organization of hospitals, health-care centers, and physicians who pledge to provide travelers with physicians who speak their language, meet IAMAT standards, and adhere to a fixed fee schedule similar to that in the United States. When medical assistance is needed, the traveler can telephone the nearest center listed in the IAMAT directory to obtain a list of local physicians. The U.S. Centers for Disease Control and Prevention Web site (http://www.cdc.gov/travel) provides information on required vaccinations, prevention of foodborne diseases, and other tips for travelers.[15]

Advice from Remote Sources

Advice is also available by telephone, by mail, and through the Internet. Many reliable agencies and groups operate toll-free hotlines and/or Web sites through which callers can obtain information or pose questions to knowledgeable parties. Some hospitals, organizations, and individual practitioners sponsor phone lines through which consumers can select tape recordings on various topics. Several managed-care companies offer phone-based counseling performed by nurses, access to prerecorded information, or self-help publications.

A few commercial services, accessible through the Internet or by phone, provide direct contact with physicians, pharmacists, or others who answer questions. The

---

☑ **Consumer Tip**

Emergency Information

Persons who are subject to epilepsy, severe allergies, diabetes, or other ailments that may require urgent attention should wear a bracelet identifying the condition or carry an emergency medical identification card that lists the person's name, next of kin, medical problems, medications taken, and doctor's name.

The technology now exists for posting detailed medical records on personal home pages on the World Wide Web that could be accessed with a password available from a bracelet or another source. The information could include the patient's medical history, current medications, and hospital discharge summaries, as well as graphic images such as electrocardiograms and x-ray pictures. This information could prove handy in an emergency or when a traveler is admitted to a hospital far from home.[16]

---

charges for such services are then billed through a credit card or on one's phone bill. Critics of these services have warned that their advice has limited value because the person giving advice is unable to physically examine the caller. These services may provide useful information, but they are not suitable for personal diagnosis. Scientific studies concerning the quality and cost-effectiveness of commercially offered health advice have not been published.

BASIC MEDICAL CARE

The belief that people should have regular health examinations has been popularized by the medical profession, and a large segment of the public in the United States regards an annual examination as advisable. The traditional assumption has been that routine examinations can detect diseases in their early stages so that treatment can prevent suffering and save lives. High blood pressure and certain cancers are among the diseases that may be influenced significantly if detected early. Annual screening examinations also help physicians to get better acquainted with their patients and provide good opportunities for patient education and reassurance.

On the other hand, most authorities doubt that complete annual physical examinations of symptom-free adults are cost-effective in terms of either money or physician time. The fact that such examinations may be financed by third parties (insurance companies, employers, or government agencies) and that the examining physician may not be the patient's personal physician (which can cause wasteful duplication of services) adds to the problem.

Consumers Union's medical consultants[17] believe that a screening test should satisfy three basic requirements:

1. It should be able to detect a serious or potentially serious disease before symptoms make the individual aware that something is wrong.
2. There should be good reason to expect treatment begun at that early stage to produce a better outcome than treatment begun after symptoms have appeared.
3. The procedure should be utilized for those most likely to benefit from it.

The AMA Council on Scientific Affairs[18] has noted that while scientific organizations may differ somewhat on the recommended content and frequency of periodic examinations, most groups agree that they are valuable, especially when combined with fitness evaluation and counseling on nutrition, exercise, accident prevention, and other aspects of a healthy lifestyle. Evaluations should also be targeted to the individual patient's risk factors.

History and Physical Examination

A thorough health evaluation consists of four phases: (1) a medical history, (2) a physical examination, (3) clinical or laboratory tests, and (4) a report to the patient. It is likely to take 30 to 90 minutes and cost from $90 to $200 for the doctor's time plus additional amounts for diagnostic tests. Internal medicine specialists tend to charge more than family practitioners.

The history should cover more than 100 detailed questions about past medical problems, current symptoms, social and family history, and health habits. It is obtained most efficiently with a questionnaire completed by the patient (or parent) or administered by a member of the physician's staff. Before the physician sees the patient, an assistant also measures height, weight, temperature, pulse rate, respiratory rate, blood pressure, and, sometimes, visual acuity. The physician then reviews the questionnaire and asks further questions.

A "complete" physical examination usually includes the following:

GENERAL APPEARANCE: Nutritional status and physical deformities are noted.
EYES: Appearance, movement, pupillary reflexes, and visual fields are checked. An ophthalmoscope is used to examine the insides of the eyes. A tonometer may be used to measure internal eye pressure.

EARS: An otoscope is used to inspect eardrums and external canals. Hearing is tested with audiometer.
NOSE: The inside is inspected for polyps or deviated septum.
ORAL CAVITY AND PHARYNX: Dental caries, tumors, and other indications of disease are noted.
NECK: Palpation is used to detect enlargement of lymph nodes or thyroid gland. Veins are inspected for distention. A stethoscope may be used to listen for arterial murmurs.
LUNGS: A stethoscope is used to hear breath sounds.
HEART: Pulse rate and rhythm are noted. Heart is palpated for abnormal rhythms. A stethoscope is used to check heart sounds.
BREASTS: Inspection and palpation are done to detect tumors.
OTHER LYMPH NODES: Armpits and groin are palpated.
BACK: Percussion with fist may be used to detect kidney tenderness. The spine is examined for abnormal curvature.
ABDOMEN: Deep palpation is used to detect tumors or enlarged organs such as the liver and spleen. A stethoscope is used to hear bowel sounds and arterial murmurs.
SKIN: Various parts of the body are examined for evidence of infection, inflammation, and cancer.
SEX ORGANS, MALE: Inspection, palpation, and a check for hernias are performed.
SEX ORGANS, FEMALE: External genitalia are inspected. Cervix is visualized with a vaginal speculum. Uterus and ovaries are palpated with two fingers inserted into the vagina and the other hand pressing on the abdomen.
RECTUM AND ANUS: Rectum and prostate are palpated with gloved finger. Anal area is inspected for hemorrhoids. Sigmoidoscopic examination may be performed.
LEGS: Varicose veins and swelling of the legs are noted.
FEET: Pedal pulses are palpated.
BONES AND JOINTS: Swelling or deformities are noted.
NEUROLOGIC EXAM: Knee jerk, ankle jerk, and other reflexes are noted.

Laboratory Tests and Procedures

A urinalysis and complete blood count are commonly ordered as part of a routine physical evaluation. Whether other tests are ordered varies according to the age of the patient, the style of the physician, the patient's history, and the physical findings. The commonly performed tests include:

URINALYSIS: The urine is tested for the presence of sugar, protein, cells, crystals, and other sediment. The presence of sugar might indicate diabetes. White blood cells might indicate infection. Red blood cells might indicate tumor or inflammation within the urinary system. Protein or other sediment may indicate kidney disease.
COMPLETE BLOOD COUNT: Hemoglobin is measured and red blood cells are examined to determine the presence of anemia. White blood cells are counted and examined to help diagnose various infections or leukemia. The platelet count is related to the ability of the blood to clot.
BLOOD SUGAR (GLUCOSE): Abnormal elevations are a sign of diabetes.

BLOOD LIPID PROFILE: Measurement of total cholesterol, high-density lipoproteins (HDL), and triglycerides can help determine the risk of cardiovascular disease.

BLOOD CHEMISTRY SCREENS: Various tests are available to measure kidney function, liver function, certain enzyme activities, and many abnormal metabolic states. Computerized equipment can perform many tests at one time, often at less cost to the patient than a few tests done singly. One common test panel, a chemistry profile, typically has 24 components.

ULTRASENSITIVE TSH: This blood test reflects the function of the thyroid gland. (TSH stands for thyroid-stimulating hormone.)

OCCULT BLOOD: Feces may be examined for blood that is not apparent. Because bleeding can be intermittent, specimens are usually collected for 3 consecutive days. Positive results do not always indicate cancer; they may be caused by bleeding gums, heavy use of aspirin, a nonmalignant polyp, diverticulitis, hemorrhoids, or other conditions.

PAPANICOLAOU (PAP) TEST: This is primarily a screening test for uterine cervical cancer, but it may also indicate the presence of infection and the status of certain hormones.

ELECTROCARDIOGRAM (ECG): This enables abnormal rhythms and certain other heart problems to be diagnosed by analyzing electrical patterns of the heart. Stress tests (ECGs performed during exercise) are discussed in Chapter 15.

Although screening tests provide considerable information at relatively low cost, they are not hazard-free. Minimal departures from "normal" can occur in healthy individuals, and "false positive" reports can result from errors in the testing or reporting procedures. The *Harvard Medical School Health Letter*[19] has observed:

The needless worry generated by an abnormal result, as well as the more expensive and sometimes risky diagnostic tests that are apt to follow, raises legitimate doubt about ordering too many tests on healthy people. Nobody has yet devised a solution to the problem of having too much information.

Many tests are ordered because the doctor is afraid of missing something and being sued. Sometimes tests are ordered because the doctor fears that, without them, the patient will feel that not enough is being done. Financial considerations may play a role; it has been shown that doctors who own testing facilities are more likely to order tests than doctors who do not.

Frequency of Examinations

Individual consumers must decide whether to invest in complete evaluations and how often to do so. Infants and young children should be checked annually. For symptom-free young adults, once every 5 years is reasonable. Complete examinations might be practical every 3 to 5 years after age 40, every 2 to 3 years after age 50, and annually after age 60. However, it is not unreasonable to have annual checkups.

Those who consult their physician several times a year for problems can achieve the equivalent of periodic complete examinations if their physician examines a few extra parts of the body during each visit. This system can be both effective and economical.

At specific ages, certain medical procedures have special significance because they may prevent problems or detect potentially serious problems that are treatable in their early stages. The U.S. Preventive Services Task Force (USPSTF) was created in 1984 to determine what types of periodic physical examinations, laboratory tests, immunizations, counseling, and other measures are science-based and cost-effective. Its 1989 and 1996 reports reflect the views of public health officials and hundreds of other experts. The 1996 report[20] covers interventions for more than 80 potentially preventable diseases and conditions. Its principal findings were:

- Effective interventions that address personal health practices are likely to substantially reduce the incidence and severity of disease and disability. Preventive advice need not be confined to visits devoted entirely to prevention but can be dispensed during almost any visit.

- The clinician and the patient should share decision-making. Rather than having a uniform policy for all patients, doctors should educate their patients and consider individual preferences in deciding which interventions to recommend.

- Clinicians should be more selective in ordering tests and providing preventive services. Although certain tests can be highly effective in reducing mortality and morbidity, many others in common use have neither been proven nor disproven. The latter category includes screening tests for detecting diabetes, anemia, thyroid malfunction, and glaucoma in individuals who have no symptoms and are not considered high risk.

Table 5-3 summarizes the panel's recommendations for people who are not at high risk. The counseling recommendations are related to the leading causes of death and disability in each age group. Consumers who wish additional detail should examine the task force report.

Some physicians treat problems as they arise and spend little time educating their patients about prevention. McCall[12] has noted that if preventive advice and care are not incorporated into a doctor's everyday dealings with patients, they may never take place, because many people only go to a doctor when they are sick.

Cancer Screening Tests

Because breast cancer occurs in one out of nine women, it is important to have periodic screening tests. Demonstration projects indicate that one third of breast cancers occur in women between ages 35 and 49 and that most of these cancers can be detected by mammogram. Mammography uses x-rays to examine the female breast. Recent improvements have resulted in much lower radiation doses and better detection ability. The American Cancer Society recommends that women age 40 or older undergo mammography every year. However, women whose sister or mother developed breast cancer before menopause should begin sooner, particularly if genetic testing results show changes in breast cancer susceptibility genes (BRCA1 and/or BRCA2).

A 1995 meta-analysis of 13 studies concluded that mammography screening of women ages 50 to 74 significantly reduces the death rate from breast cancer and that the most cost-effective interval between examinations is 2 years.[21] Mammography involves brief discomfort when the breasts are compressed between plastic plates to permit maximum examination with minimum exposure to the radiation. This discomfort can be minimized by scheduling the test for the week after a menstrual period, when the breasts are their smallest and least tender.

The American Cancer Society also recommends that women examine their breasts monthly. Literature illustrating the procedure can be obtained from a physician or an office of the Society, but it is best to review the technique under direct supervision of a physician. Monthly frequency is important to ensure familiarity with one's breasts so that changes can be noticed—and also for early detection of tumors. Women who menstruate should examine their breasts 2 or 3 days after a period, when the breasts are least likely to be swollen or tender. Those who no longer menstruate should choose a regular day, such as the first day of the month, for the examination. The USPSTF[20] has concluded that there is insufficient evidence to recommend for or against self-examination for breast cancer.

Testicular cancer, although much less common than breast cancer, is still the most common cancer in males between the ages of 15 and 34. It is easy to detect and has a high cure rate, even though half the cases are not discovered until the cancer has spread beyond the testicles. Testicular self-examination is a 1-minute, monthly self-examination best done after a bath or shower when the scrotum is most relaxed. Each testicle should be rolled gently between the thumb and fingers of both hands to look for hard lumps or enlargement. Because the cure rate is so high, however, the USPSTF[20] has concluded that there is insufficient evidence to recommend for or against routine screening or self-examination for testicular cancer.

The American Cancer Society recommends an annual pelvic examination and Pap test for all women who are sexually active or have reached age 18. If three or more consecutive tests are normal, the frequency may be decreased at the discretion of the physician.

Prostate cancer, the second most common cause of death from cancer among men, claims about 40,000 lives per year. For detecting it in its early stages, a prostate-specific antigen (PSA) test plus a digital rectal examination is more effective than the rectal examination alone.[22] The American Cancer Society recommends that PSA screening be performed annually after age 50 (or age 45 for African-Americans or individuals with a father or brother who had the disease), but this recommendation is controversial.[23] PSA values of 4.0 nanograms per milliliter (ng/mL) or higher are considered abnormal, but elevation is common in cases of prostatitis (inflammation) or benign enlargement.

Most physicians recommend that individuals with high values have further investigation, including a rectal examination, ultrasound testing, possibly a prostate biopsy, and follow-up PSA tests to see whether the level remains stable or rises (a likely sign of cancer). Asymptomatic prostate cancer is very common as men get older (ranging from about 22% at age 50 to about 54% over age 80), and aggressive treatment has a high complication rate. Only a small percentage of these latent cancers progress to a point where they become a problem, however, and it is not known whether early detection and treatment actually saves lives. Research is also needed to determine whether PSA testing is sufficiently valid in detecting curable cancers and whether widespread use of the test will lead to unnecessary treatment of an excessive number of cancers that would have remained clinically insignificant. Long-range studies to resolve these issues are under way but will take more than 10 years to complete. The USPSTF[20] does not recommend routine PSA screening. Woolf[24] recommends that patients be fully informed of the potential benefits and harm that can result from testing and treatment. A free PSA test[25] or a PSA density test (which compares PSA with prostate size)[23] may help determine whether a high PSA level warrants further investigation.

Screening for colon cancer is done with three types of tests: (1) digital rectal examination, in which the doctor inserts a gloved finger into the rectum to see whether anything feels abnormal; (2) fecal occult blood test; and (3) sigmoidoscopy or colonoscopy. The American Cancer Society and the USPSTF recommend testing for hidden (occult) blood in the stool annually after age 50. Specimen-collection materials can be obtained from the office of a physician whose staff will perform the test when the specimens are returned. Although test kits are available for home use (see Chapter 9), the American Cancer Society warns that the test should not be used alone for cancer screening.[26] A sigmoidoscope is a slender, flexible, hollow, lighted tube about the thickness of a finger. It is inserted through the rectum up into the colon. This allows the doctor to look at the inside of the rectum and part of the colon for cancer or for polyps (some of which can become cancerous). The sigmoidoscope may be connected to a video camera and video display monitor so the doctor can look closely at the inside of the colon. Polyps are small growths that can become cancerous. The test may be somewhat uncomfortable but should not be painful. Because the instrument is only 60 centimeters (around 2 feet) long, the doctor can see about half of the colon. A colonoscope is similar but long enough to reach the full length of the colon, and the examination is done with intravenous sedation. After age 50, for those at average risk, the American Cancer Society recommends an annual fecal occult blood test plus flexible sigmoidoscopy every 5 years, or colonoscopy every 10 years. More frequent examinations are recommended for people who have a family history of cancer or have had a polyp or other condition that places them at higher risk.[26]

Immunizations

Immunizations should be part of routine health care obtained through one's personal physician (or, in some instances, through a local health department). Long-lasting protection is available against measles; mumps;

Table 5-3
PERIODIC INTERVENTIONS FOR ROUTINE HEALTH CARE

Birth through 10 Years

Screening	**Parent Counseling**	**Preventive Procedures**
Height and weight	Breastfeeding	Birth: ophthalmic antibiotics
Blood pressure	Baby bottle tooth decay	Immunization against diphtheria,
Hemoglobinopathy screen (birth)	Nutrient intake, especially iron-rich foods (infants and toddlers)	tetanus, pertussis, polio, mumps, measles, rubella, hepatitis B,
Phenylalanine level (birth)	Age 2 or older: limit dietary fat and cholesterol; maintain caloric balance;	*Haemophilus influenzae* type b, varicella-zoster
Thyroid function test (birth)	emphasize grains, fruits, vegetables	Regular visits to dental care
Vision screen (age 3–4)	Regular physical activity	provider
Hearing and tuberculin test for high-risk groups	Adverse effects of tobacco products and passive smoking	Floss, brush with fluoride toothpaste daily
	Injury prevention*	Fluoride supplements for children in nonfluoridated areas (see Chapter 7)

Ages 11 through 24 Years

Screening	**Parent and Patient Counseling**	**Preventive Procedures**
Height and weight	Dietary counseling: Limit fat and cholesterol; maintain caloric balance;	Immunization against diphtheria, tetanus, measles, mumps,
Blood pressure	emphasize grains, fruits, vegetables;	rubella, hepatitis B, varicella-zoster
Papanicolaou (Pap) test (females)	maintain adequate calcium intake (females)	Regular toothbrushing and dental visits
Chlamydia screen (females older than 20)	Selection of exercise program	Fluoride supplements for children under 17 in nonfluoridated areas
Assessment for problem drinking	Avoidance of tobacco products	Multivitamin with folic acid for women who might become pregnant
	Avoidance of alcolol and drug abuse	
	Prevention of unintended pregnancy and sexually transmitted diseases	
	Injury prevention*	

---

*Injury-prevention measures include age-appropriate advice about preventing falls, fires, burns, childhood poisoning, bicycle and motor vehicle injuries, drowning, gunshot injuries, and violent behavior.

German measles (rubella); poliomyelitis; tetanus (lockjaw); whooping cough (pertussis); diphtheria, chickenpox (varicella); hepatitis B; and *Haemophilus influenzae* type b (HIB), a bacterium that can cause meningitis with death or neurologic damage to young children. Immunization against all of these is recommended by the American Academy of Pediatrics, the American Academy of Family Practice, and the Advisory Committee on Immunization Practices of the U.S. Centers for Disease Control and Prevention.

All states now require proof of immunization or other evidence of immunity against some of these diseases for admission to school. However, the requirements vary from state to state, and exemptions may be granted for medical, moral, or religious reasons. Keeping an immunization diary will help to ensure that one's protection is up-to-date.

In recent years, various individuals and groups that promote scientific practices have claimed that pertussis vaccine is prone to cause seizures and other neurologic complications. However, three studies totaling about 230,000 children and 713,000 immunizations have found no causal relationship between pertussis vaccine and any type of permanent neurologic illness.[27] Claims that MMR (measles, mumps, and rubella) is a cause of autism are unsubstantiated.[28]

Immunization is also important for adults. Those unprotected against any of the diseases just discussed (except whooping cough and HIB) should consult their physicians. Tetanus boosters should be administered every 10 years. Flu shots (which give only seasonal protection) and immunization against pneumococcal pneumonia are recommended for high-risk patients, elderly individuals, and certain institutional populations.

Table 5-3

PERIODIC INTERVENTIONS FOR ROUTINE HEALTH CARE - *CONT'D.*

Ages 25 through 64 Years

Screening	Counseling	Preventive Procedures
Blood pressure	Dietary counseling: limit fat and cholesterol; maintain caloric balance; emphasize grains, fruits, vegetables; maintain adequate calcium intake (females)	Tetanus-diphtheria booster every 10 years
Height and weight		Regular toothbrushing, flossing, and dental visits
Total cholesterol (males ages 45–64, females ages 45–64)		Multivitamin with folic acid for women who might become pregnant
Pap test and clinical breast examination (women)	Regular physical activity	Varicella vaccine for those who have not had chickenpox, zoster, or prior immunization
Mammogram every 1–2 yrs (women age 50–69)	Avoidance of tobacco products	
	Avoidance of alcohol and drug abuse	
Fecal occult blood test and/or sigmoidoscopy (age 50 or older)	Prevention of unintended pregnancy and sexually transmitted diseases	
Check for problem drinking	Injury prevention*	

Ages 65 and Older

Screening	Counseling	Preventive Procedures
Symptoms of coronary artery disease	Dietary counseling as above	Tetanus-diphtheria booster every 10 years
Blood pressure	Regular physical activity	Influenza vaccine annually
Height and weight	Avoidance of tobacco products	Pneumococcal vaccine
Fecal occult blood test and/or sigmoidoscopy	Avoidance of alcohol and drug abuse	Varicella vaccine for those who have not had chickenpox, zoster, or prior immunization
Mammogram every 1–2 yrs plus clinical breast exam	Prevention of sexually transmitted diseases	
Pap test	Discussion of estrogen replacement therapy (for females)	Regular toothbrushing, flossing, and dental visits
Vision screening	Injury prevention*	Cardiopulmonary resuscitation (CPR) training for household members
Test for hearing impairment		
Check for problem drinking		

Modified from the report of the U.S. Preventive Services Task Force.[20]
Additional interventions were recommended for people at high risk for various diseases.

Smallpox is now considered eradicated worldwide, so that vaccination is no longer given. Polio may soon be eradicated.[29]

Medical Imaging

X-ray films can yield valuable diagnostic information. Because ionizing radiation is potentially dangerous, however, the possible benefits should be weighed against the risk involved in its use. In most cases the physician is in the best position to do this, but the following points may help patients avoid unnecessary radiation:

- If the physician suggests x-ray films, the patient should understand why they are needed. One should not be afraid to ask questions.
- The patient should ask whether a lead-lined shield is available to protect the reproductive organs.
- When changing physicians, the patient should request that recent x-ray reports be sent to the new physician. It can also help to keep a list of one's x-ray examinations, to avoid duplication and to help enable comparisons between current and previous films.
- Chest x-ray films are no longer considered appropriate for screening individuals without symptoms.
- The developing fetus is especially sensitive to radiation. X-ray films of the abdominal and pelvic regions of pregnant women should be postponed if possible, especially during the first 3 months of pregnancy. Some physicians prefer to avoid pelvic films during the last half of any menstrual cycle lest the woman be pregnant.

Advances in diagnostic scanning have enabled physicians to obtain a great deal of precise, detailed information about internal body structures. The procedures described here do not invade the body and pose no risk or little risk compared to invasive procedures (such as arteriography). They require expensive equipment and can be costly.

Computerized axial tomography uses an x-ray source focused on specific planes of the body and rotated to obtain pictures from multiple angles. The data are fed into a computer and processed to create a cross-sectional depiction of density that resembles a photograph. The procedure is commonly referred to as a CT scan or CAT scan. Used selectively, it is invaluable and has replaced many invasive diagnostic procedures that were dangerous and often less reliable. Figure 5-1 shows a CT scan of the head.

Conventional x-ray procedures and CT scans use a machine to generate and project x-rays through the body to produce a visual image. In *radionuclide imaging*, this set-up is reversed: radioactive chemicals are introduced into the body and taken up by various body structures. These structures then emit gamma rays that produce an image on a special camera outside the body. Radionuclide imaging can detect tumors, infections, circulatory blockage, and other types of problems. The parts of the body commonly scanned are the bones, brain, heart, thyroid gland, gallbladder, liver, kidneys, and lungs. Within hours or days the radioactive substances lose most of their radioactivity or are excreted from the body.

Single photon emission computerized tomography (SPECT) is a specialized form of nuclear scanning that produces images similar to those of a CT scanner.

Positron emission tomography (PET) combines the use of radioactive substances and computers to produce vivid color-coded pictures. PET scans are useful for studying diseases of the heart and brain. However, they are very expensive and are used primarily in research settings.

Magnetic resonance imaging (MRI)—sometimes called *nuclear magnetic resonance (NMR)*—uses radiofrequency waves, a very strong magnetic field, and a computer to produce cross-sectional images. In some cases the picture can differentiate between adjacent soft tissues that might look the same on an x-ray film. To produce the MRI picture, the patient is placed inside a large magnetic coil. When the magnetic field is turned on, it causes hydrogen nuclei (protons) within the body to line up in one direction. Then selected radiofrequency waves flip these particles in another direction. When the waves are turned off, the particles realign, releasing an electromagnetic signal that the computer translates into an image. The technique involves no radiation but it cannot be used with patients who have a pacemaker, metallic artificial joint, or other metallic implant. Another holographic system can take data from a CT or MRI scanner and produce a bright, three-dimensional

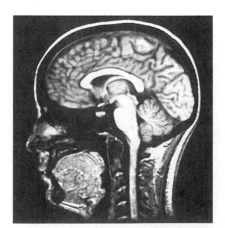

FIGURE 5-1. CT scan shows a cross-section of the head with extraordinary anatomical detail.
(Photo courtesy of GE Medical Systems)

anatomic image.[30] Figure 5-2 shows a patient about to undergo an MRI scan.

Ultrasonography is done with a device that transmits sound waves through body tissues, records the echoes as the sounds encounter structures within the body, and transforms the recordings into a photographic image. No radiation is involved. The variety and usefulness of diagnostic ultrasound procedures has increased rapidly.[31] A few practitioners, mainly chiropractors, claim that spinal ultrasound enables them to follow the progress of their treatment by detecting muscle inflammation or spasm. No published scientific study supports this contention.

Magnetic source imaging (also called *biomagnetic imaging*) uses a device that converts magnetic fields into electrical signals that are amplified and displayed on a computer screen for interpretation. It is used mainly for pinpointing abnormal brain function in epileptics and for diagnosing other disorders of the brain.

SURGICAL CARE

Surgery is defined as any operative or manual procedure for the diagnosis or treatment of a disease, injury, or deformity. Contemporary surgery in the United States is very good, probably the best in the world. Improvements in preoperative preparation, anesthesia, surgical techniques, and postoperative supervision have greatly reduced the discomfort and dangers that were a part of most operations in the past. But surgery should never be taken lightly. Any operation carries some risk, both from the surgical procedure and from the anesthetic. To be justified, surgery must be appropriate and the benefits must significantly exceed the hazards.

Preparation for Surgery

Surgical procedures can be categorized as emergency (as soon as an operating room is available), urgent (should be done within a few days), or elective (can wait from several days to several months). Contemplation of surgery should involve discussion of the patient's health problem, the general nature of the operation, its risks and possible benefits, whether equivalent nonsurgical treatment is available, the type of anesthesia to be used, how much postoperative discomfort to expect, how long it takes before normal activities can be resumed, and any allergies or other relevant health problems. During this discussion it is also advisable to bring up any special fears or concerns related to the surgery. Before surgery takes place, the patient (or a close relative if the patient is unable to do so) will be asked to sign a statement verifying that this

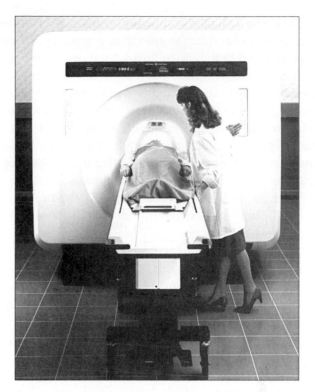

FIGURE 5-2. Patient about to undergo MRI scanning.
(Photo courtesy of GE Medical Systems)

information has been provided. This "informed consent" discussion also provides an opportunity to assess the surgeon's personality.

The best safeguard in selecting a competent surgeon is probably referral by a primary physician familiar with the surgeon's work. If this is not available, or if further investigation is desired, the following questions suggested by Bradley[32] may be useful:

- Are you board-certified in your surgical specialty?
- Are you a Fellow of the American College of Surgeons? This credential, designated by the initials FACS, requires board certification, 2 years of community practice, and a peer-review process in which local surgeons judge the candidate's ethics and personality and make first-hand observations of competence in the operating room.
- How many times have you performed the operation proposed for me?
- How do your results compare with those of other surgeons?
- What complications have you encountered with this operation, how often do they occur, and how do you manage them?
- Is the hospital equipped and staffed to handle a serious complication? Are consultations readily available?

Unnecessary Surgery

Few issues called to the attention of consumers in the United States have aroused the heat that surrounds the question of unnecessary surgery. During the early 1970s it was noticed that the number of operations performed was rising faster than the growth in population. Critics have charged that 10% to 20% of the operations performed annually in the United States are unnecessary. Criticism has been directed primarily against elective (not urgent) surgery, with hysterectomy; tonsillectomy; dilation and curettage (D&C); cesarean section; and back, knee, and prostate operations among the leading suspects. Dr. Sidney Wolfe has called unnecessary operations "the greatest single curse in medicine."

Studies by John E. Wennberg, M.D.,[33] professor of epidemiology at Dartmouth Medical School, have shown that surgical rates are closely related to the density of surgeons and the number of beds in many communities. Dr. Wennberg has also noted that hospital admission rates for nonsurgical conditions can vary just as widely and that questionable local trends tend to decrease when studies are done. He believes that considerable research is needed to determine what practice patterns may be optimal.

One strategy to reduce the volume of unnecessary surgery has been to encourage or require patients covered by insurance programs to consult a second surgeon when elective surgery is recommended. Under these plans the second surgeon is not permitted to do the operation and thus has no possible financial incentive for agreeing that surgery is needed. Eugene McCarthy, M.D., professor of public health at Cornell University Medical Center, has studied the effects of second-opinion programs on the rates of surgery and concluded that many operations were done unnecessarily. Others counter that disagreement by a consultant does not guarantee that an operation is unnecessary. Many other studies have been done to determine the effects of second-opinion programs on the quality of care and on overall health-care costs.[34] Some insurance plans offer second-opinion coverage to their subscribers.

Other strategies to reduce surplus surgery involve the development and publication of criteria that can be used to measure the appropriateness of surgery. The criteria can then be used for preoperative screening (a preventive measure) or for postoperative review, either of which can be performed by hospital committees or outside agencies. As managed-care and precertification programs have increased, the use of second-opinion programs has dropped sharply.[35]

Physician responsibility. Each hospital accredited by the Joint Commission on Accreditation of Healthcare Organizations is required to maintain several active committees of physicians to assess the quality of care at the hospital. A utilization review committee determines the appropriateness of hospital admissions and lengths of hospital stay, a tissue committee reviews operative work, and audit committees look for defective or unnecessary care. A physician whose work is judged to be substandard can have privileges curtailed or terminated. Nonaccredited hospitals may lack such committees.

Patient responsibility. Although the ultimate responsibility for preventing unnecessary surgery lies with medical experts, consumers can take a number of steps to protect themselves.

If you need to consult a surgeon, preference should be given to one who is board-certified and on the staff of an accredited hospital. If surgery is recommended, a reasonable explanation of what it entails and why it is recommended should be sought. Ask whether a medical alternative is available and consider getting a second opinion from another surgeon. Alper[10] suggests that if one's primary physician has been selected with care, the physician's opinion may be as valuable as that of a second surgeon, or even more valuable:

Capable personal physicians who are familiar with the surgeon's work will not let their patients be stampeded into an unnecessary operation. They will ask the surgeon to justify the procedure to themselves as well as to the patient.

Ambulatory Surgery

Hundreds of different operations can be done in an outpatient setting. These include sterilization procedures, laparoscopic cholecystectomy (gallbladder removal), some hernia repairs, D&C, oral surgery, breast biopsy, tonsillectomy, cataract removal, and various forms of plastic and orthopedic surgery. When appropriate, same-day surgery in a hospital outpatient facility, freestanding clinic, or doctor's office can save time and money, prevent family disruptions, and reduce the psychologic stress of having an operation. To be suitable for outpatient surgery, one must be in good general health and have adequate help available for postoperative care at home. Ambulatory surgical facilities are discussed in Chapter 10. Coronary bypass surgery (Chapter 15), cosmetic surgery (Chapter 20), therapeutic abortions (Chapter 21), and refractive surgery (Chapter 22) are discussed elsewhere.

Laser Surgery

Laser surgery is a rapidly developing technology that has great potential. *Laser* is an acronym for "light amplification by stimulated emission of radiation." The laser beam is an intense and narrow beam of light that has one wavelength. Laser beams can be focused to cut, coagulate, or vaporize small areas of tissue with minimal bleeding or disturbance to neighboring tissues. In some cases the "laser scalpel" can slice as thin as the width of a cell without damaging surrounding tissues. Medical laser devices include a source of electricity, mirrors to direct the beam, a crystal or gas that is stimulated to emit the light, and tubing to deliver the energy. Lasers are classified according to their light source. The carbon dioxide laser is effective for cutting tissue. The argon laser is especially useful for sealing off blood vessels and destroying cancerous tumors; it heats tissues and acts somewhat like a welder. The YAG laser can be directed through fiberoptic instruments to reach less accessible places in the body. The excimer laser delivers energy in the form of rapid pulses, which allows greater control over the depth of tissue being cut and does not heat healthy tissue near the target area.

Lasers are commonly used to treat problems of the retina of the eye (bleeding, glaucoma, and retinal tears),[36] blockages in coronary arteries, skin blemishes (moles, freckles, and various birthmarks),[37] gynecologic disorders (genital warts, blocked fallopian tubes, endometriosis), tumors and bleeding in the digestive tract, and many other diseases and conditions. Many laser procedures are conducted on an outpatient basis. Additional information about treatment procedures, risks, and benefits and recommendations for surgeons can be obtained from the American Society for Laser Medicine and Surgery,.

Gallbladder Surgery

Abdominal (open) cholecystectomy typically requires a 5-day hospital stay and about 1 month to recover. Laparoscopic laser cholecystectomy (popularly called "keyhole laser surgery") is faster, less invasive, and often can be done as an outpatient procedure with return to full activities within 1 week. During the procedure the instruments are inserted through four small cuts in the navel and the abdominal wall and manipulated while the operators observe their progress through a video monitor. An AMA Diagnostic and Therapeutic Technology Assessment has concluded that laparoscopic laser cholecystectomy is an appropriate treatment for uncomplicated gallstones.[38] The laparoscopic procedure, first performed in 1987, has become much more common than the open procedure, and the total number of cholecystectomies has risen sharply. Most patients who have gallstones never develop symptoms. For this reason, experts generally recommend against surgical treatment before symptoms appear, except for patients with an unusual x-ray finding that indicates a high risk of developing gallbladder cancer.[39] It is not known how many of the "extra" operations were done on a backlog of symptomatic patients who had viewed the open method as too disabling and how many were done on people with "silent" gallstones. Authorities have also warned against routinely doing the operation on patients with symptoms that "might be related" to gallstones, but the relationship is not clear-cut.

Male Circumcision

Circumcision has been practiced for religious reasons since ancient times and for health reasons for more than a century. It is discussed here because its benefits have not been firmly established. In the United States most newborn males are still circumcised, although in recent years the rate appears to be falling. Circumcision may decrease the incidence of cancer of the penis, a rare condition that occurs almost exclusively in uncircumcised men. Poor hygiene and certain sexually transmitted diseases also correlate with the incidence of cancer of the penis. The exact incidence of postoperative complications of circumcision (local infection and bleeding) is unknown but appears to be from 0.2% to 0.6%. The American Pediatric Association[40] has concluded:

Existing scientific evidence demonstrates potential medical benefits of newborn male circumcision; however, these data are not sufficient to recommend routine neonatal circumcision. In the case of circumcision, in which there are potential benefits and risks, yet the procedure is not essential to the child's current well-being, parents should determine what is in the best interest of the child. . . . It is legitimate for parents to take into account cultural, religious, and ethnic traditions, in addition to the medical factors, when making this decision. Analgesia is safe and effective in reducing the procedural pain associated with circumcision; therefore, if a decision for circumcision is made, procedural analgesia should be provided. If circumcision is performed in the newborn period, it should only be done on infants who are stable and healthy.

QUALITY OF MEDICAL CARE

The medical system in the United States unquestionably provides the best care in the world. Most physicians are well trained and practice in an ethical manner. However, there are valid concerns about the quality, distribution, and cost of health services. The problem areas include incompetence, questionable credentials, negligence, financial abuses, overutilization, impersonal care, and iatrogenic illness.

Incompetence

Incompetence can be the result of drug addiction, alcoholism, mental illness, senility, or failure to keep abreast of new medical developments. The AMA has developed a model "impaired physician" law, which has been adopted in some form by most states. The physician is first asked to seek help voluntarily. Next, hospital staffs are encouraged to find ways to care for their errant colleague. Failing that, county medical societies must step in. If a physician is not attached to a hospital or medical society, the state licensing board must act. State medical societies in every state operate programs to rehabilitate impaired physicians. For example, in Georgia a committee of recovered alcoholic or drug-addicted physicians reaches out to problem physicians to offer a treatment plan.

To keep abreast of medical developments, physicians talk with colleagues, read medical journals, attend meetings, and participate in other types of educational programs. Some authorities believe that continuing education should be formal and mandatory. Many states require a minimum number of hours per year for license renewal.

Promiscuous use of injections may be a sign of incompetence. Some injections should not be given, and others should be used sparingly. For example: antibiotics can usually be given by mouth; male hormones are unlikely to cure impotence; vitamin shots are inappropriate therapy for fatigue; and cortisone injections into joints can cause long-term harm if given too often.

The number of unfit and unethical physicians is unknown. During the past few years, the percentage of physicians using unsubstantiated diagnostic and therapeutic methods has risen significantly in response to misleading promotion of "alternative" and "complementary" methods (see Chapter 8).

Impersonal Care

Patients have a right to receive much more from physicians than mere attention to scientific therapy. Intelligent consumers want compassion and concern. They also want the right to participate in the treatment by knowing what is wrong and how it should be handled.

It appears, however, that some physicians are more concerned with the number of patients they see than the quality of their interaction with patients. Such physicians may consider medical practice to be an episodic, impersonal affair. They spend little time with patients, attending to their immediate complaints in a rapid, mechanical fashion without allowing time for questions or for complaints about other ailments. Rarely do they take the time to form a relationship and inquire about the patient's lifestyle in order to suggest improvements of a preventive nature. Many people contribute to this situation by seeking medical care only when they are ill.

Many physicians do not educate their patients sufficiently about treatment alternatives, drug side effects, and self-care. Many also fail to take cost into account when they prescribe drugs, order tests, or refer patients to specialists. With drugs, this can occur when a generic equivalent is available or when equally effective brand-name drugs differ in price.

Occasional lateness is inevitable, but some physicians are habitually late in keeping scheduled appointments. These doctors may attempt to justify their lateness by stating that urgent cases and emergencies make their schedule unpredictable and that some patients take longer than expected. However, doctors can minimize waiting time by leaving room in their daily schedules for patients who must be seen on short notice or who need extra time. A well-trained receptionist can usually determine how much time is needed by asking the patient about the nature of the problem.

If a doctor falls significantly behind schedule, patients in the waiting room should be apprised of this fact so they can decide whether to wait, leave and return later, or reschedule for another day. Patients can do their part by scheduling extra time if they think their visit will require more than an average amount of time.

Several years ago the Shawnee Mission (Kansas) Medical Center found a novel way to approach this problem. After surveys showed that their patients' main complaint was wasting time in the waiting room, the doctors began lending beepers to those who wished to use nearby shopping facilities and be paged when the office was ready for them.[41]

Malpractice

Every doctor makes mistakes. Those that are serious enough to cause damage may lead to malpractice suits. Diagnostic error is the leading cause of suits. Foreign objects (such as a sponge) left in patients during surgery are another common cause. Malpractice allegations also arise from burns resulting from the application of heat, chemicals, or x-rays. Among the suits that are settled, those for misdiagnosis of fractures and dislocations are the most common.

Contrary to popular belief, the physicians who are sued the most are not necessarily those who are incompetent. Top-notch specialists, who attract a high percentage of complicated cases, inevitably have many patients with unfavorable treatment outcomes. Such patients are more likely to file suit. Nearly all physicians carry malpractice insurance. Most hospitals require their medical staff to carry it, and some states require it for licensure.

Fear of malpractice suits has caused most physicians to practice "defensive medicine." This term refers to ordering tests that are not really necessary for medical purposes but may protect the doctor from later being accused of negligently overlooking something. Following minor accidents, for example, x-ray films often are ordered for "legal reasons."

Financial Abuse

Many insurance companies base their coverage on the physician's "usual and customary fee." Some physicians charge insured patients more than uninsured ones but represent to the insurance companies that the higher fee is the usual one, when in fact it is not.

Another illegal procedure is the "unbundling" of claims, whereby a practitioner bills separately for procedures that normally are covered by a single fee. An example would be a podiatrist who operates on three toes and submits claims for three separate operations. Other forms of fraud include upcoding (charging for a more complex service than was performed), miscoding (using a code number that does not apply to the procedure), charging for a service that was not performed, deliberately ordering unnecessary tests for the purpose of financial gain, and compensation (kickback) for making a referral.[42]

Insurance-industry and government officials estimate that fraud losses from all sources (not just physicians) total as much as $100 billion per year (10% of health-care dollars). However, no basis for these estimates has been publicly revealed and the dollar amount lost cannot actually be quantified.[43]

Questionable Credentials

According to a 1995 article in *Medical Economics* magazine, more than 75 boards not affiliated with the American Board of Medical Specialties (ABMS) or the American Osteopathic Association (AOA) have issued certificates to thousands of physicians.[44] Although a few of these self-designated boards are run legitimately and may eventually achieve ABMS or AOA recognition, most do not require residency training in their specialty. The author stated that "some physicians use fringe board certification to attract patients, who usually don't know the difference. . . . And only a handful of states restrict the advertising of board certifications or specialties."

Iatrogenic Illness

The word *iatrogenic* is derived from the Greek words *iatros* (physician) and *genesis* (production). It is broadly applied to any adverse condition produced in a patient as the result of diagnostic procedures or treatment. Dr. Ralph Greene,[45] clinical professor of pathology at Northwestern University Medical School, noted that the incidence of iatrogenic illness was growing despite and because of the growth of medical knowledge, technologic advances, and the use of new drugs to treat previously incurable illnesses. His book *Medical Overkill* included the following points:

- If people have enough tests, abnormal results that occur by chance may lead to extensive, expensive, and occasionally dangerous follow-up testing.
- Doctors sometimes order tests because they fear legal liability if they do not.
- All effective forms of treatment have the potential for troublesome side effects.
- New treatments may have unforeseeable adverse long-term consequences.
- Nearly half of our hospital beds are occupied by patients who could be treated just as well or better at home.
- Hospital-acquired infections are a serious enough problem that hospitalization should be avoided whenever possible.
- Hospitalized patients should do as much as possible to avoid becoming the victim of a careless error. They should, for example, know the names and purposes of prescribed medications and know their blood type so they can check the labeling of blood being transfused.

Some degree of iatrogenesis is obviously inevitable. The patient's best protection, Greene concludes, is to become well informed, to choose the most competent physician available, and to speak up when doubts arise.

DISCIPLINING OF PHYSICIANS

The agencies involved in the surveillance and disciplining of physicians include medical societies, hospitals, managed-care organizations, state licensing boards, and agencies that administer or oversee government-funded insurance programs.

Medical societies have the ability to reprimand or expel members. Such action may be embarrassing or lower a physician in the eyes of colleagues, but it does not curtail the right to practice medicine.

Hospital officials have the ability to reduce, suspend, or revoke a physician's treatment privileges at their particular hospital. This could be devastating to a surgeon in a one-hospital community. But practitioners who work primarily in private offices or who have privileges at another hospital are affected less. Physicians who belong to neither a medical society nor a hospital staff are unaffected by the disciplinary efforts of these organizations.

◆ **Personal Glimpse** ◆

The Essence of a Doctor?

Reared in poverty, Freddie Brant quit school after the fifth grade. After four years in the Army during World War II he found that jobs were scarce for a man with only a fifth-grade education; so he joined the paratroops. In 1949, along with a fellow paratrooper, Brant was sentenced to seven years in the penitentiary for bank robbery. He began his "medical education" working in the prison hospital. After he was released, Brant continued his education by working for four years as a laboratory and x-ray technician for Dr. Reid L. Brown of Chattanooga, Tennessee. There he picked up not only more medical lore but also the diplomas of his employer.

Posing as Dr. Reid L. Brown, he obtained a license by endorsement and served for three years at a State Hospital in Texas. One day, while stopping at the village of Groveton, Texas, he treated the injured leg of a child. Groveton had long been without a doctor and its people were clamoring for medical care.

"Dr. Brown" soon became established as the town physician and as a community leader. He might still be carrying on his thriving practice in Groveton, Texas, had he not run afoul of a computer. By coincidence he ordered drugs from a pharmaceutical firm used by the real Dr. Reid Brown. Its computer gagged when it discovered orders on the same day from two physicians with identical names. Following an investigation, Freddie Brant was charged with forgery and with false testimony.

Brant's exposure caused great consternation in Groveton, but its citizens rallied around him. He was not convicted. A Chicago newspaper said that justice was thwarted because of a "lava flow of testimonials to the effect that Freddie Brant was a prince of a medical man, license or no license." The paper said that the people of Groveton should have known that Reid Brown was not a doctor because he did too many things wrong. He made house calls for five dollars and charged only three dollars for an office visit. He approved of Medicare and would drive for miles to visit a patient, often without fee if the patient was poor. Besides, his handwriting was legible.

What were the reasons for Freddie Brant's success as an impersonator? The main ones were his readiness to refer any potentially complicated case to doctors in nearby towns, a personality that inspired confidence, and a willingness to take time to listen to his patients.

Robert C. Derbyshire, M.D.[46]

Agencies that administer Medicare and Medicaid have the ability to terminate a practitioner's participation in these programs in cases of fraud or overutilization. A managed-care organization can terminate participation of a provider who fails to meet the organization's standards. Such actions have considerable impact on physicians accustomed to seeing many patients under these programs.

State licensing boards have the authority to revoke or suspend a practitioner's license. This is a powerful action, but several factors hamper the effectiveness of state boards. A state board cannot take action unless it receives a complaint, and patients and professional colleagues often are afraid that making a complaint might involve them in an unpleasant confrontation or even a lawsuit. Equally important, many state boards have insufficient staff and funds to do their job properly.

Until recently, medical licensing laws have been rather weak. During the 1960s most revocations resulted from narcotics offenses and other felonies. Incompetence was not even a ground for action in most states. Today it is grounds for revocation in most states. Revocation by one state does not necessarily stop a physician from practicing in another. In many states disciplinary action in another state is not a reason for revocation. Moreover, because the physician's livelihood is at stake, the courts are inclined to offer considerable protection. The situation noted long ago by Derbyshire[47] is still true today:

The best efforts [of the boards] are often hampered by the capriciousness of the courts, which do not hesitate to substitute their judgment for that of the boards. They often issue stay orders in cases in which the boards have revoked the licenses of physicians. Furthermore, these stay orders permit the defendant to continue his [predatory behavior] during the long delays before his appeal is finally heard.

In response to public and medical society pressure, licensing laws have been tightened in many states during the past several years. Although court interference and underfunding remain problems, actions against physicians by state licensing boards have increased. The Federation of State Medical Boards states that the number of disciplinary actions against medical and osteopathic physicians totaled 1871 in 1984; 2183 in 1985; 2501 in 1986; 2873 in 1987; 2815 in 1988; 2957 in 1989; 3250 in 1990; 3140 in 1991; 3370 in 1992; 3707 in 1993; 4155 in 1994; 4397 in 1995; 4432 in 1996; 4467 in 1997; 4529 in 1998; and 4569 in 1999. The 1999 figure includes 1664 license losses or suspensions, 1153 license restrictions, and 1021 other prejudicial actions. The number of serious actions per thousand physicians averaged 9.35 and ranged from 1.10 in Delaware to 18.60 in Arizona.[48] State boards also take informal actions that significantly affect the behavior of the doctors involved. Some physicians not included in these totals were subjected to federal actions that excluded them from Medicare participation or revoked or restricted their narcotic license.

The Public Citizen Health Research Group (HRG)[49] has published the names of 20,125 medical and osteopathic physicians who were subjected to a total of 38,589 formal disciplinary actions by state medical boards or federal agencies from 1990 through December 1999. Some actions were not related to the quality of patient care, but most were for serious practice-related matters such as overprescribing, incompetence, negligence, and alcohol or drug abuse. HRG believes that many state boards still are underfunded, understaffed, slow-moving, and overly lenient.[50]

The Office of the Inspector General administers two agencies that collect adverse information about physicians and other health-care providers.[51] The information is not available to the general public but can be accessed by government agencies, credentialing organizations, and certain other parties.

The National Practitioner Data Bank (NPDB), which began operating in 1990, was mandated by the Health Care Quality Improvement Act of 1986. Its purpose is to hinder the movement of "problem practitioners" from one facility or state to another. Licensing boards are required to report all actions that revoke, suspend, or restrict a license for reasons related to the practitioner's professional competence or conduct. Professional societies must report all professional review actions that adversely affect the membership of a physician or dentist. Hospital administrators must report disciplinary actions that negatively affect a doctor's clinical privileges for more than 30 days and must query the Data Bank when appointing or reappointing medical and dental staff. Malpractice insurance carriers are required to report all settlements against physicians, dentists, and other licensed health-care providers. The information is available to state licensing boards; hospitals and other health-care entities; professional societies; certain federal agencies; and plaintiffs (or their attorneys) in a malpractice suit.

The Healthcare Integrity and Protection Data Bank (HIPDB), which became operational in 1999, was mandated by the Health Insurance Portability and Accountability Act of 1996. Its purpose is to combat fraud and abuse in health insurance and health-care delivery. It collects information about licensure and certification actions, criminal convictions, exclusions from federal and state health-care programs, civil judgments (other than malpractice actions) related to health care, and other adjudicated actions or decisions. The information can be accessed by health plans and federal and state agencies.

Ethical Dilemmas

Explosive progress in medical technology and increased emphasis on individual rights have raised troublesome new ethical questions and intensified old ones. Some examples follow.

What is the value of life? Who is to decide when it shall start and when it shall stop? Should life be terminated when pain is great or if the cost of prolonging it places a heavy financial burden on the family or on society? To what extent should individuals determine whether their existence should be continued? Chapter 23 explores these questions.

Suppose physicians have provided all possible medical assistance to a patient. Should the patient be kept alive by means of special equipment when it is obvious that recovery is impossible? For how long? Suppose the expense vastly exceeds what the patient or patient's family can afford. What happens then? If a hospital has equipment to keep alive only ten comatose patients, what happens when the 11th and 12th arrive? Who should be permitted to live? The 10 who got there first? The youngest? The healthiest? The richest? Who should make these decisions, and how should they be made?

Should individuals have the right to sell their own body parts? Should a pregnancy be terminated because it is an inconvenience to the woman? Or because some government decides to limit population size? Should test-tube fertilization and surrogate motherhood be permitted? How should the use of scarce resources be allocated? Should surgical procedures costing tens or hundreds of thousands of dollars be financed by tax or insurance dollars?

Should individuals who appear to be mentally ill but have not harmed anyone be hospitalized against their will? Can physicians determine who is dangerous and who is not? Should psychotic individuals be forced to take tranquilizers to improve their mental state if they do not want to? Is psychosurgery ever justified? Does our society have adequate safeguards so that nonconforming individuals and political dissidents cannot be classified as mentally ill to interfere with their freedom?

How confidential are medical records? Should the results of health examinations be centralized and computerized? Who should have access to such information? Insurance companies? Employers? Should patients have a right to inspect their own records, even when physicians believe that this would be detrimental to their welfare? Should a family member be informed of a serious problem if the patient objects? How should extremely sensitive data be handled, such as the results of AIDS tests or genetic tests that indicate a tendency toward cancer?

Medical progress depends on experimentation. Who should be selected for experiments? Should people be allowed to volunteer as control subjects even if it means they may be deprived of an effective treatment? (This does not apply to new cancer treatments, which are tested by comparing them to older ones rather than to placebos.) Should institutionalized mental patients or prison inmates be allowed to volunteer? Can such people actually exercise free choice? To what extent should animal experimentation be used? Do experiments in which genes are manipulated pose special risks to society?

Which should take precedence, producing and operating expensive equipment (such as kidney dialysis machines) for the benefit of a small number of persons, or upgrading basic medical care for a large number of underprivileged citizens?

Many of these issues have been addressed by guidelines issued by the American Medical Association[14] and other professional organizations. Some (such as entitlement to one's own medical records) have been answered by state or federal laws and guidelines. Some hospitals have an ethicist or ethics committee that gives advice in specific cases.

THE INTELLIGENT PATIENT

Good medical care should be a partnership between patient and physician. The intelligent patient learns to consult a physician at appropriate times (see Chapter 9), makes careful observations when symptoms occur, communicates efficiently and openly, strives to understand the nature of any ailment and its treatment, and takes appropriate action if a grievance arises. McCall[12] advises that "by making a habit of learning about every disorder you develop, every drug that's prescribed, and every intervention that's proposed, you get, in effect, a low-cost second opinion."

Effective Communication

When consulting a doctor, try to present a detailed and well-organized account of present symptoms and relevant past history. Before contacting the doctor, it may help to draw up a list to guide your presentation. If there is more than one problem, start with the most important one. If you have a particular concern, bring it up at the beginning of your visit. If medications are being taken, either write down their names and dosages or bring the original bottles to the appointment. Since patients typically forget much of what they are told in a doctor's office, taking notes or utilizing a tape recorder (with the doctor's permission) might be helpful.[52]

Physicians know much more about medicine than laypeople do but are not always good communicators. They may be authoritarian or even patronizing. Patients should not accept this behavior. Consumers have the right to be partners in their care and to receive a clear explanation of the physician's findings and proposed treatment. There is no good reason why a physician cannot provide this. A friendly comment that you want to be able to follow the physician's advice properly usually establishes the desired relationship.

Emanuel and Emanuel[53] have described four types of doctor-patient relationships. In the *paternalistic* model, the doctor decides what is best and the patient assumes this is correct. In the *informative* or *consumer* model, the doctor provides the facts, and the patient's values then determine what is done. In the *interpretive* model, the doctor helps to clarify the patient's values and helps the patient select the medical interventions consistent with those values. In the *deliberative* model, the doctor promotes health-related values in addition to guiding the choice of interventions. The Emanuels believe that the consumer model "reduces the physician's role to that of a technician" and that the deliberative model represents "the essence of doctoring" by physicians who really care about their patients.

It is important that feelings of fear, embarrassment, or even resentment not be permitted to create a barrier between patient and physician. Put these feelings to good use by sharing them with the physician. Someone who fears an examination or is shy about body parts should say so. Discomfort during an examination is something else the physician wants to know about. If the physician makes a sound or comment that causes concern, ask what it means. Don't let fear or embarrassment stop you from mentioning a symptom or a problem that is bothering you. McCall[12] suggests that if you wish to discuss something that you do not want to appear in your medical record, ask the doctor not to write it down.

If in doubt about a diagnosis or treatment plan, discuss these doubts. If a particular treatment is objectionable, the physician may be able to suggest an acceptable alternative. If necessary, a consultation with another physician should be requested. Similarly, if the physician suggests consultative action, the patient should appreciate this concern and be receptive to the proposal.

Some consumer advocates recommend questioning doctors closely about the need for diagnostic tests and about alternatives to whatever treatment is proposed. However, challenging everything is likely to antagonize the doctor and could result in dismissal as a patient. The best approach is to select a doctor who makes sensible and cost-effective recommendations without prodding. Questions can then be used to enhance your understanding rather than trying to out-think the doctor.

Be sure to have a clear understanding of fees involved. This matter is usually handled by the receptionist.

Access to Medical Records

Some authorities believe that unlimited access to medical records helps patients to become better informed and more involved in their care. Others believe that access should be limited where the records may contain information that could be misinterpreted or otherwise harmful. Many physicians use a large number of abbreviations, including some of their own, which could make many records incomprehensible to their patients (or even to other physicians). Some physicians concerned about confidentiality do not record information about alcoholism, drug abuse, or AIDS in the patient's chart but keep it in a separate file to which only the physician has access.

Most states have laws granting patients access to their records held by doctors and hospitals. A few more mandate access to hospital records only. The AMA[14]

states: (a) notes made in treating a patient are primarily for the physician's own use and constitute his or her personal property, and (b) when asked by the patient, a physician should provide a copy or a summary of the record to the patient or to another physician, an attorney, or other person designated by the patient. Most physicians readily furnish copies on request, except in cases where they believe that a summary would be more meaningful.

Johnson and Wolfe[55] maintain: (a) any withholding of actual medical records is paternalistic, (b) checking one's records may improve one's understanding and may also reveal errors that could prove detrimental to insurance coverage, and (c) employers who self-insure may maintain a database with inappropriate access to employee medical records. The Medical Information Bureau provides more than 600 insurance companies with access to information about people who have applied for life or health insurance. A copy of your record can be obtained for a nominal fee through the bureau's Web site at http://www.mib.com.

In December 2000 the Clinton Administration proposed rules to limit the extent to which health plans, health-care clearinghouses, and certain health providers can share medical information.[56] The rules, scheduled to take effect in 2 to 3 years, would, for example, make it illegal for health insurance companies to share medical information with entities such as mortgage companies that could use the information to deny a loan and employers who might want to check medical records before hiring an employee. Violations could trigger civil and criminal penalties that range from $100 per incident to 10 years in prison and up to $250,000 in fines for obtaining protected information under false pretenses. The 1996 Health Insurance Portability and Accountability Act required that privacy rules be issued. This law does not cover Internet sites that seek personal medical information.

Telephone Tips

Proper telephone use can do a great deal to make the physician's life easier while helping the patient to receive better service. Before calling the office, take a moment to organize your thoughts. What is the problem? When did it begin? If there is a pain, does it come and go or is it steady? Does anything bring it on or relieve it? If there is an infection or any other reason to suspect a fever, the temperature should be taken. Try to decide whether the problem is urgent. Before calling, write down a one-sentence description of your problem, your reason for calling, a symptom list, and no more than three questions that you may have.[57]

 Consumer Tip

Consultations

Diagnostic proficiency is directly related to the range and depth of the doctor's experience with any particular illness. If you're informed you have a problem and that it is rare or unusual, one that appears serious or that involves a considerable amount of treatment or medication, you might want to ask your doctor the following questions:

- What is your experience with this problem?
- Would a consultation be warranted with a doctor who has had more experience with this problem?

David R. Stutz, M.D.[54]
Bernard Feder, Ph.D.
The Savvy Patient

Most physicians receive many more phone calls a day than could possibly be handled alone. So when you call, don't start by asking to speak with the physician. The receptionist or nurse is trained to assemble the information needed for a preliminary evaluation of the situation. This person usually knows which matters to handle alone and which ones the physician must handle personally. After talking to the receptionist or nurse, if you still believe it is necessary to speak with the physician, that is the time to ask.

When you telephone, have a pad and pencil handy to write down any instructions. Human memory is notoriously faulty. Call as early in the workday as possible.

That way the physician can handle the problem most efficiently, because the physician's assistants are on duty to help and hospitals and laboratories are able to give their best services.

When calling for a prescription refill, know the phone number of the drugstore. The request should be made during the physician's office hours and before you are down to the last pill. That way the physician can review the office record to see whether the medication is still needed, whether the dosage should be changed, and so on. Such a review makes medical care safer. If you telephone outside of office hours, many physicians (especially those covering another's practice) order only

---

◆ Personal Glimpse ◆

Future Scenario

The integrated system of the future will assume responsibility for the health status of communities. When healthy individuals first enter the system, a comprehensive health status profile will be placed in the computer database. Extensive provider networks will provide easy access to care when it is needed. A new generation of information systems will monitor clinical progress and track outcomes, as the patient moves along the continuum. Whether the patient sees a primary care physician or sees a specialist, his or her electronic medical record will be accessible to all caregivers. The information system will connect remote practice sites, laboratories, imaging centers, home health agencies, surgery centers, insurers, and hospitals in comprehensive community health information networks. Bureaucracies will be leveled. Costly duplicate systems between medical groups and hospitals will be eliminated. Paper, postage, and phones will give way to the electronic superhighway.

Let's eavesdrop on a scene that is happening right now in the upper Northwest.

A physician in Washington is preparing for his next patient visit. With a click of his mouse, he calls up the patient's electronic medical record. He checks his e-mail for lab results and imaging reports. He sees that these have been received and with a click of his mouse, he sends them to the patient's electronic medical record and to the patient's personal health Web site and record. He notes that there was a referral to a consultant. He checks his e-mail for the consultant's progress notes and finds them. He is now ready to see the patient. In the exam room, after hearing the patient's complaint, he pulls his palm top from his pocket and enters a few keystrokes. He calls up some specific information dealing with the patient's condition first. Then he moves to the

prescription writer and checks both for potential adverse drug interactions and for formulary coverage under the patient's health plan. Then he taps in an order. "Mrs. Jones," he says, "I just prescribed a medication that will help you. Which pharmacy is the most convenient?" He punches send and the prescription goes via the Internet to the pharmacy she names. A record of the prescription goes automatically into the patient's electronic medial record. The doctor wants the patient to see another specialist. He e-mails a referral request to a staff member, who completes and submits an online form. The managed care authorization takes 3 minutes to receive. The confirmation goes to the practice and the specialist over the Internet in a matter of seconds. In minutes, the primary care office receives its authorization number, and the consultant gets all the information needed to bill for the consult. Just before the patient leaves, the physician says, "Be sure to check my Web site for more information on your treatments when you get home. Also, you can view the potential side effects of the drugs you will be taking and the results from your recent lab tests on your personal Web site."

After the patient leaves, the physician dictates a note that is entered by voice recognition software directly in the electronic chart. He then logs onto the hospital's Intranet to check his patients. For one patient in intensive care, he calls up the direct feed from the bedside monitors. He adjusts the medication for the patient, sending an order to the nurse. Even as the physician is tending to his business online, his back office staff are ordering supplies, submitting claims, checking eligibility and performing other tasks all in a paperless environment. This is how medicine will be practiced in the 21st century.

John D. Cochrane, M.H.A.[58]
E-Healthcare Connections

enough medication for a few days. That is the safest way in the absence of medical records, but it does increase the cost of medication.

Some physicians have begun to offer e-mail access. The "Personal Glimpse" box on page 96 indicates how electronic communication is likely to reshape the nature of medical practice.

Handling a Grievance

If you choose a physician carefully and communicate effectively, it is unlikely that a serious grievance will develop. However, should you believe that a physician has overcharged for services or treated you in an incompetent, unethical, or unprofessional manner, there are measures that can be taken.

The grievance should first be discussed directly with the physician or a staff member. It may turn out to be based on a simple misunderstanding. Or it may be possible to negotiate a satisfactory resolution. If not, the next step could be a complaint to the local medical society. Some people hesitate to do this, thinking that "doctors will always stick up for each other." Although physicians do have sympathy for each other, this feeling is balanced by an antipathy toward seriously unethical conduct, which reflects on the medical profession as a whole. Moreover, if other complaints against the same individual have been received, the society may already be suspicious of that physician.

If the physician is on the staff of a hospital, a complaint can also be made to the hospital administrator. Health maintenance organizations also have procedures for investigating complaints. Contacting the Better

Business Bureau is unlikely to be effective because that organization ordinarily refers medical complainants to the local medical society.

If these measures fail to resolve the concern, the next step should be a complaint to the state licensing board. Although the board will give priority to matters of incompetence, fraud, and illegal behavior, it may also take action in less serious situations.

If one believes a significant injury has resulted from negligence or carelessness, an attorney may be consulted to determine whether a malpractice suit is appropriate.

SUMMARY

Intelligent consumers should locate and use a primary physician (or medical group) who provides care that is scientific, considerate, and compassionate. They should take an active role in dealing with health professionals. They should endeavor to understand the nature of any health problem they experience and the mechanisms and potential hazards of treatment. They should not hesitate to ask questions about fees or request consultations for complicated problems. Good medical care should be a partnership between patient and physician. It should include preventive approaches and periodic examinations, as well as effective two-way communication.

REFERENCES

1. Lipman, M. Speak up to your doctor. Consumer Reports on Health 3:46, 1991.
2. Barzansky B, Jonas HS, Etzel SI. Educational programs in U.S. medical schools, 1999–2000. JAMA 284:1114–1120, 2000.
3. Starr P. The Social Transformation of American Medicine. New York, 1982, Basic Books Inc, Publishers.
4. Lasagna L. The Doctor's Dilemma. New York, 1962, Harper & Brothers.
5. Gevitz N. The D.O.'s: Osteopathic Medicine in America. Baltimore, 1982, The Johns Hopkins University Press.
6. Osteopathic medicine. American Osteopathic Association fact sheet, June 1, 2000.
7. Gevitz N. Sectarian medicine. JAMA 257:1636–1640, 1987.
8. Barrett S. Dubious aspects of osteopathy. Quackwatch Web site, Jan 29, 2000.
9. Eldridge J, Buono D. 150 Careers in the Health Care Field. New Providence, R.I., 1993, U.S. Directory Service.
10. Alper PR. Avoiding the "marginal" medic. In Barrett S, Jarvis W, editors. The Health Robbers: A Close Look at Quackery in America. Amherst N.Y., 1993, Prometheus Books.
11. Why do I need a doctor? I'm not sick! Executive Health's Good Health Report 32(4):5, 1996.
12. McCall TB. Examining Your Doctor: A Patient's Guide to Avoiding Harmful Medical Care. New York, 1995, Birch Lane Press.
13. Barrett S. Physician credentials: How can I check them?. Quackwatch Web site, Aug 6, 2000.

It's Your Decision

You are moving to a new community and want to find a competent physician, dentist, or other health professional. What would you do?

How would you know whether you have found the right person?

When you visit a physician for a physical examination, what should you expect it to include? What kinds of laboratory tests should be performed? Why? Should such an examination occur yearly?

What should the cost be? What questions should you ask the physician about the findings of the examination?

A doctor has advised you to have surgery (hernia repair, gallbladder removal, hysterectomy, or tonsillectomy) within the next few weeks. What action should you take to decide about the surgery?

14. AMA Council on Ethical and Judicial Affairs. Code of Medical Ethics, 2000 Edition. Chicago, 2000, American Medical Association.

15. Centers for Disease Control and Prevention. Health Information for International Travel, 1999–2000. Washington, D.C., 1999, US Government Printing Office.

16. Doyle DJ. Surfing the Internet for patient information: The personal clinical Web page. JAMA 274:1586, 1995.

17. Those costly annual physicals. Consumer Reports 45:601–606, 1980.

18. AMA Council on Scientific Affairs. Medical evaluations of healthy persons. JAMA 249:1626–1633, 1983.

19. Bennett W. A primer on routine lab tests. Harvard Medical School Health Letter 10(12):4–6, 1985.

20. U.S. Preventive Services Task Force. Guide to Clinical Preventive Services, 2nd edition. Baltimore, 1996, Williams & Wilkins.

21. Kerlikowske K and others. Efficacy of screening mammography: A meta-analysis. JAMA 273:149–154, 1995.

22. Catalona WJ and others. Measurement of prostate-specific antigen in serum as a screening test for prostate cancer. New England Journal of Medicine 324:1156–1161, 1991.

23. Prostate cancer: Detection and symptoms. American Cancer Society Web site, accessed Nov 27, 2000.

24. Woolf SH. Screening for prostate cancer with prostate-specific antigen. New England Journal of Medicine 333:1401–1405, 1995.

25. Catalona WJ and others. Evaluation of percentage of free serum prostate-specific antigen to improve specificity of prostate cancer screening. JAMA 274:1214–1220, 1995.

26. Colorectal cancer: Early screening. American Cancer Society Web site, accessed Nov 28, 2000.

27. Cherry JD. 'Pertussis vaccine encephalomyelopathy': It is time to recognize it as the myth that it is. JAMA 263:1679–1680, 1990.

28. Taylor B and others. Autism and measles, mumps, and rubella vaccine: No epidemiological evidence for a causal association. Lancet 353:2026–2029, 1999.

29. Foege WH. Polio eradication—How near? JAMA 275:1682–1683, 1996.

30. Skolnick AA. New holographic process provides noninvasive 3-D anatomic views. JAMA 271:5–7, 1994.

31. AMA Council on Scientific Affairs. Medical diagnostic ultrasound instrumentation and clinical interpretation. Report of the Ultrasonography Task Force. JAMA 265:1155–1159, 1991.

32. Bradley EL III. A Patient's Guide to Surgery. Yonkers, N.Y., 1994, Consumer Reports Books.

33. Wennberg JE. Variations in medical practice and hospital costs. Connecticut Medicine 49:444–453, 1985.

34. Crane M. Second opinions: Where are the savings? Medical Economics 64:(3):174–194, 1987.

35. Crane M. Are third parties denying patients the surgery they need? Medical Economics 68(7):79–82, 1991.

36. Patlak M. Light for sight: Lasers beginning to solve vision problems. FDA Consumer 24(6):15–18, 1990.

37. Lewis R. Erasing skin marks with lasers. FDA Consumer 26(2):23–26, 1992.

38. AMA Diagnostic and Therapeutic Technology Assessment: Laparoscopic cholecystectomy. JAMA 265:1585–1586, 1991.

39. NIH Consensus Development Panel on Gallstones and Laparoscopic Cholecystectomy. JAMA 269:1018–1024, 1993.

40. Task Force on Circumcision. Circumcision policy statement. Pediatrics 103:686–693, 1999.

41. Beeper-tagged patients roam till summoned. Medical World News, Feb 14, 1983.

42. Barrett S. Insurance fraud and abuse. Quackwatch Web site, Aug 16, 2000.

43. Testimony of William J. Mahon, Executive Director, National Health Care Anti-Fraud Association, before the U.S. Senate Special Committee on Aging, March 21, 1995.

44. Terry T. Visit Vegas! Get your boards while you're there. Medical Economics 72(3):26–36, 1995.

45. Greene R. Medical Overkill. Philadelphia, 1983, George F. Stickley Co.

46. Condensed from Derbyshire RC. The make-believe doctors. In Barrett S, Jarvis W, editors. The Health Robbers: A Close Look at Quackery in America. Amherst N.Y., 1993, Prometheus Books.

47. Derbyshire RC. Medical Licensure and Discipline in the United States. Baltimore, 1969, The Johns Hopkins University Press.

48. Summary of 1999 board actions. Federation of State Medical Boards, April 4, 2000.

49. Wolfe S and others. 20,125 Questionable Doctors. Washington, D.C., 2000, Public Citizen Health Research Group.

50. Wolfe S. 13,012 questionable doctors. Public Citizen Health Research Group Health Letter 12(4):1–3, 1996.

51. Fact sheet for the general public. Chantilly, Va., 2000, National Practitioner Data Bank, National Integrity and Protection Data Bank.

52. How Is Your Doctor Treating You? Consumer Reports 60:81–88, 1995.

53. Emanuel EJ, Emanuel LL. Four models of the physician-patient relationship. JAMA 267:2221–2226, 1992.

54. Stutz DR, Feder B. The Savvy Patient: How to Be an Active Participant in Your Medical Care. New York, 1991, Consumer Reports Books.

55. Johnson D, Wolfe SM. Medical Records: Getting Yours: A Consumer's Guide to Getting and Understanding Medical Records, ed 5. Washington, D.C., 1995, Public Citizen Publications.

56. Secretary, US Department of Health and Human Services. Standards for privacy of individually identifiable health information. Federal Register 65:82461–82829, 2000.

57. Kemper DW and others. Healthwise Handbook: A Self-Care Manual for You. Boise, Idaho, 1995, Healthwise, Inc.

58. Cochrane JD. Vision. Brochure. Second Annual Symposium on E-Healthcare Strategies for Physicians, Hospitals & Integrated Delivery Systems. La Quinta, Calif., 2000, E-Healthcare Strategies.

Chapter Six

MENTAL HEALTH CARE

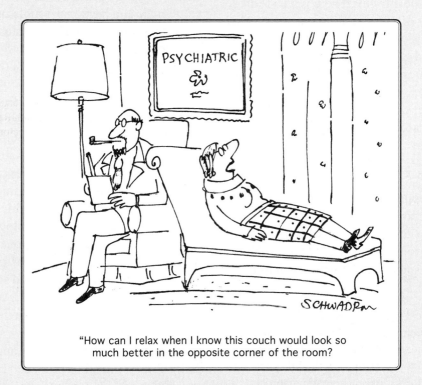

"How can I relax when I know this couch would look so much better in the opposite corner of the room?

More than one in every four Americans suffer from an emotional or behavioral problem so severe it interferes with their ability to keep up with their daily routines, do their jobs, care for their families, or relate to others as they once did. No one, regardless of age, gender, education, or income, is immune.

DIANNE HALES
ROBERT E. HALES, M.D.[1]

Theories about how people become emotionally ill are exceeded in number only by the available remedies for making them well again.
LEWIS R. WOLBERG M.D.[2]

Although excellent help is available for mental and emotional problems, selecting suitable treatment can be difficult. There is a wide array of practitioners, many of whom are incompetent. This chapter outlines the various types of practitioners, their treatment methods, and guidelines for distinguishing between proper and improper treatment. It also describes questionable self-help methods marketed to the public. Organizations that can provide additional information are listed in the Appendix.

WHO SHOULD SEEK HELP?

Professional help is appropriate when a mental, emotional, or behavioral problem significantly interferes with someone's ability to function, or when symptoms exceed an individual's tolerance. The common problems for which help is advisable can be grouped into eight categories:

DEPRESSION: persistent feelings of sadness or hopelessness; low self-esteem; frequent insomnia; loss of interest in activities; loss of appetite; weight loss; suicidal feelings

ANXIETY: intense anxiety that interferes with ability to function; phobias; panic attacks; psychosomatic disorders

RIGIDITY: obsessive thoughts or actions; self-defeating behavior

IMPULSIVITY: intense flightiness; alcohol abuse; periodic violent behavior

IMPAIRED SOCIABILITY: excessive shyness; socially inappropriate behavior; strong feelings of discomfort in social situations; abnormal dependency; generalized distrust of people

COPING DIFFICULTY: marital conflicts; parenting difficulties; school adjustment; prolonged grief reactions; excessive job stress

UNREALITY: depersonalization (e.g., feelings that one's body is changing in size); delusions (rigidly held false beliefs); hallucinations (e.g., hearing voices)

REPEATED FAILURE: an overall "batting average" in life that remains well below a person's ability

MENTAL HEALTH PRACTITIONERS

Many types of practitioners profess to treat mental, emotional, and personal problems. The training, professional standards, and legal status of the different types vary considerably.

Psychiatrists are physicians (M.D.s or D.O.s) who have completed at least 3 years of specialized training in psychiatry after graduation from medical or osteopathic school. *Child psychiatrists* have a minimum of 4 years of psychiatric training, including 2 years in adult psychiatry and 2 in child psychiatry. *Geriatric psychiatrists* are psychiatrists who have acquired additional certification by passing an examination in geriatric psychiatry. Certification is available from the American Board of Psychiatry and Neurology.

Psychologists have undergone training in the study of human behavior. Students of psychology study the mental, emotional, biologic, and social basis for human behavior, as well as theories that account for individual differences and abnormal behavior. They are also instructed in research methodology, statistics, psychologic testing, and a variety of skills applicable to their specialty if they intend to practice. The major recognized specialties are counseling, clinical psychology, school psychology, and industrial-organizational psychology.

Psychologists commonly work in private individual or group practices, community mental health centers, mental hospitals, general hospitals, schools, rehabilitation centers, and residential facilities for emotionally disturbed children. Payment for treatment by a psychologist is deductible as a medical expense for federal income tax purposes and is covered by many insurance plans.

In most states, licensing or certification for independent practice as a psychologist requires: (a) a doctoral degree (Ph.D. or Psy.D.) from an accredited training program, (b) additional years of supervised clinical experience, and (c) passage of an examination. The *National Register for Health Services Providers in Psychology*, published by the Council for the National Register, lists licensed psychologists whose doctoral degrees and supervised experience meets the Register's standards. A few states allow persons with master's level training to work as associates or assistants under the supervision of licensed or certified professionals. In 1995 the American Psychological Association's Council of Representatives resolved to promote educational programs and legislation to enable psychologists to prescribe psychotropic medications. Psychiatric organizations oppose this on grounds that a full medical education is necessary to understand the intricacies of prescribing powerful drugs.

Psychoanalysts are practitioners who have undergone personal psychoanalysis and completed several additional years of part-time training in the theories and specialized techniques of psychoanalysis. Most are psychiatrists, but some are trained in psychology, social work, or another nonmedical discipline.

Social workers practice in private offices as well as under the auspices of public, voluntary, and proprietary agencies and institutions. They are licensed or otherwise regulated in all states. The National Association of Social Workers (NASW) states that clinical social workers provide more than half of the counseling and therapy services in the United States. Certification in clinical social work or another specialty is available from the Academy of Certified Social Workers (ACSW). This requires (a) a master's or doctoral degree from a school of social work accredited by the Council on Social Work Education, (b) 2 years or 3000 hours of postgraduate experience under supervision of a master's level social worker, and (c) passage of a written examination. The *NASW Register of Clinical Social Workers* lists clinical social workers who meet the requirements for Qualified Clinical Social Worker (QCSW) or Diplomate in Clinical Social Work (DCSW). Both of these require 2 years of supervised clinical work plus either licensure, certification based on an examination, or ACSW membership. The DCSW credential requires an additional 3 years of professional experience plus completion of a clinical assessment examination. NASW also offers two other credentials: (1) School Social Work Specialist, which requires 2 years of postgraduate supervised school social work experience, plus an examination; and (2) Academy of Baccalaureate Social Workers (ACBSW), which is similar to ACSW but does not require a master's degree.

Certified *clinical mental health counselors* work in agencies, schools, colleges, and independent practice.

They must have a master's degree in counseling or a related discipline plus 2 years of experience after receiving the master's degree. They must also pass a written examination and adhere to a code of ethics. Currently 41 states plus the District of Columbia license or certify counselors. Those working in states that do not regulate counselors typically seek certification by the National Board for Counselors. The major professional organization is the American Mental Health Counselors Association.

Specialists in psychiatric nursing are registered nurses (R.N.s) who usually hold a master's degree from a program that lasts $1^1/_2$ to 2 years, but the term "psychiatric nurse" may also be applied to any nurse who has worked in a psychiatric setting. The American Nurses Association certifies psychiatric nurses on two levels. Certification as a psychiatric and mental health nurse requires a bachelor's degree in nursing, 2 years (with a minimum of 1600 hours) of experience in a mental health setting, current clinical practice, and passage of an examination. Certification as a clinical specialist requires a master's degree in psychiatric nursing (or equivalent training), 500 hours of supervised clinical experience, and passage of an examination. The *Directory of Specialists in Psychiatric Mental Health Nursing* provides names of clinical specialists in psychiatric nursing. Some psychiatric nurses conduct their own groups or serve as co-therapists in mental hospitals and clinics. Master's-level psychiatric nurses may function as psychotherapists in community mental health centers. Some have set up private practices, providing both individual and family therapy.

Marriage and family therapists are licensed or certified in 42 states. Clinical membership in the American Association for Marriage and Family Therapy (AAMFT) requires appropriate master's- or doctoral-level training plus 2 years of clinical graduate experience with couples and families under the supervision of an AAMFT-approved supervisor. Training programs in the United States and Canada are accredited by AAMFT's Commission on Accreditation for Marriage and Family Therapy Education.

Sexual therapists specialize in the treatment of sexual problems that can be helped by simple techniques and increased communication between sexual partners. They may or may not be able to deal with underlying emotional problems that require additional psychotherapy. Certification is available from the American Association of Sex Educators, Counselors and Therapists (AASECT), an interdisciplinary interest group. Certification as a sex therapist requires: (a) a master's or doctoral degree, (b) licensure or certification in an appropriate professional discipline, (c) 90 hours of specialized education, (d) 90 hours of sex-therapist training, (e) 500 hours of supervised therapy, (f) 100 to 200 hours of individual or group supervision, and (g) 12 hours of structured group experience focused on attitudes about sexuality. Certification as a sex counselor has similar requirements but can be obtained with a bachelor's degree. AASECT publishes a register of those it has certified.

Because sexual therapy is neither defined nor regulated by law, anyone can adopt the title of "sex therapist" or "sexual counselor." For this reason it is important to check the reputation of a prospective therapist. Those practicing at university-affiliated clinics can be presumed competent. Information about other therapists may be obtained from your family physician, the local medical society, or a local family service agency.

Substance abuse counselors offer evaluation, counseling, case management, and various other services to individuals who abuse alcohol or other drugs. Some counselors have entered the field without a college education. However, associate, bachelor's, or master's degree programs are required for many jobs. To become a National Certified Addiction Counselor (NCAC), candidates must hold current state certification or licensure as an alcoholism and/or drug abuse counselor, have 6000 hours or 3 years of full-time of supervised experience, and pass a written examination administered by the National Association of Alcoholism and Drug Abuse Counselors.

There are many other types of mental health practitioners whose activities are not defined by law or regulated by licensure. Included in this category are caseworkers, social-work aides, clergymen, art therapists, music therapists, dance therapists, school counselors, crisis-intervention personnel, and a wide variety of self-proclaimed therapists. Some have sound training, but others do not.

There are several reasons why finding a suitable therapist for a mental or emotional problem may be more difficult than finding one for a physical problem or for general medical care:

1. There is a wide range of types of practitioners.
2. Some types of practitioners lack standardization of training and credentials.
3. Many different approaches may be used by practitioners within each professional group.
4. The person seeking help may have no idea which type of treatment approach is most appropriate.
5. Compatibility between patient and therapist is more important in psychologic treatment than it is in the treatment of physical problems.

6. A sizable number of practitioners use questionable practices, some of which may be difficult to recognize.

PSYCHOTHERAPY

Psychotherapy can be defined as any type of persuasive or conversational approach designed to help patients. Although there are hundreds of techniques and schools of thought, most have in common a wish to understand the patient and help the patient change emotional or behavioral patterns.

Psychodynamic treatments are based on the premise that childhood experiences exert an unconscious influence that actively shapes people's current feelings and behavior. In *analytically oriented psychotherapy,* also called *exploratory therapy,* patients say what comes to mind (free association) and are helped to understand their feelings, mental mechanisms, and relationships with people. Insights are used to help patients develop healthier ways of dealing with feelings and life situations. This type of therapy typically involves one or two 50-minute sessions per week for a few months (short-term therapy) or years (long-term therapy). It is especially appropriate for people who communicate well and are motivated to change. *Psychoanalysis* is a more intensive form of psychodynamic therapy in which free association is done while lying on a couch. It usually requires three to five sessions per week for several years. Few people can afford its high cost. *Interpersonal therapy* focuses on current relationships in order to help people deal with unrecognized needs and feelings and improve their interpersonal and communication skills. Used mainly for depression, it typically involves 12 to 16 sessions.

Supportive therapy is a conversational approach intended to maintain or restore an individual's highest level of functioning. Therapists give advice and reassurance, make suggestions, and discuss alternative behaviors and problem-solving techniques. Depending on the nature of the problem, treatment ranges from a single session, or a few sessions over a period of weeks or months, to long-term care over many years.

Cognitive therapy, which typically involves 15 to 25 weekly sessions, is aimed at relieving symptoms rather than resolving underlying conflicts. It is used for the treatment of depression, anxiety disorders (mainly panic and phobias), anger management, personality disorders, and marital therapy. Therapeutic efforts center on decreasing faulty perceptions and negative attitudes. This is done by identifying how the patient reacts to life situations and helping the patient test the validity of these reactions. For example, someone who assumes that bad things never happen to good people might feel intensely unworthy in the face of an adverse event. The therapist attempts to modify this tendency by persuading the patient that adverse events occur for many reasons, most of which have nothing to do with the worth of the person.

Behavioral therapy (also called behavior modification) aims to replace maladaptive patterns with healthier ways of behaving. The therapist first analyzes the behaviors that cause stress, limit satisfaction, and affect important areas of the patient's life. Treatment techniques can include: (a) systematic desensitization (mastery of fears through gradual exposure to circumstances that provoke anxiety), (b) relaxation training, (c) exposure (gradual exposure to a feared object or situation without use of a relaxation technique), (d) flooding (maintaining exposure to feared situations until the anxiety dissipates), (e) reinforcement (rewarding behavior that is more mature), (f) modeling (copying a behavior demonstrated by the therapist), (g) social skills training, (h) paradoxical intention (temporary encouragement of behavior the patient wishes to stop), and (i) aversive therapy (associating an unpleasant stimulus with undesirable behavior). Behavioral therapy usually involves fewer than 25 sessions.

Biofeedback is a relaxation technique that can help people learn to control various autonomic functions. The patient is connected to a machine that continuously signals the heart rate, degree of muscle contraction, or other indicator. The patient is instructed to relax so that the signals decrease to a desirable level. The patient may ultimately learn to control the body function subconsciously without the machine.

Biofeedback was popularized before it had scientific support, and it is still abused by fringe practitioners. Nevertheless, it has gained a measure of respectability.[3] It has been used to help patients control pain, anxiety, phobias, hypertension, sleep disorders, and some stomach and intestinal problems. Specialized techniques have been used to treat abnormal heart rhythms, epilepsy, Tourette syndrome (multiple tics), fecal incontinence, and Parkinson's disease. Most people who go through biofeedback training use it to acquire relaxation skills that could also be learned without electronics. Most qualified practitioners are psychologists, but some have backgrounds in other health disciplines. Untrained individuals with or without a professional degree can easily obtain a biofeedback device and set up shop. Some promoters allege that "repatterning" a person's brain waves can foster effortless learning, health, creativity, and prosperity; others claim to achieve similar effects by causing the left and right halves of the brain to function more synchronously. No scientific evidence supports such claims.

In *group therapy* several people, usually eight to ten, meet with a therapist for discussion. Groups may be homogeneous (composed of people with similar problems or backgrounds) or heterogeneous. The discussion may focus on specific topics or may deal with whatever comes up. Group discussions often help people feel less alone in their feelings and provide a "laboratory" for analysis of an individual's behavior in a group situation. Reticent individuals may find group sessions, in which they can sit and listen, preferable to individual sessions, which may be relatively silent.

In *marriage counseling*, husband and wife meet individually or together with a therapist to help them identify current marital conflicts. Acting as a referee, the therapist helps the couple communicate more effectively to negotiate solutions to their dispute. In *family therapy* the therapist meets with the family as a group to help resolve current family conflicts. *Sexual therapy* is most appropriate for couples who basically get along well but have a problem with sex. Couples with a sexual problem whose general relationship is poor will probably be better off with marital counseling or individual psychotherapy.[4]

Hypnosis is a temporary condition of intense concentration during which suggestibility is greatly enhanced. This state may be used to increase the patient's control over a symptom or behavior. Hypnosis is not a treatment in itself but may accelerate the treatment process in properly selected cases. It has also been used for anesthesia during childbirth and dental procedures and for relief of headaches and other painful conditions. Because not everyone is amenable to hypnosis, the therapist should have adequate training in both the procedure and the selection of patients.

Expressive or creative activities, such as art, music, drama, poetry, or dance, are included in comprehensive treatment programs at hospitals and partial-hospital facilities.

DRUG THERAPY

Drugs are commonly prescribed for the treatment of anxiety states, depression, psychosomatic disorders, and psychoses. These drugs can affect both mental and physical functioning. Some take effect at once, some take several days to work, and some continue to work long after their use is discontinued.

Antianxiety agents (sometimes referred to as minor tranquilizers) are used to treat anxiety states, psychosomatic disorders, and alcohol addiction (during the

Historical Perspective

"Animal Magnetism"

The concept of a dreamlike or hypnotic state during which cures of symptoms are attempted has existed since ancient times. During the eighteenth century it was popularized by Austrian-born Franz Anton Mesmer (1733–1815), who acquired three doctoral degrees, including one in medicine. Mesmer derived his concept of "animal magnetism" from astrology and believed that a magnetic force from the planets influenced physical ailments. He assumed that this force was composed of invisible waves in gas form. He developed a doctrine of mental healing that contrasted with methods of physical healing. Although the theory of animal magnetism was unfounded, Mesmer's strong personality and suggestive approach helped some patients who had hysterical or psychosomatic symptoms.

After being accused of practicing magic, Mesmer was forced to leave Austria in 1778. He resumed practice in Paris but was labeled by his medical colleagues as an imposter and charlatan. In 1784 the French government appointed a commission of physicians and scientists (including Benjamin Franklin) to investigate. Mesmer's popularity waned after the commission attributed his cures not to "animal magnetism" but to an as yet unknown physiologic cause. Today hypnosis plays a modest role in the treatment of emotional problems, and the word "mesmerize" means to hypnotize, spellbind, fascinate, or enthrall.

detoxification process). Americans have been accused (with some justification) of being a "drugged society" because of their high use of alcohol and medications such as *Valium* (an antianxiety agent) and *Prozac* (an antidepressant). Although most people who receive antipsychotic medications probably need them, it is clear that physicians often prescribe antianxiety agents or antidepressants when it would be more appropriate to help patients identify and correct what is troubling them. Physicians are not entirely to blame for this, however; patients often press for instant and total relief.

Antipsychotic agents (sometimes referred to as major tranquilizers) are used mainly to treat psychotic reactions (thought disorders manifested by hallucinations, delusions, or loss of contact with reality). Since the early 1950s these drugs have revolutionized the field of psychiatry. Many patients who otherwise would have required lengthy (even lifelong) hospital stays are now able to improve or recover quickly. In addition, large

numbers of previously institutionalized patients have been able to return to their communities. This has been a mixed blessing, however, because it has increased the number of homeless individuals in communities that lack adequate programs for helping the chronically mentally ill.

Antidepressants are available to counteract severe depressions (those manifested by loss of appetite, weight loss, severe insomnia, feelings of hopelessness, or psychomotor retardation or agitation). These drugs usually require from a few days to several weeks to take effect. They are not appropriate for countering the minor upsets that are part of ordinary living. Some antidepressants and antipsychotic drugs can be prescribed as a single bedtime dose. This method reduces the cost of the medication, may aid sleep, and reduces the likelihood of annoying side effects.

Antimanic agents, most notably lithium products, are used for bipolar illness (sometimes called manic-depressive psychosis).

Anti-obsessive-compulsive agents are used to treat patients with uncontrolled repetitive thoughts or actions.

Antianxiety agents and several other types of drugs are commonly prescribed for insomnia. Although occasional use of a "sleeping pill" may be appropriate, habitual use is not. People with frequent insomnia should seek professional help to correct the cause or to develop better sleep habits.

All psychoactive drugs have the potential for adverse reactions, some serious and some not. In each case the value to the patient must be weighed against the nuisance or danger involved. The most common side effects are drowsiness, agitation, dry mouth, tremor, and muscle stiffness. Some of these disappear with reduced dosage, continued use, or medication to counter them. Others are a reason to switch to another drug.

One complication of particular concern is tardive dyskinesia, an involuntary movement disorder characterized by twitching and tongue-thrusting, which can occur with a prolonged high dosage of antipsychotic medications. Although uncommon, it is often irreversible. Because the dangers of psychosis far outweigh the risk of tardive dyskinesia, there is no reason to withhold antipsychotic medication from individuals who are psychotic. However, it is poor medical practice to prescribe these drugs for nonpsychotic anxiety.

The danger of addiction to psychiatric drugs has been grossly exaggerated by the media, particularly in the motion picture *I'm Running as Fast as I Can*. The central character in this film is an anxiety-ridden woman who takes huge amounts of *Valium*, suddenly stops taking the drug, and becomes severely ill with convulsions.

Although addiction develops occasionally with normally prescribed dosages of *Valium* and similar antianxiety drugs, the ordinary precaution of tapering off a dosage, rather than stopping suddenly, will prevent a withdrawal reaction from occurring.

Methylphenidate (Ritalin), a drug used to treat attention deficit disorder (ADD) or attention deficit hyperactivity disorder (ADHD) in children, has also been in the news. In 1996 *Newsweek* reported that 1.3 million children between the ages of 5 and 14 were taking it.[5] Although *Ritalin* can be very effective against these conditions, many children receiving it are suffering from other problems for which it is not appropriate.

ELECTROCONVULSIVE THERAPY

Electroconvulsive therapy (ECT), also referred to as EST (electroshock therapy) and shock treatment, involves producing a convulsion by giving a brief stimulus to the brain. To receive the treatment, the patient lies down and is rendered unconscious either by an electrical stimulus or by a short-acting barbiturate given intravenously. To protect against injury, a curare-like drug is also given so that the patient's muscles do not contract during the convulsion. Electrodes are applied to one or both temples and a small amount of current is transmitted to induce the convulsion. After the treatment the patient usually remains unconscious for about 15 to 30 minutes. A series of treatments may cause memory difficulty that clears up in a few weeks except for memories of some events during the months close to the period of treatment. However, the ability to remember other things or to retain new information is rarely impaired.[6,7]

ECT can be dramatically successful in certain types of severe depression and is sometimes helpful in severe psychotic reactions. However, it is seldom appropriate unless medication alone fails to produce results. Because most patients respond favorably to medication or psychotherapy, psychiatrists who give ECT to a large proportion of their patients should be viewed with suspicion.

PSYCHOSOMATIC DISORDERS

From time to time everyone experiences symptoms that are physical reactions to tension. Common examples are headaches, diarrhea, constipation, nausea, dizziness, muscle cramps, dry mouth, cold hands, indigestion, excessive sweating, and palpitations of the heart. Whether treatment is needed depends on the severity and frequency of the symptoms. They may require no treatment, self-medication with an over-the-counter product, medical care, or psychiatric treatment.

These psychosomatic (psychophysiologic) reactions are mediated through the autonomic nervous system and are related to the action of adrenaline and related hormones on various parts of the body. Diarrhea before an examination, for example, is caused by increased intestinal motility. Tension headaches are caused by muscular tension in the back of the neck. Indigestion may be caused by excessive production of acid in the stomach.

The symptoms of acute anxiety attacks—sweating, rapid heartbeat, palpitation, and a feeling of dread—are caused by release of adrenaline. Anxiety can also trigger hyperventilation syndrome, in which a feeling of shortness of breath is accompanied by lightheadedness and numbness of the hands and feet. On the more serious side, asthma, high blood pressure, backache, and ulcerative colitis can have significant emotional components.

Psychophysiologic reactions may be treated with: (a) drugs that prevent the hormones from affecting the target organs, (b) antianxiety drugs or behavioral therapy to reduce tension, (c) psychotherapy to attack the underlying causes of the tension, or (d) a combination of these. A large percentage of the ailments for which people seek medical attention are significantly related to tension.

Excessive intake of caffeine is a common cause of symptoms that resemble those of chronic anxiety. Many people don't realize that in addition to being present in coffee, caffeine is also found in tea, some soft drinks, and certain pain-relievers and cold remedies. Caffeine's effect can last up to 18 hours in sensitive individuals. In people who become physically dependent on it, withdrawal during the night can cause headaches and grogginess in the morning.

SELECTING A THERAPIST

Four basic questions should be considered during the process of seeking mental health treatment: (1) What type of help is wanted? (2) Which practitioners can provide such help? (3) Are they available in the community? and (4) How much can the patient afford to pay?

If medication is desired, one should see a physician. Most nonpsychiatric physicians can competently prescribe antianxiety agents and antidepressants for patients who are not severely disturbed. For antipsychotic drugs, a high dosage of antidepressants, or any type of long-range treatment, it is best to consult a psychiatrist. Information about the training and credentials of psy-

◆ **Personal Glimpse** ◆

An Attack from Within

An acute anxiety attack is of sudden onset and may even begin without any apparent precipitating event. The patient is suddenly extremely apprehensive. He is aware of palpitations. Perspiration becomes profuse and breathing is difficult. . . . The patient often fears that a medical calamity is taking place within his body. Particularly during the first such attack, the patient is apt to feel that he will faint, or die, or lose control of himself or of his mind. In the severe anxiety attack, the patient literally reaches a panic state where he feels overwhelmed and completely helpless. He is aware of a tremendously strong impulse to run away from wherever he is. He knows not from what he runs, nor even clearly where safety lies. Even following the attack, the patient remains chronically fearful lest he suffer another such unpleasant attack. This, of course, creates . . . additional anxiety which only tends to aid in the precipitation of further attacks.

O. Spurgeon English, M.D.
Stuart M. Finch, M.D.[8]

chiatrists can be obtained from the biographic directory of the American Psychiatric Association, the local medical society, or the psychiatrist directly. Certification by the American Board of Psychiatry and Neurology is a good indication that a psychiatrist is qualified to administer medication, but this certification is not as useful a guideline in selecting a psychotherapist. Some analytically oriented psychiatrists are not motivated to become certified because they believe the board is primarily oriented toward biologic psychiatry.

If a conversational form of treatment is preferred, names may be obtained from a personal physician, cleric, school counselor, friend, local medical or psychiatric society, local psychologic association, or the local Yellow Pages. Psychoanalytic institutes located in some major cities and the departments of psychiatry at medical schools and hospitals can provide names of psychiatrists and psychologists who specialize in psychotherapy. Psychiatrists who have trained at university hospitals are more likely to be primarily interested in psychotherapy than those who have trained at state hospitals. "Do you do psychotherapy primarily?" is a good screening question when seeking conversational treatment from a psychiatrist. Most national professional organizations publish a biographic membership directory, and most certifying organizations publish a directory of the professionals they have certified. Some of

these publications are available at public, hospital, and medical-school libraries. Credentials can also be checked by contacting the national professional organizations listed in the Appendix.

The current cost of psychotherapy with a private practitioner is usually $60 to $150 for a 50-minute session. Psychiatrists tend to charge more than nonpsychiatrists. In many communities, people who cannot afford private care can receive treatment at a mental health clinic where fees are based on the ability to pay. Most psychotherapy at community clinics is done by psychologists and social workers. A limited amount of counseling is available without charge to students through the student health service at most colleges and universities. Insurance coverage for psychotherapy is usually not generous. It typically covers 50% to 80% of the insurance company's allowable cost per session, with a low dollar limit on total cost per year.

Psychiatrist Ronald Pies[9] recommends consultation with a physician whenever mental problems are associated with any of the following symptoms: blackouts; memory lapses (such as trouble recalling recent events); persistent headaches; significant unintentional weight loss; numbness; tingling or other strange sensations; generalized weakness; dizzy spells; significant pain of any sort; difficulty walking; shortness of breath; seizures of any type; inability to control urination; unduly rapid or forceful heartbeats; frequent, heavy sweating; tremor; or slurred speech.

A survey by *Consumer Reports* magazine drew 4100 responses from readers who had sought professional help for emotional problems between 1991 and 1994. Their reasons for seeking therapy included depression, anxiety, panic, phobias, marital or sexual problems, problems with children, job problems, grief, stress-related ailments, and alcohol or drug problems. (Few reported that they had a chronic, disabling condition such as schizophrenia or manic-depressive psychosis.) Almost all felt they had been helped, with those who initially felt the worst reporting the most progress. Significantly more improvement was reported with long-term therapy than with short-term therapy. Overall, the respondents felt that psychiatrists, psychologists, and social workers were equally effective, and that marriage counselors were less so. Those who relied on their family doctors were more likely to receive medication and be less satisfied than those who sought specialized care.[10] This result mirrors research findings that most people who seek treatment benefit from it and, for most problems, the most important factor in psychotherapy is the patient-therapist match rather than the type of treatment sought.[11,12]

How much therapy is "enough" depends largely on the patient's personality and the nature of the problem. Obvious symptoms tend to diminish fairly quickly, but personality change usually takes longer. How can progress of therapy be measured? One sign is lessening of symptoms such as anxiety or depression. Another is mastery or better management of stressful situations that previously had caused difficulty. However, symptom-relief can be temporary, and other types of improvement may not be obvious until many months have elapsed. Hales and Hales[1] state that although there are no consistent indications that therapy is on course, there are "red flags" that suggest when it is not. These include a sense that the therapist doesn't understand the problem, difficulty communicating or confiding, dreading each session, feeling "stuck," and feeling that the therapist is behaving unethically. Negative feelings do not necessarily mean that the treatment is not working. People who feel they are not making progress should discuss their concern with the therapist. Ethical violations (some of which are discussed later in this chapter) are a reason to switch therapists.

HOSPITAL CARE

Psychiatric hospital care is needed in four basic situations: (1) the patient is considered dangerous to self (either suicidal or not eating enough to sustain life), (2) the patient is considered dangerous to others, (3) the patient is so malfunctional that community care is not possible, or (4) specialized treatment available only on an inpatient basis is needed.

Many communities have day-care or "partial-hospitalization" programs where patients spend 6 to 8 hours per day in a therapeutic atmosphere. Some hospitals have night-care programs. In some communities, halfway houses ease the transition from hospital to community living.

Patients who are judged sufficiently dangerous to themselves or others can be committed involuntarily to either inpatient or outpatient treatment. Contrary to popular opinion, court decisions and state laws tend to define "dangerousness" rather narrowly. As a result, commitment against a person's will can be difficult to initiate or sustain.

A type of advanced directive may be used to provide seriously mentally ill people who are in remission with a way to consent to treatment if they become too sick or upset to do so. These documents describe when and how treatment should be implemented if the patient becomes incompetent to make a rational voluntary decision.

QUESTIONABLE "SELF-HELP" PRODUCTS

Many tapes, books, and devices have been marketed with claims that they inspire people to function better mentally, improve relationships with others, relieve anxiety or depression, or achieve other desirable emotion-related goals. Gerald Rosen, Ph.D.,[13] former chairman of the American Psychological Association's Task Force on Self-Help Therapies, has noted the following:

- Although some of these materials may be helpful, most have not been tested for validity.
- Many self-help materials are promoted with extravagant and ethically questionable claims.
- The fact that a technique is useful as part of a therapy program does not mean it will work as a self-help measure. Self-help books are more likely to be helpful during periods of therapy than at other times.
- Few self-help books offer protection against failing to comply with instructions. Should failure occur, readers may inappropriately blame themselves, become skeptical that they can be helped, and fail to seek professional help.

Subliminal Tapes

Thousands of videotapes and audiotapes purported to contain repeated messages are being marketed with claims that they can help people lose weight, stop smoking, enhance athletic performance, quit drinking, think creatively, raise IQ, make friends, reduce pain, improve vision, restore hearing, cure acne, conquer fears, read faster, speak effectively, handle criticism, relieve depression, enlarge breasts, and do many other things. At least one company has offered subliminal tapes for children, including a toilet-training tape for toddlers. Many tapes contain music said to promote relaxation. Most are claimed to contain messages that are inaudible or barely audible, but some are barely or fully audible. Videotapes may feature images, said to be relaxing, combined with repeated visual messages shown so briefly that they cannot be seen at normal playing speed.

Many researchers have found that subliminal tapes provide no benefit to the user. One who tested tapes from several companies concluded that they contained no embedded messages that could conceivably influence behavior.[14] A research team tested volunteers for a study of tapes said to improve memory and self-esteem, but switched the tapes for half of the participants (to create a control group). Regardless of the tape used, about half of the volunteers claimed to achieve the results they were told to expect—but objective tests of memory and self-esteem showed no change.[15] A National Research Council committee has concluded that although many people claim that subliminal self-help tapes contribute to self-improvement, there is no scientific evidence to support such claims.[16] Thus there is no reason to believe that musical tapes with subliminal messages can do anything more for physical or mental well-being than listening to ordinary music. Moore[17] states that there is no scientific evidence that inaudible messages are unconsciously or subconsciously perceived or can influence behavior.

Biofeedback Gadgets

Battery-operated skin-temperature monitors ($20 to $80) and devices that measure muscle or brain wave activity ($200 to $400) have been marketed through the mail for home use. The *Harvard Health Letter* has warned that such devices have not been systematically evaluated and are likely to "have a short working life before they wind up in a closet or attic, gathering dust."[3] Tests on home biofeedback devices claimed to help people manipulate their alpha waves have shown that the devices actually responded to the user's eye movements or to interference from household electrical currents.

Self-Help Instructional Programs

Many entrepreneurs are using cable television infomercials to promise that their instructional materials can increase self-confidence, improve people's performance, and bring success in various ways. A recent article in *Forbes* magazine noted that "inspirational" programs may serve a useful purpose if they enable someone to act more decisively.[18] However, the programs have not been validated by scientific studies and probably will not help most people who buy them.

"Brain Wave Synchronizers"

Several companies have marketed gadgets that deliver flashing lights and sounds through modified eyeglasses and headphones. The devices are hazardous because flashing lights can trigger epileptic seizures in susceptible individuals, including some with no history of seizures. In 1992 the FDA was informed that a device of this type (the *Relaxman Synchroenergizer*) had caused a 21-year-old woman to have her first seizure. The device had been marketed with unsubstantiated claims that it could improve digestion and sexual function and control pain, habits, and addictions. In 1993 the FDA initiated a seizure of the manufacturer's entire supply, which a judge subsequently ordered destroyed.[19] The FDA also stopped the marketing of *InnerQuest Brain Wave Synchronizer,* which had been claimed to provide diet control, stress relief, pain relief, and increased mental capacity.[20] In 1995 the FTC and four state attorneys general settled complaints against Zygon International, Inc., which had claimed that users of *The Learning Machine* would learn foreign languages overnight, quadruple their reading speed, expand their psychic powers, build self-esteem, and replace bad habits with good ones.[21] The device cost about $300. Beyerstein[22] has debunked claims that various devices help people by synchronizing the two sides of the brain or increasing the frequency of alpha waves (a type of brain wave).

Bach Remedies

Ellon USA, Inc., of Lynbrook, New York, markets an "emergency rescue formula" for "calming and stabilizing emotions" and a line of 38 "flower remedies" said to alleviate negative emotions. These homeopathically prepared (highly dilute) products were developed about 60 years ago by Edward Bach, a British bacteriologist and homeopath, who—according to the company's literature—"believed that the only way to cure illness was to address the underlying emotional causes of disease." The flower remedies can be selected using Ellon's 116-item "self-help questionnaire." Someone who feels overwhelmed with work, for example, is advised to take the product called *Elm,* whereas someone who has strong opinions and is easily incensed by injustices is advised to use *Vervain.* Another company describes its *Rescue Remedy* as "the one product you need to take care of all kinds of emergency emotional stress." Its catalog has depicted the product as useful for (a) a woman under stress because her computer "froze" (b) a mother coping with a cranky toddler, (c) the partner of a doubles tennis player who missed a few shots, (d) participants in a minor auto accident, and (e) a man racing to board a plane who suddenly realizes he forgot to pack his suit and left his keys and ticket at home.

Dietary Supplements, Herbs, and Hormones

Many products marketed as "dietary supplements" are claimed to improve mental functioning. Kava and valerian are said to relieve anxiety; St. John's wort and s-adenosyl-methionine (SAMe) are marketed for the relief of depression; ginkgo biloba is claimed to improve memory; secretin is claimed to be effective against autism; and many vitamin concoctions are recommended for treating Down syndrome, hyperactivity, autism, and other childhood conditions. For those that show promise, there has not been enough research to determine whether they are safe and whether they are as effective as prescription drugs. In other cases, there is no substantiation whatsoever. In addition, most herbal products sold in the United States are not standardized, which means that determining the exact amounts of their ingredients can be difficult or impossible. This subject is covered further in Chapter 12.

QUESTIONABLE PRACTICES

Many types of practitioners who profess to treat mental, emotional, and personal problems are engaged in questionable practices. Because terms such as therapist, psychotherapist, and counselor are not defined by law, anyone may use these titles. The fields of sensitivity training, sexual counseling, marriage counseling, hypnosis, and encounter groups contain many self-proclaimed therapists who have little or no training. Other types of unqualified practitioners ply their trade under titles such as astrolotherapist, autohypnotist, palmist, past-life therapist, reader-adviser, transformational counselor, metaphysician, graphologist (handwriting analyst), and character analyst. Some have certificates from diploma mills or correspondence courses.

Some practitioners with reputable training and credentials use methods that are unscientific or unethical. Some have personal problems that interfere with proper care of their patients, and some deliberately exploit their patients. The trouble with improper mental health treatment is not merely lack of efficacy. A disillusioning experience can cause the patient to stop seeking help or can trigger a personal disaster such as suicide.

Sensitivity Training/Encounter Groups

Sensitivity training began in the 1950s with training groups (T-groups) whose purpose was to help community leaders ease social tensions in their communities. This was accomplished by an intense small-group experience that encouraged self-disclosure and expression of strong feelings while focusing on the attitudes and interactions of group members. The process was not intended for the treatment of emotionally disturbed individuals.

Over the years similar groups have proliferated under such names as marathon groups, growth centers, encounter groups, and human-relations laboratories. Their stated purpose is to help people experience personal growth by learning to express feelings more openly. They may have supportive or aggressive confrontations. Some groups emphasize physical comfort or contact such as touching. Meetings of this type can be very upsetting to people who are not self-confident enough to handle the confrontation and emotional expression that can take place. Depression, psychosis, personality disorganization, severe anxiety reactions, and physical injuries have resulted from improperly conducted meetings.

Consumers should generally be wary of groups whose participants are encouraged to express strong feelings to virtual strangers.

Meditation

Meditation is generally defined as a class of techniques intended to influence an individual's consciousness or tension level through the regulation of attention. It may involve lying quietly or sitting in a particular position, attending to one's breathing (as in yogic practice), adopting a passive attitude, attempting to be at ease, or repeating a word aloud or to oneself (transcendental meditation). A National Research Council committee has concluded that people who meditate regularly may have a more restful lifestyle and that relaxation techniques might be appropriate for stress-reduction or as a component of other treatments. (Breathing exercises, for example, may be useful in behavioral approaches to treating panic attacks.) However, the committee found no scientific evidence that stress is reduced more effectively by meditation than by simple quiet resting or that meditation alone provides lasting benefits, such as reducing high blood pressure or other unhealthy responses to stress.[15]

Megavitamin Therapy

During the early 1950s a few psychiatrists began adding massive doses of nutrients to the treatment of severe mental problems. The original substance used was vitamin B_3 (nicotinic acid or nicotinamide), and the therapy was termed "megavitamin therapy." Since that time the treatment regimen has been expanded to include other vitamins, minerals, hormones, and diets, any of which may be combined with conventional drug therapy or ECT.

Today the treatment is called "orthomolecular psychiatry," a term meaning "the treatment of mental disease by providing an optimum molecular environment for the mind, especially substances normally present in the human body." Proponents claim that abnormal behavior is caused by molecular imbalances that are correctable by administration of the "right" nutrient molecules at the right time. (*Ortho* is Greek for "right.") They also claim that their treatment is effective against many diseases. During the 1980s, for example, the Princeton Brain Bio Center (not affiliated with Princeton University), in Skillman, New Jersey, touted its "nutritional" treatment for alcoholism, allergies, arthritis, autism, epilepsy, hypertension, hypoglycemia, migraine headaches, depression, learning disabilities, retardation, mental and metabolic disorders, skin problems, and hyperactivity.[23] Its services included laboratory tests that most physicians would not consider necessary or useful for diagnosing these disorders.

A special American Psychiatric Association task force investigated the claims of the megavitamin and orthomolecular therapists. Its 1973 report noted that these psychiatrists used unconventional methods not only in treatment but in diagnosis. The report's conclusion, perhaps the most strongly worded statement ever published by a scientific review body, stated:

This review and critique has carefully examined the literature produced by megavitamin proponents and by those who have attempted to replicate their basic and clinical work. It concludes in this regard that the credibility of the megavitamin proponents is low. Their credibility is further diminished by a consistent refusal over the past decade to perform controlled experiments and to report their new results in a scientifically acceptable fashion.

Under these circumstances this Task Force considers the massive publicity which they promulgate via radio, the lay press and popular books, using catch phrases which are really misnomers like "megavitamin therapy" and "orthomolecular treatment," to be deplorable.[24]

The Research Advisory Committee of the National Institute of Mental Health reviewed pertinent scientific data through 1979 and agreed that megavitamin therapy was ineffective and could be harmful. After the U.S. Defense Subcommittee looked into this therapy, it was removed as a treatment covered by CHAMPUS, the insurance program for military dependents.

Various claims that megavitamins and mega-minerals are effective against psychosis, learning disorders, and mental retardation in children were debunked in reports by the nutrition committees of the American Academy of Pediatrics in 1976 and 1981 and by the Canadian Academy of Pediatrics in 1990.[25] Both groups have warned that there is no proven benefit in any of these conditions and that megadoses can have serious toxic effects. The 1976 report concluded that a "cult" had developed among followers of megavitamin therapy.[26] That description is still appropriate.

The Feingold Diet

In 1973 Dr. Benjamin Feingold, a pediatric allergist from California, proposed that salicylates, artificial colors, and artificial flavors caused hyperactivity in children. Hyperactivity is now medically classified as attention deficit disorder (ADD) or attention deficit hyperactivity disorder (ADHD). To treat or prevent this condition,

ADDITIVES (800) 321-3287
can trigger
ADD (Attention Deficit Disorder)

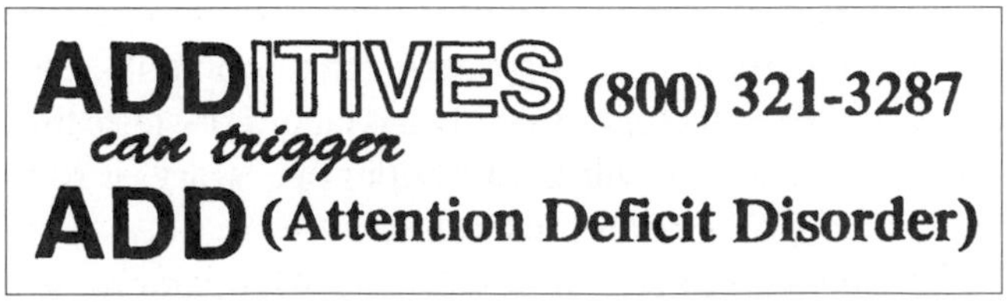

FIGURE 6-1. Feingold Association bumper sticker.

Feingold suggested a diet that was free of such chemicals. His followers now claim that asthma, bedwetting, ear infections, eye-muscle disorders, seizures, sleep disorders, stomach aches, and a long list of other symptoms may respond to the Feingold program and that sensitivity to synthetic additives and/or salicylates may be a factor in antisocial traits, compulsive aggression, self-mutilation, difficulty in reasoning, stuttering, and exceptional clumsiness.[27]

Adherence to the Feingold diet requires a drastic change in family lifestyle and eating patterns. Homemade foods prepared "from scratch" are necessary for many meals. In addition, many nonfood items such as mouthwash, toothpaste, cough drops, perfume, and some over-the-counter and prescription drugs are prohibited. Feingold strongly recommended that the hyperactive child help prepare the special foods and encouraged the entire family to participate in the dietary program. The *Feingold Cookbook* states: "A successful response to the diet depends on 100 percent compliance. The slightest infraction can lead to failure: a single bite or drink can cause an undesirable response that may persist for seventy-two hours or more."

Many parents who have followed Feingold's recommendations have reported improvement in their children's behavior. But carefully designed experiments have shown that the percentage of children who may become hyperactive in response to food additives is at best very small, and that improvement, if any, appears related to changes in family dynamics, such as paying more attention to the children.[28,29] Experts have also noted that the foods recommended in Feingold's book *Why Your Child Is Hyperactive* (1975) included some that were high in salicylates and excluded others that were low in salicylates.

Because the Feingold diet does no physical harm, it might appear helpful in some cases, because of its impact on the family. The potential benefits, however, must be weighed against the harmful effect of teaching children to blame food ingredients for their difficulties when other factors are responsible. There is additional potential for harm in creating situations where a child's eating behavior is regarded as peculiar by other children.

The Feingold Association of the United States's newsletter has reported claims that schoolchildren and their teachers were experiencing ill effects from chemicals used in construction, furnishing, maintenance, pest control, and classroom activities at their schools. It has been claimed, for example, that one child was disciplined for reacting to his teacher's perfume, another became abusive toward his mother because of the school's newly painted lunchroom, and another required tutoring because of a reaction to a leak in the school's oil furnace. Allegations like these are similar to the unsubstantiated claims made by clinical ecologists (see Chapter 8).

Consumption of sugar and aspartame (an artificial sweetener) have also been blamed for hyperactivity, but well-designed studies have found no evidence supporting such claims.[30,31]

Questionable Treatments for Learning Disabilities and/or Autism

Several approaches to learning disabilities, mental retardation, and autism have been identified as unproven and controversial.

Auditory Integration Training (AIT) was developed as a treatment for autism by Guy Berard in France in the 1960s and was introduced into the United States in 1991. It has also been advocated for children and adults with learning disabilities, attention deficit disorder, depression, migraine headaches, and many other conditions. Proponents claim that individuals with these disorders often have hearing that is disorganized, hypersensitive, different between the two ears, or otherwise abnormal. The first step in AIT is an audiogram that determines the auditory thresholds to more frequencies than are typically measured during hearing tests. Suitable individuals then undergo "training sessions"— typically two half-hour sessions per day over a 10-day period—that involve listening to music that has been computer-modified to remove frequencies to which they supposedly are hypersensitive. The American Academy of Pediatrics and the American Academy of Audiology have warned that no well-designed scientific studies demonstrate that AIT is useful.[32,33] AIT devices do not have FDA approval for treating autism, attention deficit disorder, or any other medical problem. In 1997, the FDA banned the importation of the Electric Ear or any other AIT device made by Tomatis International, of Paris, France.

Doman-Delacato treatment, also known as "patterning," was developed during the mid-1950s and offered at the Institutes for Human Potential in Philadelphia, Pennsylvania. Its proponents claim that the great majority of cases of mental retardation, learning problems, and behavior disorders are caused by brain damage or "poor neurological organization." The treatment is based on the idea that high levels of motor and sensory stimulation can train the nervous system and lessen or overcome handicaps caused by brain damage. Parents following the program may be advised to exercise the child's limbs repeatedly and use other measures said to increase blood flow to the brain and decrease brain irritability. In 1982 the American Academy of Pediatrics issued a position paper concluding that "patterning" has no special merit, that its proponents' claims are unproven, and that the demands on families are so great that in some cases there may be actual harm in its use.[34]

Eye movement desensitization and reprocessing (EMDR) is promoted for the treatment of post-traumatic stress, phobias, learning disorders, and many other mental and emotional problems. The method involves asking the client to recall the traumatic event as vividly as possible and rate certain feelings before and after visually tracking the therapist's finger as it is moved back and forth in front of the client's eyes. EMDR resembles various traditional behavioral therapies for reducing fears in that it requires clients to imagine traumatic events in a gradual fashion in the presence of a supportive therapist. However, controlled research has shown that EMDR's most distinctive feature (visual tracking) is unnecessary and is irrelevant to whatever benefits the patient may receive. Recent reviews have concluded that the data claimed to support EMDR derive mostly from uncontrolled case reports and poorly designed controlled experiments and that the theory of EMDR clashes with scientific knowledge of the role of eye movements.[35,36]

Facilitated communication is a process in which a "facilitator" supports the hand or arm of a severely handicapped person who spells out a message using a typewriter, a computer keyboard, or other device containing a list of letters, numbers, or words. It is alleged to help individuals strike the keys they desire without influencing the choice of keys. Some speech therapists and other special-education providers are using this procedure for nonverbal individuals with autism or severe mental retardation. Proponents claim that it enables such individuals to communicate. However, many scientific studies have demonstrated that the procedure is not valid because the outcome is actually determined by the "facilitator."[37] In one study, for example, autistic patients and facilitators were shown pictures of familiar objects and asked to identify them under three types of conditions: (1) assisted typing with facilitators unaware of the content of the stimulus picture, (2) unassisted typing, and (3) a condition in which the participants and facilitators were each shown pictures at the same time. In this last condition the paired pictures were either the same or different, and the participant's typing was "facilitated" to label or describe the picture. No patient gave a correct response when the facilitator had not been shown the picture. The researchers concluded that the facilitators were not aware that they were influencing the patients.[38] The American Psychological Association has denounced facilitated communication and warned that using it to elicit accusations of abuse by family members or other caregivers threatens the civil rights of both the impaired individual and those accused.[39] In 1994 the FTC settled charges that two companies had made false and unsubstantiated claims about "facilitated communication" devices they had marketed.

Neural Organization Technique (NOT) is based on the notion that learning disorders, childhood psychoses, mental retardation, cerebral palsy, bedwetting, and colorblindness are related to muscle imbalances caused by misaligned skull bones. NOT, a variation of cranial therapy (described in Chapter 7), was developed by New York chiropractor Carl Ferreri and has been taught to hundreds of other chiropractors. Its proponents claim to correct "blocked neural pathways" by "adjusting" the bones of the skull with pressure to various parts of the head. NOT came to public attention when chiropractors subjected children to it in a "research" project sponsored by school officials in California. A 1988 report in *Hippocrates* magazine described how children with epilepsy, Down syndrome, cerebral palsy, dyslexia, and various other learning disorders were forced to endure painful pressure against their skull, roof of the mouth, and eyes. One parent complained that pressure against her son's eye sockets had caused a seizure.[40] In 1991 a jury ordered Ferreri to pay $565,000 in damages to seven children and their parents who had filed suit for physical and emotional pain related to the treatment. Two other chiropractors involved in the case settled out of court for a total of $207,000.

Neuro Emotional Technique (NET) is another chiropractic approach focused on "releasing patients' emotional blocks stored in the body's memory." Its developer, Scott Walker, D.C., of Encinitas, California, describes NET as "a body-mind way, a non talk-it-out way, of dealing with emotional aberrations." Its proponents claim that everyone has such blocks and that the body "replays" these old memories, which can adversely affect health. The practitioner uses muscle testing (applied kinesiology) to "isolate a troublesome event"; asks the patient to hold in mind a "snapshot" of the emotional state while the chiropractor adjusts the patient's spine and acupuncture points; and prescribes supplement products and homeopathic remedies.

Optometric visual training is based on the idea that learning can be improved by exercises that improve coordination of the eye muscles or improve hand-eye coordination. Its proponents assume that the basic problem that leads to reading disability is some deficit in the visual system. The American Academy of Pediatrics and the American Academy of Ophthalmology have criticized this approach and cautioned that no eye-muscle defects can produce the learning disabilities associated with dyslexia.[41] (Dyslexia is a reading disorder characterized by omissions, faulty word substitutions, and impaired comprehension. It is not due to mental retardation, lack of schooling, or brain damage.)

Neurolinguistic Programming

Neurolinguistic programming (NLP) is a variable system of procedures purported to enable people to communicate more effectively and influence others. It is said to involve modifying the patterns or "programming" created by interactions among the brain (neuro), language (linguistic), and the body that produce both effective and ineffective behavior. Proponents claim that NLP has cured phobias, allergies, and other problems in one or a few brief sessions. Its core postulates are: (a) people are most influenced by messages that reflect how they internally represent whatever they are doing and (b) this representation is reflected by eye-gaze patterns, posture, tone of voice, and language patterns. The internal representation can be visual (picturing what they are involved with), auditory (hearing it sounded out), or can involve other senses. Proponents claim, for example, that someone experiencing a mental image might use the words "I *see*," whereas someone in an auditory mode might say "that *sounds* right to me." Scientific studies have demonstrated no correlation between eye movements and visual imagery, reported thoughts, or language choices. A National Research Council committee has found no significant evidence that NLP's theories are sound or that its practices are effective.[42]

Past-Life Therapy

"Past-life therapy" is based on the notion that psychologic disorders arise from the influence of traumas and personality traits from previous lives intruding on the subconscious. Proponents of this approach use hypnosis, meditation, or guided imagery to "regress" the patient to alleged earlier incarnations ("past lives") that, when recalled, lead to resolution of the patient's problems. There is, however, no scientific evidence that this theory is valid.

Experiments have shown that "past-life" reports during hypnotic trances are related to the subject's suggestibility and proneness to fantasize. In one study, 35 out of 110 subjects who were asked to regress to times before their birth enacted "past lives." In most of these cases, their past-life personalities were the same age and race as themselves. In another experiment, half of the subjects were informed by researchers that previous incarnations were often a different sex or race and had lived in exotic cultures. Those who received this advice were significantly more likely to incorporate one or more of the suggested characteristics into their past-life descriptions. In another experiment, researchers found that subjects who gave information specific enough to be checked were much more often incorrect than correct. Spanos[43] and Baker[44] have observed that past-life reports obtained from hypnotically regressed subjects are fantasy constructions of imaginative persons absorbed in make-believe situations and responding to regression suggestions—and that those who believe in reincarnation are the most likely to believe that such fantasies are related to an actual past life.

Stimulation of False Memories

If sexual abuse during childhood is a factor in a person's upset, it is unlikely to be forgotten. However, patients who are suggestible or eager to please their therapist may "remember" childhood events that did not actually take place. Usually it is the therapist who stimulates this process, either deliberately or unwittingly. Occasionally, however, the patient (possibly inspired by a book or television talk show) initiates the problem and the therapist fails to help sort fact from fantasy. Critics are using the term "false memory syndrome" (FMS) to describe the mental state generated in these situations.

Some therapists encourage their patients to confront and possibly sue the alleged perpetrator. The False Memory Syndrome (FMS) Foundation was formed in 1992 to deal with the problem of adults who mistakenly believe that they were victims of incest or child abuse. The foundation has been contacted by thousands of distressed families for advice on how to cope with sudden attacks by angry children who accused them of misdeeds that may not have taken place. Gardner[45] refers to the burgeoning number of FMS cases as "the mental health crisis of the 1990s."

Thought Field Therapy

The founder of thought field therapy (TFT) psychologist Roger J. Callahan, Ph.D., claims that TFT "provides a code to nature's healing system. . . . addresses . . . fundamental causes, balancing the body's energy system and allowing you to eliminate most negative emotions within minutes and promote the body's own healing ability." The Callahan Techniques web site also recommends dietary supplementation for persons who "suffer from multiple environmental sensitivities and even allergies which aggravate psychological problems." During TFT sessions, the therapist uses sequences of finger taps on "acupressure points" (primarily of the

hands, face, and upper body) and the patient does repetitive activities (repeats statements, counts, rolls the eyes, hums a tune) while visualizing a distressing situation.

TFT is claimed to be nearly 100% effective in treating depression, phobias, and other psychologic problems. It is based on the notion that acupressure points are related to blockages ("perturbations") of "body energy" associated with physical or emotional illness. Proponents claim that the finger-tapping releases the blockages and increases the body's energy flow. TFT's advanced techniques include muscle-testing (a variation of applied kinesiology) and "voice technology," in which the practitioner analyzes the patient's voice over the phone and determines where the patient should tap. "Voice technology" training for practitioners costs $100,000.

Critics have noted that TFT's underlying theories clash with established scientific knowledge and that studies alleging benefit have been poorly designed.[46] In 1999, the Arizona Board of Psychologist Examiners reprimanded a psychologist for using TFT and voice technology in his psychology practice, and the American Psychological Association's Continuing Education Committee notified continuing education providers that TFT courses will no longer be approved for continuing education credits.

Dianetics and "Purification"

Dianetics, a method promoted by the Church of Scientology, is described by its proponents as "an exact pastoral counseling technology for the location and elimination of unwanted emotional conditions and physical problems that are of spiritually induced origin."[47] In 2000, a Scientology web site listed 46 Dianetics Foundations in the United States and 221 in other countries.

Dianetics was developed by L. Ron Hubbard (1911–1986), a prolific science-fiction writer who founded the Church of Scientology.[47] Hubbard's *Dianetics: The Modern Science of Mental Healing* was originally published in 1950, has undergone several revisions, and is now called *Dianetics: The Modern Science of Mental Health*.[46] It is widely advertised as "the owner's manual for the human mind" and said to have sold over 14 million copies.[49] Individuals who return an inquiry card from the book may receive thousands of follow-up solicitations for Scientology publications and seminars.

According to Hubbard, the "analytical" (conscious) mind is a perfect recorder, computer, and solver of problems. It is incapable of error except when interfered with by "engrams," recordings made by the "reactive" (unconscious) mind when the analytic mind is turned off by traumatic events. Hubbard's book states that engrams stored in the reactive memory bank cause neuroses, psychoses, and psychosomatic disorders. The goal of Dianetics is to "clear" (erase) all engrams from the reactive bank. This is accomplished through a procedure called "auditing," in which the auditor may use an "E-Meter" to help the patient recall traumatic events and "drain them of their charge" so that they "no longer have power over the person."[50]

Time magazine has described the E-Meter as "a simplified lie-detector . . . designed to measure electrical changes in the skin while subjects discussed intimate details of their past."[51] In 1963 the FDA seized more than 100 E-meters at the headquarters of the Founding Church of Scientology in Washington, D.C. During the lengthy litigation that followed, a judge concluded:

Hubbard and his fellow Scientologists developed the notion of using an E-Meter to aid auditing. Substantial fees were charged for the meter and for auditing sessions using the meter. They repeatedly and explicitly represented that such auditing effectuated cures of many physical and mental illnesses. An individual processed with the aid of the E-meter was said to reach the intended goal of "clear" and was led to believe that there was reliable scientific proof that once cleared, many, indeed, most illnesses would automatically be cured. Auditing was guaranteed to be successful. All this was and is false.[52]

Upholding the FDA's charges that the E-Meter was misbranded, the judge ordered that future use of the E-Meter be confined to "bona fide religious counseling" and that the device be prominently labeled with this warning notice:

The E-Meter is not medically or scientifically useful for the diagnosis, treatment, or prevention of any disease. It is not medically or scientifically capable of improving the health or bodily functions of anyone.[53]

The copyright page of *Dianetics* states that the E-Meter "is not intended or effective for the diagnosis, treatment or prevention of any disease, or for the improvement of health or any bodily function."[48]

HealthMed, a chain of clinics run by Scientologists, offers a "purification program" of saunas, exercise, high doses of niacin, and other vitamins and minerals. The program, designed by Hubbard, is said to rid the body of "chemicals and poisons" that can dull awareness, mental acuteness, emotions, and "make a person feel dead, dull and lifeless."[54]

In addition to espousing its own approaches, the Church of Scientology has actively criticized others. In 1969 it and Thomas Szasz founded the Citizens Commission on Human Rights™ (CCHR) "to investigate and expose psychiatric abuses of human rights." CCHR is reported to have 120 chapters in 28 countries.[55] Its targets have included *Prozac* (the most widely prescribed antidepressant drug), electroconvulsive therapy, psychosurgery, the use of *Ritalin* for hyperactivity in children, and "psychotherapist sex crimes."[56] In 1990 CCHR petitioned the FDA to withdraw *Prozac* from the market, claiming that it is addictive and causes suicide, violent behavior, and abnormal body movements. The FDA rejected the petition.[57] A 1995 CCHR booklet urged readers to write to their legislators to demand that psychiatric centers and programs be removed from their community.[58] At a 1995 convention, the president of the Church of Scientology International announced plans to "eradicate" psychiatry by the year 2000.[59]

Routine Personality Testing

Psychologic tests allow the practitioner to sample a client's behavior in standardized ways. There are three broad types: (1) "intelligence" tests, which tend to test achievement rather than intelligence per se; (2) aptitude tests, which are used for vocational counseling and personnel selection; and (3) personality tests, which assess emotional or social aspects of a person's life. Objective personality tests, like the Minnesota Multiphasic Personality Inventory (MMPI), ask directly about the client's feelings and experiences. Projective personality tests, like the Rorschach inkblot test, elicit reactions to a series of ambiguous stimuli.

Personality tests are intended to reveal aspects of a person's view of self and others, along with interpersonal and emotional tendencies. Some psychologists use them routinely as part of their evaluation or treatment methods. However, most psychiatrists and many psychologists believe that the information gained is not cost-effective in terms of time, effort, and fees. Critics charge that (a) personality tests are unlikely to reveal useful information that is not obtainable by talking with the patient; (b) projective personality tests may reflect the characteristics of the person who does the scoring rather than those of the person tested; (c) the testing process can convey an incorrect message that the therapist can extract information and provide treatment to a patient who does not participate actively in the treatment process; and (d) there is little research evidence that projective personality testing leads to more accurate diagnosis or better treatment outcomes. A recent review concluded that projective tests, such as the Rorschach test, Thematic Apperception Test, Draw-a-Person Test

(DAP), Bender-Gestalt Test, Rozenzweig Picture-Frustration Study (PFS), and Sentence Completion Test (SCT), are unlikely to contribute information that cannot be obtained from simpler tests or from other sources.[60]

Psychic Counseling

Many entrepreneurs offer "psychic" advice by telephone. In the typical operation, callers dial a "900" number and are charged $2 to $4 per minute for the advice. In 1993 ABC-TV's "Prime Time Live" aired the results of a 3-month investigation of a lucrative "psychic hotline." One undercover investigator had no prior knowledge of occult matters. After being hired, she underwent a few days of training in tarot cards, astrology, and numerology. She then used her intuition (plus code words written on tarot cards) to formulate her responses to callers. She reported being instructed to permit suicidal callers to run up their bill before referring them to a legitimate suicide hotline. Another undercover investigator, posing as a prospective investor, interviewed a company director who said, "Most of the people's personal lives—who work for us—are just total shambles. How they could even give the stuff out is incredible."

Lester[61] described his visits to an astrologer, a palm-reader, and a "psychic," each of whom complimented him, made predictions, and gave specific advice. Based on his experience and reports by others, he concluded: (a) psychics and astrologers see themselves as performing counseling, and (b) their clients may be people who do not wish to think of themselves as having psychologic or psychiatric problems. Novella[62] has noted:

The common ploy used by psychics (often called the Jean Dixon effect) is to make dozens of predictions knowing that the more that are made, the better the odds that one will hit. When one comes true, the psychic counts on us to forget the ninety-nine percent that were way off. This makes the correct predictions seem much more compelling than they really are.

No systematic study of the impact of "psychic" or astrologic advice has been published in the scientific literature. But the Associated Press has reported an example of a disastrous outcome allegedly tied to such advice. In 1994 Orange County, California, filed for bankruptcy after its treasurer had lost $1.7 billion in highly speculative bond investments. The treasurer's top aide testified to a grand jury investigating the matter that the treasurer had consulted a psychic and relied on interest-rate forecasts from a mail-order astrologer while making the ill-fated investments.[63]

Mismanagement of Psychotherapy

Psychotherapy should not only help patients resolve problems but, in most cases, should also help foster independence from the therapist. Just as children must learn to handle situations without always running to their mother, patients must learn to handle upset feelings between sessions without the direct help of the therapist. Therapists who permit or encourage frequent telephone calls encourage overdependence. Therapists who receive many such calls from many patients are likely to have an underlying problem, such as a neurotic need to have people depend on them, which impairs their ability to treat patients.

A more subtle example of this problem is the therapist who cannot adhere to a schedule. Patients are scheduled for particular times, but sessions are allowed to run considerably overtime when patients are upset or

> **Consumer Health Insight**

Boundary Violations

Signs that a therapist is improperly crossing the patient-therapist boundary include:

- Repeatedly touching or hugging the patient
- Nontherapeutic contact outside of the therapist's office
- Hiring the patient or using the patient as an unpaid volunteer
- Talking about other patients
- Disclosing personal problems or intimate details of personal life, such as sexual experience
- Giving or accepting a valuable gift or loan
- Addressing the patients with a pet name
- Dressing seductively
- Ignoring mounting unpaid bills for treatment
- Offering not to charge or to greatly reduce the fee for sessions, even when the patient can afford the cost
- Permitting a patient to run errands or do other small favors for the therapist
- Using data from a therapy session (such as inside knowledge of a good investment) for personal gain
- Spending time—and wasting the patient's money—talking about the therapist's problems
- Promoting the therapist's religious belief system
- Promoting involvement in a social or political cause that the therapist is fond of
- Offering to join the patient in an investment or business venture
- Encouraging patients to engage in cultlike behavior with the therapist as a guru

Simplistic Advice

A deep understanding of a patient's dynamics may enable a therapist to give beneficial advice. But sometimes therapists give advice without considering the complexity of the patient's situation. Such ill-conceived action may be the result of inadequate training, poor therapeutic technique, or an emotional problem of the therapist. The following composite cases illustrate this point.

A 60-year-old businessman complained of insomnia and depression. Worry about his business was keeping him awake. The physician advised him to take a vacation to "get away from it all so you can stop worrying." The man went to a seaside resort but found he could not relax. He thought that his business would suffer from his absence, and idleness merely served to intensify his worrying.

A 35-year-old junior executive sought treatment for headaches and abdominal fullness. The physician correctly diagnosed that these were bodily reactions to tension, which was generated primarily at work. The patient believed he was being asked to do more than his share but was afraid to speak up about it. The physician encouraged the man to express his resentment, but failed to discuss how to do this in a constructive manner. The patient "told off" his boss and quit in a huff—a decision he later regretted.

A middle-aged couple who consulted a counselor spent the first two sessions berating each other for one thing after another. Seeing only the hostility in the relationship, the counselor advised them to get a divorce. A more qualified therapist would have realized that they could not have remained together for many years without a positive side to their relationship. The therapist should have terminated the verbal slugfest, explored the positive aspects of the relationship, identified the issues in conflict, and tried to help the couple resolve them.

A 30-year-old homemaker sought help to understand why she became angry with important people in her life, particularly her husband. The therapist encouraged discussion of her childhood, analyzed similarities between her father and her husband, and said: "You get angry with your husband when he reminds you of your father." Feeling that this information justified her resentment, the patient acted more nastily toward her husband, and their relationship deteriorated. Actually, the marital situation had been far more complex than the therapist realized. He should have explored the patient's contribution to the marital friction and helped her learn better ways to handle her feelings. Joint sessions with the patient and her husband might have helped the therapist understand the situation better.

appear to be talking about particularly meaningful material. Although an occasional brief extension may be justified, a general policy of this type encourages patients to manipulate the therapist to gain more attention. Other signs that a therapist is improperly crossing patient-therapist boundaries are listed in the box on page 115.

The most malignant type of therapist behavior is probably sexual exploitation. Although it is not unusual for therapist and patient to feel a personal or physical attraction toward each other, acting on such feelings is not therapeutic.[64] A composite case history illustrates what can happen:

An unmarried 27-year-old woman entered therapy to overcome shyness, feelings of inadequacy, and fear of involvement with men. Few men had seemed interested in her, and she had rarely dated. As therapy proceeded, she developed an intense fondness for the therapist, based largely on the fact that he was the first man who had spent time with her on a regular basis. At this point, instead of helping her learn how to attract suitable dates, the therapist suggested that sex with him would help her become more comfortable with men. She consented, hoping that marriage to the therapist would result. Her eventual disillusionment was a shattering experience that led to suicide.

Nearly all psychiatrists believe that sexual contact with a patient is inappropriate and usually harmful. Several states have laws forbidding such contact. In some states it is a criminal offense, and in others it is considered malpractice and can lead to a loss of license. In 1990 a California jury awarded $1.5 million to a woman who said she had been exploited by a psychiatrist who had treated her. Testimony during the trial indicated that they had begun dating after almost 2 years of treatment. The patient said that although she was extremely happy during the beginning of their affair, she became severely depressed when it ended.[65] In 1993 the American Psychiatric Association's board of trustees declared that "sexual activity with a current or former patient is unethical."

SUMMARY

Although excellent help is available for the treatment of mental and emotional problems, selecting a suitable therapist can be difficult. Some people respond best to a conversational approach, some to medication, and some to both. Before seeking treatment, it is advisable to understand the types of help available and the training that various types of practitioners undergo. Although most practitioners with accredited training are competent, some engage in practices that are unscientific or reflect underlying problems of their own. For this reason, consumers should also be able to recognize the common signs of inappropriate therapy.

REFERENCES

1. Hales D, Hales RE. Caring for the Mind: The Comprehensive Guide to Mental Health. New York, 1995, Bantam Books.
2. Wolberg LR. The Technique of Psychotherapy. New York, 1977, Grune & Stratton.
3. Biofeedback. Harvard Medical School Health Letter 15(10):1–4, 1990.
4. Callan J. Your Guide to Mental Health. Philadelphia, 1982, George F. Stickley Co.
5. Hancock L. Mother's little helper. Newsweek 127(12):51–56, 1996.
6. Task Force on Electroconvulsive Therapy. The Practice of Electroconvulsive Therapy: Recommendations for Treatment, Training, and Privileging. Washington D.C., 1990, American Psychiatric Association.
7. Devanand JP and others. Does ECT alter brain structure? American Journal of Psychiatry 151:957–970, 1994.
8. English OS, Finch SM. Introduction to Psychiatry. New York, 1954, WW Norton & Co. Inc.
9. Pies RW. Inside Psychotherapy: The Patient's Handbook. Philadelphia, 1983, George F. Stickley Co.
10. Mental health: Does therapy help? Consumer Reports 60:734–739, 1995.
11. Gabbard GO. Are all psychotherapies equally effective? The Menninger Letter 3(1):1–2, 1995.
12. Seligman EP. The effectiveness of psychotherapy: The Consumer Reports study. American Psychologist 50:965–974, 1995.
13. Rosen G. Quoted in Barrett S, Jarvis WT. The Health Robbers: A Close Look at Quackery in America. Amherst, N.Y., 1993, Prometheus Books.
14. Merikle PM. Subliminal auditory messages: An evaluation. Psychology and Marketing 5:355–372, 1989.
15. Greenwald AG, Spangenberg ER, Pratkanis AR. Double-blind tests of subliminal self-help audiotapes. Psychological Science 2:119–122, 1991.
16. Bjork RA and others. In the Mind's Eye. Enhancing Human Performance. Washington D.C., 1991, National Academy Press.
17. Moore TE. Subliminal perception: Facts and fallacies. Skeptical Inquirer 16:273–281, 1992.
18. Gubernick L, Mao P. The happiness hucksters. Forbes Oct 9, 1995, pp 82–88.
19. Stehlin IB. Unapproved devices seized. FDA Consumer 29(7):32–33, 1995.
20. Unapproved 'brain wave' devices condemned after seizure reports. FDA Consumer 28(2):41–43, 1994.
21. Four attorneys general, FTC reach settlement with Zygon International, manufacturer of "The Learning Machine." NAAG Consumer Protection Report, Mar/Apr 1996, pp 10–11.
22. Beyerstein BL. Brainscams: Neuromythologies of the New Age. International Journal of Mental Health 19(3):27–36, 1990.
23. Princeton BrainBio Center. Brochure distributed to patients. Skillman, N.J., 1983, The Center.

It's Your Decision

Should you or a family member need help with an emotional or mental problem, which of the following would you do?

Reason

- ☐ Check the Yellow Pages _____
- ☐ Ask a local physician for help _____
- ☐ Check with a religious counselor _____
- ☐ Call the local health department _____
- ☐ Discuss the matter with spouse or friend _____
- ☐ Take large amounts of vitamins _____
- ☐ Other: (specify) _____ _____

Should you or a family member have an alcohol problem, what action(s) would you take?

Reason

- ☐ Check with religious counselor _____
- ☐ Call one of the self-help groups in the community _____
- ☐ Talk with a family relative or friend _____
- ☐ Talk with family member about obtaining help _____
- ☐ Call your local physician _____
- ☐ Other: (specify) _____ _____

24. Lipton M and others. Task Force Report on Megavitamin and Orthomolecular Therapy in Psychiatry. Washington D.C., 1973, American Psychiatric Association.
25. Nutrition Committee, Canadian Paediatric Society. Megavitamin and megamineral therapy in childhood, Canadian Medical Association Journal 143:1009–1013, 1990.
26. Committee on Nutrition, American Academy of Pediatrics. Megavitamin therapy for childhood psychoses and learning disabilities. Pediatrics 58:910–912, 1976.
27. The Feingold Association of the United States. The Feingold Handbook. Alexandria, Va., 1986.
28. Wender EH, Lipton MA. The national advisory committee report on hyperkinesis and food additives—final report to the Nutrition Foundation. Washington D.C., 1980, The Nutrition Foundation.
29. Barrett S. The Feingold diet: Dubious benefits, subtle risks. Quackwatch web site, May 2, 2000.
30. Wolraich ML and others. Effects of diets high in sucrose or aspartame on the behavior and cognitive performance of children. New England Journal of Medicine 330:301–307, 1994.
31. Wolraich ML and others. The effect of sugar on behavior or cognition in children: A meta-analysis. JAMA 274:1617–1621, 1995.
32. American Academy of Pediatrics Committee on Children with Disabilities. Auditory integration training and facilitated communication for autism. Pediatrics 102:431–433, 1998.
33. Executive Committee, American Academy of Audiology. Position statement: Auditory integration training. Audiology Today 5(4):21, 1993.
34. American Academy of Pediatrics. Policy statement: The Doman-Delacato treatment of neurologically handicapped children. Pediatrics 70:810–812, 1982.
35. Lilienfeld SO. EMDR treatment: Less than meets the eye. Skeptical Inquirer 20:25–31, 1996.
36. Lohr JM, Tolin DF, Lilienfeld SO. Efficacy of eye movement desensitization and reprocessing: Implications for behavior therapy. Behavior Therapy 29:126–153, 1998.
37. Mulick JA and others. Anguished silence and helping hands: Autism and facilitated communication. Skeptical Inquirer 17:270–280, 1993.
38. Wheeler DL and others. An experimental assessment of facilitated communication. Mental Retardation 31:49–59, 1993.
39. American Psychological Association. Facilitated communication not a scientifically validated technique for individuals with autism or mental retardation. News release, August 24, 1994.
40. Cooke P. The Crescent City cure. Hippocrates 2(6):61–70, 1988.
41. Metzger RL, Werner DB. Use of visual training for reading disabilities. Pediatrics 73:824–829, 1984.
42. Druckman D, Swets JA, editors. Enhancing Human Performance. Washington D.C., 1988, National Academy Press.
43. Spanos NP. Past-life hypnotic regression: A critical view. Skeptical Inquirer 12:174–180, 1988.
44. Baker RA. Hidden Memories: Voices and Visions from Within. Amherst, N.Y., 1992, Prometheus Books.
45. Gardner M. The false memory syndrome. Skeptical Inquirer 17:370–375, 1993.
46. Guadiano BA, Herbert JD. Can we really tap our problems away? A critical analysis of thought field therapy. Skeptical Inquirer 24(4):29-33, 2000.
47. US Churches of Scientology. New viewpoints. Los Angeles, 1976, The Church.
48. Hubbard LR. Dianetics: The Modern Science of Mental Health. Los Angeles, 1985, Bridge Publications.
49. Church of Scientology International. The story that Time couldn't tell. Los Angeles, 1991, The Church.
50. Workbook on How to Use Dianetics. Los Angeles, 1992, Golden Era Productions.
51. Behar R. The thriving cult of greed and power. Time 137(18):50–57, 1991.
52. United States v Hubbard E-Meter, 333 F(supp)357, 1971.
53. Food Drug Cosmetic Reports. United States v Hubbard E-Meter, p 842, Mar 12, 1973.
54. Hubbard LR. Clear Body, Clear Mind. Los Angeles, 1990, Bridge Publications.
55. What Is CCHR? Citizens Commission on Human Rights web site, Aug 2000.
56. The rise of senseless violence in society: Psychiatry's role in the creation of crime. Los Angeles, 1992, Citizens Commission on Human Rights.
57. FDA denies Scientology petition against Prozac. FDA Talk Paper, Aug 1, 1991.
58. Creating racism: Psychiatry's betrayal. Los Angeles, 1995, Citizens Commission on Human Rights.
59. Jentzsch H, cited in Scientology News, issue 38, 1995, p 4.
60. Lilienfeld SO. Projective measures of personality and psychopathology. How well do they work? Skeptical Inquirer 23(5):32–39, 1999.
61. Lester D. Astrologers and psychics as therapists. American Journal of Psychotherapy 36:56–66, 1982.
62. Novella R. The power of coincidence. The Connecticut Skeptic 1(4):5, 1996.
63. Reckard ES. A psychic aided bond decisions? Philadelphia Inquirer, Dec 29, 1995.
64. Gutheil TG, Gabbard GO. The concept of boundaries in clinical practice: Theoretical and risk-management dimensions. American Journal of Psychiatry 150:188–196, 1993.
65. Rubsamen D. Psychiatrist's seduction of patient results in $1.5 million jury verdict. Psychiatric News, p 15, Mar 15, 1990.

DENTAL CARE

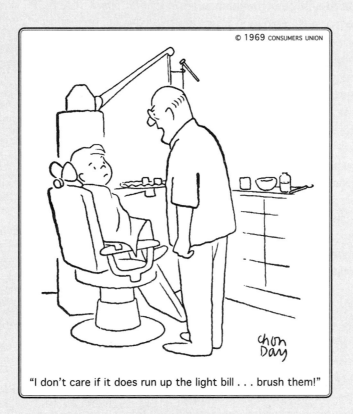

"I don't care if it does run up the light bill . . . brush them!"

The majority of dentists work in the privacy of their own office, where they usually are not subject to review by knowledgeable colleagues. This situation, plus the fact that the harm done by poor dental care may not become apparent for many years, makes it difficult for consumers to evaluate the quality of the treatment they receive.

JOHN E. DODES, D.D.S.[1]

Key Concepts
KEEP THESE POINTS IN MIND AS YOU STUDY THIS CHAPTER

- Good teeth contribute not only to appearance but to the quality of life as well.
- The key to dental health is prevention; the cornerstone of prevention is an adequate amount of fluoride.
- Community water fluoridation is the most effective and cost-effective way to obtain adequate fluoride intake.
- With proper care, teeth should last a lifetime. Self-care should involve daily brushing and flossing. The frequency of dental visits should be based on an assessment of the frequency of cavity formation, the rate of calculus formation, the condition of the gums, and any other special problem.
- Dentists who routinely recommend removal of mercury-amalgam fillings or teeth that have undergone root canal therapy are not trustworthy and should be avoided.

Dental diseases are among the most prevalent ailments in the United States. The total cost of dental services in 1998 was about $54 billion. Tooth decay (caries) affects almost everyone, and periodontal disease results in greater tooth loss than any other cause. Although proper care enables most teeth to last a lifetime, about 20% of Americans older than 45 and half of those older than 65 are toothless. Misconceptions about dental disease are common. Misinformation is spread by advertisers, food faddists, the media, and misguided or poorly informed health professionals.

This chapter covers the causes, prevention, and treatment (both appropriate and inappropriate) of dental problems. It also contains a brief discussion of smokeless tobacco products. Dental insurance is covered in Chapter 24.

DENTISTS

Dentists are licensed practitioners who hold either a doctor of dental surgery (D.D.S.) degree or the equivalent doctor of dental medicine (D.M.D.) degree. Becoming a dentist requires a minimum of 2 years of predental college work followed by 4 years of dental school. However, almost all students entering dental school have a baccalaureate degree. There are 54 accredited dental schools in the United States. The first 2 years of dental school consist largely of basic and preclinical sciences. The last 2 years are spent primarily in dental practice under faculty supervision. State licensure is then acquired by passing national and state board examinations. Dentists who wish to specialize spend 2 or more years in advanced training. To become board-certified they must then pass an examination administered by a specialty board recognized by the American Dental Association (ADA). The eight recognized specialties are:

DENTAL PUBLIC HEALTH: Prevention and control of dental disease and promotion of community dental health

ENDODONTICS: Prevention and treatment of diseases of the root pulp and related structures (root canal therapy)

ORAL AND MAXILLOFACIAL PATHOLOGY: Diagnosis of tumors, other diseases, and injuries of the head and neck

ORAL AND MAXILLOFACIAL SURGERY: Tooth extractions; surgical treatment of diseases, injuries, and defects of the mouth, jaw, and face

ORTHODONTICS AND DENTOFACIAL ORTHOPEDICS: Diagnosis and correction of tooth irregularities and facial deformities

PEDIATRIC DENTISTRY: Dental care of infants and children

PERIODONTICS: Treatment of diseases of the gums and related structures

PROSTHODONTICS: Treatment of oral dysfunction through the use of prosthetic devices such as crowns, bridges, and dentures.

The ADA estimates that during 1995, 151,000 dentists were professionally active in the United States, with about 139,000 in private practice. About 75% of dentists are ADA members.

AUXILIARY DENTAL PERSONNEL

Dentists are assisted by three categories of personnel: dental assistants, dental hygienists, and dental laboratory technicians.

Dental assistants have been part of the dental health-care team since 1885. The duties they may legally perform vary from state to state and can depend on the extent of their training. They may include preparing patients and materials, sterilizing instruments, keeping records, and taking x-ray films. Many assistants are trained by the dentists who employ them. Others have taken a short commercial course or received special training for expanded functions. Assistants must pass a special examination to be allowed to take x-ray films. Registered Dental Assistants (RDAs) have additional training and are permitted to polish teeth. Registered Dental Assistants in Extended Functions (RDAEFs) are legally permitted to apply sealants.

Dental hygienists provide clinical and educational services in private dental offices, schools, industrial plants, and public health and other government agencies. Their activities include performing oral prophylaxis (cleaning and polishing teeth), taking and processing x-ray films, conducting caries screening, and teaching oral health care. The training of dental hygienists takes 2 years for an A.A. or A.S. degree. They then can become registered by passing a state licensing examination. The scope of dental hygiene practice varies from state to state and has gradually expanded.

Dental laboratory technicians are trained to construct and repair oral appliances such as crowns, bridges, and dentures. Some train by apprenticeship, and others attend educational programs of 1 to 2 years. Some of these programs are accredited, but others are not. Many junior or community colleges include a dental technology program as part of their vocational training. Dental laboratory technicians usually work under a dentist's direction, either in the dentist's office or in a commercial laboratory. Those who work independently, selling directly to the public, are referred to as *denturists*. Denturism is illegal in most states.

TOOTH DECAY

Tooth decay (caries) is caused by bacteria in the mouth that produce acids harmful to tooth enamel. It is a highly complex phenomenon that also involves the interaction of hereditary factors, specific cariogenic bacteria, nutritional factors, dietary habits, oral hygiene, and time. Some medications and abused drugs can also cause

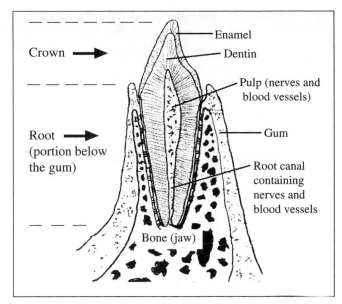

FIGURE 7-2. Schematic cross-section of an incisor tooth in its bony socket.

caries. Animal studies suggest that caries can be controlled by reducing the number of decay-producing bacteria in the mouth. The greatest intensity of caries occurs during adolescence.

Although most people know that sugar consumption has an effect on dental caries, few know how it actually works in the decay process. The amount of sugar in the diet is not as important as the frequency of eating, the acid-buffering capacity of the saliva, whether the sugar is in a food that sticks to the teeth, the availability of fluoride, or the individual's oral-hygiene practices.

Food faddists teach that honey, raw sugar, and other "natural" sweets are nutritionally superior, and that white sugar is bad because it is "empty calories." They also suggest that natural sugars are less apt to produce tooth decay. Both of these ideas are false. The vitamin content of natural sugars is minuscule. Honey is at least as cariogenic as refined sugar (sucrose) in the same concentration. The faddists' suggestion to substitute granola for conventional presweetened cereals is also foolish. (Granolas are made with oats, honey, dried fruit, and brown sugar.)

Decay-causing germs make no distinction between sugars from different sources. They digest them all and produce acids that attack (demineralize) the tooth enamel. The more frequently a person eats between meals, and the longer fermentable carbohydrates remain in contact with the teeth (as sticky sweets are most prone to do), the more the teeth are subjected to demineralization. However, remineralization (healing) occurs between periods of exposure to acids. The amount of

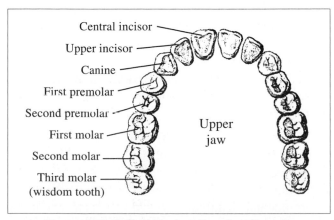

FIGURE 7-1. Schematic drawing of adult teeth.
Modified from Thibodeau GA, Patton KT.
Anatomy and Physiology, ed 3. St. Louis, 1996, Mosby.

decay depends upon the balance between demineralization and remineralization.[2] Remineralization is greatly aided by the presence of fluoride ions.

Cases have been reported of tooth damage in users of vitamin C (ascorbic acid) tablets who chew rather than swallow them. Ascorbic acid is strong enough to erode tooth enamel over a period of time.[3]

Dental Sealants

Sealants are thin plastic coatings that can protect the chewing surfaces but not the sides of the back teeth (molars) from decay. Sealants fill the pits and fissures of the chewing surfaces and harden soon after application. They usually last for years and can be reapplied if necessary. They are most effective for children between the ages of 5 and 14 when applied soon after the permanent teeth erupt. Friedman[4] and other caution that sealants should be used only for defective areas:

Not all pits and fissures need to be sealed but only those in which the sharp dental probe sticks firmly. Because molars are most likely to develop cavities, many dentists recommend sealing the . . . chewing surface whether or not defective; however, this creates an additional expense that may not be necessary.

FLUORIDATION

Fluoride is a mineral found naturally in most water supplies. When sufficient quantities of fluoride are available, especially during the process of tooth development, the resultant teeth are stronger and more resistant to decay.[5] Fluorides also work topically to prevent decay. This occurs through fluoride in saliva (due to ingested fluoride) and through applications of fluoride toothpaste, mouth rinse, or gel.

In the early 1900s a Colorado dentist named Frederick McKay suspected that something in water caused brown stains on the teeth of members of his community. The mottled teeth also were remarkably free of decay. By 1931 a new technique for water analysis enabled Dr. McKay to identify excessive fluoride as the cause. Subsequent testing determined that the ideal concentration for prevention of caries without mottling is approximately one part of fluoride per million parts of water.[6] The first community fluoridation program began in 1945 in Grand Rapids, Michigan. Today more than 135 million people in the United States are served by fluoridated water and an additional 10 million have protective levels of naturally occurring fluoride in their water. Recognition of fluoride's importance to dental health has led to dramatic declines in the prevalence and severity of tooth decay. Government surveys have

found that the percentage of children with caries-free permanent teeth rose from 28% in 1971–1974 to 36.6% in 1979–1980 and 49.9% in 1986–1987.[7,8]

Unfounded Criticism

Strident claims have been made that fluoridation causes cancer, birth defects, Down syndrome, allergies, and a wide variety of other maladies. But none of these claims has held up to scrutiny by qualified scientists.[9–11] National Council Against Health Fraud president William T. Jarvis, Ph.D., has noted:

These charges seem to grow out of a mentality of distrust. Antifluoridation groups are led by many of the same people who oppose immunization, pasteurization, sex education, mental health programs, and other public health advances. Most are closely connected with sellers of alternatives to medically accepted products and services. The so-called "health food" industry justifies its existence by declaring that our conventional sources of food, water, and health care are not trustworthy.

Too much fluoride can cause fluorosis, which, in its mildest form, causes small, white, virtually invisible opaque areas on teeth. Severe fluorosis causes brownish mottling, which occurs mainly in areas where the natural level of fluoride is considerably greater than 1 part per million. (Severe fluorosis also occurs in certain diseases, but this is not relevant to fluoridation.)

"Lifesavers Guide to Fluoridation," a pamphlet by John Yiamouyiannis, Ph.D., has been distributed in many communities considering fluoridation. The pamphlet cites 250 references to back up claims that fluoridation is ineffective and unsafe. However, experts from the Ohio Department of Health traced the references and found that almost half had no relevance to community water fluoridation and that many others actually support fluoridation but were selectively quoted and misrepresented.[12]

Consumers Union has concluded:

The simple truth is that there's no "scientific controversy" over the safety of fluoridation. The practice is safe, economical, and beneficial. The survival of this fake controversy represents one of the major triumphs of quackery over science in our generation.[10]

In 1990 an article in *Newsweek* suggested that fluoridation was ineffective and dangerous.[13] The article was triggered by unauthorized release of preliminary data from an experiment at the National Institute of Environmental Health Sciences in which rats and mice were exposed to a high dosage of fluoride. A few of the animals had developed bone cancer. However, a thorough review by a U.S. Public Health Service expert

Table 7-1

Supplemental Fluoride Dosage (Milligrams of Fluoride per Day)*

Age (years)	Concentration of fluoride in water (parts per million)		
	0.0 to 0.3	**0.3 to 0.6**	**Over 0.6**
Birth to 6 months	None	None	None
6 months to 3 years	0.25	None	None
3 to 6 years	0.50	0.25	None
6 to 16 years	1.00	0.50	None

*2.2 mg of sodium fluoride contains 1 mg of fluoride. Includes nursing infants who usually consume little exogenous water. Commercial formulas contain no fluoride. Recommended by the American Dental Association and the American Academy of Pediatrics Committee on Nutrition.[14]

panel concluded that the data were insignificant and that fluoridation posed no risk of cancer or any other disease.[15,16] Dr. Stephen Barrett called the *Newsweek* article "the most irresponsible analysis of a public health topic ever published by a major national news outlet."[17]

Fluoridation Alternatives

Fluoridation reduces the incidence of cavities 20% to 40% in children and 15% to 35% in adults.[18] The reduction is less than it was 20 to 40 years ago, probably because of improved dental hygiene and widespread use of fluoride toothpaste. Children in areas with negligible amounts of fluoride in the drinking water should be given fluoride drops or tablets prescribed by a physician or dentist. Table 7-1 gives the recommended dosage. Children who drink adequately fluoridated water should not be given supplements.

When the recommended supplement schedule is followed conscientiously from birth through early adolescence, the level of caries protection approaches that of water fluoridation. However, because few parents have sufficient motivation to carry out such a program, water fluoridation is vastly superior as a public health measure.

Topical methods apply fluoride directly to the surfaces of the teeth. They have merit but are not as effective as ingested fluorides. Fluoride toothpastes and mouth rinses are available for individual use; and gels, pastes, and solutions are available for administration by dentists. Topical fluoride methods can be used in nonfluoridated communities and also offer additional caries protection in fluoridated communities.

Water fluoridation, which costs about 50 cents per person per year, is considerably more economical than other methods of fluoride administration. Every dollar invested saves an estimated $80 in dental treatment costs.[18] The most rigorous study of preventive dentistry intervention measures ever done was the National

Preventive Dentistry Demonstration Program, which monitored nearly 30,000 children, ages 5 to 14, for four years. It concluded that the most effective and cost-effective way to prevent tooth decay is to drink fluoridated water from birth and have sealants applied as recommended.[19]

Periodontal Disease

"Periodontal disease" is the general term for inflammatory and degenerative diseases of the gums and other structures that surround the base of the teeth. A common cause of tooth loss between the ages of 30 and 70, it is usually triggered by accumulation of plaque below the gum line.

There are several types of periodontal disease, all resulting from bacterial infection that attacks the gums, bone, and ligaments that hold the teeth in the jaw. Without adequate bone and connecting fibers, the teeth loosen and are lost. Because this damage is irreversible, it is imperative that early signs of periodontal disease be recognized and treated. The earliest stage is gingivitis, which develops when plaque irritates the gums, making them red, tender, swollen, and likely to bleed. The next stage, periodontitis, occurs when toxins destroy the tissues anchoring the teeth to the bone. Gums become detached from the teeth, forming pockets that fill with more plaque. In advanced cases the gums are red and swollen and ooze pus (pyorrhea), painful abscesses may occur, and the teeth lose more attachments because the supporting bone is destroyed. Without treatment the person's teeth can fall out or require removal by a dentist.

Brushing, flossing, and periodic dental care are the first lines of defense against periodontal disease—as they are against caries. Adequate daily oral hygiene can prevent or minimize periodontal disease. Gingivitis is evidenced by redness or bleeding of the gums without discomfort. Pink coloring on the toothbrush bristles may be the first clue that gingivitis is present. The ADA states that more than half of the people older than 18 have at least the early stage of periodontal disease.[21]

Preventive cleaning by a dentist or dental hygienist is advisable at least once a year to remove calculus (also called tartar or scale), prevent gingivitis, and reduce the risk of periodontal disease. Yet many people won't go to a dentist unless they have troublesome symptoms. Properly performed professional cleaning is a meticulous procedure in which all the tartar, above and below the gumline, is carefully removed with metal instruments called scalers. An ultrasonic device can be used to remove calculus, but its use should be followed with hand-scaling to ensure that the teeth are clean and smooth. The teeth are polished after the scaling.

In the late 1970s an oral hygiene program called the Keyes technique was widely promoted as a nonsurgical alternative for treating advanced periodontal disease. The technique includes microscopic examination of the plaque and cleaning the teeth and gums with a mixture of salt, baking soda, and peroxide. At least three well-designed studies have shown that surgical treatment is more effective. A recent study found that although the baking soda mixture helped maintain oral health, it was no more effective than ordinary toothpaste. The researchers also found that people using the baking soda regimen were three times as likely to stop their program because it was inconvenient. It seems unlikely that the Keyes technique can contribute more toward healthy gums than can brushing with ordinary toothpaste and using dental floss.[1]

SELF-CARE

Although individuals can greatly influence their oral health, many people do not take dental problems seriously until it is too late. Losing teeth may not be as serious as losing an eye, a hand, or a foot, but people who lose their teeth are handicapped. Dentures are not as comfortable or functional as normal, healthy teeth and can cause difficulty in eating, as well as adverse effects on personality.

Brushing and Flossing

Teeth should be cleaned to remove plaque—the soft, sticky, colorless film of bacteria that is constantly forming on their surface. Acids produced by these bacteria are a major factor in both tooth decay and periodontal disease. The quantity and destructive character of plaque change with the passage of time. It takes about 24 hours for plaque to become sufficiently concentrated to begin causing damage. Pits, fissures,

and areas between the teeth where toothbrushes cannot reach provide hideouts for plaque and thus are the sites of most dental problems.

One thorough daily cleaning, involving both brushing and flossing, is usually sufficient to break up the colonies of bacteria that are continuously being built. A fluoridated dentifrice should be used. Brushing after meals is primarily for the purpose of dislodging food particles and should be accompanied by thorough rinsing of the mouth. Surface plaque can be identified with a disclosing solution or tablet. These dye the plaque bright red and highlight areas that are missed when cleaning the teeth. If plaque is allowed to remain on the teeth, it can harden to form calculus. Calculus is a gum irritant and can host bacteria that cause periodontal disease. Brushing with a dentifrice can reduce the amount of calculus above the gumline but not below it. Once calculus has built up, professional scaling is necessary to remove it.

Myth of "Detergent Foods"

The idea that eating crunchy foods such as apples and popcorn helps to clean the teeth by removing plaque is a myth. Even official government publications have made this claim. Although coarse foods may provide exercise for the teeth and gums, they are not a substitute for oral hygiene. Studies on a variety of foods have shown that, at best, chewing can affect plaque on the upper third of the teeth. Areas under the gums where periodontal disease occurs are completely unaffected.

DENTAL PRODUCTS

The ADA performs independent reviews of commonly used commercial dental products. Those judged to be safe and effective are permitted to carry a statement of ADA acceptance on their packages and in their advertising (see Figure 7-3).

Dentifrices

Dentifrices commonly contain abrasives, binding agents, sudsers, coloring agents, moisturizers, sweeteners, preservatives, and water. Many contain a fluoride compound. A dentifrice should be abrasive enough to prevent plaque and stain accumulation but not so harsh that it injures teeth or gums. The more abrasive toothpastes have little effect on the hard enamel in teeth, but cementum, the soft layer of the tooth just under the gum, is more vulnerable. As a person gets older, the gums may recede and expose the cementum to possible damage by abrasion. Some products can also irritate the gums themselves.

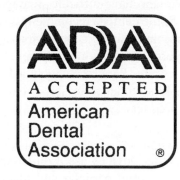

FIGURE 7-3. The ADA Seal of Acceptance. This logo, which signifies that a product meets ADA standards of safety and effectiveness, can be displayed in ads and on product labels and packages. About 400 over-the-counter products and 900 professional products are involved. Participating manufacturers must submit the products for expert evaluation and agree to have their advertising preapproved. Since 1994, this program has been administered by the ADA Council on Scientific Affairs.

Fluoride dentifrices inhibit dental caries even in adults. They are not a substitute for the fluoridation of community drinking water but are a useful adjunct. Many have been accepted by the ADA Council on Dental Therapeutics as "an effective decay preventive dentifrice that can be of significant value when used in a conscientiously applied program of oral hygiene and regular professional care." Dentists can recommend fluoride-containing products that are within the proper range of abrasiveness based on their patients' individual needs. *Consumer Reports*[22] advises brushing twice daily with a fluoride toothpaste.

Some dentifrice advertisements make claims about whitening and brightening of teeth. The basic color of the teeth is determined early in life and cannot be made whiter. Claims that toothpaste can remove calculus or retard new calculus formation also are questionable. Abrasive toothpastes may remove minor tooth discoloration caused by substances taken into the mouth, but these toothpastes can easily damage the softer parts of the teeth. Toothpastes containing urea peroxide or hydrogen peroxide can exert bleaching action. However, the wisest course of action for consumers who are concerned about tooth discoloration is to discuss the matter with their dentist.

If gums recede so that cementum is exposed, the teeth can become sensitive. Use of a dentifrice that contains potassium nitrate (e.g., *Sensodyne*) lessens this sensitivity in some people.[23]

Fluoride Mouth Rinses

The ADA Council on Dental Therapeutics has accepted several nonprescription fluoride mouth rinses as "effective decay-preventive rinses that can be of significant value when used regularly in conjunction with a decay-preventive fluoride dentifrice in a conscientiously applied program of oral hygiene and regular professional care." These can be helpful to people who live in nonfluoridated communities or whose teeth are very susceptible to decay.

Toothbrushes

Most dentists suggest a flat brushing surface with tufts of approximately equal length throughout the brush and a head small enough for comfort, regardless of the number of rows. The head of the brush must be small enough to reach all important surface areas of the mouth. Soft nylon bristles are flexible, clean teeth efficiently, and usually do not damage the gums. These bristles can make contact below the gum margin to help remove plaque. Toothbrushes with hard bristles should not be used because they can damage the teeth and gums, especially when combined with a highly abrasive toothpaste. The type of toothbrush is much less important than the way it is used. To be effective, a brush must be manipulated properly.

Electric toothbrushes are useful but are not panaceas. Careful manual brushing can be just as effective as mechanical brushing, although some studies report that certain electric toothbrushes, such as *Interplak* and *Rotadent*, remove plaque more efficiently than manual brushing. An electric toothbrush is particularly helpful for people with poor coordination caused by mental or physical disabilities, patients with orthopedic bands on their teeth, or people who are unwilling to spend sufficient time for proper brushing by hand.

Consumers Union's consultants advise replacing one's toothbrush every 4 to 6 weeks because worn bristles are less effective at removing plaque. They also state that commercially marketed ultraviolet "toothbrush sterilizers" have no practical value because there is no danger from using a toothbrush that carries germs from one's own mouth.[24]

Dental Floss and Toothpicks

Dental floss comes waxed or unwaxed. Although many dentists recommend the unwaxed type as better for removing plaque, people with tightly spaced teeth may find it easier to use the waxed type. The important point is to use floss daily in the manner prescribed by the dentist or dental hygienist. Floss holders are available for people who have difficulty manipulating the floss by hand. Some dentists recommend a toothpick (sometimes a specially shaped one such as *Stim-u-dent*) or a rubber interdental tip as a supplement to dental floss. In 1993, *Consumer Reports*[25] concluded that *Glide* dental floss had less tendency to shred than two Johnson & Johnson products.

Dental Irrigators

Oral irrigating devices use a direct spray of water to remove loose food particles and other large materials from around the teeth. Oral irrigators cannot substitute for either brushing or flossing, but patients with orthodontic bands, a fixed bridge, or excessive spacing between the teeth may find them helpful. Incorrect use of an irrigating device can injure oral tissues. For this reason, persons using such devices should get instructions from their dentist about proper use.

Mouthwashes

Advertising has suggested that mouthwashes are effective against bad breath (halitosis), can help clean the teeth, prevent or treat colds and sore throats, and help control dental plaque. Many such promotions have been misleading.

Mouthwashes can freshen the breath for a few minutes (sometimes as much as an hour), but they cannot prevent infectious diseases.[26] Some mouthwashes have a high alcohol content, which can cause excessive drying of the mouth. People who are troubled with bad breath should understand that this is a symptom whose cause, whether oral or systemic, should be ascertained. Common causes of bad breath are poor oral hygiene; postnasal drip; gum disease; tobacco use; and consumption of aromatic substances such as garlic, onions, and certain alcoholic beverages. Halitosis may also be a symptom of infections, tumors, diabetes, and various other diseases.

For many years—until stopped by federal enforcement actions—manufacturers suggested in their ads that mouthwashes can help prevent or cure infections. It is true that antiseptic mouthwashes can kill some germs on contact, but this has no practical significance. Germs in the tiny crevices in the mouth and within infected tissues cannot be reached or washed out. Germs that are washed off the surface of infected areas are quickly replaced.

The plaque-control situation is less clear-cut. In 1986 the FDA approved *Peridex* mouth rinse, a prescription drug that contains 0.12% chlorhexidine, as safe and effective in helping to control plaque. Chlorhexidine can reduce plaque below the gumline. In 1987 the ADA

Council on Dental Therapeutics concluded that: "Listerine Antiseptic has been shown to help prevent and reduce supragingival (above the gumline) plaque accumulation and gingivitis when used in a conscientiously applied program of oral hygiene and regular professional care. It has not been shown to have a therapeutic effect on periodontitis." *Listerine* does not affect plaque below the gumline and is not nearly as effective as *Peridex*. Mouthwashes are not substitutes for brushing and flossing and are appropriate mainly for individuals under dental care in which other measures are unable to control gingivitis.

Plax, another mouthwash claimed to reduce plaque, uses sodium benzoate as its principal ingredient. Consumers Union's dental consultants have stated that *Plax* has not been shown to produce a clinically meaningful reduction in plaque.[27]

Surveys have found an increased risk of oral cancers among regular users of alcohol-containing mouthrinses. This subject is being investigated because cancers of the mouth and pharynx are more common among people who drink large amounts of alcoholic beverages. However, no cause-and-effect relationship has been proven, and an FDA advisory panel has concluded that the surveys were not properly designed. A National Cancer Institute[28] survey, for example, did not determine how frequently people used mouthwash or the reasons for its use, which might have been to cover up tobacco or alcohol use.

Sugarless Gum

Chewing gum that contains sugar can contribute to tooth decay. Thus sugar-free gum is a better choice for people who chew gum frequently. Certain gums that contain xylitol are marketed with claims that it decreases the incidence of decay. John E. Dodes, D.D.S., an expert on dental quackery, states that this claim is not supported by solid scientific evidence.

Do-It-Yourself Bleaching

Dentists have been bleaching teeth in their offices for decades. This is a legitimate procedure that requires care to ensure that the patient is not injured by the caustic bleaching agent. In 1996, *Rembrandt Lighten Bleaching Gel* became the first dentist-dispensed whitening product for home use to earn the ADA Seal of Acceptance.

Some nonprescription products marketed for home use have been ineffective and even dangerous. The FDA has ruled that bleaching products containing carbamide or hydrogen peroxide are "drugs" because they alter the structure of the tooth. In 1991 the agency ordered 20 manufacturers to stop selling them until they were demonstrated to be safe and effective. A case was reported of an Illinois boy who had permanently damaged his teeth with seven applications of bleach over a 2-month period. The bleach gradually stripped off the enamel, making the teeth darker instead of whiter.[29]

Pain Relievers

People with toothaches sometimes seek temporary relief by applying a nonprescription pain reliever to the teeth. These products usually contain clove oil, anesthetics, and aspirin. Clove oil is a powerful germicide. It is uncertain whether the relief it provides is due to a local anesthetic effect or its irritant activity. Anesthetics such as benzocaine and butane sulfate can provide minor relief from pain, if the decayed area of the tooth is exposed and accessible. Aspirin does not provide topical anesthesia. It should never be packed into a carious tooth or placed onto the adjacent gum, because its acidic nature can traumatize a nerve ending and ulcerate the mucous membrane of the mouth. Ibuprofen (*Advil, Nuprin*), taken internally, can be effective against dental pain.

DENTAL RESTORATIONS

The most common material used to restore decayed teeth is silver amalgam, a mixture of an alloy of silver, tin, copper, and zinc, and an equal amount of mercury. Tooth-colored plastic (composite) fillings can be used in front teeth or for small, visible back fillings. Amalgam fillings are less expensive, more durable, and easier to replace than composite fillings.[30] If much tooth structure has been lost as the result of decay or an accident, then a cast restoration is used, preferably gold.

A cemented restoration that covers only part of the tooth is called an *inlay* or *onlay*. Cast metal, porcelain, and composite plastic materials can be used for this purpose. When not enough tooth is present to hold an inlay, a *crown* is needed. This restores the entire tooth that is visible above the gumline. Crowns are usually made of a combination of metal (preferably gold or palladium alloy) and porcelain. A front crown, sometimes called a *cap*, is usually solid porcelain.

When teeth are missing, teeth on either side of the space can be crowned and artificial teeth (a bridge) can be permanently fastened to the crowns. A bridge cemented to adjacent teeth is called a fixed bridge. Fixed bridgework is generally superior to removable bridgework, but there are situations where it cannot be used.

The "Maryland Bridge," a type of fixed bridge developed by researchers at the University of Maryland, uses special materials that bond metal to tooth structures. This method enables the dentist to replace missing teeth with a cemented restoration, without placing crowns on the adjacent teeth. It costs less than a conventional fixed bridge, but it is not as durable.

"Drill-less Fillings"

The *Caridex* is a trademarked device that uses a warm solution of sodium hydroxide, sodium chloride, sodium hypochlorite, and aminobutyric acid as its active ingredient to soften decay so that it is easily scraped from the tooth with a metal instrument. This procedure is safe and allows some patients to be treated without an injection of anesthetic. However, most cavities are not sufficiently exposed, so drilling is still needed for the great majority of patients. The *Caridex* is very slow and therefore increases the cost of performing a filling.

Bonding

Bonding is a popular method of correcting cosmetic problems in patients with healthy gums and an adequate tooth structure to which bonding material can be applied. Most dentists employ this procedure. Bonding is not an alternative to crowning. Crowns are needed if teeth are badly broken down or must anchor a bridge.

To prepare a tooth for bonding, an acid solution is applied to increase adhesion. A liquid plastic is then painted on, and a paste made of plastic and finely ground quartz, glass, or silica gel is layered onto the tooth. Each layer is hardened in minutes either chemically or by shining a very bright light on the plastic. Finally the bonded surface is polished. Cosmetic results can also be achieved by bonding very thin plastic or porcelain veneers to the acid-etched tooth enamel.

Bonding usually is painless and faster and cheaper than crowning. However, it is not permanent and may need to be repeated after several years, because the bonding material wears away. Some dentists claim to specialize in "cosmetic dentistry," but this is not a recognized specialty.

ENDODONTICS (ROOT CANAL THERAPY)

Teeth are hollow and contain living, sensitive tissue commonly called the "nerve" but referred to by dentists as the *pulp*. In infections of the pulp caused by decay or accidents, the pulp can be removed and replaced with an inert material (gutta-percha). Endodontics is expensive (typically several hundred dollars per tooth) but should be painless. Teeth often need an artificial crown and post (to increase retention of the crown) following root canal therapy, but millions of teeth have been saved through this therapy alone. Claims that endodontically treated teeth become a focus of infection or disease in other parts of the body have been refuted by meticulous research.[31]

Sargenti root canal therapy is a treatment that may save a tooth, but is much less predictable than standard endodontic treatment. It is performed with a paste that is easier and faster to place than gutta-percha. However, the paste contains paraformaldehyde, which, when it contacts water, forms formaldehyde (a preservative used in embalming fluid). The pressure needed to reach the tip of the root can force the paste into surrounding tissues where it can cause serious injury. The FDA has banned interstate marketing of Sargenti-type pastes, but pharmacists can prepare them for dentists in their community.

Proponents of the Sargenti method have formed the American Endodontic Society, which has little or no standing within the scientific dental community. The recognized endodontic specialty group is the American Association of Endodontists. In 1991 the ADA Council on Dental Therapeutics abandoned its long-held neutral position on the Sargenti method and resolved:

In view of the fact that sufficient data have not been submitted to the Council on Dental Therapeutics to establish the safety of paraformaldehyde-containing root canal filling materials and that the FDA has not approved any products with this formulation, the council cannot recommend use of these products at this time.[32]

In 1993 an FDA dental advisory panel concluded that data submitted by the company wishing to market the paste were not sufficient to warrant FDA approval. Sargenti died in 1999.

ORTHODONTICS

The goal of orthodontics is to improve the health and function of the mouth as well as the patient's physical appearance. Twenty million adults and children receive orthodontic treatment annually; many others with correctable malocclusions do not. The ADA recommends consultation with an orthodontist for children 4 to 7 years old if the family dentist suspects that the teeth are badly aligned. There is no age limit for orthodontic treatment, provided oral tissues are basically healthy.

Before beginning treatment the orthodontist obtains facial measurements, x-ray films, and plaster casts to aid in diagnosis and treatment planning. Some orthodontists also use computer analysis. Teeth responsible for overcrowding may have to be extracted. Braces are prepared, cemented or bonded to the teeth, and wired together. Slight pressure is then maintained on the bands and wires so that the teeth are gradually brought into alignment. Some discomfort may be present during the first few days after braces are applied, but severe pain normally does not occur during orthodontic treatment. When proper occlusion has been achieved, the braces are removed and a retaining appliance is substituted. The average length of treatment is 18 to 24 months for children and adolescents. Adult treatment, which is more likely to involve removable appliances, generally takes longer. A full course of orthodontic treatment can cost $2000 to $3000 or more.

DENTURES

The preparation of dentures is a complex procedure best performed by a dentist with the help of a dental laboratory technician. Poorly fitted dentures can cause serious problems, including difficulty in eating and speaking, disturbances of the temporomandibular joint (TMJ), and irreversible destruction of bone needed for denture support. Constant irritation from an ill-fitting denture, if continued over a long period, can cause open sores or inflammation. Full lower or upper dentures typically cost about $500 to $1000 each. Poorly fitted dentures can cost the patient more in the long run, when the damage they cause must be corrected.

Denturists

Denturists are a relatively small number of technicians who provide dentures directly to the public and are seeking to be licensed independently from dentists. Denturism is illegal in most states. Denturists in Maine, Arizona, and Colorado can practice under the supervision of a licensed dentist. Denturists are allowed to practice independently only in Oregon, Idaho, Montana, and Washington. However, in a 1991 study, investigators hired by the Arizona Dental Association found that only three out of the state's 13 denturists advised callers to see a dentist before visiting them.[33]

Denturists assert that they can fit dentures as competently as dentists and more cheaply. However, Canadian data indicate that fees charged by denturists in that country are similar to those charged by dentists. The major objection to denturism is that complete examination of the mouth and proper fitting of the teeth often require skills that denturists lack. Denturists are not competent to diagnose cancers or other diseases within the mouth, to screen for underlying disease, or to recognize when structural problems of the mouth (such as unseen broken-off roots of teeth) can lead to injury if not corrected before the installation of dentures. In 1991 an Arizona dental board noted that complaints concerning the state's denturists were many times more common than complaints about the state's dentists.[33]

The ADA is strongly opposed to denturism and has encouraged dental societies to sponsor community programs in which professionally acceptable dentures can be offered to financially disadvantaged individuals at a reduced cost. Programs of this type exist in most states. In addition, low-cost care may be available from dentists whose fees are comparable to those of denturists. Nearly half of dentists responding to a 1994 ADA survey reported that they offered free or discounted care to people with low incomes.[34]

Cleaning and Repair

If plaque accumulates on dentures, it can cause mouth odors and lead to the formation of calculus that can irritate the soft tissue of the mouth. Therefore, dentures should be brushed daily with a commercially available denture cleaner.

Some people have used laundry bleach (liquid sodium hypochlorite) or baking soda as denture cleaners. Although laundry bleach partially removes beverage and tobacco stains, it has the potential to burn tissues inside the mouth. It can also tarnish metal denture parts and fade the color of the plastic material. Baking soda has been found to be less effective than the better commercial cleaners. White vinegar can soften calculus on a denture.

In time dentures may loosen and need rebuilding or repair. Adhesives, repair kits, and reliner kits are available to the public, but the do-it-yourself approach to denture repair is hazardous. The FTC has warned major manufacturers of denture adhesives that it is unlawful to advertise that (a) a denture adhesive will remedy biting and chewing problems of denture wearers (unless retention is their only dental problem) or that (b) a denture adhesive will enable all denture wearers to eat foods that are hard to bite, such as apples and corn-on-the-cob.[35]

Dental Implants

Implants are artificial root substitutes that are placed within the jaw bone to anchor artificial teeth. They are usually made of titanium. The cost typically ranges from $800 to $1800 per implant for the surgical phase, plus the cost of the replacement teeth. For many years implants that were not sufficiently tested in the laboratory were used in patients, often with disastrous results. Today there are implant systems that provide a good chance of success with little danger of serious complications. The best researched of these is the osteointegrated Bränemark implant, which was developed in Sweden.

An important factor in the success of implants is to minimize chewing pressure on them for 3 to 6 months. This can be accomplished by hiding the base of the implant under the gum until the bone has healed sufficiently. Then surgery is performed to expose the implant for attachment of the artificial teeth. Consumers should carefully investigate the experience of any dentist they consult and request complete information about the type of implant and possible complications. An oral surgeon or periodontist is likely to have the best surgical skills for placing implants, but some general dentists have sufficient training to do the surgery properly.

DENTAL X-RAY PROCEDURES

X-ray films are a necessary part of modern dental practice. Usually they involve little radiation and are inexpensive, but so many are obtained that dental films are second only to chest examinations in frequency and overall cost. America's annual bill for dental radiographs is more than $1 billion.

Because any exposure to radiation involves some risk, the dental profession has worked hard to minimize exposure. This has been accomplished by: (a) reducing exposure time by combining high-voltage equipment with high-speed film, (b) using collimators to reduce the area of the exposure, (c) filtering out unnecessary radiation, (d) eliminating unnecessary repetition of x-ray films, and (e) using lead aprons to shield the rest of the body.

Dentists typically obtain full-mouth radiographs of all the teeth at the beginning of the patient's care and every 3 to 5 years thereafter. However, a history and clinical examination should be completed before deciding what type of dental radiography, if any, should be obtained. A full set normally consists of two to four bite-wing x-ray films, which show the areas between the teeth and the parts of the teeth that are outside of or just below the gums, and 14 periapical films, which reveal the deeper dental structures that include the tips of the roots of two or three teeth per film.

For bite-wing and periapical views, the film is placed inside the patient's mouth and the x-ray source is a stationary machine. Panoramic views are obtained with a machine that swings the x-ray camera around the head, enabling all the teeth to be included in a single picture. This procedure is quicker and more comfortable for the patient because the film is positioned outside the patient's mouth. Unfortunately, the resultant picture is not as detailed. Therefore bite-wing and periapical films are used to diagnose decay and periodontal disease, whereas panoramic films are appropriate for detecting diseases and infections in the jaw bones, orthodontic problems, and impactions (unerupted teeth).

Children and adults generally do not need an x-ray examination each time they see a dentist if they are not at high risk for decay and show no other signs of dental disease. Young children rarely need x-rays because baby teeth usually are spaced so that all surfaces are visible to the naked eye. Bite-wing x-ray films are appropriate annually for most patients and may be obtained more frequently if rampant caries exists. On such a schedule the diagnostic benefit clearly outweighs the risk of radiation that is involved. What little risk exists is greatly reduced by the use of a lead apron. An expert panel has concluded that the adult guidelines need no alteration during pregnancy because the amount of radiation reaching the pelvis is insignificant.[36]

If recent films are available, it may not be necessary to obtain new ones. Dental radiographs often yield more information when compared with previous films. Thus, if consulting a new dentist, bring previous films or have them forwarded to the new dentist.

QUESTIONABLE PROCEDURES

Many teeth that are extracted because of decay could have been saved by modern dental treatment: either a carefully performed large filling or root canal therapy followed by a crown. Dentists often overstate the dangers posed by third molars ("wisdom teeth"). Extraction is appropriate if they cause pain, form cysts, cause problems by pushing into other teeth, or are partially erupted and prone to cause gum infections. If none of these conditions exists, wisdom teeth should be left alone. Only 6% of wisdom teeth are diseased, and fewer than 1% cause trouble with the roots of adjacent teeth.

Both competence and conflicts of interest play a role in inappropriate extractions. Some general dentists extract teeth instead of referring the patient to a specialist who can save them. The fact that insurance policies generally pay more for extractions than they do for fillings may be a factor. Oral surgeons also have conflicting interests when they realize that a patient has been inappropriately referred for an extraction. If they refer the patient for root canal therapy, they will not only lose the surgical fee but may also stop getting referrals from the general dentist. Dodes and Schissel[37] believe that most oral surgeons faced with this situation perform the extractions.

Some dentists use a laser device to "drill" cavities and advertise that this method is quicker, more precise, and less apt to require anesthesia than normal drilling. In 1997 the FDA approved the erbium:YAG laser for drilling teeth to remove tooth decay to prepare cavities for fillings and to roughen enamel to improve bonding of restorations.[38] Lasers also have some proven uses in dental surgery.[39] However, they cannot be used for drilling teeth with fillings already in place, because the filling may heat up and damage the tooth,[38] and, in many patients, a regular drill is still required to get through the enamel on molars.[40] Nor can they be used to prepare crowns or inlays.

Some dentists are using low-power lasers (like those in laser pointers), and some are using high-power radio waves to cut nerve endings to treat headaches. There is no scientific support for either treatment.

Overuse of "conscious sedation" is another problem. Nearly all dental work can be done with local anesthesia, which entails almost no risk and is much less costly. Local anesthesia permits dentists to do complex procedures slowly and carefully, without having to worry that the longer they take, the greater the risk. Some dentists routinely sedate patients with an intravenous medication such as diazepam or fentanyl. Dodes and Schissel state that dentists who do this feel pressured to work quickly and, as a result, take shortcuts and do inferior work.[37]

DENTAL QUACKERY

Dodes[1] and Jarvis[41] have noted that a significant number of dentists have gone overboard in espousing pseudoscientific theories, particularly in the area of nutrition. "Holistic dentists" typically claim that disease can be prevented by maintaining "optimum" overall health or "wellness." In the dental office this usually involves recommendations for expensive dietary supplements or a plastic bite appliance. Dodes has remarked that "wellness" is "something for which quacks can get paid when there is nothing wrong with the patient."

Some practitioners use hair analysis, computerized dietary analysis, or a blood chemistry screening test as a basis for recommending supplements to "balance the body chemistry" of their patients. Hair analysis is not a reliable tool for measuring the body's nutritional state (see Chapter 12). Computer analysis can be useful for determining the composition of a person's diet and can be a legitimate tool for dietary counseling. Dentists receive training in the nutritional aspects of dental health; However, few are qualified to perform general dietary counseling, and computerized "nutrient deficiency tests"

Historical Perspective

The Legacy of Weston Price

Much of "holistic dentistry" is rooted in the activities of Weston A. Price, D.D.S. (1870–1948), a dentist who maintained that sugar causes not only tooth decay but physical, mental, moral, and social decay as well. Price made a whirlwind tour of primitive areas, examined the natives superficially, and jumped to simplistic conclusions. While extolling their health, he ignored their short life expectancy and high rates of infant mortality, endemic diseases, and malnutrition. While praising their diets for not producing cavities, he ignored the fact that malnourished people don't usually get many cavities.

Price knew that when primitive people were exposed to "modern" civilization they developed dental trouble and higher rates of various diseases, but he failed to realize why. Most were used to "feast or famine" eating. When large amounts of sweets were suddenly made available, they overindulged. Ignorant of the value of balancing their diets, they also ingested too much fatty and salty food. Their problems were not caused by eating "civilized" food but by *abusing* it. In addition to dietary excesses, the increased disease rates were due to (a) exposure to unfamiliar germs, to which they were not resistant, (b) the drastic change in their way of life as they gave up strenuous physical activities such as hunting, and (c) alcohol abuse.

Price also performed poorly designed studies that led him to conclude that teeth treated with root canal therapy leaked bacteria or bacterial toxins into the body, causing arthritis and many other diseases. This "focal infection" theory led to needless extraction of millions of endodontically treated teeth until well-designed studies, conducted during the 1930s, demonstrated that the theory was not valid.

Melvin Page, D.D.S., one of Price's disciples, coined the phrase "balancing body chemistry" and considered tooth decay an "outstanding example of systemic chemical imbalances." Page ran afoul of the Federal Trade Commission by marketing a mineral supplement with false claims that widespread mineral deficiencies were an underlying cause of goiter, heart trouble, tuberculosis, diabetes, anemia, high and low blood pressure, hardening of the arteries, rheumatism, neuritis, arthritis, kidney and bladder trouble, frequent colds, nervousness, constipation, acidosis, pyorrhea, overweight, underweight, cataracts, and cancer. Page also claimed that milk was "unnatural" and was the underlying cause of colds, sinus infections, colitis, and cancer.

Hal A. Huggins, D.D.S., who describes himself as one of Page's students, promoted "balancing body chemistry" so vigorously that in 1975 the American Dental Association Council on Dental Research denounced the diet that he recommended. Huggins has also crusaded against mercury-amalgam fillings, marketed mineral products with false claims that they would help the body rid itself of mercury, and advised removal of endodontically treated teeth. Another Price follower is George A. Meinig, D.D.S., whose book *Root Canal Cover-up Exposed* was published in 1994.

The Price-Pottenger Nutrition Foundation of La Mesa, California, is the repository for many of Price's manuscripts and photographs. It was founded in 1965 as the Weston Price Memorial Foundation and adopted its current name in 1972. Its newsletter, book catalog, and information service promote food faddism, megavitamin therapy, homeopathy, chelation therapy, and many other dubious practices.

---

are not legitimate (see Chapter 12). The blood chemistry tests, usually obtained from a reputable laboratory, are legitimate but misinterpreted. Instead of accepting the laboratory's range of "normal" values, "holistic dentists" use a much narrower range and tell patients that anything outside that range means they are out of balance and need treatment.

Disorders of the temporomandibular joint (TMJ, jaw joint) and facial muscles can cause facial pain and restrict opening of the mouth. Clicking alone is not considered a problem. Allegations that TMJ problems can affect scoliosis, premenstrual syndrome, or sexual problems are not supported by scientific evidence. Scientific studies show that 80% to 90% of patients with TMJ pain will get better within three months if treated with nonprescription analgesics, moist heat, and

exercises. Dodes[1] warns that correction of a "bad bite" can involve irreversible treatments such as grinding down the teeth or building them up with dental restorations:

The most widespread unscientific treatment involves placing a plastic appliance between the teeth. These devices, called mandibular orthopedic repositioning appliances (MORAs), typically cover only some of the teeth and are worn continuously for many months or even years. When worn too much, MORAs can cause the patient's teeth to move so far out of proper position that orthodontics or facial reconstructive surgery is needed to correct the deformity.

Proponents of "cranial osteopathy," "craniosacral therapy," "cranial therapy," and similar methods claim that the skull bones can be manipulated to relieve pain (especially TMJ pain) and remedy many other ailments. They also claim that a rhythm exists in the flow of the fluid that surrounds the brain and spinal cord and that diseases can be diagnosed by detecting aberrations in this rhythm and corrected by manipulating the skull. Proponents include dentists, physical therapists, osteopaths, and chiropractors. The theory underlying craniosacral therapy is erroneous because the bones of the skull are fused to each other, and cerebrospinal fluid does not have a palpable rhythm. In a recent test, three physical therapists who examined the same 12 patients diagnosed significantly different "craniosacral rates."[42]

Auriculotherapy is a variation of acupuncture based on the notion that the body and organs are represented on the surface of the ear. Proponents claim it is effective against facial pain and ailments throughout the body. Its practitioners twirl needles or administer small electrical currents at points on the ear that supposedly represent diseased organs. Courses on auriculotherapy are popular among "holistic" dentists. Complications from unsterile and broken needles have been reported.

Some dentists claim to specialize in the treatment of bad breath. Dodes and Schissel have warned that such dentists have no special expertise and are primarily interested in increasing their income by selling unproven products. One such product is *OXYFRESH*, sold through multilevel marketing with unsubstantiated claims that it eliminates mouth odors, cleans teeth, and "conditions" gums. The active ingredient is chlorine dioxide, which is also used as an algicide in swimming pools.

Some dentists assert that facial pain, heart disease, arthritis, chronic fatigue, and various other problems are caused by infected "cavitations," within the jaw bones, that are not detectable on x-ray examination or treatable with antibiotics. Advocates call this condition "cavitational osteopathosis" or "neuralgia-inducing cavitational osteonecrosis (NICO)" and claim they can cure the patient by locating and scraping out the affected tissues. They may also remove all root-canal-treated teeth and most of the vital teeth close to the area where they say an infection exists. There is no scientific evidence to support this assertion or the diagnostic and treatment methods based on it.[43] Proponents have formed the American Academy of Biological Dentistry.

The Mercury Scare

Mercury is a component of the amalgam used for "silver" fillings. The other major ingredients are silver, tin, copper, and zinc. When mixed, these elements bond to form a strong, stable substance. Very sensitive instruments can detect billionths of a gram of mercury vapor in the mouth of a person with amalgam fillings.

Some dentists claim that the mercury in amalgam fillings is toxic and causes a wide range of problems, including multiple sclerosis, arthritis, headaches, Parkinson's disease, and emotional stress. They recommend that amalgam fillings be replaced with either gold or plastic ones and that vitamin supplements be taken to prevent trouble during the process. These dentists typically use an industrial mercury detector to indicate that "toxic" amounts of mercury are being released. To use the device, the dentist asks the patient to chew vigorously for 10 minutes, which may cause tiny amounts of mercury to be released from the fillings. Although this exposure lasts just a few seconds and most of the mercury is exhaled rather than absorbed by the body, the machine gives a readout that the dentist interprets as dangerous.[44]

The most commonly used device multiplies the amount of mercury it detects in a small sample of air by a factor of 8000. This gives a reading for a cubic meter, a volume far greater than the human mouth. The proper

◆ **Personal Glimpse** ◆

Toxic Television

In 1990 CBS-TV's "60 Minutes" aired a half-hour program called "Poison in Your Mouth," which suggested that mercury-amalgam fillings were dangerous. The most powerful segment featured a woman who said that her symptoms of multiple sclerosis had disappeared overnight after her fillings were taken out. The fact that multiple sclerosis normally has ups and downs was not mentioned during the program. Nor did the program mention that the removal process temporarily raises the body's mercury load and could not possibly cause an overnight cure.[45] The broadcast induced many viewers to seek replacement of their fillings with other materials.

Consumer Reports responded with an article that concluded: "Given their solid track record and a risk that's still conjecture, amalgam fillings are still your best bet."[51] A few months later, a reader responded:

My mother, who was diagnosed with Lou Gehrig's disease more than two years ago, had her mercury fillings removed immediately after the show aired. After she had spent $10,000 and endured more than 18 hours of dental work so painful she once fainted in the waiting room, her condition did not improve. The pain was outweighed only by the monumental disappointment she and the whole family experienced as we lived through one more false hope.

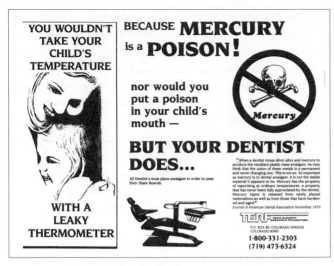

FIGURE 7-4. Misleading flyer from Hal A. Huggins, D.D.S., the leading anti-amalgamist. Whereas the mercury in thermometers is pure, the mercury in amalgam fillings is chemically bound and is not released into the body in significant amounts. Also, no toxic effects have been reported in cases where a thermometer has broken while someone's temperature is being taken.

way to determine mercury exposure is to measure blood and urine levels, which indicate how much has been absorbed by the body. Scientific testing has shown that the amount of mercury absorbed from fillings is only a small fraction of the average daily intake from food and is far below the level that exerts any adverse health effect.[46,47] In 1992 an extensive review by the U.S. Public Health Service[48] concluded that it was inappropriate to recommend restricting the use of dental amalgam. The ADA Council on Ethics, Bylaws, and Judicial Affairs considers the unnecessary removal of silver-amalgam fillings "improper and unethical."[49]

The most outspoken advocate of "mercury-amalgam toxicity" has been Hal A. Huggins, D.D.S., of Colorado Springs, Colorado (see Figure 7-4). Huggins has also targeted root canal therapy, claiming that it can make people susceptible to arthritis, multiple sclerosis, amyotrophic lateral sclerosis, and other autoimmune diseases. As with amalgam fillings, there is no objective evidence that teeth treated with root canal therapy have any adverse effect on the immune system or any other system or part of the body. Huggins's dental license was revoked in 1996. During the revocation proceedings the administrative law judge concluded (a) Huggins had diagnosed "mercury toxicity" in all patients who consulted him in his office, even some without mercury fillings; (b) he had also recommended extraction of all teeth that had had root canal therapy; and (c) Huggins's treatments were "a sham, illusory and without scientific basis."[50]

SMOKELESS PRODUCTS

Chewing tobacco and snuff contain tobacco leaf and various sweeteners and flavorings. Nicotine from the tobacco is absorbed into the bloodstream and produces mental effects described by users as relaxing or stimulating. The popularity of these products—especially among teenagers—is related to advertising that associates use of the products with macho images and athletic prowess.

Smokeless tobacco can cause bad breath, decreased ability to taste, tooth discoloration and decay, and recession of the gums (especially where the tobacco is habitually placed). Smokeless products contain three types of chemicals known to produce cancer in animals: polycyclic aromatic hydrocarbons, nitrosamines, and polonium 210, which is radioactive. A 1988 study found that 46% of 423 professional baseball players who had used smokeless products within the previous week had precancerous changes (leukoplakia) in their mucous membranes.[52] Smokeless tobacco causes about 6000 deaths per year from cancer.[53] Although this number is far less than the total death rate attributable to cigarette smoking, Dr. Gregory Connolly, director of the dental division of the Massachusetts Department of Public Health, calls smokeless tobacco use "a chemical time bomb ticking in the mouths of hundreds of thousands of boys in this country."

The nicotine content of smokeless tobacco makes it highly addictive. Some users even keep it in their mouth while sleeping. A study conducted at East Carolina University found that only one of 41 participants at "quit-smokeless-tobacco" clinics was able to stop for more than 4 hours. Other chemicals are believed to pose risks to the developing baby when smokeless products are used during pregnancy.

The Comprehensive Smokeless Tobacco Health Education Act of 1986 requires manufacturers of chewing tobacco and snuff to include the following warnings on package labels:

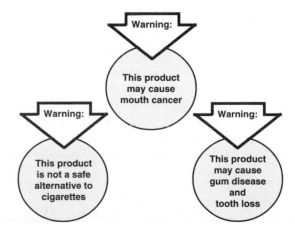

Rep. Henry Waxman (D-CA), who played a major role in passage of the law, expressed hope that the warning labels would make it obvious to children that "smokeless tobacco products are not bubblegum."

CHOOSING A DENTIST

Good dentists take a personal interest in patients and their health. They are prevention-oriented but not faddists. They use x-ray films and probably suggest a full-mouth study unless suitable films are available from the patient's previous dentists. According to Dodes:

Dental work can last a lifetime but, unfortunately, this is not always the case. In a good dentist's office the vast majority of work lasts a very long time, while in the office of Dr. Poorwork the majority of dental work falls out or decays out in a few years. The price of dental work is not the best way to judge quality; rather, pay attention to the time the dentist takes to do the work. High-quality dentistry cannot be done assembly-line style; it takes time and meticulous attention to detail.

A thorough dental examination includes inspection of the teeth, gums, tongue, lips, inside of the cheek, palate, and the skin of the face and neck, plus palpation of the neck for abnormal lymph nodes and enlargement of the thyroid gland. In adults a periodontal probe should be inserted between the gums and teeth to detect abnormally large crevices. Good dentists also chart their findings in detail. The frequency of maintenance care (including calculus removal and x-ray examinations) should be based on an assessment of the frequency of cavity formation, the rate of calculus formation, the condition of the gums, and any other special problem.

Once current treatment has been completed, the patient should be placed on a recall schedule and notified when the next checkup is due.

Friedman[4] warns that flamboyant advertising is likely to signify an emphasis on mass production rather than quality care. When the fees charged per service are low, the number of services performed may be greater than needed, resulting in higher overall cost. He also states that dentists who advertise "twilight sleep," cosmetic dentistry, and one-visit comprehensive treatment are seldom interested in long-term maintenance care that does not generate high income. He recommends avoiding dentists who use intravenous sedation; recommend automatic amalgam replacement; or "specialize" in cosmetic dentistry or in treating headaches, backaches, myofacial pain, or TMJ problems.

It makes sense to become acquainted with a family dentist before an emergency arises. You should not be embarrassed to ask about fees and payment plans. Most dentists prefer patients to initiate discussion of fees because patients know more about their own financial situation.

Consumers Research[54] offers these questions for judging a dentist's skills after you have received treatment:

- How does your bite feel?
- Is any of the dental work irritating your gum?
- Does the treated tooth look like a tooth?
- Does dental floss or your tongue catch on the tooth?
- Did the dentist take time to polish your fillings?
- Do you feel pain when drinking hot or cold liquids?
- Was any debris left in your mouth after treatment?
- Does the dentist use a water spray to cool your teeth while drilling?

In 1996, a reporter on assignment for the *Reader's Digest* visited 50 dentists in 28 states and found that their fees, examinations, and recommendations varied widely. The visits cost from $20 to $141. The reporter brought along his own x-ray films and told the dentists he had ample insurance coverage. Only 21 of the 50 dentists conducted cancer screening as recommended by the American Dental Association, and only 14 did the recommended periodontal screening. Before embarking on the study, the reporter was checked by Dr. Dodes and three other dentists who agreed that he had only one immediate problem (one molar needed filling

---

☑ **Consumer Tip**

Suggestions for Choosing a Dentist

- Friends, neighbors, or co-workers may be asked to recommend dentists with whom they are pleased.
- If there is a dental school in the area, faculty members may be able to suggest practitioners in the community.
- The dental department of a nearby hospital with an accredited dental service should be able to offer suggestions.
- The local dental society or an ADA Directory, copies of which can be found in dental school libraries and many public libraries, may be helpful.
- Your family physician may be able to recommend a dentist.
- Visiting a prospective dentist's office before making an appointment may reveal whether it is clean and run efficiently.
- Avoid dentists who purport to be "holistic" or who sell vitamins, use acupuncture or "electro-diagnosis," or say that fluoridation or mercury-amalgam filings are dangerous.

It's Your Decision

1. Your gums have started to bleed when you brush your teeth. Which of the following actions should you take?

	Reason
_____ Stop brushing your teeth	_____
_____ Use a new toothbrush	_____
_____ Try a different toothpaste	_____
_____ Try using a mouthwash	_____
_____ Floss your teeth daily	_____
_____ Use a dental stimulant	_____

2. A dentist has suggested that all your silver-amalgam fillings should be replaced with other fillings because of health dangers from the mercury found in your fillings. The dentist also states that you need to take vitamin supplements while this change is taking place. Should you follow this advice or look for another dentist? Why?

---

or a crown), and that work on another tooth might be advisable. Only 12 of the dentists agreed with this appraisal, and 15 failed to note a problem with the molar. One dentist recommended crowning all of the reporter's teeth, at a cost of $13,440. Other estimates ranged from $500 to $29,850. The reporter also visited a dental school clinic where a student and a department chairman independently recommended capping both teeth, which would cost $460. When asked how consumers can protect themselves from overtreatment and overcharging, an ADA adviser suggested seeking a second or third opinion so they can have comfort with the practitioner's recommendations, particularly if there is a lot of work to be done. The reporter replied: "I got 50 opinions, and I am not comforted."[55]

In 1997, ABC-TV's "Prime Time Live" conducted a similar investigation in which, after evaluation by an expert panel, two patients with completely healthy mouths were examined by six dentists. One patient was given estimates for $645, $1175, $1195, $2220, $2323, and $2563. The other received estimates for $2135, $2410, $2829, $3140, $3190, $3700, $4061, and $7960. No program was broadcast, but the figures were made public by one of the review panel members.[56]

SUMMARY

A combination of nutrition, oral hygiene, and professional care will enable most people to maintain their teeth in good condition throughout their life. Adequate amounts of fluoride during childhood will help make teeth resistant to decay. The most efficient way to accomplish this is through water fluoridation and the use of fluoridated toothpaste.

Daily brushing and flossing of the teeth can prevent tooth decay and periodontal disease. Professional care may include administration of sealants, removal of calculus (tartar), restoration of decayed or missing teeth, and cosmetic measures.

Most dentists provide competent care, but consumers should be alert to the signs of dental quackery. Dentists who practice "holistic" or "biological" dentistry should be avoided.

REFERENCES

1. Dodes J. Dubious dental care. New York, 1991, American Council on Science and Health.
2. Rovin S. Tooth decay: A delicate balance. Nutrition Forum 1:22–23, 1984.
3. Dannenberg JL. Vitamin C enamel loss. Journal of the American Dental Association 105:172, 1982.
4. Friedman JW and others. Complete Guide to Dental Health: How to Avoid Being Overcharged and Overtreated. New York, 1991, Consumer Reports Books.
5. Newbrun E. Effectiveness of water fluoridation. Journal of Public Health Dentistry (special issue):49(5)279–289, 1989.
6. McClure FJ. Water Fluoridation: The Search and the Victory. Washington D.C., 1970, US Department of Health, Education, and Welfare.
7. National Institute of Dental Research. The National Survey of U.S. School Children: 1986–1987. NIH Publication No. 89-2247. Washington, D.C., 1989, US Government Printing Office.
8. White BA and others. Issues in the economic evaluation of community water fluoridation. Journal of Dental Education 53:646–657, 1989.
9. Barrett S, Rovin S, editors. The Tooth Robbers: A Pro-Fluoridation Handbook. Philadelphia, 1980, George F Stickley Co.
10. Fluoridation. Consumer Reports, 43:392-396, 480–482, 1978.
11. Newbrun E. Fluorides and Dental Caries, ed 3. Springfield, Ill, 1986, Charles C Thomas.
12. Wulf C and others. Abuse of the Scientific Literature in an Antifluoridation Pamphlet, ed 2. Columbus, Ohio, 1988, American Oral Health Institute.
13. Begley S. Don't drink the water? Brush your teeth, but the fluoride from your tap may not do much good—and may cause cancer, Newsweek 115(6):60–61, 1990.
14. American Academy of Pediatrics Committee on Nutrition. Fluoride supplementation for children: interim policy recommendations. Pediatrics 95:777, 1995.
15. Review of Fluoride Benefits and Risks, Report of the Ad Hoc Subcommittee on Fluoride of the Committee to Coordinate Environmental Health and Related Programs. Washington D.C., 1991, US Public Health Service.
16. Schultz D. Fluoride: Cavity fighter on tap. FDA Consumer 26(1):34-38, 1992.
17. Barrett S. Fluoridation attacked unfairly. Nutrition Forum, 7:15, 1990.
18. Facts about fluoride, 1991, American Dental Association.

19. Fluoridation of community water systems. JAMA 267:3264–3265, 1992.

20. Weisfeld VD, editor. Preventing tooth decay: Results from a four-year national study. Special Report Number Two, 1983, Robert Wood Johnson Foundation, Princeton, N.J.

21. Periodontal diseases. Chicago, 1988, American Dental Association.

22. Which toothpaste is right for you? Consumer Reports 63:11–15, 1998.

23. American Dental Association Council on Dental Therapeutics. Accepted Dental Therapeutics. Chicago, 1984, American Dental Association.

24. A toothbrush tanning booth? Consumer Reports on Health 2:40, 1990.

25. A tough dental floss with a big price tag. Consumer Reports 58:693, 1993.

26. Mouthwashes. Consumer Reports 57:607–610, 1992.

27. Plax retracts, Plax 'pre-brushing dental rinse' promises less than it used to. What does it deliver? Consumer Reports on Health 3:21, 1991.

28. Winn DM and others. Mouthwash use and oral conditions in the risk of oral and pharyngeal cancer. Cancer Research 51:3044–3047, 1991.

29. Sears C. FDA orders tooth bleaches off market. American Health 11(1):22, 1992.

30. Bradbard L. Dental amalgam: Filling a need or foiling health? FDA Consumer 27(10):22–25, 1993.

31. American Association of Endodontists. Root canal therapy safe and effective: Focal infection ghost rises from the grave. Endodontics Fall/Winter 1994.

32. McCann D. CDT won't recommend Sargenti paste. ADA News, Oct 21, 1991.

33. McCann D. Cameras capture unlicensed dentist. ADA News, July 15, 1991.

34. Jacob JA. Survey measures free, discounted dental care provided by dentists. ADA News 27(4):22, 1996.

35. FTC warns pharmaceutical companies on unfair ads for denture products. File No 792 3155, June 18, 1979.

36. Matteson SR and others. The selection of patients for x-ray examinations: Dental radiographic examinations. HHS publications FDA 88-8273 and 8274. Washington D.C., 1988, US Government Printing Office.

37. Dodes JE, Schissel MJ. The Whole Tooth. New York, 1997, St. Martin's Press.

38. Kurzweil P. Dental more gentle with painless 'drillings' and matching fillings. FDA Consumer 33(3):18–22, 1999.

39. Lewis R. Lasers in dentistry. FDA Consumer 29(1):15–18, 1995.

40. A tale of two lasers. Consumer Reports, 56:538, 1991.

41. Dodes J, Jarvis WT. Dubious dental care. In Barrett S, Jarvis WT, editors. The Health Robbers: A Close Look at Quackery in America. Amherst, N.Y., 1993, Prometheus Books.

42. Wirth-Pattullo V, Hayes KW. Interrater reliability of craniosacral rate measurements and their relationship with subjects' and examiners' heart and respiratory rate measurements. Physical Therapy 74:908–16, 1994.

43. Dodes JE, Schissel M. Cavitational osteopathosis, NICO, and "biological dentistry." Quackwatch Web site, July 14, 2000.

44. The mercury-amalgam scare. In Barrett S and others. Health Schemes, Scams, and Frauds. New York, 1990, Consumer Reports Books.

45. Barrett S. Toxic television: The mercury amalgam scam. Priorities for Health, pp 35–37, Fall 1991.

46. Mackert JR. Dental amalgam and mercury. Journal of the American Dental Association 122:54–61, 1991.

47. Mackert JR Jr, Berglund A. Mercury exposure from dental amalgam fillings: Absorbed dose and the potential for adverse health effects. Critical Review of Oral Biology and Medicine 8:410–436, 1997.

48. Benson JS and others. Dental Amalgam: A Scientific Review and Recommended Public Health Strategy for Research, Education and Regulation. Washington, D.C., 1993, US Public Health Service.

49. Berry JH. Questionable care: What can be done about dental quackery? Journal of the American Dental Association 115:679–685, 1987.

50. Connick N. Initial decision in the matter of the disciplinary proceedings regarding the license to practice dentistry in the State of Colorado of Hal A. Huggins, D.D.S., Feb 29, 1996.

51. The mercury in your mouth. Consumer Reports 56:316–319, 1991.

52. Ernster VL and others. Smokeless tobacco use and health effects among baseball players. JAMA 264:218-224, 1990.

53. Rodu B, Cole P, Tomar SL. Would a switch from cigarettes to smokeless tobacco benefit public health? Priorities 7(4):24–30, 1996.

54. How to choose a dentist. Consumers Research, March 1997, pp 20–24.

55. Ecenbarger W. How honest are dentists? Reader's Digest, Feb 1997, pp 50-56.

56. Dodes J. Coverage questioned (letter to the editor). ADA News, Sept 15, 1997.

"ALTERNATIVE" METHODS

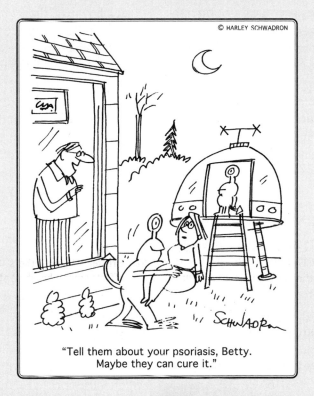

"Tell them about your psoriasis, Betty. Maybe they can cure it."

Every system—be it based on the position of the stars, the pattern of lines in the hand, the shape of the face or skull, the fall of the cards or the dice, the accidents of nature, or the intuitions of a "psychic"—claims its quota of satisfied customers.

RAY HYMAN, PH.D.[1]

All of us are exposed daily to many ideas about health, some of which are accurate and some not. . . . When you are well, unless you are taken in to an extreme degree, what you believe may not matter much. But if you have a health problem—particularly a serious one—misplacing your trust can seriously harm you or others who rely upon your judgment.

STEPHEN BARRETT, M.D.
VICTOR HERBERT, M.D., J.D.[2]

Erythromycin is an alternative to penicillin, but a pogo stick is not an alternative to an automobile.

JOHN E. DODES, D.D.S.
MARVIN J. SCHISSEL, D.D.S.[3]

"Alternative medicine" has become the politically correct term for questionable practices formerly consigned to the categories of health fraud and quackery. Alternative medicine defines itself by what it is *not*. It is *not* part of standard (science-based) medicine in the United States. The science-based medical community is committed to testing its theories and practices and accepts the accountability required by consumer protection laws. A primary feature of the scientific process is willingness to examine new ideas. However, the openmindedness of science is not empty-headedness. Enough is known about many "alternative" practices to evaluate their worth. Some services referred to as "alternative" or "complementary" may be appropriately used as part of the art of patient care or as self-care. Relaxation techniques and massage are examples. But procedures linked to belief systems that reject science itself have no place in responsible medicine.

A complete listing of "alternative" methods would be a monumental task, if not an impossible one. This chapter focuses on methods that have been widely publicized. Chapters 6, 7, 12, 13, 15, 16, 17, 18, and 23 cover additional practices related to mental health, dental care, nutrition, weight control, cardiovascular disease, arthritis, cancer, AIDS, and aging. Chapter 3 discusses the general characteristics of quackery and health fraud.

DEFINITIONAL PROBLEMS

The dictionary definition of the noun "alternative" is a choice between mutually exclusive possibilities. Until the late 1980s, in standard medical usage it referred to choices among effective treatments. In some cases they were equally effective (for example, the use of radiation or surgery for certain cancers); in others the expected outcome differed, but there were reasonable tradeoffs between risks and benefits. During recent years, however, the word "alternative" has been applied to a multitude of unsubstantiated approaches.

In a widely publicized 1993 report, researchers from Harvard Medical School defined "unconventional therapies" as "medical interventions neither taught widely in U.S. medical schools nor generally available at U.S. hospitals."[4] Subsequently the authors, the news media, and many government officials began using the words "unconventional" and "alternative" interchangeably. Later the Harvard group defined "alternative medicine" as "practices explicitly used for the purpose of medical intervention, health prevention, or disease prevention which are not routinely taught at U.S. medical schools nor routinely underwritten by third-party payers within the existing U.S. health care system."

The 1993 report stated that one out of three Americans was using unconventional care. However, this figure was inflated by counting exercise, relaxation, self-help groups, and commercial weight-loss clinics as "alternative," even though they involve practices that are medically accepted.[5] A more recent analysis of practitioner use concluded that 6.5% of Americans used both unconventional and conventional practitioners; 1.8% used only unconventional services; 59.5% used only conventional care; and 32.2% used neither.[6]

"Alternative" methods do not lend themselves to simple classification. A report prepared by proponents under the auspices of the National Institutes of Health Office of Alternative Medicine has categorized "alternative medicine" into six "fields of practice": (1) mind-body interventions, (2) bioelectromagnetic applications, (3) alternative systems of medical practice, (4) manual healing methods, (5) herbal medicine, and (6) diet and nutrition in the prevention and treatment of chronic disease.[7] However, a few methods encompassed by these fields have scientific support and should not be classified as "alternative."

Skrabanek and McCormick[8] have suggested that the distinguishing features of "alternative medicine" are (a) it does not derive from a coherent or established body of evidence, and (b) it is not subjected to rigorous assessment to establish its value.

Critics are concerned that "alternative" methods are promoted as equivalent or superior to standard methods even though they are not. Barrett and Herbert[9] have proposed that alternatives be classified as genuine, experimental, or questionable. Under this system, *genuine* alternatives are comparable methods that have met science-based criteria for safety and effectiveness; *experimental* alternatives are unproven but have a plausible rationale and are undergoing responsible investigation; and *questionable* "alternatives" are groundless and lack a scientifically plausible rationale. In line with this proposal, this textbook places the word "alternative" in quotes when referring to methods that are unproven and scientifically implausible. Classifying proven therapies as "alternative" is advantageous to proponents who suggest that if some work, the rest deserve equal consideration and respect.

Whether something should be classified as "alternative" depends not only on the method itself but also on how it is used and what claims are made for it.

☑ Consumer Tip

Questions to Use for Evaluating "Alternative" Methods

- Of what does the method consist?
- Is it testable? Can its effects be measured?
- Do its theories or practices clash with what is known?
- Is it based on vitalistic theory?
- Is it claimed to be a complete system of diagnosis and/or treatment?
- Is its scope said to be limited or unlimited?
- What evidence is there that it helps? Has scientific testing proven that it is more effective than doing nothing or using a placebo?
- What evidence is there that it harms? Has it been demonstrated that its potential benefit exceeds any potential for harm?
- Do its practitioners use standard diagnostic terminology? Are the conditions it claims to treat recognized by medical science?
- Are its practitioners adequately trained to make standard diagnoses and to stay within their scope?
- If you cannot answer all the above questions, how can you obtain the necessary information?

Spinal manipulation, for example, can be useful in properly selected cases of low-back pain. But manipulating the spine once a month for "preventive maintenance" or to promote general health—as many chiropractors recommend—is questionable. Relaxation techniques have a limited but acceptable role in the treatment of anxiety states. But meditation for the purpose of "balancing" one's "life energy" is another matter. Consideration of herbal products is even more complicated (see Chapter 12). The vast number of available products include some that have proven usefulness, some that are toxic, and many that have no plausible medical use.

When challenged about the lack of scientific evidence supporting questionable methods, their advocates typically claim that they lack the money or time to do research. However, preliminary research is simple to carry out and can be incorporated into clinical practice. The principal ingredients are careful clinical observations, detailed record-keeping, and long-term follow-up "to keep score." "Alternative" practitioners rarely do these things. Should scientific studies be performed and come out negative, proponents claim that the studies were conducted improperly or that the evaluators were biased.

"Alternative" advocates often cite a 1978 Office of Technology Assessment (OTA) report which stated that "only 10 to 20 percent of procedures currently used in medical practice have been shown to be efficacious by controlled trial."[10] The sole basis for this statement was a survey of the prescribing practices of 19 British family physicians over two 1-week periods in 1960 and 1961.[11] Since the OTA report was published, the percentage of medical treatments validated by controlled trials has increased. Many other practices have a logical basis and are supported by careful observations. A recent analysis concluded that 90 (82%) of the treatments prescribed for 109 hospitalized British patients were based on controlled studies or other persuasive evidence.[12] Most alternative procedures are supported by little more than wishful thinking.

Practitioners of "complementary" or "integrative" medicine claim to synthesize standard and alternative methods, using the best of both. However, no published data indicate the quality of such care or the extent to which they burden patients with medically useless methods. Typically these practitioners employ a "heads-I-win, tails-you-lose" strategy in which they claim credit for any improvement experienced by the patient and blame standard treatments for any negative effects. The result may be to undermine the patient's confidence in standard care, reducing compliance or causing the patient to abandon it altogether.[13]

The "integrated" concept has been further criticized by Arnold Relman, M.D., former editor of *The New England Journal of Medicine*:

There are not two kinds of medicine, one conventional and the other unconventional, that can be practiced jointly in a new kind of "integrative medicine." Nor . . . are there two kinds of thinking, or two ways to find out which treatments work and which do not. In the best kind of medical practice, all proposed treatments must be tested objectively. In the end, there will only be treatments that pass that test and those that do not, those that are proven worthwhile and those that are not.[14]

Many "alternative" approaches are rooted in *vitalism*, the concept that bodily functions are due to a vital principle or "life force" distinct from the physical forces explainable by the laws of physics and chemistry. Non-scientific health systems based on this philosophy maintain that diseases should be treated by "stimulating the body's ability to heal itself" rather than by "treating symptoms." Homeopaths, for example, claim that illness is due to a disturbance of the body's "vital force," which they can correct with special remedies, whereas acupuncturists claim that disease is due to imbalance in the flow of "life energy" (*chi* or *qi*), which they can balance by twirling needles in the skin. Many chiropractors claim to assist the body's "Innate Intelligence" by adjusting the patient's spine. Naturopaths speak of "Vis Medicatrix Naturae." Ayurvedic physicians refer to *prana*. And so on. The "energies" postulated by vitalists are not objectively measurable.

Although vitalists often pretend to be scientific, they really reject the scientific method with its basic

Historical Perspective

Folk (Traditional) Medicine

Webster's *New Collegiate Dictionary* defines folk medicine as "traditional medicine as practiced non-professionally by people isolated from modern medical services and involving especially the use of vegetable remedies on an empirical basis." Traditional medicine is largely primitive medicine, which assumes that supernatural forces are responsible for both the cause and cure of disease. Even herbal remedies may be said to harbor either good or evil spirits, so that believers can explain failures or successes in supernatural terms.

Curanderas, popular among Mexican-Americans, are regarded as specialists in the folk medicine of their people. The conditions they treat include *mal ojo* ("evil eye"), *mal air* ("bad air" due to evil spirits or other forces believed to inhabit the air), *bilis* (anger), *susto* (fright), and diseases of "hot and cold imbalance." Their ministrations include prayers, religious objects, herbs, and dietary measures.

Powwow, centered in rural Pennsylvania, combines prayer and laying on of hands. They may touch an afflicted part lightly, rub the surrounding area vigorously, or pass their hands over the entire body while praying either quietly or aloud. Some practitioners sell charms, spells, potions, and other paraphernalia. Some prescribe and sell herbs and teas.

Root doctors, found mainly in southeastern states, are consulted by people who believe they have been "hexed" or have had unduly bad luck. The "doctor" listens to their story and either prepares a token, charm, powder, or other special object ("root") that can help them fulfill their wishes or helps them undo the hex.

Voodoo, a religion indigenous to Haiti, is also practiced in southern Louisiana and elsewhere in the United States where Haitians have migrated. Derived from ancestor worship, it invokes spirits to explain and influence the course of events. It includes an elaborate system of folk medical practices. Voodoo "queens" and "doctors" also sell charms, magical powders, and amulets promised to help cure illness, and grant other desires.

Folk medicine, even when known to be erroneous, is not generally considered quackery so long as it is not done for gain. Thus self-treatment, family home treatment, neighborly medical advice, and the non-commercial activities of folk healers should not be labeled as quackery. State laws against practicing medicine without a license are rarely enforced against folk healers.

However, folk medicine and quackery are closely connected because folk medicine often provides a basis for commercial exploitation. For example, herbs long gathered for personal use have been packaged and promoted by modern entrepreneurs, and practitioners who once served their neighbors voluntarily or for gratuities may market themselves outside their traditional communities.

Folk beliefs may influence the ability or willingness of a patient to cooperate with or respond to scientific treatment. Some science-based programs have enlisted folk healers to help gain the trust of people who have little knowledge of medical care. DeSmet[15] has noted that some folk remedies have therapeutic benefits, some may provide psychosocial benefits, and others (such as azarcón powder, rattlesnake meat, and certain herbal teas) can produce serious adverse reactions. Young[16] has noted that scientific medicine discards inferior therapies as science advances, but folk medicine and quackery continue to use these as long as a demand persists.

assumptions of material reality, mechanisms of cause and effect, and testability of hypotheses. They regard personal experience, subjective judgment, and emotional satisfaction as preferable to objectivity and unbiased evidence.

It is often suggested that people seek "alternatives" because doctors are brusque, and that if doctors were more attentive their patients would not look elsewhere. It is true that doctors sometimes pay insufficient attention to the emotional needs of their patients. But some people's needs exceed what scientific health care can provide. A Canadian study of children attending an outpatient clinic found that word of mouth, fear of drug side effects, and persistence of a medical problem were more significant than dissatisfaction with conventional medicine in influencing their parents' decision to seek "alternative" care.[17] A New Zealand study of 148 cancer patients using "alternative" approaches found that most were satisfied with conventional medicine and used alternative therapy only as a supplement.[18]

Misleading publicity also plays an important role. Few media outlets place "alternative" methods in proper perspective; and most reports feature the claims of proponents and satisfied customers. A writer who monitored print and broadcast media for the National Center for Homeopathy concluded that, during 1994 and 1995, only 9% of more than 1000 mentions of homeopathy were critical.[19] Critical analyses of acupuncture, ayurveda, chelation therapy, chiropractic, macrobiotics, and naturopathy are even scarcer.

ACUPUNCTURE, QIGONG, AND CHINESE MEDICINE

"Chinese medicine," often called "Oriental medicine" or "traditional Chinese medicine (TCM)," encompasses a vast array of folk medical practices based on ancient cosmologic beliefs.[20] It holds that the body's vital energy (*chi* or *qi*) circulates through 14 channels, called *meridians*, that have branches connected to bodily organs and functions.[21] Illness is attributed to imbalance or interruption of *chi* (Figure 8-1). Practices such as acupuncture and Qigong are claimed to restore balance.

Traditional acupuncture, as now practiced, involves the insertion of stainless steel needles into various body areas. A low-frequency current may be applied to the needles to produce greater stimulation. Other procedures used separately or together with acupuncture include moxibustion (burning of floss or herbs applied to the skin); injection of sterile water, procaine, morphine, vitamins, or homeopathic solutions through the inserted needles; applications of laser beams (laserpuncture); placement of needles in the external ear (auriculo-

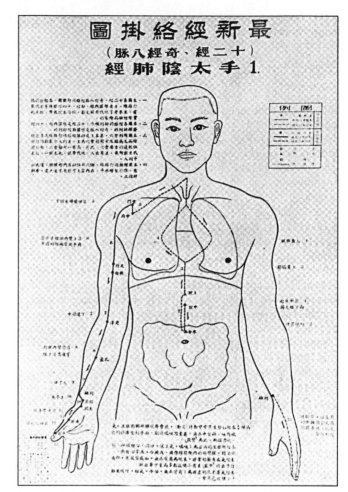

FIGURE 8-1. Acupuncture chart. This chart identifies the locations for treating the lungs. The lung "meridian" is shown running along the inner arm and into the sholulder.

therapy); and acupressure (use of manual pressure). Treatment is applied to "acupuncture points," which are said to be located throughout the body. Skrabanek[22] has noted that originally there were 365 such points, corresponding to the days of the year, but the number identified by proponents during the past 2000 years has increased gradually to over 2000. Some practitioners place needles at or near the site of disease, whereas others select points on the basis of symptoms. In traditional acupuncture a combination of points is usually used.

Qigong is also claimed to influence the flow of "vital energy." Internal Qigong involves deep breathing, concentration, and relaxation techniques used by individuals for themselves. External Qigong is performed by "Qigong masters" who claim to cure a wide variety of diseases with energy released from their fingertips. However, scientific investigators of Qigong masters in China have found no evidence of paranormal powers and some evidence of deception. They found, for example, that a patient lying on a table about

8 feet from a Qigong master moved rhythmically or thrashed about as the master moved his hands. But when she was placed so that she could no longer see him, her movements were unrelated to his.[23]

Some acupuncturists espouse the traditional Chinese view of health and disease and consider acupuncture, herbal medicine, and related practices to be valid approaches to the full gamut of disease. Others reject the traditional approach and merely claim that acupuncture offers a simple way to achieve pain relief. The diagnostic process used by practitioners of Chinese medicine may include questioning (medical history, lifestyle), observations (skin, tongue, color), listening (breathing sounds), and pulse-taking. Six pulse aspects said to correlate with body organs or functions are checked to determine which meridians are "deficient" in *chi*. (Medical science recognizes only one pulse, corresponding to the heartbeat, which can be felt in the wrist, neck, feet, and several other places.) Some acupuncturists state that the electrical properties of the body may become imbalanced weeks or even months before symptoms occur.[24] These practitioners claim that acupuncture can be used to treat conditions when the patient just "doesn't feel right," even though no disease is apparent.

The conditions claimed to respond to acupuncture include chronic pain (neck and back pain, migraine headaches), acute injury-related pain (strains, muscle and ligament tears), gastrointestinal problems (indigestion, ulcers, constipation, diarrhea), cardiovascular conditions (high and low blood pressure), genitourinary problems (menstrual irregularity, frigidity, impotence), muscle and nerve conditions (paralysis, deafness), and behavioral problems (overeating, drug dependence, smoking). However, the evidence supporting these claims consists mostly of practitioners' observations and poorly designed studies.[25] A controlled study found that electroacupuncture of the ear was no more effective than placebo stimulation (light touching) against chronic pain.[26] In 1990 three Dutch epidemiologists analyzed 51 controlled studies of acupuncture for chronic pain and concluded that "the quality of even the better studies proved to be mediocre. . . . The efficacy of acupuncture in the treatment of chronic pain remains doubtful."[27] They also examined reports of acupuncture used to treat addictions to cigarettes, heroin, and alcohol, and concluded that claims that acupuncture is effective as a therapy for these conditions are not supported by sound clinical research.[28]

Acupuncture anesthesia is not used for surgery in the Orient to the extent that its proponents suggest. In China physicians screen out patients who appear to be unsuitable. Acupuncture is not used for emergency surgery and often is accompanied by local anesthesia or narcotic medication.

How acupuncture may relieve pain is unclear. One theory suggests that pain impulses are blocked from reaching the spinal cord or brain at various "gates" to these areas. Another theory suggests that acupuncture stimulates the body to produce narcotic-like substances called *endorphins*, which reduce pain. Other theories suggest that the placebo effect, external suggestion (hypnosis), and cultural conditioning are important factors. Melzack and Wall[29] note that pain relief produced by acupuncture can also be produced by many other types of sensory hyperstimulation, such as electricity and heat at acupuncture points and elsewhere in the body. They conclude that "the effectiveness of all of these forms of stimulation indicates that acupuncture is not a magical procedure but only one of many ways to produce analgesia [pain relief] by an intense sensory input." In 1981 the American Medical Association Council on Scientific Affairs[30] noted that pain relief does not occur consistently or reproducibly in most people and does not operate at all in some people.

In 1985 George A. Ulett, M.D., Ph.D., Clinical Professor of Psychiatry, University of Missouri School of Medicine, stated that "devoid of metaphysical thinking, acupuncture becomes a rather simple technique that can be useful as a nondrug method of pain control."[31] He believes that the traditional Chinese variety is primarily a placebo treatment, but electrical stimulation of about 80 acupuncture points has been proven useful for pain control.[32,33] In a recent book he stated:

The concept of *meridians* is important only as a hypothetical construct invented for the support of a metaphysical theory involving the manipulation of *chi*. . . . Believers in unconventional healing methods that lack any proven scientific basis have attributed great physiological significance to *chi* and to these imaginary conduits, and have used the *meridian* concept to support arcane beliefs such as reflexology, tongue diagnosis, and *chakras*.[34]

Improperly performed acupuncture can cause fainting, local hematoma (due to bleeding from a punctured blood vessel), pneumothorax (punctured lung), convulsions, local infections, hepatitis B (from unsterile needles), bacterial endocarditis, contact dermatitis, and nerve damage. The herbs used by acupuncture practitioners are not regulated for safety, potency, or effectiveness. There is also risk that an acupuncturist whose approach to diagnosis is not based on scientific concepts will fail to diagnose a dangerous condition.

The data on adverse effects are conflicting. A survey of 1135 Norwegian physicians revealed 66 cases of

The Limitations of Accreditation

In the United States, educational standards are set by a network of agencies approved by the U.S. Office of Education (USOE) or the Council on Recognition of Postsecondary Accreditation (CORPA). Accreditation constitutes public recognition that an educational program meets the administrative, organizational, and financial criteria of a reviewing body recognized by one of these agencies. USOE or CORPA do not accredit individual schools, but they approve the national and regional agencies that do so. Almost all such agencies are voluntary and nongovernmental. Accreditation enables credits to be transferable from one school to another and is used as a basis for entering various professions.

Accreditation has been a powerful impetus to quality education. But in recent years the system has been compromised by USOE recognition of agencies that oversee unscientific teachings. USOE recognition is supposed to mean that an accrediting agency is "a reliable authority as to the quality of training offered."[35] However, the criteria are primarily organizational. To achieve recognition, the agency must be national or regional in scope and must have appropriate bylaws, procedures, institutional and public representation, "reliability," and autonomy. Individual schools, in turn, must meet criteria set by the recognized agency. The criteria do not include scientific validity. Although much of what is taught in chiropractic, naturopathic, and acupuncture schools is questionable, agencies for each have been recognized. While the naturopathic agency was undergoing evaluation for renewal, a USOE official actually said that if astrologers could get the required paperwork in order, they too could get an agency approved.[36]

infection, 25 cases of punctured lung, 31 cases of increased pain, and 80 other cases with complications.[37] A parallel survey of 197 acupuncturists, who are more apt to see immediate complications, yielded 132 cases of fainting, 26 cases of increased pain, eight cases of pneumothorax, and 45 other adverse results.[37] On the other hand, a 5-year study involving 76 acupuncturists at a Japanese medical facility tabulated only 64 adverse event reports (including 16 forgotten needles and 13 cases of transient low blood pressure) associated with 55,591 acupuncture treatments. No serious complications were reported. The researchers concluded that serious adverse reactions are uncommon among acupuncturists who are medically trained.[38]

In 1971 an acupuncture boom occurred in the United States because of stories about visits to China by various American dignitaries. Entrepreneurs, both medical and nonmedical, began using flamboyant advertising techniques to promote clinics, seminars, demonstrations, books, correspondence courses, and do-it-yourself kits. Today some states restrict the practice of acupuncture to physicians or others operating under their direct supervision. In 20 states people who lack medical training can perform acupuncture without medical supervision. The U.S. Food and Drug Administration (FDA) now classifies acupuncture needles as Class II medical devices and requires labeling for one-time use by practitioners who are legally authorized to use them.[39] This classification merely addresses safety and does not authorize marketing them with health claims. Acupuncture is not covered under Medicare.

An attempt is being made to set standards through voluntary certification by the National Commission for the Certification of Acupuncturists (NCCA). Several thousand practitioners have become certified, and some states have adopted the NCCA examination as all or part of their criteria for licensing. The credentials used by acupuncturists include C.A. (certified acupuncturist), M.A. (master acupuncturist), D.A. (diplomate of acupuncture), and O.M.D. (doctor of Oriental medicine). These credentials are not recognized by the scientific community. In 1990 the U.S. Secretary of Education

☑ Consumer Tip

Be Wary of Acupuncture

- Acupuncture is an invasive procedure (penetrates the skin). Although the complication rate is low, acupuncture can cause serious complications.
- Many practitioners of acupuncture do not have adequate training and use unscientific approaches to the diagnosis and treatment of health problems.
- There is no evidence that acupuncture can influence the course of any organic disease.
- Pain relief from acupuncture, if it occurs, is likely to be short-lived.
- Consumers who wish to try acupuncture should choose a practitioner who is medically trained and does not espouse "Chinese medicine" or any other nonscientific approach described in this chapter.

recognized the National Accreditation Commission for Schools and Colleges of Acupuncture and Oriental Medicine as an accrediting agency. However, such recognition is not based on the scientific validity of what is taught but upon other criteria.

The National Council Against Health Fraud (NCAHF) has concluded: (a) acupuncture is an unproven modality of treatment; (b) its theory and practice are based on primitive and fanciful concepts of health and disease that bear no relationship to scientific knowledge; (c) research has not demonstrated that acupuncture is effective against any disease; (d) perceived effects of acupuncture are probably due to a combination of expectation, suggestion, counter-irritation, conditioning, and other psychologic mechanisms; (e) the use of acupuncture should be restricted to appropriate research settings; (f) insurance companies should not be required by law to cover acupuncture treatment; (g) licensure of lay acupuncturists should be phased out; and (h) consumers who wish to try acupuncture should discuss their situation with a knowledgeable physician who has no commercial interest.[25]

In 1997, a Consensus Development Conference sponsored by the National Institutes of Health and several other agencies concluded that "there is sufficient evidence . . . of acupuncture's value to expand its use into conventional medicine and to encourage further studies of its physiology and clinical value."[40] The panelists also suggested that the federal government and insurance companies expand coverage of acupuncture so more people can have access to it. These conclusions were not based on research done after NCAHF's position paper was published. Rather, they reflected the bias of the panelists who were selected by a planning committee dominated by acupuncture proponents.[41] Wallace Sampson, M.D., who edits the *Scientific Review of Alternative Medicine*, has described the conference "a consensus of proponents, not a consensus of valid scientific opinion."

REFLEXOLOGY

Reflexology, often called zone therapy, is based on the notion that pressing on the hands or feet can help relieve pain and remove the underlying cause of disease in other parts of the body. Most proponents claim that (a) the body is divided into 10 zones that begin or end in the hands and feet; (b) each organ or part of the body is represented on the hands and feet; (c) the practitioner can diagnose abnormalities by feeling the feet; and (d) massaging or pressing each area can stimulate the

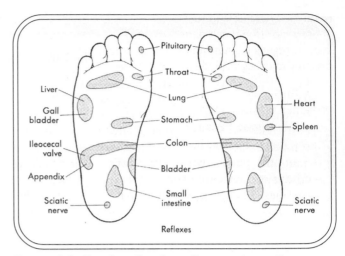

FIGURE 8-2. Simple reflexology diagram. According to proponents, pressing on the shaded areas influences the parts of the body listed.

flow of energy, blood, nutrients, and nerve impulses to the corresponding body zone. Their fees typically range from $35 to $100 per session.

One prominent proponent claims that foot reflexology can cleanse the body of toxins, increase circulation, assist in weight loss, and improve the health of organs throughout the body. Other proponents have reported success in treating earaches, anemia, bedwetting, bronchitis, convulsions in an infant, hemorrhoids, hiccups, deafness, hair loss, emphysema, prostate trouble, heart disease, overactive thyroid gland, kidney stones, liver trouble, rectal prolapse, undescended testicles, intestinal paralysis, cataracts, and hydrocephalus (a condition in which an excess of fluid surrounding the brain can cause pressure that damages the brain). One practitioner even claims to have lengthened a leg that was an inch shorter than the other. Figure 8-2 shows a simple reflexology chart.

CHIROPRACTIC

Chiropractic is a broad spectrum of practices based mainly on two notions: (1) spinal problems cause or help cause most ailments and (2) spinal manipulation can prevent or remedy a wide range of health problems. Louis Sportelli, D.C., a former chairman of the American Chiropractic Association's board of governors, has described chiropractic's basic theory as follows:

Chiropractic is a branch of the healing arts . . . based on the premise that good health depends, in part, upon a normally functioning nervous system. Body structure such as cells and organs function by the impulses carried through nerves. When these nerve impulses travel unhampered, the organs and cells of the body are able to function normally. When there is an interference (too much or not enough nerve supply), the tissues or organs cannot function properly and a state of malfunction may begin, predisposing the body to a disease state.[42]

Chiropractic is unique among nonscientific approaches because all 50 states license its practitioners. It is also unique because a small percentage of practitioners have rejected its vitalistic theories. Chiropractors can help people with certain musculoskeletal ailments, but the problems described below are widespread and, in some cases, integral to chiropractic philosophy and practice.

Historical Perspective

Various forms of spinal manipulation have been noted throughout recorded history.[43] The "discovery" of chiropractic was announced in 1895 by Daniel David ("D.D.") Palmer, a grocer, spiritualist, and "magnetic healer" who practiced in Davenport, Iowa. Palmer believed that he had restored the hearing of a deaf janitor by "adjusting" a hump on his spine. Even though the nerve that controls hearing is inside the skull and does not traverse the spine, Palmer concluded that the basic cause of disease was nerve interference caused by displaced vertebrae.[44] He originally declared that such misalignments cause abnormal tension ("tone") in the nearby nerves and that disturbed nerve tone causes 95% of all diseases. Later he elaborated a biotheology holding that: (a) "Innate Intelligence," or "nerve energy," flows throughout the nervous system and controls every bodily activity not under voluntary control; (b) even slight spinal misalignments hinder this flow, causing people to become ill; and (c) manual manipulation ("adjustment") of the spine is the remedy. He rejected the germ theory and had an aversion to drugs, surgery, and medical diagnosis.

Palmer referred to spinal "misalignments" as "luxations." A few years later a disciple began calling them "subluxations," a term that became central to chiropractic theory and is still used today. The word "chiropractic" was derived from the Greek words *cheir* (hand) and *praktikos* (practice).

Soon after his "discovery," Palmer opened a school to teach his methods to others. The basic entrance requirement, as it was in many medical schools around the turn of the century, was the ability to pay tuition.[45] One of the first students was Palmer's son, Bartlett Joshua ("B.J."), who became chiropractic's developer. In 1906 D.D. Palmer was convicted of practicing medicine without a license and spent 23 days in jail. After his release, B.J. denied him access to the school grounds and wound up purchasing D.D.'s interest in the Palmer

School of Chiropractic. At that time about 100 chiropractors were practicing. Today there are about 60,000.

Between 1913 and 1933, 40 states passed laws to license chiropractors; the remaining states gradually followed suit, with Louisiana being the last in 1974. Chiropractors have lobbied successfully in most states for laws that force insurance companies to pay for some of their services. In 1972 Congress legislated coverage under Medicare for "treatment by means of manual manipulation of the spine to correct a subluxation demonstrated by x-rays to exist." The International Chiropractors Association states that passage of this bill was spurred by more than 10 million letters received by members of Congress.[46] Data from the U.S. Department of Commerce indicate that the total reported income for chiropractic offices and clinics rose from $6.76 billion in 1994 to $7.68 billion in 1998.[47] The x-ray requirement was recently eliminated.

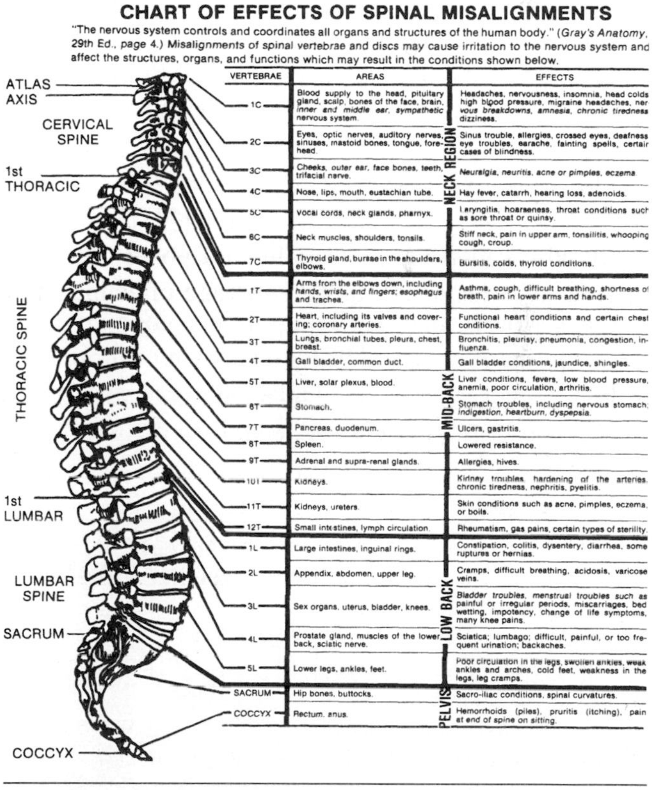

FIGURE 8-3. Chart from a chiropractic brochure. Many chiropractors use charts to reinforce the idea that spinal problems are a major cause of disease. This chart claims that "spinal misalignments" can cause more than 100 health problems, including allergies, amnesia, crossed eyes, deafness, gallbladder conditions, hernias, jaundice, and pneumonia. Other charts showing how nerves connect from the spine to the body's organs are used to persuade patients that regular spinal care is essential for good health.

Chiropractic Philosophy

National Council Against Health Fraud founder William T. Jarvis, Ph.D., whose doctoral thesis involved the study of chiropractic, notes that "chiropractic's uniqueness is not in its use of manipulation but in its theoretical basis for doing so." He describes chiropractic as "a conglomeration of factions in conflict, bound together only by opposition to outside critics."[48]

Although philosophy and treatment methods vary greatly from one chiropractor to another, there are two main types: "straights" and "mixers." Straights tend to regard "subluxations" as the primary cause of ill health and spinal "adjustments" as the remedy. Many straights disparage medical diagnosis, some even claiming that their sole responsibility is to examine and adjust the spine. Mixers, who are more numerous, acknowledge that germs, hormones, and other factors play a role in disease; however, they tend to regard mechanical disturbances of the nervous system as the *underlying* cause (through lowered resistance). Besides spinal manipulation they may use nutritional methods and various types of physiotherapy, such as heat, cold, traction, exercise, massage, and ultrasound. Mixers are more likely to diagnose medical conditions in addition to spinal abnormalities and to refer patients to medical practitioners for treatment.

Both straights and mixers may claim that the nervous system is the master of all body functions, regulating everything from major organs to intricate cellular activities. This statement is untrue. However, charts and other materials relating the spine to the full range of illnesses can still be found in many chiropractic offices (see Figure 8-3). Thus, whereas nearly all chiropractors manipulate the spine as their primary treatment method, their rationales and techniques vary considerably.

Many chiropractors claim that their services are preventative and arise from a philosophy of wellness rather than sickness. The 1996 video produced to commemorate chiropractic's 100th anniversary said that, in the next 100 years, chiropractors will be "the leaders of health care."[49]

The two largest chiropractic organizations are the American Chiropractic Association (ACA, mixers), with about 23,000 members, including 6000 students, and the International Chiropractors Association (ICA, straights), with about 7000 members, including 3000 students. The two groups have considered merging, but they are unable to agree upon the definition and scope of chiropractic. The World Chiropractic Alliance, which is smaller than the ACA and ICA, states that its mission is "promoting a subluxation-free world."

About 300 chiropractors belong to the National Association for Chiropractic Medicine, a reformist group that has openly renounced D.D. Palmer's basic theories. Its members limit their practice to musculoskeletal problems and have denounced the questionable methods used by many of their colleagues. The group's application form includes a pledge to "openly renounce the historical chiropractic philosophical concept that subluxation is the cause of disease."

Chiropractic's academic research community, a small network of faculty members at some of the chiropractic schools, is attempting to place chiropractic on a scientific basis by determining which practices are valid and which are not. Magner[36] has noted, however, that their negative findings appear to have little effect on what other chiropractors do.

The Elusive "Subluxation"

Medical doctors and chiropractors use the word "subluxation" differently. The medical meaning is incomplete or partial dislocation—a condition, visible on x-ray films, in which the bony surfaces of a joint no longer face each other exactly but remain partially aligned. Most partial dislocations occur in areas other than the spine and are the result of injury. Spondylolisthesis, a partial dislocation of a spinal bone, usually is congenital and causes no symptoms. Because the ligaments connecting the spinal bones are quite strong, vertebral dislocations rarely occur after birth and are unlikely without severe injury that would require surgical treatment, not manipulation.

Chiropractors disagree on how their "subluxations" should be defined. Some describe them as "bones out of place" and/or "pinched nerves"; some speak of

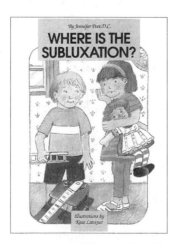

FIGURE 8-4. Chiropractic storybook. The story is about a little girl who was told she had a subluxation and searched in vain under her bed and in her toybox to find it. She finally learned its location when the chiropractor said it was a bone in her neck that was "not lined up with the other ones." The chiropractor explained: "Subluxations make your body sick. Each time I push on your back, the bones are adjusted closer to their normal position. This opens up the pathways, so that your brain may talk properly with your body. As your subluxations are corrected, you become healthier." The booklet was written by Jennifer Peet, D.C., and published in 1992.

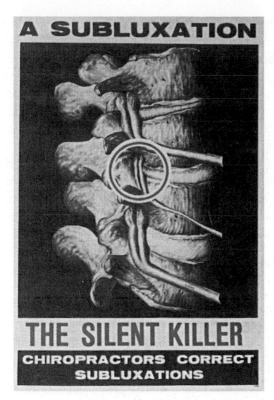

FIGURE 8-5. Poster for chiropractic offices. A distributor calls it "the most powerful single visual aid available."

"fixations" and/or loss of joint mobility; some occupy a middle ground that includes any or all of these concepts; and a few renounce chiropractic's subluxation concepts completely. A 1996 article listed 255 terms that "either relate to, are synonyms for, or have been used or cited as a description of" a subluxation or vertebral subluxation complex plus 41 synonyms for "sacroiliac subluxation."[50] Figures 8-4, 8-5, and 8-6 show how some chiropractors market the subluxation concept.

Chiropractors also disagree on whether their "subluxations" are visible on x-ray films. Those who claim that "nerve interference" results in too much or not enough "nerve supply" have never specified how this could be measured by scientific instruments.

The notion that nerve interference is a major cause of disease clashes with established anatomic facts. During the early 1970s Dr. Edmund Crelin, a prominent anatomist at Yale University, subjected subluxation theory to an actual test.[51] After collecting the spines of six people who had died a few hours earlier, he twisted them with instruments and observed the spaces between the vertebrae through which the spinal nerves passed. No nerve compression occurred, regardless of the force applied. In a later memorandum he commented further:

Only 24 of the 43 pairs of nerves that pass from the brain and spinal cord to various parts of the body could ever be impinged upon in the [vertebral openings] by the excessive dis-

placement of vertebrae. Why these 24 pairs should be causing disease, exclusive of all the others, defies a rational explanation. . . .

Complete severance of spinal nerves to the heart, glands (salivary, thyroid, liver, pancreas, etc.) and smooth muscles of the lungs, stomach, intestines, etc., has only transient effects. The gland cells and smooth and cardiac muscles not only survive, but function normally. They surely do not become diseased.[52]

Chiropractors differ among themselves about how to find "subluxations." Several studies in which many chiropractors have examined the same patient have found that the diagnoses and proposed treatments differed greatly from one practitioner to another.[53,54] Some physical therapists, athletic trainers, osteopaths, and medical doctors use manipulative techniques. Their intent, however, is not to correct misaligned bones. As noted by Stephen M. Levin, M.D, a prominent orthopedist who teaches manipulation:

The prevailing scientific viewpoint is that manipulation relieves pain and secondary muscle spasm by restoring the mobility of joints that have a mechanical malfunction. When I meet with scientifically oriented chiropractors, including educators at some of their better schools, we talk the same language.[55]

Chiropractors also differ greatly about how treatment should be done. More than 100 "technique systems" have been advocated. Thomas F. Bergman, D.C., who edits the journal *Chiropractic Technique*, has stated:

A challenge for the future is to classify and place all chiropractic techniques into a framework that allows determination as to whether any of them has a basis in fact. . . . Studies designed to compare effectiveness . . . have not been done. . . . No technique system has been demonstrated to be more or less effective than any other for any condition.[56]

Professional Preparation of Chiropractors
In 1973 the USOE approved the Council on Chiropractic Education (CCE) to accredit chiropractic schools. Admission to a CCE-accredited school requires 2 years

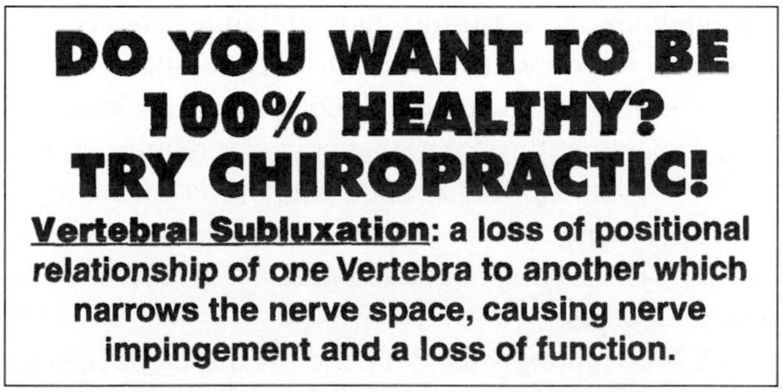

DO YOU WANT TO BE 100% HEALTHY? TRY CHIROPRACTIC!

Vertebral Subluxation: a loss of positional relationship of one Vertebra to another which narrows the nerve space, causing nerve impingement and a loss of function.

FIGURE 8-6. Portion of a recent chiropractic newspaper ad.

of prechiropractic college education with at least a C average. To receive the doctor of chiropractic (D.C.) degree, students must complete a minimum of 4200 hours of study over a 4-year period. Courses include anatomy, biochemistry, microbiology, pathology, public health, diagnosis and x-ray examination, related health sciences, and chiropractic principles and practice. Seventeen chiropractic schools in the United States have CCE accreditation.

In 1968 a comprehensive study by the U.S. Department of Health, Education, and Welfare concluded that chiropractic education does not prepare its practitioners to make an adequate diagnosis and provide appropriate treatment.[57] Although chiropractic schools have improved considerably since that time, the majority still teach subluxation theory, and a few still instruct students to treat "subluxations" rather than diseases or "conditions."[58]

Chiropractic schools do not provide the depth of diagnostic and therapeutic training that physicians receive. Whereas most medical school faculties are large and contain experts in every aspect of medical practice, chiropractic schools have few or no physicians on their faculty. Whereas the patients studied by medical students encompass the full range of disease, the vast majority seen by chiropractic students seek help for musculoskeletal problems. Although many of their courses are based on standard medical textbooks, chiropractic students lack much of the experience needed to make the information meaningful.[59] Chiropractic instruction in such subjects as pediatrics, obstetrics, and gynecology is usually limited to the classroom, with little or no actual patient contact and no experience with hospitalized patients.[59] One school, for example, has used only rubber models to teach students how to perform pelvic and rectal examinations.[36] Critics charge that because much of chiropractic is based on a false premise, neither length of study nor accreditation of its schools can ensure that those who graduate will practice competently.

After graduation many chiropractors take courses to help build their practices. These courses teach efficient office management, but some have taught unethical methods of recruiting and retaining patients. For example, one practice-building text provides detailed instructions for persuading all comers to have monthly spinal examinations.[60] Another suggests telling patients that "the best health insurance you'll ever buy is regular adjustments of your spine, releasing nerve pressures."[61] These books were authored by chiropractic college presidents.

A 1986 report by the Office of the Inspector General (OIG)[62] concluded that "practice-building courses,

popular with many chiropractors, advocate advertising techniques which suggest the universal efficacy of chiropractic treatment for every ailment known to humans." It also concluded that despite evidence of an increased emphasis on science and professionalism in the training and practice of chiropractors, "there also exist patterns of activity and practice which at best appear as overly aggressive marketing—and, in some cases, seem deliberately aimed at misleading patients and the public regarding chiropractic care." A subsequent OIG report noted that the two most common reasons for disciplinary actions by state chiropractic boards are billing abuses (relating to utilization or fees) and advertising abuses.[63]

Manipulation for Low-Back Pain

Several recent studies have examined whether spinal manipulation can relieve low-back pain. In 1991 a RAND Corporation[64] report concluded:

- Data from 22 controlled studies support the use of manipulation for acute low-back pain in patients showing no signs of lower-limb nerve root involvement.
- An appropriate trial of manipulation is two weeks each of two different types of manipulation, after which, if there is no improvement, therapy should be discontinued.
- Scientific reports provide no help in deciding when spinal manipulative treatment should be stopped, with respect to either improvement or worsening of symptoms. It is not clear how many, if any, manipulations are necessary after a patient has become pain-free.
- The frequency of complications from spinal manipulation for low-back pain has not been studied systematically. Although the risk appears small when compared to the large number of manipulations performed, no firm conclusions may be drawn because there are few data in the scientific literature.

In 1994 the Agency for Health Care Policy and Research (AHCPR) reached similar conclusions. Its panel of experts judged manipulation useful for controlling symptoms while awaiting the spontaneous recovery that occurs within 1 month in most patients with low-back problems.[65]

Although chiropractors have promoted these reports as endorsements of chiropractic, they are not. They merely support the use of manipulation in carefully selected patients. Only a few of the research studies on which their conclusions were based involved manipulation by chiropractors; most were done by medical doctors and physical therapists whose practices are not identical to those of chiropractors.[35] Most chiropractors manipulate the vast majority of patients who walk through their door, some use techniques that have not

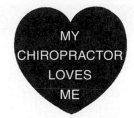

FIGURE 8-7. Chiropractic promotional materials. Many chiropractors use messages that reinforce the idea of a special bond between themselves and their patients. The bumper sticker was distributed by the American Chiropractic Association. The heart sticker is from a company that sells novelty items to chiropractors. Several companies sell birthday cards and other greeting cards with chiropractic themes.

been studied scientifically, and many chiropractors emphasize a technique that is more vigorous (and therefore potentially less safe) than the controlled manipulation used by other practitioners. Paul M. Shekelle, M.D., Ph.D., who headed the RAND study, said later that it is not known whether spinal manipulation is better than or even as good as modern back-pain therapies that emphasize keeping the patient active.[66] He has also rebuked the chiropractic profession for six "common misinterpretations" of RAND's findings.[67] The word "chiropractic" does not appear in the text of AHCPR report.

Several workers' compensation studies have found that patients treated by chiropractors were more satisfied and returned to work sooner than patients treated medically. However, these studies did not scientifically validate what the chiropractors did and were not designed for that purpose. Experts who located 16 studies published from 1966 through 1990 concluded that, although most contained data appearing to favor chiropractic, their authors did not evaluate whether the patients had comparable problems. In addition, the duration and costs of disability and time lost from work are influenced by factors other than effectiveness.[68]

Carey and others[69] have compared the cost of low-back pain treatment by family physicians, orthopedists, and chiropractors in North Carolina. The median total charges were $545 by urban chiropractors, $383 by orthopedists, $348 by rural chiropractors, $214 for rural primary-care physicians, and $169 for urban primary-care physicians. Although chiropractors charged less per visit, their treatment was costlier because they saw their patients about five times as often.

Antitrust Suits

In 1976 various chiropractors began a series of lawsuits against the AMA, other professional organizations, and several individual critics, charging that they had conspired to destroy chiropractic and to illegally deprive chiropractors of access to laboratory, x-ray, and hospital facilities. Most of the defendant groups agreed in out-of-court settlements that their physician members were free to decide for themselves how to deal with chiropractors.

In 1987 a federal judge concluded that during the 1960s "there was a lot of material available to the AMA Committee on Quackery that supported its belief that all chiropractic was unscientific and deleterious." The judge also noted that chiropractors still took too many x-rays. However, she ruled that the AMA had engaged in an illegal boycott. She concluded that the dominant reason for the AMA's antichiropractic campaign was the belief that chiropractic was not in the best interest of patients. But she ruled that this did not justify attempting to contain and eliminate an entire licensed profession without first demonstrating that a less restrictive campaign could not succeed in protecting the public.[70] Although chiropractors trumpet the antitrust ruling as an endorsement of their effectiveness, the case was decided on legal grounds (restraint of trade) and was not an evaluation of chiropractic methods.

Problems for Consumers

Critics have expressed many additional concerns:

- Although musculoskeletal disorders are the problems that chiropractors treat most often, many suggest that the scope of chiropractic treatment is much broader. Ted Koren, D.C., who publishes a large line of brochures and other practice-building supplies, includes fever, croup, bedwetting, ear infections, sore throat, eye problems, cough, asthma, bronchitis, poor concentration and 34 other problems on a "partial list" of childhood conditions within chiropractic's scope.[71] He also advises chiropractors they can double their practice "practically overnight" by having patients read the list and asking: "Do you know of any children, perhaps your own, or those of relatives or friends, that have any of the problems in this list?"[72]
- Many chiropractors use dubious diagnostic methods such as inappropriate muscle-testing (see "applied kinesiology" in Chapter 12), hair analysis (see Chapter 12), thermography (see Glossary), leg-length tests, and various gadgets alleged to detect subluxations.

An Undercover Investigation

In 1994 ABC's "20/20" reported on visits to 17 chiropractors who had made it known through advertising or other means that they treated children. In one segment, an infant named Blake was taken by his mother to nine chiropractors in the New York metropolitan area, accompanied by a "friend" who was carrying a hidden camera. Blake had had recurring ear infections, a problem that a pediatrician said could be managed with antibiotics and would eventually be outgrown. Every chiropractor found a problem, and all said they could help and recommended care ranging from several weeks to a lifetime. The first found "a misalignment between the second and third bones in his neck." The second said it was "on the right side of his neck between the first and second bones." The third, using muscle-testing, found "weakness in the adrenal glands." The fourth said there was a subluxation because one of Blake's legs was shorter than the other. The fifth claimed he could diagnose the boy's problem by pulling on *his mother's* arm while she touched the boy on the shoulder. The sixth chiropractor did a similar test by pulling on the mother's legs while Blake lay on top of her back. After diagnosing "jamming of the occiput (the back bone of the skull)," the

chiropractor said he corrected it by "lifting" Blake's occiput with his thumbs. He also said: (a) Blake needed work on his immune system, (b) learning disorder might be a problem, (c) both mother and son had "eyes that don't team too well," and (d) the cameraman, whom the chiropractor incorrectly assumed was the boy's father, had the same eye problem.

The same program also reported on visits to eight Wisconsin chiropractors by a 5-year-old boy with chronic ear infections so severe that medical doctors wanted to insert tubes in his ears to drain them. All eight chiropractors found problems, but not usually the same ones. One diagnosed a pinched nerve in the boy's neck. Another said his left leg was shorter than his right. Another said his right leg was shorter than his left. Another diagnosed zinc deficiency. Another chiropractor blamed the boy's ear problems on "food sensitivities" and advised avoiding corn, cow's milk, and white flour. Another gave similar dietary advice but said that the main diagnosis was a "subluxation" in the top vertebra. Another said the boy didn't have an ear problem but had scoliosis—a diagnosis disputed by a pediatrician and a radiologist who reviewed this chiropractor's findings.

- Many chiropractors claim that treating subluxations improves general health and is important throughout life. For example, in 1995 an ACA board member stated: "I treat my patients as if each spinal adjustment has a virtually unlimited potential in improving their health. My father adjusted me on the day that I came home from the hospital, and I did the same with my children."[73] Samuel Homola, D.C., a scientifically oriented chiropractor, says that vague claims like "manipulating the vertebrae to restore and maintain health" close many doors to chiropractors in the nation's health-care system.[74]
- Patients who rely on exaggerated chiropractic claims may delay obtaining more appropriate care.[75]
- Although not qualified by training to understand the use of prescription drugs, many chiropractors discourage their use.[76]
- Many chiropractors prescribe unnecessary vitamins, irrational "dietary supplement" formulations, and/or homeopathic products, most of which are sold to patients at two or three times their wholesale cost.[2,77] A 1998 survey by the National Board of Chiropractic Examiners[78] found that 90.4% of 3177 full-time practitioners who responded said they had used "nutritional counseling, therapy or supplements" within the previous 2 years and that 53.1% said they had prescribed homeopathic remedies.
- Many chiropractors x-ray some or all of their patients to look for "subluxations." About 10% of chiropractors still obtain 14x36-inch full-spine x-ray films, which yield little

or no diagnostic information but subject the patient's reproductive organs to high levels of radiation.
- Many chiropractors say that immunizations are ineffective and do not recommend them to their patients. In 1992, 36% of 178 chiropractors who responded to a survey agreed that "there is no scientific proof that immunization prevents infectious disease" and 23% said they were uncertain. In the same survey, 41% agreed that "immunization campaigns have not substantially changed the incidence of any infectious diseases in the 20th century" and 29% said they were unsure. Referring to efforts at health-care reform, the study's authors noted that "continued opposition to immunization and other procedures supported by scientific evidence may become a significant obstacle to assimilation of the chiropractic profession into the revised health care system."[79] The American Chiropractic Association and the International Chiropractors Association oppose compulsory immunization.
- Many chiropractors suggest unnecessary "spinal adjustments" for "preventative maintenance" or for treating nonexistent conditions. Many use scare tactics to do so.[36,37] During the 1970s the Lehigh Valley [Pa.] Committee Against Health Fraud asked 35 local practitioners how often people who feel well should have their spine checked. Most answers ranged from 4 to 12 times per year.[80]
- Manipulation, particularly of the neck, can be dangerous. In 1992 researchers at the Stanford Stroke Center asked

486 California members of the American Academy of Neurology how many patients they had seen during the previous 2 years who had suffered a stroke within 24 hours of neck manipulation by a chiropractor. The survey was sponsored by the American Heart Association. The 176 neurologists who responded said that they had treated 56 such patients, all between the ages of 21 and 60. One patient had died, and 48 were left with permanent neurologic deficits such as slurred speech, inability to arrange words properly, and vertigo (severe dizziness). The neurologists also reported treating 46 cases of nerve or muscle injury.[81] Although the percentage of chiropractic patients who are seriously injured is small, injury caused by an unnecessary manipulation is inexcusable. Assendelft, Bouter, and Knipschild reviewed 295 published reports of complications and concluded (a) it is difficult to estimate the incidence of complications of spinal manipulation because they are underreported in the scientific literature, (b) information about the risk of stroke should be included in an informed consent procedure for neck manipulation that involves thrusting, and (c) practitioners using rotatory manipulation should be avoided.[82]

During 1989, William M. London, Ed.D., visited 23 chiropractors in Ohio and Florida who had advertised free consultations or examinations. Each one espoused subluxation theory either during the consultation or in waiting room literature, and all but two recommended periodic preventive maintenance. Seventeen performed examinations. Of these, three identified subluxations (at differing locations), three said his left leg was shorter than his right leg, and two said his right leg was shorter than his left. Seven recommended treatment, and one treated him with a motorized roller device before examining him.[83]

 Consumer Tip

Avoiding Chiropractic Trouble

Consumer Reports[84] advises people to be suspicious of any chiropractor who does the following:

- Takes full-spine or repeated x-rays.
- Fails to take a comprehensive history and do a clinical examination to determine the cause of your trouble.
- Claims that the treatment will improve immune function, benefit organ systems, or cure disease.
- Offers to sell you vitamin cures, nutritional remedies, or homeopathic remedies.
- Solicits children or other family members.
- Advises against the immunization of children.
- Wants you to sign a contract for long-term care.
- Promises to prevent disease through regular checkups and spinal adjustments

---

The Vertebral Subluxation Research Institute taught chiropractors how to convert "research volunteers" into "lifetime chiropractic patients." Its chiropractor clients were instructed to use telemarketing and other approaches to ask people to volunteer for "a nationwide study on spinal conditions." During the first office visit they would be examined and given a brochure ("The Silent Killer") explaining the supposed dangers of subluxations. During the second visit—during a "report of findings"—they would be advised to have their subluxations treated.[85] A 1995 pamphlet from Koren Publications warns that only a chiropractic spinal checkup can tell whether "you and your family are carrying the silent killer, the vertebral subluxation complex."[86]

The terms "chiropractic" and "chiropractic treatment" are ambiguous and are not synonymous with "spinal manipulation." Chiropractic is both a philosophy and a treatment approach. Chiropractic treatment may include a wide variety of dubious measures in addition to appropriate or inappropriate manipulation. Thus, the potential usefulness of spinal manipulation may not counterbalance the unscientific philosophy or methods commonly embraced by chiropractors. The National Council Against Health Fraud considers chiropractic to be "a major consumer health problem."[87]

NATUROPATHY

Naturopathy, sometimes referred to as "natural medicine," is a system of healing said to "assist nature." Naturopaths claim to remove the underlying cause(s) of disease and to stimulate the body's natural healing processes.[88] They maintain that diseases are the body's effort to purify itself and that cures result from increasing the patient's "vital force" by ridding the body of waste products and "toxins." The American Association of Naturopathic Physicians[89] claims: "Naturopathic medicine has its own unique body of knowledge, evolved and refined for centuries." Although naturopaths say they emphasize prevention, they tend to oppose immunization.

Like many chiropractors, most naturopaths believe that virtually all diseases are within the scope of their practice. They offer treatment at their offices and at spas where patients may reside for several weeks. Their methods include fasting; "natural food" diets; vitamins; herbs; tissue minerals; cell salts; manipulation; massage; exercise; colonic irrigation; acupuncture; natural childbirth; minor surgery; and applications of water, heat, cold, air, sunlight, and electricity. They may use radiation for diagnosis but not for treatment.

In naturopathic practice "detoxification" plays a prominent role. As stated by Bastyr University president Joseph E. Pizzorno, Jr., N.D.:

An important theme in naturopathic medicine is recognition and correction of endogenous and exogenous toxicity. Liver and bowel detoxification, elimination of environmental toxins, correcting the metabolic function that causes the buildup of non-endproduct metabolites—all are important ways of decreasing toxic load.[90]

The most comprehensive naturopathic publications, *A Textbook of Natural Medicine* [91] (for students and professionals) and *Encyclopedia of Natural Medicine* [92] (for laypersons), recommend special diets, vitamins, minerals, and/or herbs for more than 70 health problems ranging from acne to AIDS. For many of these conditions, daily administration of 10 or more products is recommended—some in dosages high enough to cause toxicity.

The term "naturopathy" was coined in 1895 by John Scheel, a practitioner in New York City. In 1902 he sold rights to the term to Benedict Lust, who had come to the United States in 1892 to promote the Kneipp Water Cure, a form of hydrotherapy. Lust was largely responsible for naturopathy's growth in this country.[93] He acquired chiropractic, osteopathic, naturopathic, and homeopathic medical degrees; operated treatment facilities; founded several schools; operated a publishing company; and formed the American Naturopathic Association. Another prominent developer of naturopathy was Bernarr Macfadden, who promoted "physical culture" (see Chapter 14).

Before 1961, the doctor of naturopathy (N.D.) degree could be obtained at several chiropractic schools; now it is available from three full-time naturopathy schools and a few correspondence schools. Training at the full-time schools follows a pattern similar to that of chiropractic schools: 2 years of basic science courses and 2 years of clinical naturopathy. Two years of preprofessional college work are required for admission. In 1987 the U.S. Secretary of Education approved the Council on Naturopathic Medical Education as an accrediting agency for the full-time schools. As with acupuncture and chiropractic schools, this recognition is not based on the scientific validity of what is taught. The largest naturopathy school is Bastyr University in Seattle. In addition to its N.D. program, Bastyr offers M.S. programs in nutrition and acupuncture and a B.S. program in Natural Health Sciences, with majors in nutrition and Oriental medicine. Bastyr also provides health-food retailers and their employees with home-study programs that espouse "natural" approaches for the gamut of disease.

Naturopaths are licensed as independent practitioners in 11 states and may legally practice in a few others. The American Association of Naturopathic Physicians has about 500 names in its online directory. The total number of practitioners is unknown but includes chiropractors and acupuncturists who practice naturopathy. Naturopathic services are not covered by Medicare or most insurance policies.

In 1968 the U.S. Department of Health, Education, and Welfare (HEW) recommended against coverage of naturopathy under Medicare. HEW's report concluded:

Naturopathic theory and practice are not based upon the body of basic knowledge related to health, disease, and health care which has been widely accepted by the scientific community. Moreover, irrespective of its theory, the scope and quality of naturopathic education do not prepare the practitioner to make an adequate diagnosis and provide appropriate treatment.[57]

Although some aspects of naturopathic education have improved in recent years, this conclusion is still valid.

NATURAL HYGIENE

Natural Hygiene, an offshoot of naturopathy, is a philosophy of health and "natural living" that denounces most medical treatment and advocates eating a "raw food" diet of vegetables, fruits, and nuts. It also advocates periodic fasting and "food combining" (avoiding food combinations it considers detrimental).[94] Its best-known advocates are Harvey and Marilyn Diamond, authors of *Fit for Life* (discussed in Chapter 13). An American Natural Hygiene Society (ANHS) brochure states:

Natural Hygiene rejects the use of medications, blood transfusions, radiation, dietary supplements, and any other means employed to treat or "cure" various ailments. These therapies interfere with or destroy vital processes and tissue. Recovery from disease takes place in spite of, and not because of, the drugging and "curing" practices.

According to ANHS's magazine *Health Science*, the Natural Hygiene movement was founded during the 1830s by Sylvester Graham but declined until "resuscitated" from "almost dead" by Herbert M. Shelton (1895-1985). ANHS was founded in 1948 by Shelton and several associates and now has about 6500 members. Its headquarters is in Tampa, Florida. The society has been active in promoting certification of "organic foods" and opposing compulsory immunization, fluoridation, and food irradiation. *Health Science* lists 20 practitioners on its "professional referral list." Most are chiropractors, but a few hold a medical, osteopathic, or naturopathic degree.

IRIDOLOGY

Iridology is based on the belief that each area of the body is represented by a corresponding area in the iris of the eye (the colored area around the pupil), as shown in Figure 8-8. According to this viewpoint, a person's state of health and disease can be diagnosed from the color, texture, and location of various pigment flecks in the eye. Iridology practitioners claim to diagnose "imbalances" that can be treated with vitamins, minerals, herbs, and similar products. Some also claim that the eye markings can reveal a complete history of past illnesses as well as previous treatment. One textbook, for example, states that a white triangle in the appropriate area indicates appendicitis, but a black speck indicates that the appendix had been removed by surgery. Iridology charts—dozens of which exist—vary somewhat in the location and interpretation of their iris signs. Sclerology is similar to iridology but interprets the shape and condition of blood vessels on the white portion (sclera) of the eyeball.

Proponents of iridology attribute its development to Ignatz von Peczely, a Hungarian physician who, during his childhood, had accidentally broken the leg of an owl and noticed a black stripe in the lower part of the owl's eye. Nonadherents suggest that von Peczely may have developed his theory to pass time while he was imprisoned after the 1848 Hungarian revolution. After his release from prison he allegedly saved the life of his mother with homeopathic remedies, recalled the inci-

dent of the owl's eye, and began studying the eyes of his patients.

Bernard Jensen, D.C., the leading American iridologist, states that "Nature has provided us with a miniature television screen showing the most remote portions of the body by way of nerve reflex responses."[95] He also claims that iridology analyses are more reliable and "offer much more information about the state of the body than do the examinations of Western medicine." However, in 1979 he and two other proponents failed a scientific test in which they examined photographs of the eyes of 143 persons in an attempt to determine which ones had kidney impairments. (Forty-eight had been diagnosed with a standard kidney function test, and the rest had normal function.) The three iridologists showed no statistically significant ability to detect which patients had kidney disease and which did not. One iridologist, for example, decided that 88% of the normal patients had kidney disease, while another judged that 74% of patients sick enough to need artificial kidney treatment were normal.[96] More recently, five leading Dutch iridologists failed a similar test in which they were shown stereo color slides of the right iris of 78 people, half of whom had gallbladder disease. None of the five could distinguish between the patients with gallbladder disease and the people who were healthy. Nor did they agree with each other about which was which.[97]

Russell S. Worrall, O.D., an assistant clinical professor of optometry at the School of Optometry, University of California, Berkeley, has noted:

Many of the conditions detected by practitioners of iridology are "diseases" whose existence has been disputed or discredited by scientific investigation. . . . It would be difficult to agree on a standard diagnosis where the existence of the disease itself is in dispute.[98]

Worrall also points out how incorrect "diagnoses" by iridologists can have serious consequences, as illustrated by the case of an accountant who consulted a chiropractor who practiced iridology:

During the course of treatment an iridology workup was recommended. The results indicated, among many other health problems, the presence of cancer. Overwhelmed, the patient spent the day in torment. Unable to consult his family physician . . . he finally sought my advice. After a lengthy discussion, I was able to allay his fears. . . . He wondered how an intelligent person such as himself could be caught up in such a deep emotional web over such a diagnosis. The story fortunately had a pleasant ending. However, the outcome could have been much more serious since the patient is also suffering from a heart condition, which was not noted on the iridology evaluation!

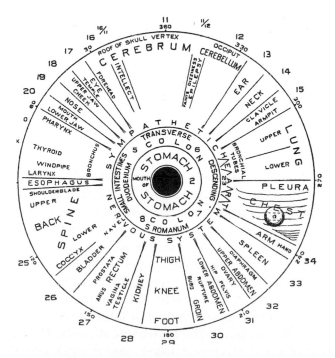

FIGURE 8-8. Iridology chart of the left eye developed by a prominent naturopath more than 70 years ago.

In 1981 the AMA Council on Scientific Affairs noted that iridology charts are similar in concept to those used years ago in "phrenology," the pseudoscience that related protuberances of the skull to the mental faculties and character of the individual. Regarding iridology's appeal, the council stated:

Iridology may stimulate interest among those turning to alternative methods of managing disease processes, and it does offer the dual attraction of simplicity and mystery without the inconvenience, and sometimes positive discomfort, that often accompanies diagnostic medical procedures; nevertheless, iridology has not yet been established as having any merit as a diagnostic technique.[30]

Stalker and Glymour[99] have noted:

Chiropractors, iridologists, reflexologists, tongue diagnosers, zone therapists, and many others all claim to treat or diagnose the whole from some anatomical part. Of course, they differ about which part, but that does not seem to bother either them or the editors of holistic books.

HOMEOPATHY

Homeopathy originated in the late 1700s when Samuel Hahnemann (1755–1843), a German physician, began formulating its basic principles. Hahnemann was justifiably distressed about bloodletting, leeching, purging, and other "heroic" medical procedures of his day that did far more harm than good. He was also critical of medications like calomel (mercurous chloride), which many physicians considered a "cure-all" and prescribed in doses that caused mercury poisoning. Thinking that these treatments were intended to "balance the body's 'humors' by opposite effects," he developed his "law of similars," a notion that diseases can be cured by administering substances that would, if given to healthy people, cause the same symptoms as the disease. The word "homeopathy" is derived from the Greek words *homoios* (similar) and *pathos* (suffering or disease).

Although ideas like this had been espoused by Hippocrates in the fourth century BCE and by Paracelsus, a fifteenth-century physician-alchemist, Hahnemann was the first to use them in a systematic way. He and his early followers conducted "provings" in which they administered herbs, minerals, and other substances to healthy people, including themselves, and kept detailed records of what they observed. Later these records were compiled into lengthy reference books called *materia medica*, which are still used to match a patient's symptoms with a "corresponding" homeopathic remedy. Whorton has noted:

Hahnemann seems to have overlooked the fact that people regularly experience "symptoms," unusual physical and emotional sensations, whether taking drugs or other stimulants, or not—especially if they have been forewarned that the experimental pills they have been given might, nay probably will, cause symptoms and that the symptoms might be mild and take several days or weeks to manifest themselves. . . . As provings by the master and his followers accumulated, homeopathic handbooks . . . grew thick with interminable symptom lists.[100]

Hahnemann also declared that diseases represent an impairment of the body's ability to heal itself and that only a small stimulus is needed to begin the healing process. To him, disease was chiefly a disturbance of the body's "spirit." At first he prescribed small doses of accepted medications. But later he used enormous dilutions and theorized that the smaller the dose, the more powerful the effect—a principle he called the "law of infinitesimals." This principle is the opposite of what pharmacologists have demonstrated in dose-response studies.

Far-Fetched Claims

Many homeopaths maintain that certain people have a special affinity to a particular remedy (their "constitutional remedy") and will respond to it for a variety of ailments. Such remedies can be prescribed according to the person's "constitutional type"—named after the corresponding remedy in a manner resembling astrologic typing. The "Ignatia Type," for example, is said to be nervous and often tearful, and to dislike tobacco smoke. The typical "Pulsatilla" is a young woman, with blonde or light-brown hair, blue eyes, and a delicate complexion, who is gentle, fearful, romantic, emotional, and friendly but shy. The "Nux Vomica Type" is said to be aggressive, bellicose, ambitious, and hyperactive. The "Sulfur Type" likes to be independent. And so on.

Homeopathic products are derived from minerals, plant substances, and several other sources. If the original substance is soluble, one part is diluted with either 9 or 99 parts of distilled water and/or alcohol and shaken vigorously; if insoluble, it is finely ground and pulverized in similar proportions with powdered lactose (milk sugar). One part of the diluted medicine is diluted, and the process is repeated until the desired concentration is reached. Dilutions of 1:10 are designated by the Roman numeral X (1X = 1/10, 3X = 1/1000, 6X = 1/1,000,000). Similarly, dilutions of 1:100 are designated by the Roman numeral C (1C = 1/100, 3C = 1/1,000,000, and so on). Most remedies today range from 6X to 30X, but products of 30C or more are marketed.

A 30X dilution means that the original substance has been diluted 10^{30} times. Assuming that a cubic centimeter of water contains 15 drops, 10^{30} is greater than the number of drops of water that would fill a container more than 50 times the size of the Earth. Robert L. Park, Ph.D., a professor of physics at the University of Maryland, has noted that since the least amount of a substance in a solution is one molecule, a 30C solution would have to have at least one molecule of the original substance dissolved in a minimum of 10^{60} molecules of water. This would require a container more than 30 billion times the size of the Earth. Another critic has calculated that if everyone on earth were to ingest three doses of a 30C product each day for 200 billion years, the chance that anyone would encounter a single molecule of the original substance would be infinitesimal.[101]

According to the laws of chemistry, there is a limit to the dilution that can be made without losing the original substance altogether. This limit, which is related to Avogadro's number (6.023×10^{23}), corresponds to homeopathic potencies of 12C or 24X (1 part in 10^{24}). Hahnemann himself realized there is virtually no chance that even one molecule of original substance would remain after extreme dilutions. But he believed that the vigorous shaking ("succussion") or pulverizing with each step of dilution leaves behind a spirit-like essence, "no longer perceptible to the senses," that cures by reviving the body's "vital force." Barrett and Herbert[2] have pointed out that if this were true, every substance encountered by a molecule of water might imprint an "essence" that could exert powerful and unpredictable medicinal effects when ingested by a person.

Many proponents claim that homeopathic products resemble vaccines because both provide a small stimulus that triggers an immune response. This comparison is not valid. The amounts of active ingredients in vaccines are much greater and can be measured. Moreover, immunizations produce antibodies whose concentration in the blood can be measured, but homeopathic products produce no measurable response.

Hahnemann's theories have never been accepted by scientifically oriented physicians, who charge that homeopathic remedies are placebos (inert substances). However, because homeopathic remedies were actually less dangerous than those of nineteenth-century medical orthodoxy, many medical practitioners began using them. At the turn of the century homeopathy had some 14,000 practitioners and 22 schools in the United States alone. As medical science and medical education advanced, homeopathy declined sharply, particularly in America, where its schools either closed or converted to responsible methods. The last pure homeopathic school in the United States closed during the 1920s.[102]

Homeopathic preparations were given legal status by the 1938 Federal Food, Drug, and Cosmetic Act, which was shepherded through Congress by Senator Royal Copeland, a homeopathic physician. One provision of this law recognized as drugs all substances included in the *Homœopathic Pharmacopœia of the United States*. Now in its ninth edition, this book lists more than 1200 substances and how they should be prepared for homeopathic use.[103] It states that inclusion of a substance means that it has been judged safe and effective. However, the symptoms or diseases for which it should be used are not identified; that is decided by the practitioner or manufacturer. Listing of the substances does not mean that either the law or the FDA recognizes them as effective.[104]

The basis for inclusion in the *Homœopathic Pharmacopœia* is not modern scientific testing, but homeopathic "provings," many of which took place more than 100 years ago. Yet Jeremy Sherr,[105] a British homeopath who wrote *The Dynamics and Methodology of Provings,* states that these provings had no consistency because "every homeopath had a different method." Some used a single dose; others dosed as often as three times a day for months; and potencies ranged from the undiluted original substance to dilutions as high as 200C. (The number 100^{200} is vastly greater than the estimated number of molecules in the universe.)

The 2000 directory of National Center for Homeopathy lists about 550 licensed practitioners. About 200 are physicians, and the rest are mostly dentists, veterinarians, nurses, chiropractors, and naturopaths. Consumers interested in homeopathic self-treatment can obtain guidance through lay study groups, books, and courses sponsored by the center. Most homeopathic practitioners still rely on *materia medica* in choosing among the thousands of remedies available.

About 50 American physicians who prescribe homeopathic remedies practice anthroposophical medicine (also called anthroposophically extended medicine), a difficult-to-describe system based on the occult philosophy of Rudolf Steiner (1861-1925). Steiner's teachings encompassed (a) a system of body movements termed "eurythmy"; (b) a peculiar educational approach that stresses art, drama, spiritual development, and "science" based on occult concepts; (c) a fanciful theory of medicine; and (d) "biodynamic" agriculture, a type of "organic" farming.[106] Anthroposophical "remedies" are marketed in the United States through Weleda Inc. of Spring Valley, New York. According to a Weleda brochure, each plant used to prepare remedies is "selected for its unique 'personality,' revealed in form, color, pattern of growth, with consideration of its beneficial properties" and is "harvested when its growth forces

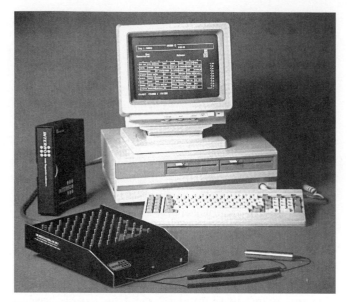

FIGURE 8-9. *Interro* device. Ampules containing homeopathic solutions may be placed in the metal honeycomb in the foreground to determine their alleged suitability for treating the patient.

are strongest." Proponents also state that "seasonal changes" and "solar, lunar and planetary influences" are factors in determining when to harvest the plants.

Electrodiagnosis

Some physicians, dentists, and chiropractors use "electrodiagnostic" devices to help select the homeopathic remedies they prescribe. These practitioners claim they can determine the cause of any disease by detecting the "energy imbalance" causing the problem. Some also claim that the devices can detect whether someone is allergic or sensitive to foods, vitamins, and/or other substances. The procedure, called electroacupuncture according to Voll (EAV), electrodiagnosis, or electrodermal screening, was begun during the 1950s by Reinhold Voll, M.D., a West German physician who developed the original device. Subsequent models include the *Vegatest, Dermatron, Accupath 1000,* and *Interro.*

Proponents claim these devices measure disturbances in the flow of "electro-magnetic energy" along the body's "acupuncture meridians." Actually, they are fancy galvanometers that measure electrical resistance of the patient's skin when touched by a probe.[107] Each device contains a low-voltage source. One wire from the device goes to a brass cylinder covered by moist gauze, which the patient holds in one hand. A second wire is connected to a probe, which the operator touches to "acupuncture points" on the patient's foot or other

hand. This completes a circuit, and the device registers the flow of current. The information is then relayed to a gauge that provides a numerical readout. The size of the number depends on how hard the probe is pressed against the patient's skin. Recent versions, such as the *Interro* (Figure 8-9), make sounds and provide the readout on a computer screen. The treatment selected depends on the scope of the practitioner's practice and may include acupuncture, dietary change, and/or vitamin supplements, as well as homeopathic products.

Regulatory agencies have seized several types of electroacupuncture devices but have not made a systematic effort to drive them from the marketplace. In 1991 the Australian College of Allergy issued a position paper stating that the use of a *Vegatest* device has no scientific basis and "may lead to inappropriate treatment and expense to the patient and community."[108]

Questionable Research

In 1988 a French scientist working at a prestigious laboratory claimed to have found that high dilutions of substances in water left a "memory" that would provide a rationale for homeopathy's "law of similars." However, a subsequent investigation by experts revealed that the research had been improperly carried out.[109]

In 1990 an article in *Review of Epidemiology* analyzed 40 randomized trials that had compared homeopathic treatment with standard treatment, a placebo, or no treatment. The authors concluded that all but three of the trials had major flaws in their design, that only one of those three had reported a positive result, and that there was no evidence that homeopathic treatment has any more value than a placebo.[110] No valid research has ever found a homeopathic product more effective than standard medication.[111]

In 1994 the journal *Pediatrics* published an article claiming that homeopathic treatment had been demonstrated to be effective against mild cases of diarrhea among Nicaraguan children.[112] The claim was based on findings that, on certain days, the "treated" group had fewer loose stools than the placebo group. However, Sampson and London[113] noted (a) the study used an unreliable and unproved diagnostic and therapeutic scheme, (b) there was no safeguard against product adulteration, (c) treatment selection was arbitrary, (d) the data were oddly grouped and contained errors and inconsistencies, (e) the results had questionable clinical significance, and (f) there was no public health significance because the only remedy needed for mild childhood diarrhea is adequate fluid intake to prevent or correct dehydration.

Proponents represent the few "positive" studies as proof that "homeopathy works." Even if positive results could be consistently reproduced (which has not happened), the most that the study of any homeopathic product for a specific disease could prove is that it was effective against that disease. It would not validate homeopathy's basic theories or prove that homeopathic treatment is useful for other diseases.

A Multitude of Products

Thousands of homeopathic products are available from practitioners, health-food stores, drugstores, multilevel distributors, and manufacturers who sell directly to the public. Homeopathic remedies appeal to some people who are afraid of potent drugs. Manufacturers cater to this fear by claiming that their remedies are "the safer alternative" and "work without side effects." Many proponents claim that homeopathy not only cures but "removes the predisposition to disease." A booklet in Bastyr University's training program for health-food retailers advises that medically prescribed drugs may interfere with the action of a homeopathic remedy.[114]

Some homeopathic manufacturers market 12 highly diluted mineral products called "cell salts" or "tissue salts." These are claimed to be effective against a wide variety of diseases, including appendicitis (ruptured or not), baldness, deafness, insomnia, and worms. Their use is based on the notion that mineral deficiency is the basic cause of disease. However, many are so diluted that they could not correct a mineral deficiency even if one were present. Development of this approach is attributed to nineteenth-century physician W.H. Schuessler.

Promoters of homeopathic remedies sometimes recommend products called "glandulars" or "glandular extracts." The theory behind their use—like the magical thinking of primitive tribes—is that enzymes or other substances found in animal organs will strengthen or rejuvenate human body processes that involve similar substances. (See "doctrine of signatures" in Glossary.) Thus an extract of animal pancreas might be recommended to strengthen a person's pancreas, an animal heart extract might be suggested for the human heart, and so on. When these substances are present in homeopathic dilution, they have no effect on the body. Even in higher concentration when taken by mouth, they are digested by the stomach and intestines. Because they are proteins, they are broken down into their component amino acids so that no "glandular substances" actually reach the cells they are supposed to help.

Many homeopathic products have been marketed with illegal claims of efficacy against serious diseases.

In 1983, for example, Biological Homeopathic Industries (BHI) of Albuquerque, New Mexico, marketed *BHI Anticancer Stimulating, BHI Antivirus, BHI Stroke*, and 50 other types of tablets that the company claimed were effective against serious diseases. In 1984 the FDA forced BHI to stop distributing several of the products and to tone down its claims for the rest.[115] However, the company has continued to make illegal claims. Its 1991 *Physicians' Reference* inappropriately recommends products for glaucoma, heart failure, hepatitis, paralysis, syphilis, kidney failure, blurred vision, and a multitude of other problems.

During 1988 the FDA took action against companies marketing "diet patches" with false claims that they could suppress one's appetite. The largest, Meditrend International, of San Diego, had instructed users to place one or two drops of a "homeopathic appetite control solution" on a patch and wear it all day affixed to an "acupuncture point" on the wrist to "bioelectrically" suppress the appetite control center of the brain.[116]

In 1991 the U.S. Postal Service challenged the marketers of a homeopathic product called *Oncor*, which had been claimed to alleviate impotence and increase sexual desire in men. An administrative law judge concluded that the product was neither safe nor effective and that the television infomercial used to promote it had been falsely represented as an independent talk show.

During the past several years many other companies have offered dubious homeopathic products for over-the-counter sale. Some examples are: *Arthritis Formula, Bleeding, Candida Yeast Infection, Candida-Away, Cardio Forte, Epilepsy Drops, Exhaustion, Flu, Gall-Stones, Gonorrhea, Heart Tonic, Herpes, Kidney Disorders, Prostate Pain, Whooping Cough, Thyro Forte*, and *Worms*.

In most states homeopathy can be practiced by any physician or other practitioner whose license includes the ability to prescribe drugs. Three states—Arizona, Nevada, and Connecticut—have separate homeopathic licensing boards. The Nevada situation is notable because some of its practitioners acquired homeopathic licenses after other states revoked their medical licenses for cancer quackery.

Lack of Consumer Protection

Public protection regarding drugs is based on a framework of federal laws and regulations that require drugs to be safe, effective, and properly labeled. However, the FDA has not applied these rules to homeopathic products. Because most are supposed to contain no detectable amount of any active ingredient, it is impossible to test whether their ingredients are those stated on their labels. They have been presumed safe, but unlike most other drugs, they have not been proven safe or effective against disease by scientific means (such as double-blind testing). If the FDA were to require such proof for homeopathic drugs to remain on the market, the industry would not survive unless the U. S. Congress granted it new privileges.

In 1987 *Consumer Reports* concluded:

Unless the laws of chemistry have gone awry, most homeopathic remedies are too dilute to have any physiological effect. . . .

Consumers Union's medical consultants believe that any system of medicine embracing such remedies involves a potential danger to patients whether the prescribers are M.D.s, other licensed practitioners, or outright quacks. Ineffective drugs are dangerous drugs when used to treat serious or life-threatening disease.

Moreover, even though homeopathic drugs are essentially nontoxic, self-medication can still be hazardous. Using them for a serious illness or undiagnosed pain instead of obtaining proper medical attention could prove harmful or even fatal.[117]

In 1994 *Consumer Reports* urged Congress to "remove the blanket exemption from drug laws enjoyed by homeopathic remedies" and recommended that remedies marketed as treatments for specific illnesses be removed from drugstore shelves unless they are tested and proven safe and effective.[118] A few months later the authors of this textbook and 38 other prominent critics of quackery and pseudoscience petitioned the FDA to require that all over-the-counter (OTC) homeopathic drugs meet the same standards of safety and effectiveness as nonhomeopathic OTC drugs. The petitioners also asked the FDA Commissioner to issue a public warning that although the agency has permitted homeopathic remedies to be sold, it does not recognize them as effective.[119,120] The FDA has not yet reached a decision.

PSYCHIC HEALING

The term "psychic healing" refers to an alleged ability to treat illness without using any type of drug, surgery, or other curative agent that is physical, measurable, or explainable by currently accepted scientific methods or theories. Psychic healing is also referred to as *faith healing, paranormal healing, divine healing, miracle healing, spiritual healing, shamanistic healing, mental healing, psi healing,* and *the laying-on of hands,* although these terms are not interchangeable.

Faith-healing practices are based on a belief that religious faith can bring about recovery, or that prayer

and faith in a healer can result in a cure through divine intervention. A high degree of confidence in the efficacy of the healer is usually thought to be the central element in faith healing.[121] However, nonreligious individuals sometimes feel healed or act as healers, and some procedures take place in secular settings.[122] Spiritual healers postulate that humans can influence supernatural beings or forces. Some secular healers claim to have an intrinsic power of their own—such as a healing touch—which they may attempt to demonstrate by Kirlian photography (described later in this chapter) or other means.

Attempts at healing by faith and magic have been made throughout history. Ancient medicine functioned with the belief that diseases were caused by demons. Early Assyrian tablets describe methods of curing illnesses by driving out demons with magic, charms, incantations, and rituals. In the famous Greek temples of Aesculapius, religious methods of healing were employed. Christian history is replete with examples of widespread belief in the efficacy of faith healing. Shrines such as Lourdes in France still attract large numbers of people who hope to be cured by an intense religious experience.

Evangelical Healers

Many evangelical faith healers attract large followings. All claim to possess a gift of "miracle healing," but some express faith in the medical profession as well. Some appear to hold sincere beliefs, whereas others engage in clear-cut fraud motivated by greed.

Kathryn Kuhlman, for many years the queen of faith healers in the United States, was an energetic woman who attracted large crowds to her healing services. A typical service would last several hours, during which Kuhlman would preach, pray, announce that individuals with various afflictions had been healed, and urge them to come forward to acknowledge their healing.

◆ **Personal Glimpse** ◆

Fatal "Healing"

During the early 1970s, the parents of Wesley Parker, an 11-year-old diabetic boy in San Bernardino, California, threw away their son's insulin after he was treated by a faith healer. The preacher had led the parents to believe that the boy had been healed. After Wesley died, his parents were found guilty of involuntary manslaughter and sentenced to 5 years' probation. Their story was dramatized in the movie *Promised a Miracle.*

She claimed that she herself did not heal, but was merely an instrument of the Holy Spirit. A number of medical doctors would "certify" her healings. Close evaluation of her work, however, was unfavorable. William Nolen, M.D., a Minnesota surgeon, was permitted to attend one of her services as an usher. Afterward he examined or interviewed many people who claimed to have been healed during the service. Not one person with organic disease had actually been helped.[123] Ms. Kuhlman died in 1976, not long after undergoing open heart surgery.

In 1981, Oral Roberts opened the City of Faith, a $250 million medical center where "prayer and scientific medicine can be merged." Roberts, who claimed to receive messages from God, had a large following of "prayer partners" who received computer-generated letters about once a month from the Oral Roberts Evangelistic Association in Tulsa, Oklahoma. He promoted the idea that money donated to him (which he called seed-faith) could bring to its donors rich rewards from God. He invited the prayer partners to indicate their spiritual and health needs so that he could pray for them in a special prayer tower at Oral Roberts University. The mailings, which asked for donations, offered objects such as a prayer cloth, prayer rope, prayer plaque, or prayer coin "to touch and hold when you need a miracle." In 1989 Roberts announced that unfilled beds—a problem from the beginning—had forced him to close the school and shut down his hospital. At its peak the 777-bed facility had only 148 inpatients.

Several years ago magician James Randi and associates intercepted radio transmissions that proved that faith healer Peter Popoff was not getting information about the ailments of his audiences from God, as he claimed, but from his wife, who was backstage. The investigators also saw that people capable of walking were placed in wheelchairs before televangelist W.V. Grant's performances, so that later he could help "cripples" walk. After extensive investigations, Randi concluded:

I honestly see a strong parallel between the rock concert, the pro wrestling scene and the faith healing phenomenon. . . . No one ever stops to ask out loud the one most important question: is it for real?

Claims made by faith healers are nothing more than hollow boasts, and do not stand up to examination. Prepared culturally to expect miracles, convinced they are helpless without supernatural intervention, and bullied into supporting their gurus far beyond their means, the pathetic victims of the healers become a disillusioned subculture playing a dangerous game. . . . They are the dupes of clever, glib, highly organized swindlers who are immune from justice and are confidently aware of that fact.[124]

Christian Science

In about 1850, Phineas Parkhurst Quimby of Maine used Anton Mesmer's ideas of animal magnetism (see Chapter 6) to develop his own healing approach. Quimby would place his hands on a sick patient's head and abdomen and encourage supposed magnetic healing forces to flow through them. He claimed that diagnosis and cure resulted from the individual's faith in him. He professed that conventional medicine was useless, that disease itself was "error," and that only health was "truth."

In 1862 Quimby treated Mary Baker Glover for a spinal problem that had failed to respond to orthodox medical care. The water massage and hypnotism that he used apparently had a positive effect. On awakening from her trance Glover found herself cured. She concluded, however, that her cure was not due to Quimby but to "truth in Christ." In 1875 she published *Science and Health*, which described her theories about religion based on the Bible and some of Quimby's ideas. She said that God was the author and that she was only the writer. In 1877 she married for the third time, becoming Mary Baker Eddy, and named her new philosophy Christian Science. The Church of Christ, Scientist was founded in 1879.

Mary Baker Eddy represented herself as the supreme healer and as infallible as Christ. She claimed to be able to perform miracles and said she had healed many people with crippling disabilities. She demanded absolute obedience to her system as well as to her person. She could not bear to be contradicted or found wrong. In her determination to justify herself on all counts, she frequently twisted evidence and facts to her purposes. Her writings contain numerous contradictions.

Christian Science contends that illness is an illusion caused by faulty beliefs, and that prayer heals by replacing bad thoughts with good ones. Christian Science practitioners work by trying to argue the sick thoughts out of the patient's mind. Consultations can take place in person, by telephone, or even by mail. Individuals may also be able to attain correct beliefs by themselves through prayer or concentration.

A pamphlet of the Christian Science Publishing Society states that "every student of Christian Science has the God-given ability to heal the sick." To become a practitioner, an individual takes 2 weeks of "primary class instruction" from a qualified teacher. The course is based on questions and answers from *Science and Health*. When training is completed, "C.S." may be placed after the person's name. After 3 years of full-time practice, a practitioner may apply for the 6-day "normal class." Completion merits the degree of

Bachelor of Christian Science (C.S.B.) and certifies the person as a teacher who may give primary instruction to 30 pupils a year. Since 1971 the number of practitioners and teachers listed in the *Christian Science Journal* has fallen from about 5000 to about 1800, and the number of churches has fallen from about 1800 to about 1300.

Devout Christian Scientists do not use medications and usually eschew medical aid. They are opposed to vaccination, immunization, and quarantine for contagious diseases, although official church policy advises members to comply with state laws. A physician or midwife may be used during childbirth. A physician may also be used to set a broken bone if no medication is administered.

The weekly magazine *Christian Science Sentinel* publishes several "testimonies" in each issue. To be considered for publication, an account must merely be "verified" by three individuals who "can vouch for the integrity of the testifier or know of the healing." Believers have claimed that prayer has produced recovery from anemia, arthritis, blood poisoning, corns, deafness, defective speech, multiple sclerosis, skin rashes, total body paralysis, visual difficulties, and various injuries. Most of these accounts contain little detail, and many of the diagnoses were made without medical consultation. The church also publishes *The Christian Science Monitor,* a daily newspaper.

Christian Scientists may legally practice in all states. Medicare and some insurance companies cover care given by Christian Science practitioners, and their services are also tax-deductible as a medical expense for federal income-tax purposes. It is not known how many members continue to fully accept Mary Baker Eddy's premise that disease is an illusion, or how many continue to visit practitioners instead of physicians. Eyeglasses, hearing aids, and dental treatment are used by some members who still maintain that illness is the consequence of mental error.

Rita Swan, Ph.D., whose 16-month-old son Matthew died of meningitis in 1977 under the care of two Christian Science practitioners, quickly collected allegations of 75 deaths and 95 serious injuries to children of Christian Scientists.[125] Angered by her experience, she formed Children's Healthcare Is a Legal Duty, Inc. (CHILD) to work for legal reforms that could protect children from inappropriate treatment by faith healers.[126] She also sued the church but lost the case. During the proceedings, church officials testified that the church had no training, workshops, or meetings for practitioners that included any discussion on how to evaluate the seriousness of a child's condition.[127] A 1993 lawsuit following the death of an 11-year-old boy resulted in a $1.5 million judgment against the boy's mother and stepfather and two Christian Science practitioners. Press reports indicate that the boy died after passing into diabetic coma while the mother prayed at his bedside and the practitioner took notes about his condition.[128]

A study published in 1989 compared alumni records from Principia College, a Christian Science school in Elsah, Illinois, with records from the University of Kansas in Lawrence, Kansas. Even though Christian Science tenets forbid the use of alcohol and tobacco, the death rates among those who had graduated from Principia between 1934 and 1948 were higher than those of their University of Kansas counterparts (26.2% vs. 20.9% in men, and 11.3% vs. 9.9% in women).[129] A subsequent study comparing Christian Scientists and Seventh-day Adventists (who also are admonished to abstain from cigarettes and alcohol) found even greater differences in the death rates.[130]

In August 1996 a federal court judge ruled that Medicare and Medicaid payments for Christian Science nursing violate the Constitutional principle of church-state separation. The ruling came in response to a suit by CHILD and two individuals. About 500 Christian Science nurses practice in the United States. When the suit was filed, CHILD noted in a news release that these nurses are neither licensed nor trained in science-based nursing. The release also stated:

Christian Science nurses cannot take a pulse, use a fever thermometer, give an enema or even a backrub. They have no training in recognizing contagious diseases. They have been retained to attend sick children and have sat taking notes as the children suffered and died, but have not called for medical care nor recommended that parents obtain it. The notes of these . . . nurses indicate that they observed children having "heavy convulsions," vomiting repeatedly, and urinating uncontrollably. They have seen the children moaning in pain and too weak to get out of bed. They have seen their eyes roll upward and fix in a glassy stare. One Christian Science nurse force-fed a toddler as he was dying of a bowel obstruction.

Although the courts ruled in CHILD's favor, Senator Orrin Hatch (R-UT) rescued the Church by engineering passage of a law providing for Medicare payment for "religious non-medical health care."

Intercessory Prayer

In 1988, Witmer and Zimmerman[131] reported that their thorough search of the scientific literature had located only three controlled examinations of the effects of prayer by third parties on people who were unaware of the prayers. Of these, one (described on page 161) claimed benefit but was poorly designed, whereas the others found no benefit and were well designed.

Surprised by the small number of published studies, Witmer and Zimmerman asked 38 journal editors whether they had ever received but rejected a manuscript on the subject of intercessory prayer. They also asked the editors to ask their readers whether they knew of any such study, published or unpublished. No editor or reader responded affirmatively.

The study most often cited as evidence that third-party prayer is effective was carried out in the coronary care unit at San Francisco General Hospital. The study compared 192 patients who were prayed for by Christians located outside the hospital with 201 patients who served as controls.[132] The published report stated that the prayed-for group had fewer complications. However, the author's tabulation was not valid because he scored interrelated complications separately and therefore gave them too much weight. The average length of hospital stay, which was not subject to this type of scoring error, was identical for the treatment and control groups.[131]

Although some studies have found that churchgoers tend to be healthier and to live longer than nonchurchgoers, church attendance itself is unlikely to be responsible for the difference.[133]

Psychic Surgery

Most "psychic surgeons" practice in the Philippines, but a few have toured the United States. They purport to penetrate the body with their bare hands without leaving a skin wound. "Blood" appears when the skin is "cut," and "diseased organs" are removed from the patient's body. However, skilled observers have noted that the illusion of surgery is created with sleight of hand.[123,134] The blood is a red dye (sometimes concealed in a false thumb), and the "diseased organs" are dye-soaked animal parts or cotton wads that are palmed. The American Cancer Society has concluded that "all demonstrations to date of psychic surgery have been done by various forms of trickery" and noted that several practitioners have been prosecuted for theft and/or practicing medicine without a license.[135]

Evaluation of Faith Healing

Many cures attributed to faith healing are actually cases of spontaneous remission (including some in which the original diagnosis was in error), but physicians recognize that faith can affect the condition of many sick people. This is especially true in the case of psychosomatic or hysterical disorders. Such ailments can sometimes be relieved by the ministrations of a faith healer—or, for that matter, by the reassurances of a medical doctor.

It has been suggested that some people with psychosomatic ailments that do not respond to medical care need "an inner sense of forgiveness or cleansing" that only a ritual can produce.[122] However, Reverend Lester Kinsolving[125] points out that although faith healers give some people a mental lift, there is a psychologic danger:

Believers who are not helped may blame themselves. They may become sicker or severely depressed by such contemplations as: "Faith always heals; I'm not healed; I'm being punished! What have I done wrong? What's wrong with me?"

Other problems with faith healers include failure to screen out or refer people who need medical treatment, a tendency to disparage medical care, failure to keep adequate records, lack of objective effort to evaluate what they do, and lack of legal restraints. The extreme potential for danger is illustrated by what happened with the Faith Assembly Church, an Indiana-based religious sect that relied on faith healing rather than doctors. In the mid-1980s the Fort Wayne *News-Sentinel* documented that at least 103 persons—most of them children—had died since 1973 because they or their parents had followed the church's teachings.

Dr. Louis Rose, a British psychiatrist, investigated hundreds of alleged faith-healing cures. As his interest became well known, he received communications from healers and patients throughout the world. He sent each correspondent a questionnaire and sought corroborating information from physicians. After nearly 20 years, he concluded, "I have been unsuccessful. . . . I have yet to find one 'miracle cure'; and without that (or, alternatively, massive statistics which others must provide) I cannot be convinced of the efficacy of what is commonly termed faith healing."[136] His published analysis of 95 purported faith cures indicates:

- In 58 cases it was not possible to obtain medical or other records; therefore the claims remained unconfirmed.
- In 22 cases records were so much at variance with the claims that further investigation would be pointless.
- In two cases the evidence in the medical records suggested that the healer may have contributed to amelioration of an organic condition.
- In one case demonstrable organic disability was relieved or cured after the healer's intervention.
- In three cases the individual improved but relapsed.
- Four cases showed a satisfactory degree of improvement, although re-examination and comparison of medical records revealed no change in the organic state.
- In four cases there was improvement when healing was received concurrently with standard medical treatment.
- One patient examined before and after treatment by the healer gained no benefit and continued to deteriorate.

Many people with chronic or incurable diseases desperately reach for help from any source. Faith healers appeal to such people's need for hope. C. Eugene Emery, Jr., a science writer for the *Providence Journal*, has closely examined the work of Reverend Ralph DiOrio, a Roman Catholic priest whose healing services attract thousands. In 1987 Emery attended a service and recorded the names of nine people who had been blessed and nine others who had been proclaimed cured. DiOrio's organization provided 10 more cases that supposedly provided irrefutable proof of the priest's ability to cure. During a 6-month investigation, Emery found no evidence that any of these individuals had been helped.[137]

Therapeutic Touch

Therapeutic touch (TT) was developed during the 1970s by Dolores Krieger, Ph.D., R.N., who for many years was a nursing professor at New York University. Proponents claim that it is possible to use one's hands to detect when someone is ill, pinpoint areas of pain, reduce anxiety, and stimulate the sick person's recuperative powers. Most practitioners are nurses, many of whom consider themselves "holistic." Proponents claim that at least 43,000 nurses have been trained in its use. About 1100 belong to Nurse Healers—Professional Associates International, which Dr. Krieger established in 1977.

As taught by Krieger, TT involves four steps: (1) "centering," a meditative process said to align the healer with the patent's energy level; (2) "assessment," said to be performed by using one's hands to detect forces emanating from the patient; (3) "unruffling the field," said to involve sweeping "stagnant energy" downward to

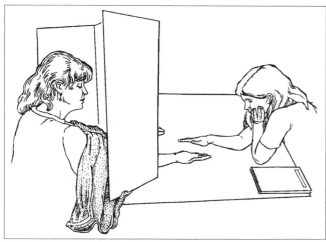

Figure 8-10. Emily Rosa testing whether a therapeutic touch practitioner can detect the presence of her hand. (Drawing by Pat Linse, Skeptics Society.)

prepare for energy transfer; and (4) transfer of "energy" from practitioner to patient. The "healer's" hands are held a few inches away from the body.

Critics who reviewed more than 800 reports have concluded that no well-designed study demonstrates any health benefit from TT. In 1998, the *Journal of the American Medical Association* published this conclusion together with the results of testing whether TT practitioners could detect the "energy field" they claim to manipulate. During the testing, the practitioners rested their forearms and hands, palms up, on a flat surface. The experimenter (Emily Rosa, who was 9 when the study began and 10 when it ended) then hovered her hand, palm down, a few inches above one of the subject's palms. A cardboard screen and a draped towel were used to prevent the subjects from seeing which hand was selected (see Figure 8-10). The practitioners correctly located Emily's hand only 122 (44%) out of 280 trials, which was no better than would be expected by guessing. The authors concluded that TT claims are groundless and that further use of TT by health professionals is unjustified.[138]

Kirlian Photography

Many TT practitioners and other psychic healers claim that they effect changes in the body's "energy field" demonstrable with Kirlian photography, which allegedly reveals the body's "aura." During this procedure the object (such as a person's hand) is placed on photographic paper or film in an apparatus that generates a high-voltage, low-amperage, high-frequency electric current. The film is then exposed by air glow that occurs when electrical discharges pass between the subject and apparatus through the photographic material.

Randi[134] has demonstrated that the pictures reflect the amount of finger pressure applied to the camera, as well as the amount of electrical grounding produced by contact between the apparatus and the subject's body. Other researchers have demonstrated that the photographic images are also affected by perspiration and many other factors.

OCCULT PRACTICES

The word "occult" refers to that which is mysterious, hidden, or obscure. It involves divination, incantation, and magic. Occult endeavors include auric healing, color healing, dowsing, exorcism, extrasensory perception (ESP), humanistic mysticism, I Ching consultation, Krishna consciousness, numerology, palmistry, phrenology, pseudoreligious ceremonies, rune casting, tarot divination, and various types of witchcraft. Many persons with severe psychiatric disorders deeply identify with occult or mystical beliefs.

For some people, occultism can be a source of support and may help reduce anxiety. People who are lonely or timid, for example, may find that the sharing of occult beliefs provides them with companionship or an intriguing hobby. However, cult members may be vulnerable to exploitation by unscrupulous leaders. Occultism can also be a breeding ground for psychosis.

Spiritualism and the "New Age"

The spiritualist movement began in 1848 when Margaret and Kate Fox claimed they were able to communicate with the dead. Through a series of rapping noises, the "spirits from beyond" gave advice, made predictions, and consoled loved ones. The Fox sisters performed in large arenas and charged clients for the opportunity to communicate with spirits. Soon after the Fox sisters began performing, thousands of mediums around the world claimed similar abilities. Years later Margaret Fox admitted that she and her sister had been perpetrating a hoax.

Although many mediums have been exposed as fake by Harry Houdini, James Randi, and other magicians, their activities persist. "Trance-channeling" is a recent fad. "Channeling" can be defined as the communication of information to, or through, a live person (the medium, or channel) from a nonphysical source, such as an angel, an extraterrestrial, or the spirit of a former human. One well-known practitioner is J.Z. Knight, who claims that a 35,000-year-old spirit named Ramtha uses her body to speak words of wisdom. Another proponent is actress Shirley MacLaine, who claims that channeling provides useful information about "past lives." The Committee for the Scientific Investigation of Claims of the Paranormal (CSICOP), which has offered to test trance-channelers under laboratory conditions, has warned:

> [We] find it surprising that trance-channelers have been allowed to make uncorroborated and unverified claims, charge people hundreds or thousands of dollars for public and private audiences, and offer advice on business and personal matters without providing evidence that they indeed have contact with discarnate beings. Many people have been harmed by such practices. . . . We suggest that the public be extremely cautious about these claims.[139]

Aligned with spiritualism is the New Age movement, whose loosely defined philosophy includes such things as: "human potential, holistic health, recycling, organic foods, grassroots activism, practical spirituality, meditation, ecology, appropriate technology, feminism and progressive politics . . . a form of utopianism, the desire to create a better society, a 'new age' in which humanity lives in harmony with the cosmos."[140] *Time* magazine described New Age as "a whole cornucopia of beliefs, fads [and] rituals" to which some followers subscribe and others do not.[141] New Age methods

---

◆ Personal Glimpse ◆

The Appeal of Channeling

Channeling offers wisdom without work, philosophy without contemplation, salvation without sacrifice. There is no demand for either the commitment or the conformity that cults or religious sects require. There is no proscription of hedonistic activities such as is commanded by most mainstream religions. There are no temptations to be avoided, no sins to eschew.

Channelers provide religious teaching.... Their basic theme is that we are spiritual and immortal beings in a universe that is essentially spiritual.... We create our own realities, and so if we want to be happy, we simply need to create a happy reality. There is no need for us to follow a guru, for we are as gods, each one of us. Indeed, Ramtha speaks like some positive-thinking inspirational author of pop psychology books who tells people to get in charge of their lives and to start enjoying themselves. . . .

Choose among traditional religion with its guilt-inducing prohibitions, channeling with its almost total preoccupation with making people feel good about themselves and their place in the universe, and the modern scientific materialistic view that seems to deny even the possibility of postmortem survival. For many it is a very easy choice. Channelers provide a hedonistic, narcissistic message that is predigested and therefore requires no wrestling with philosophical enigmas, no lifelong quest for truth. This is much in keeping with the times we live in. It requires only that we turn our minds off.

There is a clear danger in seeking advice from channels. It diverts people from trying to grapple with their difficulties in a rational and realistic way. If one has real problems and real distress, the pastiche of pop psychology and metaphysics offered up by the channelers might prove as deleterious in its effects as the fake treatments proffered by medical quacks.

James E. Alcock[142]

164   Part Two   Health-Care Approaches

include crystal healing (said to help the body balance and realign its "energy fields"), therapeutic touch, healing through mental imagery, pendulum diagnosis, pyramid healing, and dozens of others.

"Cold reading" is a factor in most contacts between "psychic" practitioners and their clients. This process can lead a client to conclude that a practitioner ("reader"), met for the first time, knows all about the individual's personality and problems. According to Hyman, the most powerful technique involves encouraging the client to reinterpret the reader's general statements in terms of the client's own vocabulary and life.[1] Other techniques include (a) using the client's reactions to general statements to formulate more specific ones, (b) posing questions that will be perceived as "hits" when they apply, but are not counted when they do not apply, and (c) rephrasing what the client says, relying on the fact that people often reveal things without remembering that they did so.

M. Lamar Keene,[143] a former professional psychic, has warned that some American psychics exchange information with each other about some of their clients but pretend to derive this information psychically.

ASTROLOGY

Astrology as applied to health and illness involves the use of a horoscope to determine the diseases and infirmities to which one is allegedly predisposed. Celestial patterns at the time of birth are said to indicate potential illness, which may be triggered by subsequent transit of the planets over sensitive areas of the natal chart. "Medical astrologers" may claim, for example, that a part of the body is prone to weakness at certain times, or that particular times may be ideal for surgery or fertility planning. Some also give dietary advice.

People are convinced of astrology's value because it "works." By this they mean that it supplies them with feedback that "feels right"—that convinces them that the horoscope provides a basis for understanding themselves and ordering their lives. It has personal meaning for them.[144]

Many experiments have demonstrated that people are likely to believe that a personality sketch fits them well, even when it was not compiled with them in mind. More than 40 years ago psychologist Bertram Forer[145] administered a personality test to the students in one of his courses. A week later he gave each a typed personality sketch with the student's name on it—the "results" of the tests. Unknown to the students, however, each one actually received an identical list of statements that Forer had copied from an astrology book:

- You have a great need for other people to like and admire you.
- You have a tendency to be critical of yourself.
- You have a great deal of unused capacity which you have not turned to your advantage.
- While you have some personality weaknesses, you are generally able to compensate for them.
- Your sexual adjustment has presented problems for you.
- Disciplined and self-controlled outside, you tend to be worrisome and insecure inside.
- At times you have serious doubts as to whether you have made the right decision or done the right thing.
- You prefer a certain amount of change and variety and become dissatisfied when hemmed in by restrictions and limitations.
- You pride yourself as an independent thinker and do not accept others' statements without satisfactory proof.
- You have found it unwise to be too frank in revealing yourself to others.
- At times you are extroverted, affable, sociable, while at other times you are introverted, wary, reserved.
- Some of your aspirations tend to be pretty unrealistic.
- Security is one of your major goals in life.

After reading the sketch, students were asked to rate how well it revealed their basic personality characteristics. On a scale of 0 (poor) to 5 (perfect), 34 out of 39 rated it 4 or better, and 16 of these rated it as perfect. Many other investigators have confirmed and added to these findings.

People's tendency to accept vague, ambiguous, and general statements as descriptive of their unique personality is known as "the Barnum effect."[146] Named after P.T. Barnum, it applies to any form of personality assessment, including interviews, standard psychologic tests, palmistry, tarot cards, and handwriting analysis ("graphology"). French and others[147] have noted:

The typical horoscope is a mix of general statements and rather more specific ones. People tend to be impressed by the specific details that appear to fit (and pay less attention to those that do not), while the general Barnum-type statements provide readily acceptable "padding."

CSICOP has asked all American newspapers that publish astrology columns to carry a disclaimer that, "Astrological forecasts should be read for entertainment value only. Such predictions have no reliable basis in scientific fact." More than 60 papers have done so, and a few others have reported CSICOP's request as a news item.

BIORHYTHMS

Creation of biorhythm theory is attributed to Wilhelm Fleiss, a German surgeon who was a close friend of

Sigmund Freud, the developer of psychoanalysis. In the 1890s Fleiss postulated that behavior was determined by innate "male" and "female" rhythms of the body. Current theory postulates three cycles: a 23-day physical cycle, a 28-day emotional cycle, and a 33-day intellectual cycle. The physical cycle influences tasks involving physical strength, endurance, energy, resistance, and confidence. The emotional curve is important in areas of high emotional content: sensibility, nerves, feelings, intuition, cheerfulness, moodiness, and creative ability. The intellectual cycle is particularly important in pursuits requiring cognitive activity: intelligence, memory, alertness, logic, reasoning power, reaction, and ambition. The three-cycle pattern repeats itself only once every 23 x 28 x 33 days (58.1 years).

Proponents claim: (a) each cycle begins at the exact moment of birth and oscillates up and down with absolute precision throughout life; (b) when the cycles are high, people are likely to be at their best; when they are low, the opposite is true; and (c) on critical days, when the cycles are changing, people are easily distracted and most prone to accidents.

Bainbridge[148] performed nine statistical studies using a Biolator calculator that provided quick measurement of cycles. He concluded that biorhythm theory is "without value." In another study, he asked 108 students whether their biorhythms, which he calculated for them on a particular day, were valid. The majority said yes. Unknown to them, however, he had determined their values by flipping a coin. Hines[149] subsequently reviewed more than 20 years' worth of studies and found no evidence to support the claims of biorhythm theory.

The human body has real, objectively measurable, biologic rhythms that have nothing to do with the aforementioned "biorhythms." Growth hormone and cholesterol production, for example, tend to peak while people are asleep at night. The science of repetitive and cyclic biologic rhythms is called *chronobiology*.

Transcendental Meditation

During transcendental meditation (TM), the meditator sits comfortably with eyes closed and mentally repeats a Sanskrit word or sound (mantra) for 15 to 20 minutes twice a day. Although the teacher supposedly chooses the mantra to fit each individual, investigators have noted that people with similar sociocultural characteristics often receive the same mantra. The process can be learned for an initiation fee that covers two introductory lectures, an initiation, and four small-group meetings. The cost has been about $1000 for adults and $600 for college students.[150]

TM is claimed to help people think more clearly, improve their memory, recover immediately from stressful situations, reverse their aging process, and enjoy life more fully. Its leaders have also claimed that "stress is the basis of all illness" and that TM is "the single most effective thing you can do to improve all aspects of health and to increase inner happiness and learning ability."[151] Meditation may temporarily relieve stress—as would forms of relaxation—but the rest of these claims have no scientific basis.

The TM movement was launched in India in 1955 by the Maharishi Mahesh Yogi, who had studied mysticism for many years. In 1958, according to Bloomfield and others, the Maharishi "proclaimed the possibility of all humanity's attaining enlightenment" and inaugurated a "World Plan" intended to encompass "every individual on earth."[152] Shortly thereafter he embarked on a world tour to spread his teachings.

Eric Woodrum,[153] a sociologist who spent a year as a participant-observer of TM activities, has described three phases of the early TM movement. From 1959 to 1965 TM was promoted as the most important component of a program of spiritual evolution and mental detachment (nirvana). During the late 1960s the movement expanded rapidly as it won major publicity by identifying with aspects of the counterculture. Since 1970 the movement has emphasized alleged practical, physiologic, material, and social benefits of TM for conventional persons, with few other-worldly references. Woodrum concluded that average meditators regarded TM as a useful mental exercise and paid little or no attention to its quasireligious belief system. Members of the inner movement, however, think in metaphysical terms and state that TM can transform the world. TM leaders maintain that large groups of people meditating together produce "the Maharishi Effect," which can reduce the incidence of crime and auto accidents. Investigators have debunked this claim by checking statistics in cities where the phenomenon had allegedly occurred.

In the mid-1970s the Maharishi began professing he could teach advanced meditators to levitate (rise and float in apparent defiance of gravity). Although thousands of people paid $3,000 each for lessons, the best they could demonstrate was cross-legged "hopping" to about 1 foot above ground level.

In 1987 a jury awarded $137,890 to an ex-devotee who contended that TM organizations had falsely promised that he could learn to levitate, reduce stress, improve his memory, and reverse the aging process. In 1988 an appeals court ordered a new trial. In 1991, the *Des Moines Register* reported that the case had been settled out of court for about $50,000.

Chapter 6 contains additional information about meditation.

Maharishi Ayur-Ved

Ayurvedic medicine is rooted in four Sanskrit books called the *Vedas*—the oldest and most important scriptures of India, shaped sometime before 200 BCE. These books attributed most disease and bad luck to demons, devils, and the influence of stars and planets. Proponents state that the body's functions are regulated by three "irreducible physiological principles," called *doshas*, whose Sanskrit names are *vata, pitta,* and *kapha*. Like the "sun signs" of astrology, these terms are used to designate body types as well as the traits that typify them. The *doshas* supposedly regulate body functions. *Vata*, for example, is said to "govern all bodily functions concerning movement" and to accumulate during cold, dry, windy weather. Through various combinations of *vata, pitta,* and *kapha*, 10 body types are possible. However, one's *doshas* (and therefore one's body type) can vary from hour to hour, season to season, and questionnaire to questionnaire.

Like astrologic writings, ayurvedic writings contain long lists of supposed physical and mental characteristics associated with each body type. One source, for example, states that *vata* individuals are "usually lightly built with excellent agility" and "love excitement and change"; *vata* balance produces mental clarity and alertness; and *vata* imbalance can produce anxiety, weight loss, constipation, high blood pressure, arthritis, weakness, and restlessness.[154]

Ayurvedic proponents claim that the symptoms of disease are always related to "imbalance" of the doshas, which can be determined by feeling the patient's wrist pulse or completing a questionnaire (see Figure 8-11). Some proponents claim that the pulse can be used to detect diabetes, cancer, musculoskeletal disease, asthma, and "imbalances at early stages when there may be no other clinical signs and when mild forms of intervention may suffice."[155] "Balance" is supposedly achieved through a multitude of procedures and products, many of which are said to be specific for specific body types.

Followers of the Maharishi Mahesh Yogi state that much of ayurvedic medicine was lost until the Maharishi reconstituted it in the early 1980s. The "revived" version has been termed Maharishi Ayurveda, Maharishi Ayur-Veda and, most recently, Maharishi Ayur-Ved. However, these names are often used interchangeably.

The full Maharishi Ayur-Ved program for "creating healthy individuals and a disease-free society" has 20 components: development of higher states of consciousness through advanced meditation techniques, use of primordial sounds, correction of "the mistake of the intellect," strengthening of emotions, Vedic structuring of language, music therapy, enlivening of the senses, pulse diagnosis, psychophysiologic integration, neuromuscular integration, neurorespiratory integration, purification (to remove "impurities due to faulty diet and behavioral patterns"), dietary measures, herbal food supplements, other herbal preparations, daily behavioral routines, prediction of future imbalances, religious ceremonies, nourishing the environment, and promoting world health and world peace. Most of these cost several hundred dollars, but some cost thousands and require the services of an ayurvedic practitioner. An investigative report in the *Journal of the American Medical Association* stated that the ayurvedic movement's marketing practices reveal what appears to be "a widespread pattern of misinformation, deception, and manipulation of lay and scientific news media."[156]

America's most prominent spokesperson for ayurveda is Deepak Chopra, M.D., an endocrinologist who, in 1984, was encouraged by the Maharishi to learn

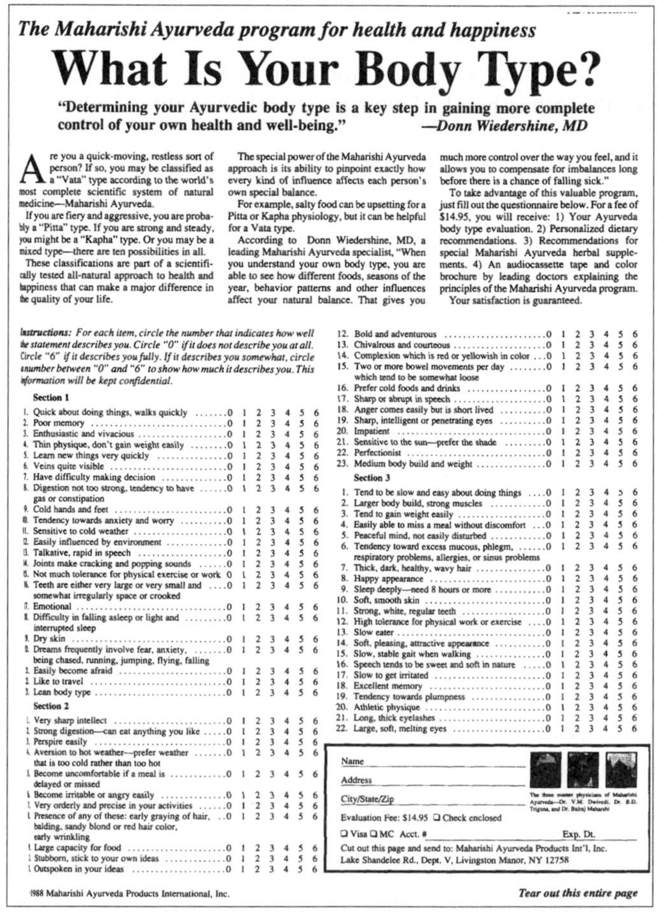

FIGURE 8-11. Ad from the March 1988 *Vegetarian Times* magazine. For $14.95 plus a completed questionnaire, readers could learn their "body type" and which foods and herbs would help them maintain "balance."

about ayurveda. During the following year Chopra became director of the Maharishi Ayurveda Health Center for Stress Management in Lancaster, Massachusetts. He also founded and became president of the American Association for Ayurvedic Medicine and Maharishi Ayur-Veda Products International (MAPI), which sells instructional materials and herbal products. In the early 1990s he severed his ties with these organizations and the TM leadership, became a consultant to a hospital-based program in California, and founded another company that markets his publications plus products similar to those of MAPI.

Chopra has written many books and gained considerable public exposure through appearances on major television talk shows. An article in *Forbes* magazine called him "the latest in a line of gurus who have prospered by blending pop science, pop psychology, and pop Hinduism."[157] One of his books, *Ageless Body, Timeless Mind*, is reported to have sold over 1 million copies. He promises "perfect health" to those who—through ayurvedic methods—can harness their consciousness as a healing force. He claims that "remaining healthy is actually a conscious choice."[158] He maintains:

If you have happy thoughts, then you make happy molecules. On the other hand, if you have sad thoughts, and angry thoughts, and hostile thoughts, then you make those molecules which may depress the immune system and make you more susceptible to disease.

Yoga Therapy

Yoga encompasses a large number of religious and quasireligious practices claimed to produce unexcelled health, well-being, and mental serenity. Yoga is based on ancient Indian beliefs about human existence. Its philosophy postulates five "sheaths" of existence: the physical body, the vital body, the mind, the higher intellect, and the abode of bliss (universal consciousness). The vital body is said to be composed of *prana*, "life energy" that flows through invisible channels. Disease is said to arise through imbalance of the three lower sheaths. In the healthy state the positive energy of the highest sheath percolates through the lower ones and brings total harmony and balance to all of the individual's faculties.

Modern proponents state that infections, injuries, and other problems with a strong physical basis should be handled by conventional medicine, but psychosomatic ailments and degenerative disorders require more.[159] The recommended exercises include yogic breathing, meditation, other relaxation techniques, bending, stretching, holding various postures, dietary measures, and "emotion culturing" (evoking positive emotions and diffusing negative ones). Hatha yoga's effects can include physical and mental relaxation, slow breathing, lowered blood pressure, reduction in metabolic activity, decreased heartbeat, and control of involuntary muscles.

Visual Training

"Vision therapists" claim to strengthen eyesight through a series of exercises and the use of eyeglasses. They emphasize exercising hand-eye coordination, watching a series of blinking lights, focusing on a string of objects, and sleeping in a certain position. Promoters say this regimen can improve school and athletic performance, increase I.Q., and help overcome learning disabilities. Training sessions may take place once or twice a week and can cost $1000. However, according to the *Mayo Clinic Health Letter*, there is no scientific evidence that the approach works.[160]

Some optometrists claim that vision therapy is valuable for children with learning disabilities. The American Academy of Pediatrics and several other professional groups have stated that muscle exercises have no proven value for learning disabilities.[161] A committee of the National Research Council concluded that although certain visual abilities may improve with practice, visual training has not been proven to enhance athletic ability.[162]

Other "Alternative" Practices

Inglis and West,[163] Segen,[164] and Raso[165,166] have identified more than 1000 "alternative therapies," including:

ALEXANDER TECHNIQUE: A manipulative "bodywork" system that aims to reduce stress and to prevent and treat various disorders by correcting poor postural habits.

AROMATHERAPY: A system based on the notion that inhaling the odors of plant oils can relieve stress and help heal hundreds of diseases and conditions.[167] Some proponents say that the oils represent the "life force" of plants.

FELDENKRAIS METHOD: An exercise system claimed to reprogram the brain so the whole body-mind system works more efficiently.

MAGNET THERAPY: Various systems of using magnets to "balance energy" within the body. Some proponents claim to be influencing the flow of energy along acupuncture meridians. Others claim to be balancing positive and negative magnetic energy that is detected with a device.

POLARITY THERAPY: A system of manipulation, stretching exercises, clear thinking, and diet, which claims to restore health by removing blocks and balancing the flow of "life energy" between the positive (head) and negative poles (feet) of the body.

RADIONICS AND RADIESTHESIA: Practices based on claims that vibrations emanating from nature can be detected with pendulums, dowsing rods, black boxes, and other devices.

REIKI: A system whose practitioners are said to harness and transmit "universal life energy" by placing their hands in specific positions on or near the body, or through absentee healing. One form of reiki, The Radiance Technique, is claimed to be useful for mental, emotional, physical, and spiritual balancing.

ROLFING: A system of massage and manipulation that seeks to liberate the body so it is able to align itself "properly with respect to gravity."

In 1987 the magazine *New Age Journal* reported that almost 100% of its readers who responded to a questionnaire had used "alternative" health methods and that 97% would be willing to choose such methods for treatment of a potentially life-threatening illness. The respondents reported using the following methods with mostly satisfactory results: acupressure (used by 42%), acupuncture (33%), aromatherapy (26%), chiropractic (56%), colonic irrigation (21%), crystal healing (25%), "energy therapy" (25%), Feldenkrais bodywork (13%), herbal medicines (47%), homeopathy (47%), iridology (19%), macrobiotic diet (26%), meditation (85%), mental imagery (70%), polarity therapy (24%), reflexology (38%), rolfing (19%), and yoga (53%). Despite the popularity of these methods among the respondents, 73% of the respondents said that an alternative practice had been harmful and 57% felt that closer regulation was needed—preferably by "experts in various holistic therapies." The methods most often judged harmful were chiropractic, acupuncture, colonic enemas, fasting, and various "natural" diets. Nearly all the respondents felt that "maintaining an emotional, physical, and spiritual balance" and "maintaining a positive attitude" were vital to good health, but only 57% thought it was important to have regular checkups by a medical doctor.[168]

UNSCIENTIFIC MEDICAL PRACTICES

A small percentage of physicians are rendering diagnoses and prescribing treatments considered invalid by the vast majority of physicians. Some of these practices have just a few proponents, whereas others have several hundred. Many of these practitioners feel alienated from scientific medical practices and promote their beliefs to the public through publications, lectures, and talk show appearances. The approaches described in this section rest on faulty medical reasoning rather than a vitalistic rationale.

Fad Diagnoses

Years ago many nervous or tired people were said to have adrenal insufficiency, a serious glandular disorder that is actually quite rare. The vast majority of these people were not only misdiagnosed but were also treated with adrenal gland extract, a potentially harmful substance they did not need. Today a diagnosis of hypoglycemia (low blood sugar) is sometimes used to explain certain symptoms of nervousness or fatigue. Doctors who are true believers in hypoglycemia are apt to diagnose it in large numbers of their patients. However, it is actually quite rare and should be diagnosed only after careful interpretation of blood glucose tests.

A diagnosis of functional hypoglycemia should not be considered unless a person who consumes a balanced diet gets symptoms 2 to 4 hours after eating, develops blood glucose levels below 45 mg per 100 ml whenever symptoms occur, and is immediately relieved of symptoms when the blood glucose level is raised. Bennion[169] cautions that the commonly performed glucose tolerance test is not reliable for evaluating most cases of suspected hypoglycemia. Low blood glucose levels without symptoms occur commonly in normal

---

◆ **Personal Glimpse** ◆

Recipe for a New Fad Disease

- Pick any symptoms—the more common the better.
- Pick any disease—real or invented. (Real diseases have more potential for confusion because their existence can't be denied.)
- Assign lots of symptoms to the disease.
- Say that millions of undiagnosed people suffer from it.
- Pick a few treatments—Including supplements will enable health-food stores and chiropractors to get in on the action.
- Promote your theories through books and talk shows.
- Don't compete with other fad diseases. Say that yours predisposes people to the rest or vice versa.
- Claim that the medical establishment, the drug companies, and the chemical industry are against you.
- State that the medical profession is afraid of your competition or trying to protect its turf.
- If challenged to prove your claims, say that you lack the money for research, that you are too busy getting sick people well, and that your clinical results speak for themselves.

persons fed large amounts of sugar. These incidents have no diagnostic significance.

Clinical ecology is based on beliefs that multiple symptoms are triggered by hypersensitivity to common foods and chemicals. Advocates of this belief system describe themselves as "ecologically oriented" and consider their patients to be suffering from "environmental illness," "multiple chemical sensitivity (MCS)," "allergy to everything," or "twentieth-century disease," which can mimic almost any other illness. Clinical ecologists speculate that (a) although various substances alone may not cause trouble, low doses of different substances can add to or multiply each other's effects; (b) hypersensitivity develops when the total load of physical and psychologic stresses exceeds a person's tolerance; and (c) hypersensitivities may be related to "immune system dysregulation" that can be difficult to diagnose and treat.[170]

According to proponents, potential stressors include practically everything that modern humans encounter, such as urban air, diesel exhaust, tobacco smoke, fresh paint or tar, organic solvents and pesticides, certain plastics, newsprint, perfumes and colognes, medications, gas used for cooking and heating, building materials, permanent press and synthetic fabrics, household cleaners, rubbing alcohol, felt-tip pens, cedar closets, tap water, and electromagnetic forces. The signs and symptoms are said to include depression, irritability, mood swings, inability to concentrate or think clearly, poor memory, fatigue, drowsiness, diarrhea, constipation, sneezing, runny or stuffy nose, wheezing, itching of the eyes and nose, skin rashes, headaches, muscle and joint pains, frequent urination, pounding heart, swelling of various parts of the body, and even schizophrenia.

To diagnose "ecologically related" disease, practitioners take a history that emphasizes dietary habits and exposure to environmental chemicals they consider harmful. Various nonstandard tests and elimination and rotation diets are used with the hope of identifying foods that cause problems. In severe cases, patients may spend several weeks in an environmental control unit designed to remove them from exposure to airborne pollutants and synthetic substances that might cause adverse reactions.

Generally patients are instructed to modify their diet and to avoid substances such as scented shampoos; aftershave products; deodorants; cigarette smoke; automobile exhaust fumes; and synthetic fibers contained in clothing, furniture, and carpets. Extreme restrictions can include staying at home for months and avoiding physical contact with family members. "Ecologically ill" patients may think of themselves as immunologi-

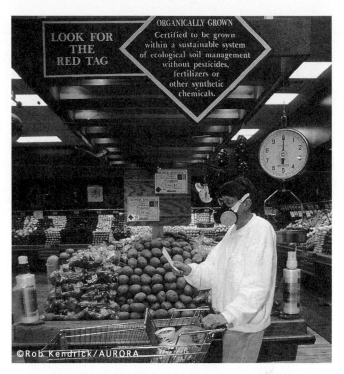

Figure 8-12. Some "MCS" patients wear a mask to filter the air they breathe when away from home.

cally disabled in a hostile world of dangerous foods and chemicals and an uncaring medical community. In many cases their life becomes centered around their illness.

The American Academy of Allergy, Asthma, and Immunology (AAAAI), the nation's largest professional organization of allergists, has warned:

Although the idea that the environment is responsible for a multitude of health problems is very appealing, to present such ideas as facts, conclusions, or even likely mechanisms without adequate support, is poor medical practice.[171]

Clinical ecologists base their diagnoses primarily on the results of "provocation" and "neutralization" tests, which are performed by having the patient report symptoms that occur within 10 minutes after suspected harmful substances are placed under the tongue or injected into the skin. If any symptoms occur, the test is considered positive, and lower concentrations are given until a dose is found that "neutralizes" the symptoms. Double-blind testing conducted by researchers at the University of California has demonstrated that these procedures are not valid. Eighteen patients each received three injections of suspected food extracts and nine of normal saline over a 3-hour period. The tests were conducted in the offices of proponents who had been treating them. In unblinded tests these patients had consistently reported symptoms when exposed to food extracts and no symptoms when given saline injections. But during the experiment they reported as many symptoms following saline injections as they did after food extract injections, indicating that their symptoms were nothing more than placebo reactions. "Neutralizing" doses were equally effective whether they were food extracts or saline. The symptoms included nasal stuffiness, dry mouth, nausea, fatigue, headaches, and feelings of disorientation or depression.[172]

In 1991 a jury in New York State awarded $489,000 in actual damages and $411,000 in punitive damages to the estate of a man who committed suicide after several years of treatment by a prominent clinical ecologist. Testimony at the trial indicated that although the man was a paranoid schizophrenic who thought "foods were out to get him," the doctor had diagnosed him as a "universal reactor" and advised that, to remain alive, he must live in a "pure" environment, follow a restrictive diet, and take supplements.[173]

"Candidiasis hypersensitivity" is an alleged condition with multiple symptoms that may include fatigue, depression, inability to concentrate, hyperactivity, headaches, skin problems (including hives), abdominal pains and bloating, constipation, diarrhea, respiratory symptoms, and problems of the urinary and reproductive organs. Its leading proponent, William J. Crook, M.D., claims that if a careful checkup does not reveal a cause for such symptoms, and a medical history includes antibiotic usage, "it's possible or even probable that your health problems are yeast-connected."[174]

The proposed treatment program includes food supplements, special diets, and treatment with antifungal drugs. Proponents claim that the diagnosis is confirmed if the patient improves after taking antifungal drugs. However, AAAAI regards the concept of candidiasis hypersensitivity as "speculative and unproven," and notes that everyone has some of its supposed symptoms from time to time. In a strongly worded position paper AAAAI has warned that some patients who take the inappropriately prescribed antifungal drugs will suffer side effects, and that overuse of these drugs could lead to the development of resistant germs that endanger everyone.[171] In 1990 a double-blind trial found the antifungal drug nystatin was no better than a placebo for relieving systemic or psychologic symptoms attributed to "candidiasis hypersensitivity syndrome."[175]

Many physicians accustomed to rendering the aforementioned "fad diagnoses" have added "chronic fatigue syndrome" (CFS) to their list. This is a controversial diagnosis that may be appropriate only for a small percentage of people who experience chronic fatigue. Because no cause has been discovered, some doctors wonder whether CFS actually is a disease.

According to criteria developed by the U.S. Centers for Disease Control and Prevention, the diagnosis should not be made unless unexplained severe fatigue persists or recurs for at least six months and is accompanied by at least four of the following: (1) impaired memory or concentration, (2) sore throat, (3) tender lymph nodes in the neck or armpits, (4) muscle pain, (5) pain in several joints, (6) new headaches, (7) unrefreshing sleep, and (8) malaise after exertion.[176] Other likely causes of fatigue must be carefully ruled out. Testing for antibodies to the Epstein-Barr virus (the causative agent of mononucleosis) is not useful for evaluating severe fatigue because 80% of healthy adults have positive antibody tests, presumably from mild or inapparent infection at an earlier age. No treatment has been proven effective for chronic fatigue syndrome,

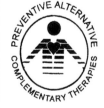

Figure 8-13. Excerpt from a 1996 flyer from an osteopathic physician whose radio advertisements invite people who have been advised to have coronary bypass surgery to consult him first. There is no published scientific evidence that chelation therapy can render bypass surgery unnecessary or can help people with any of the conditions listed in the ad. The experience to which the ad refers is not a trustworthy substitute for scientific testing.

although antidepressant drugs may help relieve certain symptoms.

Consumer Reports[177] advises conservative measures: a balanced diet, adequate sleep, avoidance of excess stress, gradually increasing exercise without overdoing it, and—above all—patience. Calling CFS "a magnet for quacks," the magazine warns that "some practitioners create CFS patients by finding the syndrome in people who clearly don't have it." In 1990 its medical writer visited three "CFS specialists" and said he had been tired for 8 months. The first said the reporter's system was "sluggish" and needed to be "detoxified." He charged $185 and recommended blood tests costing $922.50. The others ordered Epstein-Barr tests and said the results were abnormal. One prescribed a drug used to treat heroin addiction, and the other recommended vitamin injections to "bolster the immune system." Experts said that neither the tests, the diagnosis, nor the recommended treatments were appropriate.

Another diagnosis becoming popular among supplement promoters is "parasites," which may be "treated" with laxatives and other "intestinal cleansers," colonic irrigation, plant enzymes, dietary measures, and homeopathic remedies. Yet another, "leaky gut syndrome," is described by proponents as a condition in which the intestinal lining becomes irritated and porous so that unwanted food particles, "toxins," bacteria, parasites, and "Candida" enter the bloodstream and result in "a weakened immune system, digestive disorders, and eventually chronic and autoimmune disease." Treatment of this alleged condition can include dietary changes (such as not eating protein and starch at the same meal); "cleansing" with herbal products; "reestablishing good balance" of intestinal bacteria; and supplement concoctions claimed to strengthen and repair the intestinal lining.[178]

Lyme disease is also being overdiagnosed. The actual disease is a spirochetal infection acquired through a tick bite and is easily curable with antibiotics. However, some doctors are applying this diagnosis to patients with chronic nonspecific symptoms, such as headaches, fatigue, achiness, mental confusion, or sleep disturbances. The recommended treatment may include long-term antibiotic therapy, hyperbaric oxygen, colloidal silver, dietary supplements, and/or herbs, none of which have any proven value for such symptoms.[179]

Chelation Therapy

Chelation therapy involves injection of disodium EDTA into the bloodstream. The therapy is claimed to be effective against kidney and heart disease, arthritis, Parkinson's disease, emphysema, multiple sclerosis,

---

◆ Personal Glimpse ◆

Court Sides with Science

In 1991 a federal court judge in Georgia dismissed a claim asserted by a woman who suffered a stroke following surgery in 1989 for partial blockage of her left carotid artery. The woman had charged that her neurosurgeon had committed malpractice by failing to inform her that a chelation therapy was a possible alternative to the surgery. Georgia's informed consent law requires physicians, before performing surgery, to inform their patients of the risks and of "practical alternatives . . . which are generally recognized and accepted by reasonably prudent physicians." The judge ruled that the plaintiff had failed to prove that this standard had been violated.[180] Chelation therapy is a series of intravenous infusions containing an artificial amino acid (EDTA) and various other substances. Proponents claim chelation is an alternative to surgery because it can remove atherosclerotic plaque from the body's arteries.

In explaining his reasoning, the judge noted that chelation therapy is not taught in medical schools, is not FDA-approved for treating blocked arteries, and has been criticized as unproven by the American Medical Association, American Heart Association, American College of Cardiology, and American College of Physicians. Even the doctors who testified as expert witnesses on the woman's behalf had admitted that chelation therapy is unpopular and not recognized as effective against cardiovascular disease by the great majority of physicians.

---

gangrene, psoriasis, and many other serious conditions. However, no controlled trial has shown that chelation therapy can help any of them, and manufacturers of EDTA do not list them as appropriate for EDTA treatment.[181] A course of treatment, consisting of 20 to 50 intravenous infusions, can cost thousands of dollars. Chelation therapy for the conditions just listed is not covered by Medicare or most other insurance policies. Chelation therapy with calcium EDTA is one of several legitimate methods for treating cases of lead poisoning, but the protocol differs from the one just described. Some chelation therapists submit fraudulent insurance reports using a procedure code for standard infusion therapy or claiming that they treated lead poisoning.

Chelation therapy is heavily promoted as an alternative to coronary bypass surgery. It is sometimes claimed to be a "chemical Roto-Rooter" that can clean out atherosclerotic plaque from the body's arteries. It is not.[182] In 1985, after reviewing pertinent literature, the

American Heart Association's Task Force on New and Unestablished Therapies concluded that there was no scientific evidence to demonstrate any benefit.[183] Since that time no well-designed study has demonstrated any benefit against heart disease, and three studies found no benefit against intermittent claudication, a condition in which impaired circulation to the legs causes pain when the person walks. In 1999, the Federal Trade Commission obtained a consent decree barring the leading chelation therapy organization from advertising that chelation is effective against cardiovascular disease or any other disease of the circulatory system.[184]

Inspired by the claims for chelation therapy, many entrepreneurs have marketed a multitude of vitamin and homeopathic concoctions claimed to do the same thing as chelation therapy when taken by mouth. The FDA has stopped some manufacturers from marketing these products, but others are still doing so. Some falsely portray atherosclerosis as a simple buildup of fatty-cholesterol sludge that their products dissolve. As Chapter 15 explains, the buildup includes fibrous tissue that is not easily removed.

"HOLISTIC MEDICINE"

The term "holistic" (also spelled "wholistic") is used in both scientific and nonscientific circles. However, considerable confusion surrounds its use. Scientific practitioners regard holistic medicine as treatment of the "whole patient," with due attention to emotional factors as well as the patient's lifestyle. But most who label their approach holistic use methods that are nonscientific, *narrow* in focus, and *less* likely to be individualized to fit their patients. (Whereas scientific practitioners obtain a thorough history to understand the patient's total clinical picture, ayurvedic practitioners focus on "body-types," chiropractors tend to focus on the spine, and so on.) Stalker and Glymour, who have studied the holistic movement closely, consider it "a pablum of common sense and nonsense offered by cranks and quacks and failed pedants who share an attachment to magic and an animosity to reason."[100]

Some people espouse the holistic approach as an important modern development in the health-care field. Critics reply that good physicians have always considered their patients as whole beings and that the term *holistic* is a dangerous banner under which practitioners of nonscientific methods rally. Many chiropractors, for example, have organized "holistic" or "wellness" centers that offer "natural" treatments and "preventive" services, but the recommended methods typically include unnecessary vitamin supplements and spinal

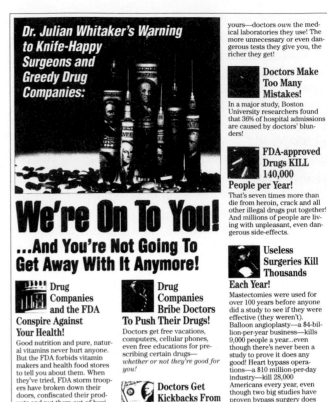

FIGURE 8-14. Portion of an ad for *Health & Healing,* a newsletter that advocates "alternative" methods. Most statements in the ad are either false or misleading.

adjustments for everyone. In contrast, wellness programs run by scientific practitioners emphasize attention to risk factors. These programs offer help with smoking cessation, counseling to promote weight control and dietary balance, and exercise methods that increase heart strength and endurance. Because the "holistic" label is a potential source of public confusion, informed observers have urged scientific practitioners to abandon it.[185]

Supportive Organizations

"Alternative" practitioners tend to be politically and emotionally supportive of one another, and many have banded together in professional groups. Some of these are limited to physicians, some accept all types of health-care providers, and some admit laypersons as well. Some of the professional groups publish a journal and operate a "specialty board" that certifies practitioners but lacks standing within the scientific community. Some groups are campaigning for laws to prevent state licensing boards from disciplining their members for using unscientific practices.

The International Academy of Preventive Medicine (IAPM) was founded in 1971 "to create an atmosphere conducive to open discussion of preventive medical practices among physicians, dentists, Ph.D.'s, and health-related professions." Subsequently it merged with a similar group, the International College of Applied Nutrition, to form the International Academy of Nutrition and Preventive Medicine (IANPM). IANPM, which has about 400 members, publishes the *Journal of Applied Nutrition* and operates the International Association of Clinical Nutritionists. The journal's largest financial supporter is the National Nutritional Foods Association, a group that represents health-food industry manufacturers, distributors, and retailers.

The American Holistic Medical Association (AHMA) was founded in 1978 by physicians who supposedly wished to use nontraditional methods as adjuncts to traditional ones. It has about 600 members, all of whom are medical or osteopathic physicians. Other "holistic" groups include the Holistic Dental Association (about 200 members), American Holistic Nurses Association (about 2700 members), and American Holistic Veterinary Medical Association (about 400 members). AHMA sponsors conferences and publishes a bimonthly magazine called *Holistic Medicine*. AHMA is closely affiliated with the American Holistic Medical Foundation, whose primary purpose is to raise funds for research and educational projects. However, it appears to have raised little money and sponsored no significant research. The topics covered at AHMA conferences have included acupuncture theory, anthroposophic medicine, ayurvedic medicine, balancing body chemistry, homeopathy, "nontraditional methods of diagnosis," "nutritional therapy," and many other approaches that the scientific community considers invalid. Many exhibitors at these meetings offer questionable products and services. AHMA recently announced plans to set up "board certification."

The American College of Advancement in Medicine (ACAM) consists mainly of medical and osteopathic physicians who practice chelation therapy. Most members also advocate megavitamins and questionable dietary practices for a wide variety of ailments. ACAM's political arm, the American Preventive Medical Association (APMA), was formed in 1992.

The Foundation for the Advancement of Innovative Medicine (FAIM) was formed in 1986 and incorporated in 1989 "as a voice for innovative medicine's professionals, physicians, patients, and suppliers." Headquartered in Suffern, New York, it has about 3000 members. Its professional members, about 60 of whom have been identified in the group's publications, include medical doctors, osteopaths, chiropractors, dentists, psychologists, and social workers, almost all of whom practice in New York or New Jersey.

Megavitamin proponents have formed the Orthomolecular Medical Society, which has about 300 members. "Clinical ecologists" have formed the American Academy of Environmental Medicine (originally called the Society for Clinical Ecology) and the American Academy of Otolaryngic Allergy.

The International Association of Dentists and Physicians, founded in 1991, is open to all types of licensed or "certified" health-care providers. Described as a "minority trade association," it hopes to set standards for unconventional methods that will be recognized by insurance companies, regulatory agencies, and the courts.

The International Association for New Science (IANS) was formed to promote research and education into "topics and phenomena which cannot be explained by traditional science, yet may have the potential for significant benefit to the health and conditions for humanity and the planet Earth."[186] The topics includes "new medicine" (e.g., acupuncture, homeopathy, therapeutic touch, herbology, color and sound therapy, iridology, vibrational medicine), "new psychology" (e.g., past lives, reincarnation, spirit possession, astrology, numerology, and mental effects from environmental toxins), "nonphysical dimensions" (e.g., ghosts, spiritual possessions, channeling), radionics, auras, dowsing, and "alternative energy."

Consumers Union has suggested that state licensing boards systematically evaluate the work of medical and osteopathic physicians who engage in megavitamin therapy, clinical ecology, chelation therapy, homeopathy, or other unscientific methods, to determine whether they are qualified to remain in practice.[187]

"MEDICAL FREEDOM" LAWS

During the past century, as scientific health-care advanced, many laws were passed to protect the public from methods that are ineffective or promoted with misinformation. "Alternative" advocates are campaigning to weaken or overturn these laws. Within the past few years, several states have passed "Medical Freedom of Choice" bills. These prevent or make it difficult for their licensing boards to discipline practitioners who use a nonstandard treatment that does not directly threaten the life or health of the patient.[188] A federal "Access to Medical Treatment Act" has been introduced to prevent the FDA from interfering with the sale and distribution of unproven drugs and devices.

Proponents claim that these types of laws increase individual freedom without increasing consumer risk. This is untrue. The basic principle of our health-related consumer-protection law is that products cannot be marketed until proven safe and effective by scientific testing. Doctors who wish to test a new product can obtain FDA permission by showing reasonable preliminary evidence of safety and potential usefulness. This policy is not oppressive; it simply requires these doctors to act in a responsible manner. "Medical freedom" laws facilitate the sale of worthless treatments, permit marketing of products whose safety has not been tested, and make it difficult to prevent unscientific practitioners from exploiting patients.

The NIH Center for Complementary and Alternative Medicine

In 1991, at the urging of a former Congressman who had used "alternative" therapies after undergoing conventional treatment for Lyme disease and prostate cancer, Senator Tom Harkin (D-IA) spearheaded passage of a law ordering the National Institutes of Health (NIH) to foster research into unconventional practices. To carry out the law's intent, the NIH established an office of unconventional medicine, which was later renamed the Office of Alternative Medicine (OAM). The NIH also appointed an advisory committee that included the former congressman and advocates of acupuncture, "energy medicine," homeopathy, ayurvedic medicine, and dubious cancer therapies. A few qualified researchers have served as advisers but have had little influence on its output.

In 1992 about 200 "alternative" proponents attended a workshop to help develop a research agenda for OAM. The outcome was a 420-page report, published in 1995, that promotes a large number of unscientific methods plus a few that have scientific support.[189] The report states that NIH has not endorsed the practices it describes and warns that "many of the therapies described have not been subjected to rigorous scientific investigation to prove safety or efficacy." However, many proponents represent it as NIH-endorsed.

The OAM's first director, Joseph J. Jacobs, M.D., spent most of his time gathering information, developing working relationships with proponents, and interacting with the news media. In 1994 he resigned, charging that Harkin and others had interfered with his ability to carry out the OAM's mission in a scientific manner.[190] During his 2-year tenure the OAM distributed 42 grants of about $30,000 each for research projects and two $840,000 grants to set up research centers at Bastyr University and at a mental health facility that treats drug abusers with acupuncture.[191] None of these projects have

produced any meaningful research. A subsequent director, Wayne Jonas, M.D., minimized press contacts and awarded large grants to set up research centers affiliated with medical schools.[192] He also developed a database of relevant journal articles. In 1996 Jonas stated that his office had stopped distributing many types of information that had not been reviewed by experts to assure its validity. However, people who inquire about specific methods are not given information about their lack of proven effectiveness. In 1998, Congress transformed OAM into the National Center for Complementary and Alternative Medicine (NCCAM), giving it more independence and a larger budget.

"Alternative" proponents have trumpeted the involvement of NIH as evidence that whatever they espouse is valid. Its main impact so far has been as a magnet for the press. The resultant press reports have contained little criticism and featured the views of proponents and their satisfied patients. Few reporters make any effort to determine whether the "alternative" or "complementary" methods they mention are useful, promising, or nonsensical. In 2000, the White House appointed a Presidential Commission on CAM to make recommendations for further study. The majority of its members appear to advocate questionable methods. Even if these goings-on generate some useful research, the benefits are unlikely to outweigh the publicity bonanza already given to worthless methods.[193]

It's Your Decision

1. Your back hurts after playing volleyball. At the suggestion of a friend, you see a chiropractor who examines you, obtains an x-ray film, manipulates your spine, and advises you to return the next day for a full report. The next day you feel completely normal but keep the appointment anyway. The chiropractor is pleased but says he has discovered that you have a curvature of your spine that may make you prone to further difficulty. He recommends weekly visits for a few weeks followed by monthly checkups and adjustments for "preventative maintenance." What should you do?

2. One of your male relatives has recurrent chest pains (angina) due to impaired coronary artery circulation. After having an angiogram, he was advised to have bypass surgery. A local chelation therapist advertises that people advised to have coronary bypass surgery should see him instead. Your relative has scheduled an appointment to see the chelationist. What should you do?

SUMMARY

"Alternative" practitioners espouse a wide variety of theories and methods not based on scientific evidence. Some of these practitioners seem sincere in their beliefs, whereas others are clear-cut frauds. In some cases they mix effective methods with ineffective ones. In some cases their methods may relieve symptoms related to tension. In many cases they claim credit for spontaneous improvements. Some "alternative" practitioners know their limitations; others will attempt to treat any ailment. The vast majority make no effort to test the validity of what they do. The National Center for Complementary and Alternative Medicine was established through the influence of political insiders rather than any scientific merits of "alternative medicine." Consumers should be wary of the practitioners described in this chapter and use them cautiously, if at all. Current consumer-protection laws need strengthening rather than weakening.

REFERENCES

1. Hyman R. "Cold reading": how to convince strangers you know all about them. The Zetetic, pp 18–37, Spring/Summer 1977.
2. Barrett S, Herbert V. The Vitamin Pushers. How the "Health Food" Industry Is Selling America a Bill of Goods. Amherst N.Y., 1994, Prometheus Books.
3. Dodes JE, Schissel MJ. Holistic dentistry: Onward to the Middle Ages. Journal of the Colorado Dental Association 73(2):12–14, 44–45.
4. Eisenberg DM and others. Unconventional medicine in the United States. New England Journal of Medicine 328:246–252, 1993.
5. Gorski T. Do the Eisenberg data hold up? Scientific Review of Alternative Medicine 3(2):62–69, 1998.
6. Druss BG, Rosenheck RA. Association between use of unconventional therapies and conventional medical services. JAMA 282:651–656, 1999.
7. Berman BM, Larsen DB, editors. Alternative Medicine: Expanding Medical Horizons. A Report to the National Institutes of Health on Alternative Medical Systems and Practices in the United States. Washington, D.C., 1995, US Government Printing Office.
8. Skrabanek P, McCormick J. Follies and Fallacies in Medicine. Amherst, N.Y., 1990, Prometheus Books.
9. Barrett S, Herbert V. Questionable cancer therapies. In Holland JF and others, editors. Cancer Medicine. Baltimore, 1996, Williams & Wilkins.
10. Office of Technology Assessment of the Congress of the United States. Assessing the Efficacy and Safety of Medical Technologies. Washington, D.C., 1978, US Government Printing Office.
11. White KL. Evidenced-based medicine (letter to the editor). Lancet 346:837–838, 1995.
12. Ellis J and others. Inpatient general medicine is evidence based. Lancet 346:407–410, 1995.
13. Zwicky JF, Hafner AW, Barrett S, Jarvis WT. Reader's Guide to "Alternative" Health Methods: An Analysis of More than 1,000 Reports on Unproven, Disproven, Controversial, Fraudulent, Quack, and/or Otherwise Questionable Approaches to Solving Health Problems. Chicago, 1993, American Medical Association.
14. Relman AS. A trip to Stonesville. The New Republic, Dec 14, 1998.
15. De Smet PAGM. Is there any danger in using traditional remedies? Journal of Ethnopharmacology 32:43–50, 1991.
16. Young JH. Folk into fake. Western Folklore, 44:225–239, 1985.
17. Spigelblatt L and others. The use of alternative medicine by children. Pediatrics 94:811–814, 1994.
18. Clinical Oncology Group. New Zealand cancer patients and alternative medicine. New Zealand Medical Journal 100:110–113, Feb 25, 1987.
19. Oelman M. Homeopathy in the news. Homeopathy Today 16(4):3, 1996.
20. Porkert M, Ullmann C. Chinese Medicine. New York, 1988, William Morrow & Co.
21. Tai D. Acupuncture & Moxibustion. St. Louis, 1987, Mosby.
22. Skrabanek P. Acupuncture: Past, present, and future. In Stalker D, Glymour C, editors. Examining Holistic Medicine. Amherst, N.Y., 1985, Prometheus Books.
23. Kurtz P, Alcock J, and others. Testing psi claims in China: Visit by a CSICOP delegation. Skeptical Inquirer 12:364–375, 1988.
24. Introduction to oriental medicine. Seattle, 1991, John Bastyr College Publications.
25. Sampson W and others. Acupuncture: The position paper of the National Council Against Health Fraud. Clinical Journal of Pain 7:162–166, 1991.
26. Melzack R, Katz J. Auriculotherapy fails to relieve chronic pain: A controlled crossover study. JAMA 251:1041–1043, 1984.
27. Ter Reit G, Kleijnen J, Knipschild P. Acupuncture and chronic pain: A criteria-based meta-analysis. Clinical Epidemiology 43:1191–1199, 1990.
28. Ter Reit G, Kleijnen J, Knipschild P. A meta-analysis of studies into the effect of acupuncture on addiction. British Journal of General Practice 40:379–382, 1990.
29. Melzack R, Wall PD. The Challenge of Pain. New York, 1983, Basic Books Inc, Publishers.
30. American Medical Association Council on Scientific Affairs. Reports of the Council on Scientific Affairs of the American Medical Association, 1981. Chicago, 1982, The Association.
31. Ulett GA. Acupuncture update 1984. Southern Medical Journal 78:233–234, 1985.
32. Ulett GA. Beyond Yin and Yang: How Acupuncture Really Works. St. Louis, 1992, Warren H. Green.
33. Ulett GA, Johnson MB. Two kinds of acupuncture. Digest of Chiropractic Economics 36(1):25–27, 1993.
34. Ulett GA. Alternative Medicine or Magical Healing. St. Louis, 1996, Warren H. Green.
35. Department of Education, Office of Postsecondary Education. Nationally Recognized Accrediting Agencies and Associations. Criteria and Procedures for Listing by the U.S. Secretary for Education and Current List. Washington, D.C., 1995, U.S. Department of Education.
36. Magner G. Chiropractic: The Victim's Perspective. Amherst, N.Y., 1995, Prometheus Books.
37. Yamashita H and others. Adverse events related to acupuncture. JAMA 280:1563–1564, 1998.
38. Norheim JA, Fennebe V. Adverse effects of acupuncture. Lancet 345:1576, 1995.
39. Acupuncture needle status changed. FDA Talk Paper T96-21, April 1, 1996.
40. Acupuncture. NIH Consensus Statement 15:(5), Nov 3-5, 1997.

41. Sampson WI. On the National Institute of Drug Abuse Consensus Conference on Acupuncture. Scientific Review of Alternative Medicine 2(1):54-55, 1998.

42. Sportelli L. Introduction to Chiropractic, 7th edition. Palmerton, Pa., 1983, PracticeMakers Products.

43. Lomax E. Manipulative therapy: A historical perspective from ancient times to the modern era. In Goldstein M, editor. The Research Status of Spinal Manipulative Therapy. Monograph 15, 1975, National Institute of Neurological and Communicative Disorders and Stroke.

44. Palmer DD. The Chiropractor's Adjuster: A Text-Book of the Science, Art and Philosophy of Chiropractic. Portland, Ore., 1910, Portland Printing House Company.

45. Smith RL. At Your Own Risk: The Case against Chiropractic. New York, 1969, Pocket Books.

46. Williams SE. Chiropractic Science & Practice in the United States. Arlington, Va., 1991, International Chiropractors Association.

47. 1992 Census of Service Industries. Washington, D.C., 1995, US Department of Commerce.

48. Jarvis WT. Chiropractic: A skeptical view. Skeptical Inquirer 12(4):47–55, 1987.

49. From Simple Beginnings (videotape). Chiropractic Centennial Foundation, 1996.

50. Rome PL. Usage of chiropractic terminology in the literature: 296 ways to say "subluxation": complex issues of the vertebral subluxation. Journal of Chiropractic Technique 8:49–60,1996.

51. Crelin E. A scientific test of the chiropractic theory. American Scientist 61:574–580, 1973.

52. Crelin E. Discussion of the newspaper advertising of Richard T LaBarre, D.C., in the Bethlehem Globe-Times 1974–1975, prepared for the district attorney of Northampton County, Pa., in 1976.

53. Barrett S. How five chiropractors diagnosed a healthy child. Pediatric Management 4(11):31, 1993.

54. Brown M. Chiro: How much healing? How much flim-flam? Quad-City Times, Davenport, Iowa, Dec 13, 1981.

55. Levin S. Interview by Dr. Stephen Barrett, 1989. In Barrett S and others. Health Schemes, Scams, and Frauds. New York, 1990, Consumer Reports Books.

56. Bergman TF. Chiropractic technique: An overview. In Lawrence DJ, editor. Advances in Chiropractic, Volume 2. St. Louis, 1996, Mosby.

57. Cohen W. Independent Practitioners under Medicare: A Report to Congress. Washington, D.C., 1968, US Department of Health, Education, and Welfare.

58. What we teach. The Chiropractic Journal 8(1):34–36, 1993.

59. Nelson CF. Chiropractic scope of practice. Journal of Manipulative and Physiological Therapeutics 16:488–497, 1993.

60. Williams SE. Dynamic Essentials of the Chiropractic Principle, Practice and Procedure. Marietta Ga., (undated, circa 1991, purchased 1999), Si-Nel Publishing Co.

61. Parker JW. Textbook of Office Procedure and Practice Building for the Chiropractic Profession, 4th edition. Fort Worth, 1975, Parker Chiropractic Research Foundation.

62. Moran MC and others. Inspection of Chiropractic Services Under Medicare. Chicago, 1986, US Department of Health and Human Services.

63. Kusserow RP. State Licensure and Discipline of Chiropractors. Office of Inspector General, Jan 1989.

64. Shekelle PG and others. The Appropriateness of Spinal Manipulation for Low-Back Pain. Part I: Project Overview and Literature Review. Santa Monica, Calif., 1991, RAND.

65. Bigos SJ and others. Acute Low Back Pain Problems in Adults. Clinical Practice Guideline No. 14. Rockville, Md., 1994, Agency for Health Care Policy and Research.

66. Shekelle PM. Spine update: Spinal manipulation. Spine 19:858–861, 1994.

67. Shekelle PM. RAND misquoted. ACA Journal of Chiropractic 30(7):59–63, 1993.

68. Assendelft WJJ, Bouter LM. Does the goose really lay golden eggs? A methodological review of workmen's compensation studies. Journal of Manipulative and Physiological Therapeutics 16:161–168, 1993.

69. Carey TS and others. The outcomes and costs of care for acute low back pain among patients seen by primary care practitioners, chiropractors, and orthopedic surgeons. New England Journal of Medicine 333:913–917, 1995.

70. Getzendanner S. Memorandum opinion and order in Wilk et al v AMA et al, No. 76 C 3777, US District Court for the Northern District of Illinois, Eastern Division, August 27, 1987.

71. Koren T. Chiropractic brings out the best in you. Philadelphia, 1995, Koren Publications, Inc.

72. Koren T. How to get 5 to 10 new patients a week without leaving your office. Philadelphia, 1996, Koren Publications, Inc.

73. Lynch RP Jr. Passion: Where has it gone? Journal of the American Chiropractic Association 32(11):5–6, 1995.

74. Homola S. Seeking a common denominator in the use of spinal manipulation. Chiropractic Technique 4:61–63, 1992.

75. Modde PJ. Malpractice is an inevitable result of chiropractic philosophy and training. Legal Aspects of Medical Practice, pp 20–23, Feb 1979.

76. Chiropractic: Still not recommended. In Barrett S and others. Health Schemes, Scams, and Frauds. New York, 1990, Consumer Reports Books.

77. Katzenstein L. "Nutrition" against disease: A close look at a chiropractic seminar. Nutrition Forum 5:25–28, 1988.

78. Christenson MG. Job Analysis of Chiropractic: A Project Report, Survey Analysis, and Summary of the Practice of Chiropractic within the United States. Greeley, Colo., 1998, National Board of Chiropractic Examiners.

79. Colley F, Haas M. Attitudes on immunization: A survey of American chiropractors. Journal of Manipulative and Physiological Therapeutics 17:584–590, 1994.

80. Barrett S. The spine salesmen. In Barrett S, Jarvis WT, editors. The Health Robbers: A Close Look at Quackery in America. Amherst N.Y., 1993, Prometheus Books.

81. Lee KP and others. Neurologic complications following chiropractic manipulation: A survey of California neurologists. Neurology 45:1213–1215, 1995.

82. Assendelft WJJ, Bouter LM, Knipschild PG. Complications of spinal manipulation: Review of the literature. Journal of Family Practice 42:475–480, 1996.

83. London W. Free chiropractic spinal exams, consultations and literature: An empirical investigation. Presented at the American Public Health Association National Convention, Chicago, Oct 24, 1989.

84. Chiropractors. Consumer Reports 59:383–390, 1994.

85. How to win patients and influence people. Consumer Reports on Health 3:11, 1991.

86. Referring others (pamphlet). Philadelphia, 1995, Koren Publications, Inc.

87. Position paper on chiropractic. Loma Linda, Calif., 1985, National Council Against Health Fraud.

88. Pizzorno JE Jr. What is a naturopathic physician? Let's Live 56(2):64, 1988.

89. American Association of Naturopathic Physicians. Twenty questions about naturopathic medicine (flyer). Seattle, 1989, The Association.

90. Pizzorno JE Jr. Naturopathic medicine. In Micozzi MS, editor. Fundamentals of Complementary and Alternative Medicine. New York, 1996, Churchill Livingstone.

91. Pizzorno JE Jr, Murray MT, editors. A Textbook of Natural Medicine, 2nd Edition. Philadelphia, 1999, WB Saunders Company.

92. Pizzorno JE Jr, Murray MT. Encyclopedia of Natural Medicine, 2nd Edition. Rocklin, Calif., 1998, Prima Publishing & Communications.

93. Cody G. History of naturopathic medicine. In Pizzorno JE Jr, Murray MT, editors. A Textbook of Natural Medicine. Seattle, 1985–1996, John Bastyr College Publications.

94. Raso J. Natural hygiene: Still alive and dangerous. Nutrition Forum 7:33–36, 1990.

95. Jensen B. Iridology simplified. Escondido, Calif., 1980, Iridologists International.

96. Simon A and others. An evaluation of iridology. JAMA 242:1385–1387, 1979.

97. Knipschild P. Looking for gall bladder disease in the patient's iris. British Medical Journal 297:1578–1581, 1988.

98. Worrall RS. Iridology: Diagnosis or delusion? Skeptical Inquirer 7(3):23–35, 1983.

99. Stalker D, Glymour C. Engineers, cranks, physicians, magicians. New England Journal of Medicine 308:960–964, 1983.

100. Whorton JC. The first holistic revolution: Alternative medicine in the nineteenth century. In Stalker D, Glymour C, editors. Examining Holistic Medicine. Amherst, N.Y., 1985, Prometheus Books.

101. Betz W. Homeopathic logic and tactics. Presentation at World Skeptics Congress: Science in the Age of (Mis)information, Buffalo, N.Y., June 21, 1996.

102. Kaufman M. Homeopathy in America. Baltimore, 1971, The Johns Hopkins University Press.

103. Homœopathic Pharmacopœia of the United States (HPUS) Revision Service. Washington D.C., 1988–1994, Homeopathic Pharmacopœia Convention of the United States.

104. FDA. Conditions under which homeopathic drugs may be marketed. FDA Compliance Policy Guide 7132.15, 1988.

105. Sherr JY. The Dynamics and Methodology of Provings. West Malvern, England, 1994, Dynamis Books.

106. Raso J. Mystical Diets: Paranormal, Spiritual, and Occult Nutrition Practices. Amherst, N.Y., 1993, Prometheus Books.

107. Barrett S. "Electrodiagnostic devices." Quackwatch Web site, July 25, 2000.

108. Katelaris CH and others. Vega testing in the diagnosis of allergic conditions. Medical Journal of Australia 155:113–114, 1991.

109. Maddox W, Randi J, Stewart WW. "High-dilution" experiments a delusion. Nature 334:287–290, 1988.

110. Hill C, Doyon F. Review of randomized trials of homeopathy. Review of Epidemiology 38:139–142, 1990.

111. Sampson W. Does homeopathy work? Healthline 15(2):10–11, 1996.

112. Jacobs J and others. Treatment of acute childhood diarrhea with homeopathic medicine: A randomized clinical trial in Nicaragua. Pediatrics 93:719–725, 1994.

113. Sampson W, London W. Analysis of homeopathic treatment of childhood diarrhea. Pediatrics 96:961–964, 1995.

114. Ullman RW. Introduction to homeopathy. Seattle, 1991, Bastyr College.

115. Barrett S. Homeopathy: Is it medicine? Nutrition Forum 4:1–6, 1987.

116. Fringe medicine. In Barrett S and others. Health Schemes, Scams, and Frauds. New York, 1990, Consumer Reports Books.

117. Homeopathic remedies: These 19th century medicines offer safety, even charm, but efficacy is another matter. Consumer Reports 52:60–62, 1987.

118. Homeopathy: Much ado about nothing? Consumer Reports 59:201–206, 1994.

119. Barrett S and others. Petition regarding homeopathic drugs. FDA Docket #94P–0316/CP 1.

120. Skolnick A. FDA petitioned to 'stop homeopathy scam.' JAMA 272:1154–1155, 1994.

121. Ireland RR. Powwow: Faith healing Pennsylvania style. Pennsylvania Medicine, pp 32–35, Aug 1973.

122. Jarvis W. Faith healing: Taming the therapeutic miracle. Unpublished manuscript, 1977.

123. Nolen W. Healing: A Doctor in Search of a Miracle. New York, 1974, Random House Inc.

124. Randi J. The Faith Healers. Amherst, N.Y., 1987, Prometheus Books.

125. Kinsolving L, Barrett S. The miracle merchants. In Barrett S, Jarvis WT, editors. The Health Robbers: A Close Look at Quackery in America. Amherst, N.Y., 1993, Prometheus Books.

126. Swan R. Faith healing, Christian Science, and the medical care of children. New England Journal of Medicine 309:1639–1641, 1983.

127. Swan R, Swan D. Civil suits against Christian Science providers; no standards established. CHILD Newsletter, No 1, 1991.

128. Christian Scientists challenged. Physicians Financial News 14(3):23, 1996.

129. Simpson WF. Comparative longevity in a college cohort of Christian Scientists. JAMA 262:1657–1658, 1989.

130. Comparative mortality of two college groups. CDC Mortality and Morbidity Weekly Report 40:579–582, 1991.

131. Witmer J, Zimmerman M. Intercessory prayer as medical treatment? An inquiry. Skeptical Inquirer 15:177–180, 1991.

132. Byrd RC. Positive therapeutic effects of intercessory prayer in a coronary care unit population. Southern Medical Journal 81:826 829, 1988.

133. Sloan RP, Bagiella E, Powell T. Religion, spirituality and medicine. Lancet 353:664-667, 1999.

134. Randi J. Flim-flam! Psychics, ESP, Unicorns and Other Delusions. Amherst N.Y., 1982, Prometheus Books.

135. American Cancer Society. Unproven methods of cancer management: "Psychic surgery." CA—A Cancer Journal for Clinicians 40:184–188, 1990.

136. Rose L. Faith Healing. Baltimore, 1971, Penguin Books.

137. Emery CE. Are they really cured? Providence Sunday Journal Magazine, Jan 15, 1989.

138. Rosa L, Rosa E, Sarner L, Barrett S. A close look at therapeutic touch. JAMA 279:1005–1010, 1998.

139. Kurtz P and others. CSICOP on trance-channelers. The Pseudoscientific Monitor, p 4, Nov 1987.

140. Adolph J. What is new age? In The 1988 Guide to New Age Living. Brighton, Mass., 1988, Rising Star Associates.

141. New age harmonies. Time Magazine 130(23):62–72, 1987.

142. Alcock JE. Channeling. In Stein G, editor. The Encyclopedia of the Paranormal. Amherst, N.Y., 1996, Prometheus Books, pp 153–159.

143. Keene ML. The Psychic Mafia. Amherst, N.Y., 1999, Prometheus Books.

144. Dean G, Mather A, Kelly IW. Astrology. In Stein G, editor. The Encyclopedia of the Paranormal. Amherst, N.Y., 1996, Prometheus Books, pp 47–99.

145. Forer BR. The fallacy of personal validation: A classroom demonstration of gullibility. Journal of Abnormal and Social Psychology 44:118–123, 1949.

146. Dutton DL. The cold reading technique. Experientia 44:326–332, 1988.

147. French C and others. Belief in astrology: A test of the Barnum effect. Skeptical Inquirer 15(2):166–172, 1991.

148. Bainbridge WS. Biorhythms: Evaluating a pseudoscience. Skeptical Inquirer 3(2):40–56, 1978.

149. Hines T. Biorhythms. In Stein G, editor. The Encyclopedia of the Paranormal. Amherst, N.Y., 1996, Prometheus Books, pp 125–129.

150. Raso J. Alternative healthcare, ayurveda, and neo-Hinduism. Nutrition Forum 11:31–42, 1994.

151. World Plan Executive Council. The transcendental meditation television special: Home video version, 1986, The Council.

152. Bloomfield HH and others. TM: Discovering Inner Energy and Overcoming Stress. New York, 1975, Dell Publishing Co.

153. Woodrum E. The development of the transcendental meditation movement. The Zetetic, pp 38–48, Spring/Summer 1977.

154. Chopra D. Growing younger: A practical guide to lifelong youth. Alexandria, Va., 1994, Time Life Video.

155. Sharma HM, Brihaspati DT, Chopra D. Maharishi ayur-veda: Modern insights into ancient medicine. JAMA 265:2633–2636, 1991.

156. Skolnik A. Maharishi Ayur-Veda: Guru's marketing scheme promises the world eternal 'perfect health.' JAMA 266:1741–1750, 1991.

157. Moukheiber Z. Lord of immortality. Forbes 153(8):132, 1994.

158. Chopra D. Creating Health: Beyond Prevention, Toward Perfection. Boston, 1987, Houghton Mifflin Co.

159. Monro R and others. Yoga for Common Ailments. New York, 1990, Simon & Schuster Inc.

160. "Visual therapy": A waste of your time and money. Mayo Clinic Health Letter 5(2):2, 1987.

161. Silver LB. The "magic cure": A review of the current controversial approaches for treating learning disabilities. Journal of Learning Disabilities 20:498–504, 512, 1987.

162. Swets JA and others. Enhancing Human Performance: Issues, Theories, and Techniques. Washington D.C., 1988, National Academy Press.

163. Inglis B, West R. The Alternative Health Guide. New York, 1983, Alfred A Knopf.

164. Segen JC. Dictionary of Alternative Medicine. Stanford, Conn., 1998, Appleton & Lange.

165. Raso J. "Alternative" Healthcare: A Comprehensive Guide. Amherst, N.Y., 1994, Prometheus Books.

166. Raso J. Dictionary of Metaphysical Healthcare. Self-published, 1998.

167. McCutcheon L. What's that I smell? The claims of aromatherapy. Skeptical Inquirer 20:35–37, 1996.

168. Health survey: The results. New Age Journal 4(5):57–58, 1987.

169. Bennion LJ. Hypoglycemia: Fact or Fad? New York, 1983, Crown Publishers Inc.

170. Barrett S, Gots R. Chemical Sensitivity: The Truth about Environmental Illness. Amherst, N.Y., 1998, Prometheus Books.

171. American Academy of Allergy, Asthma & Immunology. Position statements on clinical ecology and candidiasis hypersensitivity syndrome. Journal of Allergy and Clinical Immunology 78:269–273, 1986.

172. Jewett DL, Fein G, Greenberg MH. A double-blind study to determine food sensitivity. New England Journal of Medicine 323:429–433, 1990.

173. Medical malpractice: Treatment of paranoid schizophrenia by "clinical ecology"—wrongful death—punitive damages. New York Jury Verdict Reporter 10(23):1–2, 1991.

174. Crook W. The Yeast Connection: A Medical Breakthrough. Jackson, Tenn., 1985, Professional Books.

175. Dismukes W. A randomized, double-blind trial of nystatin therapy for the candidiasis hypersensitivity syndrome. New England Journal of Medicine 323:1717–1723, 1990.

176. Fukuda K and others. The chronic fatigue syndrome: A comprehensive approach to its definition and study. Annals of Internal Medicine 121:953–959, 1994.

177. Chronic fatigue: All in the mind? Consumer Reports 55:671–675, 1990.

178. Barrett S. Be wary of "fad" diagnoses. Quackwatch Web site, July 9, 2000.

179. McSweegan E. Lyme disease: Questionable diagnosis and treatment. Quackwatch Web site, June 29, 2000.

180. Moore J v Baker RP, US District Court for the Southern District of Georgia, Brunswick Division, Sept 5, 1991.

181. Margolis S. Chelation therapy is ineffective for the treatment of peripheral vascular disease. Alternative Therapies 1(2):53–57, 1995.

182. Green S. Chelation therapy: Unproven claims and unsound theories. Quackwatch Web site, Dec 14, 2000.

183. Questions and answers about chelation therapy. Dallas, 1985, 2000, American Heart Association.

184. Medical association settles false advertising charges over promotion of "chelation therapy." FTC news release, Dec 8, 1998.

185. Sampson WI. Wolves in sheep's clothing? In Barrett S, Jarvis WT, editors. The Health Robbers: A Close Look at Quackery in America. Amherst, N.Y., 1993, Prometheus Books.

186. Flyer for International Forum on New Science. Fort Collins, Colo., 1996, International Association for New Science.

187. What can be done? In Barrett S and others. Health Schemes, Scams, and Frauds. New York, 1990, Consumer Reports Books.

188. Barrett S. Pro-quackery legislation. Quackwatch Web site, Oct 7, 2000.

189. Berman BM, Larson DB, and others. Alternative Medicine: Expanding Medical Horizons. A Report to the National Institutes of Health on Alternative Medical Systems and Practices in the United States. Washington, D.C., 1995, US Government Printing Office.

190. Marshall E. The politics of alternative medicine. Science 265:2000–2002, 1994.

191. Kolata G. Inquests outside mainstream, medical projects rewrite rules. New York Times, June 18, 1996, pp A1, B7.

192. Villaire M. OAM sets goals for eight new centers; centers provide initial details. Alternative Therapies 2(2):20, 22, 90, 1996.

193. Barrett S. Be wary of "alternative" health methods. Quackwatch Web site, June 7, 2000.

SELF-CARE

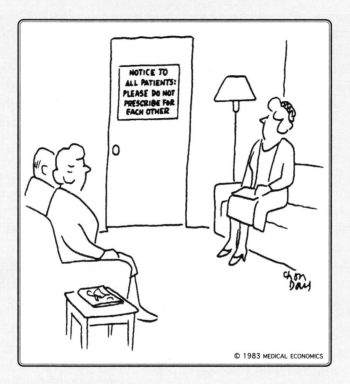

© 1983 MEDICAL ECONOMICS

The way you live profoundly affects your chance of getting certain diseases. Even so, many people seem to have the attitude that they can lead whatever kind of crazy existence they want . . . and when they get sick, simply go to the doctor and get fixed.

TIMOTHY B. MCCALL, M.D.[1]

You can do more for your health than your doctor can . . . you can save money and time. . . . You can learn to treat many medical problems at home. . . . Most . . . visits (to the doctor) are made for relatively minor medical problems . . . as many as 70 percent of visits to the doctor have been termed "unnecessary."

DONALD M. VICKERY, M.D.[2]
JAMES F. FRIES, M.D.

Self-care (also called "self-help") encompasses individual activities that augment or substitute for professional care. The American "self-care movement" was stimulated in the 1970s by accelerating health-care costs and public interest in achieving a healthier lifestyle. These factors have encouraged people to seek greater control over their own health and to educate themselves for greater participation in their own care. This chapter describes the purposes of self-care activities and focuses on health promotion, self-diagnosis, home medical tests, home treatment of chronic diseases, self-help publications, and self-help groups. Chapter 19 suggests how to stock a "home pharmacy" for self-management of minor illnesses, injuries, and certain emergency situations.

PURPOSES OF SELF-CARE

No definition of medical self-care has been universally accepted. Barofsky[3] divided self-care activities into four types: (1) *regulatory* (e.g., eating, sleeping, bathing); (2) *preventative* (exercising, brushing one's teeth), (3) *reactive* (responding to symptoms without medical input), and (4) *restorative* (complying with prescribed treatment). Vickery[4] stresses individual actions with respect to health problems.

During the 1970s and early 1980s some self-care advocates sought to help laypersons become as independent as possible of conventional medical care by teaching them how to perform tasks normally considered within the practice of medicine. Some mothers were taught, for example, how to examine their children's throat and ears to determine whether an infection warranted medical attention. However, this so-called "activated patient" movement appears to have waned because it was neither practical nor cost-effective.

Today the emphasis is on helping consumers become better informed in order to work more cooperatively with physicians.

The largest survey of organizations sponsoring self-care educational programs was sponsored by the U.S. Centers for Disease Control and Prevention and conducted in 1984 by researchers at the University of North Carolina.[5] After an extensive search they mailed questionnaires to 2284 organizations and received 920 responses, 147 of which said they had no self-care activities. Follow-up investigation indicated that about two thirds of the nonresponders had no current telephone listing or had discontinued their phone service. Thus it

---

◆ Personal Glimpse ◆

Reasons for Self-Care

- People want control over their own body and life.
- Consumers realize that they are exposed to many health risks related to lifestyle, environmental conditions, and failure to follow preventative practices.
- Medical costs continue to escalate.
- Consumers may lower their medical expenses by making fewer visits to doctors.
- Advertising of over-the-counter drugs, devices, and equipment encourages self-diagnosis and self-medication.
- Increased awareness of women's health resulting from the women's movement.
- Inability of community health agencies to meet the special needs of patients with chronic illnesses.
- Many consumers are dissatisfied with the quality of medical care: impersonal services, lack of communication, unnecessary surgery, and other problems.

<table>
<tr><td colspan="2">**Table 9-1**</td></tr>
</table>

AIMS OF SELF-CARE PROGRAMS[5]

Increase wellness or health status	94%
Reduce an established risk factor	86%
Prevent onset of illness or injury	79%
Prevent further deterioration or spread of existing illness	63%
Diagnose and assess symptoms or signs of common illness	59%
Alleviate pain, discomfort, and disability	58%
Develop advocacy skills	50%
Prevent iatrogenic (treatment-induced) disease	28%

Table 9-2

SCOPE OF SELF-CARE INSTRUCTION[5]

Lifestyle modification/health promotion	92.5%
Chronic illness conditions	65.9%
Health-care consumer information	58.4%
Acute illness conditions	54.3%
Physical examination skills	37.2%
Dental health skills	22.8%
Alternative therapies	20.7%

appeared that at least half of the groups originally listed were no longer operating. Tables 9-1 and 9-2 summarize the aims and scope of the 723 groups whose responses were compiled. The most common instructional areas were lifestyle modification/health promotion and chronic disease management. Fewer than half of the programs had laypersons serving as instructors.

Kemper and others[6] have summarized the results of 15 self-care intervention studies published between 1979 and 1990. In each case the participants were given one or more handbooks, booklets, or other educational materials and followed to see how their decisions compared with those of a control group. All but one of the studies demonstrated a reduction in visits to physicians, although some of the reductions were not statistically significant. A recent study found that distributing information to both elderly patients and their doctors improved the quality of patient-provider interactions and led patients to be more satisfied with their care.[7]

Public interest in self-care has also stimulated the marketing of questionable products. Many companies sell questionable devices claimed to promote fitness, reduce stress, improve mental functioning, protect against alleged environmental hazards, or provide other

"self-care" benefits. Table 9-3 comments on several such products. Sales of dietary supplements, herbs, and homeopathic products have also increased considerably.

HEALTH PROMOTION

Maintaining a healthy lifestyle can reduce the odds of becoming seriously ill and lower the cost of health care. Prudent consumers avoid tobacco products, eat sensibly, maintain a reasonable weight, exercise appropriately, use alcohol moderately or not at all, take appropriate safety precautions, and utilize appropriate professional care. Table 9-4 on page 183 summarizes the results of a 1995 survey in which adult Americans were asked about their health-promotion practices.

Cigarette smoking is by far the leading cause of preventable death and is a major cause of heart disease, cancer, and many other diseases (see Chapters 15 and 17).[8] Exposure to environmental tobacco smoke ("passive smoking") increases the risk of developing heart disease and can exacerbate several other diseases. Tobacco use is also an important preventable cause of spontaneous abortions, low birthweight, and infant deaths.[8,10] Smokeless tobacco results in cancer deaths.

A sensible diet will provide all the vitamins, minerals, fiber, and other nutrients that most people need. This can be achieved by consuming moderate amounts of a wide variety of foods. Attention should also be paid to the amount of dietary fat, which, if excessive, can raise blood cholesterol levels and increase the risk of coronary heart disease. Healthful diets can be achieved by following the Food Guide Pyramid system described in Chapter 11. Women should pay special attention to their calcium intake to decrease the risk of osteoporosis (see Chapter 21).

Weight is determined by the relationship between calories consumed and energy expended by the body. Mild obesity is not harmful, but being 20% overweight can contribute to high blood pressure and increase the incidence or risk of diabetes, heart and blood vessel diseases, osteoarthritis, and several other problems (see Chapter 13). To lose weight one must eat less or exercise more, but most people need to do both.

Regular exercise can increase strength, endurance, flexibility, motor fitness, and cardiorespiratory efficiency. It can also lower blood pressure, improve blood cholesterol levels, help with weight control, help lower abnormal blood sugar levels, reduce stress, improve sleep, help prevent osteoporosis, and increase longevity. Aerobic exercise is best, but even nonvigorous exercise provides considerable benefit (see Chapter 14).

Moderate drinking (no more than one drink per day

for women and two drinks per day for men) is associated with a lower-than-average risk of coronary heart disease, but higher levels of alcohol intake raise the risk for high blood pressure, stroke, myocarditis (inflammation of the heart muscle), certain cancers, accidents, violence, suicides, birth defects, and mortality (deaths). Too much alcohol can lead to dependency (addiction) and cause cirrhosis of the liver, inflammation of the pancreas, and damage to the brain and heart. Major birth defects, including fetal alcohol syndrome, have been attributed to heavy drinking by the mother while pregnant. Although there is no conclusive evidence that an occasional drink is harmful to the fetus or to the pregnant woman, a safe level of alcohol intake during pregnancy has not been established. Based on these observations, the National Research Council,[11] the American Medical Association,[12] and other authorities[13] have recommended that women who are pregnant or trying to conceive should not drink alcoholic beverages. People planning to drive a car, engage in another activity that requires attention or skill, or use certain medications are also advised to abstain.

Table 9-3

QUESTIONABLE SELF-CARE PRODUCTS FROM MAIL-ORDER CATALOGS

Device/Cost	Ad Claims	Remarks
Body Fat Tester ($99.95)	Uses infrared light passing through biceps muscle to gauge percentage of body fat "to track progress toward healthy percent-fat goals."	The amount of fat over the biceps may not reflect the amount in other parts of the body. Even if it did, few people will benefit from knowing their percentage of body fat.
Magnetic EMF Sensor ($99)	The Environmental Protection Agency has classified electromagnetic fields as a probable human carcinogen. EMF sensor will quickly alert you to EMF sources . . . guiding your family away from areas of possible health risk at home and at work.	The earth's electromagnetic field cannot be avoided. The small amounts of EMF radiation from high-voltage lines, electric blankets, and other sources have no proven health significance.
Massaging Hair Brush ($24.95)	Cordless vibrator eases tension, stimulates the flow of nutrients to each hair bulb, and decreases the likelihood of hair loss caused by reduced circulation	Massaging the scalp will not prevent hair loss.
Mini Water Dispenser ($19.95)	"Even slight dehydration impairs coordination and thinking and brings on fatigue. . . . Our mini replica of an office water cooler holds exactly 8 glasses of water. Drink from it throughout the day and when done you'll know you've done right!"	Under most circumstances thirst is an appropriate guide to the amount of water people need. Drinking a minimum of eight glasses of water daily has no proven health benefit.
Mustard Bath ($12.95 for 4 baths)	Blended with essential oils to increase circulation, open pores, stimulate sweat glands, relieve congestion, and help rid the body of toxins.	A warm bath can be relaxing and soothing. Adding aromatic oils conveys no health benefit and does not cause the body to expel "toxins."
Chlorine Filter for Shower ($49)	One shower can cause as much absorption of chlorine as drinking eight glasses of chlorinated water. Chlorine can cause dry skin, brittle hair, and can be a risk to health.	Showering in ordinary tap water poses no health risk. Any dryness of the skin is likely to be related to the frequency of showering and the type of soap used.
Vibrating Acupressure Eye Massager ($9.99)	Vibrating foam pads stimulate seven acupuncture points. Blood circulation increases, fatigue and tension headaches vanish; also helps minimize eye wrinkles and bags.	There is no evidence that "acupoints" function as claimed. A few minutes of relaxation may be beneficial. The device is superfluous.
Video Vision WorkOut ($89)	Videotapes, depth perception tools, and vision-testing charts enable user to undertake a disciplined eye exercise program that may reduce, postpone, or eliminate the need for corrective lenses.	Exercising the eyes does not deter the changes in the eyes (presbyopia) that reduce the ability to focus as one gets older.

Table 9-4

USE OF VARIOUS HEALTH-PROMOTING BEHAVIORS BY AMERICAN ADULTS (1995)*

Behavior	Importance[a]	% Using
Do not smoke	9.78	72
Avoid smoking in bed	9.24	92
Wear seat belt	9.16	73
Avoid driving after drinking	9.03	84
Smoke detector in home	8.53	93
Socialize regularly	8.31	83
Frequent strenuous exercise	8.20	40
Drink alcohol moderately	8.15	90[b]
Avoid home accidents	8.07	80
Limit fat in diet	7.82	52
Maintain proper weight	7.71	19
Obey speed limit	7.65	48
Annual blood pressure check	7.62	85
Control stress	7.58	69
Consume fiber	7.41	57
Limit cholesterol in diet	7.15	45
Adequate vitamins/minerals	7.12	58
Annual dental exam	7.08	75
Limit sodium in diet	7.04	47
Get 7–8 hours sleep/night	6.71	59

*Data excerpted from *The Prevention Index 1996 Summary Report*[10]
[a]Derived by averaging responses from 103 experts who, in 1983, rated the relative importance of these behaviors on a scale of 1 to 10.
[b]Includes 37% who said they abstain.

Safety belts reduce the incidence and severity of injury from automobile accidents. Helmets can help protect a person against head injury when riding a bicycle or motorcycle. Smoke detectors should be installed in every residence; they are important because the warning they provide may enable people to escape a fire before it is too late. Homes with a fuel-burning appliance or fireplace should have at least one carbon monoxide detector, ideally in a hallway or sleeping area.[14] Homes should also be checked for excessive radon (see Chapter 17). Appropriate precautions should be taken to avoid sexually transmitted diseases (see Chapter 21) and overexpose to sunlight (see Chapter 20).

Preventative medical care includes immunizations and periodic examinations to look for conditions that can be significantly influenced if detected early. For example, the incidence of heart disease can be reduced by modifying abnormal levels of cholesterol and blood pressure (see Chapter 15). The U.S. Preventive Services Task Force has published detailed information about the types of physical examinations, laboratory tests, immunizations, counseling, and other measures that are

cost-effective (see Chapter 5). Self-examinations of the breasts, testicles, and skin to detect cancer are also advisable.

A combination of nutrition, good eating habits, oral hygiene, and professional care will enable most people to maintain their teeth in good condition throughout their life. Adequate amounts of fluoride during childhood will help make teeth resistant to decay. The most efficient way to accomplish this is through water fluoridation and the use of fluoridated toothpaste. Daily brushing and flossing of the teeth can prevent tooth decay and periodontal disease. Professional care may include administration of sealants, removal of calculus (tartar), restoration of decayed or missing teeth, and cosmetic measures. These subjects are discussed in Chapter 7.

Smoking Cessation Methods

Although cigarette smoking involves a powerful chemical addiction and behavior patterns that are difficult to break, more than 40 million Americans have quit, 90% of them without formal medical intervention.[15] No matter how long a person has smoked, stopping is still beneficial.[16] During the first day, nicotine and carbon monoxide levels decrease in the body, and the heart and lungs begin to repair the damage caused by cigarette smoke. "Smoker's cough" usually disappears within a few weeks, energy and endurance may increase, and the senses of taste and smell may return to normal. A decade after stopping, the risk of dying from cardiovascular disease declines to the level of the nonsmoker. However, damage to some organs may be irreversible.

Smokers seeking to quit can benefit from understanding the extent to which physical dependence, habit, and anxiety reduction contribute to their urge to smoke and from knowing some basic strategies to help cope with each of these factors. Inexpensive educational

Historical Perspective

Bogus Vaccination Kits

In the late 1980s home-immunization kits consisting of alcohol, water solutions, and sugar pills were allegedly sold by an Idaho naturopath as protection against polio, scarlet fever, smallpox, measles, mumps, tetanus, whooping cough, and diphtheria. Apparently these kits were manufactured by a company in Twin Falls, Idaho, and sold to naturopaths, parents, and regional distributors in many states. The FDA did not approve these kits and warned that they did not afford protection from the diseases.[17]

materials and courses are available from the American Cancer Society, American Heart Association, American Lung Association, Seventh-day Adventist Church, community hospitals, and other local agencies. The U.S. Public Health Service offers many publications in print and online.

Most strongly motivated people can quit regardless of the method used. Many profit-oriented smoking cessation companies claim high success rates but do not follow up all patients for at least 1 year; do not verify abstinence by checking nicotine products in the saliva, urine, or blood; and report on small numbers of highly selected and motivated individuals.

In 1994 Law and Tang[18] analyzed 188 randomized controlled trials involving interventions intended to help people stop smoking and found that only 88 had used biochemical confirmation. The highest reported success rates were for heart attack survivors and healthy men at high risk of heart disease who were medically advised to quit. The authors also concluded (a) nicotine-replacement therapy was important in helping smokers addicted to nicotine, (b) hypnosis was unproved, (c) acupuncture had little or no effect, and (d) it made little difference whether cessation occurred gradually or suddenly. Recent reviews have concluded that physician advice[19] and self-help materials[20] have generally small but beneficial effects and that nicotine-replacement products approximately double the cessation rate.[21,22] Nicotine-replacement products are available by prescription and over-the-counter (see Chapter 19).

Commercial self-help products should be regarded skeptically. Graduated filters that remove nicotine and products that guide gradual reduction of the number of cigarettes smoked per day have not been proven effective. Dietary supplements, herbs, and homeopathic remedies have no scientific support and should be considered useless.

SELF-DIAGNOSIS

Everyone practices self-diagnosis to some extent. It would be impractical and a waste of medical expertise to have physicians deal with every cough, twinge, ache, and sore. However, individuals must be able to distinguish between minor and major problems to determine when professional help is needed. Most conditions appropriate for self-treatment have symptoms that are easily recognized, occasional, and temporary. Examples include the common cold, simple headaches, occasional indigestion, muscle aches and pains, slight burns, cuts and bruises, occasional sleeplessness, some skin infections, diarrhea, itching, and mild allergic reactions.

Self-diagnosis of a serious or chronic condition is another matter. Both overdiagnosis and underdiagnosis can lead to trouble. For example, a person who misdiagnoses a minor ache as arthritis may become needlessly upset, or someone who assumes that shortness of breath is the result of a bad chest cold when it is actually caused by heart failure may fail to seek timely corrective treatment. Even when self-diagnosis of a serious or chronic condition is correct, health may be threatened if a physician is not consulted. A physician's therapeutic resources far surpass any that are available to a layperson.

The FDA's classic survey of health practices and opinions asked nearly 3000 randomly selected adults whether they had ever had various serious ailments and who had diagnosed them. Almost everyone who reported heart trouble, high blood pressure, and diabetes had been diagnosed by a physician. But a sizable percentage of

---

 Consumer Tip

Using Home Tests Wisely

These suggestions can help consumers who are considering the use of home health tests:

- Consult with a doctor or other health-care professional before buying a test, and ask which brand to purchase.
- Check the expiration date because chemicals lose their potency with time and the results could be affected.
- Store products as directed; they may be affected by hot or cold temperatures. Don't leave a temperature-sensitive product in a car trunk or near a sunny car window in hot weather.
- Read labels and package instructions carefully. If questions remain, call the toll-free number if one is listed on the package or consult your doctor or the pharmacist at the place of purchase.
- Understand the limitations and purposes of the test. Remember that no test is 100% accurate.
- Follow instructions carefully. Use a stopwatch if precise timing is necessary.
- When collecting a urine specimen with a container not from a kit, wash the container thoroughly, and rinse out all traces of detergent—preferably with distilled water.
- Know what to do when results are positive, negative, or unclear. It may be advisable to repeat the test or consult a physician.
- Keep test kits containing potentially poisonous chemicals or a sharp instrument out of the reach of children.

those reporting arthritis (20%), asthma (22%), allergies (28%), and hemorrhoids (32%) had made the diagnosis themselves without consulting a health professional.[23]

People are less likely to recognize or seek help for illnesses that develop slowly, whereas illnesses with acute symptoms, such as severe abdominal pain, high fever, or excessive bleeding, are more easily recognized and brought to the physician's attention. The reasons for not seeking needed medical care include:

- Concern about cost
- Fear of being told that you are seriously ill or need surgery
- Inability to recognize symptoms of illnesses
- Fear of embarrassment
- Distrust of the medical profession
- Apathy about your health
- Belief that illness is punishment for improper behavior
- Belief that it is shameful to be ill
- Lack of transportation
- Too busy; unable to get away from work

A physician should be consulted when (a) a symptom or condition is too severe to be endured (e.g., severe abdominal or chest pain), (b) an apparently minor symptom persists for a few days with no easily identifiable cause, (c) symptoms return repeatedly for no apparent reason (e.g., digestive distress), or (d) there is doubt about the nature of the condition.

If you are unsure about whether a visit is needed, telephoning may help. If the symptoms are outlined, the nurse or receptionist (consulting with the doctor if necessary) will advise whether a visit to the office should be scheduled. Some HMOs provide a telephone consultation service for this purpose.

HOME MEDICAL TESTS

Consumers spend close to $1 billion a year on in-home laboratory tests. The most common of these are for pregnancy, ovulation, and blood-sugar measurement. To gain FDA approval, an over-the-counter test must be accurate and perform at least one of three functions: (1) doctor-recommended monitoring, (2) detecting a marker for a health condition when there are no physical signs of disease, or (3) detecting a marker when signs of a condition are apparent. The manufacturer must also convince the FDA that the results can benefit consumers and that consumers will be able to judge for themselves whether the test is appropriate.[24]

Pregnancy test kits permit women to test their urine at home for signs of pregnancy.[25] Most kits are based on monoclonal antibody technology, which permits testing on the same day as the missed period, with results available in a few minutes. The test is performed by adding a few drops of urine to a test tube containing special chemicals. A "positive" test result indicates the presence of human chorionic gonadotropin (HCG), a hormone found in the urine of pregnant women.

Test results will not be accurate unless the instructions are explicitly followed. Using a test past its expiration date, exposing the specimen to the sun, or having protein or blood in urine can affect test results. The presence of a hormone-producing cancer could also cause an error.

The early stages of pregnancy cannot be diagnosed with certainty without a medical examination. If a home test is positive, a visit to a physician will probably be necessary. The doctor will probably insist on confirming the diagnosis, which means that the woman will ultimately pay for two pregnancy tests.

Ovulation-prediction tests are designed to predict the peak periods of a woman's fertility during a given menstrual cycle.[25] The results are available in a few minutes. This test determines the level of luteinizing hormone (LH) in urine, because ovulation is triggered by an increase in LH. The test may help couples with fertility problems and may be more accurate than recording basal body temperatures (another method used to predict ovulation). Fertility experts recommend taking basal body temperatures along with the test to see whether the two measures of ovulation coincide. Medical guidance is advisable. Ovulation tests must be performed for several days in a row. If menstrual periods are irregular, testing may need to be conducted for a longer period of time. Inaccurate results can occur if the woman is entering menopause or using other hormones to treat infertility.

Diabetics can test themselves at home to see whether their blood glucose (sugar) level is appropriate.[25] The tests are performed by placing a drop of blood on a chemically treated test strip, which is inserted into a device that interprets the levels of color development. The results, which are available within 1 minute, are then used to help regulate the patient's treatment. This method is superior to urine testing because it provides more current information.

The American Cancer Society and the U.S. Preventive Services Task Force recommend testing for hidden (occult) blood in the stool annually after age 50. Specimen-collection materials can be obtained from the office of a physician whose staff will perform the test when the specimens are returned. Test kits are also available for home usage. The test is conducted by placing a stool specimen in contact (for example, on a pad) with peroxide and guaiac (a chemical sensitive to blood). If the chemical turns to a specified color, occult blood is

Irritable Bowel Syndrome

Irritable bowel syndrome (IBS)—also called irritable or spastic colon—is a common functional intestinal disorder characterized by recurrent abdominal discomfort and abnormal bowel function. The discomfort often begins after eating and goes away after a bowel movement. The symptoms can include cramps, bloating, constipation, diarrhea, and a feeling of incomplete emptying. Self-care plays an essential role in its management.

IBS occurs in about one in five Americans, more commonly in women, and more often at times of emotional stress. It usually begins in late adolescence or early adult life and rarely starts after the age of 50. In severe cases, it can result in missed work days and curtailment of social activities. Although effective help is available, many people with IBS are too embarrassed, pessimistic, or afraid to seek medical care. Even worse, some people who consult a doctor receive insufficient guidance and conclude that nothing further can be done for them.

During normal digestion, foods are broken down in the stomach and small intestine so that their nutrients can be absorbed into the body. Undigested or partially digested portions—mostly in liquid form—then enter the large intestine (colon) where most of the water is reabsorbed. Movement through the intestines results from peristalsis, a wavelike contraction of muscles in the intestinal walls that propel their contents forward. When all is well, the end result is stool that is solid but soft enough to be excreted easily.

Diet, eating habits, stress, and various environmental factors can disrupt intestinal function. If the intestines squeeze too hard or not enough, the partially digested food can travel too rapidly or too slowly through the digestive system. Movement that is too fast will result in diarrhea, because not enough water is reabsorbed. Movement that is too slow can result in constipation, because too much water is absorbed. Overly hard squeezing (spasm) can result in cramps. However, the diarrhea of IBS can also occur without pain.

IBS symptoms occur after eating because of the gastrocolic reflex—increased movement of the intestinal contents in response to food entering the stomach. The strength of this reflex can be influenced by the volume and temperature of the food and the number of calories. Large meals (particularly high-fat meals) and large amounts of cold beverages can trigger IBS attacks.

Medical care should begin with a thorough history and physical examination. The extent of further evaluation depends on the patient's age, general health, and symptoms. If symptoms have been present a long time and have a typical pattern, the doctor may rely mainly on the patient's description to diagnose IBS. If symptoms are recent in origin, testing may be needed to be certain that an infection, inflammation, or tumor is not responsible for the symptoms. The tests may include blood tests, stool tests, x-ray examinations, and endoscopy (examination of the colon with a hollow tubular instrument inserted from below).

The first step in managing IBS should be to identify what triggers the symptoms. The factors to consider include food intolerances, eating habits, dietary factors, emotional stress, exercise habits, use of laxatives, and vitamin C intake. It may help to keep a diary that relates symptoms to daily activities.

Many people with IBS have difficulty digesting lactose (milk sugar). This results from a shortage of lactase, an enzyme normally produced by cells lining the small intestine. When there is not enough lactase, undigested lactose can ferment in the large intestine and cause nausea, cramps, bloating, flatulence, and diarrhea that begin about 30 minutes to 2 hours after consuming lactose-containing foods. If lactose intolerance is significant, lactase drops or tablets can be added to ordinary milk, low-lactose products can be substituted, or dairy products can be avoided (in which case the patient should take calcium supplements).

Bloating or excessive gas can also be related to eating habits and diet. Carbonated beverages can introduce gas into the intestines and cause abdominal pain. Eating or drinking rapidly, chewing gum, smoking, nervously gulping air, or wearing loose dentures can cause some people to swallow a large amount of air, some of which reaches the large intestine. Gas can also be produced by such foods as beans, onions, broccoli, and cabbage. Eating more slowly or minimizing gas-forming foods may help.

Since caffeine can increase intestinal motility, people with IBS should avoid or minimize the use of coffee, caffeinated colas, and other caffeine-containing beverages. Fructose or sorbitol (a sugar substitute) can induce diarrhea in some people. Since vitamin C supplements of 1 gram/day or more can cause diarrhea, patients with chronically loose stools should be advised to stop taking them.

Unnecessary delay in defecation should be avoided. When an urge is felt, leaving the stool in the colon may contribute to constipation because the longer the contents remain, the more fluid may be absorbed. Use of certain laxatives can perpetuate constipation because the large intestine can become dependent on them. People with IBS should not take strong laxatives.

Increasing the fiber content of the diet or taking a stool softener such as methylcellulose or psyllium may help regulate bowel movements and reduce both constipation and diarrhea. Increasing dietary fiber should be done gradually to give the body time to adjust. Prescription drugs are available to slow the movement of food through the intestines or to relieve intestinal spasm.

In patients with abdominal pain, medication, a hot bath, or a hot water bottle applied to the abdomen may relieve an acute attack. If a certain type of activity is known to trigger an attack, taking an antispasmodic drug beforehand may prevent attack. If modifiable sources of stress can be discovered, resolving them may help. Regular exercise can also help to normalize bowel action.

present. However, a positive result does not always indicate cancer. It may be caused by bleeding gums, nonmalignant polyps, heavy use of aspirin, diverticulitis, hemorrhoids, and other conditions. High doses of vitamin C can cause a false-negative result.

A home kit for testing blood cholesterol is available but may be impractical (see Chapter 15). Home collection kits for AIDS testing are discussed in Chapter 18.

SELF-TREATMENT OF CHRONIC DISEASES

Home treatment may be practical and economical for people with chronic conditions such as allergies, asthma, arthritis, diabetes, and high blood pressure, and for some patients who need kidney dialysis. Physicians should be consulted about such possibilities.

Allergic individuals who are being desensitized by allergy shots may find it practical to administer the shots themselves, or have a friend or family member administer the shots. Home administration should not be done until it is clear that the shots are well tolerated; occasionally they cause a severe reaction.

Asthmatics (and their families) can learn how to use medications to minimize the frequency and severity of acute attacks. Some patients with arthritis can receive physical therapy at home.

Two conditions in which self-testing is of great value are diabetes and high blood pressure. Patients with diabetes, particularly those taking insulin, should regularly check their blood-sugar level. Monthly testing may be enough for people whose diabetes is under control. Daily testing may be needed for a patient who has been diagnosed recently or whose disease needs very close monitoring. Accurate home-use devices are available. Although the devices are not expensive, the cost of the test strips can add up to a large amount. So the frequency of testing should be discussed with one's physician.

Individuals whose high blood pressure is being medically treated can save time and money by checking their pressure at home as part of a medical program. Checks by a physician every 3 months may be sufficient if pressure is satisfactory and stable.

Blood-Pressure Devices

For people with high blood pressure, self-monitoring is useful because people can take far more readings at home than would be practical at a doctor's office. It can also be more accurate for those who have "white-coat hypertension," a tendency toward blood pressure elevation when readings are taken by a physician or a nurse.

The blood-pressure devices for home use resemble those used by physicians. They usually include a sphygmomanometer to measure blood pressure in the arteries and a stethoscope to listen to the arterial pulsations in the arm. Blood pressure is measured in millimeters of mercury (mm Hg); two numbers are recorded. Systolic pressure, the higher reading, is the pressure when the heart contracts to pump blood through the arteries. Diastolic pressure, the lower reading, reflects the pressure recorded between heart beats. Normal systolic pressure for adults is about 120 mm Hg. Diastolic readings above 90 are considered abnormal (see Chapter 15 for more detailed information).

There are four types of blood-pressure devices:

MERCURY: A column of mercury rises in a tube as cuff pressure is increased and falls as pressure is decreased.

MECHANICAL ANEROID (WITHOUT LIQUID): A needle moves clockwise on a dial as pressure is increased and counterclockwise as pressure is decreased.

ELECTRONIC ANEROID: A microphone under the cuff is used to register arterial sounds on a dial rather than project them aurally with a stethoscope.

FINGER DEVICES: Instead of a cuff, these automatic devices are placed on the person's finger.

The mercury type is highly accurate and does not need calibration, but it is the most difficult to use. *Consumer Reports* does not recommend this type for home use. The mechanical-aneroid type requires dexterity, good hearing to use the stethoscope, good eyesight to read the dial, and some practice to use correctly. This type should be calibrated annually to maintain accuracy. There are two types of electronic devices: one with a cuff that must be manually inflated, and the other with a cuff that automatically inflates. The electronic instruments are easier to use because they provide digital readings and do not require listening to the sounds with a stethoscope. However, they require more frequent calibration to maintain accuracy.

In 1996, *Consumer Reports*[25] studied 17 devices and concluded that the mechanical aneroid monitors offered the best value because they were less expensive and, when used correctly, were generally more accurate than electronic arm models. The top-rated models were:

MECHANICAL: Marshall 104 ($25), Omron HEM-18 ($20), Walgreens 2001 ($20), Lumiscope 100-021 ($20), Sunmark 100 ($25)

ELECTRONIC WITH AUTOMATIC INFLATION: AND UA-767 ($80), Omron HEM-711 ($90), AND UA-702 ($45), Omron HEM-712C ($80)

Two electronic finger models tested by *Consumer Reports* were judged unacceptable because they performed inaccurately. Nesselroad and others reported obtaining inaccurate readings from three finger devices:

the Marshall F-89, the Omron HEM-806F, and the SunMark 165.[26]

Consumers should be aware that (a) adequate instruction in the use of a blood-pressure device is necessary to ensure accurate readings, (b) elevated readings are not adequate for a diagnosis, which can only be made by a physician, and (c) a monitor may be a good investment for a hypertensive person who is under the care of a physician. The doctor or a member of the doctor's staff can show the patient how the test should be done and how to check that the device works properly.

The coin-operated blood-pressure machines in shopping malls, supermarkets, drugstores, airports, and other places should be used with caution because their reliability is limited. The accuracy of these machines depends on how recently they have been calibrated.

SELF-HELP PUBLICATIONS

Many books offering health advice to consumers are published each year. Large bookstores typically carry several hundred of them. Computer products are also being developed at a rapid rate.

Most health-related books fit into three classifications: (1) information on a single condition or group of conditions; (2) reference works that cover the entire scope of health problems; and (3) action-oriented books that help to evaluate symptoms and determine whether medical care is needed. Dr. Stephen Barrett, who has monitored the selections of many bookstores and mail-order book clubs for more than 25 years, believes that fewer than half of the health-related books have been reliable.

Take Care of Yourself: A Consumers' Guide to Medical Care, by Donald M. Vickery, M.D., and James F. Fries, M.D.,[2] focuses on medical problems that consumers can act upon. The book includes information about preventing illness, finding a suitable doctor, avoiding medical fraud, reducing medical costs, and the home pharmacy. It features more than 100 decision charts for managing common health problems. The charts—set up as flow sheets—indicate when to self-treat and when to consult a physician. Figure 9-1 illustrates the charts for self-management of colds and sore throats.

Healthwise Handbook: A Self-Care Manual for You[27] presents similar information in a different format. It covers more than 180 problems and focuses on prevention, home care, and when to call a doctor.

The *Home Remedies Handbook* [28] was prepared by the editors of Consumer Guide with help from more than 250 medical and technical advisers. It is filled with

practical advice on self-management of about 130 common problems.

Feel Good Again: Coping with the Emotions of Illness,[29] by psychiatrist Stephen A. Green, M.D., discusses how to recognize and deal with the reactions that are common when people become ill.

A few books promoting "do-it-yourself" home testing have claimed to provide comprehensive advice on self-testing. However, most of the tests they suggested were neither practical nor cost-effective.

Several nutrition-related books contain questionnaires that supposedly enable readers to determine whether they should take dietary supplements. Such questionnaires, which cover symptoms, lifestyle characteristics, and environmental factors, invariably lead to inappropriate recommendations for supplements. The most elaborate example is the *Self-Test Nutrition Guide,*[30] by Cass Ingram, D.O., and Judy K. Gray. It contains 35 "nutritional deficiency tests," 14 "dietary intake" tests, and 9 "illnesses and syndromes" tests, with an average of 39 items per test. For all but a few, even a single positive answer is interpreted as a "mild" problem for which large doses of vitamins and other nutrients are advisable.

Thousands of self-help books, audiotapes, and videotapes have been marketed to the public with claims that they can help people function better mentally, improve relationships with others, relieve anxiety or depression, or achieve other desired emotional changes. Few of these products have been tested for reliability or effectiveness (see Chapter 6). Gambrill notes that many books of this type exaggerate people's ability to alter themselves or their environment and that failure to achieve the unrealistic goals these books offer can make people more depressed.[31]

CD-ROMs can combine the information in books with illustrations and other audiovisual aids. The AMA's *Family Medical Guide* on CD-ROM, for example, offers the text of the AMA's *Family Medical Guide* book plus interactive self-diagnosis charts, charts illustrating how parts of the body function, and pop-up screens with self-care information. Some CD-ROMs contain health appraisals that "interview" the user. However, health appraisals are more effective when they are part of an integrated health-promotion program. Stand-alone health appraisals may not do much good because the user already knows much of what they say. (For example, people told they should not smoke already "know" they should not.)

Table 9-5 lists several books that are valuable for a home health library. Several of these provide detailed

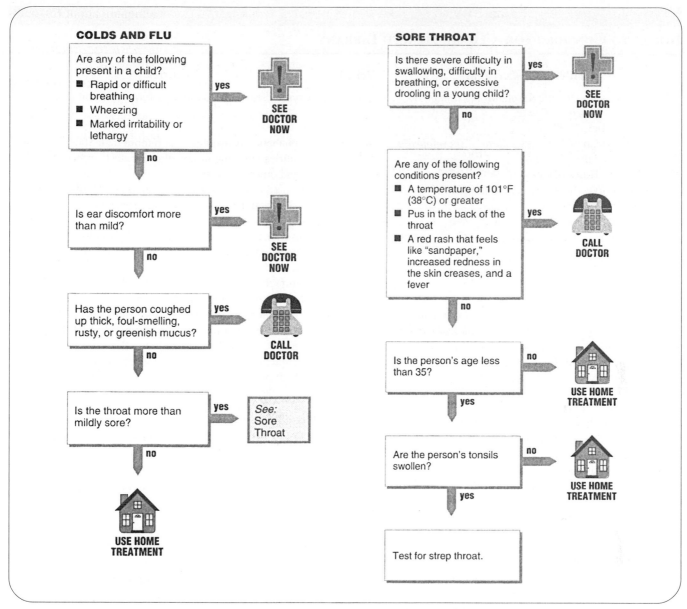

FIGURE 9-1. Decision charts for colds, flu, and sore throat. These help determine when professional help is needed.
From Vickery DM, Fries JF: *Take Care of Yourself: The Complete Illustrated Guide to Medical Self-Care,* ed 6.
© 1996 Authors and Addison-Wesley Publishing Co. (1-800-447-2226). Reproduced with permission.

guidance about self-care and when to see a doctor. Chapter 2 identifies additional sources of reliable information.

SELF-HELP GROUPS

Self-help groups provide opportunities to exchange information, share feelings, and network with others who have had similar experiences. Their services are rendered through group meetings, telephone conversations, home and hospital visits, educational seminars, practical help (such as transportation and shopping), and residential care. Katz states:

Self-help, mutual aid groups provide an accepting environment of social support that may not be available from other sources. Their help can have the intimacy and informality of the best family and neighborly assistance.

They usually bring together accurate, up-to-date information on resources and methods for coping with the problem; they often include people at different stages of dealing with it, so that newcomers can learn from the more experienced.[32]

Self-help groups range from local groups with few members to national organizations with tens of thousands of members. Some are governed by consensus, whereas others follow parliamentary procedures in

Table 9-5

BOOKS TO CONSIDER FOR A HOME HEALTH LIBRARY

Title, Publisher, Year	Price*	Features
The American Dietetic Association's Complete Food & Nutrition Guide John Wiley, 1998	24.95	Comprehensive discussion of food facts and fads
The American Medical Association Encyclopedia of Medicine Random House, 1989	45.00	Alphabetically arranged, with more than 5000 entries covering drugs, illnesses, tests, procedures, and other concepts
The American Medical Association Family Medical Guide Random House, 1994	39.95	Detailed information about more than 650 diseases, plus wellness tips and 99 decision charts
The American Medical Association Guide to Your Family's Symptoms Random House, 1994	17.00	Describes the body's workings and provides 145 decision charts for dealing with symptoms
Caring for the Mind Bantam Books, 1996	25.95	Comprehensive guide to mental and emotional problems and their treatment
The Columbia University College of Physicians and Surgeons Complete Home Medical Guide Henry Holt, 1995	19.95	Comprehensive guide to illnesses and their treatment; information on "alternative" methods is misleading and should be ignored
Complete Drug Reference Consumer Reports Books, 2001	44.00	Comprehensive guide to the uses and side effects of both prescription and nonprescription drugs
The Harvard Guide to Women's Health Harvard University Press, 1996	24.95	Over 300 entries that address questions frequently asked by women
Healthwise Handbook Healthwise, Inc., 1999	9.95	Guidelines for prevention, home treatment, and when to seek help for more than 180 problems
Healthwise for Life Healthwise, Inc., 1998	9.95	Covers over 190 health problems faced by older adults
Johns Hopkins Family Health Book Harper Family Resource, 1998	49.95	Comprehensive guide to disease prevention and treatment
Mayo Clinic Family Health Book William Morrow and Co., 1990	45.00	Comprehensive description of diseases and their treatment.
Mayo Clinic Guide to Self-Care Kensington Publishing, 1999	19.95	Advice for everyday health problems
*Merck Manual of Medical Information, Home Edition*** Pocket Books, 1999	7.99	Comprehensive guide to illnesses and their treatment.
The New Wellness Encyclopedia Houghton Mifflin Co., 1995	27.50	Focuses on preventive health measures
PDR Family Guide to Prescription Drugs Medical Economics, 1999	23.00	Lucid guide to the purposes, use, and side effects of prescription drugs
Reader's Guide to Alternative Health Methods American Medical Association, 1993	34.95	Annotated bibliography of 1000 published reports on more than 100 "alternative" methods
Take Care of Yourself Addison-Wesley Publishing, 2000	18.00	Filled with practical advice about self-care; includes over 100 decision charts
Taking Care of Your Child Addison-Wesley Publishing, 2000	19.00	Filled with practical advice about self-care; includes many decision charts
The Vitamin Pushers Prometheus Books, 1994	31.95	Basic information about food selection plus a detailed analysis of nutrition-related quackery
The Whole Tooth St. Martin's Press, 1997	23.95	User's guide for obtaining proper dental care and avoiding improper care
*Yale University School of Medicine Patient's Guide to Medical Tests*** Houghton-Mifflin, 1997	40.00	Comprehensive guide to medical tests

*Paperback prices given when available. **Full text available online.

A "Self-Help" Group Gone Awry

The People's Medical Society (PMS) was founded with the hope of helping people become better medical consumers. It was a brainchild of the late Robert Rodale, board chairman of Rodale Press and publisher of *Prevention* magazine. During 1982, he ran a series of editorials criticizing the medical establishment and promising "a grassroots campaign that will turn America's medical system on its head." The group's bimonthly newsletter occasionally contains useful suggestions, but most of its information is slanted to encourage members to distrust scientific practitioners and regard them as adversaries. Rodale Press terminated its affiliation with PMS in the late 1980s.

PMS has produced many books, booklets, reading lists, and other special reports. Some contain valuable information, but others promote unscientific methods and/or portray them as equivalent to scientific ones.

The PMS booklet *Options in Health Care*, for example, uncritically promotes the unscientific theories and practices of acupuncture, acupressure, Chinese medicine, chiropractic, homeopathy, hydrotherapy, metabolic therapy, naturopathy, orthomolecular therapy, psychic healing, and reflexology. Its book *Getting the Most for Your Health-Care Dollar* mentions these practices without the slightest hint that they are a waste of money.

PMS's bulletin on cancer-care options includes promoters of quack cancer methods in its list of sources of information. The bulletin on choosing doctors includes the dubious advice that obtaining a health-related degree through a correspondence course "does not in and of itself imply an inferior education." PMS's special report on high blood pressure contains sound advice but falsely suggests that "alternative" methods have much to offer for this condition.

PMS's reading lists include unscientific publications as well as reputable ones. For example, the bibliography on arthritis includes a book that claims that food allergy is a major cause of arthritis; a bibliography on cancer includes one boosting macrobiotic diets; and a bibliography on nutrition includes several unscientific books. The PMS report *Deregulating Doctoring* suggests that unorthodox practitioners be allowed to practice with minimal government regulation.

From time to time, PMS encourages its members to write to legislators or other officials. Some campaigns have involved antiquackery legislation (opposed by PMS), funds for organic farming (favored), licensing of nutritionists (opposed), and food irradiation (opposed).

Publicity materials describe PMS as "the largest consumer health organization in America" and state that it is run "by the people" and "for the people."[33] However, its president and board of directors are not elected, and its activities and policies appear to be determined solely by the group's president, Charles Inlander, whose salary and benefits total over $135,000 per year.

In recent years, PMS publications and local newspaper articles have stated that PMS has 125,000 members, 150,000 "supporters," and 125,000 "contributors and members." However, its tax returns do not support such figures. The financial statement filed with its California Form CT-2 lists membership fees of $148,664 for 1997 and $152,523 for 1998 and contributions of $81,056 for 1997 and $81,055 for 1998. These numbers translate into about 7500 members and either few contributors or tiny average contributions. Its main source of income is from book sales.

Although some of its stated goals are laudable, consumers should be wary of the People's Medical Society because too much of its advice is unreliable.

establishing committees and electing officers. Some are organized as service delivery systems with authority vested in a national office and an ascending hierarchy of leadership derived from people who have been helped by the group. The simplest type of national organization is a network of autonomous groups, an association supported by dues from affiliated local branches or chapters that are authorized to use its name. Some national organizations have professional staff who develop program materials for local groups and provide consultants. Some have professional advisory committees. Some organizations maintain hotlines for immediate aid to people in need. Some have outreach programs in which members make unsolicited offers of help. Some groups have formal orientation programs for group leaders and outreach volunteers. Silverman[34] states that most groups are small (10 to 20 people) and are struggling to survive.

Table 9-6 lists 20 of the largest self-help organizations, some of which are international. Others include:

Cancer
Candlelighters (childhood cancer)
Make Today Count
Reach to Recovery (breast cancer)

Family/Parenting
Adoptive Families of America
Grandparents as Parents
Stepfamily Association of America

Table 9-6

SELECTED LARGE SELF-HELP ORGANIZATIONS

Organization	Founded	Chapters	People or Problems Addressed
Al-Anon Family Groups	1951	32,000	Family members of compulsive drinker
Alcoholics Anonymous	1935	98,000	Alcohol abuse (religious/spiritual approach)
ARC	1950	1,100	Mentally retarded people and their families
Co-Dependents Anonymous	1986	3,900	Attachment to substance abusers
Cocaine Anonymous	1982	2,000	Cocaine addiction
Compassionate Friends	1969	600	Parents and siblings grieving the death of a child
Gamblers Anonymous	1957	1,800	Compulsive gambling
La Leche League	1956	3,000	Support and education for breastfeeding mothers
Narcotics Anonymous	1953	22,000	Substance abuse
National Alliance for the Mentally Ill	1979	1,200	Relatives and individuals affected by mental illness
Parents Anonymous	1970	1,000	More effective ways of raising children
Parents Without Partners	1957	350	Single parents
Rainbows	1983	7,000	Children and adults grieving a death, divorce, or other painful family transition
Recovery, Inc.	1937	700	Emotional and behavioral problems
Secular Organization for Sobriety (S.O.S.)	1986	1,200	Alcohol and drug addiction (nonreligious approach)
Stroke Connection	1979	1,800	Families and friends of stroke victims
Survivors of Incest Anonymous (S.I.A.)	1982	300	Adults victimized by childhood sexual abuse
Take Pounds Off Sensibly (T.O.P.S.)	1948	11,000	Weight control
United Ostomy Association	1962	450	People with an artificial opening in their gastrointestinal, urinary, or respiratory tract

Source: American Self-Help Clearinghouse Self-Help Sourcebook Online, December 2000.

Mental Help
Agoraphobics in Motion
Divorce Anonymous
Emotions Anonymous
Neurotics Anonymous International Liaison
Phobics Anonymous

Obesity
National Association to Advance Fat Acceptance
Weight Watchers International

Others
American Anorexia/Bulimia Association
American Association of Kidney Patients
American Parkinson's Disease Association
International Association of Laryngectomees
Mended Hearts
Meniere's Network
Moderation Management (mild to moderate problem drinking)
Multiple Sclerosis Association of America
National Headache Foundation
Phoenix Society for Burn Survivors
Resolve (infertility)
Scoliosis Association
Sickle Cell Disease Association of America
Simon Foundation for Incontinence

Some of these are listed in the Appendix of this book, and some have chapters listed in the Yellow or Blue Pages of local telephone directories. All can be located through the American Self-Help Clearinghouse sourcebook (http://www.mentalhelp.net/selfhelp) or *Encyclopedia of Medical Organizations and Agencies* (available at many libraries).

The American Self-Help Clearinghouse[35] and the National Mental Health Consumer Self-Help Clearinghouse can provide additional information and help for starting new groups. In many parts of the country, local and regional clearinghouses can provide detailed information on groups within the areas they serve. They can be located by contacting the American Self-Help Clearinghouse.

Few published studies provide objective measurement of the effectiveness of self-help groups. However, many people who participate in these groups feel they are helpful. Trojan[36] queried 232 members from 65 disease-related groups and found that most reported considerable benefit, which they attributed to support by other group members. The reported benefits included reduction of disease-related stress and better ability to relate to others. Kaminer[37] has warned that some recovery groups are too authoritative, encourage a "victim" mentality, or offer simplistic suggestions for dealing with people.

Online Support Groups

More than 1000 electronic groups have formed to share concerns and exchange information about health matters. These groups may provide practical tips and information about medical advances, but they also attract unsubstantiated testimonials and sales pitches for products.

Lamberg[38] states that the quality of postings tend to be higher on groups with moderators who organize postings into threads and screen out misinformation and advertisements. Some support groups maintain online libraries that enable members to post and download information.

SUMMARY

Self-care (also called "self-help") encompasses individual activities that augment or substitute for professional care. It includes health promotion; self-diagnosis; home treatment of chronic diseases; and the use of home medical tests, self-help publications, and self-help groups.

Health-promotion activities should include tobacco avoidance, a well-balanced diet, reasonable weight, exercising regularly, moderate (if any) alcohol intake, injury prevention measures, immunizations, brushing and flossing of the teeth, and periodic medical and dental examinations.

Most forms of health care involve at least some degree of self-care. Consumers need to distinguish between major and minor illnesses and to know when a physician should be consulted. Excellent self-help publications are available for this purpose. People with asthma, diabetes, and high blood pressure can be treated

---

◆ Personal Glimpse ◆

Self-Help Philosophy

The goal of a self-help group is to empower its members with the tools necessary to make adjustments needed to continue a life of dignity and independence. Self-help groups:

- Share a common health concern
- Govern themselves and their agenda, with success dependent on each member's feeling of ownership
- May use professionals as resource persons but not as leaders
- Provide nonjudgmental emotional support
- Gather and share accurate and specialized information
- Have a fluid membership—newcomers are helped by veterans and become veterans who may outgrow the need for a group
- Have a cause, and actively promote that cause.
- Increase public awareness and knowledge by sharing their unique and relevant information
- Charge low or no dues for involvement
- And typically struggle to survive

International Polio Network
4207 Lindell Blvd., #110
St. Louis, MO 63108

---

most effectively and inexpensively with a professionally supervised program that includes in-home testing.

Self-help groups provide opportunities to exchange information, share feelings, and network with others who have had similar experiences. Online support groups offer anonymity, convenience, and a rapid response, but they may also attract unsubstantiated testimonials, irrational advice, and sales pitches for questionable products.

It's Your Decision

You think you may be pregnant and you want to obtain confirmation of your condition. Which of the following action(s) would you take?   Reason

- ☐ Ask a friend or parent what to do   _____
- ☐ Purchase a self-diagnostic pregnancy test kit   _____
- ☐ Consult a pharmacist   _____
- ☐ Purchase a self-help book or acquire one from the library   _____
- ☐ Immediately consult a physician   _____
- ☐ Contact Planned Parenthood   _____
- ☐ Other (specify): _____   _____

REFERENCES

1. McCall TB. Examining Your Doctor: A Patient's Guide to Avoiding Harmful Medical Care. New York, 1995, Birch Lane Press.
2. Vickery DM, Fries JF. Take Care of Yourself: A Consumers' Guide to Medical Care, ed 4. Reading, Mass., 1990, Addison-Wesley Publishing Co.
3. Compliance, adherence and the therapeutic alliance: Steps in the development of self-care. Social Science and Medicine 12A(5):369–376, 1978.
4. Vickery DM. Medical self-care: A review of the concept and program models. American Journal of Health Promotion 1(1):23–28, 1986.
5. DeFriese GH and others. From activated patient to pacified activists: A study of the self-care movement in the United States. Social Science and Medicine 29:195–204, 1989.
6. Kemper DW and others. The effectiveness of medical self-care interventions: A focus on self-initiated responses to symptoms. Patient Education and Counseling 21:29–39, 1993.
7. Wasson JH and others. A randomized trial of the use of patient self-assessment data to improve community practices. Effective Clinical Practice 2(1):1–10, 1999.
8. American Council on Science and Health. Cigarettes: What the Warning Label Doesn't Tell You. The First Comprehensive Guide to the Health Consequences of Smoking. Amherst, N.Y., New York, 1997, Prometheus Books.
9. Di Franza JR, Lew RA. Effect of maternal cigarette smoking on pregnancy complications and sudden infant death syndrome. Journal of Family Practice 40:385–394, 1995.
10. The Prevention Index: 1996 Summary Report. Emmaus, Pa., 1996, Rodale Press.
11. Motulsky AG and others. Diet and Health: Implications for Reducing Chronic Disease Risk. Washington, D.C., 1989, National Academy Press.
12. AMA Council on Scientific Affairs. Fetal effects of maternal alcohol use. JAMA 249:2517–2521, 1983.
13. Nutrition and your health: Dietary guidelines for Americans, ed 4. Washington, D.C., 1995, US Departments of Agriculture and Health and Human Services.
14. CO detectors: An early warning. Consumer Reports 60:466–467, 1995.
15. Fiore MC and others. Methods used to quit smoking in the United States: Do cessation programs help? JAMA 263:2760–2765, 1990.
16. The Health Benefits of Smoking Cessation: A Report of the Surgeon General. DHHS Publication No. (CDC) 90-8416. Rockville, Md., 1990, US Deptartment of Health and Human Services.
17. Home immunization kits unapproved and ineffective. FDA Consumer 24(1):4, 1990.
18. Law M, Tang JL. An analysis of the effectiveness of interventions intended to help people stop smoking. Archives of Internal Medicine 155:1933–1941, 1995.
19. Prochazka AV. New developments in smoking cessation. Chest 117(4 Suppl 1):169S–175S, 2000.
20. Silagy C. Physician advice for smoking cessation (Cochrane Review). The Cochrane Library, 4, 2000. Oxford: Update Software.
21. Lancaster T, Stead LF. Self-help interventions for smoking cessation (Cochrane Review). The Cochrane Library, 4, 2000. Oxford: Update Software.
22. Fiore MC and others. Treating Tobacco Use and Dependence. Clinical Practice Guideline. Rockville, Md., 2000, US Dept. of Health and Human Services.
23. Food and Drug Administration. A Study of Health Practices and Opinions. Springfield, Va., 1972, National Technical Information Service.
24. Farley D. In-home tests: Make home-care easier. FDA Consumer 28(10):25–28, 1994.
25. Bringing medicine home: Self-test kits monitor your health. Consumer Reports 61(10):47–55, 1996.
26. Nesselroad JM and others. Accuracy of automated finger blood pressure devices. Family Medicine 28:189–192, 1996.
27. Healthwise Handbook: A Self-Care Manual for You. Boise, Idaho, 1999, Healthwise Incorporated.
28. Editors of Consumer Guide. The Home Remedies Handbook. Lincolnwood, Ill., 1993, Publications International.
29. Green SA and the editors of Consumer Reports. Feel Good Again: Coping with the Emotions of Illness. Yonkers, N.Y., 1990, Consumer Reports Books.
30. Ingram C, Gray JK. Self-Test Nutrition Guide. Hiawatha, Iowa, 1994, Knowledge House Publishers.
31. Gambrill E. Self-help books. Pseudoscience in the guise of science. Skeptical Inquirer 16(4):389-399, 1992.
32. Katz AH. Foreword to White BJ, Madera EJ. The Self-Help Sourcebook. Denville, N.J., 1995, American Self-Help Clearinghouse.
33. The goals and philosophy of the People's Medical Society. News from Pantheon Books, undated, released in 1988.
34. Silverman P. An introduction to self-help groups. In White BJ, Madera EJ. The Self-Help Sourcebook. Denville, N.J., 1995, American Self-Help Clearinghouse.
35. Hall B. Health information service has become a model for the nation. The New York Times, March 26, 1995, p 9D.
36. Trojan A. Benefits of self-help groups: A survey of 232 members of 65 disease-related groups. Social Science and Medicine 29:225-232, 1989.
37. Kaminer W. I'm Dysfunctional, You're Dysfunctional: The Recovery Movement and Other Self-Help Fashions. Reading, Mass., 1992, Addison-Wesley Publishing Co.
38. Lamberg L. Patients go online for support. American Medical News, April 1, 1966.

Chapter Ten

HEALTH-CARE FACILITIES

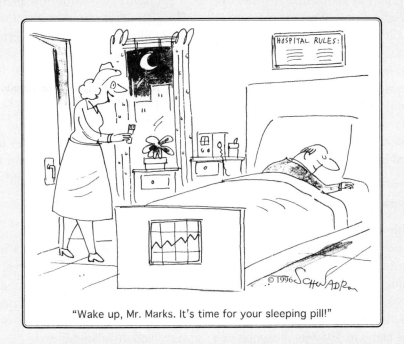

"Wake up, Mr. Marks. It's time for your sleeping pill!"

Finding a hospital is not a job for the faint of heart.
KATIE BAER, M.P.H.[1]
HARVARD HEALTH LETTER

A long stay in a nursing home can consign a resident's family to financial hardship, even poverty. But choose the wrong nursing home, and you may also consign your loved one to physical and emotional hardship.

CONSUMER REPORTS[2]

While staff members may be well-trained professionals, and hospitals may be efficiently run, in the best of circumstances most people would rather be in a familiar setting, nursed by those who know and care about them.

EDITORS OF CONSUMER REPORTS BOOKS[3]

Many types of community facilities are available to help with illnesses and infirmities. Hospitals provide inpatient treatment for acutely or seriously ill people. Nursing homes provide convalescent services as well as long-term care for the chronically ill or disabled. A myriad of home care agencies offer services ranging from help with everyday living tasks to complex medical care. Various residential arrangements offer an alternative to institutional care.

The best choice of facility depends on the type and urgency of the problem as well as insurance coverage and other financial considerations. This chapter discusses the accreditation process and focuses on outpatient clinics, ambulatory care centers, ambulatory surgery centers, hospitals, nursing homes, alternative residential facilities, and home care services.

THE JOINT COMMISSION

Accreditation of a health-care facility constitutes public recognition that it meets standards set by a recognized accrediting agency. The most prominent such agency is the Joint Commission on Accreditation of Healthcare Organizations, which was created in 1951 as the Joint Commission on Accreditation of Hospitals and assumed its current name in 1987 as its scope expanded. Its purpose is to improve quality of care by developing standards and evaluating their implementation. Its board of commissioners, which oversees standard-setting and accrediting policies, has seven representatives from the American Hospital Association, seven from the American Medical Association, three from the American College of Physicians, three from the American College of Surgeons, one from the American Dental Association, one at-large nursing representative, and six public members appointed by the board itself.

The Joint Commission accredits hospitals; substance abuse and rehabilitation programs; community mental health centers; health care networks; nursing homes and other long-term-care facilities; home care organizations; ambulatory health care organizations; and clinical laboratories. Nearly 20,000 facilities participate in the accreditation process. Accreditation is voluntary, but hospitals must be accredited to receive direct payments for services from Medicare and Medicaid or to maintain a recognized residency program for physicians. Hospitals accredited by the Joint Commission qualify for Medicare and Medicaid certification without having to undergo a government survey. In most states and the District of Columbia, Joint Commission accreditation is also recognized in whole or in part for purposes of hospital licensure. The "General Public" section of the Joint Commission's Web site (http://www.jcaho.org) describes standards, provides detailed advice on how to choose facilities, and has a searchable directory of those that have been evaluated.

OUTPATIENT MEDICAL FACILITIES

Outpatient medical facilities include private medical offices, student health services, work-related facilities, ambulatory care centers, ambulatory surgery centers, and hospital emergency departments and outpatient clinics. Table 10-1 on page 198 summarizes their advantages and disadvantages.

Private Medical Offices

Physicians practice singly and in small and large groups. Nearly all medical offices have scheduled hours and operate by appointment. Primary-care physicians who know their patients well are often in the best position to render appropriate care. Chapter 5 discusses strategies for the selection and most effective use of private physicians.

Student Health Services

At most colleges and universities, basic student health services are covered by required fees, and additional services may be covered by an insurance policy. The extent of services offered varies mainly with the size of the school. Some schools use one or more part-time physicians, whereas others maintain a full-time medical staff. At some, students seeking help are screened by a nurse or physician's assistant. It is advisable for students to know the extent of their insurance coverage and what to do if an emergency arises outside of scheduled hours.

Hospital Emergency Departments

Most hospitals have an emergency department that is open 24 hours a day, 365 days a year, and is supervised by physicians experienced in emergency medicine. These facilities give priority to people who are seriously ill or injured. People with less serious problems will usually be seen but may have a lengthy wait.

Emergency room care typically costs more than twice as much as similar care in a private medical office or ambulatory care center. However, emergency care cannot be denied because someone is uninsured or unable to pay. The Consolidated Omnibus Budget Reconciliation Act (COBRA), which Congress passed in 1986, requires that everyone who shows up for care be examined. If the situation is an emergency (or the person is a woman in labor), the hospital must provide treatment at least until the condition has stabilized.[4] Violating this law can trigger fines and loss of the hospital's accreditation (see Personal Glimpse box).

Hospital Outpatient Clinics

Many hospitals have outpatient clinics where the fees are based on the individual's ability to pay. In teaching hospitals much of this care is rendered by resident physicians. Many clinics have such a full schedule that new patients must wait months to be seen by appointment.

At hospitals that receive federal funds, low-income patients who qualify under Hill-Burton Act guidelines can obtain laboratory tests and certain other services free of charge. (This legislation, which began with the Hospital Survey and Construction Act of 1946, provides federal help in constructing and modernizing hospitals and other health-care facilities.) For full-paying patients, hospital clinic fees may be higher than those at private offices.

Other Community Clinics

Some communities have clinics run by the local health department or a nonprofit agency. Some are open to everyone, some serve only the poor. Some offer help for a wide variety of problems, while others have a narrow scope. These facilities are usually listed in the "Clinics" section of the Yellow Pages.

◆ Personal Glimpse ◆

Doctor Fined for "Patient Dumping"[5]

In December 1986, an uninsured woman gave birth in an ambulance at the side of a road after being transferred from a hospital emergency room by an on-call obstetrician. The doctor noted that the woman's blood pressure was the highest he had ever seen in a pregnant woman—a condition that can lead to life-threatening complications. He ordered the woman transferred to a public hospital 170 miles away, where a sophisticated neonatal unit was available. Within an hour after the ambulance began its trip, the woman gave birth. She then returned to the original hospital and was admitted. Fortunately, both she and the baby did well.

This incident led to the first case of a financial penalty against a doctor for violating a 1986 federal law intended to stop the practice known as "patient dumping." The doctor appealed the proposed $20,000 penalty, claiming that the transfer was done to provide superior medical care and that doctors should have the right to determine who they treat. He also said he was afraid that he might be sued for malpractice if complications arose. But others involved in the case insisted that the original hospital had adequate facilities and that it was improper to transfer a patient who was about to give birth. In 1991 a federal court of appeals upheld the fine.

Ambulatory Care Centers

Ambulatory care centers (ACCs)—also called urgent care facilities—provide walk-in care by a physician for people with minor medical emergencies, such as cut fingers, nosebleeds, sprained ankles, simple fractures, and illnesses such as a sore throat or the flu. These facilities also handle other problems that require only one visit or a small number of visits. Their staff usually consists of medical doctors (full time and part time), nurses, and clerical help. They may be owned by physicians, other private individuals, or hospitals.

Accreditation is available from the Joint Commission and the Accreditation Association for Ambulatory Health Care. The facilities are legally considered the equivalent of medical offices and are not regulated by separate licensure.

Some ACCs function as family medical centers, offering long-term care as well as episodic care. All have laboratory and x-ray facilities. Most provide prepackaged prescription services for frequently used drugs. Some participate in managed-care programs, and some have contracts to provide treatment to injured workers. The fees at ACCs tend to be comparable to those of standard medical offices and much less than those of hospital emergency departments. Many ACCs give a discount when payment is made at the time of the visit.

Most ACCs are located in small shopping centers, malls, and other busy thoroughfares. These facilities have proliferated because of (a) the high cost of hospital services, (b) the realization that people can become ill or injured at any time of the day, (c) competition for patients as a result of a surplus of physicians in some communities, (d) insurance companies' desire to reduce hospital costs by lowering reimbursements to hospitals for emergency department services, (e) the lack of physicians in some areas, (f) the tendency of physicians to refer patients to hospital emergency rooms after office hours, and (g) consumer dissatisfaction with the emergency room environment.

ACCs can provide care for injuries or illnesses that occur when one's personal physician is not available. These centers do not require an appointment and generally provide quick service. They have longer hours than most medical offices, and nearly all function 7 days a week. They provide an alternative for people who do not have a regular physician, who wish to be seen for an acute problem outside their regular physician's

working hours, or who are traveling away from home. For chronic conditions, or for conditions where familiarity with the patient is important for making a diagnosis or for designing a treatment plan, a primary physician is a better choice.

Ambulatory Surgery Centers

Ambulatory surgery centers (ASCs) comprise freestanding, independent, corporate, or hospital-owned facilities where outpatient surgery is performed after the patient has been medically evaluated elsewhere. Each year nearly 6 million operations are performed in more than 2700 outpatient surgery centers nationwide. Most operations done at ASCs cost less than they would in an inpatient hospital setting. The costs include charges for using the facility plus the fees of the attending surgeon, anesthesiologist, and pathologist. The common ambulatory procedures include:

EYE OPERATIONS: Cataract removal, eye muscle surgery, refractive surgery, foreign body removal
GYNECOLOGIC PROCEDURES: Dilation and curettage (D&C), laparoscopy, biopsies
EAR/NOSE/THROAT PROCEDURES: Tonsil and adenoid removal, drainage of fluid from the ears
ORTHOPEDIC SURGERY: Biopsies, bone grafts, joint surgery, ligament and tendon repair, treatment of broken bones

Table 10-1

ADVANTAGES AND DISADVANTAGES OF OUTPATIENT HEALTH-CARE FACILITIES

Facility	Advantages	Disadvantages
Private medical office	Maximum personal attention Relatively low cost per visit	Limited hours
Multispecialty group practice	Relatively low cost per visit Consultations may be more readily available	Same physician may not always be seen (varies with setup of group)
Student health service	Convenient location Minimal cost	Hours and scope of practice may be limited
Ambulatory care center	Cost similar to medical office, much less than hospital emergency department Open long hours No appointment needed	When care is episodic, doctor does not get to know the patient as an individual. Extra tests may be ordered because records are unavailable or physician does not know patient well
Hospital emergency department	Open 24 hours a day Able to handle serious emergencies Sophisticated equipment available	Highest cost Nonemergency cases may not receive much attention Follow-up care may be minimal Care is episodic and less personal
Hospital outpatient clinic	Fees may be reduced for individuals who cannot afford private care	Patients may have to wait a long time to be seen Tend to have high staff turnover so different doctors may be seen
Ambulatory surgery center	Surgery costs less than it would in a hospital	Unsuitable for major surgery

GENERAL SURGERY: Removal of cysts, skin lesions, and stitches; breast and muscle biopsies; hernia repair; hemorrhoid operations; and laparoscopic gallbladder removal

RECONSTRUCTIVE AND COSMETIC SURGERY: Scar revision, skin grafts, facial surgery

PODIATRIC SURGERY: Removal of bunions, corns, and warts; surgery on bone spurs.

ASCs are licensed in 43 states. About 85% are approved by Medicare. Accreditation is available from the Joint Commission, Accreditation Association for Ambulatory Health Care, and the American Association for Accreditation for Ambulatory Surgery Facilities. Some communities have overnight recovery care centers for patients who need observation for 24 to 48 hours following outpatient surgery.

HOSPITALS

Hospitals can be categorized as community or noncommunity; general or specialty; government-owned or nongovernmental; nonprofit or for-profit; and short-term (average length of stay is under 30 days) or long-term (over 30 days). In 1998 the 6021 hospitals in the United States had a total of 1,012,582 beds and an average occupancy rate of 65.4%. Of these, 5015 (83%) were community hospitals and 771 (13%) were for-profit hospitals.[6]

Regarding size: 24% of community hospitals had fewer than 50 beds, 22% had 50 to 99 beds, 26% had 100 to 199 beds, 24% had 200 to 499 beds, and 5% had 500 or more beds. Larger hospitals tend to be better equipped and staffed to provide comprehensive care.

In recent years the total number of hospitals in the United States has declined, but the number of investor-owned, for-profit hospitals has increased. Some are chains owned by corporations listed on the stock market. Many hospitals have formed various collaborative or networking ventures, a trend that is increasing rapidly in response to economic pressures. (A network is a group of hospitals, physicians, other providers, insurers, and/or community agencies that work together to coordinate and deliver a broad spectrum of services to their community.) Cost-control efforts have tightened the criteria for admission, shortened average lengths of stay, and caused many facilities to merge to achieve economies of scale and avoid duplicating services and technologies. This subject is discussed further in Chapter 25.

Accreditation

The Joint Commission grants hospital accreditation for 3 years. Its ratings are: (a) accredited with commenda-

tion, (b) accredited, (c) accredited with type I recommendations (at least one problem must be resolved), (d) provisional accreditation (pending a final inspection), (e) conditional accreditation (significant shortcomings must be corrected quickly), (f) preliminary non-accreditation, or (g) not accredited. About 80% of the hospitals in the United States are accredited. Those with fewer than 50 beds are less likely than larger hospitals to be accredited. The hospital standards include:[7,8]

- A safe, clean, uncrowded hospital with enough beds to handle the patient load.
- A well-organized administration with a chief executive and a governing body.
- Appropriate protection of the rights of patients.
- Appropriate standards for ensuring that patients are appropriately assessed and treated.
- Provision of such services as a pharmacy, a diagnostic x-ray department, a clinical laboratory, surgical facilities, nursing, and food service, each staffed and supervised by qualified professionals. (For example, the nursing services must be supervised by registered nurses, and the pharmacy must be maintained by a registered pharmacist.)
- Procedures by which physicians apply for staff membership and are evaluated in terms of experience, judgment, ability, and competence.
- Establishment of rules and regulations for the medical staff, including the maintenance of committees to review the quality of medical care of its members. (For example, a tissue committee must review the appropriateness of surgical procedures and a utilization review process must evaluate the appropriateness of patient admissions and lengths of stays.)
- Maintenance and safeguarding of complete and continuous medical records on each patient.
- Maintenance of infection-control procedures. (This is important because hospitals are potential breeding grounds for infectious organisms, and many seriously ill patients are susceptible.)
- Regularly scheduled case conferences and other educational activities for the staff.

Well-managed hospitals carefully check the credentials of their medical staff and limit privileges to areas in which the individual has appropriate training and has demonstrated competence. Active staff members have full admitting privileges, are eligible to serve on hospital committees, and can vote on hospital matters. Courtesy staff members admit or co-manage a limited number of patients per year but do not participate in hospital affairs. Consulting staff members are permitted to perform consultations and serve on certain committees. New applicants are usually appointed to the provisional staff and monitored for 1 year, after which they can apply for active, courtesy, or consulting status.

In addition to being accredited, a good hospital:

- Is likely to be a teaching hospital affiliated with a medical school and approved for the training of resident physicians, medical students, and nurses.
- Has staff members involved in research. The care is likely to be more consistently of high quality, with practitioners having the most up-to-date medical knowledge available.
- Has a wide range of diagnostic and treatment facilities and services.
- Has a wide range of specialists, most of whom are board-certified, and employs adequate numbers of registered nurses and nursing aides.
- Uses peer-review to maintain medical standards and provides high-quality educational programs for its staff.
- Has an effective tissue review committee. The committee reviews pathology reports on tissue specimens obtained during surgery to determine whether the surgery was justified. If a physician appears in error, the committee expects an explanation. A physician who performs several questionable operations might be requested to appear before the executive committee of the medical staff of the hospital. When violations are sufficiently flagrant, the physician could be barred from practice at the hospital.
- Requires consultations with other physicians when diagnoses are questionable, when great risk is involved, or when treatment procedures are in doubt.
- Holds meetings of an advisory committee to determine ways to run the hospital more efficiently and humanely.
- Provides the services of some type of ombudsman, or patient representative, who communicates with patients and is concerned with their general welfare.
- Abides by the *Patient's Bill of Rights* (see box on opposite page).
- Encourages community participation in the conduct of the hospital. It has a consumer board or a consumer representative who participates in hospital planning sessions and makes recommendations for improving services.
- Is involved in community activities, such as programs for cancer screening, smoking cessation, substance-abuse treatment, and consumer education.

Selecting a Hospital

There is no simple way for the average consumer to determine whether a hospital provides high-quality care. The effort that should be made depends upon the patient's situation. In an emergency where minutes count, the most practical choice may be the nearest hospital. If the doctor selected has only one hospital affiliation or the community has only one hospital, that hospital must be used if you want the doctor to manage your care. Choice may also be limited by one's insurance coverage. For nonemergency conditions, some investigation may be prudent.

Physicians who attend hospitalized patients are in a good position to observe the quality of nursing care

 Consumer Tip

Strategies for Hospitalized Patients

Be alert. Alertness may be needed to avoid receiving the wrong medication or undergoing a procedure intended for someone else. Ask questions; if you are too ill to do so, ask a family member or friend to assist you.

Medications. Before taking any new drug, have the nurse check your name and any drug allergies listed on your wristband. Also ask the name of the drug and check its appearance. If it doesn't look like what you have previously received or what your doctor said you would be getting, have the nurse check the order book or contact your physician.

Tests and procedures. You should be informed of the purpose of each and of any risk or discomfort that may be involved. Make sure you know about any special pretest preparations such as the use of laxatives, enemas, fasting, and the like. Be sure the test or procedure is for you and is relevant for your condition. If relevant, ask your doctor whether temperature and blood pressure checks can be postponed until morning rather than interrupting your sleep.

Too many doctors. Know who's in charge of your case. If doctors treating you provide conflicting information, raise questions and ask them to communicate with each other before they talk with you.

Speak up. If there are problems with your food, pain control, delayed responses by nurses, curt replies to your requests, or other significant difficulties, talk to the nurse, dietitian, physician, or the hospital's patient advocate or ombudsman.

Check your bill carefully. Hospital billing errors are very common. Be sure that the bill is itemized and that you understand everything listed.

and other services that the hospital provides. Thus a trustworthy personal physician is probably the best source of advice about choosing a hospital. It is also prudent to know whether the cost of a hospital stay will be covered fully or partially by one's insurance.

For unusual or serious conditions, a hospital with special equipment or staff expertise may be needed. That, too, is best determined with the help of one's personal physician. Information is also available from *U.S. News & World Report,* which publishes an annual report on the quality of care at leading tertiary care hospitals. (These are hospitals that offer highly specialized and technologically complex services in addition to more common ones.) The rankings for four of the specialties are based on a survey of 150 board-certified specialists. The rankings for the rest are based on a survey plus analyses of death rates and several other types of objective data. The top six overall were Johns Hopkins Hospital, the Mayo Clinic, Massachusetts General Hospital, Cleveland Clinic, UCLA Medical Center, and Duke University Medical Center. The latest report, which includes a searchable database of the rankings, is also available on the magazine's Web site.[9] Many states now collect and analyze information about hospital charges and performance, but the data they release may be difficult to interpret.

When a hospital has been selected, several things can be done to make one's stay more pleasant. Leeds and Strauss[10] advise inquiring about visiting hours, restrictions on who may visit, and availability of a telephone and a television set. Consideration should be given to the type of room desired. It can be difficult to share a semiprivate room with someone who is seriously ill and is noisy or requires frequent staff attention during the night. Most insurance policies cover the cost of a semiprivate room (a room with two to four beds). The extra cost of a private room would have to be paid out-of-pocket.

Problems with Inpatient Care

Hospital care can entail several types of problems for consumers. The quality of care varies considerably. Patients may receive inadequate nursing attention, which can jeopardize their health or subject them to unnecessary discomfort and inconvenience. The food may be unappetizing. Accidents, hospital-acquired infections, and other preventable complications can occur. Patients may receive the wrong drug dose or be given a drug, test, or procedure intended for someone else. In addition, hospital costs are very high and billing errors quite common.

Some of these difficulties can be prevented or overcome by prudent consumers. *Consumer Reports on Health*[12,13] stresses that patients should keep informed and speak up when necessary. People who are too ill to do this should try to have a family member or friend fulfill this role.

Ulene and Ulene[14] advise keeping a daily diary listing every service performed and everything else that happened. This record should include the names of the physicians who visited, what they said, what tests or procedures were performed, and what medications were received. The record will not only help to understand what is taking place but will also be useful for evaluating the hospital bill.

The "Strategies for Hospitalized Patients" box on page 200 summarizes actions advised by the above authorities and others.

HOME CARE SERVICES

Home care can be defined as the provision of equipment and services to the patient in the home for the purpose of restoring and maintaining the patient's maximum level of comfort, function, and health.[16] Home care is

---

A HOSPITAL PATIENT'S BILL OF RIGHTS

A declaration of the rights of hospitalized patients was published in 1972 by the American Hospital Association and revised in 1992.[11] A document embodying these rights is usually distributed as part of the admissions process. The exact wording is up to the hospital, but patients are basically entitled to:

1. Considerate and respectful care.
2. Complete information about diagnosis, treatment, prognosis, and the names of the physicians, nurses, and others handling the patient's case.
3. Information that enables the patient to give informed consent before any procedure or treatment starts.
4. An advance directive (such as a living will, health care proxy, or durable power of attorney for health care) with the expectation that the hospital will honor the intent of these directives to the extent that the law allows.
5. Privacy in the conduct of case discussion, consultation, examination, and treatment.
6. Confidentiality of communications and records.
7. Review and interpretation of their hospital records.
8. Reasonable responses to requests for services.
9. Information about the existence of business relationships among the hospital, educational institutions, other health-care providers, or payers that may influence the patient's care.
10. Consent or decline to participate in proposed research studies.
11. Reasonable continuity of care when hospital care is no longer appropriate.
12. Know the cost of hospital care and what hospital rules and regulations apply to the patient's conduct while a patient.

not a single service. It is a wide range of services with two common goals: to keep the home intact and to improve quality of life by providing help in the home. It encompasses everything from help with everyday tasks of living to advanced medical care. As of March 2000, the National Association for Home Care (NAHC) had identified 7747 Medicare-certified home care agencies, 2288 Medicare-certified hospices, and more than 10,000 others that are not certified.[16] NAHC has also estimated that about 10 million Americans need home care and that the total spent for purchased or compensated home care services in 1999 was about $36 billion. However, most home care services are provided by family members, friends, or other uncompensated caregivers.

Most hospitals offer home care services. Many patients are discharged earlier because home care can be achieved at a much lower cost. Professional home care services can include medical and skilled nursing care; speech, respiratory, physical, or occupational therapy; intravenous drug therapy; nutrition or dietary services; personal care (help with bathing, dressing, and eating); and hospice services for the terminally ill (covered in Chapter 23). Charges are usually on a "per-visit" basis, although they may be on an hourly basis. NAHC estimates that the median cost per home call visit in 1999 was about $27 for registered nurses, $18 for licensed practical nurses, $44 for therapists, $12 for home care aides, and $40 for medical social workers. Federal law requires that home health aides whose employers receive reimbursement by Medicare complete at least 75 hours of classroom and practical training by a registered nurse and pass a competency test. Training may be administered at the home health-care agency and should include basic home nursing, personal care, safety, food, and nutrition.

Sources of information about home care include (a) physicians; (b) hospital-based social and home care offices; (c) the Visiting Nurse Association (check local telephone directory); and (d) organizations such as the National Association for Home Care, Foundation for Hospice and Homecare, and American Federation of HomeCare Providers. Private agencies may be listed in the Yellow Pages under the headings "Home Health Services" or "Nurses."

The following questions can be helpful when selecting a home care agency:[17,18]

- How long has the agency been serving the community?
- Is the agency certified by Medicare? If so, you can review its Medicare Survey Report.
- Is the agency licensed?

- Is the agency accredited by the Community Health Accreditation Program, the Joint Commission on Accreditation of Healthcare Organizations, and/or the National Homecaring Council Division of the Foundation for Hospice and Homecare?
- Does the agency provide literature explaining its services, eligibility requirements, fees, and funding sources?
- How does the agency select and train its employees?
- Are the agency's nurses required to evaluate the patient's home care needs? If so, what does this entail? Are the patient's physicians and family members consulted?
- Is the patient's treatment documented with a detailed plan? Is a copy of this plan given to the patient or the patient's family?
- Do supervisors oversee the care? If so, how often do they visit, who can be contacted with questions and complaints, and how are problems resolved?
- Does the agency take time to educate family members on the type of care being provided?
- What procedures are in place to handle emergencies?

An agency's reputation can also be checked by consulting physicians, hospital discharge planners, community leaders, the local health department, the local Area Agency on Aging, clients of the agency, or others familiar with its operation. General information may be obtained from the National Consumers League and the National Association of Area Agencies on Aging.

NURSING HOMES

A nursing home is a nonhospital facility with an organized professional staff that provides continuous nursing and other health-related psychosocial and personal care services to patients who are not acutely ill but require continued inpatient care.

Nursing homes accept patients for reasons of infirmity, advanced age, illness, injury, convalescence, chronic physical disability, and mental incompetence. They generally do not admit patients suffering from a communicable disease, alcoholism, drug addiction, or acute mental illness.

There were few nursing homes in the United States before 1935. In that year the Social Security Act made federal funds available to the impoverished aged, giving impetus to the development of nursing homes. In 1965 amendments to the Social Security Act created Medicare and Medicaid, which pay a large percentage of the cost of nursing home care. To receive payments under these programs, a facility must meet federal certification standards.

In 1997, an estimated 1.6 million people resided in more than 17,000 certified nursing homes throughout the United States.[19] About two thirds of these were for-profit. About 90% of nursing home residents were at least 65 years old, and about 36% were at least 85 years old.[20] Typical costs ranged from $3000 to $6000 per month. Approximately 44% of people using nursing homes after age 65 start as private payers, 27% start and end as Medicaid recipients, and 14% "spend down" their assets to become eligible for Medicaid benefits.[21]

In 1991, Kemper and Murtaugh[22] estimated that 43% of persons who were 65 in 1990 would enter a nursing home some time before they die, that half of these would spend at least 1 year there, and that 21% would spend at least 5 years there.

From both humanitarian and cost-containment perspectives, long-term care for elderly persons with chronic health problems is a significant societal problem. Most elderly Americans cannot afford nursing home care for even 1 year. Consequently, many chronically ill elderly have their assets depleted to the point where they qualify for Medicaid coverage. People who contemplate placing an elderly person in a nursing home need to know what facilities are available, how to judge their quality, how to deal with problems, and whether an alternative facility is suitable.

Types and Levels of Care

Three general types of services are available in nursing homes. *Nursing care* requires the professional skills of an RN or LPN. It includes administering oral medications and injections and carrying out procedures ordered by attending physicians. Posthospitalization stroke, cardiac, and orthopedic care are available with related services, such as physical and occupational therapy, dental services, dietary consultation, laboratory and x-ray services, and a pharmaceutical dispensary. *Personal care* services include help with walking, getting in and out of bed, bathing, dressing, and eating, as well as preparation of special diets as prescribed by a physician. *Residential care* involves general supervision and a protective environment, including room and board. The facility may also provide for the social and spiritual needs of the resident.

Nursing homes can be licensed for up to three levels of care:

SKILLED NURSING: Continuous nursing service on a 24-hour basis, with emphasis on restoring the patient's functional status.
INTERMEDIATE CARE: Supervision by a registered nurse for at least one 8-hour shift per day for patients capable of performing some activities of daily living (eating, toileting, dressing, bathing, and getting from one location to another). The level of nursing care is less than that provided by skilled nursing facilities.

CUSTODIAL CARE: Care in which room, board, and other non-medical personal assistance are required, generally on a long-term basis, for individuals who are relatively functional.

Quality-of-Care Problems

The minimal standards for nursing home licensure pertain to facilities, staffing, and services. Many qualified homes participate in peer review in consultation with state affiliate members of the American Health Care Association and the Long-Term Care Council of the Joint Commission.

Despite periodic inspections, nursing homes vary considerably within the established criteria. In addition, conformity with the law does not guarantee the skill of the staff, the provision of a friendly atmosphere, or the quality of the care rendered. Flagrant abuse in facilities that provide care for the elderly continues to be evident in many homes.

In 1986 the Institute of Medicine (IOM), a component of the National Academy of Sciences, published the results of its $2^1/_2$-year study of nursing homes.[23] Many good facilities were found; however, poor-quality facilities outnumbered very good ones. The IOM stated that in many government-certified facilities, residents received very inadequate—sometimes shockingly deficient—care likely to hasten a patient's deterioration. They found evidence of discrimination against low-income patients, patterns of lax enforcement, and repeated noncompliance with quality standards.

Congress responded to this report by including provisions pertaining to nursing homes in the 1987 Omnibus Budget Reconstruction Act (OBRA-87). Regulations for implementation were issued in 1990 but were not finalized until 1994.[24] These rules include staffing requirements, comprehensive patient assessment within 14 days after admission, and measures involving patient rights. The rules also forbid restraining patients with drugs, belts, or vests unless medical necessity has been established.

Deficiencies in nursing home care are tabulated in the Federal Online Survey Certification and Reporting System (OSCAR). Staff members of *Consumer Reports* have analyzed 4 years' worth of Health Care Financing Administration (HCFA) inspection reports and visited 53 nursing homes and 27 assisted-living and board-and-care facilities. In 1995 the magazine stated:

- The quality of care at thousands of the nation's nursing homes is poor or questionable at best. Facilities allow life-threatening bedsores to develop, violate residents' dignity, fail to produce required care plans to assure a decent quality of life, improperly use physical restraints such as vests and waist belts, and fail to meet basic standards for sanitary food preparation.

- About 40% of facilities certified by the HCFA have repeatedly violated federal standards over the last four inspection surveys, including standards covering critical aspects of patient care.
- The political influence of the nursing-home industry and the erratic enforcement of state and federal laws permit nursing homes to continue to operate despite repeated violations of health, safety, and nutrition standards.
- Government agencies set up to assist the public—area agencies on aging, and state and local departments of elder affairs—provide little or no useful information about specific facilities.
- State inspection reports, which detail how well or poorly a facility treats its residents, are not readily available to consumers. Some nursing homes hide their inspection reports in violation of the law; state licensing agencies may provide them, but often too late to help make a decision.[18]

The General Accounting Office recently concluded that (a) each year, more than one fourth of the homes had deficiencies that caused actual harm to residents or placed them at risk of death or serious injury; (b) the most frequent violations causing actual harm included inadequate prevention of pressure sores, failure to prevent accidents, and failure to assess residents' needs and provide appropriate care; (c) although most homes were found to have corrected the identified deficiencies, subsequent surveys showed that problems often returned; (d) about 40% of the homes that had such problems in their first survey between July 1995 to October 1998 had them again in their last survey during the period; (e) most sanctions initiated by HCFA against non-compliant nursing homes were never implemented; (f) the threat of sanctions appeared to have little effect on deterring homes from falling out of compliance again because homes could continue to avoid sanctions' effect as long as they kept correcting their deficiencies; and (g) fines are potentially a strong deterrent, but the usefulness of civil monetary penalties is hampered by a backlog of administrative appeals coupled with a legal provision that prohibits collection of the penalty until the appeal is resolved.[25]

Cost Considerations
It has been said that good nursing homes are expensive, but poor ones are not cheap. The Better Business Bureau advises consumers to be wary about signing a life-care contract. It cannot be canceled, and the necessary intensive care, if needed, may not be provided. The Bureau also suggests caution if a large initial deposit or pledge of assets is required for admission. When the

person's resources are depleted, it may be impossible to leave if the facility proves unsatisfactory. If a deposit must be made, explore the possibility of arranging monthly payments rather than liquidating assets. In 1997 the average basic daily charge for private-pay nursing home residents was $136 for skilled care, $107 for intermediate care, and $97 for residential care.

Institutional care may be paid for by Medicare, Medicaid, health insurance, or private funds. Medicare covers skilled nursing care for up to 100 days (20 days fully and all but $99 a day for 80 more days) per benefit period in a Medicare-certified nursing home, provided: (a) the care begins within 30 days of a stay of at least 3 continuous days in an acute-care hospital and (b) a physician certifies that skilled nursing care is required every day for the same condition that caused the hospitalization. A new benefit period begins when the patient has not had inpatient or skilled-nursing care for 60 consecutive days. Medicare does not pay for care in custodial or intermediate care facilities.

Medicaid, a federal-state program, covers long-term care in all three types of facilities for people whose income and total assets are low enough to qualify. However, because Medicare pays considerably more than Medicaid, nursing homes prefer Medicare patients, and Medicaid patients may have to wait months or even years to gain admission. If a Medicaid patient must be transferred to a hospital, there may not be a place to return to afterward, even though the law requires nursing homes to readmit such a patient to the next available bed.

Medicaid coverage is arranged through the local welfare office. In 1998 Medicaid paid $40.6 billion and Medicare paid about $10.4 billion toward the cost of nursing home care for about 1.6 million elderly Americans in nursing homes.

Health insurance and prepaid health-care plans sometimes include nursing home care as a benefit. The care usually is referred to as *extended care*. The cost may be high. Inquiry should be made about the criteria for coverage.

Selecting a Nursing Home
Locating a suitable facility can require considerable time, effort, and patience. There is no easy solution to finding an extended-care facility that provides quality services. However, the following steps can help.

1. Prepare a list of nursing homes that appear suitable. The following sources may provide the desired information: the local health department, local medical society, Social Security district office, welfare and family assistance office, local council of social agencies or

social service referral center, hospital social service department ("discharge planner") physicians, clergy, relatives, friends, and possibly the Yellow Pages. If the community has prepared a directory of nursing homes and helping agencies, its use will save time in making this list.

2. Telephone several homes to determine the types of services they provide and whether they have the level of care needed. Friends, neighbors, physicians, and the local health department may be asked for recommendations and reactions to the facilities under consideration.

3. Visit several homes to inspect the facilities, review inspection reports, verify implementation of the Nursing Home Patient's Bill of Rights (see box below), and obtain information about fees and payment schedules. An initial guided tour should be scheduled, but additional unannounced visits should be made. State licensing agencies are supposed to provide copies of inspection reports, but *Consumer Reports* advises that if the latest report is not available at the facility itself, assume it has something to hide and cross it off your list.

4. Complete information about costs, payment policies, and other details should be obtained. These should include daily and monthly room rates and extra charges for services and supplies (for physician, physical therapist, private nursing services, medications, laundry, haircuts, and special diets). Also find out when payment is expected. If required in advance, the policy concerning refunds for unused portions should be discussed. Higher costs for services may mean that facilities have more nurses and other staff members. However, they do not guarantee better care.

5. Before signing a contract for admission to a nursing home, it is advisable to have an attorney review it. A good contract should include (a) permission for the patient or family to purchase supplies, medications, and equipment on the open market if so desired; (b) a clear statement of the behavior or financial condition that will precipitate eviction; and (c) a refund for unused time when a patient is discharged, dies, or is evicted for behavior problems. It is undesirable for a contract to (a) absolve the home from financial liability for injury or theft; (b) waive the right to be informed in advance of changes in patient care or charges for services; (c) guarantee to pay all costs of litigation, including a nursing home attorney, if the home is sued; or (d) bar cancellation of a life-care contract (unless a trial period of at least 60 days of residence is permitted).

6. After narrowing the choices of nursing homes to one or two, an unannounced visit should be made at a mealtime to determine the quality of the food and how it is served. An evening or night visit might be advisable as well. These visits will provide opportunities to judge the quality of care when the staff is not primed to impress visitors and to raise questions and concerns that may have arisen since the first visit. Observe the activities and talk with the patients: Do they seem interested in life? Does the staff show concern for the patients?

Anticipating and Handling Problems

Laws alone cannot ensure quality care. Family members or other concerned parties must not only be discriminating in selecting places for elderly and chronically ill persons, but also should observe the quality of patient care after admission and take action when services appear inadequate. Federal regulations require nursing homes to record and periodically update a management plan for each patient. Concerned parties can request a copy of the plan of care and monitor its

---

A NURSING HOME PATIENT'S BILL OF RIGHTS

To achieve Medicare and Medicaid certification, nursing homes must meet federal standards that include offering these rights to their residents:

- The right to choose your own doctors and to help plan your course of treatment.
- Freedom from physical and mental abuse and from any restraints not medically required.
- Use of pharmacologic drugs by prescription and only for the symptoms for which they are prescribed.
- The right to privacy.
- Confidentiality of records.
- The right to services tailored to the resident's individual needs and advanced notice before room or roommate is changed.
- The right to voice grievances.
- The right to organize and participate in resident groups.
- The right to participate in social, religious, and community activities.
- The right to examine the most recent report of the facility and to review plans to correct deficiencies.
- Any other right established by the Secretary of Health and Human Services.

Table 10-2

SCOPE AND RELATIVE COST OF LONG-TERM CARE FACILITIES AND SERVICES

Type	Scope	Relative Cost
Boarding facility	Room, meals, housekeeping services, and possibly personal care services	Moderate
Congregate housing	Apartment complexes that offer meals, housekeeping, and health-care services	Moderate
Day care	Supervised lunch, recreational and social activities, and other services for ambulatory patients	No fee, sliding scale, or full fee (expensive)
Domiciliary care	Supervised residential programs for elderly, physically impaired, mentally ill, or mentally retarded people	Low to moderate; may be covered by Medicaid
Emergency response system	Portable or wall-mounted devices that can signal a monitoring service that contacts an appropriate agency or family member for help (see Chapter 22)	Moderate; costs include an installation fee plus a monthly charge for the monitoring
Home health care	Wide range of health and personal services	Varies; may be based on ability to pay
Home visitor/ companion	Volunteers visit ailing seniors	None
Home-delivered meals	Delivery of prepared food, usually weekdays only; typically called "Meals on Wheels"	Low or nominal
Hospice	Full range of services for the terminally ill (see Chapter 23)	Expensive but usually covered by Medicare
Life-care community	Housing and services that range from independent living to skilled nursing care. Apartments for "well elderly" typically include close medical monitoring, dietary and housekeeping services; social, recreational, and spiritual services; and nursing care when needed	Expensive; large entry fee plus monthly fees based on extent of services
Nursing home	Three levels of service: skilled, intermediate, and custodial	Depends on level of care, but all are expensive
Personal care facility	Custodial care in which the facility supplies individual rooms and supportive services in return for a monthly fee	Expensive but usually less than nursing home
Respite care	Short-term care in the home or an institution to temporarily relieve the home caregiver; may be used to help in recovery from illness or enable a family to take a vacation	Varies
Rest home	Custodial care; may include the services of a visiting nurse	Moderate
Senior centers	Social, recreational, and educational activities	Nominal
Shared housing	House or apartment occupied by a few people, each with his or her own bedroom; supervised by a public or private agency; may provide services such as cleaning, shopping, cooking, and nurse visits	Low to moderate; may be based on ability to pay
Special housing	Apartment buildings specially designed for the elderly	Eligibility and rent usually based on ability to pay
Telephone reassurance	Homebound individual "checks in" or is contacted by a designated person or agency at specified times	None
Transportation service	Transportation to medical appointments and other essential activities	Free or nominal

implementation. The *Johns Hopkins Medical Letter*[26] has suggested the following actions to prevent unnecessary use of restraints:

- If legally responsible for the resident, tell the administrators that you want no restraint to be used until you or your physician provide informed consent.
- Request an explanation from the administrator that details the specific reasons when a restraint is the only recourse.
- Ask for an estimate of when the restraint will be removed, reinforcing the notion that restraints should be used as little as possible.
- Spend as much time as you can participating in the resident's care. Restraints may be applied if a patient being tube-fed through the nose pulls out the tube; offering to feed the patient might circumvent this problem.
- When shopping for a nursing home, inquire about the policy regarding the use of restraints.

Problems that arise should be discussed with the nursing staff and, if necessary, with the nursing home administrator. If this is unsuccessful, complaints can be made to the local Social Security office, the patient's caseworker (if covered by Medicaid), a nursing home ombudsman, the state licensing board, the local Better Business Bureau, or an attorney.

Alternatives

Before deciding about nursing home care, it is advisable to determine the level of care needed and whether an alternative is available. A physician, public health nurse, social worker, or family members may help with these determinations. The needed care may include 24-hour care, daily medical supervision, minimal assistance with daily activities (help with shopping, cleaning, and cooking meals), or other services. The term "assisted living facility" is often used to describe boarding homes, supervised individual apartments, and personal-care facilities that offer help with activities of daily living in a homelike atmosphere.[27] The legal definition, scope of services, and regulation of these facilities vary from state to state. The cost depends largely on the amount of services offered and can be quite expensive.[28]

Table 10-2 describes various types of community assistance and their relative costs.

Summary

Many types of community facilities are available to help with illnesses and infirmities.

Outpatient medical facilities include private medical offices, student health services, work-related facilities, ambulatory care centers, ambulatory surgical centers,

and hospital emergency departments and outpatient clinics.

Inpatient facilities include hospitals and nursing homes. A wide variety of home care services may enable disabled individuals to avoid institutionalization.

More than 20,000 facilities are accredited by the Joint Commission on Accreditation of Healthcare Organizations and other accrediting agencies.

The best choice of facility depends on the type and urgency of the problem as well as insurance coverage and other financial considerations. Prudent consumers know the pitfalls of the various facilities and try to avoid them.

References

1. Baer K. How to pick the right hospital. Harvard Health Letter, Special Supplement, July 1995.
2. Nursing homes: When a loved one needs care. Consumer Reports 60:518–528, 1995.
3. Editors of Consumer Reports Books. Foreword to Nassif JZ. The Home Health Care Solution. Yonkers, N.Y., 1985, Consumer Reports Books.
4. Isaacs SL, Swartz AC. The Consumer's Legal Guide to Today's Health Care: Your Medical Rights and How to Assert Them. Boston, 1992, Houghton Mifflin Co.
5. Patient dumping case goes to court. Public Citizen Health Research Group Health Letter 7(5):3, 1991.
6. Health, United States, 2000. Hyattsville, Md., 2000, National Center for Health Statistics Web site, Dec 15, 2000.
7. Brook RH and others. Quality of ambulatory care. Medical Care 28:392–407, 1990.
8. Hospital accreditation: What it means and how it works. Oakbrook, Ill., 1996, Joint Commission on Accreditation of Healthcare Organizations.
9. America's Best Hospitals. U.S. News & World Report, July 17, 2000.
10. A patient's bill of rights. Chicago, 1992, American Hospital Association.
11. Leeds D, Strauss JM. Smart Questions to Ask Your Doctor. New York, 1992, HarperCollins.
12. Lipman MM. Surviving a stay in the hospital. Consumer Reports on Health 3:30, 1991.
13. Avoiding hospital blunders: Knowing the risks and speaking up can help you stay safe. Consumer Reports on Health 12(6):1–5, 2000.

14. Ulene A, Ulene V. How to Cut Your Medical Bills. Berkeley, Calif., 1994, Ulysses Press.

15. Scott WC and others. Home care in the 1990s. JAMA 263:1241–1244, 1991.

16. Basic statistics about home care (1999). National Association for Home Care Web site, accessed Dec 6, 2000.

17. A consumer's guide: How to choose a home health care agency. Washington, D.C., 1996, National Association for Home Care.

18. Can your loved ones avoid a nursing home? Consumer Reports 60:656–662, 1995.

<u>19</u>. Gabrel CS. An overview of nursing home facilities: Data from the 1997 National Nursing Home Survey. Advance Data No. 311, March 1, 2000.

20. Brown E Jr. Facts and Trends: The Nursing Facility Sourcebook. Washington, D.C., 1996, American Health Care Association.

21. Spillman BC, Kemper P. Lifetime patterns of payment for nursing home care. Medical Care 33:280–296, 1995.

22. Kemper P, Murtaugh CM. Lifetime use of nursing home care. New England Journal of Medicine 324:595–600, 1991.

23. Institute of Medicine Committee on Nursing Home Regulation. Improving the Quality of Care in Nursing Homes. Washington, D.C., 1986, National Academy Press.

24. Health Care Financing Administration. Medicare and Medicaid Programs: Survey, Certi-fication, and Enforcement of Skilled Nursing Facilities and Nursing Facilities. Final Rule. Federal Register 59:56116–56252, 1994.

<u>25</u>. Nursing Homes: Additional Steps Needed to Strengthen Enforcement of Federal Quality Standards (Letter Report, 3/18/99, GAO/HEHS-99-46).

26. Restraints on nursing home restraints. The Johns Hopkins Medical Letter, Health After 50 2(9):6, 1990

27. Citro J, Hermanson S. Assisted living in the United States. AARP Web site, March 1999.

28. Is assisted living the right choice? The promise and the pitfalls of a residential option designed to fill the gap between independent living and nursing-home care. Consumer Reports 66(1):26–31, 2001.

Part III

Nutrition and Fitness

Chapter Eleven

BASIC NUTRITION CONCEPTS

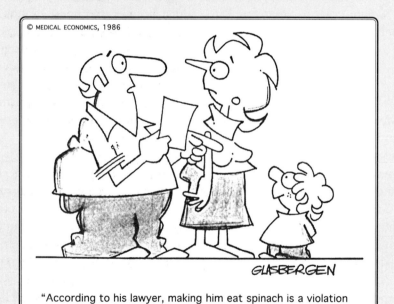

© MEDICAL ECONOMICS, 1986

GLASBERGEN

"According to his lawyer, making him eat spinach is a violation of his civil rights. He's suing us for a million dollars."

The wide variety of great-tasting nutritious foods available today gives us more options for healthful eating than ever before. . . . Eating is a fun and enjoyable part of life. There's no reason good nutrition can't be too.

DORIS DERELIAN, PH.D., R.D.[1]
PRESIDENT, AMERICAN DIETETIC ASSOCIATION

Good nutrition is neither complicated nor restrictive. Unless you have a severe metabolic disorder or other specific nutrition-related health problem, you can enjoy virtually every food . . . so long as you practice moderation, variety and balance.

VICTOR HERBERT, M.D., J.D.
TRACY STOPLER KASDAN, M.S., R.D.[2]

Key Concepts

KEEP THESE POINTS IN MIND AS YOU STUDY THIS CHAPTER

- The fundamental principles of healthy eating are moderation, variety, and balance.
- A sensible diet based on the Dietary Guidelines for Americans and the USDA Food Guide Pyramid system will usually provide adequate amounts of essential nutrients.
- Food product labels must disclose the amounts of fat and several other significant nutrients.
- Consumers seeking nutrition advice should choose their sources carefully.

Nutrition is the science of food and how the body uses it in health and in disease. A working knowledge of basic nutrition will help you make intelligent food choices and protect yourself against the vast array of misinformation you will encounter. This chapter discusses major food components, essential nutrients and their food sources, dietary guidelines, food labeling, and sources of reliable nutrition information. Nutrition quackery and weight control are covered in the following two chapters. The relationships between diet and heart disease are analyzed in Chapter 15.

MAJOR FOOD COMPONENTS

The major nutrient components of food are proteins, carbohydrates, fats, vitamins, minerals, and water. Proteins, carbohydrates, and fats supply energy (calories) and are needed in relatively large amounts. They are called *macronutrients* and are conveniently measured in grams. (*Makros* is a Greek word that means large.) Practically all foods contain mixtures of proteins, fats, and carbohydrates, although they are commonly classified according to the predominant macrocomponent.

Vitamins and minerals are needed in relatively small amounts for specific purposes, mainly to help regulate body functions. They are called *micronutrients* and are usually measured in milligram (mg) or microgram (μg) amounts. Water is the major component in both foods and the human body, which is about 60% water.

The body's digestive system breaks food down into molecules small enough to be absorbed through intestinal walls into the bloodstream. The absorbed substances are metabolized and used for energy, growth and repair, and many other body functions.

Proteins

Proteins, the body's main structural component, are used to make bone, connective tissue, muscle, skin, hair, and cell membranes. Proteins also function as enzymes, hormones; antibodies; and as part of hemoglobin, which transports oxygen to the tissues.

The proteins in food are too large to be absorbed through the intestinal wall, so they are broken down during digestion into their component amino acids. These are absorbed from the small intestine and reassembled as needed into the thousands of proteins needed by the body. Amino acids not used for this purpose are used for energy. There are about 20 amino acids in the foods we eat, eight or nine of which are essential in the diet because the body cannot manufacture them. The essential amino acids are isoleucine, leucine, lysine, methionine, phenylalanine, threonine, tryptophan, and valine; for infants, histidine also is essential.

Protein sources are considered *complete* (of high quality) if they supply all of the essential amino acids in adequate amounts and *incomplete* (of poor quality) if they do not.

Carbohydrates

Carbohydrates are excellent sources of energy and supply about half the calories consumed in the average American's diet. Humans can digest two types of carbohydrates: starches and sugars. Sucrose, the predominant sugar, is composed of glucose and fructose. Lactose (milk sugar) is also a significant dietary sugar. Cellulose, a carbohydrate that is indigestible by humans, is a component of dietary fiber and is not an energy source for humans.

Starches are found in all grains from which breads, cereals, and pasta are made, and also in rice, potatoes, and other vegetables. Starches and most types of dietary fiber are *complex carbohydrates* composed of long chains of glucose molecules. Sugars, such as table sugar (sucrose), honey, and corn syrup (including high-fructose corn syrup), contain one or two sugar molecules and are called *simple carbohydrates*.

Glucose has been called the universal sugar because it is the basic form of food energy. All carbohydrates must be metabolized to glucose so that the energy in its molecular bonds can be used by the body. Glucose circulates in the blood and is stored in the form of glycogen (animal starch), mainly in the liver and some in the muscles. However, most extra calories are stored as fat, a more concentrated form of stored energy than glycogen. If carbohydrate is not supplied in the diet, the body must use a less efficient process (described in Chapter 13) to break down fats and proteins for energy.

Many food faddists claim that sucrose is a "deadly poison," while complex carbohydrates are safer and more desirable. Foods that contain complex carbohydrates are an important part of a balanced diet. However, as noted by Stare, Aronson, and Barrett:

It is ridiculous to claim that one type of digestible carbohydrate is dangerously inferior to the others when all become glucose in the body anyway. All edible carbohydrates are safe when eaten in moderate amounts.[3]

Dietary fiber. Dietary fiber (also called bulk or roughage) refers to plant components that are resistant to digestion by human gastrointestinal secretions. It includes a heterogeneous group of carbohydrate compounds (cellulose, hemicellulose, mucilages, pectin, and gums) and also a noncarbohydrate, lignin. All foods of vegetable origin contain fiber in various quantities. Whole-grain foods are a major source of dietary fiber. Bran has 9% to 12% crude fiber; dry beans, lentils, and soybeans have over 4%; roasted nuts have 2.3% to 2.6%. Most fruits and vegetables contain 0.5% to 1% of fiber.

Fiber in the intestinal tract holds water, improving the body's reservoir for hydration. It also makes the feces bulkier (heavier) and softer, which enables them to pass more quickly and easily through the intestines. Low-fiber diets often result in constipation. Epidemiologic data provide evidence that prolonged lack of dietary fiber is associated with gastrointestinal, circulatory, and metabolic problems such as diverticulitis (inflamed outpouches in the large intestine), varicose veins, deep vein thrombosis, hemorrhoids, increased blood cholesterol levels, obesity, and diabetes.

Naturally occurring fiber in food is usually a mixture of water-*soluble fibers* (pectins, gums, and mucilages), *insoluble fibers* (cellulose and lignin), and combinations of insoluble and soluble fiber (hemicellulose). Oat bran and oatmeal contain relatively large amounts of soluble fiber, and whole wheat contains relatively large amounts of insoluble fiber.

Epidemiologic studies have found relationships between the amount of fiber in the diet and the incidence of various diseases.[4] Since foods high in fiber have a variety of fiber components and tend to be low in fat, it is difficult to design studies that can test for specific effects of fiber. Much research needs to be done to determine which components, if any, might be most useful and the amounts of these components that would

be optimal. However, it is known that increasing the amount of soluble fiber may help lower high blood-cholesterol levels and that increasing total dietary fiber is useful in treating constipation and hemorrhoids.[5] It is uncertain whether fiber has specific benefits in weight control.[5]

All major scientific groups that have issued dietary guidelines agree that it is desirable for one's overall diet to contain adequate amounts of dietary fiber. The Food and Drug Administration (FDA)[6] does not believe there is adequate evidence to permit manufacturers to claim that the amount of fiber in *individual* food products can help prevent cancer or lower the risk of cardiovascular disease, but it does allow claims involving fiber-containing foods as part of a healthful diet (see Table 11-6, page 229). Chapter 15 covers the importance of soluble fiber in the treatment of high cholesterol levels.

A study prepared for the FDA by the Federation of American Societies for Experimental Biology (FASEB) recommends that healthy adults consume 20 to 35 g of fiber per day, which corresponds to approximately 10 to 13 g per 1000 calories of food. The report concluded that achieving this level of intake is feasible by selecting ordinary foods that are currently available and that many Americans already did so.[7] Fiber intake can be increased by eating more whole-grain breads and cereals, fruits, vegetables, legumes, and nuts. But even fiber that occurs naturally should be eaten in moderation. A high-fiber diet can cause one to feel stuffed or bloated; can cause diarrhea; and can interfere with the absorption of iron, copper, zinc, and calcium. Purified fibers and fiber supplements are generally not recommended for individuals who are able to obtain fiber from food.[5,8]

Fats (Lipids)

Lipid is the general term for fatty substances, including triglycerides (fats and oils), phospholipids (such as lecithin), and sterols (including cholesterol). In common usage, fats are lipids that are solid at room temperature, and oils are lipids that are liquid at room temperature.

The fats commonly found in foods and in the body are triglycerides. Their molecules are composed of glycerol (an alcohol) plus three chainlike fatty acids. Fatty acids differ in the length of their molecular chains and their degree of saturation with hydrogen. Those filled to capacity with hydrogen are called *saturated* fatty acids. Chains that have room for two hydrogen atoms are called *monounsaturated* fatty acids. Those with room for four or more hydrogen atoms are called *polyunsaturated*. Linoleic acid, which is polyunsaturated, is the only lipid nutrient recognized as essential for humans. Lipids in the diet contain many other fatty acids, but these can be synthesized from other substances and are not essential.

Triglycerides can contain combinations of fatty acids of all types. The dominant fatty-acid type determines the characteristics of the triglyceride. Oils tend to be richer in polyunsaturates, but palm oil and coconut oil are saturated. Other saturated fats originate from animals or are vegetable oils with hydrogen added by hydrogenation, but fish oils are largely polyunsaturated. When oils are hydrogenated, they become pasty. The process changes some unsaturated fatty acids to saturated ones and rearranges others from their natural cis-configuration to trans-fatty acids.

Cholesterol, an important component of cell membranes, is transported through the bloodstream in three main cholesterol-protein combinations: *high-density lipoprotein* (HDL—"good cholesterol"), *low-density lipoprotein* (LDL—"bad cholesterol"), and *very-low-density lipoprotein* (VLDL). Actually, HDL and LDL are not types of cholesterol but are fat-protein compounds that transport cholesterol through the blood. HDL tends to carry cholesterol away from the arterial walls, and LDL tends to deposit it there. When cholesterol is attached to a lipoprotein, the entire complex is properly referred to as HDL- or LDL-cholesterol. However, the terms HDL and LDL are more commonly used. VLDL is related to blood triglyceride levels. Chapter 15 thoroughly discusses the relationships between dietary factors, lipoproteins, and heart disease.

Vitamins

Vitamins are organic (carbon-containing) substances required in tiny amounts to promote one or more specific biochemical reactions. Only tiny amounts are necessary because vitamins are catalysts (substances that initiate or speed up chemical reactions but remain unchanged while performing their tasks repeatedly). Vitamins do not provide energy directly but are part of the enzyme systems needed to release energy from carbohydrates, fats, and proteins. There are 13 known vitamins for humans: four are fat-soluble (A, D, E, and K) and nine are water-soluble (C and the eight B-complex vitamins: thiamin [B_1], riboflavin [B_2], niacin, B_6, B_{12}, folic acid, biotin, and pantothenic acid). Since patients can survive for many years without becoming ill on intravenous feedings fortified with these substances, it appears that no vitamins remain to be discovered.

Vitamins must be obtained from food because the human body cannot manufacture them, but a few are also made within the body. Vitamin D is made in the skin when it is exposed to sunlight, and biotin and vitamin K are made by bacteria in the large intestine.

Vitamin deficiency diseases are rare in the United States because vitamins are plentiful in the food supply, both naturally and through fortification. Population groups at risk for deficiency are identified in Chapter 12.

Minerals

Minerals are inorganic compounds needed in relatively small amounts to help regulate body functions, aid in growth and maintenance of body tissues, and act as catalysts for the release of energy. The 17 essential minerals may be categorized as *major minerals* (macrominerals) or *trace minerals* (microminerals). The macrominerals are those present in the body in amounts exceeding 5 g: calcium, phosphorus, magnesium, sodium, potassium, chloride, and sulfur. Sodium, potassium, and chloride are called *electrolytes* because, in solution, they help to conduct electrical currents. The essential trace minerals are chromium, cobalt, copper, fluoride, iodide, iron, manganese, molybdenum, selenium, and zinc.

HUMAN NUTRIENT NEEDS

Three sets of guidelines are available to help people make intelligent dietary choices. The Dietary Guidelines for Americans (DGA) provide practical advice for healthful food choice. The Reference Dietary Intakes

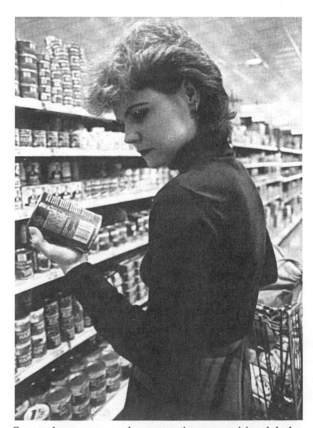

Smart shoppers pay close attention to nutrition labels.

(DRIs) define what is known about the ranges of safe and adequate consumption of individual nutrients. The U.S. Department of Agriculture (USDA) Food Guide Pyramid addresses both nutrient adequacy and disease prevention.

Dietary Guidelines for Americans (DGA)

The DGA, developed jointly by the U.S. Department of Health and Human Services and the USDA, provide recommendations based on current scientific knowledge about how dietary intake may reduce risk for major chronic diseases and how a healthful diet may improve nutrition. The guidelines form the basis of federal food, nutrition education, and information programs. They address the question, "What should Americans eat to have the best chance of staying healthy?" Federal law requires the guidelines to be reviewed every 5 years. The first four versions were published in 1980, 1985, 1990, and 1995.[9] DGA 2000[10] contains 10 guidelines, three more than the 1995 version. Organized under three basic

---

TABLE 11-1

DIETARY GUIDELINES FOR AMERICANS 2000

AIM FOR FITNESS

Aim for a healthy weight.

- If you are at a healthy weight, aim to avoid weight gain. If you are already overweight, first aim to prevent further weight gain, and then lose weight to improve your health.
- Build a healthy base by eating vegetables, fruits, and grains (especially whole grains), with little added sugar.
- Select sensible portion sizes.
- Get moving. Get regular physical activity to balance calories from the foods you eat.
- Set a good example for children by practicing healthy eating habits and enjoying regular physical activities together.
- Keep in mind that even though heredity and the environment are important influences, your behaviors help determine your body weight.

Be physically active each day.

- Engage in at least 30 minutes (adults) or 60 minutes (children) of moderate physical activity most, preferably all, days of the week.
- Become physically active if you are inactive.
- Maintain or increase physical activity if you are already active.
- Stay active throughout your life.
- Help children get at least 60 minutes of physical activity daily.
- Choose physical activities that fit in with your daily routine; or choose recreational or structured exercise programs; or both.
- Consult your health care professional when starting a new vigorous physical activity plan if you have a chronic health problem, or if you are over 40 (men) or 50 (women).

BUILD A HEALTHY BASE

Let the Pyramid guide your food choices.

- Build a healthy base: Use the Food Guide Pyramid to help you make healthy food choices that you can enjoy.
- Build your eating pattern on a variety of plant foods, including whole grains, fruits, and vegetables.
- Also choose some low-fat dairy products and low-fat foods from the meat and beans group each day.
- It's fine to enjoy fats and sweets occasionally.

Choose a variety of grains daily, especially whole grains.

- Build a healthy base by making a variety of grains the foundation of your diet.
- Eat 6 or more servings of grain products daily (whole grain and refined breads, cereals, pasta, and rice). Include several servings of whole grain foods daily for their good taste and their health benefits. If your calorie needs are low, have only 6 servings of sensible size daily.
- Eat foods made from a variety of whole grains—such as whole wheat, brown rice, oats, and whole-grain corn—every day.
- Combine whole grains with other tasty, nutritious foods in mixed dishes.
- Prepare or choose grain products with little added saturated fat and moderate or low amounts of added sugars. Also, check the sodium content on the Nutrition Facts package label.

Choose a variety of fruits and vegetables daily.

- Enjoy five a day—eat at least 2 servings of fruit and at least 3 servings of vegetables each day
- Choose fresh, frozen, dried, or canned forms and a variety of colors and kinds.
- Choose dark-green leafy vegetables, bright-orange fruits and vegetables, and cooked dry beans and peas often.

headings, they are intended for healthy children (age 2 or above) and adults. The full text is available on the Agriculture Department's Web site and as a 40-page booklet. Table 11-1 provides a summary.

Dietary Reference Intakes (DRIs)

The DRIs are nutrient-based reference values for use in planning and assessing diets. They are an expansion of the Recommended Dietary Allowances (RDAs) that the National Academy of Sciences has published since 1941. They are being determined by the Standing Committee on the Scientific Evaluation of Dietary Reference Intakes of the Food and Nutrition Board, Institute of Medicine (IOM), National Academy of Sciences, with help from Health Canada.

The DRIs will be released in a series of seven reports. The first report, published in 1997, covers nutrients related to bone health (calcium, phosphorus, magnesium, vitamin D, and fluoride).[11] The second, which covered folate and other B vitamins, was released in 1998.[12] The third, published in 2000, is about antioxidants (vitamin C, vitamin E, selenium, and carotenoids).[13] The others will cover macronutrients (e.g., protein, fat, carbohydrates); trace elements (e.g., iron, zinc); electrolytes and water; and other food components (e.g., fiber, phytoestrogens).

The RDAs have been the benchmark of nutritional adequacy in the United States.[14] More than 20 years ago, they were defined as: "The levels of intake of essential nutrients that, on the basis of scientific knowledge, are judged by the Food and Nutrition Board to be adequate to meet the known nutrient needs of practically all healthy persons." Since that time, scientific knowledge about the roles of nutrients has expanded dramatically.

TABLE 11-1

DIETARY GUIDELINES FOR AMERICANS 2000 – CONT'D.

Keep food safe to eat.

- Clean. Wash hands and food-contact surfaces often.
- Separate. Separate raw, cooked, and ready-to-eat foods while shopping, preparing, or storing.
- Cook. Cook foods to a safe temperature.
- Chill. Refrigerate perishable foods promptly.
- Check and follow the label.
- Serve safely. Keep hot foods hot (above 140°F) and cold foods cold (below 40°F)
- When in doubt, throw it out.

CHOOSE SENSIBLY

Choose a diet that is low in saturated fat and cholesterol and moderate in total fat.

- Limit use of solid fats, such as butter, hard margarines, lard, and partially hydrogenated shortenings. Use vegetable oils as a substitute.
- Choose fat-free or low-fat dairy products, cooked dried beans and peas, fish, and lean meats and poultry.
- Eat plenty of grain products, vegetables, and fruits daily.
- Use the Nutrition Facts Label to help you choose foods lower in fat, saturated fat, and cholesterol.

Choose beverages and foods that limit your intake of sugars.

- Choose sensibly to limit your intake of beverages and foods that are high in sugars.

- Get most of your calories from grains (especially whole grains), fruits and vegetables, low-fat or non-fat dairy products, and lean meats or meat substitutes.
- Take care not to let soft drinks or other sweets crowd out other foods you need to maintain health, such as juices and low-fat milk or other good sources of calcium.
- Remember the simple tips to keep your teeth and gums healthy.
- Drink water often.

Choose and prepare foods with less salt.

- Choose sensibly to moderate your salt intake.
- Choose fruits and vegetables often. They contain very little salt unless it is added in processing.
- Read the Nutrition Facts Label to compare and help identify foods lower in sodium— especially prepared foods.
- Use herbs, spices, and fruits to flavor food, and cut the amount of salty seasonings by half.
- If you eat restaurant foods or fast foods, choose those that are prepared with only moderate amounts of salt or salty flavorings.

If you drink alcoholic beverages, do so in moderation.

- If you choose to drink alcoholic beverages, do so sensibly.
- Limit intake to one drink/day for women or two/ day for men, and take with meals to slow alcohol absorption.
- Avoid drinking before or when driving, or whenever it puts you or others at risk.

Many studies have examined relationships between diet and chronic disease. The Food and Nutrition Board has responded to these developments by changing its basic approach to setting nutrient reference values.

The DRIs reflect a shift in emphasis from preventing deficiency to decreasing the risk of chronic disease through nutrition. The RDAs were based on the amounts needed to protect against deficiency diseases. Where adequate scientific data exist, the DRIs will include levels that can help prevent cardiovascular disease, osteoporosis, certain cancers, and other diseases that are diet-related. Instead of a single category, the DRIs will encompass at least four:

1. ESTIMATED AVERAGE REQUIREMENT (EAR): The intake that meets the estimated nutrient need of 50% of the individuals in a specific group. This figure will be used as the basis for developing the RDA and can be used by nutrition policy-makers to evaluate the adequacy of nutrient intakes for population groups.
2. RECOMMENDED DIETARY ALLOWANCE (RDA): The intake that meets the nutrient need of almost all (97% to 98%) of the healthy individuals in a specific age and gender group. The RDA should be used in guiding individuals to achieve adequate nutrient intake aimed at decreasing the risk of chronic disease. It is based on estimating an average requirement plus an increase to account for the variation within a particular group. If individual variation in requirements is well defined, the RDA is set at 2 standard deviations above the EAR, which means it should be high enough to meet the needs of at least 97% to 98% of the population. If sufficient data are not available, the RDA is set at 1.2 x EAR.
3. ADEQUATE INTAKE (AI): When sufficient scientific evidence is not available to estimate an average requirement, AIs will be set. These are derived through experimental or observational data that show a mean intake which appears to sustain a desired indicator of health, such as calcium retention in bone. The AIs should be used as a goal for individual intake where no RDAs exist.
4. TOLERABLE UPPER INTAKE LEVEL (UL): The maximum intake by an individual that is unlikely to pose risks of adverse health effects in almost all healthy individuals in a specified group. The UL is not intended to be a recommended level of intake, and there is no established benefit for individuals to consume nutrients at levels above the RDA or AI. The term "tolerable upper intake level" was chosen to avoid implying a possible beneficial effect. For most nutrients, it refers to total intake from food, fortified food, and supplements.

The DRIs are intended to apply to the healthy general population. RDAs and AIs are dietary intake values that should minimize the risk of developing a condition or sign associated with that nutrient in question and that has a negative functional outcome. They refer to average daily intake over 1 or more weeks. They may not be sufficient to supply individuals who are already malnourished or who have a disease state marked by increased requirements. Individuals in these categories, or who have increased sensitivity to developing adverse effects associated with higher intakes, should be guided by qualified medical and nutrition personnel.

Intake less than the RDA does not necessarily mean that a given individual is not getting enough of that nutrient. Healthy individuals who meet the AI have a low risk of inadequate intake. However, an intake well below the RDA or AI would be a reason to assess the individual's nutritional status through laboratory testing or clinical examination. The IOM expects future publications to provide more detailed advice on how the DRIs should be interpreted and used.

In many cases, various levels of intake can have different benefits. One level may be related to the risk of deficiency, for example, while another level can influence the risk of chronic disease. Therefore, "nutrient adequacy" should be expressed in terms of "Adequate for what?" For this reason, the DRIs are far more elaborate than the RDAs and cannot be expressed in a simple table of values.

A sensible diet of foods, as described in Figure 11-1, can provide adequate amounts of all essential nutrients. Most individuals do not need supplementary vitamins, minerals, protein, or amino acids. However, as noted later in this chapter, a few nutrients may need special attention. Table 11-2 identifies the functions and best food sources of the major nutrients.

Biochemical Individuality
RDAs are recommended daily *averages*. They are neither requirements nor minimums, and they do take into account the differing needs of individuals. Stare, Aronson, and Barrett have noted:

Intakes equivalent to half the RDA are usually adequate. . . . Anyone who advises healthy persons to take doses of vitamins and minerals higher than the RDA "to be sure they get enough" is bypassing the collective wisdom of the scientific nutrition community.[3]

Victor Herbert, M.D., a member of the 1980–1985 RDA committee, has noted:

To promote supplements, health hustlers misrepresent the concept of "biochemical individuality" (our genetic blueprint) to imply that individuals should consume more than the RDAs in case they have greater-than-average needs. . . . RDAs are deliberately set higher than virtually all normal people

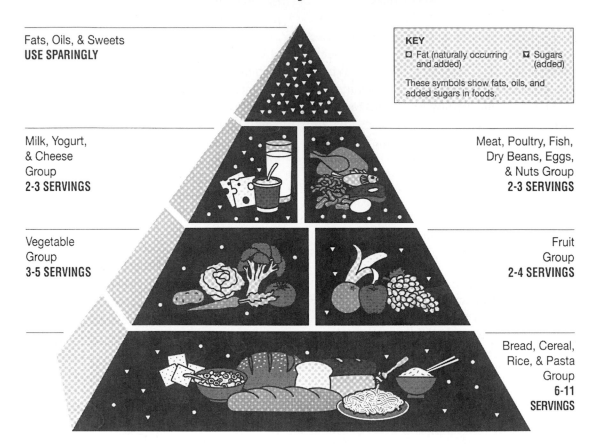

Food Guide Pyramid
A Guide to Daily Food Choices

Fats, Oils, & Sweets
USE SPARINGLY

KEY
□ Fat (naturally occurring and added)   ☑ Sugars (added)

These symbols show fats, oils, and added sugars in foods.

Milk, Yogurt, & Cheese Group
2-3 SERVINGS

Meat, Poultry, Fish, Dry Beans, Eggs, & Nuts Group
2-3 SERVINGS

Vegetable Group
3-5 SERVINGS

Fruit Group
2-4 SERVINGS

Bread, Cereal, Rice, & Pasta Group
6-11 SERVINGS

How many servings are right for me?

The pyramid shows a range of servings for each food group. The number of servings that are right for you depends on how many calories you need, which in turn depends on your age, size, and activity level. Almost everyone should have the lowest number of servings in the ranges.

The following calorie level suggestions are based on recommendations of the National Academy of Sciences and on calorie intakes reported by people in national food-consumption surveys.

For adults and teens:

1600 calories is about right for many sedentary women and some older adults.

2200 calories is about right for most children, teenage girls, active women, and many sedentary men. Women who are pregnant or breastfeeding may need somewhat more.

2800 calories is about right for teenage boys, many active men, and some very active women.

Sample Diets for a Day at Three Calorie Levels

	Lower about **1600**	Moderate about **2200**	Higher about **2800**
Bread group servings	6	9	11
Vegetable group servings	3	4	5
Fruit group servings	2	3	4
Milk group servings	2–3[a]	2–3[a]	2–3[a]
Meat group (ounces)[b]	5	6	7
Total fat (grams)	53	73	93
Total added sugars (tsp.)	6	12	18

[a]Teenagers, young adults to age 24, and women who are pregnant or breastfeeding should have three servings.

[b]This figure represents the number of ounces of meat or meat equivalents that should be counted (see Table 11-3).

FIGURE 11-1. Food Guide Pyramid and suggested daily calorie levels. After estimating your appropriate calorie level, use the worksheet and Table 11-3 on pages 220–221 to judge the quality of your diet.

Table 11-2

FUNCTIONS AND FOOD SOURCES OF MAJOR NUTRIENTS

Nutrient	Major Functions in Body	Best Food Sources
Protein	Forms cell structure; supports growth, maintenance, and repair of tissue; needed for enzymes and hormones	Meat, poultry, fish, dry beans, eggs, nuts Milk, yogurt, and cheese
Carbohydrate	Serves as primary energy source; can provide fiber for proper digestive function	Bread, cereal, rice, and pasta Fruits and vegetables
Fat	Serves as concentrated energy source; supplies essential fatty acid; carries fat-soluble vitamins	Milk group: whole-milk products Meat group: meats, nuts, peanut butter Other sources: butter, margarine, oils, salad dressing, fried foods, and many processed foods
Vitamins and minerals	Perform various functions to help regulate body processes; necessary to obtain energy from foods	Fruits and vegetables: vitamins A, C, folic acid Bread group: B vitamins Milk group: calcium, phosphorus, riboflavin Meat group: B vitamins, iron, zinc
Water	Transports nutrients; helps regulate body temperature; aids in digestion	Water and other beverages Fruit and vegetable groups Milk group: milk

---

require in order to encompass the range of individual variations. . . . In other words, biochemical individuality has been taken into account.[15]

Many supplements are supposedly formulated to meet the "special" needs of athletes, executives, or others categorized by age or lifestyle factors. The intended target group is suggested by the product's name (for example, *Coach's Formula, Exec-30, Teenplex, Ger-E-Time*). A few products designed for men, women, or individuals over age 50 are rationally formulated. However, the idea that many segments of the American population have "special needs" that make supplementation *advisable* has no scientific foundation (see Chapter 12).

FOOD-GROUP SYSTEMS

The fundamental principles of healthful eating are *moderation, variety,* and *balance.* Healthful eating should also be psychologically satisfying and pleasing to the senses. A diet is balanced if it contains appropriate amounts of each nutrient. Food guides enable consumers to select foods from groups of nutritionally related foods rather than having to calculate the amount of each nutrient in each individual portion. Such guides, which specify the size and number of servings needed daily from each group to provide nutritional adequacy, have been published since 1916 by the USDA and various nongovernmental agencies.[16]

The Basic Four Food Groups system, devised in the mid-1950s, recommended a minimum number of servings from four food groups: two servings of milk and milk products; two of meat, poultry, eggs, dry beans, or nuts; four of fruits and vegetables; and four of grain products.[3] In 1979 the USDA issued a daily food guide that included a fifth group: fats, sweets, and alcoholic beverages. This group, also referred to as "extras," was said to be appropriate for consumption if one's basic needs were being met with the nutrient-rich foods from the other four groups.

In 1989 the USDA revised its daily food guide to incorporate the principles of the U.S. Dietary Guidelines and published its recommendations as "A Pattern for Daily Food Choices." This plan designates fruits and vegetables as separate groups and recommends more servings of fruits, vegetables, and grains. Diets based on this plan get the bulk of their calories from carbohydrates and are limited in fat. The same principles were then used to construct a "Food Guide Pyramid" that was published in final form in 1992 (see Figure 11-1).[17] The pyramid gives more space to grains, fruits, and vegetables than to meat and dairy groups. This differs from previous charts, which gave equal space to all of the food groups, even though fewer portions of meat and

HOW TO RATE YOUR DIET

To rate your diet, complete Steps 1 through 3 for a few days. Step 1 can be done from memory, but would be more accurate if done as you go along. Step 2 will indicate whether your diet is generally well balanced and nutritionally adequate. Step 3 will evaluate its fat content. To determine the number of grams of fat for each food you list, use the nutrition labels on packaged foods and Table 11-3 for the other foods.

Step 1

Jot down everything you ate yesterday for meals and snacks   *Grams of fat*

(blank lines)

Total [ ]

Step 2

Did you have the number of servings from the five food groups that are right for you? (See Figure 11-1 to determine the appropriate number of servings.)

	Circle the servings right for you	Servings you had
Bread group servings	6 7 8 9 10 11	[ ]
Vegetable group servings	3 4 5	[ ]
Fruit group servings	2 3 4	[ ]
Milk group servings	2 3	[ ]
Meat group (ounces)	5 6 7	[ ]

How did you do? Not enough? About right?

Step 3

Add up your grams of fat listed in Step 1. Did you have more fat than the amount right for you?

	Grams right for you	Grams you had
Fat	53 73 93	[ ]

How did you do? Not enough? About right?

Step 4

Decide what changes you can make for a healthier diet. Start by making small changes, like switching to low-fat or nonfat salad dressings or adding an extra serving of vegetables. Make additional changes gradually until healthy eating becomes a habit. Chapter 15 provides detailed advice on lowering the fat content of your diet.

Modified from USDA Human Nutrition Service: *The Food Guide Pyramid.*[17]

dairy products were recommended. The featured nutrients are:

BREADS, CEREALS, RICE, AND PASTA GROUP: Complex carbohydrates, vitamins, minerals, fiber
VEGETABLE GROUP: Vitamins A and C, folic acid, minerals, fiber
FRUIT GROUP: Vitamins A and C, potassium
MEAT, FISH, DRY BEANS, EGGS, AND NUTS GROUP: Protein, B vitamins, iron, zinc
MILK, YOGURT, AND CHEESE GROUP: Protein, vitamins, calcium, other minerals

Evaluating Your Diet

To estimate the adequacy of your diet, determine the approximate number of calories you consume per day and the recommended number of servings in each food group (see Figure 11-1) for your daily calorie level. Then use Worksheet 11-1 and Table 11-3 to estimate how many servings you have been consuming and how much fat your daily diet contains.

Proteins and carbohydrates contain four calories per gram, while fat contains nine calories per gram. To

Table 11-3

FAT CONTENT OF COMMON FOODS

	Servings	Grams of fat		Servings	Grams of fat
Bread, Cereal, Rice, and Pasta Group			***Vegetable Group***		
Bread, 1 slice	1	1	Vegetables, cooked, ¹/₂ cup	1	Trace
Hamburger roll, bagel, English muffin, 1	2	2	Vegetables, leafy, raw, 1 cup	1	Trace
Tortilla, 1	1	3	Vegetables, nonleafy, raw, chopped, ¹/₂ cup	1	Trace
Rice, pasta, cooked, ¹/₂ cup	1	Trace	Potatoes, scalloped, ¹/₂ cup	1	4
Plain crackers, small, 3–4	1	3	Potato salad, ¹/₂ cup	1	8
Breakfast cereal, 1 oz.	1	See label	French fries, 10	1	8
Pancakes, 4" diameter, 2	2	3			
Croissant, 1 large (2 oz.)	2	12	***Meat, Poultry, Fish, Dry Beans, Eggs, and Nuts Group***		
Doughnut, 1 medium (2 oz.)	2	11	Lean meat, poultry, fish, cooked	3 oz	6
Danish, 1 medium (2 oz.)	2	13	Ground beef, lean, cooked	3 oz*	16
Cake, frosted, ¹/₁₆ average	1	13	Chicken, with skin, fried	3 oz*	13
Cookies, 2 medium	1	4	Bologna, 2 slices	1 oz*	16
Pie, fruit, 2-crust, ¹/₆ 8" pie	2	19	Egg, 1	1 oz*	5
			Dry beans and peas, cooked, ¹/₂ cup	1 oz*	Trace
Fruit Group			Peanut butter, 2 tbsp.	1 oz*	16
Whole fruit: medium apple, orange, banana	1	Trace	Nuts, ¹/₃ cup	1 oz*	22
Fruit, raw or canned, ¹/₂ cup	1	Trace	*Ounces of lean meat to which these items are equivalent		
Fruit juice, unsweetened, ³/₄ cup	1	Trace			
Avocado, ¹/₄	1	9	***Milk, Yogurt, and Cheese Group***		
			Skim milk, 1 cup	1	Trace
Fats, Oils, and Sweets			Nonfat yogurt, plain, 8 oz.	1	Trace
Butter, margarine, 1 tsp.	1	4	Lowfat milk, 2 percent, 1 cup	1	5
Mayonnaise, 1 tbsp.	1	11	Whole milk, 1 cup	1	8
Salad dressing, 1 tbsp.	1	7	Chocolate milk, 2 percent, 1 cup	1	5
Sour cream, 2 tbsp.	1	6	Lowfat yogurt, plain, 8 oz.	1	4
Cream cheese, 1 oz.	1	10	Lowfat yogurt, fruit, 8 oz.	1	3
Sugar, jam, jelly, 1 tsp.	1	0	Natural Cheddar cheese, 1¹/₂ oz.	1	14
Cola, soft drink, 12 fl. oz.	1	0	Processed cheese, 2 oz.	1	18
Fruit drink, ade, 12 fl. oz.	1	0	Mozzarella, part skim, 1¹/₂ oz.	1	7
Chocolate bar, 1 oz.	1	9	Ricotta, part skim, ¹/₂ cup	1	10
Sherbet, ¹/₂ cup	1	2	Cottage cheese, 4% fat, 1 cup	¹/₃	5
Fruit sorbet, ¹/₂ cup	1	0	Ice cream, ¹/₂ cup	¹/₄	7
Gelatin dessert, ¹/₂ cup	1	0	Ice milk, ¹/₂ cup	¹/₃	3
			Frozen yogurt, ¹/₂ cup	¹/₂	2

Modified from USDA Human Nutrition Service: *The Food Guide Pyramid.*[16]

determine the percentages of calories of these macro-nutrients in a particular food, you can examine the label or apply the following formulas:

$$\% \text{ carbohydrate} = \frac{\text{grams of carbohydrate} \times 4}{\text{total calories per serving}}$$

$$\% \text{ protein} = \frac{\text{grams of protein} \times 4}{\text{total calories per serving}}$$

$$\% \text{ fat} = \frac{\text{grams of fat} \times 9}{\text{total calories per serving}}$$

Thus a serving of food that contains 120 calories and 4 grams of fat would have a fat content of 30%: [(4 x 9) ÷ 120] x 100. The calculation of overall dietary fat content is discussed in Chapter 15.

Various computer programs are available for dietary analysis. It should be noted, however, that they vary greatly in quality and ease of use and that measuring portion sizes and entering the data require considerable time and effort. The best programs are user-friendly and include a large database of brand-name foods.[18]

"JUNK FOOD"

Many people who use the term "junk food" allege that Americans are filling up on nutritionless foods. The term "junk food" is unpopular with nutrition scientists because all foods contain nutrients. Dr. Helen Guthrie, professor of nutrition at The Pennsylvania State University, has summarized the scientific perspective:

The term "junk food" is meaningless and should be discarded. In my opinion, there is no totally worthless food any more than there is a "perfect food" that meets all our nutritional needs. Obviously, some foods contribute greater amounts of nutrients than others do. But I cannot think of one food that doesn't have some redeeming value under the right circumstances. The problem arises when foods that contribute more calories than nutrients become so important in our diet that foods of higher nutritional value are excluded. It is equally possible to make an unbalanced selection of our most sacred nutritious foods and wind up with a diet overabundant in some nutrients yet deficient in others. In both cases, the result is a junk diet.[20]

Professionals use the terms "nutrient-dense" and "non–nutrient-dense" to describe how the nutritional value of foods compares to their caloric value. Broccoli, which is rich in vitamins and low in calories, is an example of a nutrient-dense food. Dr. William T. Jarvis has noted:

The term "junk food" is usually applied to foods that people eat for enjoyment. This conjures up remembrances of Puritanism in which anything pleasurable was regarded as a tool of the Devil. I believe that pleasurable foods can be valuable "mental health foods." There is nothing unhealthful as long as the basic principle of moderation is followed.

Fast Food

The term "fast food" applies to the speed with which a food is prepared and served rather than the nature or composition of the food. Sometimes these foods are accused of being "junk foods" or of having "empty calories." The American Council on Science and Health (ACSH) states:

Contrary to common belief, fast food has substantial nutritional value. Individuals who want to eat healthfully can incorporate fast food meals into a balanced diet by varying their fast food selections, choosing menu items that contribute to nutrient needs, and choosing meals of appropriate calorie content.[21]

ACSH acknowledges that many fast foods are high in sodium, fats, and calories, and recommends eating such foods in moderation. Individuals who eat at fast food outlets can satisfy food group and dietary guidelines by including salad selections and other low-fat items.

DIETARY GUIDELINES FOR INFANTS

In 1989 and 1994, the Gerber Products Company[22,23] published Dietary Guidelines for Infants, modeled after the 1990 DGAs. The Gerber guidelines were based on statements by the American Academy of Pediatrics' Committee on Nutrition and were prepared with the help of several nutrition experts. Their aim was to provide sufficient nourishment while fostering the development of healthful eating habits. Gerber officials have said they were prompted by a telephone survey showing that many parents were responding inappropriately to adult nutritional guidelines by giving their babies skim milk instead of whole milk. In addition, cases had been reported

---

◆ **Personal Glimpse** ◆

Did You Know?

Diet has always had a vital influence on health. Until as recently as the 1940s, diseases such as rickets, pellagra, scurvy, beriberi, xerophthalmia and goiter (caused by lack of adequate dietary vitamin D, niacin, vitamin C, thiamin, vitamin A, and iodine, respectively) were prevalent in this country and throughout the world. Today, thanks to an abundant food supply, fortification of some foods with critical trace nutrients, and better methods for determining and improving the nutrient content of foods, such "deficiency" diseases have been virtually eliminated in developing countries. . . .

As the diseases of nutritional deficiency have diminished, they have been replaced by diseases of dietary excess and imbalance—problems that now rank among the leading causes of death, touch the lives of most Americans, and generate substantial health care costs. . . .

In addition to five of these causes that scientific studies have associated with diet (coronary heart disease, some types of cancer, stroke, diabetes mellitus, and atherosclerosis), another three—cirrhosis of the liver, accidents, and suicides—have been associated with excessive alcohol intake. . . . Dietary excesses or imbalance also contribute to other problems such as high blood pressure, obesity, dental diseases, osteoporosis, and gastrointestinal diseases.

C. Everett Koop, M.D.[19]
Surgeon General
U.S. Public Health Service

of older children who failed to grow properly because of overzealous, medically unsupervised dietary treatment for high cholesterol levels.

In 1997 the American Academy of Pediatrics issued a position statement recommending breastfeeding for nearly all infants. The statement recommends that breastfeeding continue for at least 12 months and thereafter for as long as mutually desired. The following information is adapted from the Gerber guidelines with No. 1 modified to reflect the Academy's recommendations. The guidelines are applicable whether the child is breast-fed or bottle-fed.[24]

1. *Build to a variety of foods.* Children below the age of 2 are not "little adults." Unlike adults, they do not require variety to secure nutrition during the first 6 months or so of life. Except for fluoride and vitamin D (in the absence of sunlight), human milk alone provides the vitamins, minerals, carbohydrates, fats, and proteins needed for normal growth and development during early infancy. In the first 6 months, water, juice, and other foods are generally unnecessary for breastfed infants. Vitamin D and iron may need to be given before 6 months of age in selected groups of infants (vitamin D for infants whose mothers are vitamin D-deficient or those infants not exposed to adequate sunlight; iron for those who have low iron stores or anemia). Infants weaned before 12 months of age should receive iron-fortified infant formula rather than cow's milk.

Most babies are ready to start supplemental foods at approximately 6 months of age. Single-grain cereal is often the first one added. Other single-ingredient foods can be added gradually until the baby is eating a variety of foods. New foods should be added one at a time, at intervals of a few days. This allows the baby to get used to the flavor of the food and can reveal whether a food might not agree with the baby.

Fluoride should not be administered to infants during the first 6 months after birth, whether they are breastfed or formula-fed. During the period from 6 months to 3 years of age, infants require fluoride supplementation only if the water supply is severely deficient in fluoride (less than 0.3 ppm). This should be discussed with the child's doctor.

2. *Pay attention to your baby's appetite to avoid overfeeding or underfeeding.* Although healthy infants can vary considerably from one another in their caloric intake, appetite is likely to be the most efficient way to determine what an infant needs. Most infants instinctively know how much food they need and will not undereat or overeat unless pressured. Babies should be fed when hungry but should not be forced to finish the last few ounces of formula or food. The baby's

physician can check whether growth and development are progressing normally.

3. *Babies need fat.* Although low-fat and low-cholesterol diets are widely recommended for adults, they are not appropriate for children under the age of 2. Nutritional requirements are higher during infancy than during any other period. At the same time, stomach capacity is limited, so food sources must provide sufficient calories and nutrients in a small volume. Infants require fat in their diet for normal growth and development.

4. *Introduce fruits, vegetables, and grains, but don't overdo high-fiber foods.* Infants and young children who eat a highly varied diet will consume enough fiber for their needs. A diet high in fiber may be too low in calories and may interfere with absorption of iron, calcium, magnesium, and zinc.

5. *Babies need sugars in moderation.* Sugar, which exists in several forms, is a source of calories and makes some foods taste better. Breast milk, the ideal food for infants, contains 5% to 9% lactose, which is similar to table sugar but much less sweet. Other foods in a balanced diet may contain moderate amounts of sugar, but excessive amounts can crowd out more nutritious foods. Sugar has not been shown to cause hyperactivity, diabetes, obesity, or chronic diseases later in life. Sugar is linked to tooth decay, but good dental hygiene, proper bottle-feeding practices, and adequate fluoride intake will reduce the likelihood. Bottles of milk or juice or a pacifier dipped in honey should not be used to put a baby to sleep, because prolonged contact with their natural sugars can cause tooth decay. Artificially sweetened foods should be avoided because they lack the calories that growing babies need.

6. *Babies need sodium in moderation.* Salt also increases the palatability of some foods. Although the amount of sodium in the diet of a small percentage of adults is related to high blood pressure, the sodium content of an infant's diet has not been shown to cause high blood pressure in later life. Even though healthy infants can tolerate a range of sodium intakes without apparent ill effects, moderation in sodium intake is urged.

7. *Choose foods with iron, zinc, and calcium.* Infants are born with enough stored iron for 4 to 6 months. During this period, human milk or cow milk–based formulas usually supply sufficient amounts of zinc and calcium. After that, iron is more likely than any other nutrient to be lacking in the infant's diet. For this reason, special efforts should be made to provide infants with iron during the first 2 years. In addition to breast milk, the best sources are meats and poultry, iron-fortified formula, and iron-fortified infant cereal. Dietary

sources of zinc include oat cereals, meats and poultry, wheat germ, egg yolk, and cheddar cheese. Calcium is abundant in milk and other dairy products.

VEGETARIANISM

Vegetarians are individuals who restrict or eliminate foods of animal origin (meat, poultry, fish, eggs, milk) from their diet. The main reasons people choose a vegetarian alternative are: (a) they think it is healthier, (b) they think it is more "natural," (c) they think it is more "ecologic" because it takes less energy to produce vegetarian food than animal products, and (d) they are following religious or moral dictates. Dingott and Dwyer[25] have classified vegetarians into four categories:

VEGANS OR STRICT VEGETARIANS: Eat no animal products at all.

LACTOVEGETARIANS: Consume milk and other dairy products in addition to plant foods. This form of vegetarianism is common among Seventh-day Adventists.

LACTO-OVO-VEGETARIANS: Eat no meat, poultry, or fish, but do eat eggs and milk products.

SEMIVEGETARIANS: Eat no red meat, but do include small amounts of poultry or fish in their diet.

Data on the prevalence of vegetarianism in the United States are conflicting. A 1992 independent study commissioned by *Vegetarian Times* magazine found that about 5% of those surveyed described themselves as vegetarian, but most of them ate poultry and fish and occasionally ate red meat. A 1992–93 survey commissioned by the National Live Stock and Meat Board found that 95% of the responders in 2000 randomly selected households classified themselves as "red meat eaters," 5% classified themselves as "red meat avoiders," and about 2% classified themselves as "vegetarians." When their diets were analyzed, however, fewer than 1% consumed no red meat and a smaller percentage ate no meat, poultry, or fish during the 2-week reporting period.[26] USDA data indicate that per-capita consumption of red meat and of eggs has fallen during the past 25 years, while poultry and fish consumption have risen considerably. As a result, the combined total of meat and poultry has risen, and the combined total of meat, poultry and fish is at record levels.[27]

Possible Benefits of Vegetarianism

Dingott and Dwyer[25] state that vegetarianism based on sound nutrition principles can be a healthful lifestyle, but neither vegetarians nor omnivores have a monopoly on healthful eating. Similar health benefits can be gained from well-selected diets of either type. The following are possible advantages of a vegetarian diet.

- Vegetarians, especially those who abstain from all animal foods, tend to eat less fat and have a lower body weight for their height than nonvegetarians do.
- Vegetarians have less constipation than meat-eaters.
- Vegetarianism, as practiced by Seventh-day Adventists, has been associated with lower death rates from certain cancers (although abstention from tobacco and alcohol may be responsible for this).
- Vegetarianism may be associated with a lower incidence of atherosclerotic heart disease, high blood pressure, and diabetes. Lower body weight and/or nondietary factors may be contributory factors.

Possible Risks of Vegetarianism

It is possible to obtain all the nutrients required for proper growth and health while adhering to a vegetarian diet. To avoid deficiencies, however, careful attention must be paid to food selection. Dr. William T. Jarvis has encountered many tragedies in which cultlike adherence to a vegetarian ideology led people to starve themselves or their children to death or to substitute an ineffective "diet cure" for proven medical treatment.[28]

Foods of both animal and vegetable origin provide protein. However, proteins vary in nutritional quality because they differ in the kinds and amounts of amino acids they contain. Proteins from meat, fish, poultry, milk, and eggs rate the highest because they supply all of the essential amino acids in about the same proportions as those needed by the body. The proteins from some legumes (particularly soybeans and chickpeas) are close in nutritional quality to those from animal sources. Combining a small amount of animal protein with plant foods helps to improve the overall protein quality of the diet. High-quality protein can also be obtained by consuming plant foods that are complementary; in other words, the essential amino acids insufficient in one food are provided by another food with an adequate amount. Succotash is an example of a high-quality mixture of complementary foods (corn and lima beans).

Unless they choose a proper balance of foods, strict vegetarians are at risk for several deficiencies, especially vitamin B_{12}. They also risk deficiencies of riboflavin, calcium, iron, and the essential amino acids lysine and methionine. Vegetarian children not exposed to sunlight are at risk for vitamin D deficiency. Zinc deficiency can occur in vegans because the phytic acid in whole grains binds zinc, and there is little zinc in fruits and vegetables. Since B_{12} is present only in animal foods and a limited number of specially fortified foods, vegans should probably take B_{12} supplements prescribed by a physician.

Strict vegetarianism is not desirable for children under the age of 5 because it is difficult for vegans to meet children's high requirements for protein and some other nutrients. Growing adolescents may have difficulty getting adequate caloric and nutrient intake from a vegan diet. Vegetarianism is not a good idea for pregnant or lactating women. Excellent summaries of the special problems of vegetarian eating have been published by the American Academy of Pediatrics,[29] the National Institute of Nutrition (Canada),[30] and the American Dietetic Association.[31]

What Vegetarians Should Eat

Stare, Aronson, and Barrett[3] advise vegetarians to select a variety of items daily from each of the following groups:

PROTEIN GROUP: Dried beans and peas, lentils, nuts, and eggs.

GRAIN AND CEREAL GROUP: Whole grain and enriched breads, cereals, pasta, crackers, and other grain products.

FRUIT AND VEGETABLE GROUP: All fruits and vegetables, including a citrus fruit daily and a leafy green or bright yellow vegetable every other day.

MILK AND MILK PRODUCTS GROUP: Milk, yogurt, cheese, and other foods made with milk. This group is especially important for infants, children, and pregnant and nursing women because milk is the single best dietary source of calcium.

NUTRIENTS OF SPECIAL CONCERN

Certain nutrients should be of special concern to consumers. Iron (Chapter 19), fluoride (Chapter 7), folic acid (folate), and calcium are insufficient in the diets of some segments of the population. Sodium is consumed in excessive amounts by many persons.

Folic Acid

Several studies have shown that women who have adequate folic acid intake during the months before and after conception have about half the incidence of neural tube defects (NTDs) among their offspring.[32,33] These birth defects include spina bifida and other abnormalities caused by failure of the spinal column to close during the first month after conception, which leaves parts of the spinal cord exposed. The amount needed to reduce the risk is 0.4 mg (400 μ) per day, which is the adult RDA. The U.S. Centers for Disease Control and Prevention recommends that all women of childbearing age who are capable of becoming pregnant should consume 0.4 mg of folic acid per day.[34] Folic acid is found naturally in liver, green leafy vegetables, legumes, wheat germ, yeast, egg yolk, beets, whole wheat bread, fortified cereal, and citrus fruits and juices. Although well-balanced diets provide adequate amounts of folic acid, some women still fall below the recommended

amount. In 1993 the FDA approved health claims for supplement labels stating that women who consume adequate amounts of folate may reduce the risk of having a child with an NTD. In 1996 the agency published a final rule ordering folic acid fortification of most enriched grain products. Fortification is also expected to reduce the incidence of heart disease by lowering abnormal blood levels of homocysteine (see Chapter 15).

Calcium

Calcium, along with fluoride and vitamin D, is essential for the proper formation and maintenance of bones and teeth. Osteoporosis (thinning of the bones) is a common disease in the aged, especially in women (see Chapter 21). Although hormonal problems may be more important than diet in the development of osteoporosis, the significance of maintaining adequate dietary calcium, fluoride, and vitamin D should not be overlooked.[10] A 1994 National Institutes of Health Consensus Statement warned that a large percentage of Americans were failing to meet recommended guidelines for optimal calcium intake.[35]

Milk is the most common source of calcium, but cheese, yogurt, and other foods made with milk also provide significant amounts. Sardines and canned salmon, if eaten with the bones, are rich in calcium. Dark green leafy vegetables such as spinach and broccoli contain some calcium in absorbable form. It is difficult to ingest adequate amounts of absorbable calcium if dairy products are eliminated from the diet. Women should discuss with their physicians how to ensure adequate intake of calcium through intake of dairy products and/or supplementation. This is especially important for lactose-intolerant individuals who restrict their intake of milk to avoid the unpleasant symptoms of irregular lactose digestion.

Sodium

The relationship of sodium intake to high blood pressure (hypertension) is of concern because hypertension is an important risk factor in coronary heart disease and stroke. However, sodium intake has not been proven to cause hypertension to develop.[36] Current data suggest that approximately 80% of Americans are not genetically predisposed to hypertension. One third of the remaining 20% appear to be sensitive to sodium; they may be exposed to a higher risk if they consume excess amounts of sodium. Treatment of people with medically diagnosed hypertension will include sodium restriction for those who are salt-sensitive. This subject is discussed in Chapter 15.

The average American consumes approximately 10 to 12 g (2 to 2½ teaspoons) of salt per day, of which 3 g occur naturally in foods, 4 to 6 g come from salt or salt-containing ingredients added during food processing, and 3 to 4 g is discretionary intake (from the salt shaker). Since salt is about 40% sodium, this amounts to 4 to 5 g of sodium daily. Food labels (see below) list a Daily Value of 2.4 g per day for sodium, the amount contained in 6 g of salt. The National Research Council and various government agencies have concluded that reducing salt intake to 3 g per day (which would require eliminating the use of salt in cooking and at the table) would not be harmful. Most people, however, are not willing to do this. Habits, cultural preferences, and culinary customs are difficult to change.

Significant amounts of sodium are contained in cured and processed meats, salted snacks, pickled and canned foods, and many frozen convenience foods. Even the small amounts of baking powder, flavor enhancers, and other additives in some foods contain sodium. Many manufacturers have reacted to recent health advice by producing more low-salt and no-salt products. Consumers who wish to limit their salt intake should check food labels. Sodium is also present in antacids, laxatives, and other drugstore items. When a household water-softening system replaces calcium ("hardness") with sodium, having a kitchen faucet for untreated water is another prudent strategy for sodium reduction.

NUTRITION LABELING

The USDA regulates the labeling of meat and poultry products. The FDA regulates the labeling of nearly all other foods. Modern nutrition labeling began in 1974 when these agencies established voluntary rules requiring nutrition information on the labels of products that contained added nutrients or that carried nutrition claims. In 1993 new rules were published to provide for consistent, scientifically based labeling for nearly all processed foods.[37-39]

The new rules, which took effect in 1994, provided a basic format for the nutrition panel, which must be titled "Nutrition Facts." This panel must not only list the significant nutrients in the product, but also must indicate how the amounts of certain ingredients are related to recommended levels. These relationships are expressed as "% Daily Values." The product label must also disclose the amount per serving of saturated fat, cholesterol, dietary fiber, and other nutrients important to consumers. Other provisions include customary serving sizes and definitions for descriptive terms such as "light," "low fat," and "high fiber."

Daily Values (DVs) are derived from two sets of reference values: Reference Daily Intakes (RDIs) and Daily Reference Values (DRVs), neither of which appear on the labels themselves. The RDIs cover 12 vitamins and 7 minerals. The DRVs, which are used for fat, carbohydrates, protein, fiber, sodium, and potassium, are based on a diet containing 60% carbohydrate, 10% protein, 30% fat (including 10% saturated fat), and 11.5 g of fiber per 1000 calories. Daily Values for cholesterol, sodium, and potassium are the same regardless of calorie level.

For labeling purposes, Percent Daily Values are based on a diet of 2000 calories. This approximates the maintenance level for postmenopausal women, the group most often targeted for weight reduction. Where space permits, the label must include DVs for both

---

Table 11-4

DAILY VALUES (DVs) FOR FOOD LABELS[14,37]

Nutrient	Daily Value	Nutrient	Daily Value	Nutrient	Daily Value
Total fat*	< 65 g	Iron	18 mg	Pantothenic acid	10 mg
Saturated fat*	< 20 g	Vitamin D	400 IU	Phosphorus	1000 mg
Cholesterol*	< 300 mg	Vitamin E	30 IU	Iodine	150 µg
Sodium*	2400 mg	Vitamin K	80 µg	Magnesium	400 mg
Potassium*	3500 mg	Thiamin	1.5 mg	Zinc	15 mg
Total carbohydrate*	300 g	Riboflavin	1.7 mg	Selenium	70 µg
Fiber*	25 g	Niacin	20 mg	Copper	2 mg
Protein*	50 g	Vitamin B_6	2 mg	Manganese	2 mg
Vitamin A	5000 IU	Folate	400 µg	Chromium	120 µg
Vitamin C	60 mg	Vitamin B_{12}	6 µg	Molybdenum	75 µg
Calcium	1000 mg	Biotin	300 µg	Chloride	3400 mg

*Based on 2000 calories a day for adults and children over age 4.

2000- and 2500-calorie diets, and manufacturers are permitted to indicate DVs for other calorie levels. Table 11-4 lists the DVs for adults and children over the age of 4. Figure 11-2 illustrates the "Nutrition Facts" panel required on most food labels. Table 11-5 defines the conditions under which terms such as "light" or "low-fat" are legally permitted.

The FDA intends to propose RDIs for infants, children under age 4, and pregnant women.

The FDA estimates that about 90% of processed food should carry nutrition information. In addition, uniform point-of-purchase nutrition information should accompany many fresh foods, such as fruits, vegetables, raw fish, meat, and poultry. Although this is voluntary, it will be mandated if fewer than 60% of retailers fail to comply voluntarily. Similar labeling rules may be proposed for restaurant, delicatessen, and institutional foods.

Approved Health Claims

A "health claim" is defined as any type of communication in labeling that is intended to suggest "a direct beneficial relationship between the presence or level of any substance in the food and a health or disease-related condition." Health claims will be permitted only if (a) a food substance is associated with a disease or health-related condition for which the general U.S. population or an identified subgroup is at risk, (b) the claim is made in the context of the product's relationship to overall diet, (c) the claim is supported by publicly available scientific evidence (including well-designed and properly conducted experiments), and (d) there is significant agreement among qualified experts that the claims are supported by such evidence. In addition, the claims must be "complete, truthful, and not misleading." The FDA does not permit health claims to be based on "preliminary evidence." And any claim that a single

FIGURE 11-2.
Sample food label.

Serving sizes, stated in both household and metric measures, reflect the amounts that people actually eat.

The nutrients required on the nutrition panel are those considered most important to the health of today's consumers, most of whom need to worry about getting too much of certain items (such as fat) rather than too few (as was the case years ago with certain vitamins and minerals).

Fats, carbohydrates, and proteins are the nutrients that provide energy (calories).

Calories from fat are shown to help consumers meet dietary guidelines, which recommend that people get no more than 30% of their calories from fat.

% Daily Value shows how a food fits into the overall daily diet. Some daily values are maximums, as with fat, while others are minimums, as with carbohydrates.

The Daily Values are based on daily diets of 2000 and 2500 calories. Individuals should adjust these values to fit their own calorie intake. (Moderately active people consume about 15 calories per day for each pound of body weight.)

Nutrition Facts

Serving Size 1/2 cup (114g)
Servings Per Container 4

Amount Per Serving

Calories 260   Calories from Fat 120

	% Daily Value*
Total Fat 13g	**20**%
Saturated Fat 5g	**25**%
Cholesterol 30mg	**10**%
Sodium 660mg	**28**%
Total Carbohydrate 31g	**11**%
Dietary Fiber 0g	**0**%
Sugars 5g	
Protein 5g	

Vitamin A 4%	•	Vitamin C 2%
Calcium 15%	•	Iron 4%

* Percent Daily Values are based on a 2,000 calorie diet. Your daily values may be higher or lower depending on your calorie needs:

		Calories:	2,000	2,500
Total Fat	Less than		65g	80g
Sat Fat	Less than		20g	25g
Cholesterol	Less than		300mg	300mg
Sodium	Less than		2,400mg	2,400mg
Total Carbohydrate			300g	375g
Dietary Fiber			25g	30g

Calories per gram:
Fat 9 • Carbohydrate 4 • Protein 4

Table 11-5

LEGAL DEFINITIONS OF DESCRIPTIVE TERMS FOR FOOD LABELS

FREE OR WITHOUT: An amount that is nutritionally trivial and unlikely to have a physiologic consequence.

CALORIE FREE: Fewer than 5 calories per serving.

SUGAR FREE: Less than 0.5 g per serving of monosaccharides and/or disaccharides.

SODIUM FREE OR SALT FREE: Less than 5 mg per serving. A claim made for a food normally free of or low in a nutrient must indicate that the situation exists for all similar foods. For example: "spinach: a low-sodium food." Labels of foods containing insignificant amounts of ingredients (such as baking soda or sodium ascorbate) commonly understood to contain sodium must use an asterisk to refer to a note below the ingredient list that the amount of added sodium is trivial.

LOW OR LITTLE: Low enough to allow frequent consumption without exceeding the dietary guidelines. Generally less than 2% of the Daily Value for the nutrient. A claim of "very low" can be made only about sodium.

LOW CALORIE: Less than 40 mg per serving and per 100 g of food. May be used for meal-type products with 120 calories per 100 g of food.

LIGHT (OR LITE): Contains one-third fewer calories than the referenced food. Products deriving more than half their calories from fat must have their fat content reduced by 50% or more with a minimum reduction of more than 3 g per serving. The percentage of reduction of calories and/or fat must be specified immediately proximal to the claim. May not be used for foods or nutrients meeting the requirements for a "low" claim. The term "light" can be used for a salt substitute if it contains at least 50% less sodium than ordinary table salt. Other use of "light" must specify whether it refers to look, taste or odor, unless the meaning of the term is obvious and fundamental to the product's identity. (Thus, light brown sugar would require no explanation).

LESS (OR FEWER), LOWER, OR REDUCED: Contains at least 25% less of a nutrient (or calories) than the referenced food. May not be used for foods or nutrients meeting the requirements for a "low" claim.

MORE: Contains at least 10% more of a desirable nutrient than does a comparable food. The terms "fortified," "enriched," or "added" may be used instead under appropriate circumstances.

HIGH, RICH IN, OR EXCELLENT SOURCE: Contains 20% or more of the RDA or DRV.

GOOD SOURCE: Contains 10% to 19% of the RDA or DRV. Can also be described as "contains" or "provides."

FAT FREE: Less than 0.5 g of fat per reference amount and serving size, and no added ingredient that is a fat or oil. The term "fat free" may not be used for a food that is inherently free of fat unless there is an accompanying statement that all foods of this type are inherently fat free. Labels of foods containing insignificant amounts of ingredients (such as nuts) commonly understood to contain fats are permitted to use an asterisk to refer to a note below the ingredient list that the amount of added fat is trivial.

LOW FAT: Contains 3 g or less of fat per reference amount, per serving size and per 100 g of product. May not be used for foods inherently low in fat unless accompanied by a disclaimer that all foods of this type are inherently low in fat. May be applied to meal-type products if the meals also derive 30% or fewer of their calories from fat.

(PERCENT) FAT FREE: Only for foods that meet the FDA definition of low fat.

REDUCED OR LESS FAT: Reduced fat content by 25% or more, with at least 3 g less per reference amount and per serving size.

SATURATED FAT FREE: May be used for all products that are fat free. Labels of products that are not fat free but contain less than 0.5 g of saturated fat per reference amount must disclose the amount of total fat.

LOW IN SATURATED FAT: 1 g or less per serving, with not more than 15% of calories from saturated fat and 1% or less of total fat as trans-fatty acids. Labels of foods containing insignificant amounts of ingredients commonly understood to contain saturated fats must state that the amount of saturated fat is trivial. Meal-type products must also derive less than 10% of their calories from saturated fat.

REDUCED OR LESS SATURATED FAT: At least 25% less saturated fat per serving than the reference food. When these terms are used the label must indicate the % reduction and the amount of saturated fat in the reference food. The reduction must be at least 1 g.

CHOLESTEROL FREE: Less than 2 mg of cholesterol and 2 g or less of saturated fat per serving. Labels of foods containing insignificant amounts of ingredients commonly understood to contain cholesterol must state that the amount of cholesterol is trivial.

LOW IN CHOLESTEROL: 20 mg or less per serving and per 100 g of food, and 2 g or less of saturated fat per serving.

REDUCED OR LESS CHOLESTEROL: At least 25% less cholesterol per serving than its comparison food. The label of a food containing more than 13 g of total fat per serving or per 100 g of the food must disclose that fact.

LOW SODIUM: Less than 140 mg per serving and per 100 g of food (a little less than half a cup).

VERY LOW SODIUM: Less than 35 mg per serving and per 100 g of food.

LIGHT IN SODIUM: Contains at least 50% less sodium than an appropriate comparison food.

FRESH: Can only be linked to raw food, food that has not been frozen, heated, processed, or preserved. (Low-level irradiation is permissible.)

FRESHLY: Can be used with a verb such as "prepared," "baked," or "roasted" if the food is recently made and has not been heat-processed or preserved. "Freshly frozen" may be used for foods that are quickly frozen while fresh.

LEAN: Meat or poultry product with less than 10 g of fat, less than 4 g of saturated fat, and less than 95 mg cholesterol per 100 g.

EXTRA LEAN: Meat or poultry product with less than 5 g of fat, less than 2 g of saturated fat, and less than 95 mg cholesterol per 100 g.

food (as opposed to overall dietary composition) or food component (such as a vitamin, mineral, or other entity portrayed as a dietary supplement) can prevent, cure, mitigate, or treat a disease or symptom would render the product subject to regulation as a drug and would not be appropriate for labeling of a food.

Table 11-6 lists the types of permissible food-related health claims. For each, the FDA has documented the supporting evidence and issued model claims. Government officials believe that use of such statements will provide food companies with an incentive to improve the nutritional quality of many types of products.

Table 11-6

EXAMPLES OF MODEL HEALTH CLAIMS PERMISSIBLE IN FOOD LABELING

FRUITS AND VEGETABLES AND CANCER

- Low-fat diets rich in fruits and vegetables (foods that are low in fat and may contain dietary fiber, vitamin A, and vitamin C) may reduce the risk of some types of cancer, a disease associated with many factors. Broccoli is high in vitamins A and C and is a good source of dietary fiber.

FIBER-CONTAINING GRAIN PRODUCTS, FRUITS, AND VEGETABLES AND CANCER

- Low-fat diets rich in fiber-containing grain products, fruits, and vegetables may reduce the risk of some types of cancer, a disease associated with many factors.

DIETARY FAT AND CANCER

- Eating a healthful diet low in fat may help reduce the risk of some types of cancers. Development of cancer is associated with many factors, including a family history of the disease, cigarette smoking and what you eat.

DIETARY SATURATED FAT AND CHOLESTEROL AND RISK OF CORONARY HEART DISEASE

- While many factors affect heart disease, diets low in saturated fat and cholesterol may reduce the risk of this disease.

FRUITS, VEGETABLES, AND GRAIN PRODUCTS THAT CONTAIN FIBER, PARTICULARLY SOLUBLE FIBER, AND RISK OF CORONARY HEART DISEASE

- Development of heart disease depends on many factors. Eating a diet low in saturated fat and cholesterol and high in fruits, vegetables, and grain products that contain fiber may lower blood cholesterol levels and reduce your risk of heart disease.

SOY PROTEIN AND HEART DISEASE

- Diets low in saturated fat and cholesterol that include 25 grams of soy protein a day may reduce the risk of heart disease. One serving of (name of food) provides _____ grams of soy protein.[40]

SOLUBLE FIBER FROM CERTAIN FOODS AND RISK OF CORONARY HEART DISEASE

- Soluble fiber from foods such as [name of soluble fiber source, and, if desired, name of food product], as part of a diet low in saturated fat and cholesterol, may reduce the risk of heart disease. A serving of [name of food product] supplies __ grams of the [necessary daily dietary intake for the benefit] soluble fiber from [name of soluble fiber source] necessary per day to have this effect.

PLANT STEROL AND PLANT STANOL ESTERS AND CORONARY HEART DISEASE

- Diets low in saturated fat and cholesterol that include two servings of foods that provide a daily total of at least 3.4 grams of plant stanol esters in two meals may reduce the risk of heart disease. A serving of [name of the food] supplies ____ grams of plant stanol esters.[41]

SODIUM AND HYPERTENSION

- Development of hypertension or high blood pressure depends on many factors. [This product] can be part of a low-sodium, low-salt diet that might reduce the risk of hypertension or high blood pressure.

CALCIUM AND OSTEOPOROSIS

- Regular exercise and a healthy diet with enough calcium help teen and young adult white and Asian women maintain good bone health and may reduce their risk of osteoporosis later in life.

FOLATE AND NEURAL TUBE DEFECTS

- Healthful diets with adequate folate may reduce a woman's risk of having a child with a brain or spinal cord defect.

DIETARY SUGAR ALCOHOL AND DENTAL CARIES

- Full claim: Frequent between-meal consumption of foods high in sugars and starches promotes tooth decay. The sugar alcohols in [name of food] do not promote tooth decay. Shortened claim (on small packages only): Does not promote tooth decay.

Manufacturers who want to use wording that differs from the FDA's model claims can petition for FDA approval. Although preapproval is not required, claims that are not preapproved can trigger regulatory action if the FDA considers them misleading.

RELIABLE INFORMATION SOURCES

The dissemination of nutrition advice is poorly regulated by law. For this reason, consumers seeking nutrition advice should be very careful in selecting their advisers. Reliable information can be obtained from nutrition or medical professionals, professional organizations, and publications identified in the remainder of this chapter and in the Appendix. Unreliable sources are identified in Chapter 12.

Your personal physician is probably the most convenient person from whom to obtain advice on nutrition. Medical doctors are often criticized for not knowing enough about nutrition. The American Council on Science and Health disagrees:

Not all physicians are nutrition experts, just as not all are specialists in cardiology or community medicine. However, the practicing physician has sufficient knowledge of the biochemical and physiological principles of nutrition, and has access to many resources which can aid in answering patients' questions. Most people who read about a "new nutritional discovery" don't have enough knowledge to figure out whether it's a real scientific development or a piece of quack nonsense. Physicians do have the expertise to make this kind of judgment and to evaluate the technical research on which popular reports are based. If you have a question that your doctor can't answer, he or she can refer you to someone who can.[42]

✓ Consumer Tip

Many organizations evaluate and publish accurate information about nutrition. Some communicate primarily with health and nutrition professionals, while others primarily serve the public. The following organizations are generally reliable:

> American Council on Science and Health
> American Dietetic Association
> American Institute of Nutrition
> American Medical Association
> American Society for Clinical Nutrition
> Council on Agricultural Science and Technology
> International Food Information Council
> Institute of Food Technologists
> International Life Sciences Institute/Nutrition
>   Foundation
> National Center for Nutrition and Dietetics
> National Council Against Health Fraud, Inc.
> Quackwatch
> USDA Food and Nutrition Information Center
> U.S. Food and Drug Administration

Nutrition Professionals

Many accredited colleges and universities offer nutrition courses based on scientific principles and taught by qualified instructors. A bachelor's degree requires 4 years of full-time study that qualify a graduate for entry-level positions in dietetics or foodservice, often in a hospital. A master's degree in nutrition requires 2 more years of full-time study beyond the undergraduate level. People who wish to become nutrition researchers usually pursue a Ph.D. in biochemistry. This requires at least 2 more years of study plus a dissertation based on original laboratory research. Those wishing to concentrate on teaching or educational research usually seek a degree of Ph.D. or Ed.D. in nutrition education. With few exceptions, a nutrition-related degree from an accredited university signifies a broad background in nutrition science and a thorough grasp of nutritional concepts.

In addition to an academic degree, most legitimate nutritionists seek professional certification. There are two professional associations restricted to qualified nutrition scientists. Active membership in the American Institute of Nutrition (AIN) is open to respected scientists who have published meritorious original research on some aspect of nutrition, who are presently working in the field, and who are sponsored by two AIN members. Nominees are considered by a membership committee, a council of officers, and the membership. The clinical arm of AIN is the American Society for Clinical Nutrition (ASCN), whose requirements are similar but include clinical research. All ASCN members are also members of AIN, and about 70% of them are physicians. These requirements, plus an enforceable code of professional responsibility, make it highly unlikely that a promoter of quackery will become (or remain) a member of either of these organizations.

Nutritionists at the doctoral level may also seek certification by the American Board of Nutrition as specialists in clinical nutrition (M.D.s only) or human nutrition sciences (M.D.s and Ph.D.s). To obtain this credential, they must pass both written and oral examinations on a wide range of topics. Currently there are about 300 board-certified nutrition specialists in the United States. Most are affiliated with medical schools and hospitals, where they conduct clinical research and offer consultation to primary-care physicians.

Registered dietitians (R.D.s) are specially trained to translate nutrition research into appropriate diets. Compared to physicians, they usually know less about basic biochemistry, physiology, and metabolism, but more about the nutrient content of specific foods. The R.D. certification is usually sought by bachelor- and

---

It's Your Decision

1. You plan to obtain a quick dinner at a fast food outlet. How can you ensure a nutritious food intake?

2. You have heard that many Americans are not eating properly. How can you check whether your diet contains adequate amounts of all the nutrients you need? Should you take a vitamin/mineral supplement just to be on the safe side? If you are not sure what to do, how can you locate a professional person to help you?

---

master-level nutrition graduates. To qualify, they must have appropriate professional experience and pass a written test concerning all aspects of nutrition and foodservice management. To maintain their credential, they must also participate regularly in continuing-education programs approved by the American Dietetic Association (ADA).

Most of the country's 60,000 active R.D.s work in hospitals. Typically they counsel patients and conduct classes for pregnant women, heart and kidney patients, diabetics, and other persons with special dietary needs. Dietitians are also employed by community agencies such as geriatric, day care, and drug/alcohol abuse centers. Some dietitians do research. Others engage in private practice where they counsel physician-referred patients. The ADA also has a certification process for advanced-level practitioners and for specialists in renal (kidney), pediatric, and metabolic nutrition.

About 40 states have enacted laws to license or certify dietitians and/or nutritionists. Some of these laws restrict the use of titles, whereas others restrict who is permitted to do nutritional assessment and counseling. Although holding such a credential is a good sign, in some states the standards are not high enough to prevent unqualified individuals from becoming licensed.

Other Sources

The National Institute for Dental Research, the National Institute of Allergy and Infectious Diseases, the National Cancer Institute, and the National Institute of Arthritis, Metabolism and Digestive and Kidney Diseases all have educational material about nutrition as it applies to their areas of interest.

State and local dietetic associations are usually eager to be helpful. Dial-A-Dietitian services to answer telephone inquiries are available in a number of cities. Other local sources include accredited colleges and medical schools, USDA Extension Services of land-

grant universities, home economists at USDA county cooperative services (for information on food preparation), state health departments, some local health departments, and state or county medical societies. Available local sources are listed in the Yellow or blue pages of the telephone directory.

The National Center for Nutrition and Dietetics, cosponsored by the American Dietetic Association, operates a consumer hotline that permits callers to speak with a registered dietitian, listen to recorded nutrition messages, or leave their name and address for a free brochure. The American Dental Association and several other organizations listed in the Appendix provide information about nutrition as it applies to their areas of special interest.

Table 2-3 lists newsletters and magazines that provide reliable nutrition information. Some cover nutrition only, while others cover health topics with occasional articles on nutrition.

SUMMARY

The basic principles of nutrition are moderation, variety, and balance. These can be achieved by daily selection of appropriate numbers of moderate-sized portions from each of the food groups. The Food Guide Pyramid enables consumers to select foods from groups rather than having to calculate the amount of each nutrient in each individual portion of food. The Dietary Guidelines for Americans provide additional advice about moderating dietary fat (to help prevent heart disease) and consuming adequate amounts of fiber. Vitamin deficiencies are rare in the United States, but many women do not consume enough iron or calcium in their diet. Vegetarian diets can be a healthful alternative to those that include meat, but must be constructed carefully to avoid nutrient deficiencies. Many qualified professionals can provide consumers with reliable information and advice about diet and nutrition. Nutrition labeling enables consumers to ascertain the nutrient contents of most foods.

REFERENCES

1. Derelian D. Foreword to the American Dietetic Association 1995 nutrition trends survey. Chicago, 1995, The Association.
2. Herbert V, Kasdan TS. What is a healthy food plan? In Herbert V, Subak-Sharpe GJ, editors. Total Nutrition: The Only Guide You'll Ever Need. New York, 1995, St. Martin's Press.
3. Stare F, Aronson V, Barrett S. Your Guide to Good Nutrition. Amherst, N.Y., 1991, Prometheus Books.
4. Fiber: Strands of protection. Consumer Reports on Health 11(8):1–5, 1999.

<u>5</u>. Kava R. Dietary fiber. New York, 1997, American Council on Science and Health.

<u>6</u>. Food and Drug Administration. Food labeling: Proposed rules. Federal Register 56:60366–60878, 1991.

7. Pilch SM and others. Physiological Effects and Health Consequences of Dietary Fiber. Washington, D.C., 1987, Federation of American Societies for Experimental Biology.

8. AMA Council on Scientific Affairs. Dietary fiber and health. JAMA 262:542–546, 1989.

<u>9</u>. Appendix I: History of the Dietary Guidelines for Americans. In Garza C and others. Report of the Dietary Guidelines Advisory Committee on the Dietary Guidelines for Americans. Washington, D.C., Feb 2, 2000.

<u>10</u>. Food and Nutrition Board. Dietary Reference Intakes for Calcium, Phosphorus, Magnesium, Vitamin D, and Fluoride. Washington, D.C., 1997, National Academy Press.

<u>11</u>. Food and Nutrition Board. Dietary Reference Intakes for Thiamin, Riboflavin, Niacin, Vitamin B6, Folate, Vitamin B12, Pantothenic Acid, Biotin, and Choline. Washington, D.C., 1998, National Academy Press.

12. Food and Nutrition Board. Dietary Reference Intakes for Vitamin C, Vitamin E, Selenium and Carotenoids. Washington, D.C., 2000, National Academy Press.

<u>13</u>. Nutrition and Your Health: Dietary Guidelines for Americans, 2000. Washington, D.C., 2000, US Departments of Agriculture and Health and Human Services.

14. Sims LS. Uses of the Recommended Dietary Allowances: A commentary. Journal of the American Dietetic Association 96:659–662, 1996.

15. Herbert V, Barrett S. The Vitamin Pushers: How the "Health Food" Industry Is Selling America a Bill of Goods. Amherst, N.Y., 1994, Prometheus Books.

16. Welsh S and others. A brief history of food guides in the United States. Nutrition Today 27(6):6–11, 1992.

<u>17</u>. USDA Human Nutrition Service. The Food Guide Pyramid, ed 5. House and Garden Bulletin No. 252. Washington, D.C., 2000, US Departments of Agriculture and Health and Human Services.

18. Lee RD and others. Comparison of eight microcomputer dietary analysis programs with the USDA nutrient data base for standard reference. Journal of the American Dietetic Association 95:858–867, 1995.

19. Guthrie HA. There's no such thing as "junk food," but there are junk diets. Healthline 5(10):11–12, 1986.

20. Koop CE. The Surgeon General's Report on Nutrition and Health. DHHS (PHS) Publication No. 88–50210. Washington, D.C., 1988, Superintendent of Documents.

21. American Council on Science and Health. Fast food and the American diet. New York, 1985, The Council.

22. Fineberg L and others. Dietary guidelines for infants (professional version). Fremont, Mich., 1989, Gerber Products Company.

23. Coletta FA and others. Dietary guidelines for infants. Pediatric Basics No. 69, Fremont, Mich., Summer 1994, Gerber Products Company.

<u>24</u>. AAP Work Group on Breastfeeding. Breastfeeding and the use of human milk. Pediatrics 100:1035–1039, 1997.

<u>25</u>. Dingott S, Dwyer J. Benefits and risks of vegetarian diets. Nutrition Forum 8:45–47, 1991.

26. Eating in America Today: A Dietary Pattern and Intake Report/ Edition II. Chicago, 1995, National Live Stock and Meat Board.

27. Putnam JJ, Duewer LA. U.S. per capita food consumption: Record high meat and sugars in 1994. Food Review 18(2):2–11, 1995.

<u>28</u>. Jarvis WT. Why I am not a vegetarian. Priorities 9(2):32–43, 1997.

29. American Academy of Pediatrics. Nutritional aspects of vegetarianism, health fads, and health diets. Pediatrics 59:460–464, 1977.

30. Risks and benefits of vegetarian diets. Nutrition Today 25(2):27–29, 1990.

31. Havala S, Dwyer J. Position of the American Dietetic Association: Vegetarian diets. Journal of the American Dietetic Association 93:351–355, 1993.

32. Czeizel AE, Dudas I. Prevention of the first occurrence of neural-tube defects by periconceptual vitamin supplementation. New England Journal of Medicine 327:1832–1835, 1992.

33. Werler MM and others. Periconceptual folic acid exposure and risk of occurrent neural tube defects. JAMA 269:1257–1261, 1993.

34. Centers for Disease Control and Prevention. Recommendations for the use of folic acid to reduce the number of cases of spina bifida and other neural tube defects. Morbidity and Mortality Report 41:1–7, 1992.

35. Optimal calcium intake. NIH Consensus Statement 12(4):1–31, 1994.

36. Midgley JP and others. Effect of reduced dietary sodium on blood pressure: A meta-analysis of randomized controlled trials. JAMA 275:1590–1597, 1996.

37. Food and Drug Administration. Food labeling. Federal Register 58(3):631–691, 2065–2964, 1993. Summarized in The new food label (FDA Backgrounder BG–94–2, April 1994).

38. Barrett S. New food regulations issued. Nutrition Forum 10:25–30, 1993.

<u>39</u>. A Food Labeling Guide. FDA Center for Food Safety and Nutrition, revised June 1999.

<u>40</u>. Food and Drug Administration. Food labeling: Health claims; Soy protein and coronary heart disease. Federal Register 64:57699–57733, 1999.

<u>41</u>. Food and Drug Administration. Food labeling: Health claims; Plant sterol/stanol esters and coronary heart disease; Interim final rule. Federal Register 65:54685–54739, 2000.

42. Meister KA. How much does your doctor know about nutrition? ACSH News & Views 1(6):4–5, 1980.

Chapter Twelve

NUTRITION FADS, FALLACIES, AND SCAMS

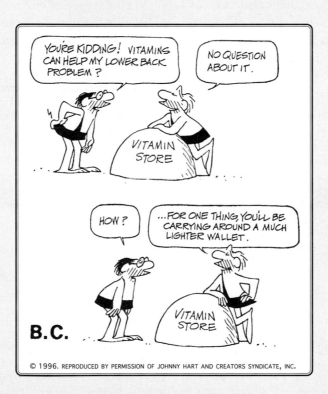

© 1996. REPRODUCED BY PERMISSION OF JOHNNY HART AND CREATORS SYNDICATE, INC.

Nutrition seems to be like politics: everyone is an expert.
HAROLD J. MOROWITZ, PH.D.[1]

The very term "health food" is a deceptive slogan. All food is health food in moderation; any food is junk food in excess. Did you ever stop to think that your corner grocery, fruit market, meat market, and supermarket are also health-food stores? They are—and they generally charge less than stores that use the slogan.
VICTOR HERBERT, M.D., J.D.[2]

Erroneous nutrition concepts lead Americans to waste billions of dollars annually and sometimes to jeopardize their health. Most Americans probably are harmed to some degree by nutrition fads and fallacies. At the core of this problem are individuals and groups whose collective efforts can be referred to as the health-food industry. However, pharmaceutical manufacturers and large food companies also foster and exploit public confusion about nutrition. This chapter illustrates how misinformation is used to promote vitamin and mineral supplements, "health foods," "organic" foods, "natural" foods, herbs, related products, and dietary fads. This chapter also discusses the activities and backgrounds of some of the leading promoters of nutrition misinformation. Facts and fads related to weight control are covered in the next chapter.

FOOD FADDISM AND QUACKERY

Sociologist Robert Schafer and food scientist Elizabeth A. Yetley[3] have defined food faddism as an unusual, enthusiastically adopted pattern of food behavior. These authors report that faddism is expressed by (a) beliefs that specific foods have special curative properties, (b) elimination of certain foods from the diet in the belief that harmful elements are present, or (c) emphasis on "natural" foods. They also state that food faddists use foods not as ends in themselves but as a means of achieving a stable and predictable life pattern. Olson[4] has noted that food faddism persists because food has an emotional rather than an intellectual value to the average person. Beal[5] has classified eight types of food faddists, as shown in Table 12-1.

Table 12-1

EMOTIONAL NEEDS OF FOOD FADDISTS

Type of Faddist	Need Served by Fad
Miracle-seeker	Patterning need to establish stability regarding health, energy, and so on. Accomplished by diets intended to forestall aging or restore organism to health. Ego defense need to re-establish positive self-concept and feeling of self-worth.
Anti-establishmentarian	Self-realization need to express self in a manner consistent with self-concept and value system.
Super health-seeker	Ego defense need to forestall aging process. Accomplished by diet intended to give super health. Self-realization need to present front of strength and health.
Distruster of medical profession	Ego defense need to establish control over own destiny and not be dependent on unknown others.
Fashion-follower	Ego defense and patterning need to establish an identity to gain approval and acceptance from others.
Authority-seeker	Self-realization need for recognition of self-competency, provided by apparent knowledge in area of food information.
Truth-seeker	Patterning need to process existing claims concerning nutrition.
One concerned about uncertainties of living	Patterning need for anchors and stability concerning the world.

From Beal VA: Food faddism and organic and natural foods. Reprinted courtesy of the American Dietetic Association.[5]

TABLE 12-2

30 TIPS TO HELP SPOT VITAMIN PUSHERS AND FOOD QUACKS

1. When talking about nutrients, they tell only part of the relevant story.
2. They claim that most Americans are poorly nourished.
3. They recommend "nutrition insurance" for everyone.
4. They say that if you eat badly, you'll be OK as long as you take supplements.
5. They say that most diseases are due to faulty diet and can be treated with "nutritional" methods.
6. They allege that modern processing methods and storage remove all nutritive value from our food.
7. They claim that diet is a major factor in behavior.
8. They claim that fluoridation is dangerous.
9. They claim that soil depletion and the use of pesticides and "chemical" fertilizers result in food that is less safe and less nourishing.
10. They claim you are in danger of being "poisoned" by ordinary food additives and preservatives.
11. They charge that the recommended dietary allowances (RDAs) have been set too low.
12. They claim that under stress, and in certain diseases, your need for nutrients is increased.
13. They recommend "supplements" and "health foods" for everyone.
14. They say it is easy to lose weight.
15. They claim that sugar is a deadly poison.
16. They oppose pasteurization of milk and fluoridation of water.
17. They recommend a wide variety of substances similar to those found in your body.
18. They claim that "natural" vitamins are better than "synthetic" ones.
19. They suggest that a questionnaire can be used to indicate whether you need dietary supplements.
20. They promise quick, dramatic, miraculous results.
21. They routinely sell vitamins and other "dietary supplements" as part of their practice.
22. They use disclaimers couched in pseudomedical jargon.
23. They use anecdotes and testimonials to support their claims.
24. They offer phony "vitamins."
25. They display credentials not recognized by responsible scientists or educators.
26. They offer to determine your body's nutritional state with a single laboratory test.
27. They claim they are being persecuted by orthodox medicine and that their work is being suppressed because it's controversial.
28. They warn you not to trust your doctor.
29. They sue to intimidate their critics.
30. They encourage patients to lend political support to their treatment methods.

From Barrett S, Herbert V. *The Vitamin Pushers: How the "Health Food" Industry Is Selling America a Bill of Goods.*[6]

Faddists use propaganda techniques that play on people's fears, hopes, and prejudices. One technique is to make the respondent hate a perceived enemy and love and support a cause. Many aspects of food faddism become social movements that represent symbolic rebellions against authority, society at large, or some imagined enemy.

Whorton[7] suggests that the term *faddism* is misleading because it connotes little more than temporary foolishness. Instead, he suggests, the high levels of devotion, asceticism, and zeal associated with certain health ideologies makes it more appropriate to call them "hygienic religions."

Promoters of nutrition quackery are skilled at arousing and exploiting fears and false hopes. Four basic myths are used to encourage the use of "health foods" and dietary supplements:

1. It is difficult if not impossible to get the nourishment you need from ordinary foods.
2. Vitamin and mineral deficiencies are common.
3. Virtually all diseases are caused by faulty diet.
4. Virtually all diseases can be prevented or remedied nutritionally.

Table 12-2 lists 30 misleading statements used by "vitamin pushers" and food quacks. The "Science of Foolology Box" on page 236 recounts how a fictional character anticipated some of these approaches more than 80 years ago.

DIETARY SUPPLEMENTS

In ordinary use the terms "dietary supplement" or "food supplement" refer to any food substance, or mixture of such substances, consumed in addition to or in place of food. The most commonly used supplements are vitamins and minerals. Many products sold as supplements contain substances not needed in the human diet.

The Dietary Supplement Health and Education Act of 1994 defines "dietary supplement" as any product (except tobacco) that contains at least one of the

Historical Perspective

The Science of Foolology[8]

One evening at Mory's, Dink Stover sits listening to Ricky Rickets discourse on how he plans to become a millionaire in 10 years. That certain route to wealth lies in "making an exact science" of beguiling the foolish. "What's the principle of a patent medicine?" Ricky asks rhetorically, and then answers himself. "Advertise first, then concoct your medicine." "All the science of Foolology," he elaborates, "is: first, find something all the fools love and enjoy, tell them it's wrong, hammer it into them, give them a substitute and sit back, chuckle, and shovel away the ducats. Why, Dink, in the next 20 years all the fools will be feeding on substitutes for everything they want . . . and blessing the name of the foolmaster who fooled them."

Ricky's prediction [made in a fictional work published in 1912!] contained much truth. Many blessings, and ducats too, have enriched critics of the regular diet who have provided some substitute promoted to preserve and restore health.

James Harvey Young, Ph.D.

following: (a) a vitamin, (b) a mineral, (c) an herb or botanical, (d) an amino acid, (e) a dietary substance "for use to supplement the diet by increasing total dietary intake," or (f) any concentrate, metabolite, constituent, extract, or combination of any of the aforementioned ingredients. Herbs, of course, are not consumed for a nutritional purpose and often are marketed with therapeutic claims. The supplement industry, which lobbied vigorously for passage of this act, included them in this definition to weaken the FDA's ability to regulate their marketing.

Vitamins are sold individually and combined with other vitamins and/or minerals. Multivitamin-mineral combinations may contain as many as 50 ingredients, but some ingredients, such as bioflavonoids, inositol, rutin, and para-aminobenzoic acid (PABA), are not needed in the human diet. Herbs are sold individually, in herbal mixtures, and combined with vitamins, minerals, and/or amino acids. The variety of products sold as dietary supplements (including many that contain no essential nutrients) is huge. Altogether, several hundred companies market about 30,000 such products.

Americans spend over $9 billion a year for supplement and herbal products. Most people who use multivitamins think they are getting "nutrition insurance," but many erroneously believe that extra vitamins can

provide extra energy, improve general health, and protect against stress. Most who supplement with individual nutrients believe that these products have medicinal value.[8] In a recent survey, users of vitamin and mineral supplements, herbs, and "specialty supplements" said they took them to ensure good health; improve energy or stamina; prevent or treat common illnesses like colds and the flu; improve memory or mental sharpness; prevent or treat more serious medical conditions; reduce anxiety, stress, or tension; slow down the aging process; improve mood or alleviate depression; lose weight or control appetite; improve sexual function or pleasure; and/or help with menopause (women only).[9]

Multivitamins vary greatly in the types and amounts of their individual ingredients. Many products contain amounts that exceed the RDA. Vitamin A is present in amounts up to 25,000 IU (international units), or five times its RDA; vitamin D is present in amounts up to 1000 IU, $2^1/_2$ times its RDA; vitamin B_6 as high as 500 mg, 250 times the RDA; vitamin E up to 1000 IU, 100 times its RDA; and vitamin C up to 1000 mg, 11 times its RDA. Single supplement tablets of vitamin C may contain as much as 2000 mg. Dosages this high are unnecessary, costly, and sometimes harmful. Most mineral supplements contain below-RDA amounts, but a few contain slightly more.

It is not legal to market any product with therapeutic claims unless satisfactory evidence of safety and effectiveness is presented to the FDA. However, many products are marketed as "dietary supplements" even though they are nutritionally insignificant or are intended for treating a health problem. Intended therapeutic uses seldom appear on product labels but are communicated in other ways to retailers and prospective customers. Thus, although customers are led to believe that various "supplements" can function as drugs, the FDA cannot regulate them as drugs.

Several scientific and professional groups have recommended that the FDA limit the dosage of certain ingredients in over-the-counter (OTC) vitamin and mineral products. However, the FDA is unable to implement these suggestions because the Proxmire Amendment to the Food, Drug, and Cosmetic Act prevents the agency from regulating the dosages of vitamin products that are not inherently dangerous. The amendment was passed in 1976 after a massive lobbying campaign spearheaded by the health-food industry.[10]

Curiously, the American public is not highly confident that dietary supplements are safe or accurately labeled. A recent survey found that (a) only 41% were very confident about the safety of vitamin and mineral supplements, (b) 34% believed the information on the labels was very accurate, (c) 24% were very confident that herbal products are safe, (d) and 32% believed herbal products were very accurately labeled. In addition, 12% of herbal products and 13% of specialty supplement users experienced adverse reactions to these products.[9]

"Nutrition Insurance"

Most nutrition authorities agree that healthy individuals can get all the nutrients they need by eating sensibly. Most Americans believe this too, but many worry that their eating habits place them at risk for deficiency. The fear of not getting enough nutrients is promoted vigorously, not only by food faddists and health-food industry publicists, but also by major pharmaceutical manufacturers and trade associations. Faddists tend to stress unscientific ideas that people cannot get sufficient nourishment from ordinary foods, while the drug companies use more subtle suggestions that various people may not be getting enough. Both groups fail to suggest how to obtain nutrients from foods or how to tell whether you are getting enough. Dr. Paul Thomas,[11] a former staff scientist for the Food and Nutrition Board, says that taking supplements is more like gambling than insurance (see "Personal Glimpse" box).

One of the main arguments used to support recommendations for "insurance" by vitamin supplements is that reputable health and nutrition surveys have found that intakes of some vitamins by some segments of the population are below the RDAs. Dr. Alfred E. Harper,[12] a former chairman of the Food and Nutrition Board, has explained why the above argument is misleading:

◆ Personal Glimpse ◆

Nutrition Insurance or Nutrition Roulette?

Those who recommend that healthy people supplement their diet with extra vitamins and minerals often call it a form of dietary insurance. I disagree. When you purchase insurance, the benefits and costs of the policy are detailed and you chose a specific level of protection. The terms of a dietary insurance policy, though, can never be known, much less specified. Taking supplements without a clear need is more analogous to playing the lottery. You hope to win some money, and ideally the jackpot, by buying lottery tickets. You won't hurt yourself unless you buy more tickets over time than you can afford, but you are not likely to win anything either, especially the big prize.

Paul R. Thomas, Ed.D., R.D.[11]

- The RDAs are set high enough to encompass the needs of individuals with the highest requirements. Using them directly as standards for evaluating the adequacy of individual nutrient intakes would be like setting the standard for a person's height at 7 feet and concluding that all those under 7 feet have suffered growth retardation.
- Surveys often identify vitamin A as a "problem nutrient." However, when the results of dietary surveys are based on measurements of nutrient intakes for a single day, many people who consume adequate amounts of vitamin A over a longer period of time are classified as having a "low" intake. Since vitamin A is stored efficiently in the liver, a surplus consumed on one day will provide a reserve that is available on subsequent days.

Another factor in the low values found in surveys is that people tend to under-report the amount they eat.[13] Even under highly controlled conditions, the under-reporting of caloric intake can be nearly 20%.[14]

The best strategy for individuals worried about the adequacy of their diet is to keep a food diary for several days and have it analyzed by a physician or registered dietitian. If a problem exists, it usually is better to correct the diet than to take supplements.[15]

Several manufacturers have pushed "meals in a can" with nutrition insurance claims like those made for vitamin pills. The major brands are *Ensure, Sustacal, Nutra-Start, Boost,* and *Resource.* The first such product (*Ensure*) was developed about 20 years ago for use in hospitals and nursing homes for people who were too ill or too weak to eat. However, they have been advertised aggressively to the general public and sold in grocery stores and pharmacies. These products cost between $1 and $2 per can and contain protein, carbohydrates, a modest amount of fat, and significant amounts of a few vitamins and minerals. However, most contain little or no fiber, and all lack carotenoids and other health-protecting plant-based chemicals.[16] Canned supplements can benefit ill people who are having difficulty consuming enough calories, but they are a waste of money for people whose appetite is not impaired.

In 1997 Abbott Laboratories agreed to settle Federal Trade Commission (FTC) charges that it made false and unsubstantiated claims in an extensive national advertising campaign that promoted *Ensure* for healthy, active adults. Several of Abbott's ads featured active, healthy people, many of whom appeared to be in their 30s or 40s. The featured adults referred to their own nutritional needs and their doctors' advice on maintaining good nutrition. The ads included statements such as, "Ensure is recommended number one by doctors as a source of complete balanced nutrition." The FTC alleged that Abbott represented without adequate

TABLE 12-3

ANALYSIS OF MISLEADING ADS THAT PROMOTE "NUTRITION INSURANCE"

Claim	Comment
Remember that the health of your eyes, teeth, bones, and internal systems depends upon a sufficient intake of these vital nutrients.[a]	Messages of this type, intended to make one nutrient-conscious, are true but misleading. They never say how to tell if one is getting enough.
No matter how hard you try, in our fast food society, it's often difficult to make sure you're getting enough essential vitamins and minerals in the food you eat.[b]	Falsely suggests that balancing one's diet is difficult.
How much of your vitamin C gets lost on the way to the table? Picking, packing, processing. All these plus transportation can lead to the destruction of part of the vitamin C in your foods.[c]	The real issues are how much remains in one's diet and whether it is enough. Most Americans consume adequate amounts of vitamin C.
It would take a computer and a good deal of conscious effort to devise a diet that each day would give all the nutrients in optimum amounts. Even well-trained nutritionists find it difficult to get complete nutrition in their diet.[d]	Falsely implies that ordinary people are at risk unless they take supplements. Food-group systems such as the Food Guide Pyramid (Chapter 12) provide for adequate amounts of nutrients and are easy to follow.
Getting a balanced diet can be tough, especially when you're busy with other things. So to avoid taking chances, take a supplement.[c]	Falsely suggests that busy people have difficulty in eating a balanced diet.
Most packaged foods have many, if not all, of the natural nutrients removed during processing and replaced with chemicals.[e]	Greatly exaggerates the amount of nutrients lost in processing; exploits public fear that our foods contain too many "chemicals."
Our soils are depleted.	Falsely suggests that adequate nutrition can be obtained only by ingesting food supplements or special foods.
"I take my vitamins every day. Just to be on the safe side." (Said by man pictured climbing a steep mountain)[c]	Misleading comparison of dangers of mountain climbing and of not taking daily vitamin pills.
Most of the water-soluble vitamins—B-complex and C—should be replaced daily. That's why a good diet is so important. Stresstabs high potency stress formula vitamins can help you to back up your diet because they concentrate on vitamins your body can't store.[f]	Water-soluble vitamins do not need to be replaced daily. The body can store them for at least several weeks. Using vitamins to "back up" a good diet is a waste of money. If a supplement is desired, there is no reason to select a "high-potency" (above-RDA) product.
Theragran-M is "fine-tuned for the way you live." (Said during a television commercial depicting attractive young people doing various athletic activities.)	Except for food intake, lifestyle characteristics have little to do with vitamin or mineral needs. The imagery falsely suggests that the product is likely to make people more vigorous.
Scientists are now studying the nutritional role of vitamins, minerals and other nutrients in helping to protect against diseases such as cancer, heart disease, and osteoporosis.[g]	The fact that various nutrients are being studied does not mean that supplementation with these nutrients has been proven beneficial.
Geritol Extend has all the vitamins the National Academy of Sciences recommends for people over 50.[h]	The Recommended Dietary Allowances (RDAs) are higher than most people need. The Academy does not recommend supplementation for everyone over 50.
Rich in Vitamin B Complex and Biotin, the "energy releasers" essential for converting food into energy.[i]	Subtly suggests that taking the product will cause users to have more energy, which is untrue.

[a]Vitamin, mineral and food supplement guide (flyer), Safeway Stores, 1979.
[b]Advertising flyer, Sears, 1979.
[c]Magazine ads, Hoffmann-La Roche, 1981-1983.
[d]Thompson RW: Why you should take vitamins and minerals (flyer), General Nutrition Corporation, 1983.
[e]Neo-Life Corporation: Sharing the new life through better nutrition... every day of your life! *Counselor*, Feb 1979, pp 3–5.
[f]Magazine ad, Lederle Laboratories, 1991-1992.
[g]Magazine ad, Council for Responsible Nutrition, 1989.
[h]Magazine ad, SmithKline Beecham, 1990.
[i]Magazine ad, E.R. Squibb & Sons, 1988.

substantiation that many doctors recommend *Ensure* as a meal supplement and replacement for healthy adults, including those in their 30s and 40s. An FTC official stated that beverage products like *Ensure* may provide a benefit for people with a medical condition that makes it difficult to eat or for people who use them in place of an occasional skipped meal. However, Abbott went too far when it suggested that doctors recommend *Ensure* for healthy, active people, like those pictured in the ads, in order to stay active and healthy.

Table 12-3 on page 236 analyzes common sales pitches for "nutrition insurance."

Perspectives on Food Processing

To promote the use of supplements, the health-food industry suggests that the processing of food removes its nourishment. It is true that processing can change the nutrient content of food, but the changes are not drastic. Only a few nutrients are affected by processing, and most losses are insignificant to the overall diet. Food processing and home food preparation can destroy certain vitamins with heat and remove some water-soluble vitamins and minerals through contact with water during cooking. Usually these are only partial losses. Moreover, the nutrients lost from certain foods between the farm and the table are readily obtainable from other foods. For example, although pasteurization of milk destroys some of its vitamin C content, milk is not a significant source of vitamin C to begin with. The chief dietary sources of vitamin C are fruits and vegetables. Some nutrient losses in processing (for example, vitamin losses during the milling of flour) are restored by enrichment. The negative effects of some food-processing operations are more than balanced by the overall positive effects, especially the continuous availability of most types of food items at reasonable cost. As noted in Chapter 11, eating moderate amounts of a wide variety of foods, including some uncooked fruits and vegetables, provides an adequate supply of nutrients.

"Stress Supplements"

Many vitamin manufacturers advertise that extra vitamins are needed to protect against "stress." While some companies list only physical stresses that supposedly increase vitamin needs, some include mental stress, overwork, and the like. Some companies market products for the "special needs" of athletes, housewives, busy executives, and smokers. Others make no health claims at all, relying only on the product's name to sell it.

"Stress-formulas" typically contain several times the RDA for vitamin C and several B-vitamins. The products manufactured by drug companies do not provide toxic amounts of these ingredients. But some marketed by health-food industry companies contain enough vitamin C to cause diarrhea, and some contain enough B_6 to cause nerve damage over a long period of time. Some formulas contain questionable food substances such as spirulina, bee pollen, and ginseng to make them appear more "complete." Herbal and homeopathic "stress formulas" are also available.

Although vitamin needs may rise slightly in certain physical conditions, they seldom exceed the RDA, and they are easily met by eating a balanced diet. Anyone really in danger of deficiency as a result of illness would be very ill and probably require hospitalization.

Some vitamin manufacturers suggest that strenuous physical activity increases the need for vitamins so that people who engage in vigorous exercise or athletics should take supplements. Strenuous exercise does increase the need for calories, water, and a few nutrients. However, the nutrient needs are unlikely to exceed the RDAs. Even if above-RDA amounts were necessary, they would be supplied by the increase in food intake normally associated with exercising. The belief that extra vitamins are useful to athletes is also tied to the idea that extra vitamins provide extra energy—which is untrue. Vitamin concoctions pitched to athletes (so-called ergogenic aids) are discussed further in Chapter 14.

Smokers tend to have lower blood levels of vitamin C than do nonsmokers. In 2000 the RDA for vitamin C was set at 75 mg for men and 90 mg for women, with an additional 35 mg for smokers. However, no evidence exists that smokers are deficient in vitamin C.[12] Regardless of whether smokers need extra vitamin C, all of these amounts are readily obtainable from food.

No scientific evidence shows that emotional stress increases one's need for vitamins. In 1982 the National Advertising Division (NAD) of the Council of Better Business Bureaus reacted to an ad by Hoffmann-La Roche and noted that the terms "stress" and "acute stress" have one meaning in science and another in popular speech. NAD wondered whether the Roche ads would give a false impression that mental stresses, both minor and acute, might raise the body's requirement for vitamin C. The company agreed and pledged to modify its future advertising.[17]

In 1985 E.R. Squibb & Sons, Inc., agreed to pay $15,000 to New York State and to stop making false and misleading claims for its *Theragran Stress Formula*. In 1986 Lederle Laboratories agreed to pay $25,000 and to stop suggesting that *Stresstabs* could reduce the effects of psychologic stress or the ordinary stress of life.

Both cases were prosecuted by New York's attorney general. In a 1985 interview, Lederle's chief of nutrition science acknowledged that "people who eat a balanced diet do not need stress vitamins—or for that matter any vitamin supplement at all."[18]

In 1990 Miles Laboratories (makers of *One-A-Day* products) signed a three-year "assurance of discontinuance" order with the attorneys general of New York, California, and Texas and agreed to pay $10,000 to each of these three states. Without admitting wrongdoing, the company pledged not to claim that (a) the average consumer needs a supplement to prevent mineral and vitamin loss, (b) vitamins can prevent or reverse lung damage caused by pollution, (c) routine daily stress depletes vitamins, and (d) routine physical exercise (such as the aerobics shown in Miles' television ad) depletes essential minerals.

In 1994 Dr. Stephen Barrett petitioned the FDA to (a) remove vitamins and other ineffective ingredients from products marketed for the prevention or relief of "stress" and (b) to issue a public warning that although the FDA has permitted "stress formulas" to be sold, it does not recognize them as effective against emotional stress or ordinary stress.[19] In 1996 the petition was denied. The Dietary Supplement Health and Education Act of 1994 requires manufacturers who make statements of "nutritional support" to indicate that such statements have not been evaluated by the FDA and that "the product is not intended to diagnose, treat, cure, or prevent any disease." The agency's denial letter to Dr. Barrett stated: "This mandatory label statement is sufficient to inform consumers that FDA has not evaluated a claim made for a dietary supplement."

"Natural" vs Synthetic Vitamins

Many promoters claim that "natural" vitamins are better than the synthetic vitamins. Such claims are unfounded. A few synthetic vitamins have slightly different structures than their natural counterparts, but these differences are of no importance inside the body. As noted by Herbert,[20] vitamins are specific molecules; the body makes no distinction between vitamins made in the "factories" of nature and those made in the factories of chemical companies. The prices of "natural" vitamins tend to be higher than those of synthetic vitamins.

Antioxidants and Other Phytochemicals

Many "antioxidant" products are marketed with claims that, by blocking the action of free radicals, they can help prevent heart disease, cancer, and various other conditions associated with aging. Figure 12-1 shows an ad with this type of message.

Free radicals are atoms or groups of atoms that have at least one unpaired electron, which makes them highly reactive. Free radicals promote beneficial oxidation that produces energy and kills bacterial invaders. In excess, however, they produce harmful oxidation that can damage cell membranes and cell contents. It is known that people who eat adequate amounts of fruits and vegetables high in antioxidants have a lower incidence of cardiovascular disease, certain cancers, and cataracts. Fruits and vegetables are rich in antioxidants, but it is not known which dietary factors are responsible for the beneficial effects. Each plant contains hundreds of phytochemicals (plant chemicals) whose presence is dictated by hereditary factors. Only well-designed long-term research can determine whether any of these chemicals, taken in a pill, would be useful for preventing any disease.

The most publicized nutrients with antioxidant properties are vitamin C, vitamin E, and beta-carotene (which

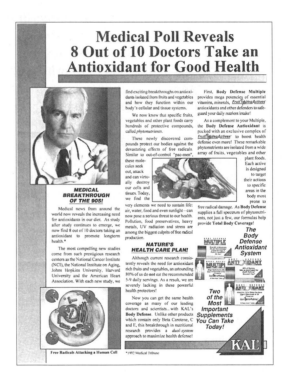

Figure 12-1. Ad that appeared in many health-food industry publications during 1994. Small print at the bottom cites a report in *Medical Tribune* (a newspaper for doctors) as the source of the "8 out of 10" statistic. No survey on antioxidant usage had actually been done; the editor had merely asked for opinions on the use of vitamin E. About 80% who responded wrote favorable comments, many of which described their recommendations to patients. No attempt was made to determine whether the respondents were typical of *Medical Tribune* readers or physicians in general, or whether they personally took supplements. The percentage of people who do or don't do something cannot be measured this way.

the body converts into vitamin A). Evidence exists that vitamin E can help prevent atherosclerosis by interfering with the oxidation of low-density lipoproteins (LDL), a factor associated with increased risk of heart disease (see Chapter 15). However, vitamin E also has an anticoagulant effect that can promote excessive bleeding. In 1993 *The New England Journal of Medicine* published two epidemiologic studies which found that people who took vitamin E supplements had fewer deaths from heart disease.[21,22] These studies did not prove that taking vitamin E was useful because they did not rule out the effects of other lifestyle factors or consider death rates from other diseases. Moreover, other studies have had conflicting results. The only way to settle the question scientifically is to conduct long-term double-blind clinical studies comparing vitamin users to nonusers and checking death rates from all causes.

At least seven large clinical trials have been reported. The first trial compared the effects of vitamin E, beta-carotene, and a placebo among heavy smokers. The researchers found no benefit from vitamin E and 18% *more* lung cancer among those who received beta-carotene. In addition, the overall death rate of beta-carotene recipients was 8% higher, and those who took vitamin E had a higher frequency of hemorrhagic stroke.[23,24] The second study found no evidence that supplementing with vitamin C, vitamin E, or beta-carotene prevented colorectal cancer.[25] The third study, which followed 22,000 physicians for 12 years, found no difference in cancer or cardiovascular disease rates between users and nonusers of beta-carotene.[26] The fourth trial, which tested a combination of beta-carotene and vitamin A, was terminated after four years because it appeared that the supplement-takers who smoked had a 28% higher incidence of lung cancer and a 17% higher death rate.[27]

More recently, a double-blind clinical trial found that taking high doses of vitamins C and E and beta-carotene did not reduce the odds of arteries reclogging after balloon coronary angioplasty.[28] Another study involved 2545 women and 6996 men 55 years of age or older who were at high risk for cardiovascular events because they had cardiovascular disease or diabetes in addition to one other risk factor. These patients were randomly assigned to receive either 400 IU of natural vitamin E or a matching placebo for an average of 4½ years. There were no significant differences in heart attacks, strokes, or death between the vitamin E and placebo groups.[29] Yet another study tested aspirin, vitamin E, and beta-carotene in the prevention of cancer and cardiovascular disease among 39,876 women aged 45 years or older. Among those randomly assigned to

receive 50 mg of beta-carotene or a placebo every other day, there were no statistically significant differences in incidence of cancer, cardiovascular disease, or overall death rate after a median of 2 years of treatment and two years of follow-up.[30]

Charles Hennekens, M.D., who participated in two of the aforementioned studies, has pointed out that even if antioxidants could provide the benefits suggested by epidemiologic studies, smoking cessation and other lifestyle factors would have a far greater effect on the rates of lung cancer and coronary heart disease.[31] The *Medical Letter* has concluded that (a) the benefits of taking high doses of vitamin E remain to be established, (b) there is no convincing evidence that taking supplements of vitamin C prevents any disease, and (c) no one should take beta-carotene supplements.[32]

The American Heart Association recommends that "the most prudent and scientifically supportable recommendation for the general population is to consume a balanced diet with emphasis on antioxidant-rich fruits and vegetables and whole grains."[33]

Research is also being done to determine whether taking supplements or eating foods rich in antioxidants can protect against age-related macular degeneration (AMD), a disease in which the central portion of the retina deteriorates so that only peripheral vision remains. A team of Australian researchers who followed 3654 subjects age 49 or older found no statistically significant association between AMD and dietary intake of either carotene, zinc, or vitamins A or C, either from diet, supplements, or both.[34] Other published studies have had conflicting results, with some finding correlations and others finding none.[34]

The negative publicity has not deterred manufacturers from continuing to market antioxidants as though they have been proven beneficial. Some have responded by hyping new mixtures of beta-carotene and other carotenoids, which, they suggest, may provide the same benefits as fruits and vegetables.

Many types of pills described as "concentrates" of fruits and/or vegetables are being marketed. Critics of these products state that it is not possible to condense large amounts of produce into a pill without losing fiber, nutrients, and many other phytochemicals.[35] Although some products contain significant amounts of nutrients, these nutrients are readily obtainable at lower cost from foods.

Amino Acid Products
Many supplement products containing amino acids are marketed as weight-loss and/or ergogenic aids despite lack of evidence that they are effective for either

purpose (see Chapters 13 and 14). The Federation of American Societies for Experimental Biology (FASEB) has sharply criticized this situation. Following extensive review of the scientific literature, FASEB experts concluded: (a) single- or multiple-ingredient capsules, tablets, and liquid products are used primarily for pharmacologic purposes or enhancement of physiologic functions rather than for nutritional purposes; (b) little scientific literature exists on most amino acids ingested for these purposes; (c) no scientific rationale has been presented to justify ingestion of amino acid supplements by healthy individuals; (d) safety levels for amino-acid supplement use have not been established; and (e) a systematic approach to safety testing is needed.[36]

MEGAVITAMIN CLAIMS VS FACTS

Claims are widespread that high dosages of vitamins and minerals can prevent or cure a great diversity of ailments. Dr. Linus Pauling, a Nobel Prize winner in chemistry and former professor of chemistry at Stanford University, was the chief theoretician for this approach, which he termed "orthomolecular" treatment (*ortho* is Greek for "right"). This approach supposedly provides the correct amounts of nutritionally "right" molecules normally found in the body. It began during the early 1950s as megavitamin therapy for schizophrenia and is also called "nutritional medicine." This section examines some megavitamin claims, the evidence against them, and the dangers involved. Megavitamin treatment for emotional problems is discussed in Chapter 6.

Pauling and Vitamin C

Controversy over the use of massive dosages of vitamin C stems largely from Pauling's publications. His 1970 book, *Vitamin C and the Common Cold*, claimed that taking 1000 mg of vitamin C daily would reduce the incidence of colds by 45% for most people, but that some needed much larger amounts. The book's 1976 revision, *Vitamin C, the Common Cold and the Flu*, suggested even higher dosages. A third book, published in 1979, claimed that high dosages of vitamin C may be effective against cancer.[37] A flyer distributed in 1991 by the Linus Pauling Institute recommended daily doses of 6000 to 18,000 mg of vitamin C, 400 to 1600 IU of vitamin E, and 25,000 IU of vitamin A, plus various other vitamins and minerals. Pauling himself reportedly took 12,000 mg of vitamin C daily and raised the amount to 40,000 mg if symptoms of a cold appeared. However, most medical and nutritional scientists strongly disagree with Pauling's views concerning vitamin C.

Experiments on the possible value of vitamin C for preventing infections have been conducted by medical investigators ever since the vitamin became commercially available during the 1930s. At least 15 well-designed double-blind studies have shown that supplementation with vitamin C does not prevent colds, and that, at best, it may slightly reduce the symptoms of a cold.[38] Slight symptom reduction may occur because of an antihistamine-like effect, but whether this has practical value is debatable. Pauling's views were based on analysis of the same studies as other scientists, but his conclusions were different.[39]

The largest clinical trials, involving thousands of volunteers, were directed by Dr. Terence Anderson, professor of epidemiology at the University of Toronto. Taken together, his studies suggest that extra vitamin C intake may slightly reduce the severity of colds, but it is not necessary to take the high doses recommended by Pauling to achieve this result. Nor is there anything to be gained by taking vitamin C supplements year-round in the hope of preventing colds.[38]

Another important study was reported in 1975 by scientists at the National Institutes of Health who had compared the effects of vitamin C pills with a placebo before and during colds. Although the experiment was designed to be double-blind, half the subjects guessed which pill they were getting. When the results were tabulated, the average number of colds reported per person was 1.27 for the vitamin group and 1.36 for the placebo group over a 9-month period. But among the half who had not guessed which pill they had been taking, no difference in the incidence or severity was found. This illustrates how people who think they are doing something effective (such as taking a vitamin) can report a favorable result even when none exists.[40]

In 1976 Pauling and Ewan Cameron, a Scottish physician, reported that most of 100 patients with terminal cancer treated with 10,000 mg of vitamin C daily had survived three to four times longer than similar patients who did not receive vitamin C supplements. However, Dr. William DeWys, chief of clinical investigations at the National Cancer Institute, found that the study was poorly designed because the patient groups were not comparable. The vitamin C patients were Cameron's, while the other patients were under the care of other physicians. Cameron's patients started taking vitamin C when he labeled them untreatable by other methods, and their subsequent survival was compared with the survival of the "control" patients after they had been labeled untreatable by their doctors. DeWys[41] reasoned that if the two groups were comparable, the lengths of time from entry into the hospital to being labeled untreatable should be similar in both groups. However, Cameron's patients were labeled untreatable much earlier in the course of their disease—which means that they entered the hospital before they were as sick as the other doctors' patients and would naturally be expected to live longer.

In 1979 the Mayo Clinic reported a double-blind study of 123 patients with advanced cancer. Half of the patients received 10,000 mg of vitamin C daily, while the others were given a placebo. No differences were found between the two groups in survival time, appetite, weight loss, severity of pain, or amount of nausea and vomiting.[42] Other well-designed studies reported in 1983 and 1985 yielded similar results.[43,44] Pauling died of prostate cancer in 1995.

Therapeutic Claims for Megavitamin E

Claims have been made that large dosages of vitamin E are effective treatment for acne, atherosclerosis, cancer, diabetes, sexual frigidity, infertility, repeated spontaneous abortions, muscular dystrophy, peptic ulcers, rheumatic fever, and fibrocystic disease of the breast. Some proponents have claimed that vitamin E will increase stamina, prolong life, and protect against the effects of atmospheric pollution. Vitamin E is added to aftershave lotions, soaps, and underarm deodorants. However, it has no proven therapeutic, nutritional, or cosmetic value for any of the these.[38]

Vitamin E deficiency symptoms in humans that are traceable only to an inadequate diet have never been reported, except in premature infants.[38] In adults, deficiency has been observed only in patients with an inability to absorb fat during the digestive process (vitamin E is fat-soluble). About 25 years ago several researchers placed human volunteers on a low-vitamin E diet for 4½ years to see whether they could produce signs of deficiency. The volunteers had minor changes in their red blood cells but experienced no symptoms.[38] Thus it is clearly irrational for healthy persons to take vitamin E supplements as protection against deficiency. Vitamin E may ultimately be shown to have a limited role in preventing and treating coronary heart disease, but much research needs to be done to determine this.

Dangers of Excess Vitamins and Minerals

Vitamins in excess of the body's needs seldom serve a useful function and can be harmful. Excess amounts of fat-soluble vitamins are stored in body fat, where they can build up to toxic levels over a period of time. Excess water-soluble vitamins are excreted through the urine, but these can still have adverse effects.

Vitamin A toxicity can result from ingesting too much vitamin A on a regular basis for months or years.

The problems that develop as body stores build up include headache, hair loss, bone malformation, bleeding tendencies, bone fracture, muscle and joint pain, vision problems, retarded growth in children, drying and cracking of the skin, and enlargement of the liver and spleen. Most adverse effects disappear after excessive intake is stopped, but permanent damage can occur to the liver, bones, and eyes. Liver damage in adults has been reported at daily doses of 25,000 IU or more.[45]

Vitamin A supplements taken early in pregnancy are hazardous to the developing fetus. A recent study concluded that among the babies born to women who took more than 10,000 IU per day in the form of supplements, about 1 in 57 had a birth defect attributable to the supplements.[46]

Prolonged excessive intake of vitamin D (usually five times the RDA or more) can cause loss of appetite, nausea, weakness, weight loss, excess urinary output, constipation, vague aches, stiffness, kidney stones, tissue calcification, high blood pressure, acidosis, and kidney failure (which can lead to death).

Doses in the range of 40 to 300 times the RDA of niacin can cause severe flushing, itching, liver damage,

◆ Personal Glimpse ◆

Vitamin A Poisoning

In 1979 a chiropractor in Peoria, Illinois, prescribed massive doses of vitamin A for Lynne Crampton, age 9, and her brother Dale, age 4. Both children suffered from ichthyosis, a congenital disorder in which the skin is scaly and resembles that of a fish. Lynne was prescribed 750,000 international units (IU) daily for several weeks, to be followed by 370,000 IU daily for 2 months. Dale was prescribed 675,000 IU daily for 2 months and then half that amount. The RDA of vitamin A is 1665 IU for 4-year-olds and 2331 IU for 9-year-olds.

Within a few months Lynne developed swelling of the brain, manifested by blurred vision and headaches. She also had musculoskeletal pain and tenderness, hair loss for 2 months, and damage to the growth centers of several of her bones. Dale developed bone pain and enlargement of his liver and spleen. Although their acute symptoms subsided after the vitamin A was stopped, both children were permanently harmed. One of Lynne's legs became several inches shorter than the other, which caused her to develop scoliosis. Dale has permanent damage to his liver and spleen. Between 1986 and 1989, suits filed against the chiropractor and the vitamin A manufacturers were settled out of court for a total of $895,000.[47]

skin disorders, gout, ulcers, and blood-sugar disorders. (Despite this, large doses administered under medical supervision can be valuable for controlling abnormal blood cholesterol levels, as described in Chapter 15.)

Excessive vitamin E (usually 400 IU or more) can cause headaches, nausea, tiredness, giddiness, inflammation of the mouth, chapped lips, gastrointestinal disturbances, muscle weakness, low blood-sugar levels, and increased bleeding tendency.

Vitamin C, in amounts upwards of 20 times the RDA, can damage growing bone, produce diarrhea, cause "rebound scurvy" (when stopped abruptly) in adults and in newborn infants whose mothers took large doses, cause adverse effects in pregnancy, produce kidney stones, and cause false urine tests for sugar in diabetics. Large doses can also produce false-negative tests for blood in the stool and thereby prevent early detection of serious gastrointestinal diseases, including cancer.[37]

Very large doses of B_6 (2000 mg or more; 1000 times the RDA) have caused symptoms resembling those of multiple sclerosis, including numbness and tingling of the hands, difficulty in walking, and the feeling of electric shocks shooting down the spine. Although most of the afflicted individuals recovered after they stopped taking B_6 supplements, some did not. In the 1980s it was discovered that more than 100 women attending a clinic specializing in treating premenstrual syndrome had developed neurologic symptoms as a result of taking vitamin B_6. Ninety-two had taken less than 200 mg (100 times the RDA) daily for more than 6 months. Twenty of them had taken less than 50 mg per day.[48] The lowest dosage on which anyone developed symptoms was 20 mg per day for 2 years; the shortest time was 2 months of 100 mg per day. All of their symptoms resolved when the B_6 was stopped.

As with fat-soluble vitamins, excess amounts of most minerals are stored in the body and can gradually build up to toxic levels. An excess of one mineral can also interfere with the functioning of others. Certain people can benefit from mineral supplements, but they should never be used without medical supervision.[38,49]

Barrett and Herbert[8] state that there are only two situations in which vitamin use at higher-than-RDA levels is legitimate: (1) treatment of medically diagnosed deficiency states—conditions rare except among alcoholics; persons with intestinal absorption defects; and the poor, especially those who are pregnant or elderly and (2) certain problems for which large doses of vitamins are used as drugs—with full recognition of any risks involved. An example is the use of niacin to improve blood cholesterol levels (see Chapter 15).

APPROPRIATE USE OF SUPPLEMENTS

In general, supplements are useful for individuals who are unable or unwilling to consume an adequate diet. Physicians commonly recommend vitamins for very young children until they are eating solid foods that contain enough vitamins. After a child reaches the age of 2, however, it is seldom necessary to continue supplements "just to be sure." In 1980 the American Academy of Pediatrics[50] stated that supplements might be appropriate as follows:

- Fluoride supplements should be given to children not drinking fluoridated water. (See Chapter 7 for dosage.)
- Children with poor eating habits and those using weight-reduction diets can be given a multivitamin-mineral supplement containing nutrients not exceeding RDA levels.
- Children on strict vegetarian diets may need supplementation, particularly of vitamin B_{12}.
- Pregnant teenagers are likely to need supplementary iron and folic acid.

The U.S. Preventive Services Task Force[51] recommends that women who might become pregnant take a daily multivitamin or multivitamin-mineral supplement that contains 0.4 mg of folic acid in order to reduce the risk of birth defects in their offspring (see Chapter 11). Although a well-balanced diet will provide adequate amounts of folic acid, the Task Force felt that, for some women, achieving adequate dietary intake might be more difficult than taking supplements.

People using prolonged weight-reduction diets, particularly diets that are below 1200 calories per day or are nutritionally unbalanced, may benefit from a multivitamin-mineral supplement.

Individuals recovering from surgery or serious illnesses that have disrupted normal eating habits may also benefit from supplementation.

Elderly persons who become sedentary or lose interest in eating may not get sufficient nutrients; they too may benefit from multivitamin-mineral supplementation. Unadvertised brands costing about 5 cents per day are available.

Because iron deficiency is not rare, a National Academy of Sciences committee has recommended that pregnant women take a 30 mg supplement daily during the second and third trimesters. Although adequately nourished women do not need supplementation, it is simpler and less costly to supplement the diet than to measure blood iron levels several times during the pregnancy. The committee also suggested that although the best way to obtain nutrients is from food, pregnant women who ordinarily do not consume an adequate diet might benefit from a multivitamin-mineral supplement containing moderate dosages of iron, zinc, copper, calcium, vitamin B_6, folic acid, vitamin C, and vitamin D.[52]

Women should be sure that their intake of calcium is adequate to help prevent thinning of their bones (osteoporosis). This can be done with adequate intake of dairy products, but some women prefer calcium supplements. Women should discuss this matter with their physician or a registered dietitian. Chapter 21 covers this subject further.

"ORGANIC" FOODS

Promoters of "organic" and "organically grown" foods suggest that these are safer and more nutritious than conventionally grown foods. The terms attempt to describe the methods by which foods are produced. "Organically grown" may be the more appropriate term because in scientific usage, "organic" refers to compounds that contain carbon, which all food substances do. The most common concept of "organically grown" food was articulated in 1972 by Robert Rodale, editor of *Organic Gardening and Farming* magazine, at a hearing conducted by New York State Attorney General Louis Lefkowitz:

Food grown without pesticides; grown without artificial fertilizers; grown in soil whose humus content is increased by the additions of organic matter, grown in soil whose mineral content is increased by the application of natural mineral fertilizers; has not been treated with preservatives, hormones, antibiotics, etc.[53]

Many scientists believe this definition is inherently misleading and cite the following facts:

- "Organic" promoters imply that their products are pesticide-free, but surveys have found no significant differences in pesticide levels between organic and conventionally grown foods. Pesticides on the outside of fruits and vegetables may be removed by washing. The tiny amounts found in some foods pose no health risk.[54,55] FDA data show that dietary intakes of pesticides are well within recognized safety standards.[56]
- Plants obtain nutrients from soil in their inorganic state. Organic fertilizers must decompose before their nutrients become available for absorption. What counts is the availability of required nutrients rather than the type of fertilizer.
- Plant nutrient content is determined primarily by heredity. Mineral levels may be affected by the mineral content of the soil, but this has no significance in the overall diet. If essential nutrients are missing from the soil, the plant will not grow. If plants grow, that means the essential nutrients are present. As noted by Ronald Deutsch,[57] this is

logical because a plant does not make its nutrients "as a generous gesture to humans but for its own growth and survival." Experiments have found no difference in the nutrient content of organically grown crops and those grown under standard agricultural conditions.[58]
- The taste of raw food is determined by the product's genetic programming, ripeness when harvested, and freshness. A large-scale test of 25 foods at the University of Florida found that many supermarket foods actually looked and tasted better than their "organic" counterparts.[59] A more recent study obtained 460 assessments of nine different fruits and vegetables and found no significant difference in taste quality between "organic" and conventionally grown samples.[60]

"Organic" agriculture is sometimes referred to as "alternative" or "sustainable" agriculture. Neither of these terms is precisely definable.[61]

Foods labeled organic nearly always cost more than their conventional counterparts. Since they cannot be told apart by their appearance, some storekeepers have labeled conventionally grown foods "organic" to increase profits.

◆ Personal Glimpse ◆

The Latest "Organic" Definition

At its April 1995 meeting the National Organic Standards Board adopted the following "definition," which addresses production methods rather than the foods themselves. Do you think it is enforceable? Will enforcement protect consumers from fraud?

Organic agriculture is an ecological production management system that promotes and enhances biodiversity, biological cycles and soil biological activity. It is based on minimal use of off-farm inputs and on management practices that restore, maintain and enhance ecological harmony. "Organic" is a labeling term that denotes products produced under the authority of the Organic Foods Production Act. The principal guidelines for organic production are to use materials and practices that enhance the ecological balance of natural systems and that integrate the parts of the farming system into an ecological whole. Organic agriculture practices cannot ensure that products are completely free of residues; however, methods are used to minimize pollution from air, soil and water. Organic food handlers, processors and retailers adhere to standards that maintain the integrity of organic agricultural products. The primary goal of organic agriculture is to optimize the health and productivity of interdependent communities of soil life, plants, animals and people.

Government Involvement

In 1974 the FTC began working on an industrywide rule to cover food advertising, including claims for "organic" and "natural" foods. Proponents of these terms attempted to persuade agency officials to define them legally and establish standards. Opponents argued that commercial use should be prohibited because such words are inherently misleading. In 1982 the Commission voted to terminate the rule-making procedure and use a case-by-case approach.

In 1980 a team of scientists appointed by the U.S. Department of Agriculture (USDA) to study "organic farming" concluded that there is no universally accepted definition of the term:

The organic movement represents a spectrum of practices, attitudes and philosophies. On the one hand are those organic practitioners who would not use chemical fertilizers or pesticides under any circumstances. These producers hold rigidly to their purist philosophy. At the other end of the spectrum, organic farmers espouse a more flexible approach. While striving to avoid the use of chemical fertilizers and pesticides, these practitioners do not rule them out entirely. Instead, when absolutely necessary, some fertilizers and also herbicides are very selectively and sparingly used as a second line of defense. Nevertheless, these farmers, too, consider themselves to be organic farmers.[62]

During subsequent years, in response to pressure from proponents, about half the states passed some type of organic certification law. In 1990 Congress passed the U.S. Organic Foods Production Act, which directs the U.S. Secretary of Agriculture to establish certification standards and procedures with help from a 15-member National Organic Standards Board. The standards were finalized in 1999. Once they are implemented, violators may face civil penalties of up to $10,000 per offense. Commenting on the bill, Larkin[63] stated:

"Organic certification" isn't the answer. It will merely create more confusion and distrust in the marketplace. Foods certified as "organic" will neither be safer nor more nutritious than "regular" foods. They will just cost more. Instead of spending money to legitimize nutrition nonsense, our government should do more to attack its spread.

Figure 12-2. Organic certification seal

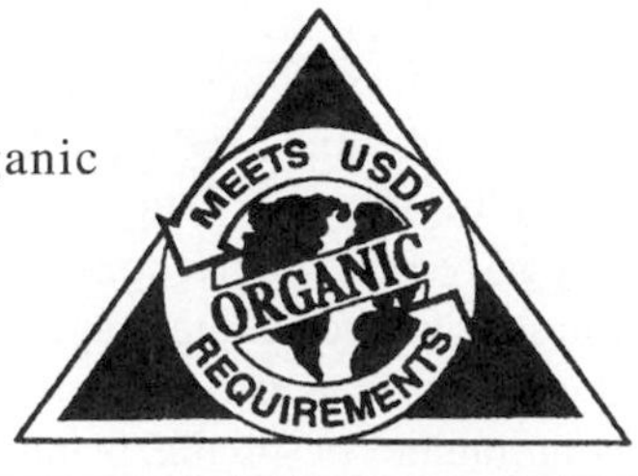

"Health Foods"

"Health foods" are claimed to be special foods that can benefit people's health. The terms *health food, natural food, organic food,* and *organically grown food* are often used interchangeably by both sellers and consumers. Vegetarian foods and foods labeled "dietetic" may also be referred to as health foods.

Nutrition authorities believe that the term "health food" is inherently misleading, because all foods are healthy when eaten in moderation and can be unhealthy when eaten in excess amounts. Stare, Aronson, and Barrett[3] have observed:

The term is merely a gimmick used to boost sales. . . . Some foods popular as "health foods" are rich in nutrients, but no food has unique health-promoting properties. All foods can contribute to health when eaten as part of a varied and balanced diet. The problem with so-called health foods is that they are promoted with false claims and usually are overpriced.

The foods eaten are not useful in the body until they are broken down into their component nutrients before being absorbed from the digestive tract; thus claims that certain foods are especially healthful should be evaluated by considering the components of these foods. Confronted with such claims, intelligent consumers should ask the following:

- What are the food's significant components and their nutritional value?
- Can special health claims made about it be scientifically justified?
- What other foods are comparable?
- How do comparable foods compare in price?

Table 12-4 lists commonly promoted "health foods," supplements, hormones, and other products sold in health-food stores.

"Natural" Foods

"Natural" foods are said to be those produced with minimal processing and without additives or artificial ingredients. The word "natural," like the word "organic," usually means that the product is higher-priced. Advocates of "natural foods" say that processing reduces nutritional value and that additives are harmful. Critics of the designation "natural" maintain that the American food supply is the safest and best the world has ever seen. They also state that "natural" cannot be meaningfully defined because there is no sharp dividing line between processed and unprocessed foods.

—*Text continued on page 251.*

TABLE 12-4

PRODUCTS COMMONLY SOLD IN HEALTH-FOOD STORES

The following are commonly promoted "health foods," supplements, and other products sold in health-food stores. Those marked with an asterisk (*) can cause difficulties. Popular herbs are discussed in Table 12-5, page 253.

Acidophilus: *Lactobacillus acidophilus* is a bacterial organism that ferments the sugars present in milk. Capsules of acidophilus are claimed to aid digestion and promote the health of the digestive tract. This is impractical, however, because oral doses of the bacteria may not survive the acidic environment of the stomach and the number and activity of the bacteria may be reduced during storage. Acidophilus preparations such as sweet acidophilus milk can be useful to persons who have difficulty digesting lactose (a condition called lactose intolerance). These widely available dairy products are produced by adding acid-tolerant strains of acidophilus bacteria to milk. Those surviving passage into the intestine will produce lactase, an enzyme that helps to digest the milk's lactose. However, individuals with lactose intolerance should have guidance from a physician, and use of lactase without the bacteria may be an alternative. Lactase-treated milk is available in supermarkets throughout the United States.

Activated charcoal: Supplements labeled "activated organic charcoal" are usually said to be made by burning "natural organic" peat moss. Charcoal supposedly absorbs intestinal gases and "serves as a powerful detoxicant" that combats "gas" and "makes you feel intestinally clean." However, this product is of little value and can add to gastrointestinal distress by interfering with the action of digestive enzymes.

*Alfalfa: Although its advocates suggest that alfalfa contains certain nutrients that more common plant foods do not, it actually has less nutritional value than most of the more popular vegetables such as broccoli, carrots, and spinach. Alfalfa has also been claimed to contain all of the essential amino acids, but this is untrue. Alfalfa contains L-canavanine, a toxic amino acid that can bring out latent immune disorders, particularly hemolytic anemia, lupus erythematosus, and rheumatoid arthritis.[8]

*Aloe vera: Unsubstantiated claims are made that aloe vera products can cure or alleviate colitis, bursitis, asthma, glaucoma, hemorrhoids, boils, arthritis, intestinal problems, acne, poison ivy, anemia, tuberculosis, cancer, diabetes, depression, multiple sclerosis, stretch marks, varicose veins, and even blindness. Aloe skin creams or gels are probably harmless; and even though it will not reverse the aging process, topical aloe may exert some skin softening and moisturizing effects. However, aloe juice is a harsh laxative that can cause gastrointestinal upset.[64]

*Bee pollen: Bee pollen is flower pollen harvested from bees. Although claimed to be a "perfect food," it contains no nutrients that are not present in conventional foods and costs much more than ordinary foods containing the same nutrients. It is also touted as an aid to athletic performance, although actual tests on swimmers and runners have shown no benefit.[65] In susceptible individuals, bee pollen can cause anaphylactic shock, a life-threatening allergic reaction in which swelling of the throat can cause suffocation.[66]

Bioflavonoids: Bioflavonoids are promoted as essential for good health. They are claimed to increase resistance to colds and the flu. Scientific tests have shown this claim to be false.[31] Bioflavonoids are sometimes referred to as "vitamin P," but they are neither vitamins nor essential for humans.

Blackstrap molasses: Blackstrap molasses is the dark, less-refined form of molasses. It is less sweet than other syrups and has an unpleasant taste. It is touted as a "wonder food" that can restore hair color and cure anemia. Blackstrap molasses is simply another form of sugar. It cannot reverse the graying of hair. It contains variable amounts of iron; consuming a few tablespoons of molasses at regular intervals can contribute significantly to iron intake. However, iron supplementation should not be done without competent medical advice.

*Bone meal: Powdered bone is claimed to be a rich source of calcium. Actually, its calcium is poorly absorbed. FDA scientists have found that some animal bone meal samples contain high levels of lead, a toxic mineral, as a result of lifelong accumulation in old animals.[67]

Boron: The mineral boron is falsely claimed to be a "supernutrient." It has been said to "end bone disease," increase muscle mass and strength, suppress menopausal hot flashes, increase sexual desire, correct and prevent arthritis, stop memory loss, and prevent or cure osteoporosis. However, there is no reliable evidence that boron supplements can do any of these things.[68] Adequate amounts of boron are readily available from food.

Brewer's yeast: Brewer's yeast is used to ferment carbohydrate in making beer. It is a source of protein and several B vitamins, but it is certainly no miracle food. Most people dislike its taste.

Carob: Carob beans have been cultivated in Mediterranean countries since ancient times. Carob is used in dog biscuits, as a flavoring agent in chewing tobacco, and as a chocolate substitute in confectionery and snack foods. It is lower in fat than chocolate and is caffeine-free, but it is similar in caloric content and does not taste like real chocolate. Claims of wondrous health benefits associated with carob intake are false.

"Catalyst-altered water": This water—also known as "Willard's Water"—is claimed to have been altered by adding special submicroscopic particles of silicone, which form a network of molecules that makes the water more "bioactive." There is no reason to believe that it has any healing properties or is significantly different from normal drinking water.

*Chelated minerals: *Chelate* means "to bind." Minerals in chelated supplements usually are bound to an amino acid,

TABLE 12-4

PRODUCTS COMMONLY SOLD IN HEALTH-FOOD STORES – *CONT'D*.

which may increase the efficiency with which they are absorbed from the intestines and excreted through the kidneys. When chelation increases absorption, it equally increases excretion, so there is no net gain. Individuals with a medically diagnosed need for mineral supplements should not take chelated forms, which are more expensive and may not be as effective.

Chitosan: is derived from chitin, a polysaccharide found in the exoskeleton of shellfish such as shrimp, lobster, and crabs. It is claimed to cause weight loss by binding fats in the intestinal tract and preventing them from being digested and absorbed. Although chitosan may decrease fat absorption, the amount in the products is too small to significantly affect cholesterol levels. There is no evidence that chitosan is effective for weight control.[69]

Chlorophyll: Chlorophyll, the pigment responsible for the green color of plants, helps "trap" the energy from sunlight, enabling the plant to synthesize carbohydrates. Claims that chlorophyll is effective against many diseases and can reduce odors are not substantiated. It can kill certain bacteria but is too weak to have practical use as an antibiotic or a toothpaste additive. Chlorophyll is sometimes said to function as the "blood" of plants, but it does not.

Choline: Not essential in the diets of humans, choline occurs in many foods. Thus, even if people required a dietary source, supplements would be unnecessary. Although research is being conducted concerning choline compounds in the treatment of certain brain disorders, use of supplements will not improve memory or "counter the aging process" as claimed by faddists.

Chromium picolinate: Chromium picolinate is a chromium-containing supplement patented by Gary W. Evans, Ph.D., and claimed to help shed fat and increase muscle mass. Independent research does not support these claims. (Patenting laws do not require proof that claims made for health products are valid.)

Cider vinegar: Vinegar made from apples has long been touted as a cure-all, often together with honey. Cider vinegar is claimed to "keep the body in balance," thin the blood, and aid digestion—none of which is true. Like the supermarket variety, cider vinegar is a condiment (flavoring agent), but the myths surrounding its use should be ignored.

Coenzyme Q_{10}: Preliminary evidence suggests that coenzyme Q_{10}, an enzyme produced in the body, may help keep atherosclerotic plaque from forming by acting as an antioxidant. But there is no evidence that coenzyme Q_{10} supplements prevent aging.[70]

Cold-pressed oils: Most vegetable oils are filtered to remove impurities and have antioxidant preservatives added to prevent rapid spoilage. "Cold-pressed" oils are processed differently but offer no health advantage over oils processed by the usual methods.[71]

Dehydroepiandrosterone (DHEA): "DHEA pills" have been promoted with false claims that they have anti-aging properties and can cause effortless weight loss. In experiments with certain strains of mice, DHEA has blocked tumors and prevented weight gain. Scientists have speculated that declining levels of this adrenal hormone after young adulthood play a role in aging. However, significant dosages can cause unwanted hair growth, liver enlargement, and other adverse effects that make its use impractical. During the mid-1980s several "DHEA" products marketed through health-food stores were found to contain little or no DHEA.[72] In 1985 the FDA ordered manufacturers to stop marketing DHEA products as weight-loss aids.

Desiccated liver: Desiccated liver in pill or powder form contains a number of nutrients. However, it has no advantage over cooked liver and is more expensive.

*Desiccated thyroid: Dried thyroid gland from a pig or cow is available as a prescription drug for treating hypothyroidism (low thyroid function), but responsible physicians rarely prescribe it because its hormonal content can vary from batch to batch; synthetic hormone pills are more reliable. Desiccated thyroid is also an ingredient in some products sold in health-food stores. Dietary supplements containing glandular substances are supposed to be processed so that they contain no active hormone. However, cases have been reported of individuals who ingested toxic amounts of thyroid hormone while self-medicating with such products.

*Dolomite: Dolomite, mined from rocks, contains calcium and magnesium, but in a poorly absorbable form. Lead, arsenic, mercury, and other contaminants have been found in dolomite samples in amounts high enough to cause nerve damage and other health problems.

Enzymes (oral): Many products containing enzymes are claimed to enhance body processes. Enzymes are proteins that act as catalysts in the body. Those present in food are treated in the digestive tract in the same way as any other protein: acid in the stomach and other digestive chemicals reduce them to smaller constituents that are no longer enzymes by the time they are absorbed into the body. The tiny amounts of amino acids oral enzymes provide make no significant nutritional contribution. Pancreatic enzymes have some legitimate medical uses in diseases that cause decreased secretion of pancreatic enzymes into the intestine, but these conditions are not appropriate for self-diagnosis or self-treatment.

Evening primrose oil: Evening primrose oil, which contains gamma-linolenic acid, may be effective against premenstrual discomfort and a few other problems. However, it has not been proven safe for long-term use and is not legally marketable with health claims in the United States. Some products have been adulterated with cheaper oils or were biologically useless due to decomposition.[73]

Fertile eggs: These eggs supposedly have been fertilized by a rooster, while the supermarket varieties have not. Fertilized eggs tend to spoil faster and cost more. Faddists claim that fertilized eggs come from hens that are happier, better adjusted, and more "alive." Nutritionally, however,

TABLE 12-4

PRODUCTS COMMONLY SOLD IN HEALTH-FOOD STORES – *CONT'D.*

they are equivalent. Some faddists claim that brown eggs are nutritionally superior to white eggs. However, egg color is hereditary and has nothing to do with nutrient composition.

Fish-oil capsules: Epidemiologic research has found that Arctic dwellers and others whose diet is rich in certain fatty acids have less heart disease than other Americans or Europeans. Other research has found that supplements of omega-3 fatty acids (found in fish oils) can help lower blood cholesterol levels and inhibit clotting, which means they may be useful in preventing atherosclerotic heart disease but harmful in promoting internal bleeding. However, it is not known what dosage is appropriate or whether long-term use is safe or effective. Most authorities believe it is unwise to self-medicate with fish-oil capsules; they should be used only by individuals at high risk for heart disease who are under close medical supervision. However, eating fish once or twice a week may be beneficial.[74] The FDA has ordered manufacturers to stop making claims that fish-oil capsules are effective against various diseases.

*Germanium: "Organic germanium" is touted as a "miracle drug" for a wide range of health problems. Proponents claim that cancer, heart disease, mental deficiency, and many other problems are due to an "oxygen deficiency" that organic germanium can eradicate. There is no scientific evidence to support these claims.[75] A few germanium compounds have been tested for anti-tumor activity, but no practical application has been found. Although many health-food stores sell germanium products, it is illegal to market them with therapeutic claims. The FDA has banned importation of germanium products intended for human consumption and has seized germanium products from several U.S. manufacturers. Germanium supplements have caused irreversible kidney damage and death.

Glandular extracts: These products, sold as "food supplements," are claimed to cure diseases by augmenting glandular function in the body. Actually, they contain no hormones and therefore have no pharmacologic effect on the body. If they did produce such an effect, they would be dangerous for self-medication.

Granola: Granola is the common term used to describe breakfast cereals and candy bars composed largely of oats plus other grains, dried fruits, seeds, and nuts. Touted as "natural" and rich in nutrients, granola products tend to be high in sugar (usually brown sugar and/or honey), fats (from vegetable oils, nuts, seeds, and coconut), and calories.

Guarana: An herb that contains a significant amount of caffeine, a fact that is sometimes omitted on product labels.

Inositol: Contrary to popular claims, supplements of inositol will not alleviate baldness, reduce blood cholesterol levels, or aid in weight loss. Inositol is not a B vitamin, and the body can manufacture all it needs. Even if it were a vitamin, supplements would be unnecessary because it is readily available in our food supply.

*Kelp: Kelp is a seaweed common in the Japanese diet. Tablets of kelp are prepared from dried seaweed and promoted in health-food stores as a weight-reduction aid; a rich source of iodide; an energy booster; and a "natural" cure for certain ailments, including goiter (enlargement of the thyroid gland). Kelp is high in iodine, a mineral needed to prevent goiter. However, iodized salt furnishes an adequate supply of this mineral at a fraction of the cost of kelp. Excess iodine can be detrimental.

Lecithin: Lecithin is manufactured by the liver and occurs in many foods, including soybeans, whole grains, and egg yolks. Claims that lecithin supplements can dissolve blood cholesterol, rid the bloodstream of undesirable fats, cure arthritis, improve brain power, and aid in weight reduction are unsupported by scientific evidence.

*Melatonin: Melatonin is a hormone produced from the amino acid L-tryptophan by the pineal gland, a small structure near the center of the brain. Its secretion increases when it is dark, which signals the body that it is time to sleep. In most people, blood levels peak near puberty and steadily decline with age. Melatonin products appear to improve some people's sleep and protect against "jet lag," but no clinical trials have been conducted. The effective dose is usually less than 0.1 to 0.3 mg, which is far below the 2 to 3 mg doses commonly sold in health-food stores. Claims that melatonin supplements can improve sex life, protect against many diseases, or reverse the aging process are un-substantiated. Adverse reactions have been reported, and it is not known whether melatonin is safe for long-term use.[76]

Octacosanol: This substance, found in wheat germ oil and many other plant oils, is not essential in the human diet. Claims that it improves stamina and endurance, reduces blood cholesterol, and helps reproduction have not been substantiated.

PABA (para-aminobenzoic acid): PABA is a vitamin for bacteria, but not for humans. It is claimed that oral dosages can prevent or reverse the graying of hair, but no scientific evidence supports this claim.

Papain: Papain, an enzyme present in papaya extract, is promoted as a cure for gum disease and an aid to digestion and weight-reduction. When taken by mouth, papain is rapidly destroyed in the digestive tract. Its only significant use is as a meat tenderizer; it can be added to meats before they are consumed and while the enzyme is still chemically active.

*Propolis: Propolis ("bee glue") is a resinous material bees collect and use to fill cracks in their hives. It has mild antibacterial properties but has not been scientifically demonstrated to have practical use as a medication. Skin inflammation has occurred among users of cosmetics containing propolis, and mouth ulcers have been reported following the use of propolis-containing lozenges.

*Protein supplements: Protein powders, tablets, and liquids have been advertised as strength-promoting and especially important to athletes. These claims are incorrect. The RDA for protein is easily obtained by eating a well-balanced diet. Supplements provide no additional benefit and,

TABLE 12-4

PRODUCTS COMMONLY SOLD IN HEALTH-FOOD STORES – *CONT'D.*

in large amounts, can cause nutritional imbalances and kidney problems.[77]

Raw milk: Raw milk is milk in its natural (non-pasteurized) state. Pasteurization is done to destroy any disease-producing bacteria that may be present. Health faddists claim that it destroys essential nutrients. Although about 10% to 30% of the heat-sensitive vitamins (vitamin C and thiamine) are destroyed in the pasteurizing process, milk is not a significant source of these nutrients. Contaminated raw milk can be a source of harmful bacteria, such as those that cause undulant fever, dysentery, salmonellosis, and tuberculosis. "Certified" milk, obtained from cows certified as healthy, is unpasteurized milk with a bacteria count below a specified standard, but it still can contain significant numbers of disease-producing organisms. The risks of raw milk are not related to mishandling; thus the only way to avoid them is not to consume the product. In 1987 the FDA ordered that milk and milk products in final-package form for human consumption in interstate commerce be pasteurized. The sale of raw milk has been banned in about half the states. It is legal within California, which harbors the largest raw-milk seller.

Resveratrol: This compound, found largely in the skins of red grapes, is touted as an antioxidant and a phyto-estrogen. Laboratory tests have demonstrated that it may help prevent cardiovascular disease and cancer, However, further studies in animals and humans are necessary to determine whether resveratrol supplementation makes sense.[78]

RNA/DNA: Supplements of these genetic materials are claimed to rejuvenate old cells, improve memory, and prevent skin wrinkling. When taken orally, they are inactivated by the digestive process. Even if they could be absorbed and reach the cells, they would not work because human cells utilize human nucleic acids, not those from lower animals. Ingesting large amounts can raise blood uric acid levels, which can cause problems.

Royal jelly: Royal jelly is food for queen bees. Claimed to increase endurance, it has been recommended for athletes. It is also advertised as rich in calcium pantothenate (claimed to be "vitamin B5"), a supposed antioxidant-antistress nutrient used also in "miracle" skin creams and hair tonics. These claims are unsubstantiated.

Rutin: A chemical related to the bioflavonoids, rutin is not a vitamin for humans. It is illegal for supplement labels to carry nutritional claims for rutin, but it is often included in multivitamins by sellers who wish to create the impression that their product is "more complete."

Sea salt: Proponents of sea salt claim that it is unrefined and therefore more nutritious than ordinary salt, but actually it is refined to remove impurities. Sea salt contains as much sodium as table salt and also variable amounts of iodine, but table salt can have the advantage of being iodized with the correct dose. Salts said to be "seawater concentrates" have been marketed with false claims that they can cure cancer, diabetes, and many other diseases.

Spirulina: Spirulina is a blue-green alga, some species of which have been used as a dietary staple in several parts of the world. Spirulina is similar to soybeans in nutrient content. It contains protein of fair quality plus some other nutrients, but nothing that cannot be obtained much less expensively and more hygienically from conventional foods. Despite proponents' claims, spirulina has no value as a weight-reduction aid or as a remedy for any disease. Law enforcement agencies have ordered several companies to stop making illegal therapeutic claims for spirulina products, but others continue to do so. Some products sold as "spirulina" contain no spirulina, and some have been found to be contaminated with insect parts, other filth,[8] and toxins called microcystins.[79]

Superoxide dismutase (SOD): SOD is an enzyme promoted as an "antioxidant" that supposedly protects body tissues against environmental contaminants, heart disease, cancer, and arthritis. The body has its own supply of functioning antioxidants, including various enzymes and vitamins C and E. Enzymes taken orally are digested in the gastrointestinal tract.

Wheat germ: Wheat germ is a source of protein, several B vitamins, vitamin E, some minerals, and fiber. It is neither a cure-all nor a dietary essential. It is amply provided in whole wheat products. As a supplement, it is relatively high in calories and cost.

Wheat grass juice: A juice, made from sprouted wheat berries, said to be high in chlorophyll and claimed to "cleanse" the body, neutralize toxins, slow the aging process, and prevent cancer. Its principal proponent, the late Ann Wigmore, attributed these supposed benefits to enzymes in the plant that supplement the body's enzymes when ingested. These claims are false. The enzymes in foods are not absorbed into the body but are digested like other proteins. Even if they could be absorbed intact, enzymes from plants would not enhance the metabolic processes of humans.

Zinc gluconate. A study published in 1996 sharply boosted sales of zinc gluconate lozenges for treating colds. The study compared 50 patients who used them with 50 who took a placebo.[80] The zinc dosage was 13.3 mg every 2 hours with an average of six per day. Blinding was not perfect, however, because the zinc lozenges tasted more astringent than the placebos. The zinc-treated patients had fewer cold symptoms but had higher frequencies of bad taste, mouth irritation, and nausea. Complete symptom resolution (as reported by the patients) took 4.4 days for the zinc group and 7.6 for the control group. The *Medical Letter* reviewed seven other studies and concluded that three had positive results and four found no benefit. It concluded: "Treatment with large doses of zinc might decrease the symptoms and shorted the duration of the common cold, but properly blinded confirmatory studies are needed. The long-term safety of taking zinc in doses higher than the Recommended Dietary Allowances has not been established."[81] (The adult RDAs are 15 mg for men and 12 mg for women.)

Purposes and Safety of Food Additives

A few basic facts about additive processing should reassure consumers. About 2800 substances are intentionally added to foods for one or more of the following reasons:

- *Maintain or improve nutritional value*: Vitamins and minerals may be added to enrich (replace those lost in processing) or fortify (add nutrients that may be lacking in the diet). In enriched bread, for example, iron, thiamin, and niacin are restored to the levels found in whole wheat, and riboflavin is added to a higher level.
- *Maintain product quality*: Preservatives are used to prevent food spoilage due to bacteria, molds, and yeast; extend shelf life; protect food against undesirable changes in color and flavor; and protect food fats from becoming rancid.
- *Aid in preparation*: Emulsifiers, stabilizers, thickeners, texturizers, and anti-caking agents improve the homogeneity, consistency, stability, texture, and "mouthfeel" of food; leavening agents affect baking results; pH control agents affect acidity and alkalinity; humectants cause moisture retention; maturing and bleaching agents and dough conditioners improve the quality of baked goods.
- *Improve taste or appearance*: Flavor enhancers, flavors, and sweeteners may alter the original taste and/or aroma or restore flavor lost in processing; colors may make foods more appealing.

The most widely used additives are sugar, salt, and corn syrup—all found naturally. These three, plus citric acid (found naturally in oranges and lemons), baking soda, vegetable colors, mustard, and pepper, account for 98% of all food additives by weight used in the United States.[82]

To promote "natural" foods, the health-food industry alleges that too many chemicals are added to our foods. The important issue, however, is not the number of chemicals, but whether they are safe and serve useful purposes. It is illogical to condemn additives with sweeping generalizations; the only proper way to evaluate them is individually. This is the responsibility of the FDA, which has paid a great deal of attention to this matter. Food additives have survived stringent evaluation procedures not applied to the great majority of natural products. To remain in use, additives must be judged not only safe but also functionally important. During the early 1980s, a USDA committee ranked food additives eighth on a list of 10 areas of food safety that deserved further research.[83]

To protect consumers, the FDA sets tolerance levels in foods and conducts frequent "market basket" studies wherein foods from regions throughout the United States are purchased and analyzed. The most recent study found that 63.7% of 9438 fruits, vegetables, and other domestic or imported foods had no detectable pesticide residues. Violative levels were found in only 0.8% of the domestic foods and 3.1% of the imported ones.[56] The agency's annual Total Diet Study found that dietary intakes of pesticides for all population groups were well within international and Environmental Protection Agency standards.

In 1997 *Consumer Reports* purchased about 1000 pounds of tomatoes, peaches, green bell peppers, and apples in five cities and tested them for more than 300 synthetic pesticides. Traces were detected in 77% of conventional foods and 25% of organically labeled foods, but only one sample of each exceeded the federal limit.[84]

Food Industry Involvement

Dr. Elizabeth Whelan,[85] president of the American Council on Science and Health, has noted:

Many of our country's largest and most respected food companies have jumped on the back-to-nature bandwagon. Today the words "natural" and "additive-free" are applied to almost every type of edible product. Even beer and candy bars (so-called "health bars") bear these magic words. . . .

Companies that exploit the growing public fear of additives may make windfall profits—but they also ignore their responsibility to the American public. Promoting accurate nutrition information and exposing food faddism would be much more commendable actions.

Many supermarkets are competing directly with health-food stores by maintaining "nutrition centers" or sections for "natural" foods and food supplements. Some manufacturers of baby foods have marketed "organic" products that cost considerably more than their standard foods.

"MEDICINAL" USE OF HERBAL PRODUCTS

Herbal remedies have been used throughout history. The Persians, Romans, Greeks, Hebrews, and Babylonians were familiar with the practice of herbal medicine. By trial and error, accident or design, people concluded that certain roots, plants, barks, and seeds possessed medicinal properties. In the second century BCE the Egyptians used myrrh, cumin, peppermint, caraway, fennel, and oil of cloves for various ailments. Licorice was especially esteemed. Sarsaparilla, the dried root of the similax, a climbing vine native to tropical regions of the Americas, was introduced in Europe in the 16th century as a tonic for venereal disease and later for chronic rheumatism, scrofula, and skin disease. In the latter part of the 19th century its use as a medicine was abandoned, but it became popular as a syrup for soft drinks.

Although a few plant substances have been used in modern medical practice, most have been replaced by products that are safer or more effective or have fewer unpleasant side effects. For example, reserpine, found naturally in snakeroot (rauwolfia), was one of the earliest effective remedies against high blood pressure and was used extensively during the 1950s and 1960s until better synthetic drugs were developed. Curare, used to paralyze muscles during surgical procedures, has been replaced by synthetic derivatives. Foxglove leaves contain digitalis, a drug used to treat heart failure and abnormal heart rhythms. But the use of dried leaves has given way to extracts and synthetic drugs whose dosages are precisely controlled.

Today, Americans spend billions of dollars per year for capsules, tablets, bulk herbs, and herbal teas used for supposed medicinal qualities. Most are purchased over-the-counter, but some are prescribed by practitioners. Many herbs contain hundreds or even thousands of chemicals that have not been completely catalogued. While some may ultimately prove useful as therapeutic agents, others could well prove toxic. Most herbal products sold in the United States are not standardized, which means that determining the exact amounts of their ingredients can be difficult or impossible. Moreover, many herbal practitioners are nonphysicians who are not qualified to make appropriate diagnoses or to determine how herbs compare to proven drugs.

Many herbal products are marketed as "dietary supplements," even though they have little or no nutritional value. No legal standards exist for their processing, harvesting, or packaging. In many cases, particularly for products with expensive raw ingredients, contents and potency are not accurately disclosed on the label. Many products marketed as herbs contain no useful ingredients, and some even lack the principal ingredient for which people buy them. Some manufacturers are trying to develop industrywide quality-assurance standards, but possible solutions are a long way off.

Herbs in their natural state can vary greatly from batch to batch and often contain chemicals that cause side effects but provide no benefit. Surveys conducted in the United States have found that the ingredients and doses of various products vary considerably from brand to brand and even between lots of the same product.[86] For example, researchers at the University of Arkansas tested 20 "supplement" products containing ephedra (ma huang) and found that half the products exhibited discrepancies of 20% or more between the label claim and the actual content, and one product contained no ephedra alkaloids. Ephedra products are marketed as "energy boosters" and/or "thermogenic" diet aids, even though no published clinical trials substantiate that they are safe or effective for these purposes. The researchers also noted that hundreds of such products are marketed and that their number exceeds that of conventional prescription and nonprescription ephedra products, which are FDA-approved as decongestants.[87]

To make a rational decision about an herbal product, it would be necessary to know what it contains, whether it is safe, and whether it has been demonstrated to be as good or better than pharmaceutical products available for the same purpose. For most herbal ingredients this information is incomplete or unavailable.

"Popularity" is not a reliable sign of effectiveness. In 1999, *Consumer Reports* asked its readers in the United States and Canada to rate the standard and "complementary" therapies they had used most often for the two most serious or bothersome medical conditions they had encountered during the previous 2 years. Prescription drugs scored significantly better than herbs for each of the reported problems where both were used.[88]

Even when a botanical product has some effectiveness, it may not be practical to use. Garlic, for example, has been demonstrated to lower cholesterol. However, prescription drugs are more potent for this purpose, and garlic has anticoagulant properties. No data are available to indicate the risk of combining garlic with other widely used products (vitamin E, ginkgo, fish oil, and aspirin) that can interfere with blood clotting.

The best source of information about herbs is the Natural Medicines Comprehensive Database, which is available online (http://www.naturaldatabase.com) and in print for $92 per year (or $132 for both versions). The online version is updated daily, while the print version is updated several times a year. The 1999 book covered 964 herbs and dietary supplements, of which only 15% had been proven safe and only 11% had been proven effective. Another excellent resource is the *Professional's Handbook of Complementary & Alternative Medicines*,[89] which provides practical advice for over 300 herbs. The widely touted *Commission E Report* and its derivative, the *PDR for Herbal Medicine*, are not as reliable or practical.

The recent entry of drug companies into the herbal marketplace may result in standardization of dosage for some products, and recent public and professional interest in herbs is likely to stimulate more research. However, with safe and effective medicines available, treatment with herbs rarely makes sense, and many of the conditions for which herbs are recommended are not suitable for self-treatment.

TABLE 12-5

12 POPULAR HERBAL PRODUCTS

Cat's claw. Although cat's claw appears to have potential for treating certain viral and inflammtory diseases, more clinical research is needed to determine its effectiveness and long-term safety.[89]

Echinacea. Test-tube evidence suggests that echinacea stimulates immune processes. Taking echinacea at the first sign of a cold may reduce the infection's duration, but most studies have not found echinacea able to prevent colds. Echinacea should not be taken by people with an autoimmune disease (such as type 1 diabetes, rheumatoid arthritis, or multiple sclerosis) or a disease that causes immune suppression.

Garlic. Allicin, a component of garlic, has been shown to inhibit the production of cholesterol by the liver. Population studies have found an association between lower cholesterol levels and increased intake of garlic, onions, and related vegetables. However, most well-designed clinical trials have not found a cholesterol-lowering benefit for garlic supplements, and its anticoagulation property may undesirably enhance that of other blood-thinners.

Ginkgo biloba. Ginkgo biloba contains compounds that can increase blood flow to the brain. A 1997 clinical trial found that patients with dementia caused by small strokes or Alzheimer's disease who took 120 mg of ginkgo extract a day scored modestly higher in mental performance tests and had a slightly delayed mental decline than those who took a placebo.[90] There is no evidence that ginkgo will cure or prevent Alzheimer's disease or will generally improve mental sharpness or memory. Ginkgo's anticoagulation property may undesirably enhance that of other blood-thinners.

Ginseng. Ginseng may help improve sleep, appetite, and work efficiency. However, it can raise blood pressure and many ginseng products contain little or none of the active ingredient.

Goldenseal. Goldenseal is claimed to have anti-inflammatory, anti-hemorrhagic, and laxative properties. It has many adverse effects; and its use is not supported by adequate research.[89]

Green tea. Epidemiologic and animal studies suggest that green tea may help prevent atherosclerosis. However, clinical trials are needed to accurately assess its usefulness.

Kava. Small studies suggest that kava may be useful for treating anxiety, stress, and restlessness. However, chronic, heavy use can cause adverse effects. Additional studies are needed.

Milk thistle. Studies suggest that milk-thistle extract may have a useful role in treating various liver diseases. However, most of the supporting research has not been well-designed.[89]

Saw palmetto. Saw palmetto may relieve symptoms of benign enlargement of the prostate gland, such as slow urine flow, which is common in older men. A 1998 review of 18 clinical trials found that about 75% of those who used saw palmetto for 2 months reported an improvement.[90] However, a survey of *Consumer Reports* readers found that about half improved, compared with about 75% of prescription drug users.[91]

St. John's wort. St. John's wort is widely promoted as an antidepressant. Its mechanism of action is unknown, and the active ingredient, if any, has not been ascertained. A few studies have found it somewhat more effective than a standard antidepressant, but none lasted more than 6 weeks, some were poorly designed, and significant side effects and adverse drug interactions have been reported. NIH is sponsoring a long-term study that should help determine whether its use is practical. St. John's wort should not be combined with standard antidepressants or used by women who are pregnant or are breastfeeding. A Good Housekeeping Institute analysis of six widely available St. John's wort supplement capsules and four liquid extracts revealed a lack of consistency of the suspected active ingredients, hypericin and pseudohypericin. The study found a 17-fold difference between the capsules containing the smallest and the largest amounts of hypericin, based on the manufacturer's maximum recommended dosage.[92]

Valerian. Valerian appears to exert mild sedative-hypnotic effects, but most supportive studies have been methodologically flawed. A U.S. Pharmacopeia expert panel has determined that there is not enough evidence to support its use for treating insomnia.[93]

The National Council Against Health Fraud believes that the FDA should correct this situation by establishing a special category of over-the-counter drugs called "Traditional Herbal Remedies." This would permit these products to be marketed with less-than-standard proof of effectiveness provided: (a) reasonable evidence exists that they are safe and effective; (b) labels identify the name and quantity of each active ingredient; (d) indications are restricted to nonserious, self-limiting conditions; (d) labels contain adequate directions for use, including a warning about inappropriate self-treatment; and (e) adverse reactions are reported.[94]

Herbal teas may have a single ingredient or may be blends of as many as 20 different kinds of leaves, seeds, and flowers. *The Medical Letter* has identified the following as potentially troublesome: buckthorn bark, burdock root, catnip, chamomile, devil's claw root, ginseng, horsetail, hydrangea, Indian tobacco, jimsonweed, juniper berries, licorice root, lobelia, mistletoe, nutmeg, pokeweed (especially the root), sassafras root bark, senna leaves, shave grass, and wormwood.[95] A 1993 FDA report stated that chaparral, comfrey, germander, jin bu huan, lobelia, ma huang, willow bark, and yohimbe have been associated with illness or injury.[96] Pennyroyal, taken with the hope of inducing menstruation or an abortion, has caused serious toxicity and death.[97]

MACROBIOTIC DIETS

Macrobiotics is a quasireligious philosophical system founded by the late George Ohsawa. (Macrobiotic means "way of long life.") The system advocates a vegetarian diet in which foods of animal origin are used as condiments rather than as full-fledged menu items. The optimal diet is achieved by balancing "yin" and "yang" foods. Ohsawa outlined a 10-stage "Zen" macrobiotic diet in which each stage is progressively more restrictive. The diet was alleged to enable individuals to overcome all forms of illness, which Ohsawa said were due to excesses in diet.

In 1971 the AMA Council on Foods and Nutrition said that followers of the diet, particularly the highest level, stood in "great danger" of malnutrition, and that several deaths had been reported.[98]

Current proponents espouse a diet that is less restrictive but still can be nutritionally inadequate. They recommend whole grains (50% to 60% of each meal), vegetables (25% to 30% of each meal), whole beans or soybean-based products (5% to 10% of daily food), nuts and seeds (small amounts as snacks), miso soup, herbal teas, and small amounts of white meat or seafood once or twice a week.

Today's leading proponent is Michio Kushi, a former student of Ohsawa, who founded and heads the Kushi Institute in Becket, Massachusetts. Institute publications recommend chewing food at least 50 times per mouthful (or until it becomes liquid), not wearing synthetic or woolen clothing next to the skin, avoiding long hot baths or showers (unless you have been consuming too much salt or animal food), having large green plants in your house to enrich the oxygen content of the air, and singing a happy song every day.

Kushi[99] claims that macrobiotic eating can help prevent cancer and many other diseases. He also presents case histories of people whose cancers have supposedly disappeared after they adopted the macrobiotic diet. Dwyer[100] states that there is no scientific evidence of benefit, and that the diet itself can cause cancer patients to undergo serious weight loss. Raso,[101] who attended a macrobiotic seminar for professionals, reported that astrologic conditions, weather conditions, and a long list of other bizarre factors were said to be relevant to diagnosing patients. Lindner[102] had a private consultation at the Institute as part of an assignment for *American Health* magazine. After examining Lindner's face,

the practitioner stated that Lindner's kidneys were weak, he was slightly hypoglycemic, and his heart was enlarged because he ate too much fruit. He was also told that deposits of fat and mucus were starting to build up on his intestines.

PROMOTION OF QUESTIONABLE NUTRITION

Food faddism is promoted through practitioners, health resorts, retail establishments, trade organizations, and media outlets. Roth[103] notes that many of the activities of food faddists parallel those of scientific nutrition advocates.

Freedom of speech and freedom of the press make it legal for anyone to make false or unproven health claims about a product as long as the claims are not made while selling the product. Most claims directed to the public about health foods and related products are not found on labels (where they would be illegal) but reach consumers through other channels of communication.

Unsubstantiated claims appear in newspapers, magazines, books, newsletters, pamphlets, lectures, and on radio and television talk shows. Many of those who make the claims have no direct connection with supplement manufacturers, while others are paid as "consultants." Retailers absorb misinformation from health-food magazines, trade publications, materials distributed by manufacturers, and seminars sponsored by trade organizations. Many health-food stores display or distribute free literature (newsletters, flyers, and article reprints) containing claims that would be illegal on product labels. Illegal oral claims are made quite often in the privacy of health-food stores, practitioners' offices, and customers' homes (by multilevel distributors, as described in Chapter 4). Products are also promoted through the use of pseudodiagnostic tests that supposedly detect vitamin and mineral deficiencies, allergies, or "imbalances."

Between 1986 and 1990 the American Dietetic Association collected more than 500 case reports of people harmed by inappropriate nutrition advice from bogus "nutritionists," health-food store operators, and others. Privacy considerations, however, prevented the association from performing a detailed analysis.

Books

In 1996 an estimated $267 million was spent for books purchased in health-food stores. The amount spent for similar books in bookstores and other outlets has not been calculated but is probably larger. Nutri-Books, the largest wholesale distributor, stocks more than 2000

Some Roots of Today's Food Faddism

Nutrition-related fads and myths have existed throughout the ages. It has been alleged that foods can sustain or interfere with general health and that many foods can cause or cure various illnesses. Although the science of nutrition offers the potential to curb faddism, the parallel development of mass communication has enabled faddists to reach vast audiences of unsuspecting people.

Food faddism's basic premise, traceable to ancient times, is that diet is the *primal* factor in health, disease, intellect, behavior, and mortality. Many cultures have believed that "we are what we eat." The ancient doctrine of correspondences held that "like is like" or that "like produces like." Thus eating a tiger's heart would produce courage, and eating its genitals would enhance virility.

The ancient Egyptians believed that all diseases were caused by what people ate and that dietary regimens were curative. They preserved corpses so that a winged creature could recognize them and carry their soul to the sun god for eternal circulation in the heavens. Believing that the anus was the center for disease and decay, the Egyptians were also preoccupied with enemas, drenches (drinking large quantities of water), and bowel movements to cleanse the colon.

The Greeks ate grasshoppers for liver disorders and believed that fevers were helped by eating seven bugs from the skin of a bear. The Romans thought lettuce cleansed the senses, garlic gave physical strength, and truffles increased sexual potency. They also believed that good health came only with sacrifice, discomfort, self-discipline, and dour attitudes—concepts still common among faddists.

"Modern" food faddism began with the preaching of Sylvester Graham (1794–1851), who mixed religion with a zeal for the natural, "uncomplicated" life. Graham was ordained as a Presbyterian minister in 1826 but was influenced by Philadelphia's Bible Christian Church. He practiced homeopathy and lectured on temperance, cholera, fresh air, bathing, and sexual restraint. He was one of the first American "health reformers" to reach large audiences. His initial focus on the evils of alcohol soon expanded to other health concerns. "The simpler, plainer, and more natural the food," he said, "the more healthy, vigorous, and long-lived will be the body." Among the prohibited foods were salt and other condiments (these and sexual excesses caused insanity), cooked vegetables (against God's law), and chicken pies (caused cholera).

Graham's most vigorous attacks were against "unnatural" substances such as meat, white-flour products, and water consumed at mealtimes. He also claimed that people did not bathe enough and needed external applications of cold water at least weekly. Partly

because of his advocacy, Saturday night baths and setting-up exercises before open windows became common practices. Although Graham died at the early age of 57, the cracker that bears his name is still with us.

James Caleb Jackson (1811–1895) was a farmer before he became a physician by apprenticeship. His health had failed due to heart and kidney trouble and dyspepsia. He attributed his recovery to drinking 30 to 40 glasses of water daily. In 1858 he opened a sanitarium to provide his "water cures" both internally and externally. At this facility women were encouraged to wear bloomers (the standard reformist dress) instead of a corset. They were also relieved of their false hair; fed fruits, Graham crackers, and bread; and urged to take naps and walks. Jackson also advocated phrenology and vegetarianism. To supplement the Graham crackers, he prepared broken bits of rock-hard baked wheat with water, which he called *Granula.* He also marketed a cereal coffee called *So Mo* and several other items. These may have been the first prominent "health foods" sold in the United States.[104]

John Harvey Kellogg (1852–1943) reportedly ate his way through medical school on a diet of apples and Graham crackers. He belonged to a Seventh-day Adventist group that had founded a religious colony and health sanitarium at Battle Creek, Michigan. He and his brother Will were probably the first to make $1 million from food faddism. Under John Harvey's leadership, the Battle Creek Sanitarium attracted hordes of wealthy clients whose intestines he "detoxified" with enemas and high-fiber diets. His 1217-page book, *Rational Hydrotherapy,* recommended a "water cure" for virtually every known ailment.

While trying to develop a dried bread product upon which his clients could exercise their teeth without breaking them, Kellogg hit upon the idea of a wheat flake. By 1899 the flakes had evolved into a cereal-based company that soon had many competitors. One was Charles W. Post, a former Kellogg patient, who ground up wheat and barley loaves, called his new product "grape nuts," and marketed it as a cure for appendicitis, malaria, consumption (tuberculosis), and loose teeth. Their enterprises were the roots of two of today's giant cereal producers: the Kellogg Company and the Post Division of General Foods (now part of Philip Morris).

Bernarr Macfadden (1868–1955) was the first faddist to use mass-media techniques to amass a fortune (see Chapter 14). He taught that medical care (which he steadfastly avoided) should be rejected in favor of "natural" methods.

D.C. Jarvis, M.D. (1881–1966), wrote that body alkalinity was the principal threat to American health

Historical Perspective

Some Roots of Today's Food Faddism - *Cont'd.*

and that honey and apple cider were the antidotes. False claims in his book—which is still widely sold—were the basis for an FDA seizure of a product called *Honegar.*

Gayelord Hauser (1895–1984) promised to add years to people's life with five wonder foods: skim milk, brewer's yeast, wheat germ, yogurt, and blackstrap molasses. He lectured frequently and was a partner in Modern Products, Inc., of Milwaukee, Wisconsin, a company that markets products bearing his name. Hauser wrote a syndicated newspaper column and more than a dozen books reported to have sold close to 50 million copies here and abroad. One book, *Look Younger, Live Longer*, led the bestseller list in 1951. That same year, the FDA seized copies of the book, claiming they were being used to promote sales of blackstrap molasses as a cure-all. The court readily agreed that the molasses was misbranded by many false claims in the book.

Adolphus Hohensee (1901–1967) began his training in nutrition with a job as a soda jerk. After dabbling in real estate (with time in jail for mail fraud) and the field of transportation (during which time he was arrested for passing bad checks), Hohensee resumed his education. In 1943 he acquired an Honorary Degree of Doctor of Medicine from a nonaccredited school and followed this with Doctor of Naturopathy degrees from two schools that he did not attend. In 1946 he acquired a chiropractic license in the state of Nevada.

A master showman, Hohensee could lecture for hours about the terrible American diet that would stagnate the blood, corrode blood vessels, erode the kidneys, and clog the intestines. He said that most people had intestinal worms, which, fortunately, could be cured by his special cleansing. He promised a long life to those who consumed his wonder products. Repeated prosecution by the FDA made him more cautious about selling his products during lectures, but his promotion of the gamut of food myths sent his audiences flocking to nearby health-food stores whose shelves just happened to be well-stocked with his product line.

In 1955, alert reporters caught Hohensee eating a meal of forbidden foods after one of his lectures. In 1962 he began serving an 18-month prison term for selling honey with false claims. But neither of these setbacks dampened his enthusiasm or that of his loyal followers.

Lelord Kordel (b. 1904), author of about 20 books, recommended high-protein foods, lecithin ("the miracle nutrient"), and high-dosage vitamin and mineral supplements for everyone. Court records state that he began producing and marketing supplements in 1941, operating under various trade names. In 1946 he was convicted of misbranding and fined $4,000. One product in the case was *Gotu Kola*, an herbal tablet said to restore youth and "produce erect posture, sharp eyes, velvety skin, limbs of splendid proportions, deep chests, firm bodies, gracefully curved hips, flat abdomens" and even "pleasing laughter." Thirteen other products were falsely claimed to be effective against various conditions including heart disease, liver troubles, tuberculosis, bone infections, and impotence.

Kordel had a brush with the FTC in 1957 and two more with the FDA in 1961. In 1963, when he was president of Detroit Vital Foods, Inc., products shipped by the company were found to be misbranded because they were accompanied by Kordel publications which falsely claimed that nutritional products could treat practically all diseases. After the appeals process ended in 1971, Kordel was fined $10,000 and served 1 year in prison. Recent catalogs from Vital Foods, Inc., describe him as "America's leading vitamin and diet expert" and claim that he has never been ill.

During the 1950s and early 1960s government agencies carried out more than 200 successful actions against misbranding. Several prominent faddists were sentenced to prison, and the courts ruled that any false message given in the context of a sale could be considered part of a product's labeling. The budding health-food industry soon reorganized to get around the law. Most supplement manufacturers stopped labeling their products as effective against specific diseases. Industry emphasis shifted somewhat from "miracle" drugs to "nutrition insurance," an approach that tends to attract little regulatory attention. "Specialization" developed whereby most publicists have no direct financial tie to the sale of specific products. This enables their claims to be protected by the doctrines of freedom of speech and freedom of the press.

---

titles, most of which promote questionable health ideas and products. Its merchandising manuals, distributed to health-food retailers, have stated:

Books and articles created the nutritional foods industry. . . . They are the number one product-promoters of our industry. Books and magazines are your "silent sales force". . . . Books tell your customers what your products will do. They ex-

plain the ways your products may be used. Very often this is information you may not be able to give—or may not be permitted to discuss. . . . Magazines pack a double wallop. Their articles sell products, and so do their ads.[105]

The health-food industry is well-organized to promote and capitalize on popular books. *Life Extension*, a bestseller in 1982 and 1983, was based on the medically unacceptable premise that the results of animal experiments can be extrapolated to help humans live to the age of 150. The book's publisher advertised that authors Durk Pearson and Sandy Shaw had appeared on the Merv Griffin Show 12 times. A Nutri-Books newsletter for health-food stores provided the dates and locations of other TV talk show appearances so that the stores would stock the book. *Health Foods Business*, which reports industry trends, noted that sales of "antioxidants, moisturizers and antiaging products" increased following publication of the book. Many companies designed new products to take advantage of the book's popularity. Pearson and Shaw now license several lines of nutritional products based on their formulations.

Similarly, publication in 1985 of *Dr. Berger's Immune Power Diet*, combined with public concern about AIDS, stimulated the health-food industry to market dozens of products that supposedly boost the immune system. *Consumer Reports* has expressed skepticism toward "immune-booster" and "life-extension" products.[70,106]

The book most widely used as a sales tool today is *Prescription for Nutritional Healing* by urologist James Balch, M.D., and his wife Phyllis A. Balch, "C.N.C." The book's jacket describes Dr. Balch as a urologist who "has helped patients to assume a portion of responsibility for their own well-being" and Mrs. Balch as a "certified nutrition consultant" who works in her husband's practice and has established a health-food store. The "C.N.C." designation is a dubious credential issued by the American Association of Nutritional Consultants, an organization whose only requirement for professional membership is payment of $50.[107] The book lists nutrients that are "essential," "very important," or "helpful"

for more than 250 health problems. Some lists contain more than 30 items. The authors recommend daily dosages of 3000 mg or more of vitamin C for everybody ("for maintaining good health") and higher doses (up to 30,000 mg/day "under a doctor's supervision") for dozens of problems. They also recommend daily dosages of vitamin A ranging from 50,000 to 100,000 IU for many conditions, and 75,000 IU for "maintaining healthy eyes." The vitamin C dosages are high enough to produce severe diarrhea; the vitamin A dosages are high enough to cause liver injury.

The most prolific publisher of unscientific health and nutrition information is Keats Publishing, of New Canaan, Connecticut. Established in 1971, it has issued more than 400 books, of which over 200 are still in print. It has also published more than 100 "Good Health Guides," booklets that focus on products or product categories.

Periodicals

It is illegal for manufacturers to make therapeutic claims for products that are not recognized by experts as safe and effective for their intended use. For example, it would be illegal for a manufacturer to claim that a vitamin C product could prevent colds or that a mineral mixture could cure impotence. However, it is legal for claims of this type to be made in articles written by "independent" authors. Many specialized magazines, newsletters, and newspapers cater to supplement manufacturers through articles promoting the ingredients of their products. Claims in these articles—no matter how farfetched—are protected by the doctrine of freedom of the press as long as there is no direct connection between the author and the manufacturer. In some

FIGURE 12-2. Ads for publications that promote the products sold in health-food stores. The cartoons remind retailers that "independent" publications can convey information that would be illegal for retailers (and product labels) to provide directly. The Nutri-Books brochure depicts how books "call out" to customers. The ad for *Nutrition News* (a newsletter) promises that "educated" customers will buy more products and that "well informed, enthusiastic employees" will sell more products.

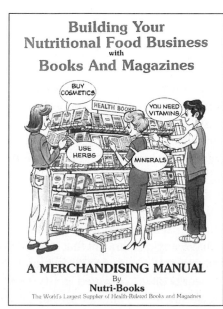

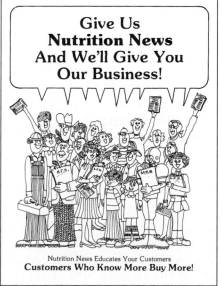

periodicals, ads for supplement products are placed on pages adjacent to articles boosting their ingredients. Figure 12-2 illustrates how retailers are encouraged to use books and periodicals to promote their products.

Health-Food Stores

Health Foods Business estimated that in 1996 there were 9789 health-food stores in America with total gross sales of $9.8 billion, including $3 billion for vitamins and other supplements.[108] No special knowledge or training is required to become a salesperson. Personnel in these stores typically obtain information by reading books and magazines that promote supplement products for the treatment of virtually all health problems. Retailers also get information from manufacturers and can attend seminars at trade shows sponsored by industry groups and trade magazines.[109] Barrett and Herbert[8] characterize health-food stores as "centers of misinformation."

Although storekeepers cannot legally "diagnose" or "prescribe," they commonly do both. Investigators from the American Council on Science and Health demonstrated this in 1983 by making 105 inquiries at stores in three states. When asked about symptoms characteristic of glaucoma, 17 out of 24 suggested a wide variety of products for a person not present; none recognized that urgent medical care was needed. Asked by telephone about a sudden, unexplained 15-pound weight loss in 1 month's time, nine out of 17 recommended products sold in their store; only seven suggested medical evaluation. Seven out of 10 stores carried "starch blockers" despite an FDA ban. Nine out of 10 recommended bone meal and dolomite, products considered hazardous because of possible lead contamination. Nine retailers made false claims of effectiveness for bee pollen, and 10 did so for RNA. The investigators concluded that most health-food store clerks give advice that is irrational, unsafe, and illegal.[110]

In 1986 dietitian Clare Aigner posed five similar questions to proprietors of 10 health-food stores in eastern Pennsylvania and concluded that only 46% of their answers were correct.[111] In 1991 Julia M. Haidet, a student at Kent State University, made 30 phone calls to 10 stores in Ohio and asked each for advice about headaches; kidney stones; and abnormal thirst, dizziness, and fatigue. She received no appropriate advice.[112]

In 1993, posing as potential customers, FDA agents visited local health-food stores throughout the United States. The investigators asked: (a) "What do you sell to help high blood pressure?" (b) "Do you have anything to help fight infection or help my immune system?" and/or (c) "Do you have anything that works on cancer?" Of 129 inquiries, 120 resulted in recommen-

dations for products. In 23 cases the retailer looked up the answer in *Prescription for Nutritional Healing* or advised the agent to refer to or purchase the book.[96]

In 1994 Jennifer E. Pumphrey, a student at Kent State University, inquired about ephedra-containing products at 10 randomly chosen health-food stores in the Cleveland metropolitan area. In each store she found an "energy booster" containing ephedra and asked: "Do you think this works?" and "Is it safe? Does it have any side effects?" At two stores she was correctly told that the products were powerful and should not be taken by people with high blood pressure. At the rest she was told that the product had no side effects. Some said it was harmless because it was herbal, natural, or "not a drug."[113]

In 1998, in Oahu, Hawaii, a researcher posing as the daughter of a cancer patient asked personnel at 40 health-food stores whether they had any product that would be effective against metastatic breast cancer. After products were suggested, if store personnel provided no further information, the researcher asked: (a) How does the product work? (b) Do you recommend any particular brand (if more than one brand available)? (c) Could I write down some prices? (d) How much of the product does my mother need to take per day? (e) Can the product(s) be taken together with the medication my mother is receiving from her physician? and (f) Is there anything else you can recommend? Personnel in 36 of the stores recommended one or more of 38 inappropriate products, the most common of which were shark cartilage (recommended by 17) and essiac (recommended by eight), and maitake mushrooms (recommended by seven).[114]

General Nutrition operates the largest chain of health-food stores in the United States and Canada. In 1999 it had about 4200 stores and total sales of about $1.4 billion. In 1984 the company, three of its officers, and two of its store managers were charged with criminal violations of the Federal Food, Drug, and Cosmetic Act. The indictment accused them of conspiring to promote and sell an evening primrose oil product with claims that it is effective against high blood pressure, arthritis, multiple sclerosis, and other diseases. The product had been promoted with newspaper and magazine articles, radio talk show discussions, flyers, and claims made by salespersons to customers. Although the company termed the product a "food supplement," the promotional claims made it a "drug" under federal law. This meant that it could not be legally marketed without FDA approval (which it lacked). In 1986 General Nutrition pleaded guilty to four counts of misbranding a drug, and its former president and a vice president pleaded guilty to one count. The company agreed to pay $10,000 to the government as reimbursement for costs of prosecution, and the former president was fined $1,000.

Settlement of this case climaxed a series of federal enforcement actions against General Nutrition. In 1985 the company had signed consent agreements with the U.S. Postal Service to stop making unsubstantiated claims for 14 of its products sold by mail. In 1986 an FTC administrative law judge ruled that ads for another product were deliberately misleading, and he concluded that "General Nutrition's unconscionable, false, and misleading advertising found in this case is not an isolated incident but part of a continuing pattern." In 1988 the FTC charges were settled by a consent agreement in which the company agreed to donate $200,000 each to the American Heart Association, American Cancer Society, and American Diabetes Association for nutrition research. The agreement also prohibited the company from making any future claim for any company-produced product that cannot be substantiated by scientific evidence.

During 1988 the FTC also obtained a consent agreement prohibiting Great Earth International, the second-largest chain of health-food stores (150 stores), from making unsubstantiated claims for its products.

In 1993 GNC agreed to pay a penalty of $2.4 million to settle FTC charges that it had made unsubstantiated claims for 41 more products. These included 15 alleged weight-control products, 18 alleged "ergogenic aids," five bogus hair-loss preventers, two alleged anti-fatigue products, and two purported disease-related products. This case appears to have persuaded GNC to stop making blatantly false claims in its ads. False claims still appear, however, in the text of articles in health-food magazines in which GNC advertises, particularly in *Let's Live*, which has been distributed free to customers enrolled in the "GNC Health Club" discount program.

Pharmacists

Pharmacists play an important role in the vitamin marketplace. Virtually every pharmacy stocks and sells supplements that are irrationally formulated, and many stock dubious herbal and homeopathic products in addition to standard drugs. Chain drugstores are more likely to do so than individually owned stores.

Although pharmacists are generally regarded as experts, surveys suggest that most give poor advice about supplement products. In 1985, for example, reporters from *Consumer Reports* magazine visited 30 drugstores in Pennsylvania, Missouri, and California. The reporters complained of feeling tired or nervous and asked whether a vitamin product might help. Seventeen were sold a vitamin product and one was sold an amino acid preparation. Only nine of the 30 pharmacists suggested that a doctor be consulted.[115]

◆ **Personal Glimpse** ◆

Dubious Corporate Ethics[116]

During the late 1970s many manufacturers began marketing "supplements" of the amino acid L-tryptophan with unsubstantiated claims. In 1989 eosinophilia-myalgia syndrome (EMS) broke out among users of these products. Previously rare, EMS is characterized by severe muscle and joint pain, weakness, swelling of the arms and legs, fever, skin rash, and an increase of eosinophils (certain white blood cells) in the blood. At least 38 people died and more than 5000 became ill, many of whom are still disabled. When the link between EMS and L-tryptophan became apparent, the FDA quickly banned its sale and more than 2000 victims (or their survivors) filed lawsuits. During a deposition, the board chairman of General Nutrition Corporation (GNC) was asked whether his company was morally obliged to test whether the products it sold were safe and effective for their intended uses:

Q. Don't you think that GNC, before it sells pills for people to take, ought to . . . determine whether there is in fact some benefit in people taking those pills? . . .

A. No . . . we should not. We are not compelled to do that.

Q. So far as you're concerned. . . it's perfectly all right for GNC to sell people pills to take even if those pills have no benefit whatsoever? . . .

A. That's not what I said. . . . The benefit to them is from their perception . . . .

Q. So in other words, it's OK for GNC to sell pills for people to take them into their bodies . . . as long as some customer is under the belief or perception that they're going to get some benefit? . . .

A. I'm telling you that it's up to the individual. . . . They make the decision how they want to supplement their diet. . . .

Q. Would you agree that your company has an obligation to test . . . products before they're sold for human consumption to determine whether they are in fact beneficial?

A. No more than a grocery store does foods coming in. We're a retailer.

Not long afterward, two dietitians examined the labels of vitamin products at five pharmacies, three groceries, and three health-food stores in New Haven, Connecticut. Products were considered appropriate if they contained between 50% and 200% the U.S. RDA and no more than 100% of others for which Estimated Safe and Adequate Daily Dietary Intakes exist. Only 16 out of 105 (15%) of the multivitamin-mineral products met these criteria.[117]

Barrett and Herbert believe that "pharmacists have as much of an ethical duty to discourage inappropriate use of vitamin and mineral supplements as physicians do to advise against unnecessary surgery or medical care."[8] Very few pharmacists do so.

Dr. Merlin Nelson,[118] a pharmacy educator, mailed a questionnaire asking pharmacists in Detroit to list their five most common reasons for recommending supplements. The most common responses included stress, colds, and athletic activity, none of which is an appropriate reason to recommend vitamins. Nelson also asked pharmacists why they promote and sell food supplements to healthy individuals who don't need them. He concluded:

The most common reason is greed. Advertising creates a demand that the pharmacist can supply and make a profit. "If I don't sell them, they'll just go to my competition down the street," is a common response. Pharmacists are apparently more interested in a sale than in the patient's welfare. . . .

Rather than just recommending a multivitamin to patients concerned about obtaining enough vitamins in their diet, pharmacists should offer sound nutritional advice or provide referrals to experts in nutrition such as registered dietitians.[119]

Chiropractors

More than 50 companies market supplements through chiropractic offices, where they typically are sold for at least twice their wholesale cost. Many of these products are intended for the treatment of disease, even though they are unproven and lack FDA approval for this use. Since it is illegal to place an unproven claim on a product label, product information is communicated separately through literature distributed at chiropractic meetings, company-sponsored seminars, and by mail.[120] In 1988 a *Consumer Reports* editor who gained entrance to a company-sponsored seminar was given a 164-page manual describing how to use the company's products to treat 142 diseases and conditions including epilepsy, heart disease, and whooping cough. The cost of a proposed treatment program for a patient whose case was presented at the meeting was over $5 per day.[121] The company has advertised regularly in several

chiropractic journals, including *Nutritional Perspectives*, the journal of the American Chiropractic Association Council on Nutrition.

The number of chiropractors engaged in unscientific nutrition practices is unknown, but several studies suggest that it is substantial. In 1988, 74% of about 2400 chiropractors who responded to a survey by the leading chiropractic newspaper reported using nutritional supplements in their practices.[122] Not long afterward, researchers at San Jose State University's Department of Nutrition and Food Science mailed a survey to 438 members of the San Francisco Bay Area Chiropractic Society.[123] Of the 100 who responded, 60% said that they routinely provide nutrition information to their patients, 38% said they provide it on request, 60% said that they treat patients for nutritional deficiencies, 19% said they use hair analysis, and 9% indicated that they used "applied kinesiology" for nutritional assessment. Neither hair analysis (see "Dubious Diagnostic Tests") nor applied kinesiology (see Chapter 8) are valid for the nutritional assessment of patients.

Unqualified "Nutrition Consultants"

Chapter 11 describes the training of dietitians and other nutrition professionals at accredited schools. During the past 15 years several nonaccredited correspondence schools have offered B.S., M.S., and Ph.D. "degrees" in nutrition. The most prominent school was Donsbach University of Huntington Beach, California, whose president, Kurt W. Donsbach, is discussed later in this chapter. The school was "authorized" to operate by the State of California, which meant only that it had assets

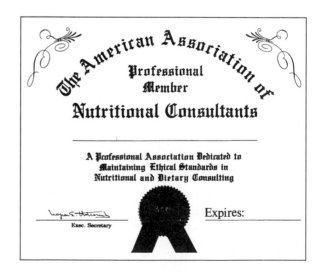

FIGURE 12-3. This attractive "credential," printed on imitation parchment and decorated with a gold seal and red ribbon, was issued to a pet hamster whose owner merely submitted the rodent's name and address and a check for $50.

of at least $50,000 and had informed the authorizing agency of its programs. Most "textbooks" required for the school's basic curriculum were books written for the general public by promoters of dubious nutrition practices. A typical degree program took less than 1 year to complete. Graduates typically refer to themselves as "nutrition consultants," a term also used by some reputable nutritionists. The school ceased operations in 1987, but some of its "graduates" are still in practice.

Bernadean University, of Van Nuys, California, offered "nutritionist" and "cancer researcher" certificates, "master's degrees," and "Ph.D. degrees" in acupuncture, reflexology, iridology, naturopathy, homeopathy, and nutrition. Dietitian Virginia Aronson took the "nutritionist" course and reported that she got high grades on all tests whether she put down correct answers or not.[124] In 1982 Bernadean was ordered to cease operations because it was not authorized by the state. However, it is still functioning. Bernadean's most prominent alumnus is "Dr." Richard Passwater, author of *Supernutrition* and several other books.

"Nutrition consultants" who wish to acquire additional "credentials" can join the American Association of Nutritional Consultants, which issues certificates suitable for framing and publishes a directory and a monthly newspaper. Its "professional membership" application asks only for the applicant's name and address plus $50. Several investigators have been able to enroll household pets (Figure 12-3).[107]

In 1993 a 32-state survey sponsored by the National Council Against Health Fraud found that 286 (46%) of 618 Yellow Page listings under the heading "Nutritionists" were spurious and 72 (12%) were suspicious. Listings were considered "spurious" if the advertiser used an invalid method of diagnosis, treatment, or nutritional assessment. Listings were rated "suspicious" if the practitioner did not comply with a request for information on credentials or methods used. Dubious nutrition practitioners were also found under the headings "Acupuncture," "Health & Diet Products," "Health, Fitness & Nutrition Consultants," "Herbs," "Holistic Practitioners," "Weight Control Services," and "Wellness Programs." Many listings under these headings were for chiropractors, homeopaths, naturopaths, "holistic" physicians, health-food stores, and distributors for multilevel companies such as Herbalife International, Nu Skin International, Shaklee Corporation, and Sunrider International. The credentials used included: C.C.N. (certified clinical nutritionist), C.N. (certified nutritionist), C.C.T. (certified colon therapist), C.M.T. (certified massage therapist), C.N.C. (certified nutrition consultant), D.C. (doctor of chiropractic), H.M.D. (homeopathic medical doctor), L.Ac. (licensed acupuncturist), M.L.D. (manual lymph drainage), N.C. (nutrition counselor), N.D. (doctor of naturopathy), N.M.D. (doctor of nutrimedicine), and O.M.D. (oriental medical doctor). Among 24 individuals identified as "Ph.D." in their ad, three were Donsbach graduates and 14 others had equally spurious credentials. Among 231 listings under the heading "Dietitians," 21 (9%) were spurious, including several from GNC stores.[125]

In response to the flaunting of dubious credentials, dietitians have gained passage of laws to regulate nutritionists in most states and the District of Columbia. Some make it illegal for unqualified persons to call themselves dietitians or nutritionists, while others define nutrition practice and who is eligible to practice. In states that regulate nutrition practice, health-food retailers are still permitted to give limited advice about diet and the use of their products but are not permitted to do nutrition assessment or counseling.

In 1996 the Distance Education and Training Council awarded accreditation to the National Institute of Nutrition Education (NINE), a correspondence school affiliated with the health-food industry. NINE was founded in 1982 and began enrollment for its "Certified Nutritionist" (C.N.) program in 1983. Several books it has used as textbooks were written by promoters of nutritional quackery.[8] Raso has identified 21 other schools that offer dubious nutrition-related correspondence programs.[126]

Dubious Diagnostic Tests

Nutrition consultants, chiropractors, and small numbers of other licensed practitioners use a wide variety of tests as a basis for recommending supplements. The most widely used include hair analysis, "muscle-testing," live-cell analysis, and Functional Intracellular Analysis.

Hair analysis is performed by obtaining a sample of hair, usually from the back of the neck, and sending it to a laboratory for analysis. The customer and the referring source usually receive a computerized printout that supposedly indicates deficiencies or excesses of minerals. Some also report supposed deficiencies of vitamins. The test usually costs from $60 to $135.

Medical authorities agree that hair analysis is not appropriate for assessing the body's nutritional state. It has limited usefulness as a screening procedure for detecting toxic levels of lead or other heavy metals. Hair analysis cannot diagnose vitamin deficiency because normally there are no vitamins in hair except at the root (below the skin surface). Nor can it identify mineral deficiencies because the lower limits of "normal" have not been scientifically established. Moreover, the mineral composition of hair can be affected by a person's age, natural hair color, and rate of hair growth, as well as the use of hair dyes, bleaches, and shampoos.[127]

When 52 hair samples from two healthy teenagers were sent under assumed names to 13 commercial hair analysis laboratories, the reported levels of minerals varied considerably between identical samples sent to the same lab and from lab to lab. The labs also disagreed about what was "normal" or "usual" for many of the minerals. Most reports contained computerized interpretations that were voluminous, bizarre, and potentially frightening to patients. Six labs recommended food supplements, but the types and amounts varied widely from report to report. One report diagnosed 23 "possible or probable conditions," including atherosclerosis and kidney failure, and recommended 56 supplement doses per day. Literature from most of the labs suggested falsely that their reports were useful against a wide variety of diseases and supposed nutrient imbalances.[128]

In 1985 the FTC secured a court order forbidding one laboratory from advertising to the public that hair mineral analysis could be used as a basis for recommending supplements. For about 10 years, this order discouraged other companies from advertising directly to consumers. However, many Web sites are now marketing the test. In 1999, researchers from the California Department of Health located nine laboratories and sent identical samples to six of them. The reported mineral levels, the alleged significance of the findings, and the recommendations made in the reports differed widely from one to another. The researchers concluded that the procedure is still unreliable and recommended that government agencies act vigorously to protect consumers.[129]

Muscle-testing is part of a pseudoscientific system of diagnosis and treatment called applied kinesiology (AK). AK is based on the notion that every organ dysfunction is accompanied by a specific muscle weakness, which enables diseases to be diagnosed through muscle-testing procedures. Its practitioners, most of whom are chiropractors, also claim that nutritional deficiencies, allergies, and other adverse reactions to food substances can be detected by placing substances in the mouth so that the patient salivates. "Good" substances will make specific muscles stronger, whereas "bad" substances will cause specific weaknesses. "Treatment" may include special diets, food supplements, acupressure, and spinal manipulation.

Applied kinesiology should be distinguished from kinesiology (biomechanics), which is the scientific study of movement. The concepts of applied kinesiology do not conform to scientific facts about the causes of disease. Controlled studies have found no difference

between the results with test substances and with placebos.[130] Differences from one test to another may be due to suggestibility, variations in the amount of force or leverage involved, and/or muscle fatigue.

Live-cell analysis is carried out by placing a drop of blood from the patient's fingertip on a microscope slide under a glass coverslip to slow down the process of drying out. The slide is then viewed with a dark-field microscope to which a television monitor has been attached. Both practitioner and patient can see the blood cells, which appear as dark bodies outlined in white. The practitioner may also make a videotape for himself and the patient. Proponents of live-cell analysis claim that it is useful for diagnosing vitamin and mineral deficiencies, enzyme deficiencies, tendencies toward allergic reactions, liver weakness, and many other health problems.

Dark-field microscopy is a valid scientific tool in which special lighting is used to examine specimens of cells and tissues. Connecting a television monitor to a microscope for diagnostic purposes is also a legitimate practice. However, experts believe that live-cell analysis is useless in diagnosing most of the conditions that its practitioners claim to detect. Lowell,[131] who has observed several practitioners, noted that they failed to clean their microscope slides carefully between patients, which meant that dirt seen under the microscope would be misinterpreted as blood components. He also noted that one practitioner reported blood cell patterns that resulted from his microscope being out of focus. Cell changes also occur as the preparation begins to dry out. Infinity², a multilevel company headquartered in Mesa, Arizona, is now marketing live-cell analysis through chiropractors, naturopaths, and "nutritional consultants." In 1995 Dr. Barrett was tested by two Infinity² distributors. One diagnosed a mild B_{12} deficiency and "maldigestion" that could weaken the immune system and cause fatigue. The other said Barrett's blood cells showed evidence of "liver toxicity," "bacterial infection," and "free radical damage." The recommended "treatment" was enzyme pills, which Infinity² markets with claims that "enzyme deficiency" is widespread among Americans. The company also maintains a telephone line for recording testimonials which are typed and "kept on file for future reference."

Functional intracellular analysis (FIA) is claimed to precisely measure an individual's nutrient status. It is marketed by SpectraCell Laboratories, Inc., of Houston, Texas, which maintains that the majority of Americans have nutrient deficiencies and that "intracellular nutrient deficiencies" even occur in over 40% of the more than 100 million Americans taking multivitamins as "insurance." The test is performed by placing lymphocytes (a type of white blood cell) from the patient's blood into petri dishes containing various concentrations of nutrients. A growth stimulant is added and, a few days later, technicians identify the dishes in which "greatest cell growth" takes place, which supposedly points to a deficiency. Properly performed lymphocyte cultures have a legitimate role in medical practice, but they are not appropriate for general screening or for diagnosing "nutrient deficiencies" in the manner used by FIA. Victor Herbert, M.D., J.D., who helped develop the use of lymphocyte cultures for nutrition-related evaluations, states that FIA merely measures the amounts of nutrients stored in the lymphocytes at the time of the test and not whether the body has a shortage.[8] He considers the test a gimmick used to promote the sale of supplements.

"Nutrient Deficiency" Questionnaires

Some nutrition consultants and retailers use computers to help them decide what to recommend. The tests usually involve completion of a dietary history and/or a questionnaire about symptoms that supposedly signify deficiency. Computer analysis of diet is a valuable tool that reputable nutritionists may find useful when appropriate computer programs are used (see Chapter 11). However, those used by the health-food industry are designed to tell everyone that they need large numbers of supplements.

In 1988 the Council for Responsible Nutrition (CRN) began advertising that stress and a fast-paced life made it advisable for women to take supplements. The ads contained a seven-question National Vitamin Gap Test with advice that a single "No" answer might indicate a need for supplements (Figure 12-4). However, the questions were so narrowly written that many people with perfectly adequate diets would give at least one negative answer.[132] The advertising campaign was launched after focus groups conducted by CRN indicated that vitamin sales had declined because people thought [correctly] they were getting sufficient nutrients from food.[8]

PROMOTERS OF QUESTIONABLE NUTRITION

Many organizations promote unscientific concepts of nutrition that can cause public confusion and lead individuals to make unwise purchases or jeopardize their health. Some of the organizations have respectable- or scientific-sounding names, and some even engage in a few activities helpful to the general public. For these reasons, they deserve close scrutiny by consumers.

Take the National Vitamin Gap Test

1. Do you: Drink 3 glasses of low-fat milk every day? YES☐ NO☐

2. Do you: Eat high fiber cereal or whole wheat bread every day? YES☐ NO☐

3. Do you: Eat fish at least twice a week? YES☐ NO☐

4. Do you: Eat 4 servings of green/yellow/red vegetables per day? YES☐ NO☐

5. Do you: Eat 2 servings of fruit per day? YES☐ NO☐

6. Do you: Limit fats, sweets and alcohol? YES☐ NO☐

7. Do you: Maintain desirable weight without periodic "dieting"? YES☐ NO☐

If you answered "No" to any of these questions, you may have one of these gaps:

Vitamin A
Vitamin C
B Vitamins
Vitamin E
Beta Carotene
Selenium
Iron
Zinc
Calcium
Magnesium
Omega—3's
Fiber

Vitamins fill the gap.

FIGURE 12-5. Vitamin Gap Test. The questions are so narrowly written that many people with an adequate diet would answer "no" to one or more questions. Someone who drinks "less than three glasses of low-fat milk each day," for example, might be obtaining milk-related nutrients by consuming equivalent amounts of yogurt, cheese, or other dairy products. Note, too, that selenium, iron, zinc, calcium, magnesium, omega-3s, and fiber are not vitamins.

National Health Federation

The National Health Federation (NHF) is a membership organization headquartered in Monrovia, California. NHF's primary theme is "freedom of choice" in health matters, but it has little interest in scientifically recognized methods. Its magazine, *Health Freedom News*, promotes dubious treatments and criticizes proven public health measures such as pasteurization, immunization, water fluoridation, and food irradiation. Speakers at NHF conventions espouse worthless cancer treatments and a wide range of other dubious practices. Government enforcement actions have been taken against at least 20 of NHF's past or present leaders (or their companies) who engaged in illegal health-related activities.[10]

NHF is active in the political arena. It presents testimony to regulatory agencies and supports legislation aimed at minimizing government interference with the health-food industry. Its letter-writing campaigns, often voluminous, typically include charges of persecution, discrimination, and conspiracy.

NHF was founded in 1955 by Fred J. Hart, president of the Electronic Medical Foundation. In 1954 a U.S. district court ordered Hart and the Foundation to stop distributing 13 electronic devices with false claims that they could diagnose and treat hundreds of diseases and conditions. Royal S. Lee, a nonpracticing dentist who died in 1967, helped Hart found NHF and served on its board of governors. In 1962 he and the vitamin company that he owned were convicted of misbranding 115 "food supplement" products by making false claims on their labels for the treatment of more than 500 diseases and conditions. In 1973 a prominent FDA official described Lee as "probably the largest publisher of unreliable and false information in the world."[10] The products contained various combinations of vitamins, minerals, herbs, and dehydrated animal organs. The company, Standard Process Laboratories, still markets many of them, primarily through chiropractors. Although unsubstantiated health claims no longer appear on the product labels, such claims are made at seminars sponsored by "independent" distributors of the products.

Kurt Donsbach, who chaired NHF's board of governors from 1975 through 1989, obtained a chiropractic degree but practiced chiropractic only briefly. During the 1960s, he worked for Lee as a "research associate." In 1970, while Donsbach operated a health-food store, agents of the Fraud Division of the California Bureau of Food and Drug observed him represent that vitamins, minerals, and herbal teas were effective against cancer, emphysema, and other conditions.

Charged with practicing medicine without a license, he pleaded guilty and paid a small fine. His subsequent health-related ventures have included books, magazines, newsletters, vitamin companies, non-accredited correspondence schools, and syndicated radio and television programs. In recent years he has operated Hospital Santa Monica, a Mexican clinic that offers dubious treatments for cancer and other serious diseases. In 1996, after a lengthy investigation by the U.S. Justice Department, he was indicted and pleaded guilty to smuggling unapproved drugs into the U.S. and not paying income tax on the money he made for selling them.[133]

Citizens for Health

Citizens for Health (CFH) was formed in 1992 in response to concerns about FDA regulation of supplement products. It appears to have grown rapidly and to have thousands of members, with state and local chapters throughout the country. An affiliated professional group, the American Preventive Medical Association (APMA), was launched the same year. Alexander G. Schauss, the first executive director of both groups, has promoted unsubstantiated theories about diet and behavior through books, lectures, and the *International Journal of Biosocial Research*, which he edited and published. He obtained a "Ph.D." degree in psychology from a nonaccredited school in 1992.

Like NHF, CFH and APMA campaigned actively for the 1994 Dietary Supplement Health and Education Act, the purpose of which was to weaken government regulation of food supplements. These groups are also promoting an "Access to Medical Treatment Act" intended to block government interference with "alternative" practitioners (see Chapter 8).

Rodale Press

Rodale Press was founded by J.I. Rodale (1898–1971), who was best known for his interests in "organic farming" and "health foods." The company, which publishes 11 magazines and 80 to 100 books a year, has a gross annual income of about $500 million. *Prevention*, its leading magazine, was launched in 1950 as a device to promote the products of its advertisers.[8] It did this by attacking ordinary foods and recommending supplements and health foods with claims that often were ludicrous. During the 1980s *Prevention* shifted toward the scientific mainstream and acquired a prominent editorial advisory board. Today the magazine emphasizes dietary improvement, appropriate exercise programs, and other health-promoting activities. Although much of its advice is accurate, its coverage of nutrition news has been unbalanced, it promotes dubious "alternative" methods, and it tends to encourage undue experimentation with dietary supplements.

Rodale's book division and the Prevention Book Club have marketed some authoritative books, but most of their nutrition-related books contain questionable ideas. Ads for the books are more blatant than the books themselves. For example, a mailer for *The Doctor's Vitamin and Mineral Encyclopedia*, by Sheldon Saul Hendler, M.D., was headlined "The World's Most Powerful Healing Vitamins and Minerals" and promised information on "a substance that reverses the aging process," a "heavy-duty smart pill" that "stops the aging process and dramatically improves your memory," and a one-a-day supplement that "could dramatically reduce your chances of breast cancer." The pertinent passages in the book reported speculations based on preliminary or anecdotal evidence.

Prominent Individual Promoters

Many individuals have developed and promoted food fads and other dubious nutrition practices. Each of the following persons has written several books and achieved notoriety during the past three decades.

Adelle Davis received a degree in dietetics from the University of California, Berkeley, and a Master of Science degree in biochemistry from the University of Southern California School of Medicine. Her four books sold a total of 10 million copies: *Let's Eat Right to Keep Fit, Let's Get Well, Let's Cook It Right,* and *Let's Have Healthy Children.* She criticized the American diet as excessively high in salt; loaded with refined sugar; and contaminated by pesticides, growth hormones, and preservatives. She claimed modern food processing destroys vital nutrients. She proposed that people eat organic fruits and vegetables, whole wheat bread, wheat germ, vitamin supplements, certified raw milk, fresh stone-ground whole-grain bread or cereal, and other "health food" products.

Several critics have noted that many of the claims Adelle Davis made were not even supported by the evidence she cited. Dr. Edward H. Rynearson, emeritus professor of medicine, Mayo Clinic, Rochester, Minnesota, made these comments about *Let's Get Well:*

She lists 2402 reference. . . . She says . . . "hundreds of studies used as source material for this book have been conducted almost entirely by doctors, perhaps 95% of whom are professors in medical schools" . . . but this simply is not true. Probably less than 10% are professors. I wrote to a number of these eminent scientists (18 responded) . . . in many instances their remarks were either misquoted or taken out of context and not one could recommend this book. . . . I checked her references. I found glaring examples of misquotations and inaccuracies.[134]

Some of the advice in Davis' books was harmful, even potentially fatal. In 1978, for example, a 2-month-old infant was given liquid potassium as recommended for colic in Davis's book *Let's Have Healthy Children.* After the second dose he became listless, stopped breathing, and was rushed to a hospital, where he died the next day. After a suit was filed against the publisher, the estate of Adelle Davis, and the manufacturer of the potassium product, the book was recalled from bookstores and the defendants settled for a total of $160,000. The book was reissued after being revised by a physician allied with the health-food industry.

Carlton Fredericks was described on some of his book jackets as "America's foremost nutritionist." He considered himself an expert and gave copious advice in books and articles for health-food publications. According to the FDA, however, he had virtually no nutrition or health science training. He graduated from the University of Alabama in 1931 with a major in English and a minor in political science. In 1937 he began writing advertising copy for a vitamin company. He also gave sales talks, adopting the title of "nutrition educator."

In 1945, after investigators found that he had been diagnosing patients and prescribing vitamins for their illnesses, Fredericks pleaded guilty to practicing medicine without a license and paid a small fine. He then obtained a master's degree in education and a Ph.D. in communications at New York University. His doctoral thesis was based on the responses of listeners to his radio programs. For 30 years, beginning in 1957, he hosted "Design for Living," a daily show on radio station WOR in New York City. Toward the end of his career, he provided "nutrition consultations" for $200 each at the offices of Robert Atkins, M.D.

Atkins, who practices in New York City, claims that "nutrition has been useful in just about every condition I have treated. . . . And there are probably herbal answers for every condition for which there is a pharmacological answer." He describes his method of practice as "complementary medicine," which he defines as a synthesis of orthodox and "alternative" medicine put together to integrate the best of both. He considers Fredericks to have been his mentor and took over Fredericks' radio program after his death in 1987.[2]

Atkins's books include: *Dr. Atkins' Diet Revolution* (1971*), Dr. Atkins' Superenergy Diet* (1977), *Dr. Atkins' Nutrition Breakthrough* (1981), *Dr. Atkins' Health Revolution* (1988), and *Dr. Atkins' New Diet Revolution*

(1992). He also markets a "Targeted Nutrition Program" in which "building blocks" are added to a "basic formula" to "help the body to create its own cures." The 17 building blocks include supplements called *Cardiovascular Formula, Heart Rhythm Formula, Hypoglycemia Formula, Anti-Arthritic Formula,* and *Urinary Frequency Formula.* A brochure from his office states that the formulas evolved from 25 years of using nutrition to treat more than 40,000 patients.

In 1986 Atkins launched the Foundation for the Advancement of Innovative Medicine (FAIM), which holds public meetings and is striving to protect "complementary" physicians from disciplinary action taken by their state medical boards.[135] In 1993 FAIM gained passage of a law that would place "alternative" practitioners on the board that regulates professional practice in New York State.

Earl Mindell, a co-founder of Great Earth International, has a bachelor's degree in pharmacy from the University of North Dakota and "Ph.D.s" in nutrition from two nonaccredited schools.[8,136] His books include *Earl Mindell's Vitamin Bible, Earl Mindell's Vitamin Bible for Kids, Unsafe at Any Meal, Earl Mindell's Herb Bible,* and *Earl Mindell's Soy Miracle.* The *Vitamin Bible* recommends self-treatment with supplements for more than 50 health problems. The book also promotes substances that Mindell calls "vitamins" B_{10}, B_{11}, B_{13}, B_{15}, B_{17}, P, T, and U. There is no scientific evidence that any of these substances are vitamins (essential to humans) or that supplements of any of them are beneficial.

Mindell is co-editor, with Richard Passwater, of Keats Publishing Company's "Good Health Guides," a large series of booklets promoting scores of questionable supplements. Mindell has also written information sheets that were distributed free of charge in many health-food stores. Although all of them warned that their information was "not intended as medical advice but only as a guide in working with your doctor," it is clear that they were used to boost sales by making claims that would be illegal on product labels. Now retired from active management of his stores, Mindell spends much of his time writing, lecturing, and appearing on talk shows. He writes a newsletter and is marketing "Soy Miracle" products with a multilevel company called FreeLife International. FreeLife flyers call Mindell "America's #1 Nutrition Expert."

Lendon H. Smith, M.D., is a pediatrician who claims that allergies, insomnia, alcoholism, hyperactivity in children, and a variety of other ailments are the result of enzyme disturbances that can be helped by dietary changes. He recommends a variety of food supplements and avoidance of white sugar, white flour, pasteurized milk, and other foods that are not "natural." His ideas were widely promoted through television appearances. His books include *Feed Your Kids Right, Feed Yourself Right,* and *Improving Your Child's Behavior Chemistry.*

In 1973 the Oregon State Board of Medical Examiners placed Smith on probation because he had prescribed medication that was "not necessary or medically indicated" for six adult patients, one diagnosed as hyperactive and the other five as heroin addicts. He remained on probation until 1981. In 1987 Smith permanently surrendered his medical license rather than face Board action on charges of insurance fraud. According to press reports, the trouble arose because he had signed documents authorizing insurance payments for patients he had not seen. The patients had actually been seen by chiropractors, homeopaths, and other nontraditional practitioners at "nutrition-oriented" clinics in which Smith had worked.[137] Lately Smith has promoted homeopathic products.

Gary Null, Ph.D., whose books bill him as "one of America's leading health and fitness advocates,"

☑ Consumer Tip

Suggestions for Consumers

The following suggestions should help consumers make healthy and economically sound decisions regarding nutrition:

- It is virtually impossible for laypersons to sort out nutrition sense from nonsense on a claim-by-claim basis. The more practical approach is to examine the overall philosophy of the individual, organization, or publication making the claim.
- Be wary of anyone who promotes the fads and fallacies identified in this chapter. Use the reliable sources of information identified in Chapter 2 and the Appendix of this book.
- Avoid practitioners who prescribe vitamin supplements for everyone or who sell them in connection with their practice.
- Be wary of any product promoted for a particular purpose that is not printed on its label. Federal laws require that health products be truthfully labeled and carry adequate directions for use. It is extremely unlikely that a product will do anything that is not claimed on its label.
- Knowledge of the basic principles of nutrition as outlined in Chapter 11 should enable you to make wise food selections.

It's Your Decision

1. You have suffered from severe tension at work and at home. You have read an advertisement for "stress vitamins." What action should you take to reach an intelligent decision about using such vitamins?

2. You visit a health-food store to buy some rice flour. While you are browsing, a clerk engages you in conversation, learns that you are troubled by occasional headaches, and suggests several herbal products to help you. The clerk also learns that your mother has arthritis and suggests several products for her. What should you do about these recommendations?

promotes dubious treatments for many serious diseases. He hosts radio and television talk shows, writes books, gives lectures, and has marketed supplement products. He has spoken out against fluoridation, immunization, food irradiation, mercury-amalgam fillings, and many forms of proven medical treatment. Null's supplement products have included *Guard-Ion* (an "antioxidant" formula claimed to help protect athletes from free radicals the body cannot control); *Candida Complex* (to bolster the body's defenses against yeast infection); *Rebalancer* (a "cleansing formulation" for adults exposed to air pollutants, pesticides, or preservatives or who have "internal metabolic imbalances"); and *Gary Null's Immune Nutrients* ("to nourish and stimulate immune function, not merely at a marginal level of preventing disease and degeneration, but . . . for optimal health").

Andrew Weil, M.D., is described on the covers of his best-selling books as "the guru of alternative medicine," "one of the most skilled, articulate, and important leaders in the field of health and healing," and "a pioneer in the medicine of the future." His advice is a mixture of sense and nonsense. The sensible part includes standard advice about diet and exercise. The nonsense includes such ideas as "improper breathing is a common cause of ill health" and the recommendation that following surgery, patients should get massive intravenous doses of vitamin C. He tends to prefer the use of "natural remedies" rather than conventional medicines. He has published nothing in scientific journals to objectively document his personal experiences with allegedly cured patients or to substantiate his claims that the nonstandard remedies he advocates are effective.[138] His "Ask Dr. Weil" Web site contains an interactive "Vitamin Advisor" questionnaire that leads to a "personalized formula of my recommended vitamins, supplements and tonics"—typically 6 to 10 products per person that would cost about $2 per day. The explanations for these recommendations are poorly reasoned.

Trade Organizations

Health-food retailers have regional and national trade organizations that provide political, legal, and educational support. The most active is the National Nutritional Foods Association, which represents about 5000 health-food retailers, distributors, and producers. Its activities include annual conventions, a newsletter, and campaigning to minimize governmental regulation of the industry. Major manufacturers and distributors of vitamins and minerals also are represented by the Council for Responsible Nutrition.

During 1991 the health-food industry became alarmed that proposed new labeling rules (see Chapter 11) would greatly reduce the number of products it could market and that proposed laws to strengthen federal enforcement agencies would weaken the industry still further. Early in 1992 the Nutritional Health Alliance (NHA) was formed to enable manufacturers, suppliers, distributors, retailers, consumers, and other supplement industry allies to coordinate their efforts to protect the industry. NHA quickly launched a campaign that generated over 1 million protest letters to Congress and spearheaded legislation intended to weaken the FDA. Citizens for Health and the National Nutritional Foods Association also played major roles in the campaign, which Dr. Barrett characterized as a "vitamin war."[139] The resultant Dietary Supplement Health and Education Act of 1994 is described in Chapter 26.

SUMMARY

Most Americans probably are harmed to some degree by nutrition fads and fallacies. Promoters of nutrition quackery are well-organized and skilled at arousing and exploiting fears and false hopes. Their most persuasive sales pitch is that everyone should take supplements to be sure of getting enough vitamins and minerals. However, it is more sensible for individuals worried about this to keep a food diary for several days and have a physician or registered dietitian determine whether any problem exists.

Supplements and "health foods" have been recommended for virtually every ailment. However, there is little or no scientific evidence to support such recommendations. Megadoses of vitamins and minerals have few legitimate uses and should never be taken without competent medical advice. Anyone who recommends supplements for everyone should be ignored.

REFERENCES

1. Morowitz HJ. Drinking hemlock and other nutritional matters. Hospital Practice 13:155–156, 1978.
2. Herbert V. Vitamin pushers and food quacks. In Barrett S, Jarvis T, editors. The Health Robbers: A Close Look at Quackery in America. Amherst, N.Y., 1993, Prometheus Books.
3. Schafer R, Yetley EA. Social psychology of food faddism. Journal of the American Dietetic Association 66:129–133, 1975.
4. Olson RE. Book review of The Vitamin Pushers. American Journal of Clinical Nutrition 63:406–407, 1996.
5. Beal VA. Food faddism and organic and natural foods. Presented at National Dairy Council Food Writers' Conference, Newport, R.I., May 1972, reported in Schafer R, Yetley EA. Social psychology of food faddism. Journal of the American Dietetic Association 66:129–133, 1975.
6. Barrett S, Herbert V. The Vitamin Pushers: How the "Health Food" Industry Is Selling America a Bill of Goods. Amherst, N.Y., 1994, Prometheus Books.
7. Whorton JC. Crusaders for Fitness. Mt. Vernon, N.Y., 1982, Consumer Reports Books.
8. Johnson O. Stover at Yale. New York, 1912, Frederick A. Stokes. Cited in Young JH. "The foolmaster who fooled them." Yale Journal of Biology and Medicine 53:555–566, 1980.
9. Consumer Use of Dietary Supplements. Emmaus, Pa., Prevention Magazine, 2000.
10. Barrett S. The unhealthy alliance: Crusaders for "health freedom." New York, 1988, American Council on Science and Health.
11. Thomas PR. Food for thought about dietary supplements. Nutrition Today 31:46–54, 1996.
12. Harper AE. "Nutrition insurance": A skeptical view. Nutrition Forum 4:33–37, 1987.
13. Welsh S. Nutrient standards, dietary guidelines, and food guides. In Ziegler EE, Filer LJ Jr, editors. Present Knowledge in Nutrition, ed 2. Washington, D.C., 1996, ILSI Press.
14. Mertz W and others. What are people really eating? The relationship between energy intake derived from estimated diet records and intake determined to maintain body weight. American Journal of Clinical Nutrition 54:291–295, 1991.
15. Barrett S. Dietary supplements: Appropriate use. Quackwatch, Web site, March 17, 2000.
16. Nutrition shortcut in a can? HealthNews 2(8):1–2, 1996.
17. NAD Case Report 12:15, 1982.
18. Barrett S and others. The Vitamin Pushers. In Barrett S and others. Health Schemes, Scams, and Frauds. New York, 1990, Consumer Reports Books.
19. Barrett S. Petition regarding "stress formulas." Filed December 1994. Docket #94P–0438/CPI.
20. Herbert V. Separating food facts and myths. In Herbert V, Subak-Sharpe GJ, editors. Total Nutrition: the Only Guide You'll Ever Need. New York, 1995, St. Martin's Press.
21. Stampfer MJ and others. Vitamin consumption and the risk of coronary disease in women. New England Journal of Medicine 328:1444–1449, 1993.
22. Rimm EB and others. Vitamin consumption and the risk of coronary disease in men. New England Journal of Medicine 328:1450–1456, 1993.
23. Alpha-Tocopherol, Beta Carotene Cancer Prevention Study Group. The effect of vitamin E and beta carotene on the incidence of lung cancer and other cancers in male smokers. New England Journal of Medicine 330:1029–1035, 1994.
24. Rapola JM and others. Randomised trial of alpha-tocopherol and beta-carotene supplements on incidence of major coronary events in men with previous myocardial infarction. Lancet 349:1715–1720, 1997.
25. Greenberg RE and others. A clinical trial of antioxidant vitamins to prevent colorectal cancer. New England Journal of Medicine 331:141–147, 1994.
26. Hennekens CH and others. Lack of effect of long-term supplementation with beta-carotene on the incidence of malignant neoplasms and cardiovascular disease. New England Journal of Medicine 334:1145–1149, 1996.
27. Omenn GS and others. Effects of a combination of beta-carotene and vitamin A on lung cancer and cardiovascular disease. New England Journal of Medicine 334:1150–1155, 1996.
28. Tardif J-C. Probucol and multivitamins in the prevention of restenosis after coronary angioplasty. New England Journal of Medicine 337:365–372, 1997.
29. The Heart Outcomes Prevention Evaluation Study Investigators. Vitamin E supplementation and cardiovascular events in high-risk patients. New England Journal of Medicine 342:145–153, 2000.
30. Lee IM and others. Beta-carotene supplementation and incidence of cancer and cardiovascular disease: The Women's Health Study. Journal of the National Cancer Institute 91:2102–2106, 1999.
31. Hennekens CH and others. Antioxidant vitamins: Benefits not yet proved. New England Journal of Medicine 330:1080–1081, 1994.
32. Vitamin supplements. The Medical Letter on Drugs and Therapeutics 40:75–77, 1998.
33. Tribble DL and others. Antioxidant consumption and risk of coronary heart disease: Emphasis on vitamin C, vitamin E, and beta-carotene. American Heart Association Science Advisory. Circulation 99:591–595, 1999.
34. Smith W and others. Dietary oxidants and age-related maculopathy: The Blue Mountains Study. Ophthalmology 106:761–767, 1999.
35. Phytochemicals. Drugstore in a salad. Consumer Reports on Health 7:133–135, 1995.
36. Anderson SA, Raiten DJ and others: Safety of Amino Acids Used as Dietary Supplements. Bethesda, Md., 1992, Federation of American Societies for Experimental Biology.
37. Cameron E, Pauling L. Cancer and Vitamin C. New York, 1979, W.W. Norton & Co.
38. Marshall CW. Vitamins and Minerals: Help or Harm? New York, 1985, Consumer Reports Books.
39. Goertzel T, Goertzel B. Linus Pauling: A Life in Science and Politics. New York, 1995, Basic Books.
40. Karlowski TR and others. Ascorbic acid for the common cold: A prophylactic and therapeutic trial. JAMA 231:1038–1042, 1975.
41. DeWys WD. How to evaluate a new treatment for cancer. Your Patient and Cancer 2(5):31–36, 1982.
42. Creagan ET, Moertel CG, and others. Failure of high-dose vitamin C (ascorbic acid) therapy to benefit patients with advanced cancer, a controlled trial. New England Journal of Medicine 301:687–690, 1979.
43. Vitamin C goes down for the count in advanced-cancer controlled trial. Medical World News, Aug 22, 1983.
44. Moertel CG and others. High-dose vitamin C versus placebo in the treatment of patients with advanced cancer who had no prior chemotherapy. New England Journal of Medicine 312:137–141, 1985.

45. Geubel A and others. Liver damage caused by therapeutic vitamin A administration: Estimate of dose-related toxicity in 41 cases. Gastroenterology 100:1701–1709, 1991.

46. Rothman KJ and others. Teratogenicity of high vitamin A intake. New England Journal of Medicine 333:1369–1373, 1995.

47. Vitamin A cases settled for record sum. Nutrition Forum 7:31, 1990.

48. Dalton K, Dalton MJT. Characteristics of pyridoxine overdose neuropathy syndrome. Acta Neurologica Scandinavia 76:8–11, 1987.

49. Stare FJ, Aronson V, Barrett S. Your Guide to Good Nutrition. Amherst, N.Y., 1991, Prometheus Books.

50. American Academy of Pediatrics Committee on Nutrition. Vitamin and mineral supplement needs of normal children in the United States. Pediatrics 66:1015–1020, 1980.

51. U.S Preventive Services Task Force. Guide to Clinical Preventive Services, ed 2. Baltimore, 1996, Williams & Wilkins.

52. King JC, Allen L and others. Nutrition during Pregnancy. Washington D.C., 1990, National Academy Press.

53. New York State public hearing in the matter of organic foods. New York City, Dec 1, 1972.

54. Newsome R. Organically grown foods: A scientific status summary by the Institute of Food Technologists' expert panel on food safety and nutrition. Food Technology 44(12):123–130, 1990.

55. Jones P. Pesticides and food safety. New York, 1989, American Council on Science and Health.

56. Food and Drug Administration Pesticide Program – residue monitoring – 1999. Washington, D.C., 1999, Food and Drug Administration.

57. Deutsch R. Family Guide to Better Food and Better Health. Des Moines, 1971, Meredith Corp.

58. Jukes TH, Barrett S. Genuine fakes. In Barrett S, Jarvis T, editors. The Health Robbers: A Close Look at Quackery in America. Amherst, N.Y., 1993, Prometheus Books.

59. Appledorf H and others. Sensory evaluation of health foods: A comparison with traditional foods. Florida Agricultural Experimental Stations Series, 5328, 1974.

60. Basker D. Comparison of taste quality between organically and conventionally grown fruits and vegetables. American Journal of Alternative Agriculture 7:129–136, 1992.

61. Pesek J and others. Alternative Agriculture. Washington D.C., 1989, National Academy Press.

62. Aldrich SA and others. Organic and conventional farming compared. Ames, Iowa, 1980, The Council for Agricultural Science and Technology.

63. Larkin M. Organic foods get government "blessing" despite claims that aren't kosher. Nutrition Forum 8:25–29, 1991.

64. Lulinski B, Kapica C. Some notes on aloe vera. Quackwatch, Web site, June 23, 1998.

65. Larkin T. Bee pollen as a health food. FDA Consumer 18(3):21–22, 1984.

66. Mirkin G. Can bee pollen benefit health? JAMA 262:1854, 1989.

67. Advice on limiting intake of bone meal. FDA Drug Bulletin, 12:5–6, 1982.

68. Nielsen FH. Facts and fallacies about boron. Nutrition Today 27(3):6–12, 1992.

69. Barrett S. Is chitosan a "fat magnet"? Quackwatch Web site, May 10, 2000.

70. Can you live longer? What works and what doesn't. Consumer Reports 57:7–15, 1992.

71. It's natural! It's organic! Or is it? Consumer Reports 45:410–415, 1980.

72. Cunningham J. DHEA: Facts vs. hype. Nutrition Forum 2:30–31, 1985.

73. Tyler VE, Foster S. The Honest Herbal, ed 4. New York, 1999, Hayworth Press.

74. Fish: The next health food? Consumer Reports 51:368–370, 1986.

75. Lowell JA. Organic germanium: Another health food store junk food. Nutrition Forum 5:53–57, 1988.

76. Herbert V, Kava R. When natural isn't safe: The lowdown on melatonin. Priorities 7(4):20–23, 1995.

77. Hammock DA. Protein. In Herbert V, Subak-Sharpe GJ, editors. Total Nutrition: The Only Guide You'll Ever Need. New York, 1995, St. Martin's Press.

78. McElderry MQB. Grape expectations: The resveratrol story. Quackwatch, Sept 1, 1999.

79. Barrett S. Algae: False claims and hype. Quackwatch, May 15, 2000.

80. Mossad SB and others. Zinc gluconate lozenges for treating the common cold. A randomized, double-blind, placebo-controlled study. Archives of Internal Medicine 125:81–88, 1996.

81. Zinc for the common cold. Medical Letter 39:9–10, 1997.

82. Lehmann P. More than you ever thought you would know about additives (3-part series). FDA Consumer 13(3):10–16, 13:(4)12–15, 13:(5)18–23, 1979.

83. Kroger M. Food safety: What are the real issues? Nutrition Forum 2:17–18, 1985.

84. Organic produce. Consumer Reports 63(1):12–18, 1998.

85. Whelan EM. The food-fear epidemic. In Barrett S, Jarvis T, editors. The Health Robbers: A Close Look at Quackery in America. Amherst, N.Y., 1993, Prometheus Books.

86. Barrett S. The herbal minefield. Quackwatch Web site, June 22, 2000.

87. Gurley BJ and others. Content versus label claims in ephedra-containing dietary supplements. American Journal of Health-System Pharmacists 57:963-969, 2000.

88. The mainstreaming of alternative medicine. Consumer Reports 65(5):17–25, 2000.

89. Fetrow CW, Avila JR. Professional's Handbook of Complementary & Alternative Medicines. Springhouse, Pa., 1999, Springhouse Corporation.

90. Le Bars PL and others. A placebo-controlled, double-blind, randomized trial of an extract of Ginkgo biloba for dementia. North American EGb Study Group. JAMA 278(16):1327–1332, 1997.

91. Wilk TJ and others. Saw palmetto extracts for treatment of benign prostatic hyperplasia: A systematic review. JAMA 280:1604–1609, 1998.

92. Good Housekeeping Institute. New Good Housekeeping Institute study finds drastic discrepancy in potencies of popular herbal supplement. News release, Consumer Safety Symposium on Dietary Supplements and Herbs, New York City, March 3, 1998.

93. United States Pharmacopeia. Valerian (Valeriana officinalis). Information Monograph. Rockville, Md., 1998, United States Pharmacopeia.

94. NCAHF position paper on over-the-counter herbal remedies. Loma Linda, Calif., 1995, National Council Against Health Fraud.

95. Toxic plant products sold in health food stores. The Medical Letter, April 6, 1979.

96. Unsubstantiated Claims and Documented Health Hazards in the Dietary Supplement Marketplace. Rockville, Md., 1993, U.S. Food and Drug Administration.

97. Anderson IB and others. Pennyroyal toxicity: Measurement of toxic metabolite levels in two cases and review of the literature. Annals of Internal Medicine 124:726–734, 1996.

98. AMA Council on Foods and Nutrition. Zen macrobiotic diets. JAMA 218:397, 1971.

99. Kushi M, Jack A. The Cancer Prevention Diet: Michio Kushi's Nutritional Blueprint for the Relief and Prevention of Disease. New York, 1983, St. Martin's Press.

100. Dwyer J. The macrobiotic diet: No cancer cure. Nutrition Forum 7:9–11, 1990.

101. Raso J. A Kushi seminar for professionals. Nutrition Forum 7:17–21, 1990.

102. Lindner L. The new improved macrobiotic diet. American Health 7(4):71–86, 1988.

103. Roth JA. Health Purifiers and Their Enemies. New York, 1977, Neal Watson Academic Publications (Prodist).

104. Deutsch RM. The New Nuts Among the Berries. Palo Alto, Calif., 1977, Bull Publishing.

105. Building your nutritional food business with books and magazines—a merchandising manual. Denver, 1982, Nutri-Books.

106. Power failure for the 'Immune Power' diet. Consumer Reports 51:112–113, 1986.

107. Barrett S. The American Association of Nutritional Consultants: Who and what does it represent? Quackwatch Web site, Dec 11, 1999.

108. Geslewitz G. 22nd annual survey of health food stores. Health Foods Business 43(4):21–34, 1997.

109. Fanning O. "Training" for health food retailers. Nutrition Forum 3:33–38, 1986.

110. Meister KM. Do health food stores give sound nutrition advice? ACSH News and Views, May/June 1983.

111. Aigner C. Advice in health food stores. Nutrition Forum 5:1–4, Jan 1988.

112. Haidet JM. Poor advice plus doubletalk: A probe of "health food" stores in central Ohio. Nutrition Forum 9:6–7, 1992.

113. Pumphrey JE. Marketing of ephedra products in health food stores. Nutrition Forum 12:33–34, 1995.

114. Gotay CC, Dumitriu D. Health food store recommendations for breast cancer patients. Archives of Family Medicine 9:692–698, 2000.

115. The vitamin pushers. Consumer Reports 51:170–175, 1987.

116. Horn JD. Deposition re L-tryptophan litigation. MDL docket number 865, U.S. District Court, District of South Carolina, Columbia Division, Aug 11, 1992.

117. Bell LS, Fairchild M. Evaluation of commercial multivitamin supplements. Journal of the American Dietetic Association 87:341–343, 1987.

118. Nelson MV, Baille G. A survey of pharmacists recommendations for food supplements in the U.S.A. and U.K. Journal of Clinical Pharmacy and Therapeutics 15:131–139, 1990.

119. Nelson MV. Promotion and selling of unnecessary food supplements: Quackery or ethical pharmacy practice? American Pharmacy NS28(10):34–36, 1988.

120. Barrett S. Chiropractors and nutrition: The supplement underground. Nutrition Forum 9:25–28, 1992.

121. Katzenstein L. Nutrition against disease: A close look at a 1987 seminar for chiropractors. Chirobase Web site, Nov 22, 1999.

122. How DCs in the USA practice. Dynamic Chiropractic 6(17):3, 1988.

123. Newman CF and others. Nutrition-related backgrounds and counseling practices of doctors of chiropractic. Journal of the American Dietetic Association 89:939–943, 1989.

124. Aronson V. Bernadean University: A nutrition diploma mill. ACSH News & Views 4(2):7, 12, 19, 1983.

125. Milner I. The color of quackery? Fingering the phony nutritionists of the Yellow pages. Nutrition Forum 11:19–22, 1995.

126. Raso J. Alternative health education and pseudocredentialing. Skeptical Inquirer 29(4):39–45, 1996.

127. Hambidge KM. Hair analysis: Worthless for vitamins, limited for minerals. American Journal of Clinical Nutrition 36:943–949, 1982.

128. Barrett S. Commercial hair analysis: Science or scam? JAMA 254:1041–1045, 1985.

129. Seidel S and others. Assessment of commercial laboratories performing hair mineral analysis. JAMA 285:67–72, 2001.

130. Kenny JJ, Clemens R, Forsythe KD. Applied kinesiology unreliable for assessing nutrient status. Journal of the American Dietetic Association 88:698–704, 1988.

131. Lowell J. Live cell analysis: High-tech hokum. Nutrition Forum 3:81–85, 1986.

132. Barrett S. Be wary of bogus vitamin questionnaires. Priorities, pp 37–40, Spring 1990.

133. United States v. Kurt W. Donsbach: Criminal case No. '96-347B, U.S. District Court, Southern District of California.

134. Rynearson EH. Americans love hogwash. Nutrition Reviews 32 (suppl):1–14, 1974.

135. Raso J. The FAIM symposium: A "complementary medicine" smorgasboard. Nutrition Forum, 8:17–22, 1991.

136. Lowell JA. An irreverent look at the Vitamin Bible and its author. Nutrition Forum 3:46–47, 1986.

137. Lund D. Lendon Smith loses license! Nutrition Forum 4:56, 1987.

138. Relman A. A Trip to Stonesville. The New Republic, Dec 14, 1998.

139. Barrett S. Proposed labeling rules stir controversy. Nutrition Forum 9:9–14, 1992.

Chapter Thirteen

WEIGHT CONTROL

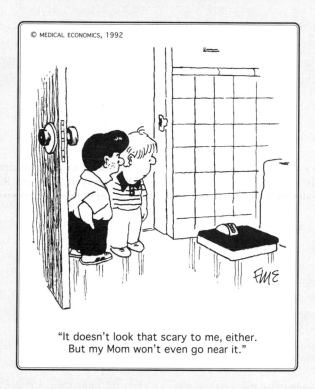

© MEDICAL ECONOMICS, 1992

"It doesn't look that scary to me, either.
But my Mom won't even go near it."

Americans brought up in a society full of technological miracles are constantly searching for the easy way out. In desperation, they are willing to try anything offered to them, wasting money, time and sometimes their own lives.

GEORGE L. BLACKBURN, M.D., PH.D.
KONSTANTIN PAVLOU, SC.D.[1]

Diets usually leave a person aggravated, discouraged, and the same size.

AMY LANOU, PH.D.[2]

Q. Can a diet pill really cause people to lose fat while they sleep?
A. If it worked you would be reading about it in the headlines of every newspaper in the country.

ANN LANDERS

Americans spend more than $32 billion a year for products and services they hope will enable them to control their weight.[3] Much of this money is wasted. The following observation, made in 1972 in the AMA's *Today's Health* magazine, is still appropriate today:

They will attend reducing clinics and join reducing programs. They will visit doctors who will write weight-reducing prescriptions for them and inject them with hormones. They will enter hospitals for fat-removing operations. They will get themselves hypnotized, and psychoanalyzed individually and in groups. They will purchase books and pamphlets extolling the virtues of high-calorie diets; low-calorie diets; high fat, carbohydrate and/or protein diets; low-fat, carbohydrate and/or protein diets; grapefruit diets; water diets; drinking men's diets; organic food diets; and sex-instead-of-supper diets. They will gulp down diet pills, blow on diet soups, chomp on diet cookies and chew on diet gum. Most of the time, for a variety of legitimate reasons, they will emerge in much the same condition as when they began: fat. And much of the time, for a variety of illegitimate reasons, they will also emerge defrauded.[4]

This chapter describes the basic principles of weight control and the various types of products, procedures, and professional services used in the attempt to achieve it. Included in this discussion are diets, pills, special foods, and gadgets, as well as medical, surgical, and psychologic procedures, clinics, and self-help groups. For additional information on exercise, exercise devices, and "spot-reducers," see Chapter 14.

BASIC CONCEPTS

The words *obese* and *overweight* are often used interchangeably. Strictly speaking, *obesity* refers to an excess accumulation of fatty tissue in the body, whereas *overweight* refers to a weight greater than that listed in an established height-weight table (Table 13-1). These terms are not mutually exclusive, because obese persons are also overweight.

Many experts define overweight as 10% above the weights in a Metropolitan Life Insurance Company table and define obesity as 20% or more above these weights. The latest National Institutes of Health (NIH) guidelines use body mass index (BMI), which is the person's weight in kilograms divided by the square of the person's height in meters. (BMI can also be calculated by multiplying one's weight in pounds by 700, dividing the result by one's height in inches, and dividing by height again.) NIH classifies adults 18 and older into six groups: underweight (BMI less than 18.5), normal (18.5–24.9), overweight (25.0–29.9), Class I obesity (30.0–34.9), Class II obesity (35.0–39.9), and Class III (extreme) obesity (40 or more). Table 13-2 illustrates representative BMI values. BMI calculators are available on http://www.consumer.gov/weightloss/bmi.htm and many other Web sites.

The causes of obesity are multiple and complex; they include glandular abnormalities (rarely), heredity, improper eating habits, insufficient physical activity, and psychosocial problems. High-fat diets are more likely than high-carbohydrate diets to produce obesity.[5]

Americans generally are getting heavier. Based on data from the 1988–1994 National Health Examination Survey (NHANES III), experts have estimated that 34.9% of adults age 20 or older were overweight, up from about 25% in a similar survey in 1976–1980. From one study to the other, the prevalence of overweight also rose from 7.6% to 13.7% among children aged 6–11 and from 5.7% to 11.5% among adolescents aged 12–17.[6]

Most people who are overweight are overfat. However, some individuals—particularly muscular young men—can exceed the listed weight without being overfat. Thus it is more precise to use the term *overfat* when referring to someone whose weight is too high because of excessive body-fat content. Gabe Mirkin, M.D.,[7] a sports medicine specialist, suggests:

The sanest definition for all these terms is this: You're fat, overweight or obese if you have an excess of body fat sufficient to impair your health or shorten your life.

Health Risks of Obesity

The concept of the height-weight table was developed many years ago by Louis Dublin, a Metropolitan Life Insurance Company statistician. After grouping policyholders by age, height, and weight, he found that those

---

Table 13-1

DESIRABLE WEIGHTS FOR AGES 25 AND OVER

Weight in Pounds (in Indoor Clothing)

	Height in Shoes	Small Frame	Medium Frame	Large Frame
	5'–2"	112–120	118–129	126–141
	5'–3"	115–123	121–133	129–144
	5'–4"	118–126	124–136	132–148
	5'–5"	121–129	127–139	135–152
	5'–6"	124–133	130–143	138–156
	5'–7"	128–137	134–147	142–161
M	5'–8"	132–141	138–152	147–166
E	5'–9"	136–145	142–156	151–170
N	5'–10"	140–150	146–160	155–174
	5'–11"	144–154	150–165	159–179
	6'–0"	148–158	154–170	164–184
	6'–1"	152–162	158–175	168–189
	6'–2"	156–167	162–180	173–194
	6'–3"	160–171	167–185	178–199
	6'–4"	164–175	172–190	182–204
	4'–10"	92–98	96–107	104–119
	4'–11"	94–101	98–110	106–122
	5'–0"	96–104	101–113	109–125
	5'–1"	99–107	104–116	112–128
	5'–2"	102–110	107–119	115–131
W	5'–3"	105–113	110–122	118–134
O	5'–4"	108–116	113–126	121–138
M	5'–5"	111–119	116–130	125–142
E	5'–6"	114–123	120–135	129–146
N	5'–7"	118–127	124–139	133–150
	5'–8"	122–131	128–143	137–154
	5'–9"	126–135	132–147	141–158
	5'–10"	130–140	136–151	145–163
	5'–11"	134–144	140–155	149–168
	6'–0"	138–148	144–159	153–173

Weights are obtained in indoor clothing, with men wearing shoes with 1-inch heels and women wearing shoes with two-inch heels. The data are based on weights associated with lowest death rates. For adults younger than 25, subtract 1 pound for each year under 25.

Source: Metropolitan Life Insurance Company (1959)[8]

---

who lived longest were the ones who maintained their weight at the average level for 25-year-olds. Because Dublin felt that there was no "ideal" weight for all individuals, he called these ranges "desirable weights." Some statisticians have criticized these weights because they involve only individuals who had qualified for life insurance and mainly reflect data from upper-middle-class white groups. But many authorities believe they are still the best figures relating weight to life expectancy.[9,10] Table 13-1 lists Metropolitan Life's 1959 "desirable weights."

Tens of millions of Americans have too much body fat. Small degrees of overfat are not harmful, but being 20% overfat is clearly a health hazard.[11] The most serious problem associated with being overfat is high blood pressure, but there are also considerably increased risks of sickness or death from diabetes; gallstones; liver, kidney, heart, and blood vessel diseases; osteoarthritis; and other problems.[12] JoAnn E. Manson, M.D., an endocrinologist at Harvard Medical School, estimates that obesity is responsible for about 300,000 deaths per year.[13]

Body fat can be estimated with fair accuracy by measuring the thickness of various skin folds with one's fingers[7,14] or a special skin caliper.[7] More accurate methods include underwater weighing, ultrasound, electromagnetic methods, bioelectrical impedance, CT scanning, neutron activation, and nuclear magnetic imaging, but these are expensive and used mainly for research purposes.

The health significance of body fat can be estimated by using the BMI. The National Institutes of Health Task Force on Prevention and Treatment of Obesity[15] has stated that individuals are obese if their BMI is 25 or more through age 34, but this may classify some muscular individuals as obese when they are not. Mild obesity carries a slightly increased risk for weight-related health problems, but BMI levels of 30 or more entail serious health risks.[16,17]

A rough indication of excessive body fat can be obtained by pinching the flesh on the back of the upper arm, midway between the shoulder and the elbow. Men who can pinch 1 inch or more and women who can pinch more than 1¼ inches are probably overfat. Perhaps the most practical method is to remove one's clothes and look into a full-length mirror.

Obese men tend to accumulate abdominal fat, whereas women tend to accumulate fat on their hips and thighs. A waist-to-hip ratio (WHR) greater than 1 indicates a high risk of adverse health consequences. WHR is determined by dividing the circumference of the waist by the circumference of the buttocks. A man with 35-inch hips and a 42-inch waist, for example,

Table 13-2

BODY MASS INDEX (BMI)

Height	Weight (Pounds)												
4'-10"	96	100	105	110	115	119	124	129	134	138	143	167	191
4'-11"	99	104	109	114	119	124	128	133	138	143	148	173	198
5'-0"	102	107	112	118	123	128	133	138	143	148	153	179	204
5'-1"	106	111	116	122	127	132	137	143	148	153	158	185	211
5'-2"	109	115	120	126	131	136	142	147	153	158	164	191	218
5'-3"	113	118	124	130	135	141	146	152	158	163	169	197	225
5'-4"	116	122	128	134	140	145	151	157	163	169	174	204	232
5'-5"	120	126	132	138	144	150	156	162	168	174	180	210	240
5'-6"	124	130	136	142	148	155	161	167	173	179	186	216	247
5'-7"	127	134	140	146	153	159	166	172	178	185	191	223	255
5'-8"	131	138	144	151	158	164	171	177	184	190	197	230	262
5'-9"	135	142	149	155	162	169	176	182	189	196	203	236	270
5'-10"	139	146	153	160	167	174	181	188	195	202	207	243	278
5'-11"	143	150	157	165	172	179	186	193	200	208	215	250	286
6'-0"	147	154	162	169	177	184	191	199	206	213	221	258	294
6'-1"	151	159	166	174	182	189	197	204	212	219	227	265	302
6'-2"	155	163	171	179	186	194	202	210	218	225	233	272	311
6'-3"	160	168	176	184	192	200	208	216	224	232	240	279	319
6'-4"	164	172	180	189	197	205	213	221	230	238	246	287	328
BMI:	20	21	22	23	24	25	26	27	28	29	30	35	40

Find your height in the left column and move across to the column containing your weight. The number at the bottom of the column is your BMI (your weight in kilograms divided by the square of your height in meters.)

would have a WHR of 1.2. The waist is measured at the level of the navel (belly button), and the hips are measured at the area of maximum protrusion of the buttocks.

With respect to health risks, the location may be more important than the total amount of body fat. In men a high WHR is associated with elevated blood-cholesterol levels and increased risk of coronary artery disease, high blood pressure, and adult-onset diabetes. These problems are related more to fatty tissue located inside the abdominal cavity than to fatty tissue located just under the skin.[18]

Preventing obesity during childhood may lower the chance of obesity in adult life. Obesity is related to both the number of fat cells and the amount of fat they contain; the more fat cells a person has, the more likely the person will become and remain obese. Excessive calorie intake tends to increase the number of fat cells in the body, particularly during childhood. When people lose weight they decrease the fat content of their cells, but not their number. Thus the more excess weight gained early in life, the more difficult it will be to lose or maintain weight.[18] Unfortunately, large surveys have shown that the incidence of obesity among American children and adolescents is high and has been increasing steadily.[19]

Difficulty with "Dieting"

The two basic factors involved in weight control are caloric intake and energy expenditure. To lose weight one must eat less or exercise more—but most people need to do both. There are about 3500 calories stored in 1 pound of body fat. Most moderately active people need

Table 13-3

APPROXIMATE CALORIC INTAKE MODERATELY ACTIVE PEOPLE NEED TO MAINTAIN WEIGHT

Weight	Daily Calories Needed
100	1500
110	1650
120	1800
130	1950
140	2100
150	2250
160	2400
170	2550
180	2700
190	2950
200	3000

Table 13-4

WEEKS NEEDED TO LOSE WEIGHT AT VARIOUS CALORIC DEFICITS

Pounds to Lose	Calorie Deficit*											
	100	*200*	*300*	*400*	*500*	*600*	*700*	*800*	*900*	*1000*	*1100*	*1200*
1	5.0	2.5	1.7	1.3	1.0	0.8	0.7	0.6	0.6	0.5	0.5	0.4
2	10.0	5.0	3.3	2.5	2.0	1.7	1.4	1.3	1.1	1.0	0.9	0.8
3	15.0	7.5	5.0	3.8	3.0	2.5	2.1	1.9	1.7	1.5	1.4	1.3
4	20.0	10.0	6.7	5.0	4.0	3.3	2.9	2.5	2.2	2.0	1.8	1.7
5	25.0	12.5	8.3	6.3	5.0	4.2	3.6	3.1	2.8	2.5	2.3	2.1
6	30.0	15.0	10.0	7.5	6.0	5.0	4.3	3.8	3.3	3.0	2.7	2.5
7	35.0	17.5	11.7	8.8	7.0	5.8	5.0	4.4	3.9	3.5	3.2	2.9
8	40.0	20.0	13.3	10.0	8.0	6.7	5.7	5.0	4.4	4.0	3.6	3.3
9	45.0	22.5	15.0	11.3	9.0	7.5	6.4	5.6	5.0	4.5	4.1	3.8
10	50.0	25.0	16.7	12.5	10.0	8.3	7.1	6.3	5.6	5.0	4.5	4.2

*Calorie deficit = calories expended minus calories consumed. Each 3500-calorie deficit produces loss of 1 pound of fat.
Most moderately active people need about 15 calories per pound to maintain their weight.   © 2001, Stephen Barrett, M.D.

about 15 calories per pound to maintain their weight (see Table 13-3).[20] To lose 1 pound of fat per week, one must consume an average of 500 fewer calories per day than are metabolized. Nutritionists recommend that diets under 1200 calories per day should not be carried out without medical supervision. Table 13-4 shows how caloric deficit is related to the rate of weight loss.

Most people who are overfat find weight control difficult or impossible to achieve. Long-term studies of overfat individuals—done mainly in hospital clinics—have found that more than 95% of those who lost weight by dieting regained it within 1 year. Dietary treatment is most likely to succeed in people who are only modestly overweight. Obese individuals tend to burn calories more slowly. They tend to be less active, which compounds the problem, because people tend to eat more when they are sedentary. They also tend to underestimate the number of calories they eat,[21,22] and to underreport their weight and overreport their height after participating in a weight-loss program.[23]

In 1993 *Consumer Reports*[24] tabulated the results of a survey that drew 95,000 responses from readers who said that they had tried to lose weight during the previous 3 years. About 19,000 had used a commercial diet program. About 25% said they had lost some weight and, 2 years after finishing their program, had been able to keep most of it off.

Evidence is accumulating that heredity may be the major factor in determining how much people weigh. When people deviate from their usual weight, metabolic adjustments tend to oppose the change. Researchers have found, for example, that significant weight loss is accompanied by increased hunger and a decrease in the body's metabolic rate.[25] Bennett has noted that the weight-control measures are not hopeless, because people's "fat thermostat" may be reset if they consume less fat and increase their habitual level of physical activity.[26]

It is not clear whether people whose weight goes up and down repeatedly (referred to as "weight cycling" or "yo-yo dieting") have higher rates of death and disease. A 32-year study of more than 3130 men and women found that weight-cyclers had a higher overall death rate and as much as twice the chance of dying from heart disease.[27] The researchers also found that people who dieted tended to vary more in weight than people who did not. Expressing concern that "the risks due to overweight may not outweigh the risks due to weight fluctuation," the researchers recommended that weight-loss programs give greater emphasis to preventing relapses. Kelley Brownell, Ph.D., the psychologist in charge of the study, said that many women who are not overweight create trouble for themselves by dieting. A 12-year study of 11,703 middle-aged and elderly Harvard University alumni has found that both weight gain and weight loss were associated with significantly increased death rates from all causes and from coronary heart disease.[28] The most likely explanation is that those who lost the most weight were more likely to have had cycles of yo-yo dieting. However, the National Task Force on the

Prevention and Treatment of Obesity[29] has concluded that the majority of studies published between 1966 and 1994 did not conclusively show that weight cycling is harmful. The task force stated that significantly obese individuals should not allow concerns about hazards of weight cycling to deter them from trying to control their weight.

Because "dieting" is usually unsuccessful, many experts believe that people's emphasis should be on fitness (readily attainable through exercise) and control of cardiovascular risk factors (abnormal blood cholesterol levels, high blood pressure, and elevated blood sugar levels).[30-32] The participants in a 1992 NIH Technology Assessment Conference concluded:

Methods whose primary goal is short-term rapid or unsupervised weight loss, or that rely on such diet aids as drinks, prepackaged foods, or pharmacologic agents but do not include education in and eventual transition to a lasting program of healthful eating and activity, have never been shown to lead to long-term success. It has been fairly said that such programs fail people, not vice-versa. Recognition of this by society and individuals and a focus on approaches that can produce health benefits independently of weight loss may be the best way to improve the physical and psychological health of Americans seeking to lose weight.[33]

The panelists also concluded: "A health paradox exists in modern America. On the one hand, many people who do not need to lose weight are trying to. On the other hand, most who do need to lose weight are not succeeding." Abernathy and Black[31] state that more emphasis should be placed on risk factors and healthy lifestyles and less on height/weight tables and body-fat percentages. *Consumer Reports* agrees:

Given the strong likelihood that any weight lost on a reducing diet will be gained back promptly, we recommend that anyone contemplating a diet think seriously about whether losing weight is necessary or desirable in the first place. . . . The majority of dieters would probably do better to forget about cutting calories, focus on exercising and eating a healthful diet, and let the pounds fall where they may.[24]

◆ Personal Glimpse ◆

A Plug for Fitness

People who have met me within the last 25 years find it hard to believe that I was once a third bigger than I am now. Like many women in their early 20s, I had become obsessed with weight and quite miserable about the extra pounds that had begun to clutter up my five-foot frame. So, like millions of others in the same boat, I tried dieting. All kinds of diets. Many commercial programs and gimmicks and a few I made up on my own. And sure, I would lose weight, but then I'd gain it back—and usually some extra pounds to boot—when I got sick and tired of feeling deprived and living on eggs and grapefruit or cottage cheese and carrots or whatever happened to be the popular weight-loss concoction of the day.

Believe me, I tried them all—even the ridiculous drinking man's diet—and all they did was result in an ever-bigger me.

Then one day I panicked. I was fat. But even more important, I realized, I was probably killing myself with my atrocious eating habits. I vowed to turn over a new leaf. I decided that if I was going to be fat, so be it, but at least I could be healthy and fat.

I gave up diets and gimmicks and cycles of starving and bingeing, and I started eating: three wholesome meals, with wholesome snacks if I was hungry between meals, and one little "no-no" each day—two cookies, a couple of spoons of ice cream, a thin sliver of cake or pie—something I loved and did not want to miss. No deprivation, no starvation, no bingeing. Only moderation.

And I put myself on a regular exercise program. Every day I would do something physically challenging: walking, cycling, skating, swimming, tennis—something that got me breathing hard (I kept thinking about how all that oxygen was restoring my cells to health) and feeling good about my body.

Losing weight wasn't part of this plan, but lose weight I did. Even though I was eating whenever I was hungry and consuming what felt like mountains of food, I lost weight: about seven pounds the first month and then about one or two pounds a month thereafter, until my weight stabilized two years later at 35 pounds lighter. And there it has stayed, give or take five pounds here or there, for a quarter-century.

Trying to lose weight fast is probably the single biggest mistake dieters make. Weight that comes off quickly nearly always comes back on even faster. You didn't gain those extra pounds in a fortnight, and you shouldn't be trying to take them off in two weeks, or even necessarily in two months or two years. The idea is to adopt an eating and exercise plan that you can go on and can stay on for the rest of your life, a program that will allow you to lose weight slowly, tone up your body gradually and eventually stabilize at a weight and shape that is right for you.

Jane Brody[34]
Personal Health Columnist
The New York Times

Table 13-5

WEIGHT-CONTROL MYTHS VS FACTS

New research findings are revising many long-held beliefs and assumptions about obesity. These examples were assembled by the Nutrition Research Center at St. Luke's-Roosevelt Hospital Center and the Nestlé Research and Development Center, Inc.

Myth: *You can't get fat on a low-fat diet.*
Fact: Restricting fat intake is useful in weight control and has distinct health advantages in terms of coronary heart disease and cancer. However, while it is more difficult to gain weight on a low-fat diet than a high-fat diet, it is by no means impossible. The net calories available to your body still count, whether they come from fat or carbohydrates. No matter what the source, if you eat more calories than you burn, the excess is stored as fat. People gain weight every day from too many calories from low-fat ice cream, cakes, cookies, mayonnaise, and margarine.

Myth: *Obesity results from psychological problems.*
Fact: For many years, some people suffering from obesity underwent treatment for emotional distress under the assumption they were anxious or depressed and ate to compensate for some inner need. This simply is not true. For example, epidemiological surveys have shown that neither manic/depressive illness nor schizophrenia is more common among obese than among lean people.

Myth: *Eating slowly will make you feel full faster, thus helping to reduce food intake during mealtime.*
Fact: There is no concrete evidence to support this claim. Recent laboratory studies in which eating rates were manipulated and food intake was measured showed no effect on the amount of food eaten.

Myth: *People who binge-eat do so because they have a deep sugar/carbohydrate craving.*
Fact: Laboratory studies have revealed that the food preferences of people with binge eating disorder, or a related "binge-purge" disorder known as bulimia, aren't very different from those of the normal population. The problem is they can't control the amount they eat. More recent studies suggest they may have a physiologic disturbance that begins at some point after the onset of the disorder and affects their sense of satiety. In other words, they may not experience the sense of fullness that normally occurs at the end of a meal until they have consumed an excessive amount of food.

Myth: *Since genetics and obesity can be linked, trying to control obesity by diet won't work.*
Fact: Despite your family history, the number of calories you consume still plays an important role in determining whether you will lose or gain weight.

Myth: *Obese people can "eat like a bird" and still not lose weight.*
Fact: Researchers at St. Luke's-Roosevelt Hospital Center have found that obese men and women tend to underreport the number of calories they actually consume. The fact is that, all things being equal, if they did eat very little, they would lose weight.

Myth: *Through diet and exercise, you will be able to change the way your body fat is distributed.*
Fact: The location of body fat may be a direct result of whether you are male or female, your genetic makeup, your age, and whether you are under stress, smoke or drink. Diet and exercise may slim you—and improve your health—but won't change fat distribution.

Myth: *Once obese people bring their weight down to a desirable level, that level can be easily maintained by eating the usual, moderate amount of calories.*
Fact: The body tends to resist intervention that lowers or raises its fat content. Scientists have found that reducing weight causes some metabolic processes to slow down so that it takes fewer calories than before to make you gain weight again. In other words, to maintain the same healthy weight, an obese person who has reduced often must eat fewer calories than someone who's never been obese. It's one reason for the high recidivism rate among dieters. The reverse is also true. Gaining weight increases energy expenditure, which means that if you've been thin, it will take more calories than ever to keep your weight up.

Myth: *Obesity is due to a simple lack of willpower.*
Fact: The bulk of research evidence shows that there is a strong genetic component to obesity, which may reflect a special vulnerability to an environment in which calorie-rich foods are relentlessly promoted. Several genes have been identified that not only influence appetite and satiety, but may also affect how efficiently the body stores food calories.

Myth: *Certain fats, such as fish oils and olive oil, are not fattening.*
Fact: Studies show that, like saturated fats, monounsaturated fats (such as olive oil, which is associated with the popular Mediterranean diet) and polyunsaturated fats (such as fish and vegetable oils) are fattening. Although there is a difference in the way various fatty acids are metabolized in the body, all fats can promote obesity and should be eaten in moderation.

The Institute of Medicine has defined successful dieting as a 5% reduction in initial body weight that is maintained for at least 1 year.[16] A recent U.S. Department of Agriculture white paper has concluded that controlled clinical trials are needed to answer questions about long-term effectiveness (weight maintenance), health detriments, and adverse effects of high-fat, low-carbohydrate and low- and very-low-fat diets.[35] The agency plans to sponsor such trials.

EATING DISORDERS

Our society's preoccupation with body image and dieting has stimulated many people to resort to extreme measures of weight control.[36] Anorexia nervosa is a life-threatening condition in which food intake is severely limited. The victims, most of whom are young women, have an intense fear of gaining weight or becoming fat, even though they are underweight. Bulimia (also called bulimia nervosa) is a disorder characterized by bingeing (episodes of eating large amounts of food) and purging (getting rid of the food by vomiting or using laxatives). In contrast with anorectics, most bulimics (a) do not get emaciated, (b) are aware that they have a problem, and (c) feel compelled to conceal it. About half of anorectics develop symptoms of bulimia, and about half of bulimics have a history of anorexia or eventually develop it.[37]

Inadequate food intake or extreme purging can cause metabolic imbalances that result in fatigue, irregular heartbeat, thinning of the bones, and cessation of menstruation. Frequent self-induced vomiting can damage the stomach and esophagus, make the gums recede, and erode tooth enamel. Studies have found that as many as 1% of females become anorectic between the ages of 12 and 18 and that about 5% of female first-year college students have a history of bulimia.[38]

Eating disorders may require psychologic and dietary counseling, as well as medical treatment for any physical ailments that have developed. If a patient's weight becomes dangerously low, hospitalization with intensive therapy is recommended. Medical treatment for anorexia may have to include tube feedings or hyperalimentation (complete nutrition through the veins) if the patient will not or cannot eat. Dietary counseling may help an anorectic individual understand the importance of nutrition and instill healthy eating behaviors. Psychologic therapy should aim for greater self-understanding, clarification of family dynamics, and the development of the patient's own individual personality. Additional information about eating disorders can be obtained from the National Association of Anorexia Nervosa and Associated Disorders and the Anorexia Bulimia Treatment and Education Center.

Eating disorders are common among participants in some of the performing arts and among athletes in sports that emphasize leanness or have weight classifications. The activities include ballet, dance, gymnastics, wrestling, judo, boxing, weightlifting, bodybuilding, figure skating, diving, horse racing, and distance running. The methods used to keep thin or to "make weight" for a competition include rubber suits, excessive heat in saunas, diuretics, laxatives, self-induced vomiting, excessive exercise, starvation, and dehydration—all of which have potentially dangerous consequences.

THE DIET AND WEIGHT-LOSS MARKETPLACE

Surveys have estimated that the percentage of overweight adults in the United States is between 25% and 64%, depending on the criteria and methods used to collect the data. Major surveys conducted during 1990 found that 44% of female high school students, 15% of male high school students, 38% of female adults (age 18 or older), and 24% of male adults reported that they were trying to lose weight.[39] A 1991 FDA telephone survey of 1431 persons 18 years or older found that 33% of the women and 20% of the men said they were trying to lose weight.[40]

Marketdata Enterprises, an independent market research and consulting firm, estimated that 1999 sales of weight-loss products and services totaled $32.22 billion. The leading categories were diet soft drinks ($13.57 billion); health clubs ($10.65 billion); artificial sweeteners ($1.61 billion); over-the counter (OTC) appetite suppressants and meal-replacement products ($1.49 billion); low-calorie prepared foods ($1.47 billion); medically supervised diet programs ($1.31 billion); commercial weight-loss center programs ($1.13 billion); and diet books, cassette tapes, and exercise videos ($1.04 billion).[3] Marketdata also noted that the number of Web-based weight-loss services has exploded, with some companies operating retail centers and others operating only online. In 1995, Marketdata concluded most dieters with money to spend were "cosmetically obese" (20 to 30 pounds to lose) rather than medically at risk and that 70% of teenage girls were dieting.

QUESTIONABLE DIETS

Most fad diets, if followed closely, will result in weight loss—as a result of caloric restriction—but they are monotonous and often dangerous to health if followed for long periods. Yet many obese individuals are sufficiently desperate or gullible to try one questionable method after another. A highly publicized diet will attract many people who try it for a short period of time, lose weight, and encourage others to do the same. Because most will regain their lost weight, the market for "new" diets is inexhaustible.

Dr. Philip L. White, former director of the AMA Department of Foods and Nutrition, warned against trying any method promised to induce weight loss of more than two pounds a week. He gave these additional tips for spotting an unreliable diet promotion:

- It suggests that a nutrient or food group is either the key to weight reduction or the primary "villain" that keeps people overweight.
- It claims to be a revolutionary new idea.
- It reports testimonials rather than documented research.
- It refers to the author's own case histories, but does not describe them in detail.
- It claims 100% success.
- The promoter claims persecution by the medical profession.[41]

The National Council Against Health Fraud warns consumers to be wary of any weight-control program that encourages the use of special products rather than learning how to make wise food choices from the conventional food supply.[42]

Most fad diets lack important nutrients or even whole food groups and are therefore nutritionally unbalanced. The three main types of unbalanced approaches to weight loss are complete fasting (starvation), supplemented fasting, and low-carbohydrate (high-protein) diets.

Complete Fasting

The most drastic way to reduce caloric intake is to stop eating. Intake of water, of course, is still necessary. Fasting has been used for weight reduction since ancient times. Losses will be greatest in heaviest subjects and least in individuals who are the lightest. A few days of fasting are unlikely to be dangerous, but prolonged fasting leads to dangerous metabolic imbalances.

Glucose is essential for the brain and is the preferred fuel for other body tissues. Glucose is obtained easily from carbohydrates, less easily from proteins, but not at all from fats. After a few days of total fasting, body fats and proteins are metabolized to produce energy. The fats are broken down into fatty acids, which can be used as fuel. If sufficient carbohydrate is not available to the body, the fatty acids may be incompletely metabolized and yield ketone bodies, causing a condition known as ketosis. This situation, if prolonged,

is hazardous because proteins must be broken down to ensure an adequate supply of glucose for the brain. During fasting, because no proteins are available from food, they are obtained from muscles and major organs such as the heart and kidneys. A prolonged fast can also lead to anemia, liver impairment, kidney stones, postural hypotension (low blood pressure), mineral imbalances, and other adverse effects.

Part of the reason for fasting's popularity is that it can produce dramatic weight loss during its early stages. As ketosis begins, large amounts of water will be shed, leading the dieter to think that significant weight reduction is taking place. However, most of the loss is water rather than fat; the lost water is regained quickly when eating is resumed. Appetite, often reduced during ketosis, also returns when a balanced diet is resumed. Claims that fasting "cleanses the body of toxic chemicals" are false.[43]

Supplemented Fasting

Medical researchers have discovered that if fasting individuals eat small amounts of protein, the protein will break down slowly to provide the glucose needed by the brain. Eating carbohydrates for this purpose does not work because it triggers an insulin response that causes intense hunger. In the early 1970s Dr. George Blackburn and colleagues at the Deaconess Hospital in Boston developed the "protein-sparing modified fast" in which fasting patients were given small amounts of high-quality protein along with noncaloric liquids, vitamins, calcium, potassium, other minerals, and sometimes glucose. Patients were initially hospitalized for 1 week of evaluation and then followed closely as outpatients. Their diets were carefully calculated. The program emphasized not only diet but also an overall approach that included exercise, instruction in nutrition, and behavior modification.

Today, modified fasting can be done safely on an outpatient basis under skilled medical supervision. But popularization of very-low-calorie (VLC) diets—by such events as Oprah Winfrey's celebrated 67-pound weight-loss (followed by her regaining a greater amount)—can lead to dangerous misuse. Experts have expressed fears that the vigorous marketing of meal-replacement drinks will encourage people to use these products inappropriately. The more meals replaced and the lower the number of calories consumed daily, the greater the risk. The risk is greatest in individuals who are not severely overweight. The FDA now requires a warning label on weight-reduction products if more than half of their calories come from protein.

VLC diets usually contain 400 to 800 calories per

day, most of them from high-quality proteins, plus vitamins and minerals, particularly potassium. Some programs use liquid formulas, whereas others utilize food sources (poultry, fish, and lean meats). Programs this drastic should be restricted to individuals who are at least 30% overweight and be administered only under close medical supervision as part of a comprehensive program. The programs should include a weekly examination by a physician familiar with the metabolic effects of VLC diets, blood tests to detect potentially dangerous metabolic abnormalities, and behavior modification. Patients in controlled investigations have typically consumed the diets for 12 to 16 weeks. Weight gain is common after the eating of food is resumed, but the gain is more likely to occur with do-it-yourself programs than with medically supervised ones.[44] Bennion and others[18] have noted that fewer than half of the people who sign up for a VLC program actually reach their goal weight. The National Task Force on the Prevention and Treatment of Obesity has said that there is no advantage to intakes lower than 800 calories per day.[45]

Low-Carbohydrate Diets
Most low-carbohydrate diets do not limit the intake of proteins, fats, or total calories. Promoters claim that unbalancing the diet will lead to increased metabolism of unwanted fat even if the calories are not restricted. This is not true, but calorie reduction is likely to occur because the diet's monotony tends to discourage over-eating. A diet that is low in both carbohydrates and calories will produce ketosis and rapid initial weight loss, as noted in the previous section.

Some promoters of low-carbohydrate diets regard carbohydrates as "the dieter's number one enemy." This designation is inappropriate, because calories from any source contribute equally to weight gain if consumed in excess. Moreover, because of their high water and fiber content, most carbohydrate foods other than table sugar contain fewer calories per volume of food than most other foods.

Table 13-6 summarizes the shortcomings of various fad diets.

The Atkins Diet
The most widely used low-carbohydrate diet is the one advocated by Robert C. Atkins, M.D., of New York City. His 1972 book *Dr. Atkins' Diet Revolution* sold millions of copies within the first 2 years. His 1992 update, *Dr. Atkins' New Diet Revolution*, has sold even more. The current plan has four steps: a 2-week "induction" period, during which the goal is to reduce carbohydrate intake to under 20 grams per day, and three periods

during which carbohydrate intake is progressively raised but kept below what Atkins calls "your critical carbohydrate level" for losing or maintaining weight. The dieter is permitted to eat unlimited amounts of noncarbohydrate foods "when hungry," but ketosis tends to suppress appetite. The plan calls for checking one's urine for ketone bodies to ensure that the desired level of ketosis is reached. Large amounts of nutritional supplements are also recommended.[46]

The AMA Council on Foods and Nutrition,[47] *Consumer Reports*,[48] and many individual experts have warned that the unlimited intake of saturated fats under Atkins' food plan can increase the dieter's risk of heart disease. A computer analysis by Anderson and colleagues found that the diet provided fewer servings of grains, vegetables, and fruits than the U.S. Dietary Guidelines recommend, which means that long-term use probably increases the risk of cardiovascular disease and cancer.[49] However, no long-term follow-up study has been published either by Atkins or by his critics.

Recently, researchers at the Bassett Research Institute in Cooperstown, N.Y., followed 18 Atkins dieters for 1 month. During the 2-week induction period, the dieters consumed 1419 calories a day, compared with 2481 calories a day before starting the diet, and lost an average of about 8 pounds. In the next phase, dieters averaged 1500 calories a day and lost an additional 3 pounds in 2 weeks. Dieters in both phases cut back on carbohydrates by more than 90%, but the actual amounts of fat and protein they ate changed little. Some patients felt tired, and some were nauseated on the plan. Most indicated that they were eager to go back to their regular diet.[50]

Researchers who compile the National Weight Control Registry analyzed the diets of 2681 members who had maintained at least a 30-pound weight loss for 1 year or more. They found that fewer than 1% had followed a diet similar to the Atkins program. Most followed high-carbohydrate, low-fat diets.[50] Chapter 12 contains additional information about Atkins.

The Scarsdale Diet
The Scarsdale Medical Diet is a carefully designed regimen that itemizes foods for every day of the week, with no substitutions allowed. The expected intake is 750 to 1000 calories per day. The plan's author, the late Dr. Herman Tarnower, suggested preliminary consultation with a physician, a daily 2-mile walk, and alteration of the 2-week periods of the basic diet with 2-week periods of a more liberal "Keep-Trim Program." Mirkin[7] states that the diet cannot be followed permanently and does not help people change their eating habits.

Table 13-6

QUESTIONABLE DIET PLANS—PAST AND PRESENT

Diet Plan	Brief Description	Comments
Atkins' New Diet Revolution	Four-phase low-carbohydrate, high-protein diet plus high-dosage dietary supplements	Unbalanced; high in fat/cholesterol; deliberately produces ketosis in induction phase
Bio-Diet	Alternates "crash" diet with binges, plus supplements	Unhealthy practice; supplements do not provide weight-loss benefits as claimed
Bloomingdale's Eat Healthy Diet	Highly restrictive diet based on false premise that certain foods are addictive	Unbalanced, can slow metabolism; semi-starvation encourages binge eating
Carbohydrate Addict's Diet	Claims to break "carbohydrate addiction" through a low-carbohydrate diet plus "reward meals"	Actual addiction to carbohydrates does not exist; "reward meals" encourage uncontrolled eating habits
Dr. Abravenel's Body-Type Diet	"Body-type" claimed to signify glandular imbalance that causes obesity; food groups are emphasized or eliminated for each "body type"	Bizarre rationale; some regimens are unbalanced and high in fat; others are well balanced
Eat Right 4 Your Type	Claims that blood type determines how people react to nutrients and therefore should guide dietary choices	Bizarre theory; some recommendations result in dietary imbalance
F-Plan Diet	Low-calorie, high-fiber diet	May be deficient in calcium; excessive fiber can cause side effects
Fat-Destroyer Foods Diet	Low-carbohydrate, high-protein diet	Unbalanced, high in fat/cholesterol, causes ketosis and other serious side effects; weight loss primarily due to temporary fluid loss
Fructose Diet	Low-carbohydrate diet with relatively large intake of fructose	Unbalanced; fructose does not provide weight-loss benefits claimed
Grapefruit Diet	Grapefruit and/or supplements before meals to "burn" fat	Based on myth that grapefruit facilitates weight loss
I Love New York Diet	Alternates "crash" diet with binges	Unhealthy practice, can slow metabolism; promises unrealistic results
Kelp, Lecithin, Vitamin B_6 and Cider Vinegar Diet	Low-carbohydrate diet plus supplements	Unbalanced; supplements do not provide weight-loss benefits claimed
Mayo Diet	Grapefruit eaten before meals to "burn" fat	Ineffective, based on myth; not connected with the Mayo Clinic
Mono-food diets	Special emphasis given to one food or food type, such as eggs, grapefruit, or fruit only	Unbalanced; can slow metabolism; nutrient deficiencies can develop
Rice Diet	Five phases, beginning with only rice and fruit	Unbalanced, can cause low blood pressure and lead to nutrient shortages
Rotation Diet	Low-calorie diet alternating with "normal" eating	Unbalanced; can slow metabolism; may promote binge eating
Southampton Diet	Low-calorie diet with "mood foods"	Promises unrealistic results; promotes nutrition nonsense
The Zone	Shuns supposedly "unfavorable" carbohydrates	Complex system based on questionable assertions about metabolism
As long as people buy them, the endless parade of questionable diet plans will continue	More of the same	Most likely unbalanced and restrictive and ultimately disappointing; may slow your metabolism and prove dangerous to health

Modified from Stare FJ, Aronson V, Barrett S: *Your Guide to Good Nutrition*[9] and *Consumer Reports* evaluations.[48]

The Beverly Hills Diet

The Beverly Hills Diet is based on bizarre notions about digestion and metabolism, including the idea that undigested food is what winds up as fat. The author, Judy Mazel, is not a nutrition professional. She claimed that for food to be digested properly, only one type (protein, fat, or carbohydrate) should be eaten each day. Her diet called for just fruit for the first 10 days, then other types of foods were added in various combinations. Three cases of severe diarrhea, muscle weakness, and dizziness on this diet were reported by Mirkin and Shore,[51] who also warned that more serious reactions would not be surprising. Harvard nutritionist D. Mark Hegsted, Ph.D.,[52] noted the diet's low protein content and called it "a sure recipe for malnutrition if you stay on it long enough."

Fit for Life Diet

Fit for Life is based on theories of "Natural Hygiene," which allege that eating foods in the wrong combination can cause health problems (see Chapter 8). The book's authors, Harvey and Marilyn Diamond, lack scientific training in nutrition but acquired credentials from the American College of Health Science, a nonaccredited correspondence school that in 1986 was ordered by a Texas court to stop granting "degrees" and calling itself a college.[53] According to the Diamonds, when certain foods are eaten together, they "rot" and "decay," creating digestive cesspools that somehow poison one's system and make one tired and fat. They recommend a low-fat, high-fiber diet with foods high in water content to "wash out the body from the inside." These ideas are nonsensical.[54] Katherine Musgrave, a University of Maine nutrition professor, did a computerized analysis of the diet and concluded that it was inadequate in calcium, zinc, and vitamins B_{12} and D.[55] Despite enormous criticism from the scientific community, the book sold close to 2 million copies. Dr. William T. Jarvis stated:

Fit for Life seems unprecedented in the amount of misinformation contained. It is appalling that such a book can become a best seller in the latter half of the 20th century. Its only socially redeeming feature is that its popularity may alert American educators of their failure to impart the most fundamental knowledge about health and nutrition to students entrusted to their care.[56]

Cabbage Soup Diet

In 1996 *U.S. News & World Report* described the cabbage soup diet as "a quick-weight-loss plan that has poured from photocopiers, fax machines, and publications such as *USA Today* in recent months."[57] Some versions are said to have been endorsed by the American Heart Association, the Cleveland Clinic, and Loma Linda University—which all three organizations deny. The diet is falsely claimed to cause weight loss of 5 to 7 pounds in 3 days and 10 to 17 pounds in 1 week. It is also claimed to be "fast" and "fat-burning," to produce abundant energy, and to "flush your system of impurities." The instructions call for unlimited amounts of a soup made from cabbage, onions, celery, tomatoes, green peppers, and Lipton Onion Soup Mix. Fruit is added on day 1, vegetables on day 2, fruit and vegetables on day 3, bananas and skim milk on day 4, beef and tomatoes or vegetables on days 5 and 6, and brown rice, fruit juices, and vegetables on day 7. The American Heart Association has stated that a small amount of weight loss may occur because of caloric restriction, but that the diet is unbalanced and does not provide adequate nutrient intake for long-term use. Nor do its instructions advise the dieter to increase exercise or modify eating habits.

Herbalife

Herbalife International is a multilevel marketing company founded in 1980. Its diet plan was based on four products: (1) a powdered protein meal substitute, (2) an herbal blend with ingredients that include small amounts of laxatives, (3) a multivitamin/multimineral/herb formula, and (4) a linseed oil formula. Initially these products and others were marketed with suggestions that they would produce rapid weight loss and that the herbs they contain were effective against a large number of serious diseases. Testimonials to this effect were spread by personal contact and frequent television specials.

In 1982 the FDA sent Herbalife a Notice of Adverse Findings, which stated that certain products were misbranded by claims that they were effective for treating many diseases, dissolving and removing tumors, rejuvenating the body, increasing circulation, and producing mental alertness. In 1985 a U.S. Senate subcommittee held hearings at which experts testified that Herbalife had made many false claims, and company officials admitted that many users had experienced headaches, diarrhea, constipation, or other adverse effects from its products.[58]

Soon afterward, the California Attorney General charged that Herbalife had made false claims for many of its products and engaged in an illegal pyramid-style marketing scheme. In 1986 the company and its president, Mark Hughes, agreed to pay $850,000 to settle these charges. The court order settling the case forbids representation without reasonable basis that Herbalife products contain herbs that can curb appetite, burn off calories, or cleanse the system.

The company's current program (the Herbalife Cellular Nutrition Health and Weight Management System) includes some ingredients that differ from its original program. Although Herbalife's literature no longer contains false disease-related claims, its products are still hyped by both the company and its distributors. A 1994 Herbalife audiotape, for example, stated that America's health was declining as a result of faulty nutrition and that somehow Herbalife products would provide special nutritional help at the "cellular level."[59] However, there appear to be no published scientific studies in which Herbalife products were tested for effectiveness. In 2000, after a 4-day drinking binge, Hughes died of an overdose of alcohol and a toxic level of the antidepressant doxepin. His blood alcohol level was 0.21%, which is more than twice the legal limit for driving a car.[60]

PRESCRIPTION DRUGS

No drug or drug product can ensure permanent weight loss. Some products can suppress appetite temporarily, but side effects or other negative characteristics limit their usefulness.

Amphetamines ("speed") were once widely prescribed as appetite suppressants. Their adverse effects and potential for addiction outweigh any usefulness as a dieting aid. Although they can temporarily curb appetite, the effect will wear off after a few months unless dangerously high doses are prescribed. Amphetamines can cause nervousness, irritability, insomnia, and fatigue. High dosages can cause abnormal heart rhythms, fainting, and psychotic reactions.

Thyroid hormone helps to control metabolism (the rate at which calories are used up by the body). However, unless a documented deficiency of this hormone exists, use of thyroid supplements is inadvisable. Small doses given to normal individuals merely suppress normal thyroid hormone production and have no metabolic effect. Large dosages will cause weight reduction, but they will also raise blood pressure and strain the heart. The FDA requires the labels on thyroid products to warn that they should not be used for obesity and that large doses produce serious and life-threatening effects.[62]

Human chorionic gonadotropin (HCG) is a hormone found in the urine of pregnant women. More than 40 years ago, Dr. Albert T. Simeons, a British-born physician, contended that it would enable dieters to subsist comfortably on a 500-calorie-a-day diet. He claimed that HCG would mobilize stored fat; suppress appetite; and redistribute fat from the waist, hips, and thighs. There is no scientific evidence to support these claims. More-over, a 500-calorie (semi-starvation) diet is likely to result in loss of protein from vital organs, and HCG can cause other adverse effects. The FDA requires labeling and advertising of HCG to state that it has not been demonstrated to be effective against obesity. Mirkin[7] states, "At one time, HCG was the most widespread obesity medication administered in the United States. Some doctors liked it because it assured them of a steady clientele. Patients had to come in once a week for an injection."

Diuretics are substances that cause water loss from the body by increasing the output of urine. They can be very valuable in the medical treatment of cardiovascular disease, but are inappropriate for use in weight-reduction programs. Any weight loss that results from water loss is temporary and will be reversed when the body is rehydrated. In addition, improper use of diuretics can cause a dangerous depletion of body sodium or potassium.

Fenfluramine (*Pondimin*), phentermine (*Ionamin*), dexfenfluramine (*Redux*), and several other prescription drugs can suppress appetite by increasing serotonin levels in the brain, which induces feelings of fullness and satisfaction.[62] In clinical studies, these drugs have helped to produce weight loss of $1/2$ to $1^{1}/_{2}$ pounds per week. However, the effect usually plateaus after 6 months and, when the drug is discontinued, most users gain weight. Many gain more weight than they lost while taking the drug. The longest study followed patients for up to 4 years and included caloric restriction, behavior modification sessions, exercise reinforcement, and physician visits.[63] These drugs can cause dry mouth, nervousness, sleep disturbances, blood pressure elevation, and many other side effects. Bennion and others[18] stated that appetite-suppressant drugs should not be used for weight control because the risk of side effects outweighs the likelihood of a lasting benefit. However, a subsequent review by Goldstein and Potvin concluded that the benefits of extended treatment appear to outweigh the risks for appropriately selected individuals who can maintain adequate weight loss with long-term drug therapy.[64]

In 1996 the FDA approved the use of dexfenfluramine for periods of up to 1 year in patients with a BMI of 30 (or 27 with other risk factors for heart disease). Researchers who did an epidemiologic study had concluded that people who use dexfenfluramine for more than 3 months have an increased risk of developing primary pulmonary hypertension, a rare but potentially fatal disease. FDA approval was based on the belief that in patients who were markedly obese, the potential benefits still outweighed the risks. However, many doctors prescribed it for people with mild obesity; unscrupulous operators made it readily available through the Internet; and some combined it with phentermine, a combination commonly referred to as "Fen-phen." In 1997, after heart-valve damage was reported among many users of Fen-phen and a few users of fenfluramine or dexfenfluramine, fenfluramine and dexfenfluramine were withdrawn from the market. (Phentermine remains because its use alone was not associated with the problem.)[65]

In 1997, the FDA approved the marketing of subitramine hydrochloride (*Meridia*), a drug that is structurally related to amphetamine. The *Medical Letter* considers it "modestly effective," but recommends against using it because it can cause dry mouth, headache, insomnia, and constipation and can elevate blood pressure and heart rate.[66] In 1999, the FDA approved the marketing of orlistat (*Xenical*), which inactivates the intestinal enzymes (lipase) needed to absorb fat from food. The amount absorbed is reduced about 30%. As a result, users who consume large amounts of fat may experience bloating, gas, and loose stools. Orlistat can also block absorption of fat-soluble vitamins (A, D, E), so that supplementation would be prudent.

Consumer Reports on Health advises that long-term use of prescription weight-control drugs is unknown and therefore they should not even be considered unless a person is extremely obese and has made serious attempts to lose weight without drugs.[67]

NONPRESCRIPTION PRODUCTS

During the 1970s an FDA advisory panel evaluated more than 100 substances that had been used in weight-loss formulas. The panel's 1979 report concluded that some had no pharmacologic activity at all, and that many were not worth considering because no shred of evidence suggested that they could be helpful. The panel judged only two ingredients safe and effective: phenylpropanolamine and benzocaine.

In 1990, after Congressman Ron Wyden (D–OR) conducted a hearing, the FDA proposed to ban arginine, caffeine, kelp, guar gum, lecithin, papaya enzymes, phenylalanine, tryptophan, vitamin B_6, and 102 other substances as ingredients in weight-loss products. The ban took effect in 1992, but the substances can still be marketed as "dietary supplements" without claims for weight control.

Phenylpropanolamine

Phenylpropanolamine (PPA), a nasal decongestant, has been the active ingredient in many OTC diet products,

including *Acutrim, Appedrine, Control, Dexatrim, Diet Ayds, Diet-Trim, Prolamine, Super Odrinex, Thinz,* and *Unitrol.* Doses high enough to suppress appetite may produce side effects such as headaches, blurred vision, excessive sweating, rapid pulse, nervousness, insomnia, dizziness, heart palpitations, and elevations in blood pressure. The drug should not be used by women who are pregnant or breastfeeding; young children; the elderly; and those in poor health, especially individuals with high blood pressure, heart disease, diabetes, or thyroid or kidney disorders. The advisory panel judged that 150 mg of PPA daily was safe, but a series of adverse case reports prompted the FDA to set the maximum sanctioned daily dosage at 75 mg.

Although the panel report was widely criticized and was not endorsed by the FDA itself, sales of PPA products quickly shot up to over $200 million a year. In 1982 *Consumer Reports* noted that mail-order manufacturers were misrepresenting the significance of the panel report and exaggerating the potency of PPA, calling it a "wonder ingredient" able to "neutralize the effect of all incoming calories," "proven safe and effective in government tests," and so on. After reviewing the transcripts of the FDA panel hearings, *Consumer Reports* concluded that (a) the studies considered by the panel had limitations in size, duration, or design; (b) PPA diet aids may suppress appetites for short periods in some individuals; (c) most of the resultant weight loss occurs during the first 2 weeks of use; and (d) PPA may undermine weight-loss efforts in the long run.[68] *Consumer Reports'* 1992 survey found that more than 30% of PPA users said they always felt hungry and 20% said they experienced side effects such as dizziness or nausea. Fewer than 5% said they were satisfied or very satisfied with their results.[24]

PPA has been an ingredient in fake pep pills. In 1981 the FDA estimated that PPA overdosage was responsible for more than 10,000 poison control cases and 1000 emergency room visits per year.[68] Cases of moderate and severe anxiety from single doses of 50 to 75 mg have been reported.[69]

The FDA plans to order the removal of PPA as an ingredient in OTC and prescription drug products and has asked manufacturers to voluntarily stop marketing them. The warning was based on estimates that 200 to 500 strokes per year among persons 18 to 49 could be associated with PPA use. A recent study by scientists at Yale University found an association between PPA use and hemorrhagic stroke in women.[70] The study did not contain enough men to estimate the risk to men, but there is no reason to believe it is lower. The FDA Web site has a page that provides comprehensive information about PPA.

Ma Huang (Ephedra)

Ma huang is an herb that contains ephedrine, a decongestant and nervous-system stimulant that can raise blood pressure. Products containing ma huang are marketed as weight-loss aids, even though they have not been proven safe and effective for this purpose. In 1997, after collecting more than 800 reports of adverse effects, the FDA proposed to establish a dosing regimen, require warning statements, and affect other aspects of labeling for "dietary supplement" products containing ephedrine alkaloids. In 1999, the U.S. General Accounting Office concluded that the FDA's concern about ephedra-containing products was justified, but the agency had relied too heavily on reports that had not been sufficiently investigated.[71] The FDA then withdrew its proposal and said it would investigate further. Independent experts who reviewed 140 of the adverse reports concluded that 31% of the cases were definitely or probably attributable to the products and 31% were possibly related. The most frequent complications were blood pressure elevation (17 reports); palpitations, abnormally fast heartbeat, or both (13); stroke (10); and seizures (7). Ten events resulted in death, and 13 produced permanent disability.[72]

Diet Teas

Many teas have been marketed with claims that they can help people lose weight. No such tea has been proven effective for this purpose. Some contain laxatives that can be dangerous if consumed in large quantities. Investigative reporter David Zimmerman has noted the cases of two women who died unexpectedly in 1991 while using *Laci Le Beau Super Dieter's Tea*, which contains senna, a powerful laxative. The FDA and the California Department of Health received about two dozen other complaints from users of the tea, most of whom complained about cramps and diarrhea. A company official told Zimmerman that (despite its name), the product was not marketed with weight-loss claims but was a flavorful tea intended to give dieters a break from the "blahs" of daily dieting. In 1984 the FDA had warned the manufacturer to stop falsely claiming that the tea might enable people to accomplish mild weight loss even while eating normally.[73]

Benzocaine

Benzocaine, a local anesthetic, is used in chewing gum, lozenges, and before-meal candies. The theory behind its use is that dulling nerve endings in the mouth can decrease a person's sense of taste and therefore decrease interest in eating. Benzocaine was also judged by the FDA panel as a safe and effective weight-loss aid, but the FDA and most medical authorities do not agree with the panel's conclusion. Mirkin[7] states:

People who lack the will to diet effectively without benzocaine can hardly be expected to put up with the drug indefinitely either. It tastes bad, creates numbness in the mouth, and removes most of the taste in all food, not just fattening food. It can discourage a worthwhile effort to learn good eating habits, and it is never an adequate substitute for those habits.

Bulk Producers

Bulking agents are indigestible, noncaloric substances that absorb water during digestion and supposedly trick the stomach into thinking it is full. The substances include alginic acid, carboxymethylcellulose, carrageenan, guar gum, karaya gum, methylcellulose, psyllium, kelp, and xanthan gum. The FDA panel judged these substances to be safe but not proven effective. Dr. Ernest Drenick of Los Angeles, who tested methylcellulose tablets in volunteers, found that they experienced no reduction in hunger or appetite. He also demonstrated with x-ray examination that methylcellulose does not actually fill the stomach but quickly passes into the small intestine. Drenick noted that there is no evidence that increasing the volume of a meal will produce satiety in obese individuals.[74]

Health-food stores have promoted two other bulking agents: glucomannan and pectin. Glucomannan is made from the fibers of a Japanese root plant. Some manufacturers of glucomannan products promoted them as effective in lowering cholesterol, eliminating ingested chemicals, aiding digestion, and reducing blood-sugar levels. However, there is no scientific evidence to support these claims. In 1980 Dr. Judith Stern of the University of California conducted a double-blind study in which the test group received 1 gram of glucomannan before meals, while the control group received a placebo. Both groups participated in a behavior modification program and lost weight, but no statistically significant difference in hunger ratings or weight loss was found between the groups.[58]

Pectin has been marketed in powder and tablet form as a wonder drug for weight reduction. It is naturally present in a number of foods such as apples, apricots, plums, the rinds of citrus fruits, and root vegetables such as carrots and radishes. Pectin has no proven value as an appetite suppressant.

In 1989 the FTC charged that Schering Corporation had marketed *Fibre Trim* with unsubstantiated claims that it is effective for weight loss, weight control, and weight maintenance. In 1991 an FTC administrative law judge[75] ruled that there was no scientific evidence to substantiate such claims. *Fibre Trim* is composed of natural fiber from citrus and grain compressed into tablets. The recommended daily dosage contains about 4 g of fiber, which is not a large amount. (Experts generally recommend 20 to 35 g per day as part of a healthful diet.) Schering's ads said the product could provide a feeling of fullness and could "take the edge off hunger." A company document estimated that 70% of *Fibre Trim*'s 1986 sales were to consumers "looking for the magic pill" and who "want a product that will do the work." The judge ordered Schering to refrain from making unsubstantiated claims that *Fibre Trim* (a) is a rich source of fiber; (b) could provide any health benefit associated with the intake of fiber; or (c) could provide any appetite-suppressant, weight-loss, or weight-control benefit.

Chitosan

Chitosan is derived from chitin, a polysaccharide found in the outer skeleton of shellfish such as shrimp, lobster, and crabs. Many sellers claim that chitosan causes weight loss by binding fats in the stomach and preventing them from being digested and absorbed. There is no evidence that chitosan is effective for weight control. A study performed at the University of California-Davis in which seven healthy young men who ingested 135 grams per day of fat for 12 days used a chitosan product marketed by Enforma Natural Products. Tests showed that the amount of fat in their feces did not significantly differ before and after using the product, even though they took more than the recommended amount.[76] Two other studies have found no significant differences in weight between subjects who took chitosan and those who received a placebo.[77,78]

Diet Candies

These products are usually caramels that may contain added vitamins and minerals. Taken before meals, they supposedly cause a rise in blood-sugar levels, which decreases appetite. Candies of this type, such as *Ayds*, contain 25 calories each and are eaten two at a time before meals. Consumers Union notes that they neither raise blood-sugar levels significantly nor suppress appetite.[79]

Starch Blockers

"Starch blockers" have been promoted as containing an enzyme extracted from beans that, when taken before meals, supposedly blocks digestion of significant amounts of dietary starch. The enzyme works in the test tube, but the body produces more starch-digesting enzymes than starch-blocker pills could possibly block. A 1982 study published in the *New England Journal of Medicine* found no evidence in the feces of pill-takers that starch digestion was actually blocked.[80] Moreover, if undigested starch does reach the large intestine, it is fermented by bacteria normally present, leading to gas production and causing digestive disturbances. Some users of starch blockers have experienced abdominal pain, nausea, vomiting, and diarrhea, probably caused by toxic contaminants in the product. In 1982 the FDA received more than 100 reports of adverse reactions, including 30 cases requiring hospitalization and one death from pancreatitis. As these reports poured in, the agency warned manufacturers to stop marketing these products and obtained injunctions against several companies that refused.

Sugar Blockers

"Sugar blockers" containing an extract of *Gymnema sylvestre*, a plant grown in India, are claimed to cause weight loss by preventing sugar in the diet from being absorbed into the body. According to Purdue University's Varro E. Tyler, Ph.D., a leading authority on plant medicine, chewing the plant's leaves can prevent the taste sensation of sweetness. But there is no reliable evidence that the chemicals they contain can block the absorption of sugar into the body or cause weight loss.

Chromium Picolinate

Health-food publications and various manufacturers have claimed that chromium picolinate supplements can melt fat away and reduce body fat without dieting or exercise. Some note that the process for synthesizing picolinates was developed at the U.S. Department of Agriculture Human Nutrition Research Center in Grand Forks, N.D., and that USDA holds the patent. However, Hank Lukaski, the research leader at the North Dakota facility, has stated that chromium picolinate has no effect on body fat.[81]

A recent computerized search of the scientific literature found no evidence that the weight-loss claims have been scientifically tested. Chromium picolinate is discussed further in Chapter 26.

Garcinia Cambogia

Hydroxycitric acid, the active ingredient in the herbal compound *Garcinia cambogia*, has been claimed to lower body weight and reduce fat mass in humans. A few studies in which hydroxycitrate was combined with other substances have supported these claims. However, a better-designed 3-month study of 135 obese individuals found no difference between those who received garcinia and those who received a placebo.[82]

Hormonal Fakery

Following the publication of *Life Extension*, by Durk Pearson and Sandy Shaw, many companies began marketing combinations of the amino acids arginine, ornithine, and tryptophan. Products of this type (*Dream Away, Super-Amino Night, Nite Diet*) were claimed to cause weight loss through growth hormone release (GHR). As noted by Lowell,[83] however: (a) amino acid pills do not cause growth hormone release; (b) growth hormone release would be unlikely to cause weight loss; and (c) if significant amounts of this hormone were released in the body, it could cause acromegaly, a disease in which the hands, feet, and face become abnormally large and deformed. In 1988 the FTC charged the makers of *Dream Away* with false advertising and asked an Arizona federal court to issue an injunction and order them to pay consumer redress.[84] A few months later the defendants agreed to place $1.1 million in an escrow account to repay *Dream Away* purchasers and pledged not to misrepresent any food, drug, or device in the future.

Cholecystokinin (CCK) is a hormone involved in the digestive process. Products said to contain CCK have been sold by mail and in health-food stores with claims that they can decrease hunger and cause sudden and dramatic weight loss. However, although injections of CCK appear to decrease hunger in test animals, doses taken by mouth have no such effect.

Dehydroepiandrosterone (DHEA) is a hormone that can reduce weight gain in some strains of mice and rats. Based on this fact, several companies have marketed DHEA products as "miracle weight-reducers." According to Cunningham,[85] people who use DHEA with the hope of losing weight could endanger their health by tampering with their hormones. Moreover, tests of three DHEA products sold in health-food stores found that one contained no DHEA at all and the others contained insignificant amounts.

In 1985 the Postal Service forced General Nutrition Corporation to stop making false claims for GHR, CCK, and DHEA products. In 1986 the FDA issued a regulatory letter ordering all manufacturers of DHEA and CCK to stop marketing the products; and in 1988 the FTC forced Great Earth International to agree to stop making unsubstantiated claims for its GHR products. These actions drove many products of this type from the marketplace, but a few still are sold.

LOW-CALORIE PRODUCTS

Many low-calorie foods and beverages are available for use by weight-conscious individuals. These include liq-

uid or powdered preparations (to which water is added) to consume instead of a meal; low-fat foods such as salad dressings made without oil; and foods and beverages made with artificial sweeteners. Well-designed studies to measure the effectiveness of such products are scarce, but some people seem to find these products helpful. Some experts, however, speculate that low-calorie and low-fat foods have been a factor in America's rising obesity rates because some people consume too much of them.[86]

FDA Definitions

According to FDA guidelines, "low-calorie" foods cannot contain more than 40 calories per serving or 0.4 calories per gram. Foods labeled "reduced calorie" are not limited in calories per serving, but they must be at least one-third lower in calorie content than similar foods that contain the usual amount of calories. Foods that are labeled "low calorie" or "reduced calorie" must also bear nutrition labeling that includes serving size and calories per serving in addition to significant nutrient values. If a standardized food is modified so that it no longer complies with the standard, the food must be labeled "imitation." Because consumers would reasonably expect food labeled "sugar-free" or "sugarless" to be reduced in calories, the label must alert them if this is not the case. If the word "light" (or "lite") appears on the label, the food is likely to be reduced in calories. Under FDA regulations (see Chapter 11), these words are permissible for foods that contain one-third fewer calories than the referenced food; any other use of the term must specify if it refers to color, taste, or odor.

FDA regulations also state that the actual number of calories in a food may be more than 20% greater than the amount claimed in advertising or on the label. In 1992 investigators from the Obesity Research Center of St. Lukes/Roosevelt Hospital Center in New York City measured the calorie levels of 40 "diet" and "health" food items to see whether they were accurately labeled. Of 20 foods that were nationally advertised, none exceeded the FDA limit. However, seven out of 12 regionally distributed items and five out of eight locally prepared items did so.[87]

Meal-Replacement Drinks

Slim-Fast, Ultra Slim-Fast, Dyna-Trim, and various other drink mixes contain protein, sugars, fiber, vitamins and minerals. A *Consumer Reports*' survey found little evidence that they are effective. Most respondents who used them replaced one meal a day or less, but one out of six used them for more than half their meals. The average weight loss was only 4% of starting weight for men and 3% for women. Two-fifths lost less than 5 pounds, and one-fifth gained 5 pounds or more. More than one third said they were "always hungry" while using the drinks, and nearly as many reported that they started to regain weight as soon as they stopped using the products.[24]

Nature's Sunshine Products, a multilevel company headquartered in Spanish Fork, Utah, markets *GlanDiet* meal-replacement powders formulated according to the bizarre theories of Elliot Abravanel, M.D., co-author of *Dr. Abravanel's Body Type and Lifetime Nutrition Plan* and *Dr. Abravanel's Anti-Craving Weight Loss Diet.* Abravanel claims there is a "dominant gland" at the root of every weight problem and that weight can be controlled by soothing the errant gland and moderating its cravings. The books advise tailoring a corrective plan to the individual's "body type," which is determined by completing a questionnaire about the person's shape, body fat distribution, food cravings, sleep patterns, and various other characteristics (see Figure 13-1). Women can be classified as "thyroid," "pituitary," "adrenal," or "gonadal" type, while men can be classified as "thyroid," "pituitary," or "adrenal." The personality traits described for each type resemble those of a typical horoscope. *GlanDiet* guidelines list "foods to eat or avoid" and

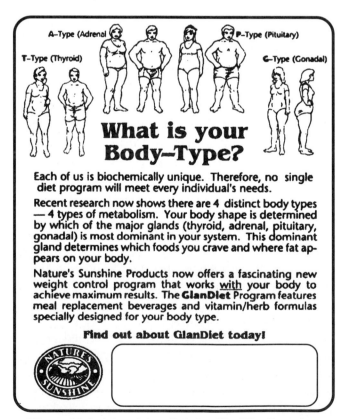

Figure 13-1. Advertising slick for GlanDiet Program.

"herbs to use when the urge to snack strikes" for each body type. All dieters are advised to begin with a 2- to 3-day "cleanse," engage in aerobic exercise, and aim for an overall calorie count of 1200/day for women or 1400/day for men. Raso[88] has noted that most people who exercise and restrict calories to such levels will lose weight with or without Nature's Sunshine products.

Artificial Sweeteners

Four artificial sweeteners currently have FDA approval: saccharin, aspartame, acesulfame potassium (acesulfame-K), and sucralose.

In 1977 the FDA announced its intention to ban saccharin after a single study found that high doses of saccharin caused bladder tumors in rats. However, considerable outcry from both scientists and the general public prompted passage of a law to prevent a ban. The FDA withdrew its proposal in 1991 but still required saccharin product labels to warn that saccharin had been determined to cause cancer in laboratory animals. The American Council on Science and Health believes that saccharin presents no health hazard at normal levels of use. A 1993 Council report notes that studies of diabetics who used large amounts of saccharin over long periods of time have shown no association between saccharin use and bladder cancer.[89] In 2000, after a National Toxicology Program review[90] concluded that saccharin poses no health hazard, Congress enacted the Saccharin Warning Elimination via Environmental Testing Employing Science and Technology Act ("SWEETEST Act") to eliminate the saccharin warning.

Aspartame is formed from the amino acids phenylalanine and aspartic acid. It is used (as *NutraSweet*) to sweeten cereals, milk shake mixes, diet drinks, and many other foods. About 180 times as sweet as table sugar (sucrose), it does not have saccharin's bitter aftertaste. In tabletop form it is marketed as *Equal.* Widespread use of aspartame has provoked some reports of headaches and various other reactions. However, a double-blind study of 40 subjects who had reported headaches following ingestion of *NutraSweet* found that the incidence of symptoms after using aspartame was not significantly different from the incidence after using a placebo.[91] Products containing aspartame are labeled with a warning against consumption by individuals with phenylketonuria, a congenital disease in which impaired metabolism can cause phenylalanine to accumulate and cause brain damage.

Acesulfame-K, marketed as *Sunette,* is used in powdered drinks, puddings, chewing gum, and tabletop sweeteners. The substance is about 200 times sweeter than sucrose and is chemically unrelated to saccharin or aspartame. Unlike saccharin, it has no aftertaste. Unlike aspartame, it is not broken down by heat or digestion and passes through the body unchanged.

Sucralose is a water-soluble, noncaloric powder made by substituting three atoms of chlorine for three hydroxyl groups on the sugar molecule. It tastes like sugar, has no calories, and is about 600 times as sweet as sugar. The FDA has approved it for use in beverages, baked goods, and other foods, and as a tabletop sweetener. The tabletop version is marketed as *Splenda*.

Fat Substitutes

Simplesse, made by the NutraSweet Company, is a low-calorie, low-cholesterol product made of natural protein from egg white or milk. It is produced by a microparticulation process that changes protein into a form that can be used to make products with the rich taste and texture of butter, cheese spreads, creamy salad dressings, mayonnaise, and ice cream.

Olestra, made by Procter & Gamble, provides no calories because it passes through the body unchanged. It is made by heating soybean oil with sugar to produce molecules composed of sucrose with six, seven, or eight fatty acid groups attached. It is similar to edible fats in most respects, including taste, but cannot be digested into smaller components because the body has no enzymes that can break it down. Olestra is marketed under the trade name *Olean.* It is approved for use in snack foods and may eventually be approved for blending with frying and cooking oils.

Although it seems likely that fat substitutes will help individuals lower the fat content of their diet, none has been proven effective as a treatment for obesity.[92] Nor is it known whether it is safe to replace large amounts of dietary fat with fat substitutes. Blackburn has warned that "fat substitution alone will not help . . . achieve a healthy weight or win the war against obesity and the chronic diseases that accompany it. That requires cutting back on calories and eating a high-fiber, low-fat, plant-based diet."[93] Critics have also expressed concerns that olestra reduces the absorption of fat-soluble nutri-

ents and medications and can cause gastrointestinal symptoms with excessive use. Products containing olestra must be labeled with this warning:

This product contains Olestra. Olestra may cause abdominal cramping and loose stools. Olestra inhibits the absorption of some vitamins and other nutrients. Vitamins A, D, E, and K have been added.

QUESTIONABLE PRODUCTS AND PROCEDURES

Many devices and procedures have been marketed with claims that they can help to reduce weight of the entire body or just in selected body parts. "Spot-reducing devices," all of which are fakes, are discussed in Chapter 14.

Body Wrapping

Many individuals operate salons in which it is claimed that clients can trim inches off the waist, hips, thighs, and other areas of the body. These facilities use wraps or garments, with or without special lotions or creams applied to the skin. The garments may be applied to parts of the body or to the entire body. Clients are typically assured that fat will "melt away" and they can lose "up to 2 inches from those problem areas in just 1 hour."[94] However, no product can cause selective reduction of an area of the body. Although wrapping may cause temporary water loss as a result of perspiration, any fluid lost will soon be replaced by drinking or eating. Figure 13-2 shows an imaginative ad inviting people to learn how to do body wrapping.

Cellulite Removers

Cellulite is a term coined in European salons and spas to describe deposits of dimpled fat found on the thighs and buttocks of many women. Widespread promotion of the concept in the United States followed the 1973 publication of *Cellulite: Those Lumps, Bumps and Bulges You Couldn't Lose Before*, by Nicole Ronsard, owner of a New York City beauty salon that specialized in skin and body care. Cellulite is alleged to be a special type of "fat gone wrong," a combination of fat, water, and "toxic wastes" that the body has failed to eliminate. Alleged "anticellulite" products sold through retail outlets and by mail include "loofah" sponges, cactus fibers, special washcloths, horsehair mitts, creams and lotions to "dissolve" cellulite, vitamin-mineral supplements with herbs, bath liquids, massagers, rubberized pants, brushes, and rollers. Many salons offer treatment with electrical muscle stimulation, vibrating machines, inflatable hip-high pressurized boots, "hormone" or "enzyme" injections, heating pads, and massage. Some operators claim that 5 to 15 inches can

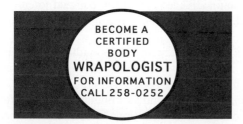

FIGURE 13-2. Local newspaper ad offering "certification" in body wrapping.

be lost in 1 hour. A series of treatments commonly costs hundreds of dollars.[95]

"Cellulite" is not a medical term. Medical authorities agree that cellulite is simply ordinary fatty tissue. Strands of fibrous tissue connect the skin to deeper tissue layers and also separate compartments that contain fat cells. When fat cells increase in size, these compartments bulge and produce a waffled appearance of the skin. Dr. Neil Solomon, former secretary of Maryland's Department of Health and Mental Hygiene, actually conducted a double-blind study of 100 people to see whether cellulite is different from ordinary fat. Specimens of regular fat and lumpy fat were obtained by a needle biopsy procedure and given to pathologists for analysis and comparison. No difference between the two was found.[96]

During the past 2 years, the most widely promoted cellulite remover has been *Cellasene*, which the manufacturer claims can "increase blood circulation, reduce fluid buildup, stimulate metabolism and reduce localized fats." The ingredients are primrose oil, dried fucus vesiculosis extract, gelatine, fish oil, glycerol, soya oil, grape seed extract, bioflavonoids, soya lecithin, fatty acids, dried sweet clover extract, dried ginkgo biloba extract, and iron oxide. The manufacturer also claims that the product works without a change in the user's diet and exercise routine. In 2000, the FTC charged the distributor (Rexall Sundown, Inc.) with false advertising, and several dissatisfied consumers filed class action suits.[96]

In 1998 the FDA approved a high-powered, handheld massage tool that consists of a treatment head and two motorized rollers with a suction device that compresses the affected tissue between the two rollers. The manufacturer is permitted to promote it for "temporarily improving the appearance of cellulite." The procedure—called Endermologie—usually takes 10 to 20 treatments to get the best results, and one or two maintenance treatments per month are required to maintain them. Without the maintenance, the benefits will soon be lost. The typical cost is $45 to $65 per session. A recently published study of 85 women between the ages of 21 to 61 found that 46 patients who completed seven sessions showed a mean index reduction in body circumference of 1.34 cm, while 39 patients who completed 14 sessions of treatments showed a mean index reduction in body circumference of 1.83 cm.[97] However, another study, involving 52 women, found no objective difference in thigh girth (at two points) or thigh fat depth (measured by ultrasound).[98]

Experts agree that no equipment, exercise, or nonsurgical treatment can remove fat exclusively from a single area of the body. The amount of fat in the body is determined by the individual's eating and exercise habits, but the distribution of fat in the body is determined by heredity. In most cases, reduction of a particular part can be accomplished only as part of an overall weight reduction program. Endermologie may temporarily improve the appearance of dimpled areas, but the procedure is time-consuming and expensive. Liposuction, which may be helpful in some cases, is discussed later in this chapter and in Chapter 20.

Gadgets and Gimmicks

Over the years, hundreds of bogus gadgets and gimmicks have been marketed with claims that they act in some special way to produce weight control or to slim various parts of the body. For example:

The *Vision Dieter* was a two-toned pair of eyeglasses claimed to control appetite if worn 2 hours a day. Its inventor reasoned that if colors could induce shoppers to buy certain products in supermarkets, they also could produce an opposite effect that would reduce food consumption.

Slim-Skins, a plastic suit with an attached hose, was alleged to slim the body if connected to a vacuum cleaner during exercise.

Astro-Trimmer and various other belts or waistbands have been falsely claimed to reduce one's waistline by applying pressure or producing extra heat loss.

Subliminal tapes have been falsely claimed to produce weight loss by reprogramming the brain.

"Walk-on-air" shoes, made of plastic and lined with springs, were claimed to make people move faster, feel better, and burn more calories.

A blue velour blanket was claimed to melt fat during sleep if wrapped around the body after the user took a shower and drank lemon water.

A machine was said to help dieters by counting the number of bites of food and sounding a bell to announce when the user had eaten enough.

Rubber pellets said to resemble maggots were to be wet and sprinkled over a forbidden food. The wriggling motion they develop was claimed to make the user want to avoid the food.

A crossbar contraption that would enable users to hang upside down was claimed to cause calories to rush to the brain where they cannot be absorbed by the intestines.

Earrings and earpieces have been claimed to curb appetite through pressure on "acupuncture points" located on the ear.

Bandaids moistened with homeopathic drops have been claimed to suppress appetite when applied to "acupuncture points" on the wrists.

"Slimming soles" are said to stimulate specific reflexology points on the feet. When slipped into a person's shoes, they allegedly cause automatic weight loss ("over 15 lbs in 6 weeks") with every step the person takes.

As far-fetched as items like these may seem, they still may attract large numbers of buyers who are desperate or gullible enough to try almost anything.

GOVERNMENT REGULATORY ACTIONS

Many weight-loss programs are marketed through direct mail, TV infomercials, and the Internet. Products typically are claimed to "neutralize food calories," "melt fat off without hunger," and cause weight loss of 10 to 20 pounds in the first week. The programs usually consist of one or more tablets or capsules plus a low-calorie diet, which is usually high in protein. Following the diet will result in modest weight loss, but the ads are worded to suggest that the pill is the key to the program. Since 1979 some of the mail-order programs have used PPA capsules.

The most prominent weight-loss scam during the 1990s was *Cal-Ban 3000*, a guar gum product claimed to virtually eliminate fat by "short-circuiting the fat-building process." Guar gum is a soluble fiber used in small amounts as a thickener in sauces, desserts, syrups, and various other foods. It has some medically recognized value as a bulk laxative, a cholesterol-lowering agent, and an adjunct to controlling blood-sugar levels in certain diabetics. But it has not been proven effective for weight control; no long-term controlled test of guar gum as a weight-control agent has been reported in the scientific literature. Although weight loss has been reported among individuals who took guar gum during studies related to cholesterol and blood-sugar control, this finding has not been consistent.

The marketing of *Cal-Ban 3000* began in 1986 and lasted 4 years despite regulatory action by the Postal Service and the Iowa Attorney General. It was widely promoted through ads showing before-and-after pictures of obese individuals who said they had lost large amounts of weight. Sales were estimated to be $10 to $20 million per year.

By 1990 the FDA was aware of complaints involving more than 100 people, at least 50 of whom needed medical intervention. The complaints included esophageal obstruction, gastric obstruction, upper and lower intestinal obstruction, nausea, and vomiting.[100] During the summer of 1990 state, local, and federal agencies conducted seizures and obtained injunctions that drove the manufacturer out of business.[101]

In 1991 the FTC charged HealthComm, Inc., and Nu-Day Enterprises, Inc., of Gig Harbor, Washington, and their owner, Jeffrey S. Bland, Ph.D., with falsely claiming that their diet program could cause weight loss by turning up the body's "heat-producing machinery" so that fat is lost as body heat instead of being stored. The Nu-Day Diet Program, which cost $59.95 for a 2-week supply, included instructional materials, a meal-replacement formula, and a fiber-containing formula said to be a "natural appetite suppressant." The Nu-Day program was promoted with a 30-minute television program entitled "The Perfect Diet," which offered "amazing true stories of people like yourself losing 20, 30, 50 pounds or more, safely, quickly and naturally." The FTC also charged that the format used to make these claims was deceptive. Although the television program appeared to be an independent consumer news show that used interviews to report on its discovery of the Nu-Day Diet, it was actually a paid ad.

The case was settled with a consent agreement in which Bland agreed to pay $30,000 for redress and to refrain from making the claims that had been challenged. The consent order also required future programs of 15 minutes or longer to display messages identifying them as paid ads for the products offered.[102] Bland, identified during the program as "one of the nation's leading nutritional biochemists," is the health-food industry's most prolific interpreter of nutrition-related scientific developments.[103] His interpretations consistently favor the use of supplements. A former chemistry professor, he has appeared frequently at trade shows, written and edited publications, produced audio and video tapes, and conducted seminars for health professionals. He has also been a research associate at the Linus Pauling Institute of Medicine and has directed its nutrient analysis laboratory.

In 1995 the FTC charged Bland and his companies with violating the consent order by making unsubstantiated weight-loss claims for several products. In addition, their *UltraClear* dietary program had been falsely claimed to reduce the incidence and severity of symptoms associated with gastrointestinal problems, inflammatory or immunological problems, fatigue, food allergies, mercury exposure, kidney disorders, and rheumatoid arthritis. The settlement agreement included a $45,000 civil penalty.

In 1994, the FTC charged that Ronald A. Gorayeb and his companies had made unsubstantiated claims for $39.95 group-hypnosis seminars held at various sites throughout the United States. One advertisement claimed that participants in a Gorayeb Weight-Loss Seminar could expect "results ranging from 30–60 lbs. in three months to 120 lbs. in a year" without willpower, hunger, or dieting. The ad also stated: (a) Gorayeb was a "certified hypno-therapist," (b) the seminars had worked for thousands, and (c) participants who felt that a single seminar did not meet their needs could attend future seminars without charge. The case was settled with a consent agreement banning unsubstantiated claims that the sessions were effective.

In 1996 the FTC charged that NordicTrack, Inc., had made unreasonable claims that 70% to 80% of those who had purchased NordicTrack cross-country ski exercisers had lost an average of 17 pounds and that 80% of those who had lost weight had maintained all their weight loss for at least 1 year. The FTC complaint stated that these figures were flawed because they did not take dietary habits into account and reflected only the experience of highly motivated purchasers who had integrated the machine into their regular exercise program. The company pledged not to make similar claims in the future unless they were backed by well-designed studies.

In 1996 the FTC announced settlements with Nutrition 21 and two other California companies charged with making unsupported claims about weight loss and health benefits for chromium picolinate. The companies had claimed that the supplement would cause significant and long-term weight loss, improve body composition by reducing body fat and building muscle, increase metabolic rate, control appetite, reduce serum cholesterol, regulate blood-sugar levels, increase energy and/or stamina, and treat and prevent diabetes.[104]

SURGICAL PROCEDURES

Surgery for weight-loss purposes is considered a radical approach. Because complication rates are quite high, this approach should be used only for individuals who are morbidly obese (100 or more pounds above desirable weight) and in danger of dying as a result. The following procedures have been used:

JAW WIRING: Wiring the jaw to prevent chewing restricts the patient to sipping beverages and liquefied foods. This leads to rapid loss of weight for the majority of individuals, but most regain their losses once the wiring is undone. Undesirable side effects can occur, such as dental decay from lack of brushing and flossing, atrophy and weakening of jaw muscles, and considerable pain.

GASTRIC BYPASS SURGERY: In some procedures, the small intestine is shortened by looping a section off from the rest to limit caloric absorption. In other procedures, the stomach is constricted and parts of the intestine are bypassed. Side effects can include diarrhea, vitamin deficiencies, anemia, protein deficiency, hair loss, impaired immunity, neurologic disorders, joint pains, kidney stones and gallstones, cardiac irregularities, and liver damage.

VERTICAL BANDED GASTROPLASTY: Procedures of this type involve creation of a pouch or other measures to reduce the size of the stomach. This limits the amount that can be eaten at one sitting. Although these procedures are safer than intestinal bypass, postoperative risks include inflammation, hemorrhage, ulceration, and certain nutritional deficiencies. Also, the patient may get around the surgery by ingesting food constantly in small amounts.

The 1991 National Institutes of Health Consensus Development Conference on Gastrointestinal Surgery for Severe Obesity concluded that vertical banded gastroplasty and gastric bypass surgery "dominate practice in the early 1990s and have advanced beyond the experimental stage."[105]

Two types of surgery may be done to remove local fat deposits for cosmetic purposes:

LIPECTOMY: A lipectomy, usually done for cosmetic purposes, removes fat from beneath the skin. If overeating resumes, the fat simply reaccumulates.

SUCTION LIPECTOMY (LIPOSUCTION): Fat is sucked out through a small hollow tube inserted into the fatty area. Proponents state that it can remove 6 pounds of fat with little or no scarring. Complications have included postoperative pain, perforation of internal organs, and fat embolism. Loss of skin elasticity limits the degree of improvement in older patients.[106]

WEIGHT-CONTROL ORGANIZATIONS

Many organizations have been established to provide both individual and group counseling for people seeking to lose weight. Some organizations are nonprofit and relatively inexpensive, whereas others are quite costly. Many hospitals and universities conduct obesity clinics. Several self-help organizations have chapters in many cities. Few scientific reports have been published about the effectiveness and complication rates of the methods described in this section.

Inexpensive Programs

TOPS (Take Off Pounds Sensibly) was started in 1948 and has over 11,000 chapters and about 275,000 members in 20 countries. The members must submit weight goals and a diet from a health professional in writing. Each group elects a nonprofessional volunteer to direct and organize its activities for 1 year. The weekly meetings include a confidential weigh-in and offer moral support, with awards for lifestyle changes and special recognition for the best losers.[16,107] Membership costs $20 per year.

Weight Watchers is a franchise started in the 1960s that now includes diet, behavior modification, and exercise. Over 1 million members attend over 29,000 weekly meetings in 29 countries worldwide. The program focuses on changing one's eating habits rather than counting calories. It attempts to help overweight people to cope with the problems that made them fat and to alter their eating habits.[16] It costs about $20 to join and about $12 per week for meetings. Lifetime members who have completed a maintenance plan and remain within 2 pounds of their weight goal can attend free monthly meetings.

Overeaters Anonymous (OA), founded in 1960, is a nonprofit organization for individuals who define themselves as compulsive overeaters. It has about 8500 groups in 50 countries. It operates on the premise that overeating is a progressive illness that cannot be cured but can be arrested. OA encourages its members to seek professional help for an individualized diet/nutrition plan and for any emotional or physical problems. Members attend weekly meetings when needed. They follow a 12-step plan similar to that of Alcoholics Anonymous. There are no dues or fees. OA's strength is its regular meetings in which members can share their successes and failures, their problems and solutions.[16]

Expensive Programs

Thousands of commercial obesity clinics and centers are operating in the United States, most of them franchised by large national organizations. Advertisements for these facilities typically promise weight loss of 20 to 30 pounds in the first month and include before-and-after pictures of clients who supposedly have accomplished this. Programs are said to be medically supervised, but the degree of supervision varies. Many clinics are administered by registered nurses. Many employ a physician to do an initial physical examination, but the client might not see the physician again. Prepackaged foods, drinks, or supplement mixtures may be used instead of all or just some meals. Some diets are balanced, whereas others cause ketosis. Fees commonly range from $25 to $75 per week, depending on the program and whether special products are purchased. In several parts of the country, dietitians who have inquired at various clinics have encountered incorrect nutrition concepts and misleading claims for many of these programs.

Diet Center and Physicians Weight Loss Center offer restrictive diet plans using ordinary foods, plus individual counseling and daily vitamin and mineral supplements.

Diet Workshop offers a four-point lifetime program: diet (1200 calories, high in protein), behavior modification, nutrition education, and exercise. Menu plans are based one the USDA Food Guide Pyramid and range from 1200 to 1800 calories per day, depending on individual needs. Meeting fees are nominal but products are expensive.[107]

◆ **Personal Glimpse** ◆

Low-Calorie Disaster[108]

In 1990 Carol Householder of Flagstaff, Arizona, testified to a Congressional subcommittee on behalf of her husband Michael, who had a doctoral degree and had been a college engineering professor. In 1985, at age 44, Michael was 6 feet tall and weighed 215 pounds. Having gained 30 pounds during the previous 5 years, he wanted to weigh approximately 180. He considered himself to be in good physical condition. He had biked, jogged, swum, played racquetball, skied, and, earlier that summer, had hiked the Grand Canyon rim to rim (25 miles). Having seen ads stating that the Nutri/System diet succeeds where other diets fail, he joined the Nutri/System program and followed its 1000-calorie-per-day diet. In about 7 weeks, he lost approximately 28 pounds.

A few days later, after jogging, he passed out for a minute or two. He discussed this with his Nutri/System adviser, who said he should eat more fruit. A week later, only 1 pound short of his goal, he suffered a cardiac arrest while returning from a jog. Although resuscitated by paramedics, he remained in a coma, hooked to life support systems, for the following 70 hours. His attending physician said that the cardiac arrest had been triggered by potassium deficiency and borderline protein deficiency.

When Michael awakened, both his long- and short-term memory had been erased. He didn't know his name. He couldn't recognize his family, and it took months for him to begin over again. He was just a fraction of his former himself, permanently unable to work and requiring supervision of all daily activities. In order to take care of him and their three children, Carol was forced to leave her job.

Jenny Craig and Nutri/System offer prepackaged foods plus counseling and support. A major drawback of this approach is that when participants stop using the prepackaged meals, they must still learn how to make proper food choices. During the early 1990s hundreds of former clients filed lawsuits claiming that the Nutri/System program caused them to develop gallstones.

Health Management Resources, Medifast, and Optifast are medically supervised, supplemented fasting programs designed for individuals who are at least 30% above their ideal body weight. The initial phase involves the use of prepackaged supplements containing 520 to 800 calories per day. The stabilization phase gradually reintroduces food, and the maintenance phase stresses lifestyle changes. These programs cost from $1500 to $3000, depending on the length of participation and the amount used of the prepackaged products.[16]

Respondents to *Consumer Reports'* 1992 survey who attended a Diet Center, Physicians Weight Loss Center, Jenny Craig, or Nutri/System facility reported average losses of 10% to 12% of their starting weight by the program's end and 6% to 7% by 6 months later. Those who used a supplemented fasting program reported initial losses of 15% to 20% and 6-month levels of 8% to 15%. Weight Watchers participants reported less weight loss but higher satisfaction from their

experience. The survey also found that about 25% of the people who used commercial programs were not overweight when they entered them, which meant that the program administrators were willing to sell unnecessary services.[24]

The NIH Technology Conference panel[109] on weight-loss methods concluded that information about program success should include the percentage of beginning participants who complete the program; the percentage of those who achieve various degrees of weight loss; the proportion of weight loss retained after 1, 3, and 5 years; and data on adverse medical or psychological effects the participants experience. A subsequent NIH obesity task force issued five consumer guidelines for choosing a program:

1. The diet should be safe and include all of the Recommended Dietary Allowances for vitamins, minerals, and protein.
2. The program should be directed towards a slow, steady weight loss unless a more rapid loss is medically indicated.
3. A doctor should evaluate health status if the client's weight goal is greater than 15 to 20 pounds, if the client has any health problems, or if the client takes medication on a regular basis.
4. The program should include plans for weight maintenance.
5. Prospective clients should receive a detailed list of all fees and costs.[15]

Marsha Hudnall,[110, 111] a dietitian who investigated several weight-control programs, found that none of them offered follow-up statistics that could be used to compare one program with another. She concluded, however, that "the relative sensibleness, low cost, and widespread availability may well make Weight Watchers the best option for many people."

A study of 31 people whose photograph and testimonial had appeared in newspaper ads for a weight-loss clinic found that 20 months later, only eight (26%) had remained within 5 pounds of their target weight. The clinic, a Midwestern affiliate of a national commercial weight-loss program, offered behavioral education with a prepackaged food regimen. The researchers caution that their data should be interpreted cautiously because their findings did not reflect the experience of clients who never met their weight loss goals.[112]

Government Investigations

During 1990 a U.S. House of Representatives subcommittee, chaired by Representative Ron Wyden (D-OR), held two hearings focused on deception and fraud in the diet industry.[108] Testimony indicated that some

---

Table 13-7

SUGGESTED "NEW LIFESTYLE LANGUAGE"

Weight Watchers International wants America's buzzwords to reflect a more reasonable way of thinking about how a healthy lifestyle can be achieved:

"What's In"	"What's Out"
Moderation	Deprivation
Healthful eating	Diets
Portion control	Calorie counting
Healthy weight range	"Ideal" weight
Self-acceptance	Self-condemnation
Increased physical activity	"No-pain, no-gain"
Support systems	"Going it alone"
Balanced food plan	Liquid diets/pills
High-carbohydrate diet	High-protein diet
Reading food labels	Ignoring contents
Small changes	Radical weight loss
Behavior modification	Uneducated change
Healthy snacking	No eating between meals
Weight management	Weight loss
Long-term weight loss	Weight cycling

Source: Weight Watchers International press release, Dec 27, 1993.

commercial programs referred to their staff as "certified" nutrition counselors, behavior therapists, and the like, even though the only certification they had was by the company offering the program. One woman described how her husband had suffered a cardiac arrest as a result of a poorly supervised program (see Personal Glimpse box on page 293).

During 1991 agents of the New York City Department of Consumer Affairs[113] called or visited 14 weight-loss centers and reported the following:

- Few of the centers warned about or discussed the safety risks of their program (or of rapid weight loss in general), even when directly asked about possible problems. One representative said her center's program was "absolutely safe," even though the health history form that prospective clients had to sign contained a warning about health risks.
- Some centers attempted to sell their services to people who did not need them, including underweight people.
- Some centers were engaged more in quackery than medicine. One clinic representative advised that filling the stomach with certain foods would speed up metabolism. Another said her clinic's maintenance program would "close up the body's fat cells."
- Some centers engaged in high-pressure sales tactics.

◆ Personal Glimpse ◆

Selling It[113]

On April 30, 1991, a sales representative from a diet center in New York City told a 5'-8" woman who weighed 130 pounds that she was 5 pounds overweight and could afford to lose 7 pounds. This ran counter to advice of the woman's personal physician, who confirmed that she already was at an ideal weight and did not need to lose any more. Moreover, the 7-pound loss would have put her several pounds beneath the ideal target weight listed on the sales repre-sentative's own chart. The program would cost $710, which amounted to $100 per pound. When the woman failed to sign up, the sales representative urged her repeatedly and offered reduced payments as an incentive.

On May 8, 1991, a 5'-8" man who weighed 178 pounds was told at another center that he should lose 18 pounds. No measurements other than weight were taken. The man worked out regularly and was very muscular. He had a low body fat content and did not need to lose weight. On the same day at another center, another man who was 5'-9" and weighed 142 pounds was urged to sign up for a program to lose 8 pounds in 2 weeks.

Following its study, the Department of Consumer Affairs implemented regulations requiring weight-loss centers to (a) display a large sign stating that rapid weight loss (more than $1\frac{1}{2}$ to 2 pounds a week) may cause serious health problems, (b) advise consultation with a physician, (c) indicate that only permanent lifestyle changes can promote long-term weight loss, and (d) inform customers that information on dropout rates and staff qualifications are available on request.

During the past several years the FTC has settled enforcement actions against Diet Center, Jenny Craig International, Nutri/System, Physicians Weight Loss Centers, Weight Watchers International, and 13 other marketers of commercial weight-loss programs, after charging them with (a) making deceptive and unsubstantiated claims about their results, (b) failing to fully disclose costs, and/or (c) using testimonials that did not reflect the typical user's experience. The settlements include four requirements:

1. Claims that a specified weight loss is typical must be based on a sample of all patients who have entered the program (or another clearly identified segment of patients).
2. Claims that weight loss is long-term must be based on sound studies that cover at least 2 years after completion of a weight-loss and maintenance program.
3. Claims of permanence must be based on a period of time recognized by experts or demonstrated by reliable survey evidence as sufficient.
4. Claims of successful maintenance must include disclosures of average weight loss and the length it was maintained, as well as the statement: "For many dieters, weight loss is only temporary."

SUGGESTIONS FOR WEIGHT CONTROL

Medical and nutrition scientists agree that the key to weight control is to establish prudent and permanent habits of exercise and control of calorie intake. For initial weight loss, they recommend a well-balanced diet with few enough calories to produce a steady loss of 1 to 2 pounds per week. A diet of 1200 to 1300 calories per day can be a good starting point; it is low enough to achieve weight reduction, yet high enough to be able to supply adequate amounts of the essential nutrients. If food selection is done properly at this caloric level, vitamin supplements are unnecessary. Additional calories can be added to the diet after one's desirable weight is achieved. Because obesity often is associated with a high-fat diet, some researchers suspect that low-fat eating offers promise as a weight-control measure. However, research in this area is only in its early stages.[114]

Table 13-8

CALORIES BURNED DURING VARIOUS PHYSICAL ACTIVITIES

Work Activities	Calories per Minute*	Recreational Activities	Calories per Minute*
Carpentry	3.8	Archery	5.2
Chopping wood	7.5	Badminton (recreation-competition)	5.2–10.0
Cleaning windows	3.7	Baseball (except pitcher)	4.7
Clerical work	1.2–1.6	Basketball half-full court (more for fastbreak)	6.0–9.0
Dressing	3.4		
Driving car	2.8	Bowling (while active)	7.0
Driving motorcycle	3.4	Calisthenics	5.0
Farming		Canoeing (2.5-4.0 mph)	3.0–7.0
Chores	3.8	Cycling (5-15 mph; 10-speed bicycle)	5.0–12.0
Haying, plowing with horse	6.7	Dancing	
Planting, hoeing, raking	4.7	Modern: moderate-vigorous	4.2–5.7
Gardening		Ballroom: waltz-rumba	5.7–7.0
Digging	8.6	Square	7.7
Weeding	5.6	Football (while active)	13.3
Hiking		Golf (foursome-twosome)	3.7–5.0
Road-field (3.5 mph)	5.6–7.0	Handball and squash	10.0
Snow: hard-soft (3.5-2.5 mph)	10.0–20.0	Horseshoes	3.8
Downhill: 5%-10% grade (2.5 mph)	3.5–3.6	Judo and karate	13.0
Downhill: 15%-20% grade (2.5 mph)	3.7–4.3	Mountain climbing	10.0
Uphill: 5%-15% grade (3.5 mph)	8.0–15.0	Pool or billiards	1.8
40-lb pack: (3.0 mph)	5.0	Rowing (pleasure-vigorous)	5.0–15.0
40-lb pack: 36% grade (1.5 mph)	16.0	Running	
House painting	3.5	12-min mile (5 mph)	10.0
Ironing clothes	4.2	8-min mile (7.5 mph)	15.0
Making beds	3.4	6-min mile (10 mph)	20.0
Metal working	3.5	5-min mile (12 mph)	25.0
Mixing cement	4.7	Skating (recreation-vigorous)	5.0–15.0
Mopping floors	4.9	Skiing	
Pick-and-shovel work	6.7	Moderate to steep	8.0–12.0
Plastering walls	4.1	Downhill racing	16.5
Sawing		Cross-country (3-8 mph)	9.0–17.0
Chain saw	6.2	Snowshoeing (2.5 mph)	9.0
Crosscut saw	7.5–10.5	Soccer	9.0
Shining shoes	3.2	Swimming	
Shoveling (depends on weight of load, rate of work, height of lift)	5.4–10.5	Pleasure	6.0
		Crawl (25-50 yd/min)	6.0–12.5
Showering	3.4	Butterfly (50 yd/min)	14.0
Stacking lumber	5.8	Backstroke (25-50 yd/min)	6.0–12.5
Standing, light activity	2.6	Breaststroke (25-50 yd/min)	6.0–12.5
Stone masonry	6.3	Sidestroke (40 yd/min)	11.0
Sweeping floors	3.9	Skipping rope	10.0–15.0
Truck and auto repair	4.2	Table tennis	4.9–7.0
Walking	7.1	Tennis (recreation-competition)	7.0–11.0
Down stairs	5.1	Volleyball (recreation-competition)	3.5–8.0
Indoors	3.1	Water skiing	8.0
Up stairs	10.0–18.0	Wrestling	14.4
Washing clothes	3.1		
Washing and dressing	2.6		
Washing and shaving	2.6		

*Calories burned depends on efficiency and body weight. Add 10% for each 15 pounds above 150. Subtract 10% for each 15 pounds below 150.

Source: Sharkey BJ. Fitness and Work Capacity. U.S. Department of Agriculture Forest Service, 1977.

Exercise

Experts agree that exercise plays a critical role in weight control. The idea that exercise is self-defeating is a myth. In most cases exercise does not increase appetite unduly.[115] Most research on humans indicates that food intake (a) does not change with moderate exercise of extended duration and (b) decreases slightly with vigorous exercise of short duration.[116]

Mirkin[7] states that the beneficial effects of exercise occur throughout the day, not just during the actual exercise periods. He recommends walking, swimming, or riding a stationary bicycle for individuals who are obese, over 40 tears old, or not used to strenuous activities. However, Gwinup[117] has shown that swimming as the sole form of exercise is generally not useful for weight control. He believes that rapid heat loss while in contact with water (especially water colder than 80 degrees F) may stimulate the appetite mechanism to increase caloric consumption.[118] Swimming in relatively warm water, or including other aerobic activities in one's exercise program, may prevent this problem.

Consumer Reports on Health[119] suggests that people wishing to lose 10 pounds or less might do best by increasing exercise without dieting. Table 13-8 shows the approximate number of calories burned during various activities. Chapter 14 contains additional information on exercise and weight control.

Behavior Modification

Successful weight control requires a permanent change in habits rather than a temporary change (such as a diet) that one adheres to until a desired weight level is reached. Various modification procedures are aimed at helping the overfat individuals change their patterns of inappropriate food consumption such as overeating, eating high-calorie foods, or snacking between meals. Those who overeat in response to tension may require psychotherapy as well. In many cases other members of the obese individual's household will have to modify

---

It's Your Decision

1. Many people on television describe how a product has helped them to lose weight. How can you determine whether the product really works?

2. You have heard about several inexpensive weight-control organizations that offer help with weight control. What information would you need to determine which one might be best?

---

behavior that stimulates overeating. Foreyt and Goodrick[120] identified these methods as useful:

SELF-MONITORING: Self-observing and recording of situational factors, thoughts, and feelings that occur before, during, and after attempting to eat and exercise prudently. Self-review enables tracking of progress. Scrutiny by a therapist may enhance self-control.

STIMULUS CONTROL: Modification of factors that stimulate inappropriate eating or exercise behavior.

GRADUATED TARGET BEHAVIORS: Gradual dietary change to avoid feelings of deprivation; gradual development of cardiorespiratory fitness to avoid the perception of exercise as punishment.

CONTINGENCY MANAGEMENT: Use of a signed contract specifying what the patient will do and the rewards for doing it.

COGNITIVE-BEHAVIORAL STRATEGIES: Movement from self-rejection to self-acceptance; focusing on ways in which thoughts, moods, diets, and social pressures affect eating control.

Stare, Aronson, and Barrett[9] offer the following tips for achieving calorie reduction:

- Use alternatives to food as rewards (for example, long walks, relaxing baths, tickets to a movie or play).
- Resist the temptation to always "clean the plate."
- If you eat moderate portions of your favorite foods, you will be less apt to crave them and overindulge.
- Do not eat while doing anything else, such as talking on the phone or watching television.
- Find nonfood outlets for release of emotional tension.

Aaron Altschul, Ph.D., of the Georgetown University Clinic, has concluded that successful dieters achieve the following:

- They know their weight; they weigh themselves often enough that they are never in doubt about where they stand in relation to their goal.
- They know what they are eating; if necessary, they keep daily records until they automatically know what they are eating every day, can anticipate heavy eating events, and can adjust their intake accordingly.
- They control their alcohol intake.
- They engage in a regular program of exercise.
- They use a personally suitable diet plan—one that they can enjoy or tolerate permanently.

SUMMARY

To lose weight, people must eat less, exercise more, or do both. Although hundreds of "miracle" products and "revolutionary" diets have been marketed, no pill, potion, or dietary plan can produce weight loss without exercise or lowering of caloric intake. To lose 1 pound of fat it is necessary to burn 3500 more calories than are taken in. Professional help may be required to clarify and modify the behavior that contributes to overeating.

The most sensible weight-loss methods aim for a steady reduction of about 1 pound a week. The diet that experts recommend most often is a balanced, low-calorie, low-fat food plan that is easily adapted for long-term maintenance. Although unbalanced diets can cause weight loss, they are usually too monotonous for long-term use and are followed by weight gain when the user returns to "normal" eating. Repeated dieting followed by weight gain ("yo-yo dieting") may increase the risk of premature death from heart disease and several other diseases, but the research on this is not conclusive. For most people, the most important factor in successful weight control is exercise.

Many people diet even though they are not overweight. The majority of people concerned about their weight would probably do better to focus on exercise, healthful eating, and minimizing cardiovascular risk factors rather than on counting calories.

REFERENCES

1. Blackburn GL, Pavlou K. Fad reducing diets: Separating fads from facts. Contemporary Nutrition, July 1983.
2. Lanou A. No body's perfect. New Century Nutrition 2(3):5, 1996.
3. The U.S. Weight Loss and Diet Control Market, ed 6. Tampa, Fla., 2000, Marketdata Enterprises.
4. Singer S. When they stop telling you it's easy to lose weight. Today's Health 50:47–49, 62, Nov 1972.
5. Dreon DM and others. Dietary fat: Carbohydrate ratio and obesity in middle-aged men. American Journal of Clinical Nutrition 47:995–1000, 1988.
6. Update: Prevalence of overweight among children, adolescents, and adults—United States, 1988–1994. Mortality and Morbidity Weekly Report 46:199–202, 1997.
7. Mirkin G. Getting Thin. Boston, 1983, Little, Brown & Co.
8. Statistical Bulletin of the Metropolitan Life Insurance Company 40:1, 1959.
9. Stare FJ, Aronson V, Barrett S. Your Guide to Good Nutrition. Amherst, N.Y., 1991, Prometheus Books.
10. Pi-Sunyer FX. Obesity. In Shils ME and others, editors. Modern Nutrition in Health and Disease, ed 9. Baltimore, 1999, Williams & Wilkins.
11. Garrison RJ and others. Cigarette smoking as a confounder of the relationship between relative weight and long-term mortality. JAMA 249:2199–2203, 1983.
12. Pi-Sunyer FX. Medical hazards of obesity. Annals of Internal Medicine 119:655–660, 1993.
13. Manson JE. Interview in Brody JE. Moderate weight gain risky for women, a study warns. New York Times, Sept 14, 1995, pp A1, B13.
14. Darden E. Your Basic Guide to Fitness. Philadelphia, 1982, George F Stickley Co.
15. Pi-Sunyer FX and others. The Clinical Guidelines on the Identification, Evaluation, and Treatment of Overweight and Obesity in Adults: The Evidence Report. Rockville, Md., 1998, National Institutes of Health.
16. Food and Nutrition Board Committee to Develop Criteria for Evaluating the Outcomes and Approaches to Prevent and Treat Obesity. Weighing the Options: Criteria for Evaluating Weight-Management Programs. Washington, D.C., 1995, National Academy Press.
17. Manson JE and others. Body weight and mortality among women. New England Journal of Medicine 333:677–685, 1995.
18. Bennion L, Bierman EL, Ferguson JM. Straight Talk about Weight Control. New York, 1991, Consumer Reports Books.
19. Troiano RP and others. Overweight prevalence and trends for children and adolescents. The National Health and Nutrition Examination Surveys, 1963 to 1991. Archives of Pediatric and Adolescent Medicine 149:1085–1091, 1995.
20. American Medical Association Council on Foods and Nutrition: The healthy approach to slimming. Chicago, 1979, The Association.
21. Mertz W and others. What are people really eating? The relationship between energy intake derived from estimated diet records and intake determined to maintain body weight. American Journal of Clinical Nutrition 54:291–295, 1992.
22. Lichtman S and others. Discrepancy between self-reported and actual calorie intake and exercise in obese subjects. New England Journal of Medicine 327:1893–1898, 1992.
23. DelPrete LR and others. Self-reported and measured weights and heights in community-based weight-loss programs. Journal of the American Dietetic Association 92:1483–1486, 1992.
24. Losing weight: What works. What doesn't. Consumer Reports 58:347–357, 1993.
25. Leibel RL, Rosenbaum M, Hirsch J. Changes in energy expenditure resulting from altered body weight. New England Journal of Medicine 332:621–628, 1995.
26. Bennett WI. Beyond overeating. New England Journal of Medicine 332:673–674, 1995.
27. Lissner L and others. Variability of body weight and health outcomes in the Framingham population. New England Journal of Medicine 324:1839–1844, 1991.
28. Min-Lee I, Paffenberger RS Jr. Change in body weight and longevity. JAMA 268:2045–2049, 1992.
29. National Task Force on the Prevention and Treatment of Obesity. Weight cycling. JAMA 272:1196–1202, 1994.
30. Berg FM. Health Risks of Weight Loss. Hettinger N.D., 1995, Healthy Living Institute.
31. Abernathy RP, Black DR. Is adipose tissue oversold as health risk? Journal of the American Dietetic Association 94:641–644, 1994.
32. Ikeda JP and others A commentary on the new obesity guidelines from NIH. Journal of the American Dietetic Association 99:918–919, 1999.
33. Fletcher SW and others. Methods for voluntary weight loss and control. National Institutes of Health Technology Assessment Conference Statement. Bethesda, Md., 1992, US Department of Health and Human Services.
34. Brody J. Condensed from Foreword to Fletcher AM. Thin for Life: 10 Keys to Success from People Who Have Lost Weight & Kept It Off. Shelburne, Vt., 1994, Chapters Publishing Ltd.
35. USDA Coordinated Nutrition Research Program on Health and Nutrition Effects of Popular Weight-loss Diets. White paper. Journal of Obesity Research (in press).
36. Kilbourne J. Still killing us softly: Advertising and the obsession with thinness. In Fallon P, Katz MA, Wooley SC, editors. Feminist Perspectives on Eating Disorders. New York, 1994, Guilford Press, pp 395–418.

37. Anorexia nervosa and bulimia nervosa. In Carlson KJ and others. Harvard Guide to Women's Health. Cambridge, Mass., 1996, Harvard University Press, pp 44–48.

38. Farley D. On the teen scene: Eating disorders require medical attention. FDA Consumer 26(2):27–29, 1992.

39. Serdula MK and others. Weight control practices of U.S. adolescents and adults. Annals of Internal Medicine 199:667–671, 1993.

40. Levy AS, Heaton AW. Weight-control practices of U.S. adults trying to lose weight. Annals of Internal Medicine 199:661–666, 1992.

41. Barrett S. Diet facts and fads. In Barrett S, editor. The Health Robbers, ed 2. Philadelphia, 1980, George F Stickley Co.

42. National Council Against Health Fraud. Commercial weight-loss programs. NCAHF position paper, Loma Linda, Calif., 1987, The Council.

43. Berg FM. "Detoxification" with pills and fasting. Quackwatch Web site, Aug 15, 1997.

44. Wadden TA, Van Italie TB, Blackburn GL. Responsible and irresponsible use of very-low-caloric diets in the treatment of obesity. JAMA 263:83–85, 1990.

45. National Task Force on the Prevention and Treatment of Obesity. Very low-calorie diets. JAMA 270:967–974, 1993.

46. Atkins RC. Dr. Atkins' New Diet Revolution. New York, 1992, M. Evans & Co.

47. White PL. A critique of low-carbohydrate ketogenic weight reduction regimens: A review of Dr. Atkins' diet revolution. JAMA 224:1415–1419, 1973.

48. Top-selling diets: Lots of gimmicks, little solid advice. Consumer Reports 63:60–61, 1998.

49. Anderson JW and others. Health advantages and disadvantages of weight-reducing diets: a computer analysis and critical review. Journal of the American College of Nutrition 19:578–590, 2000.

50. Hellmich N. Success of Atkins diet is in the calories. USA Today, Nov 8, 2000.

51. Mirkin G, Shore RN. The Beverly Hills Diet: Dangers of the newest weight-loss fad. JAMA 246:2235–2237, 1981.

52. Hegsted DM. Rating the diets. Health 15(1):21–32, 1983.

53. Kenney JJ. Fit for Life: Some notes on the book and its roots. Nutrition Forum 3:57–59, 1986.

54. Yetiv JZ. Popular Nutritional Practices. San Carlos, Calif., 1986, Popular Nutrition Press.

55. Power L. Food combining: Fit for laughs. Shape 6(5):38, 1987.

56. Jarvis WT. Notable quote. Nutrition Forum 3:59, 1986.

57. A bad diet with phony credentials. U.S. News & World Report. June 24, 1996, p 69.

58. U.S. Senate Committee on Governmental Affairs. Hearings before the Permanent Subcommittee on Investigations, May 14, 1985. Washington D.C., 1985, US Government Printing Office.

59. Barrett S, Herbert V. The Vitamin Pushers: How the "Health Food" Industry Is Selling America a Bill of Goods. Amherst, N.Y., 1994, Prometheus Books.

60. Evans D. Herbalife CEO died after 4-day binge, autopsy reveals. Bloomberg News, Aug 11, 2000.

61. FDA warns on use of two drugs for obesity. FDA Consumer 11(6):26, 1977.

62. Will a pill take your pounds off? Consumer Reports 61:15–17, 1996.

63. Weintraub M and others. Long-term weight control study: I–VII. Clinical Pharmacology and Therapeutics 51:581–646, 1992.

64. Goldstein DJ, Potvin JH. Long-term weight loss: The effect of pharmacologic agents. American Journal of Clinical Nutrition 60:647–657, 1994.

65. FDA Center for Drug Evaluation and Research. Questions and answers about withdrawal of fenfluramine (Pondimin) and Dexfenfluramine (Redux). Sept 18, 1997.

66. Subitramine for obesity. Medical Letter 40:32, 1998.

67. The great weight debate. A major medical journal says people should worry less about the weight. The government says worry more. Here's what we say. Consumer Reports on Health 11(1):4–6, 1999.

68. The new diet pills. Consumer Reports 47:14–17, 1982.

69. Dietz AJ. Amphetamine-like reactions to propanolamine. JAMA 245:601–602, 1981.

70. Horwitz AI and others. Phenylpropanolamine & risk of hemorrhagic stroke: Final report of the Hemorrhagic Stroke Project. May 10, 2000. Published on FDA Web site.

71. Dietary Supplements: Uncertainties in Analyses Underlying FDA's Proposed Rule on Ephedrine Alkaloids. Washington, D.C., 1999, General Accounting Office.

72. Haller CA, Benowitz NL. Adverse cardiovascular and central nervous system events associated with dietary supplements containing ephedra alkaloids. New England Journal of Medicine 343:1833–1838, 2000.

73. Zimmerman D. Legal snarl allows laxative to be sold as 'Dieter's Tea.' Probe 3(6):1, 4–8, 1994.

74. Drenick EJ. Bulk producers, JAMA 234:271, 1975.

75. Parker LF. Initial decision in the matter of Schering Corporation, FTC Docket No. 9232, Sept 16, 1991.

76. Stern JS and others. Chitosan does not block fat absorption in men fed a high fat diet. Obesity Research 8:91s. (Supplement 1: abstract PB94), Oct 2000.

77. Pitler MH and others. Randomized, double-blind trial of chitosan for body weight reduction. European Journal of Clinical Nutrition 53:379–381, 1999.

78. Wuolijoki E and others. Decrease in serum LDL cholesterol with microcrystalline chitosan. Methods and Findings in Experimental and Clinical Pharmacology 21(5):357–361, 1999.

79. Consumer Reports. The Medicine Show, ed 4. Mt. Vernon, N.Y., 1974, Consumers Union.

80. Bo-Linn GW et al. Starch blockers: Their effect on calorie absorption from a high-starch meal. New England Journal of Medicine 23:1413–1416, 1982.

81. Berg FM. Chromium picolinate: Scam of the hour? Healthy Weight Journal 7:54, 1993.

82. Heymsfield SB and others. Garcinia cambogia (hydroxycitric acid) as a potential antiobesity agent. JAMA 280:1596–2000, 1998.

83. Lowell J. "Growth hormone releasers" don't cause weight loss. Nutrition Forum 1:24, 1984.

84. FTC charges "weight-loss while you sleep" ads are false. FTC News Notes, Jan 18, 1988.

85. Cunningham JJ. DHEA: Facts vs. hype. Nutrition Forum 2:30, 1985.

86. Allred J. Too much of a good thing? An overemphasis on eating low-fat foods may be contributing to the alarming increase of overweight among US adults. Journal of the American Dietetic Association 95:417–418, 1995.

87. Alison DB and others. Counting calories—Caveat emptor. JAMA 270:1454–1456, 1993.

88. Raso J. The shady business of Nature's Sunshine. Nutrition Forum 9:17–23, 1992.

89. Meister KA. Low-calorie sweeteners. New York, 1993, American Council on Science and Health.

90. Fact Sheet: Report on Carcinogens, ed 9. Rockville, Md., 2000, National Toxicology Program.

91. Schiffman SS and others. Aspartame and susceptibility to headache. New England Journal of Medicine 317:1181–1184, 1987.

92. Segal M. Fat substitutes: A taste of the future? FDA Consumer 24(10):25–27, 1990.

93. Blackburn G. Physician's perspective on olestra. HealthNews 2(4):1–2, 1996.

94. Wills J. About body wraps, pills, and other magic wands for losing weight. FDA Consumer 16(9):18–20, 1982.

95. Fenner L. Cellulite: Hard to budge pudge. FDA Consumer 14(4):5–9, 1980.

96. Barrett S. Cellulite removers. Quackwatch Web site, Oct 9, 2000.

97. Chang P and others. Noninvasive mechanical body contouring: (Endermologie) A one-year clinical outcome study update. Aesthetic and Plastic Surgery 22:145-153, 1998.

98. Collis N and others. Cellulite treatment: a myth or reality: a prospective randomized, controlled trial of two therapies, endermologie and aminophylline cream. Plastic and Reconstructive Surgery 104:1110-1114, 1999.

99. The facts about weight loss products and programs. Undated flyer issued in 1993 by the FTC, FDA, and National Association of Attorneys General.

100. Lewis JH. Esophageal and small bowel obstruction from guar gum-containing "diet pills": Analysis of 26 cases reported to the Food and Drug Administration. American Journal of Gastroenterology 87:1424–1428, 1992.

101. Barrett S. The rise and fall of Cal-Ban 3000. Nutrition Today 25(6):24–28, 1990.

102. False claims barred for diet program. Nutrition Forum 9:5, 1992.

103. Fanning O. "Training" for health food retailers. Nutrition Forum 3:33–37, 1985.

104. Companies advertising popular dietary supplement chromium picolinate can't substantiate weight loss and health benefit claims, says FTC. FTC news release, Nov 7, 1996.

105. Grundy S and others. Consensus statement: Gastrointestinal surgery for severe obesity. Paper presented at the NIH Consensus Development Conference, Vol 9, No. 1, March 25–27, 1991.

106. Liposuction. Arlington Heights, Ill., 1998, American Society of Plastic Surgeons.

107. Environmental Nutrition's critique of popular weight-loss programs. Environmental Nutrition 21(1): 4–5, 1998.

108. Deception and fraud in the diet industry. Hearings before the Subcommittee on Regulation, Business Opportunities, and Energy, U.S. House of Representatives Committee on Small Business, March 26, 1990 (Part I) and May 7, 1990 (Part II). Washington D.C., U.S. Government Printing Office.

109. National Institute of Diabetes and Digestive and Kidney Diseases. Understanding Adult Obesity. NIH Publ. No. 94–3680. Rockville, Md., 1993, National Institutes of Health.

110. Hudnall M. A look at commercial dieting programs (4-part series). Environmental Nutrition 10(4):2–3, 10(5):2–3, 10(6):4–5, 10(7):5, 1987.

111. Hudnall M. How popular diet programs compare. Environmental Nutrition 10(8):4–5, 1987.

112. Fatis M and others. Following up on a commercial weight loss program: Do the pounds stay off after your picture has been in the newspaper? Journal of the American Dietetic Association 89:547–548, 1989.

113. Winner K. A Weighty Issue: Dangers and Deceptions of the Weight Loss Industry. New York, 1991, New York City Department of Consumer Affairs.

114. Datillo AM. Dietary fat and its relationship to body weight. Nutrition Today 27(1):13–19, 1992.

115. Stare FJ, Whelan EM. The Harvard Square Diet. Amherst, N.Y., 1987, Prometheus Books.

116. Franklin BA, Rubenfire M. Losing weight through exercise. JAMA 244:377–379, 1980.

117. Gwinup G. Weight loss without dietary restriction: Efficacy of different forms of aerobic exercise. American Journal of Sports Medicine 15(3):275–279, 1987.

118. Steinman D. Study finds swimming ineffective for weight control. Nutrition Forum 5:14–15, 1988.

119. Diet vs. exercise: What's best? Consumer Reports on Health 4:1–3, 1992.

120. Foreyt JP, Goodrick GK. Evidence for success of behavior modification in weight loss and control. Annals of Internal Medicine 119:698–701, 1993.

Chapter Fourteen

Exercise Concepts, Products, and Services

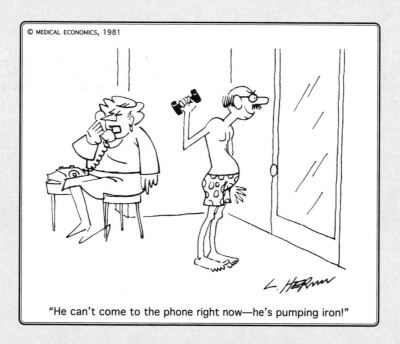

© MEDICAL ECONOMICS, 1981

"He can't come to the phone right now—he's pumping iron!"

An ideal exercise would improve your aerobic fitness, burn excess body fat, add to muscular strength and endurance, and be easy to start and sustain. However, there is no ideal exercise—at least not for everyone. So aim for a program that helps you accomplish your goals without boredom or guilt.

Consumer Reports on Health[1]

It's best to go slow as you consider taking the plunge into home exercise equipment. For every exercise bike or rowing machine that's used regularly in a basement or bedroom, another is gathering dust.

Consumer Reports[2]

Exercise is the planned, structured, repetitive physical activity done to achieve physical fitness and other specific goals. Physical fitness is the ability to carry out daily activities without undue fatigue and with ample energy left to enjoy leisure-time pursuits and meet the physical demands of emergencies.

Performance-related fitness (which includes speed, power, balance, coordination, and agility) may enhance life in many ways and can contribute to longevity. But health benefits occur with even modest levels of physical activity.

Although the principles of exercise physiology are well-developed, many people promote unscientific regimens, and many consumers waste money on products and services that have no value. Safety should also be an important consideration. This chapter elucidates the role of exercise in health and fitness and provides guidelines for choosing programs, facilities, equipment, and services. It also discusses "ergogenic aids" and the dangers of anabolic steroids.

PUBLIC PERCEPTIONS

People today generally accept the idea that exercise is good for their health, but this was not always so. Hippocrates, whose writings influenced medical thinking for more than 2000 years, considered the health of athletes precarious:

In the case of athletes too good a condition of health is treacherous if it be an extreme state; for it cannot quietly stay as it is, and therefore, since it cannot change for the better, can only change for the worse. For this reason it is well to lose no time in putting an end to such a good condition of health, so that the body can start again to reconstitute itself.[3]

The ancient Greeks knew that extreme exertion was hazardous. According to ancient legend, Philippides ran from the battlefield at Marathon to Athens, announced "rejoice, we conquer," and fell dead. Although many people perceive the ability to run a marathon as a sign of superhealth, this idea is part of folklore about strenuous exercise.

In early America common experience did not suggest that athletic prowess and good health were equivalent. Sports events were staged for entertainment, to provide opportunities for gambling, and to promote nationalism. Feats of strength by "muscle-men," 6-day bicycle races, 24-hour walking contests, dance marathons, and boxing matches with unlimited rounds were excesses with questionable health benefits. Early advocates of healthful living promoted exercise as desirable, but they emphasized posture; calisthenics (then called "gymnastics"); and relatively useless practices such as breathing deeply, waving wands, and tossing Indian clubs and medicine balls.

The need for exercise became a social concern after thousands of young men had been rejected as physically unfit for military duty in World War I. This led to the introduction of physical training activities for the general public and in the schools. In the 1920s, as the science of exercise physiology developed, school programs were called "physical education." The popularity of sporting events led educators to incorporate athletic activities into physical education, using them to foster physical development, sportsmanship, and fair play.

The 1950s were pivotal to the public perception of exercise and health. Tests during the early part of this decade revealed that American children were not as fit as European children. Findings like these led President Dwight D. Eisenhower to convene experts to propose ways to improve America's fitness level. President John F. Kennedy subsequently established the Office of Sports and Fitness (now the President's Council on Physical Fitness and Sports) in Washington, D.C. The Council's impact was limited, however, because it promoted exercise standards and fitness levels that were higher than most people could meet.

In the late 1960s cardiologist Kenneth Cooper, M.D., wrote *Aerobics*, a popular book that outlined fitness programs for adults and stressed heart-lung efficiency. As awareness of the importance of physical fitness increased, physical education became more closely related to all-around fitness and health. In the late 1970s marathon runner Jim Fixx's *The Complete Book of Running* became a bestseller and fueled a growing interest in jogging and long-distance running.

Thomas Bassler, M.D., president of the American Medical Joggers Association, had speculated that

marathon running may confer immunity from coronary artery disease. This hypothesis was refuted in cardiology journals as contrary evidence from autopsies was found. However, the idea that marathon runners were not "supermen" immune to heart disease did not hit home with the public until 1984 when Fixx, age 52, died suddenly during a 10-mile run. Fixx's father had had his first heart attack at age 35 and had died at age 42.[5] Jim Fixx's death dramatized the fact that a high degree of fitness may not overcome a strong heredity tendency toward coronary disease. (On the other hand, risk-factor modification as described in Chapter 15 is still very important because some hereditary factors are modifiable.) The most common cause of sudden death among competitive athletes is hypertrophic cardiomyopathy, a heart-muscle disease that is not related to coronary heart disease and is difficult to detect.[6]

In recent years there has been surge of interest in strength training with weights and body-building machines. Magazine racks in some stores have entire sections devoted to sports, fitness, and body improvement.

BENEFITS OF EXERCISE

Exercise offers many benefits. It can increase stamina and endurance, lower blood pressure, improve blood cholesterol levels, help with weight control, help lower abnormal blood sugar levels, reduce stress, improve sleep, and help prevent osteoporosis. Exercise can also prolong life.

The effect of exercise on longevity has been substantiated by several large studies.[7] One involved 9777 men, ages 20 to 82, who were followed for up to 18 years (average 4.9 years). The highest age-adjusted death rate from all causes was seen in men who were unfit at both examinations (122 deaths per 10,000 man-years). The lowest age-adjusted death rate was in men who were physically fit at both examinations (39.6 deaths per 10,000 man-years). Men who improved from unfit to fit between the two examinations had an age-adjusted death rate of 67.7 deaths per 10,000 man-years, which reflected a 44% reduction in all-cause mortality and a 52% reduction in cardiovascular disease mortality.[8] Although sedentary lifestyle is not the strongest of the major modifiable risk factors for heart disease, it is the most prevalent one among Americans.[9]

The U.S. Railroad Study followed what happened to more than 3000 men for 17 to 20 years. The data showed that physical activity lowered the incidence of death from coronary heart disease as well as the overall death rate.[10] The Harvard Alumni Study of 13,485 men

---

◆ **Personal Glimpse** ◆

A Demonstration of Great Strength

In 1912 Bernarr Macfadden toured midwestern cities to spark interest in his courses in "physical culture." One of the muscular youths who accompanied him was 18-year-old Forrest C. Shaklee, who became a chiropractor and later founded the Shaklee Corporation, a large company that markets "natural" products through person-to-person sales. Shaklee literature describes how young Forrest helped Macfadden's promotion:

> Parades were held on the main street of each town, and consisted of a pride of muscular youths, some musicians, and a flatbed wagon. . . . When enough of a crowd had been gathered around the flatbed, each of the youths was to exercise with a given piece of equipment. This was preceded by a discourse from Macfadden, extolling health through nature, diet and especially non-diet (he tended to look upon fasting as a blanket cure-all) and, of course, strenuous exercise . . . .
>
> The pièce de résistance of these outdoor displays was the lifting of an iron ball which appeared to weigh easily 500 pounds. Secured to the ball was a massive link chain, which one of the youths would grasp and which, with much concentration and apparent straining, he would raise gradually over his head. The crowds watching in awed silence at the beginning of the feat, would break into cheers and applause when the ball was finally raised. When it was his turn at the ball, Forrest discovered that lifting it was easily accomplished; the ball was hollow![4]

(mean age 57.5 years) found that those who reported exercising vigorously tended to live longer than those who exercised nonvigorously or not at all.[11] An 8-year study of 72,488 female nurses aged 40 to 65 years found that those who exercised more often or more vigorously had a lower incidence of stroke.[12]

The main reason most people exercise is not to prevent disease but to feel more alert and energetic. Many exercise regularly because they feel it benefits their emotional state, helps them cope with emotional stress, and makes them look better. Young men generally wish to build up their muscles and gain weight, while young women are more likely to want to lose weight "in the right places."

Many people exercise to maintain a fitness level that enables them to enjoy recreational sports, which can also serve as a social outlet. Team sports such as basketball, softball, touch football, or soccer are the focus of many people's life, even into the sixth decade. Activities such as golf, tennis, racquetball, rock climbing, backpacking, cycling, skiing, and dancing can also contribute to a basic exercise program.

Many people also find that exercise has psychologic value. Stress-management programs commonly employ exercise as a way to cope with the effects of stress. Some psychotherapists recommend it for the same reason. Exercise produces endorphins, natural chemicals that act as tranquilizers. These account for the relaxation effects of exercise and its role as an aid to sleep. Looking fit can enhance self-image, which can help people feel better about themselves. Many people who pursue bodybuilding as a lifestyle take special pride in their appearance.

TYPES OF EXERCISE

Exercise can be classified as anaerobic, aerobic, isometric, isotonic, and isokinetic. During vigorous exercise the respiratory rate increases, the lungs transmit more oxygen to the bloodstream, and the heart pumps harder and faster to convey the oxygen to the muscles.

Anaerobic exercise is so intense that respiration cannot supply all of the oxygen the body needs. The resultant "oxygen debt" permits lactic acid to build up in the muscles, impairing muscular activity until sufficient oxygen is available for recovery. (The word "anaerobic" means "without oxygen.") In high-intensity events, such as the 100-yard dash, most of the energy is supplied anaerobically.

Aerobic exercise is prolonged effort during which nearly all of the oxygen needed is supplied through breathing. Aerobic training promotes heart-lung efficiency and raises the anaerobic threshold (the activity level at which the body goes into oxygen debt).

Isometric exercise refers to muscle contractions exerted against resistance in which there is no movement of body parts. Muscles may merely be tightened or may be used to push against or pull an object that does not move. Isometric exercise can be used with minimal or no equipment and can be performed while sitting, while in bed recuperating from surgery, and in many other confining situations. It can help develop strength, but only at the angles worked. In untrained muscles it develops more rapidly than isotonics, although the latter will eventually catch up. Isometric exercises are useful for sports (primarily football) in which there is limited time to prepare for intense physical activity. They contribute nothing to cardiorespiratory fitness or flexibility. Although somewhat useful for sedentary and elderly individuals, isometrics have little value for an ongoing fitness program. Extreme exertion, whether isometric or isotonic, can temporarily raise blood pressure and slow the heart, which is dangerous for some people.

Isotonic exercise refers to the contraction of muscles, with or without resistance, in which parts of the body move. It can build strength, flexibility, and cardiovascular endurance, depending on its intensity and duration. It occurs during calisthenics, weight lifting, swimming, walking, running, and many other athletic activities. Isotonic exercise is superior to isometrics because it develops strength throughout the entire range of motion.

Isokinetic exercise employs specially designed equipment that enables pushing or pulling against constant resistance through an entire range of motion. This increases the intensity of the exercise, strengthens muscles faster with less activity, and increases endurance somewhat.

COMPONENTS OF FITNESS

Muscles become stronger through use and weaker as a result of inactivity. Regular exercise can increase strength, endurance, flexibility, motor fitness, and cardiorespiratory efficiency.

Strength is the amount of force that can be applied by a muscle or group of muscles with a single contraction. The best way to strengthen muscles is through exercise that involves gradually increased resistance. Muscles increase in size and develop strength in proportion to the amount of resistance during the exercise. The more resistance a person works against, the greater will be the strength gains.

Endurance is the ability to use muscles repeatedly for extended periods of time. Endurance-trained muscles have a better blood supply because additional capillaries develop as the muscles adapt. Regular exercise that exceeds 15 repetitions or two minutes contributes to muscular endurance, with greater endurance occurring with more repetitions or longer duration.

An extreme example of muscular endurance is seen in marathon runners, whose legs contract more than 25,000 times during a race. The fatigue these runners experience is caused much more by muscular demands than by cardiovascular-respiratory demands. Only the large muscles of the legs are capable of such repetitive performance. Muscles of the arms, abdomen, and back are much more limited, which limits the numbers of consecutive pull-ups, push-ups, or sit-ups that can be performed. Intracellular adaptations that make muscle cells more efficient and change blood profiles also occur as part of the physiologic adaption to repetitious exercise. Muscular endurance activities can be done daily.

Flexibility is the stretching ability of muscles and other soft tissues that affect the range of motion of joints. Exercise folklore holds that weightlifting causes people to become musclebound (lacking in flexibility). Flexibility can be diminished if high-resistance exercises are done without a full range of motion or if the exercise session does not include stretching. However, the combined strength and flexibility exhibited by well-trained gymnasts attests to the fact that these two qualities of muscular fitness can co-exist when training is proper. Muscles that lack flexibility are more apt to tear, while those with too much flexibility are prone to tendon rup-

ture. A significant degree of flexibility appears to be inherited. Flexibility is the most difficult feature of muscular fitness to improve.

Motor fitness refers to the ability to move quickly and efficiently. Measurable qualities are agility (the ability to change direction while in motion), speed, and coordination. Sports activities such as tennis, racquetball, squash, and dancing contribute to motor fitness. The ability to move well can help avoid accidents and enable a person to engage in enjoyable recreational activities.

Cardiorespiratory efficiency is the ability of the circulatory system to deliver oxygen-rich blood throughout the body. A circulatory system that is efficient will operate at a lower pulse rate than one that is not.

In 1998 the American College of Sports Medicine (ACSM)[13] recommended the following guidelines for healthy adults:

MODE OF ACTIVITY: Any activity that uses large muscle groups that can be continuously maintained. Examples include walking, jogging, running, swimming, skating, bicycling, rowing, cross-country skiing, rope jumping, jazzercise, dancing of various kinds, and other rhythmic activities.

FREQUENCY: 3 to 5 days a week.

INTENSITY: 55%/65% to 90% of maximum heart rate.

DURATION: 20 to 60 minutes of continuous or intermittent aerobic activity. (Intermittent means bouts of 10-minutes or more accumulated through the day.)

RESISTANCE TRAINING: Strength training of moderate intensity, with one set of 8 to 12 repetitions of 8 to 10 exercises that condition the major muscle groups 2 or 3 days per week.

FLEXIBILITY TRAINING: Sufficient to develop and maintain range of motion; a minimum of 2 or 3 days per week.

A simple way to monitor exercise is to determine the heart rate by taking your pulse. To determine the appropriate intensity of activity, subtract your age from 220 and take 60% to 90% of the remainder for the target heart rate. The American Heart Association lists the target zone for pulse beats and the average maximum heart rates at different ages, as shown in Table 14-1. As fitness increases, the target pulse rate can be increased.

In 1995 ACSM and the U.S. Centers for Disease Control and Prevention issued a consensus statement that, "Every U.S. adult should accumulate 30 minutes or more of moderate-intensity physical activity on most, preferably all, days of the week." This level can be met with activity, such as a 2-mile walk, that expends approximately 200 calories per day. (Table 14-2 indicates the rate of calorie expenditure for various activities.) This recommendation was intended to complement rather than replace the guidelines for higher-intensity exercise to develop aerobic fitness. This recommendation acknowledged that most of the disease-

Table 14-1
TARGET PULSE RATES FOR AEROBIC EXERCISE

Age (Years)	Avg. Maximum Heart Rate*	Target Zone† (Beats per Minute)
20	200	120–180
25	195	117–175
30	190	114–171
35	185	111–166
40	180	108–162
45	175	105–157
50	170	102–153
55	165	99–148
60	160	96–144
65	155	93–139
70	150	90–135

*Maximum heart rate = 220 minus your age.

†Target zone is maximum heart rate × 60% to 90%

Table 14-2

Caloric Expenditure per Minute for Various Activities and Body Weights

Activity	105–115 lbs	127–137 lbs	160–170 lbs	182–192 lbs
Golfing, hand cart	3.25	3.75	4.41	4.91
Baseball, fielder	3.66	4.16	4.91	5.41
Walking, 3 mph	3.90	4.50	5.23	5.80
Hiking, 20 lb pack, 2 mph	3.91	4.50	5.25	5.83
Rowing machine, easy	3.91	4.50	5.25	5.83
Swimming, crawl, 20 yd/min	3.91	4.50	5.25	5.83
Badminton, singles	4.58	5.16	6.16	6.75
Skating, leisurely	4.58	5.16	6.16	6.75
Calisthenics	3.91	4.50	7.33	7.91
Bicycling, 10 mph	5.41	6.16	7.33	7.85
Tennis, doubles	5.58	6.33	7.50	8.25
Aerobic dancing	5.83	6.58	7.83	8.58
Basketball, half-court	7.25	8.25	9.75	10.75
Handball	7.83	8.91	10.50	11.58
Volleyball	7.83	8.91	10.50	11.58
Jogging, 5 mph	8.58	9.75	11.50	12.66
Running, 6.5 mph	8.90	10.20	12.00	13.20
Skiing cross-country, 5 mph	9.16	10.41	12.25	13.33
Bicycling, stationary, 20 mph	11.66	13.25	15.58	17.16

Modified from Perry P. Are we having fun yet? American Health 6(2):59-63, 1987.

prevention benefits of physical activity will occur with moderate-intensity activities outside of formal exercise programs.[14] Similar recommendations have been issued by an NIH Consensus Conference,[15] the U.S. Surgeon General,[16] and the American Heart Association.[17]

Starting an Exercise Program

A basic exercise program will complement an individual's daily routine and recreational exercise. A balanced program will maintain or develop the upper body (muscle groups used to move the body with the arms), legs (muscle groups used in locomotion), trunk (abdomen and back), heart, lungs, and circulation (aerobic activity). Activities that demand high resistance do not build endurance, while low-resistance exercises do not increase muscle strength. Sports activities develop the body unevenly. Some overemphasize the legs; others, the upper body. Some contribute to cardiovascular fitness; others contribute nothing toward this important goal. Most sports activities alternate in intensity with bursts of energy and periods of relative inactivity. People with a sedentary occupation require an exercise program that includes all aspects of physical fitness.

Well-designed exercise programs have four phases: warm-up, cardiovascular, muscular (resistance exercise),

and cool-down. The warm-up phase consists of mild exercise and stretching to prepare the body for more intense activity. The cardiovascular and muscular phases are the heart of the workout. The cool-down involves activities that help the recovery process, such as walking until breathing returns to normal following intense running or stretching muscles that have been involved in high-resistance exercise. When starting a program, people who have followed a relatively inactive lifestyle should consider the following guidelines:

1. Consider whether or not to obtain a physician's advice. Authorities do not agree on who should have a health assessment. However, a health examination may be appropriate for anyone over 35 starting a vigorous exercise program for the first time. An examination is more appropriate for a sedentary person than for one who has been physically active. ACSM stated that asymptomatic, physically active persons of any age with no history of risk factors for coronary heart disease usually require little supervision.

Whether to have exercise electrocardiography (an assessment of heart function while walking on a treadmill; commonly called a "stress test") can be discussed with one's physician. The procedure costs several hundred dollars and often yields false positive results that lead to further expense and more invasive testing. The

American Heart Association[18] recommends exercise testing for people planning to start an exercise program more intense than walking at 50% to 60% of maximum heart rate (or running or jogging) if they (a) are age 40 or older and have been sedentary, (b) have symptoms such as chest pain, (c) have a heart murmur or high blood pressure, or (d) have two or more major coronary risk factors. The Association states that people under 40 who have no major risk factors or signs of heart disease do not need an exercise test and should not be restricted in their exercise program. (Chapter 15 provides additional information about exercise testing.)

2. Determine the present level of fitness so that future results can be compared using the same method of determination. The *ACSM Fitness Book*[19] provides complete information on designing an exercise program.

3. Select a type of exercise that is compatible with age and physical condition. Dr. Cooper suggests:

UNDER 30 YEARS: If there are no medical problems, the individual can participate in any type of exercise activity.

30 TO 39 YEARS: Most types of activity are permissible. However, if strenuous exercises are planned, a physician's approval may be advisable.

40 TO 59 YEARS: It is advisable to start with a walking program. After conditioning has occurred, running, jogging, and other more demanding activities may be undertaken. However, a physician's approval is advisable before starting. If approval is not given, less strenuous activities such as walking, golf, cycling, and swimming should be permissible.

60 YEARS AND OVER: The average individual should avoid jogging, running, and vigorous competitive sports. Walking, swimming, and stationary cycling will be more beneficial.

4. Be prudent about the amount of exercise performed. Do not attempt an overly intense exercise program. Progress gradually at the start. Include warm-up activities: jog in place, ride a stationary bicycle, do calisthenics for a few minutes; stretch muscles daily to improve flexibility and prevent injury (do not bounce). Cool off by doing the same activity at a slower pace for 2 to 3 minutes; then stretch again. High-resistance exercises should not be done more often than roughly every 36 hours—every other day is a practical guideline.

5. Add physical activity to your daily routine. Whenever possible, for example, walk instead of riding and climb stairs instead using an elevator or escalator.

6. It is advantageous to have specific goals that can be evaluated periodically. These could include achieving or maintaining a specified body weight, resting heart rate, blood pressure, or blood lipid profile or achieving a specified level on a field test (e.g., a 15-minute run, 25 pull-ups, 75 pounds bench-pressed).

Some experts believe that aerobics has been oversold at the expense of muscle-building. ACSM suggests that, in addition to aerobic exercise, individuals should engage in weight training at least two times per week, performing 8 to 10 different exercises to strengthen the large muscles of the chest, arms, back, and legs. When done correctly, this can increase strength, speed, flexibility, and muscle endurance. It can also improve a person's appearance and confidence.

Many people have difficulty sustaining an exercise program. Changes in schedule (e.g., vacations, special events), illnesses, bad weather, and other interruptions can scuttle a program. The key to maintaining a healthful lifestyle is not "willpower" but motivation. People are more apt to sustain an exercise program if they exercise for the sake of personal appearance (bodybuilders, weight-control enthusiasts); to maintain their ability to perform at sports (avid skiers, mountain climbers, rock climbers, tennis tournament players); to recover health (cardiac rehabilitation patients, women recovering from the effects of childbirth); because their social life centers around activities which are improved by keeping fit (bowling, golf, curling, softball); or because their job description requires that they pass periodic fitness tests (firefighter, police officers, military personnel).

Most sports activities alternate in intensity with bursts of energy and periods of relative inactivity. Table 14-3 indicates how various sports activities relate to fitness goals. This type of information can be misleading, however. For instance, the contribution that swimming makes to cardiovascular fitness can vary greatly. Competitive swimmers gain cardiovascular fitness from their intense training, but recreational swimmers may not.

Some people stop exercising out of boredom. Boredom can be prevented by careful activity selection and timing. Some people prefer certain times of the day. Some enjoy seeing the sun rise or set. Some prefer the effects of exercise in the morning, whereas others like to break up their day with a run at noon, or relax after work, or run before bedtime. Some find it helpful to use a portable tape player or radio to listen to music or a talk show, whereas others prefer the sounds of nature or other aspects of life. Some prefer to exercise with a partner or a group, whereas others prefer to do it alone. Indoor exercisers may find that watching television holds their interest. The key point is that the surroundings may make the difference between maintaining a program and giving it up.

If physical activity is substantially reduced, many of the effects of exercise training on fitness will diminish within two weeks and will disappear within 2 to 8 months if significant activity is not resumed.[16]

Table 14-3

FITNESS CONTRIBUTIONS OF VARIOUS ACTIVITIES*

Activity	Cardiorespiratory	Strength	Muscle Endurance	Flexibility
Aerobics, high-impact	VM	M	VM	M
Aerobics, low-impact	M-VM	S-M	M-VM	M
Aqua exercises	L	S-M	M	M
Basketball	VM	S-M	M	M
Bicycling	VM	M	M	S-M
Bowling	L	L	L	L
Calisthenics	S-M	S	S-M	S
Disco dancing	VM	S-M	M	M
Golf	S-M	S	S	S
Jogging	VM	S-M	M	S-M
Rope jumping	VM	M	M-VM	S
Swimming	VM	S-M	M	M
Tennis	M-VM	S-M	VM	S-M
Walking	S-M	L-S	S-M	L

*The extent of benefits from any sport depends on frequency, duration, resistance, and muscles involved.
Key: VM = very much, M = much, S = some, L = little.
Modified from Kusinitz I and others. Physical Fitness for Practically Everybody. Mt. Vernon, N.Y., 1983, Consumer Reports Books.

Table 14-4

PURPOSES AND METHODS OF STRETCHING

Goal	Purpose	How to Achieve
Warm-up for agility sports activities	To prepare the body for quick movements, abrupt changes of direction, or trunk rotation	Do mild isotonic activities until a feeling of warmth occurs. Stretch the muscles that are to be involved in the activity for which you are preparing.
Warm-up	To reduce muscular soreness caused by a previous workout	Perform static stretching for 30–60 seconds per muscle group; repeat three times.
To relieve or avoid back or neck pain	To stretch tight, overdeveloped muscles that are antagonistic to weaker, overstretched muscles	Do mild isotonic activities until a feeling of warmth occurs. Soaking in heated water may be substituted or added. Use static stretching for 30–60 seconds per muscle group. (It is equally important to strengthen weaker antagonists.)
To increase flexibility	To develop the ability to perform special movements, such as the splits of gymnasts and ballet dancers	At the end of workout sessions, do multiple sets of static stretching at 1–2 minutes per muscle group. Measure progress at regular intervals. Be patient because results come slowly.

Stretching Exercises

Stretching can help reduce muscular soreness, prepare the body for certain sports, increase flexibility, and prevent muscle spasms. There are three main types of stretches:

STATIC: Muscles should be gently stretched until tension occurs and held in that position for between 20 seconds and 2 minutes. After about 20 seconds the stretch reflex will cease, the muscle will relax, and actual stretching of the tissues can take place. The extent of actual stretching is probably more important than the length of time the position is held.

BALLISTIC: Stretching is applied by bouncing or jerking movements. This method is no longer recommended because it can produce injury.
PASSIVE: Stretching by an external force, such as a partner. This may be useful for obtaining extreme degrees of flexibility but are not appropriate for most athletic training programs.

People who do aerobic activities such as walking, jogging, running, cycling, or swimming do not normally need to stretch beforehand. They can warm up by beginning the activity slowly and gradually increasing their pace as it becomes comfortable.

Stretching can be used to reduce the soreness that occurs after doing movements to which the body is not adapted. For people preparing for sports requiring agility, stretching can also reduce the chance of soft-tissue injuries and improve physical performance.

Muscles are arranged in sets that are antagonistic to each other. Muscle spasms can occur when the strength and flexibility of antagonistic muscle groups are too far out of balance. For example, low-back pain can occur when the back muscles are considerably stronger and less flexible than the abdominals. Exercises that strengthen the abdominals and stretch the lower back can help prevent a recurrence.

The muscles should be completely warmed up before flexibility exercises are performed. For this reason, stretching fits well at the end of an exercise session. Progress can be measured with a goniometer, a device that measures the angles to which joints can be moved. Table 14-4 provides additional guidelines for stretching.

Power and Athletic Performance

In addition to the achievements previously presented, high-performance athletes must maintain power. In scientific terms, power is strength multiplied by the speed of muscle contraction—the latter is determined by heredity. Athletic performance also involves skill and experience. Because of its explosive action, power is hazardous to muscles, tendons, and ligaments. Improving or maintaining performance in leisure-time athletic pursuits can be a powerful motivation to sustain a regular exercise program.

Assessing Exercise Intensity

The demand exercise places on the heart can be measured and expressed in metabolic equivalents (METs). A MET is the amount of oxygen consumed while a person sits at rest—approximately 3.5 ml of oxygen per kg of body weight per minute. Performing a 2-MET activity will raise oxygen consumption to 7 ml/kg, while a 3-MET activity will triple the energy demand. Blair[20] lists these MET values for various common activities:

MODERATE INTENSITY (3 TO 4.9 METs): Calisthenics, golf (not riding in a cart), weightlifting, recreational volleyball, walking at 3 to 4 mph (15 to 20 minutes per mile)

HARD INTENSITY (5 TO 6.9 METs): Aerobic dance, doubles tennis, ice or roller skating, slow-paced swimming, walking at 4.5 to 5.5 mph (10.9 to 13.3 minutes per mile)

VERY HARD INTENSITY (OVER 7 METs): Running, fast-paced swimming, rope jumping, singles tennis, competitive racquetball

Figure 14-1 shows additional MET values.

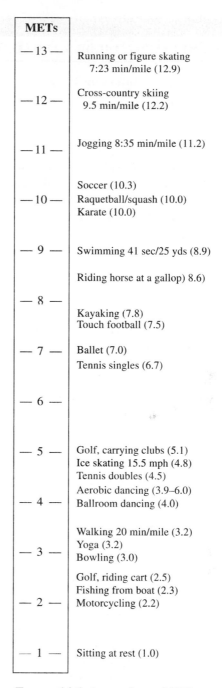

FIGURE 14-1. Approximate METs of various recreational activities.

MET values can be used to guide doctors who prescribe exercise programs for patients recovering from heart attacks or other cardiovascular problems. For example, if a 5-MET level of exertion on a stress test does not cause symptoms, it is unlikely that the heart will be strained by exercise at home.

Injury Prevention

Many people are injured yearly in sports and recreational activities. Injuries range from minor aches and pains to severe overuse syndromes, fractures, and connective

Table 14-5

EXERCISE-RELATED INJURIES AND ILLNESSES

Body Part	Injury or Symptoms	Contributing Factors	Activities
Ankle	Twists, sprains	Overtiredness	Racquet sports, volleyball, basketball
Back	Strain, soreness, muscle spasms, disc herniation	Sudden lunges or twists when tired; improper lifting technique	Running, weightlifting
Calf	Achilles tendinitis, shin splints	Overuse	Running, aerobics
Ear	Swimmer's ear (external otitis)	Inflammation due to prolonged exposure to moisture	Swimming
Elbow	Soreness at joint (tennis elbow)	Overuse and poor technique	Racquet sports
Eye	Conjunctivitis	Irritation from chlorine	Swimming
Foot	Blisters, jogger's heel (plantar fasciitis)	Overuse	Running, jumping
Head	Accidental injury	Blow to head from a fall	Cycling
Hip, groin	Pulled muscle	Overuse, changes of exercise routine	Running
Knee	Torn cartilage and other problems	Overuse, changes of exercise routine	Running, weightlifting
Neck	Tightness or soreness	Overworking of muscles	Cycling
Shoulder	Bicipital tendinitis and other types of painful conditions of the joint	Overuse or poor technique	Swimming, tennis, baseball
Thigh	Pulled hamstring muscle	Inadequate warm-up in sports involving running, jumping, or twisting	Football, racquet sports, soccer, sprints

tissue tears. The most common problems are injuries due to overuse—wear-and-tear to the muscles, ligaments, tendons, and joints (Table 14-5). The risks of injury are greater for sedentary individuals and those who thrust themselves into activities that are either too strenuous, prolonged, or frequent. As Jones and others have noted:

Excessive activity without adequate conditioning and sufficient rest equals trouble. . . . All changes in frequency, duration, and intensity of exercise should be gradual.

Serious athletes and weekend warriors alike should undergo overall strength and flexibility training in addition to the specific techniques required by the particular sport or activity. Flexibility is an important component of fitness, as is general body strength. An overuse injury is a signal that the body is working against itself. Appropriate strengthening and flexibility exercises, as well as an organized, progressive increase in the duration and intensity of exercise, will help to cure the problem and prevent its recurrence.[21]

Well-designed exercise programs include time for the body to recover. High-resistance exercises such as heavy weightlifting or intense anaerobic activities (such as sprinting, jumping, competitive tennis, or competitive swimming) require 36 to 48 hours for full recovery. Aerobic activities and light-resistance exercises can be done daily (or even twice daily). Exercise programs usually become highly individualized and may vary considerably from season to season.

Table 14-6 outlines sample programs that contribute to all-around fitness, weight control, and recreational sports ability.

Table 14-7 describes the certification requirements for various types of exercise instructors.

SPORTS MEDICINE SPECIALISTS

Most exercise-related injuries are minor and will resolve with reduced activity levels or rest. A general rule for muscle soreness or joint pain is to continue exercising at a lower level of intensity if the pain or soreness goes away after warming up. If the pain persists or worsens, the exercise program should be discontinued until activities can be comfortably resumed. A physician should be consulted if (a) pain is severe or persists; (b) movement of the injured part of the body is difficult or impossible, or (c) the injury does not appear to be healing.

When professional care is needed, the best first source is probably one's primary physician. The *Penn State Sports Medicine Newsletter*[22] has advised that the next step might be toward a primary-care physician who has a Certificate of Added Qualifications in sports medicine.

Several other types of professionals can offer advice about exercise programs, procedures, and equipment or provide services to people who are injured. Some work primarily by referral, and some practice independently:

ATHLETIC TRAINER: Athletic trainers help people plan exercise programs. They can also work under physician supervision to help treat sports injuries. Certification as an athletic trainer (A.T.C.) can be obtained by passing a written, oral, and practical examination administered by the National Athletic Trainers' Association. Eligibility for the test can be established by (a) majoring in athletic training at one of about 150 colleges and universities and completing at least 800 hours of supervised experience or (b) obtaining a bachelor's degree and completing an internship with 1500 hours of supervised experience.[23]

EXERCISE PHYSIOLOGIST (Ph.D. or M.S.): Someone who helps design exercise programs for healthy athletes, hospital patients, or fitness club clients. Many are research specialists. Those who work in health clubs generally have a master's degree.

MASSAGE THERAPIST (MASSOTHERAPIST): A certified or licensed person who may help speed up recovery by stroking and kneading muscles.

ORTHOPEDIST (M.D.): A physician who specializes in the diagnosis and treatment of problems of muscles, bones, joints, and the spine.

PHYSICAL THERAPIST (P.T. or R.P.T.): A trained and licensed individual who helps maintain and restore function to injured limbs and joints using strengthening machines, various exercises, heat, and water. Works closely with physicians in rehabilitation.

PODIATRIST (D.P.M.): A person medically trained in the prevention, diagnosis, and treatment of injuries, disease, and abnormalities of the foot and ankle.

SPORTS NUTRITIONIST (R.D.): A registered dietitian who helps with the nutritional needs of athletes.

SPORTS PSYCHOLOGIST (Ph.D. or M.S.): Someone who works with athletes and teams to provide stress relief and to help meet specific training and competition goals.

EXERCISE EQUIPMENT AND SUPPLIES

Americans spend several billion dollars a year on exercise devices. Some contribute greatly to physical fitness and safety, whereas others have little or no value. Consumers contemplating purchase or use of exercise equipment should consider whether the benefits to be derived will contribute to endurance, flexibility, strength, and cardiorespiratory efficiency. Consumers may also investigate whether similar benefits can be obtained without equipment or in a less expensive way. Most people who purchase exercise equipment waste money, largely because boredom sets in. A 1998 survey found that fewer than one third of machines bought by *Consumer Reports* readers who began exercise programs during the previous 4 years were still in use.[24]

Table 14-6

SAMPLE EXERCISE PROGRAMS

Primary Goal	Weekly Schedule
Moderate-level cardiorespiratory fitness	Aerobic exercise 3 days (every other day)
High-level cardiorespiratory fitness*	Aerobic exercise 5–7 days
Moderate-level overall fitness	Mon-Wed-Fri: aerobic exercise
	Tues-Thur: weightlifting or other resistance exercise
High-level overall fitness*	Sun-Tues-Thurs-Sat AM: distance running
	Mon-Wed-Fri AM: interval running†
	Sun-Tues-Thurs PM: lap swimming, weightlifting, or other resistance exercise
	Mon-Wed-Fri PM: raquetball, tennis, handball, or basketball
Moderate-level weight control	Daily AM: walk-jog-run
High-level weight control	Daily AM and PM walk-jog-run
High-level weight control and fitness*	Daily AM: aerobic activities
	Sun-Tues-Thurs PM: lap swimming, weightlifting, or other resistance exercise
	Mon-Wed-Fri PM: raquetball, tennis, handball, or basketball
Bodybuilding	Sun-Tues-Thurs-Sat: walk-jog-run
	Mon-Wed-Fri: high-resistance training
Recreational sport performance	Daily AM: walk-jog-run or bike
	Sun-Tues-Thurs-Sat PM: participation in specific sport
	Mon-Wed-Fri PM: supplemental training for specific sport

*High-performance programs exceed what is needed to achieve a fitness level associated with good health. However, high-level fitness may be desirable for achieving athletic prowess or for other reasons.
†Interval running involves timed, fast-pace runs over measured distances for 1.5 to 3-minute periods, with walking until recovery in-between runs.

Table 14-7

EXERCISE INSTRUCTOR CERTIFICATION PROGRAMS

Organization	*Type of Instructor* / Requirements (All Require CPR Certification)
American College of Sports Medicine http://www.acsm.org	*ACSM personal trainer, ACSM health and fitness instructor, ACSM exercise leader* Knowledge of exercise science, exercise physiology, nutrition, health-appraisal techniques, injury prevention, teaching techniques
American Council on Exercise (ACE) http://www.acefitness.org	*Group fitness instructor* Written exam on exercise physiology, anatomy, exercise programming, administrative skills, nutrition, and weight control *Personal trainer certification* Health screening, fitness testing, design and implementation of fitness programs
Aerobics and Fitness Association of America http://www.afaa.com	*Personal training, aerobics instructors, step certification* Written exam similar to ACE's. Must also do practical exam, including demonstration of a short aerobics session
Institute for Aerobics Research http://www.cooperinst.org	*Physical fitness specialist (personal trainer)* Written and practical exam on exercise physiology, anatomy, fitness assessment, and individual program planning *Group exercise leaders* Written and practical exam on leadership and group programming skill

The use of exercise equipment involves some risk. Burroughs[25] reported on 18,000 injuries that required emergency room treatment. During 1991 the U.S. Consumer Product Safety Commission identified many exercise devices with faulty springs that had caused bruises, lacerations, and other injuries to users.

It is important for consumers to clearly understand their fitness goals, to obtain expert help in using equipment, and to check the quality of items before purchasing them.

Table 14-8 compares 29 exercise products, many of which are questionable, that have been advertised in popular magazines and newspapers.

Exercise Bicycles

More than 100 brands and models of exercise bicycles are available, most costing between $150 and $2000. The best ones have rigid construction, a comfortable seat, easily adjustable height, and smooth riding action. Three types are marketed. Regular upright bikes involve pumping with the legs to turn a flywheel linked to the pedals. Resistance to pumping is provided by a strap around the wheel or a set of caliper brake pads. The tighter the strap or pads, the more difficult it is to turn the wheel, and the greater the workout. Dual-action uprights have their handlebars linked to the pedals so they move back and forth as the bike is pedaled; these provide exercise for the arms and legs. Recumbent bikes are operated by sitting in a seat resembling the bucket seat of a car; the user may be more comfortable and have less strain placed on back muscles. Training stands, which support a regular bike and add a resistance device, cost less but will not provide an aerobic workout for someone in good shape. The home exercise bikes rated highest by *Consumer Reports*[26] were:

SINGLE-ACTION ($220 to $1130): Precor M8.2E/L, Lifecycle 3500, Tunturi Motivational Electronic F460

DUAL-ACTION ($140 to $630): Schwinn Airdyne, Ross Future 950, DP Prime Fit

RECUMBENT ($350 to $965): Tunturi Motivational Recumbent, Tunturi Recumbent, PreCor 855e, and Schwinn Professional 230.

Rowing Machines

High-quality rowing machines cost at least $250. Good equipment has sturdy tubing; parts that fit snugly together; a padded, contoured seat that slides smoothly; and double-piston "oars" with adjustable tension.

Table 14-8

COMPARISON OF EXERCISE EQUIPMENT

Description	Advertising Claims	Comments
Barbells: Forms and shapes vary in size and weight; made of iron, rubber, plastic; water- or sand-filled	Tones muscles; very light; easy to store	Provides resistance exercise; especially useful with other equipment; benefits depend on types of exercise, amount of weight, and frequency of use. Loosely handled free weights are hazardous to fingers and toes.
Bull-worker: Two spring-loaded cylinders about 3 feet long with handles at each end that telescope when compressed	Isometric/isotonic exerciser; develops muscles and builds body through push, pull, and press; easy to use; takes 70 seconds a day	Benefits limited as indicated; perhaps some isometric value; limited to upper body, excluding abdominals; "70 seconds" advertising claim unreasonable
Bicycle, stationary: A bicycle without the usual wheels that registers speed and distance; can provide varying degrees of resistance; some also have rowing action	Permits aerobic fitness in home or office; promotes circulation, improves muscle tone and coordination, increases endurance	Extent of resistance and intensity will determine benefits; equipment can vary degrees of resistance
Chinning bar: Metal bar hung in doorway or attached to ceiling or wall slightly above reach	Rarely advertised; may be part of a multiple equipment system	Benefits limited to upper body strength development; strenuous for the unfit; can be made easily and cheaply in a home workshop
Chest pull/chest expander: Heavy rubber or elastic bands or springs with handles on each end	Isometric/isotonic exercise; no long, tiring workouts; tones and shapes all muscle groups in one fourth the time required for barbells and dead weights	Good isotonic trainer for upper body; provides limited resistance exercise benefits; resistance exercise can speed up strength improvement, but time requirement cannot be verified; does not provide isokinetic or isometric exercise
Cross-country ski machine: Leg glide with smooth sensation of cross-country motion; arm pulls provide resistance	Elevates heart rate to fitness level; burns more calories; exercises all muscle groups in upper and lower body	Simulates skiing; fairly good workout; requires good coordination; little strain on body, especially knees
Door gym/portable gym: Varies in complexity of equipment; includes chinning bar, tension items	Provides 30 different body-building and shaping exercises—as many as Nautilus and other costly machines; virtually all exercises offered by other expensive weight machines	Depending on type of resistance exercise, might be good weight training device; the several types of equipment do provide a variety of activities; frequency and duration of resistance exercise will determine benefits
Electronic muscle/nerve stimulator: Electropulse pads placed in various muscle areas in which three levels of electrical intensity can be applied	300 sit-ups without moving an inch; 10 miles of jogging lying flat on your back; smooth, flattened tummy, slender thighs, youthful bustline, no-sag backside, wrinkle removal, weight loss	Unrealistic claims; no aerobic conditioning; FDA has approved some electrical nerve/muscle stimulation devices for maintaining muscle tone under medical supervision—used in rehabilitation after surgery and injuries and for arthritic patients
Quick-Trim Isoelectric Exerciser or Rope Tension Gym: Lightweight dynamic tension device; heavy spring pulled and pushed by arms and leg	Firms and trims waist, hips, thighs, derriere; flattens stomach; firms and strengthens chest, arms quickly and easily; use only 5 minutes each day	Claims false or exaggerated; very limited benefits; one cannot spot-reduce or trim fat by toning a muscle beneath the fat; check quality of equipment

Table 14-8

COMPARISON OF EXERCISE EQUIPMENT - *CONT'D.*

Description	Advertising Claims	Comments
Gravity Guiding Rack System/ Portable Gravity Guide/ Gravity Inversion Boots: Simple to complex equipment; individual turns upside down, hangs by feet; uses special boots	Relieves backache, stress on spine; relieves back pain without surgery and expensive therapy; restores body flexibility and vigor; gravity flattens stomach, strengthens back and legs; totally safe	No scientific evidence to support claims; hanging upside down empties leg veins, but so does lying in bed with feet elevated; elevates blood pressure and eye pressure; use with caution, can cause injuries (originally designed as traction apparatus to relieve interdisc pressures)
Grip strengthener: Rubber ball; fairly hard substance	Builds muscles in wrist/forearm by simply squeezing ball; also exercises toes and instep; great tension reliever	Any round rubber object or other resistant substance will strengthen muscles; frequency and duration important; no evidence of tension relief
Hip Cycle, PedaBike, Lazy Slimmer: Operate pedals like bicycle while lying down or sitting in chair	Firms hips, trims thighs, shapes calves; makes exercise easier; firms abdomen, buttocks, hips	No resistance exercise, no strength; no involved abdominal, buttock or hip muslces; stationary bicycle better; note benefit limits
Jump rope: Made of cotton, nylon, polyester material, with handles	Involves cardiorespiratory efficiency (CRE); leg muscle endurance/stamina	Improves CRE; develops leg strength; excellent activity with inexpensive equipment; can be homemade; weighted ropes available
Minitrampoline: Steel frame with tough vinyl cover, 34 x 10 inches	Combines aerobic exercises to work on each muscle in body and heart; easier on knees than jogging; improves posture, balance, digestion; strengthens heart; enjoyable	No effect on digestion; good if intensity is high: probably can benefit the unfit; must work very hard for aerobic effect; hazard of losing balance and falling; some claims are conjecture; less traumatic to the body than running or jumping on hard surfaces
Multipurpose gyms. Home fitness system/portable gym/ weight training complex: Contain various weight-training items such as a sit-up/slant board and leg lifts; most popular are Nautilus and Universal	Permits full range of professional gym exercises; over 50 simple exercises from heavy body-building to general physical fitness; do leg lifts, leg curls, arm curls, and arm rowing	Provides resistive exercise that can speed up strength development and fitness; limited cardiorespiratory involvement; body parts involved depend on choice of exercises; some equipment usable in small space in home; less costly equipment and programs are available
Orthopedic inversion machine: Upside-down stretch that relaxes back and abdominal muscles	Easy, safe; strengthens muscle; supports back; painless inverted abdominal curls; perform trunk twists and hyperextensions; improves circulation; releases stress; adds energy and vitality	May strengthen back muscles with some trunk value; no evidence to support release of stress or improve circulation; high-cost item—same effect achieved at less or no cost; injury a problem (see Gravity Guiding Rack)
Pushup bars: Two individual steel bars 6 inches from floor	Provides better, quicker results than ordinary push-ups; allows greater range of motion	Resistance may quicken benefits; whether better is unproven; same results can be achieved without equipment
Rowing machine: Various styles; some collapsible, some attached to wall, have pulse meter, caloric meter, clock to track elapsed time	Strengthens heart, lungs; tones stomach, hip, thighs, and arms; increases endurance; gets rid of tension; rowing is a great all-around fitness program	Good benefits if frequency and intensity and duration maintained; needs high degree of motivation to prevent boredom from use; risky for people with back problems
Sit-up bar: Bar attached 6 inches from wall for hooking feet when exercising	Strengthens middle; shapes legs	Especially helps tone abdominals if knees in bent position; "shaping of legs" claim is puffery; with feet locked, hip flexors are involved

Table 14-8

COMPARISON OF EXERCISE EQUIPMENT - *CONT'D.*

Description	Advertising Claims	Comments
Slant board: Vinyl-covered, padded board, 12 to 14 inches wide; can be tilted up or down; person lies on it when exercising	Firms muscles; orthopedically approved	Greater benefit because of greater resistance from gravity than in flat sit-ups; use of barbells and weights increases resistance and benefits; may be part of home gym equipment; knees should be bent during use
Slim/Small Wheel: 6- to 8-inch wheel with bar through center for hands; is rolled to and from body while in kneeling position	Tightens muscles; takes off inches from waistline without dieting or weight loss; twice a day merely roll back and forth five times; equals same results as a dozen conventional sit-ups	Claims are outrageous, not substantiated; benefits limited; not for people with back or shoulder problems; mostly a latissimus dorsi exercise
Stair climber: Grasp handle and begin to step and pull, working upper body and lower body at same time	Work upper and lower body at same time; work every muscle group; for serious training	Good aerobic activity; most muscles involved; limited arm and very limited abdominal and back involvement
Stairway Stepping: 2-, 4-, 6-, and 8-inch blocks; 4-inch high platform to step; plus video	Latest in low-impact video; mix stair climbing and jazz aerobics	Good aerobic and strength activity; limited upper arm and body involvement unless weights are used; could be strenuous and should be taken in gradual steps; 6- to 8-inch steps for advanced fitness
Stomach eliminators: Crossbar or heavy spring attached; stirrups-like foot grips	Slimmer, younger look in 2 weeks; flattens stomach, strengthens chest, arms, back, thighs	Benefits limited; some back and arm strength; hazard—breakage of spring
Thigh machine: Bar 12 inches from floor, movable against some resistance by the arms and legs	Slims legs; tones and stretches all body parts; over 40 isotonic and isometric exercises	May strengthen a few muscles but does not affect all body parts or make legs slimmer
Treadmill: A flat, moving surface on rollers; permits walking at home; some lightweight and portable with adjustable speeds	Benefits thighs, legs, stomach, lower back, waist, abdomen, calves, ankles, buttocks, lungs, heart, circulation; improves muscle tone	Benefits good if motivation maintained; costly equipment especially with motor; benefits obtainable in less costly ways
Tummy Toner: Knee pad on rollers attached to steel frame with 12-inch high bar in front for hands; glide back and forward on rollers while kneeling	Helps melt away middle bulge; improves muscle tone; gradually firms muscles from rib cage and pelvis	Promotes fallacious spot-reducing concept; spot exercises can develop but not slim specific muscle groups
Tummy Trimming/Stomach Trimmer: Wide rubber/elastic belt that buttons, tightens, shapes abdominal area	Look inches slimmer instantly; flatten stomach; no diet; no exercise	Promotes fallacious spot-reducing concept; spot exercises can develop but not slim specific muscle groups
Twister: 12-inch plastic/metal circle/square rotates on ball bearings; person stands on it and twists body	Tones muscles; strengthens legs and hips; slims thighs	Benefits limited; provides some balance and trunk movement, hence some waistline effect; difficult to maintain motivation

Cross-Country Ski Exercisers

Cross-country ski machines are very popular. This equipment may help produce weight loss, stimulate interest in cross-country skiing, and strengthen and firm many muscle groups, especially in the legs. When planning to purchase a cross-country ski exerciser, look for smoothness of operation, overall stability, foot security, a fit that allows adequate adjustment for people of different height, ease of resistance adjustment, and quiet operation. *Consumer Reports* recommends choosing one with skis that move independently. It rated the Nordic Track Pro as excellent and the Precor 515E, Nordic Track Challenger, and Nordic Sport World Class Ski as very good.[27] Nordic Track no longer makes these products, but used ones may be available.

Stair Steppers and Climbers

Steppers are single-action devices that work out only the lower body. Climbers offer upper-body exercise with hand grips that can be pulled down and pushed up while stepping with the feet. With the better models, the feet move independently, which means that each leg must do the work of stepping without help from the other.

Treadmills

Motorized treadmills provide the same benefits as walking or running outdoors with less chance of injury and regardless of weather conditions. Most treadmills permit the user to control the rigor of the workout by adjusting the speed and incline of the track. Low-priced models (under $500) are inconvenient to adjust and are too short and/or too slow for jogging. Mid-priced models ($500 to $1000) offer a long platform, higher speeds, and the ability to adjust the incline conveniently. Some can be used for jogging, but they may not last long if the user weighs more than 150 pounds. High-priced models ($1600 up) are built more sturdily, are more convenient to adjust, and have more electronic gadgetry. The four rated highest in a recent *Consumer Reports* evaluation were the Image 10.6.Q ($1600), HealthRider Softstrider EX ($1000), Tunturi J660 ($2000), and Life Fitness TR-4000 ($2400).[24] Nonmotorized treadmills are not recommended because they force the user to walk in an unnatural position.

A recent study compared the exercise workload and how people felt when using an Airdyne machine, a ski simulator, an exercise bike, a rowing machine, a stairs-tepper, and a treadmill for walking. The subjects of the study were healthy, young adult volunteers who were trained to rate their perceived degree of exertion. The researchers found that the treadmill produced the highest energy expenditure (and therefore the best aerobic workout) for each level of perceived exertion.[28]

Elliptical Exercisers

These are a cross between an exercise bike and a ski machine. They provide an effective cardiovascular workout, especially for advanced beginner and intermediate exercisers. Consumer Reports recommends the Orbi-Trek ($260) and the ProForm 485e ($400).[24]

Mountain Bikes

Mountain bicycles typically have a sturdy frame; fat, knobby tires; and flat handlebars. (Road bikes have a lighter frame; skinnier, smoother tires; and drop handlebars.) The best bikes tested by *Consumer Reports* were full-suspension models costing about $1000 and front-suspension models costing $440 to $700. Although less expensive bikes are suitable for casual riding, models that provides a less jarring ride are recommended for off-road use.[29]

Bicycle Helmets

Studies have found that helmet use can substantially reduce the risk of head injury among cyclists. Yet only small percentages of children and adults wear one. Standards required by law are set by the Consumer Product Safety Commission. *Consumer Reports*[30] has investigated helmets that ranged from $8 to $35 for toddler models, $20 to $40 for youth models, and $32 to $150 for adult models. It recommends looking for the following features:

- Fitting pads that are attached with Velcro-type fasteners so that they hold the helmet in place firmly yet comfortably
- A rear stabilizer that encourages correct head position once the straps are properly adjusted
- Strap guides that lock and unlock with a hinged strap, making it easier to adjust strap length.
- Straps that move freely through slots in the front or rear of the helmet, making adjustment easier
- A buckle with a pinch guard to protect the skin under the chin.

The top rated models were *Bell Half Point* ($30) for children up to 4 years old, the *Giro Wheelie* ($35) for children from 5 to 14, and the *Louis Garneau Globe* ($50), *Trek Vapor* ($32), or *GT Gator* ($40) for adults.

Electronic Feedback

Electronic monitors found on many exercise machines (or available as an accessory) provide feedback on heart rate, speed, miles pedaled or traveled, and calories burned. Devices that report distance, speed, repetitions, elapsed time, and heart rate are usually accurate. Those that report calories burned may have a large margin of error. Generally, the more gadgetry, the higher the cost.

Portable monitors check the pulse during exercise to enable individuals to know whether they are performing at an appropriate pulse rate (usually 60% to 90% of maximum).

There are two types of monitors: (1) finger or earlobe sensor and (2) transmitter worn on the chest that broadcasts to a watch that provides the pulse readout. The finger or earlobe type is less expensive but less accurate. This equipment may be an unnecessary expense because there is another easy way to check the pulse rate. Place the first three fingers of one hand on the inside of the wrist, below where the bone connects to the thumb, and feel the beat. Count the number of pulsations for 15 seconds and multiply by 4 to get the 1-minute pulse rate.

For serious exercisers who wish to build up to and remain safely within the high end of the target range, the chest transmitter is the only one that is worthwhile. Excellent ones can be obtained for about $100. Higher-priced models can provide additional data, such as the amount of time spent within the target range.

Some fitness facilities have computers to help people make their workouts more precise and efficient. Some can create exercise programs tailored to specific goals. For example, computers can provide an exercise prescription based on a person's interests, times available, attendance, and fitness scores. Computerized devices can also be used to test muscle strength and to prescribe activities needed to increase strength. Some athletes use the devices to compare their own performances with those of champions to determine weaknesses. Professional help may be needed to utilize these approaches.

Strength-Training Equipment

There are three basic types of strength-training equipment. Free weights include dumbbells, barbells, and hand weights. Weight stacks use either discs or blocks of weights attached to a lever or pulley system. Nautilus and other machines that do not use weight stacks use pneumatic resistance, hydraulic resistance, compression of rubber, or other mechanisms within the machine. *Consumers Digest*[31] advises prospective purchasers of such equipment for home use to consider price, size (vs size of exercise area), safety (sturdy construction with no sharp edges), and quality of instructional material.

Athletic Shoes

The average person takes 10,000 steps per day. Each step exerts a force greater than the body weight on certain bones and muscles of the feet. Running more than triples that force, and various other fitness and athletic activities also increase it. Cumulative pounding, complicated by poorly fitting shoes, can cause aching feet and other foot problems. Foot problems can alter a person's gait and posture, causing pain to progress to the ankles, knees, hips, and lower back. One way to properly take care of the feet is to have proper athletic shoes.

The nature of the physical activity determines the type of shoe needed; good ones typically cost $45 to $135. They are designed to provide rigidity, durability, flexibility, proper fit, adequate cushioning (shock absorption), and comfort. Figure 14-2 illustrates the features of a good walking shoe. When buying shoes, the most important consideration should be a good fit; they should feel comfortable from the moment they are put on. These additional tips may help:

- Give preference to stores that employ a professional shoe fitter (pedorthist) or serious recreational athlete who knows about foot problems and biomechanics.
- Shop late in the day or after exercising, when your feet are largest. Don't expect athletic shoes to stretch.
- Wear the kind of socks you plan to wear when exercising.
- An old pair of athletic shoes may help a knowledgeable salesperson determine what is best for you.
- Be sure that the toe box is wide enough to permit toes to wiggle and long enough to have about half an inch of space in front of the longest toe.
- Feel inside for seams and ridges.
- Be sure that the shoes bend easily at their widest part. Running shoes need more flexibility in the toe area in order to push off; walking shoes should be more rigid to permit rolling off the toes and joints rather than bending through them.[32]
- Take a test walk or jog in the store.

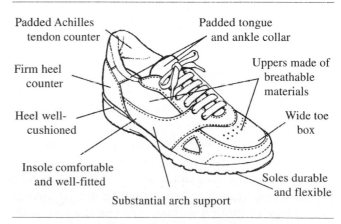

Padded Achilles tendon counter

Padded tongue and ankle collar

Firm heel counter

Uppers made of breathable materials

Heel well-cushioned

Wide toe box

Insole comfortable and well-fitted

Soles durable and flexible

Substantial arch support

FIGURE 14-2. Features of a good walking shoe.

The American Running Association maintains a database to help people choose suitable running shoes. Its Web site (http://www.americanrunning.org) has a questionnaire that can be submitted with $10 to receive a list of recommended shoes, prices, and manufacturer contacts.

The running shoes rated highest by *Consumer Reports*[33] were the *Adidas Response, Asics GEL-MC126, Adidas The Formula, New Balance M586NV,* and *Saucony Grid Jazz-i* for men, and the *Ryka 10K Stability, Etonic Pro III, Saucony Grid Stabil,* and *Asics GEL-MC126* for women.

Snug, poorly ventilated shoes and damp, sweaty socks provide a breeding ground for athlete's foot, a fungal infection that causes itching, redness, and skin peeling between the toes. To prevent this condition, daily washing of the feet with soap and water is advisable, and the feet, especially between the toes, should be dried thoroughly. Talcum powder can help to keep the feet dry after washing. A 1% tolnaftate solution or ointment can also help protect against athlete's foot. Chapter 19 discusses its treatment.

Sports Bras

A need for custom sports bras to support female athletes' breasts has not been clearly established. Studies by Hunger and Torgan[34] indicate there is no need for a special type of bra. They reviewed the 5-year injury records of women who participated in intercollegiate athletics at the University of Washington and found no breast injuries had occurred and no breast pain complaints had been made. Hunger and Torgan also surveyed 85 female athletes who participated in a variety of sports and found no relationship between breast pain and trauma and the type of bra worn. Only 10 of the women wore special sports bras; the rest used a variety of commercial bras, most of which were made from nylon or cotton and nylon with elastic. The majority said they preferred inexpensive bras that were made of absorbent material and had seamless cups, nonirritating clasps, and shoulder straps that do not slide.

Questionable Devices

Many types of exercise devices and equipment are advertised with claims that have no scientific foundation. Bogus claims regarding weight control, body shaping, and effortless muscle-building are the most common.

Continuous passive motion tables. Continuous passive motion (CPM) tables are motorized in segments so that isolated muscle groups can be moved through their range of motion without effort on the part of the user. CPM units have been used in the rehabilitation of injured athletes to restore and maintain joint motions and have revolutionized some types of orthopedic surgery.[35] They are useful during recovery from joint replacement, ligament reconstruction, and recovery from various other operations and illnesses. They provide movement that could help with joint flexibility for the elderly, sedentary people, and those with neuromuscular disorders. However, they have also been used in clinics and salons where they are claimed to provide "exercise without exercise" and to tone muscles, reduce stress, improve posture, cause weight loss, and eliminate excess water retention. These claims are unsubstantiated. Consumers should be aware that CPM units have value in therapy and rehabilitation but will not benefit healthy, active people.

"Gravity inversion" devices. So-called gravity boots are used with support systems that hold people in an upside-down position. The boots were invented in 1965 by Dr. Robert Martin, an osteopath who developed them to relieve stress on spines and joints caused by standing and sitting. Martin claimed that body inversion decompresses spinal discs, stretches back muscles, and improves overall flexibility, posture, and well-being—everything from hemorrhoids to sagging bowels. He also espoused a long-held notion that gravity produced aging, and therefore that positioning the body upside down would have an opposite effect. During the early 1980s more than a dozen companies were marketing devices for inverted exercise or plain hanging, and members of several prominent sports teams were identified as users of such equipment. There is no scientific evidence that hanging upside down has any health benefit. Critics have warned that inversion raises blood pressure conside-rably.[36] It can also be hazardous to people with glaucoma, spinal instability, or a hiatal hernia.

Abdominal toners. Many devices are claimed to enable people to "flatten" their abdomen by tightening and toning the abdominal muscles. The *Tufts University Diet & Nutrition Letter* states: (a) abdominal exercises cannot flatten a flabby stomach because they cannot spot-reduce the layer of fat between the muscles and the skin, (b) some of these devices help exercise the abdominal muscles by making it easier to do sit-ups, but others actually exercise the arms rather than the abdominal muscles, and (c) it is not necessary to spend money to "tone one's abs." Sit-ups with knees bent and hands on thighs (not behind the neck) will do an effective job.[37]

"Spot-reducers." Some products or devices are claimed to reduce or remove fat from specific parts of the body. In controlled studies that compared individuals who performed general exercises with others who performed spot exercises, both groups lost fat where it was most conspicuous, regardless of the type of exercise. Exercise does "burn off" fat and calories, but it does this throughout the body and not just in an exercised area. There is no such thing as spot-reducing.

Special garments. Many types of garments have been marketed with fanciful claims that fitness, weight-reduction, or body-shaping can be produced without any effort on the part of the wearer. Rubber sweatsuits have been claimed to cause weight loss by increasing the amount of water lost through perspiration. (Of course, when the wearer consumes water, any such weight returns.) Heat belts have been marketed with similar claims. Some have chemical heat packs to increase the temperature around the waist and have elasticized waist cinchers to fit close to the body to keep sweat from evaporating. An "effortless exerciser," a tight-fitting garment said to have been perfected by a "leading physician" (unidentified), was advertised to give a new body and new heart in just 2 easy minutes a day. The ad claimed that a hidden "muscle-girdle" that one never removes would develop the body. Advertisements informed women that the device could squeeze their hips away, firm their bustline, and put a glow in complexions that no cosmetic could match.

Electrical nerve/muscle stimulators. Electrical nerve stimulators (ENS)/electrical muscle stimulators (EMS) are sold through the mail or without prescription at $19.95 and up; professional models used in hospitals and other places are priced at $2500. Powered by a 12-volt battery, these machines stimulate nerves that cause muscles to contract. Some consumers purchase this equipment for home use; others pay $25 or more for 45-minute sessions at Futureshape, Figuretrim, Ultimate Image, Bodytone parlors, and other such establishments. The advertisements for these products stress an effortless "no-sweat workout," which is a method of moving muscles and obtaining exercise without effort. One advertisement states that users can get the equivalent of 10 miles of jogging while lying flat on their back. Other ads claim that ENS/EMS will strengthen the arm, leg, and other muscles; slim and trim the body; shape and contour the body; produce a facelift without surgery (remove wrinkles); control weight; spot-reduce; increase bust size; and remove cellulite. The *Wall Street Journal* reported that these machines are supposed to "battle hanging bellies," "deflate derrieres," and help "pooped-out pecs." The FDA stated that there was no evidence to support these claims and that users were being ripped off.[38]

Low-intensity electrical stimulation can help relieve muscle soreness and can speed recovery. ENS/EMS devices have FDA approval for use in physical therapy by trained health practitioners for relaxing muscle spasms, preventing clots in leg muscles of patients bedridden after surgery or a stroke, increasing circulation to a part of the body, increasing or monitoring the range of motion of an arm or leg, and retarding or preventing muscle atrophy resulting from disease or injury.

ENS/EMS devices can cause electrical shocks and burns. They should not be used by pregnant women or by persons with heart problems (especially those with a pacemaker), cancer, or epilepsy. Electrodes should not be placed where strong current passes though the heart, brain, or spinal cord.

The *Relax-A-Cizor* was a similar device that was claimed to reduce the waistline. Like the electrical nerve stimulator (ENS), it delivered shocks through contact pads. More than 400,000 units were sold for $200 to $400 each. In the late 1960s the FDA brought suit to stop its sale because it was dangerous. At the trial, 40 witnesses testified that they suffered varying degrees of injury while using the machine. The judge concluded that the device could cause miscarriages and aggravate many pre-existing medical conditions, including hernias, ulcers, varicose veins, and epilepsy. In 1971 a U.S. district court ruled that the device could be used only under a physician's prescription and issued a permanent injunction prohibiting its sale to the public.

EXERCISE FACILITIES

Health clubs and fitness centers are popular because they provide equipment and the opportunity for social interaction and a structured program. These range from small storefront exercise rooms to clubs that provide high-tech exercise machines, a gymnasium, a swimming pool, racquetball and tennis courts, whirlpool, sauna and steam facilities, and even an indoor track. Some clubs offer individual instruction from a personal trainer and seminars on topics such as nutrition, stress management, weight control, and smoking cessation. The cost of membership usually includes an entry fee (typically $100 to $500) plus monthly fees (typically $25 to $75).[39]

The following questions can help in selecting an exercise facility:

- What is the nature of the facility and equipment (types, condition, maintenance, sufficient for peak times, time limits on use)?
- Do the locker rooms, showers, bathrooms, and whirlpools show signs of neglect or poor sanitation?

- Does the program serve my purposes? Is it designed to meet individual needs?
- What are the costs (entry fee, rates, additional charges)?
- What is the nature of the staff (are their qualifications adequate; are they pleasant, attentive, certified by reputable organizations)?
- Is it conveniently located?
- Is there a system to assess fitness and help evaluate progress toward a goal, and is this clearly identified?
- How does the facility function at peak hours? Will the equipment desired be available?
- Are there members I can contact as references?
- Is the contract understandable? Are there hidden clauses? Can I take it home to read? Can I get a refund if I cancel? Can I bring guests?
- Are high-pressure tactics used to get me to join? Are staff members courteous and friendly?
- Does a local Y or a competitor provide appropriate facilities at a lower cost?
- Is the club well-established? (Check with the local Better Business Bureau or consumer protection agency about complaints.)
- Can the services be sampled before purchasing a membership?

Consumer Problems

People seriously interested in joining a health club should be wary of promotional gimmicks offering free time at the facilities. Deceptive practices are common throughout the health spa industry. Prospective members may be subjected to a sad commentary on the state of their physique and appearance, promised radiant results from the use of equipment, and offered a contract containing doubletalk. Other abuses include (a) misleading advertising, (b) high-pressure sales, (c) misrepresentation in sales presentations, and (d) collection practices that harass the customer. Consumers should beware of these practices:

SPECIAL REDUCED PRICE: This price is frequently the regular rate.

BAIT-AND-SWITCH: Ten treatment sessions are advertised for $10. But after arrival at the club the customer may be told that two treatments must be taken on each visit or that only limited facilities for limited hours are available under the offer. The salesperson then tries to sell a more expensive, longer-term program.

FREE VISITS: These are sometimes offered to all who sign up at registration tables. "Winners" often find that their "free visit" amounts to a high-pressure sales pitch to accept the prize of a supposed discount on an inflated membership fee.

BEFORE-AND-AFTER PHOTOGRAPHS: These are frequently staged to produce the desired effect. In some cases the person in the picture may never have visited the club, or two different people are shown in the comparison photographs.

WEIGHT LOSS WITHOUT EXERCISE: There is no evidence that devices that vibrate or shake the body actually aid in weight reduction or improve muscle tone.

PERSONAL PROGRAMS: These may prove to be standard calisthenics or other exercises that vary little from one person to another.

LAST-DAY-ONLY RATES: The last-day-only offer of a special price may be fraudulent because no price increase was being considered.

RESERVATION FORMS: Application forms may be used to deceive a prospective customer into believing that a place is being reserved; the customer may be signing a contract for long-term membership.

GUARANTEES: Guarantees of weight loss are often meaningless. The spa may be the sole judge of whether the patron followed the program to the letter and can renege on the agreement by judging that the client did not follow the "exact" program.

REASSIGNMENT CONTRACT: Difficulty may occur when a contract is sold to a third party (such as a loan company) who later demands payment of an unfulfilled contract.

CANCELLATION: Requests for cancellation of membership contracts often are denied. Apparently a high percentage of people who sign a contract discontinue using the spa in a short time, forfeiting their initial payment. Many people never use the facilities after the first few weeks.

SPA FAILURES OR NOT OPENING: After contracts are signed and money is paid, consumers may lose their investment because the spa does not operate.

These suggestions will help to decide whether to sign a contract:

- Ask members and former members their opinions of the club and its programs. If necessary, names can be obtained from the organization. If the club refuses to comply, be wary.
- Think it over for a few days; a reputable club will not press for an immediate decision.
- Read the contract carefully or get a knowledgeable person to read it to be sure you understand the provisions.
- Ask for a short-term trial program.
- Understand what happens if you are unable to use the facilities temporarily or decide to cancel the contract. In an ideal cancellation arrangement the customer gets a refund based on the proportion of time used during the contract. Under present collection practices used by some spas, however, an individual could be pressured and even sued for the full contract price—even if the spa's facilities were never used. A few clubs permit transfer of the membership but charge a fee for this.
- Try to determine whether the equipment you want to use is likely to be available at the times you would like to use it or whether the facilities are overcrowded.

Individuals who believe that they have been dealt with unjustly or improperly pressured into joining by a health club can seek help from a small claims court, local or state consumer affairs office, state attorney general, or county district attorney.

The quality of instructors or supervisory personnel at these various facilities should be reviewed carefully. Employees without adequate credentials may be calling themselves exercise leaders or specialists, or even exercise physiologists. Some college- and university-based programs offer training in recreation management that qualifies individuals for employment at a fitness facility. Some instructors are trained in physical education, exercise physiology, or physical therapy, or are former athletes or nurses. Exercise instructors should have had some experience in teaching exercises, plus coursework that includes kinesiology (muscle functions), physiology of exercise, psychology, safety, and first aid. Where weight control advice is offered, personnel should have training in nutrition from a reputable institution. Table 14-7 on page 312 describes the credentials of the instructors who work at health clubs.

Many health clubs provide personal trainers (PTs) for individuals who lack information or are too busy to plan their own fitness regimens. Planning may include a medical history and tests for fitness, body fat, flexibility, blood pressure, and heart rate. When an exercise program is prescribed, the consumer is helped to implement it, either individually or in a small group. Some clubs provide this service at no cost, and its extent may be limited. Where extensive personal attention is desired, the cost of the service may be $40 to $100 per hour. Should a person desire a personal trainer, these suggestions should be followed:

• Ask for credentials
• Ask for references, talk with references, and watch a trainer helping a client
• Be sure to feel comfortable with the trainer
• Expect the first consultation to be free; discuss fitness status assessment and type, and implementation of program
• Ask about the cost and number of sessions needed to reach the fitness goal
• Be wary of any trainer who makes unrealistic promises regarding achievement of the fitness goal

Saunas

Saunas include portable contrivances and built-in rooms that emit steam or dry heat that raises body temperature, thereby causing profuse sweating. Saunas are located in homes, health clubs, and elsewhere. Traditionally popular in Finland, they have proliferated in Europe and the United States. Their popularity is undoubtedly related to people's interest in health and to benefits they expect from applying heat (and cold) to the body.

◆ **Personal Glimpse** ◆

Consumer Beware

In San Francisco a nonmember was invited to spend an evening at a health club. He was allowed and encouraged to use every machine available. After 2 hours he was taken to a small room and subjected to a high-pressure sales pitch, while another spa employee locked the door to the building and left. Reluctantly, the young man signed a $349 contract. He later learned that he had signed a bank draft for the full amount of the contract to be withdrawn immediately from his bank account. Fortunately, the consumer action office in the city was able to have the contract rescinded.

Sauna advertisements have claimed that saunas help reduce weight sensibly, clear acne and other skin blemishes, promote fitness, and cure arthritis and bursitis. Some weight is lost when people perspire, but it is quickly replaced when water or other fluids are consumed. Acne involves the oil-producing sebaceous glands, not the sweat glands (see Chapter 20). Sweating does not "cleanse" the sebaceous glands. Soap and water probably do as much for acne and blemished skin as the increased heat. There is no indication of how fitness improvement could take place. Some people may find that heat provides temporary relief of arthritis pain, but it is not curative.

Saunas are not recommended for people with heart or respiratory problems. There are several other dangers, including heat stroke caused by the body's absorption and storage of heat and by dehydration. The maximum exposure to a sauna should be 15 minutes.

Portable sauna devices may be purchased for $300 and up. It might cost $1500 to $3000 or more to build one in a home.

"Sauna shorts" (about $20) have been claimed to retain body heat, creating saunalike warmth that causes reduction of the underlying area. This claim is fraudulent.

Hot Tubs and Whirlpools

Hot tubs and whirlpools increase blood flow by increasing the circulation of blood to body parts, thereby helping heal some injury problems. They may also help to relax muscles and reduce tension. The usual 100° to 104°F temperature makes them unsuitable for use by people with high blood pressure and related heart problems.

A survey of state epidemiologists from 49 states identified 72 whirlpool-associated outbreaks caused by

Pseudomonas bacteria during a 10-year period. These resulted in papular or pustular rashes. Other symptoms included external otitis, mastitis, conjunctivitis, fevers, malaise, and headaches. The rashes lasted 4 to 14 days. Most of these outbreaks occurred in apartments, motels, and commercial spas. Two additional outbreaks resulted in legionnaires' disease. The risk factors associated with these illnesses are not clear. However, it is believed they were related to the quantity of bacteria in the water, the type of spa construction (concrete, tile, wood, fiberglass, and types of filters), and the type and method of disinfection. It is important that the hot water in these tubs and whirlpools be disinfected adequately, including the periodic addition of an extra disinfectant agent.

Hot tubs, saunas, and whirlpools may be hazardous unless certain educational programs and environmental controls are provided. They are high-risk drowning sites for young children; Shinaberger and others[40] reported the deaths of 74 children under the age of 5 years. The causative factors included lack of supervision, neuromuscular disabilities, and entrapment by suction. To reduce the incidence of drowning, critical areas may need fencing, hard covers over them, and supervision. Press[41] noted that 158 adult deaths in hot tubs, saunas, and spas occurred from hyperthermia or drowning caused mainly by alcohol ingestion, heart disease, seizure disorders, and cocaine ingestion (alone or with alcohol). These authors recommended that people using these facilities shorten their time of exposure, lower the temperature, and adhere to the warning notices.

Home Equipment

There are several less costly alternatives to joining a health club. Local Y's have programs with membership fees around $300 yearly. Local schools and recreation centers may offer sports, exercise, and physical education programs. Another alternative is a home mini-gym. Expensive equipment is not required to achieve fitness. With some ingenuity, simple equipment can be assembled and many exercise activities can be performed. The equipment chosen can be selected according to one's goals and budget:

MINIMUM LEVEL. For less than $50 to $85—include a jump rope, $3 to $10; a sit-up bar to fit under any door, $15; a padded mat on which to perform calisthenics, $35; and a 16-pound adjustable-free dumbbell set, $15 to $25.

INTERMEDIATE LEVEL. For $250 or more—supplement the minimum-level equipment with a stationary bicycle, 100 pounds of weights with long and short bars, a weight bench with a leg lift, and a videotaped exercise program.

HIGH LEVEL. For $500 to $1000 or more—include a treadmill, ski-exerciser, stairclimber, or rowing machine for aerobic conditioning and a multipurpose machine for strength training.

Listening to music, watching television, or reading during activities can help prevent boredom. Additional motivation may be derived from the calisthenics and aerobics programs found on radio, television, and videotapes.

CHILDREN'S EXERCISE CENTERS

Some community centers, health clubs, and local Y's operate exercise centers for children. Parents and others considering their use should raise certain questions:

- Are the facilities appropriate to replace free or partially free programs provided by schools, community centers, religious institutions, recreation and parks programs, and others?
- Are they meant to augment such programs?
- Are they necessary?
- What are the benefits and hazards?
- Who determines the risks involved in use of the equipment and participation in the programs?
- Are they too advanced for some children?
- Are children being pushed into regimented and possibly harmful programs during their growth and development stages in life?
- Has the equipment been constructed with children's safety in mind?

The American Academy of Pediatrics has concluded that formal exercise programs are not necessary for normal childhood development. It has also cautioned that children and adolescents should avoid weightlifting, power lifting, and bodybuilding until they are physically mature.[42] Cook and Leit state:

Owing to an increase in children participating in competitive organized sports, there is a real concern for the health and well-being of the individual pediatric athlete. . . . Children are not small adults. They not only have a different physiologic response to exercise, but also have many cartilaginous growth areas that are susceptible to injury. Appropriate training in the pediatric athlete will help prevent injury. Conservative training programs, completed in a well-ventilated and air-conditioned area, are important. In the prepubescent, efforts should be made to make training fun, with emphasis placed on skills important to the sport rather than monotonous repetitions and intensive conditioning.[43]

EXERCISE WHILE TRAVELING

Many exercise opportunities are available to travelers. It may be advisable to plan ahead to take advantage of them. Many hotels have health clubs with equipment, a swimming pool, and/or a sauna. Local health clubs, aerobic dance clubs, or Y's are listed in telephone directories. There may also be public or private facilities for tennis, golf, racquetball, and other sports. Walking, jogging, and stairclimbing can be done without special equipment or facilities.

A set of dumbbells, which can be inflated with water, and a jump rope can be carried easily in a suitcase. If an audiotape containing music is included, a self-devised program can easily be arranged. Early morning exercise programs are available on television.

When traveling by plane, bus, or train, isometric exercise while sitting will provide limited muscle activity. Periodic standing, stretching, or walking exercises can also be managed. When traveling by car, occasional stops to walk or to stretch the various muscle groups can be beneficial.

CORPORATE FITNESS PROGRAMS

Most American corporations with 50 or more employees offer some kind of health and fitness program. Some have elaborate facilities that include a swimming pool, track, sauna, and a testing laboratory supervised by an exercise physiologist, whereas others make an area available for aerobic exercises. Some programs are run through a local Y or other community organization, whereas others have cooperative arrangements with shared facilities and consultants.

Although most programs focus on employee fitness, many have adopted a wellness program that includes weight loss and stress management instruction. In addition, there may be medical screenings, exercise testing, back care, and health education about nutrition, drug abuse, alcoholism, and smoking cessation.

The effectiveness of these programs has been demonstrated by decreased absenteeism and by savings of $1.50 to $2 per $1 invested. A 10-year program conducted by Kimberly-Clark included medical screening, exercise testing, health education, and physical fitness. Many participants increased their fitness level and reduced their weight, body fat content, serum triglyceride level, and systolic and diastolic blood pressure. These results were also reported: 70% fewer accidents, 43% less absenteeism, 76% improvement in job performance, and 76% of those in the program overcame their dependency on drugs and alcohol.

The National Aeronautics and Space Administration (NASA), with the U.S. Public Health Service, conducted a study of 259 employees, ages 35 to 55, who participated in a 1-year, 3-times-per-week exercise program. Half the participants reported better job performance and better attitude toward work, almost all said they felt better, 89% reported improved stamina, 40% said they slept better, 60% lost weight, and absenteeism was reduced by approximately 4 days per year per employee.

EXERCISE AND WEIGHT CONTROL

The American Dietetic Association[44] makes these recommendations to the general public about nutrition and physical fitness:

- A nutritionally adequate diet and exercise are major contributing factors to physical fitness and health.
- Weight maintenance and weight loss can be achieved by a combination of dietary modification, change in eating behavior, and regular aerobic exercise.
- Generally healthy individuals consuming a diet that supplies the Recommended Dietary Allowances receive all the nutrients needed for a physical conditioning program.
- The intensity, duration, and frequency of exercise should be determined according to the individual's age, physical condition, and health status.
- Habits for a nutritionally balanced diet and physical fitness should be established during childhood and maintained throughout life.
- Nothing done to the body from the outside—heating, steaming, pummeling, pounding, or jerking or jiggling by a machine—can make people lose weight.

To lose 1 pound of fat it is necessary to metabolize about 3500 more calories than are taken in. The weight-loss process can be speeded up by reducing daily food intake or increasing the number of calories burned. For example, deleting 100 calories of food daily from the regular amount ingested will enable a person to lose 1 pound after 35 days (see Table 13-3, page 275). Increasing activity to burn an additional 100 calories daily will also achieve the same results. Someone who walks for 30 minutes daily (7.1 calories per minute) will burn 213 calories. If caloric intake is not increased, about 2 pounds will be lost per month. A recent study found that the amount of fat loss is determined by the total calories expended in exercise rather than its intensity.[45] Note, however, that exercise is more important for maintaining a healthy weight than for losing weight per se.

NUTRITION FOR ATHLETES

The American Dietetic Association stated that a proper, well-balanced diet is an essential component of any fitness or sports program.[45] A good mix would contain 50% to 60% carbohydrates, 20% to 30% fat, and 15% to 20%

Table 14-9

EXERCISE MYTHS AND FACTS[46]

Myth	Facts
No pain, no gain.	Health benefits are achievable by exercising as little as 15 minutes, 3 times weekly; almost any activity has benefits. Some soreness is inevitable with programs that produce high levels of fitness, but this does not justify pain from overuse of pushing oneself too hard.
Muscle will turn into fat if you stop exercising.	Muscles grow weaker and become smaller through disuse, but they do not turn into fat.
Vitamin supplements provide extra energy.	Vitamins do not provide energy; they help regulate body processes and are readily obtainable from food.
Drinking liquids during exercise causes cramps.	Cool drinks of water are advisable during and after exercise to replace lost fluids.
Excess weight can be sweated off.	Perspiration sheds fluid, not fat; the weight lost due to perspiration is quickly regained when the body is rehydrated.
Extra protein helps build stronger muscles.	Excess protein is stored as fat; muscle-building comes through "resistance" exercising such as lifting weights.
Exercise can backfire for someone trying to lose weight, because it increases appetite and thereby leads to overeating.	Moderate exercise does not increase appetite. It mobilizes stored glycogen and decreases hunger. Only extended physical activity increases appetite.
Sugary foods eaten before or during a workout supply quick energy.	Foods eaten just before exercise mobilize the glycogen-storing mechanism of insulin, thus reducing blood glucose and temporarily impairing performance.
Spot-reducing causes more fat to be lost from that area than from the rest of the body.	Fat lost generally comes from deposits throughout the body. There is no such thing as "spot-reducing."
"Sports drinks" are the best kind of fluids for exercisers.	The best beverage is plain water. If electrolytes are lost, they can be replaced by eating food. In extremely warm weather a bit of salt should be added to the water. Many sports drinks contain salt but are needlessly costly. Ingesting salt without water increases dehydration.
Women who participate in strength-training develop oversized muscles.	Muscle strength is increased, but not necessarily size; male hormones are the reason that men are more prone to muscle enlargement.
To exercise effectively, people have to be athletic.	Most physical activities require no athletic skills. Walking provides a perfect example of this fact.
Exercise makes people tired.	Most people feel more energetic as they become more fit.

protein. Buskirk[47] states that there is little reason for the dietary pattern of a physically active person diet to differ from what is good for other healthy persons.

The energy needs of people who engage in vigorous activity range from 3000 to 6000 calories per day or more. Complex carbohydrates should compose 50% to 55% or more of their diet. A diet too low in carbohydrates prior to strenuous exercise can cause fatigue. The pregame meal should be completed $3\frac{1}{2}$ to 4 hours before competing and should be high in complex carbohydrates. Fats and proteins, which require more time for digestion, should be avoided to prevent stomach upsets or indigestion that will affect performance.

Carbohydrate loading is a regimen that combines high-carbohydrate eating with gradual tapering of exercise activity. Used to temporarily increase the amount of muscle glycogen, it is beneficial only to participants in lengthy endurance or multiple-event competitions.

Endurance athletes may need to increase their protein intake above the RDA of 0.8 per kg (54 g for a 150-pound man). The *Tufts University Diet & Nutrition Letter* stated that protein intake should be 95 g for a 150-pound man, but notes that "most athletes eat more food than nonathletes, so their higher protein needs are met automatically."[48]

Above-RDA amounts of vitamins and minerals may be needed by people who exercise vigorously, but they too will be supplied in a balanced diet containing extra calories. Thus vitamin, mineral, and protein supplementation are unwarranted for people who eat properly.

Energy Bars

Sports bars, which cost $1.25 to $2.50, contain between 100 and 300 calories, mostly from carbohydrates. Sports nutritionist Nancy Clark, R.D., states that people who exercise at an intensity that can be maintained for more than 30 minutes may benefit from consuming up to 400 calories plus 8 to 16 ounces of water before or during such exercise. She points out, however, that the same result can be achieved less expensively by eating standard foods such as bagels, bananas, or raisins.[49]

Sports Drinks

Americans spend close to $1 billion a year on sports drinks such as *Gatorade, Exceed*, and *Quickick*, with the belief that the calories and minerals they contain will help with fatigue and dehydration. Proper hydration is essential for athletic performance. Extreme exercise levels, prolonged strenuous activity, and certain environmental conditions may warrant a low-dose electrolyte-replacement beverage during endurance competition.[50] However, cool water can be used to meet the needs of most people who exercise in moderate climates. *Consumer Reports* has noted:

- For most people, sports drinks are no better than water.
- Sugars in the drinks are supposed to maintain high levels of blood sugar to prevent fatigue; however, it takes $1\frac{1}{2}$ hours of strenuous exercise to deplete energy resources.
- Deliberate replacement of lost electrolytes (primarily sodium) is not necessary for moderate exercise if a person has a normal diet. In very hot weather a pinch of salt added to meals for a few days will adequately provide for body needs.
- These drinks may taste good and cause more to be ingested than needed.
- People running marathons or involved in intense exercise for hours may benefit from a sports drink to bolster sugar levels and replace electrolytes.[51]

ANABOLIC STEROIDS

Anabolism is the phase of metabolism in which the complex materials of the body are built up from smaller simpler compounds (e.g., proteins from amino acids). Anabolic androgenic steroids are male hormones, available by prescription, that have legitimate medical uses for certain types of anemias, hereditary angioedema, protein anabolism, and certain gynecologic conditions. They are also useful as an adjunct to growth hormone therapy and for treating osteoporosis.

The use of steroids has been widespread among weightlifters, shotputters, discus throwers, football players, and participants in other sports where strength is required. Use has also been associated with endurance sports such as Nordic skiing, cycling, and distance running. Steroids have been used by both professional and collegiate athletes. Data from a 1991 survey indicated that more than 1 million Americans had abused steroids, with a median starting age of 18. The study also found that for 12- to 17-year-olds, the median starting age was 15.[52] The doses used by athletes are generally much higher than those used for medical purposes. Many steroid abusers achieve high dosage by combining several different brands, a practice called "stacking."

Steroids are obtained illegally from physicians who prescribe them knowing that they will be used by athletes and from drug dealers and other illicit nonmedical channels. The FDA has estimated that annual sales of anabolic steroids for nonmedical reasons exceed $100 million.[53] These drugs originate mainly from underground laboratories and foreign sources. The federal Anti-Drug Abuse Act of 1988 increased the penalties for those who distribute steroids or have steroids in their possession with the intent to distribute them. The Act increases fines and authorizes jail sentences of up to 6 years for convicted dealers.

The AMA Council on Scientific Affairs has reported that steroid studies show that muscle size and strength can be increased when the drug is used by those who are already training intensively and who combine this activity with a high-protein and high-calorie diet.[54] Body weight is also increased, although much is due to fluid retention. Steroids can increase energy and the ability to train more intensely with a shortened recovery period, allowing more frequent training. Many athletes report that large doses result in euphoria, lack of fatigue, greater self-confidence, and enhanced appearance. However, adverse effects include acne, genital changes, jaundice, stunted growth, sterility, liver tumors, abdominal pains, diarrhea, muscle cramps, headache, bone pains, depression, breast development in men, gallstones, high blood pressure, coronary heart disease, and kidney disease. Women who abuse steroids can develop menstrual irregularities, permanent enlargement of the

---

◆ Personal Glimpse ◆

A Steroid Disaster

A 23-year-old bodybuilder, complaining of severe groin pains, was taken to the hospital. Doctors found his liver and kidneys had stopped working. He was immediately rushed to the intensive-care unit. Four days later, he died when his heart stopped. An autopsy revealed that he was a steroid user.

Table 14-10

PERCENTAGES OF 72 CURRRENT AND FORMER STEROID USERS WHO KNEW ABOUT VARIOUS STEROID-RELATED PROBLEMS*[58]

Problem	% Who Knew
Liver disease	71
Heart disease	56
Cancer	50
Shrinking of the testicles	49
Adverse personality changes	49
Death	45
Sterility	44
Kidney disease	38
Blood pressure problems	38
Stunted growth	36

*Respondents were allowed more than one response.

clitoris, lowered voice pitch, facial hair, increased body hair, decreased breast size, and male-pattern baldness. Taken before puberty, anabolic steroids can stop bone growth and cause permanent stunting of growth. Steroid use may cause aggressive behavior in previously non-aggressive men and women or increase aggressiveness in those who tend toward aggression.

Some studies suggest that steroid use is often addictive.[55,56] The characteristic signs include craving for the substance, use of larger doses, more frequent use, inability to stop, and withdrawal symptoms. A controlled 2-week study done with 20 volunteers found that steroid administration caused distractibility, irritability, decreased energy level, insomnia, and fatigue.[57]

A Department of Health and Human Services survey of 72 current and former steroid users who began their use before age 19 found that most were aware of health problems associated with steroid use (Table 14-10). Yet many of the current users said they discounted these possibilities because: (a) they were not experiencing problems, (b) they knew others who had experienced no problems, (c) "hard" evidence was lacking, (d) they regarded the warnings as scare tactics, and/or (e) experts had been wrong in the past.[58]

Mishra[53] has warned:

Although it may be true that in combination with intensive weight training and a high-calorie, high-protein diet, steroids can augment short-term muscle gain, teens need to ask themselves: Is it worth all the short-term health effects and the possibility of long-term permanent damage? Is it worth the disgrace of being eliminated from competition, or even of being arrested?

The AMA Council on Scientific Affairs has made these recommendations:

- The nonmedical use of steroids by athletes to enhance or sustain athletic performance is inappropriate and should be discontinued.
- Dealers and distributors of anabolic steroids used for nonmedical purposes should be punished severely.
- Further research should be done on the short-term and long-term health effects of steroids.[54]

OTHER "ERGOGENIC AIDS"

Many companies are marketing concoctions of vitamins, minerals, amino acids, and other ingredients with false claims that they can increase stamina and endurance and help build stronger muscles. Many of these products are touted as "natural steroids" or "growth-hormone releasers," which they are not. Very high doses of certain amino acids have been reported to influence hormone production in laboratory animals. But no such effect from low-dose pills has been demonstrated in humans. Ads for these products typically contain an endorsement from a champion athlete or bodybuilder who attributes success to the products. Some ads contain explicit claims, while others rely on images to convey their message (see Figure 14-3 on page 328). Some of the products are also marketed as weight-loss aids (see Chapter 13). Gamma hydroxybutyrate (GHB) and clenbuterol—both of which can be deadly—have also been marketed as "steroid alternatives." (See Personal Glimpse Box on page 7.)

In 1991 researchers from the U.S. Centers for Disease Control and Prevention surveyed 12 popular health and bodybuilding magazines (one issue each) and found ads for 89 brands and 311 products with a total of 235 unique ingredients. The most frequent ingredients were amino acids and herbs. Among the 221 products for which an effect was claimed, 59 were said to produce

☑ Consumer Tip

Breathing Oxygen

Breathing oxygen before running, swimming, or cycling cannot improve sprint performance. At rest, blood leaving the lungs is nearly saturated with oxygen. Breathing pure oxygen can slightly raise the arterial oxygen level. By the time the athlete moves to the starting point and the race begins, however, body oxygen stores return to normal. Thus there is no physiologic advantage.

Faddist Underpinnings[59]

Bernarr Macfadden (1868–1955), an early proponent of exercise, advocated a variety of strange practices as well. During his youth he supposedly was sickly and unable to walk. At age 15 he discovered the gymnasium and began developing his body. He had little exposure to school before working as a physical education instructor at a school in Illinois.

Macfadden launched *Physical Culture* magazine in 1899 and developed a publishing empire that made him a multimillionaire. Concern for physical culture was timely, since there was a growing distrust of patent medicines and the health-reform movement advocated a simpler, more natural form of hygiene. Macfadden believed he had learned the true secrets of health without using scientific investigation. He advocated strenuous repetitive exercises. He concluded that health problems could be resolved by eating less and by fasting, which would give the body more time for repairs. For cancer he recommended fasting for a few days and a diet consisting of large quantities of grapes. His publishing ventures included health handbooks, romance and detective magazines, and sensationalist tabloids. Macfadden Holdings, Inc., his corporate descendant, now publishes the *National Enquirer, Weekly World News, True Romance,* and several other monthly magazines.

Interest in bodybuilding probably evolved from the strong-man vaudeville acts of the 19th century. Bob Hoffman (1899–1985) and Joe Weider (b. 1923) can be considered the chief modern popularizers. Hoffman, a prominent oarsman and weightlifter, served for 32 years as the Olympic weightlifting coach and helped found the President's Council on Physical Fitness and Sports. Weider helped found the International Federation of Bodybuilders, which promotes the sport worldwide and sponsors competitions. Both made fortunes publishing magazines and selling exercise equipment and supplement products. Both played a substantial role in spreading misinformation about protein supplements and other "ergogenic aids." In articles and ads, they falsely asserted that athletes have special protein needs, that protein supplements have special muscle-building and health-giving powers, and that the most efficient way to get enough protein is by using supplements.

In 1960 Hoffman's York Barbell Company was charged with falsely claiming that its wheat germ oil could prevent or treat more than 120 diseases and conditions, including epilepsy, gallstones, and arthritis. A supply seized by the FDA was destroyed by consent decree. In 1961 15 other York Barbell products were seized as misbranded. Additional regulatory actions took place in 1968, 1972, and 1974.

In 1984 the FTC charged that ads for two of Weider's amino-acid products had been misleading. The case was settled in 1985 when Weider and his company agreed not to falsely claim that these products can help build muscles or are effective substitutes for anabolic steroids. They also agreed to pay a penalty of at least $400,000 in refunds or for research on the relationship of nutrition to muscle development.

Although the claims forbidden by the FTC order no longer appear in Weider ads, similar messages appear in articles in his *Muscle & Fitness* magazine and are implied by endorsements and pictures of muscular athletes. Hoffman's *Muscular Development* magazine, which has a similar structure, is now published by a subsidiary of another supplement company.

---

muscle growth, 27 were said to increase testosterone levels, 17 were said to enhance energy, 15 were said to reduce fat, and 12 were said to increase strength.[60]

Barron and Vanscoy[61] evaluated many claims of this type made for 19 "natural" substances in bodybuilding magazine ads, in fact sheets for health-food retailers, and on product labels. After reviewing the scientific literature, the authors concluded: (a) muscle-building claims for Argentinean bull testes, boron, cyclofinil, dicobenzide, gamma oryzanol, *Menispermum conadense*, plant sterols (diosgenin, smilagenin, hecogenin), and saw palmetto berries were unfounded; (b) certain claims for chromium picolinate, clenbuterol, guarana, inosine, kola nut, and ma huang have scientific support, but products containing these substances are marketed in a misleading manner; (c) claims that yohimbe bark is an anabolic agent are supported by studies in animals but not humans; and (d) claims for arginine/ornithine, carnitine, and *Gymnema sylvestre* have some scientific support, but these substances have not been proven effective.

In 1992 the New York City Department of Consumer Affairs[62] warned consumers to beware of products advertised with terms like "fat burner," "fat fighter," "fat metabolizer," "energy enhancer," "performance booster," "strength booster," "ergogenic aid," "anabolic optimizer," and "genetic optimizer." Manufacturers surveyed by the department were unable to provide a single published report from a scientific journal to back the claims that their products did any of these things. City officials calculated that a supplement program recommended in the leading bodybuilding magazine (*Muscle & Fitness*) would cost more than $11 per day. Calling the bodybuilding supplement industry "an economic hoax with unhealthy consequences," they issued "Notices of Violation" to six companies and challenged federal agencies to stop the "blatantly drug-like claims" and false advertising used to promote these products. The FTC subsequently took action against General Nutrition (see Chapter 12).

During the past decade, David Lightsey, an exercise physiologist and nutritionist who coordinates the National Council Against Health Fraud's Task Force on Ergogenic Aids, has requested written documentation from more than 80 companies that market "ergogenic aids." Fewer than half sent anything, and the rest submitted studies that were poorly designed or did not actually support product claims. Lightsey also checked statements that various teams were using certain products and found the management had neither endorsed the products nor encouraged their use.[63] Lightsey believes there are two reasons why many athletes believe that various products have helped them: (1) use of the product often coincides with natural improvement due to training and (2) increased self-confidence or a placebo effect inspires greater performance. Any such "psychologic benefit," however, should be weighed against the dangers of misinformation, wasted money, misplaced faith, and adverse physical effects—both known and unknown—that can result from megadoses of nutrients.

Lulinski has noted that creatine has some potential for helping to build muscle mass, research is conflicting, side effects are common, and long-range safety and effectiveness have not been demonstrated.[64] Williams has pointed out that if any of the "dietary supplements" marketed as ergogenic aids were proven to be effective, their use by competitive athletes might be considered unethical.[65]

SUMMARY

Regular exercise can increase strength, endurance, flexibility, motor fitness, and cardiorespiratory efficiency. It can also lower blood pressure, improve blood cholesterol levels, help with weight control, help lower abnormal blood sugar levels, reduce stress, improve sleep, help prevent osteoporosis, and increase longevity. The risks of injury are greater for sedentary individuals and those who thrust themselves into activities that are either too strenuous or too prolonged.

Exercises can be classified as aerobic, anaerobic, isometric, isotonic, and isokinetic. The type and amount should be adapted to the age and fitness level of the individual. A minimum program to achieve cardiores-

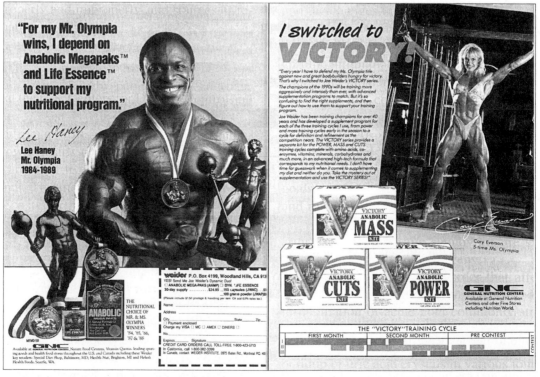

FIGURE 14-3. Ads from the leading bodybuilding magazine *(Muscle & Fitness).* Although these ads make no explicit claims, they falsely imply that the products were the key to success.

It's Your Decision

1. You have never been involved in aerobic exercise, but you now believe you can improve your health through such participation. Which of the following would you do?

   Reason

   ☐ Enroll in a local exercise center or club   _____
   ☐ Purchase an exercycle or rowing machine   _____
   ☐ Decide what you want to achieve from your exercise   _____
   ☐ Buy a book on aerobics written by an expert   _____
   ☐ Check exercise programs at the local "Y"   _____
   ☐ Start jogging/walking 2–3 miles daily   _____
   ☐ Visit your family physician for a physical examination   _____

2. You have been involved in an exercise program and want to assess whether it is the best program for you. How would you do this? Is there anyone you would seek out for help?

3. You wish to lose 10–20 pounds and believe this goal can be achieved through exercise. What type of program should you follow? Where can you find help with this decision?

piratory fitness should be 20 to 30 minutes, 3 days a week, at 60% to 90% of one's maximum heart rate.

Exercise equipment should be selected by considering potential benefits, effects on body areas, costs, and personal suitability. Advertising claims should be regarded skeptically because many devices have little or no value.

Health clubs and fitness centers are popular because they provide equipment and the opportunity for social interaction and a structured program. Prospective members should carefully scrutinize advertisements and contracts from these centers. Fitness can be usually achieved at home with less equipment and less expense. It also is possible to maintain an exercise regimen while traveling. Children's centers have been established, although their value is questionable.

Weight loss can be achieved only through a combination of dietary changes, eating behavior changes, and regular aerobic exercise. Sports drinks and energy bars can be useful, but cool water and common carbohydrate foods can provide the same benefits at much lower cost.

The use of anabolic steroids by athletes is dangerous. Protein supplements and concoctions of vitamins, minerals, and/or low doses of amino acids convey no athletic benefits and are a waste of money for people who eat properly.

REFERENCES

1. Exercising your options. Consumer Reports on Health 1:17, 19–20, 1989.
2. Health clubs: The right choice for you? Consumer Reports 61:27–30, 1996.
3. Lloyd GER, editor. Hippocratic Writings. New York, 1978, Penguin Books.
4. Spunt G: When Nature Speaks: The Life of Forrest C Shaklee, Sr., New York, 1977, Frederick Fell Publishers. (Marketed by the Shaklee Corporation to its distributors.)
5. Ullyot J. Exercise and coronary disease. Healthline 3(10):1–2, 1984.
6. Maron BJ. Sudden death in young competitive athletes: Clinical, demographic, and pathological profiles. JAMA 276:199–204, 1996.
7. Fletcher GF and others. A statement for health professionals by the Committee on Exercise and Cardiac Rehabilitation of the Council on Clinical Cardiology, American Heart Association. Circulation 94:857–862, 1996.
8. Blair SN and others. Changes in physical fitness and all-cause mortality: A prospective study of healthy and unhealthy men. JAMA 273:1093–1098, 1995.
9. Coronary heart disease attributable to sedentary lifestyle— selected states. MMWR 39:541–544, 1990.
10. Slattery ML and others. Leisure time physical activity and coronary heart disease death: The US Railroad Study. Circulation 79:304–311, 1989.
11. Lee IM, Paffenbarger RS Jr. Associations of light, moderate, and vigorous intensity physical activity with longevity. The Harvard Alumni Health Study. American Journal of Epidemiology 151:293–299, 2000.
12. Hu FB and others. Physical activity and the risk of stroke in women. JAMA 283:2961–2967, 2000.
13. Pollock ML and others. ACSM position stand on the recommended quantity and quality of exercise for developing and maintaining cardiorespiratory and muscular fitness, and flexibility in healthy adults. Medicine and Science in Sports and Exercise 30:875–991, 1998.
14. Pate RR and others. Physical activity and public health. A recommendation from the US Centers for Disease Control and Prevention and the American College of Sports Medicine. JAMA 273:402–407, 1995.
15. NIH Consensus Development Panel on Physical Activity and Cardiovascular Health. Physical activity and cardiovascular health. JAMA 276:241–246, 1996.

16. Physical Activity and Health: A Report of the Surgeon General. Washington, D.C., 1996, Superintendent of Documents.

17. Fletcher GF and others. Statement on exercise: Benefits and recommendations for physical activity for all Americans. Circulation 94:857–862, 1996.

18. Fletcher GF and others. Exercise standards: A statement for healthcare professionals from the American Heart Association. Circulation 91:580–615, 1995.

19. Kenney WL. ACSM Fitness Book, 2nd edition. Champaign, Ill., 1997, Human Kinetics Press.

20. Blair SN. Living with Exercise. Dallas, 1991, American Health Publishing Co.

21. Jones JJ and others. Managing sports-related overuse injuries. Patient Care 30:(7):55–71, 1996.

22. Choosing a sports medicine physician. Penn State Sports Medicine Newsletter 3(12):1–2, 1995.

23. Athletic trainers: First line of defense. Penn State Sports Medicine Newsletter 4(4):6–7, 1995.

24. Workouts that work. Consumer Reports 64(2):31–39, 1999.

25. Burroughs B. Allure of home exercise devices sparks big sales—and many injuries. The Wall Street Journal, p 33, April 18, 1985.

26. Exercise bikes: Good workout, good value. Consumer Reports 61:18–21, 1996.

27. Ski machines: How close to the real thing? Consumer Reports 59:587, 1994.

28. Zeni AI and others. Energy expenditure with indoor exercise machines. JAMA 275:1424–1427, 1996.

29. Wild rides . . . or tame, there are bikes that fill the bill. Consumer Reports 64(6):38–41, 1999.

30. Head cases: We checked fit, venting, and adherence to a new safety standard. Consumer Reports 64(6):42–44, 1999.

31. Health & fitness equipment buying guide. Consumers Digest 34(5):33–48, 1995.

32. Wichmann S, Martin DR. Athletic shoes: Finding the right fit. The Physician and Sportsmedicine 21:204–211, 1993.

33. Think before you run: Buy shoes that match how your feet hit the street. Consumer Reports 64:23–27, 1998.

34. Hunger LY, Torgan C. The bra controversy: are sports bras a necessity? Physician and Sports Medicine 10(11):75–76, 1982.

35. Gauthier MM. Continuous passive motion: The no-exercise exercise. Physician and Sports Medicine 15(8):142–148, 1987.

36. LeMarr JD and others. Cardiorespiratory responses to inversion. The Physician and Sportsmedicine 11(11):51–57, 1983.

37. "A flat, sexy stomach in 5 minutes flat!" (Yeah, right!). Tufts University Diet & Nutrition Letter 14(6):6–7, 1996.

38. Miller RW. EMS: Fraudulent flab remover. FDA Consumer 17(4):29–32, 1983.

39. Health clubs: The right choice for you? Consumer Reports 61:27–30, 1996.

40. Shinaberger CS and others. Young children who drown in hot tubs, spas, and whirlpools in California: A 26-year survey. American Journal of Public Health 80:613–614, 1990.

41. Press E. The health hazards of saunas and spas and how to minimize them. American Journal of Public Health 81:1034–1037, 1991.

42. News release: AAP recommends children and adolescents avoid weight lifting until physically mature. Elk Grove Village, Ill., Jan 14, 1990, American Academy of Pediatrics.

43. Cook PC, Leit ME. Issues in the pediatric athlete. Orthopedic Clinics of North America 26:(3):453–464, 1995.

44. Position of the American Dietetic Association: Nutrition for physical fitness and athletic performance for adults. Journal of the American Dietetic Association 87:933–939, 1987.

45. Gredmagin MA and others. Exercise intensity does not affect body composition change in untrained, moderately overfat women. Journal of the American Dietetic Association 95:661–665, 1995.

46. Modified from The diet/exercise link: Separating fact from fiction. Tufts University Diet Nutrition Letter 6(12):3–5, 1989.

47. Buskirk ER. Exercise. In Ziegler EE, Filer LJ Jr, editors. Present Knowledge in Nutrition, ed 2. Washington, D.C., 1996, ILSI Press.

48. How much protein do athletes really need? Tufts University Diet & Nutrition Letter 5(8):1, 1987.

49. Energy Bars: Are these fast fuelers for you? The Physician and Sportsmedicine 23(9):7–8, 1995.

50. American College of Sports Medicine. Position stand on exercise and fluid replacement. Medicine and Science in Sports and Exercise 28(1):i–vii, 1996.

51. Does Gatorade beat water? Consumer Reports on Health 3:63, 1991.

52. Yesalis CE and others. Anabolic-androgenic steroid use in the United States. JAMA 270:1217–1221, 1993.

53. Mishra R: On the teen scene: Steroids and sports. FDA Consumer 25(7):25–27, 1991.

54. American Medical Association Council on Scientific Affairs. Medical and nonmedical uses of anabolic-androgenic steroids. JAMA 204:2923–2927, 1990.

55. Leary WE. Users of steroids risk addiction, two researchers at Yale report. New York Times, Dec 8, 1989.

56. Study shows addiction with anabolic steroids. FDA Consumer 25(10):6–7, 1991.

57. Su T-P and others. Neuropsychiatric effects of anabolic steroids in male normal volunteers. JAMA 269:2760–2764, 1993.

58. Teenagers blasé about steroid use. FDA Consumer 24(10):2, 1990.

59. Barrett S, Herbert V. The Vitamin Pushers: How the "Health Food" Industry Is Selling America a Bill of Goods. Amherst, N.Y., 1994, Prometheus Books.

60. Philan RM and others. Survey of advertising for nutritional supplements in health and bodybuilding magazines. JAMA 268:1008–1011, 1992.

61. Barron RL, Vanscoy GJ. Natural products and the athlete: Facts and folklore. Annals of Pharmacotherapy 27:607–615, 1993.

62. von Nostitz G and others. Magic muscle pills!! Health and fitness quackery in nutrition supplements. New York, 1992, New York City Department of Consumer Affairs.

63. Lightsey DM, Attaway JR. Deceptive tactics used in marketing purported ergogenic aids. National Strength and Conditioning Association Journal 14(2):26–32, 1991.

64. Lulinski B. Creatine supplementation. Quackwatch Web site, Sept 17, 1999.

65. Williams MH. The Ergogenics Edge. Champaign, Ill., 1998, Human Kinetics.

PART IV

MAJOR HEALTH PROBLEMS

Chapter Fifteen

CARDIOVASCULAR DISEASE

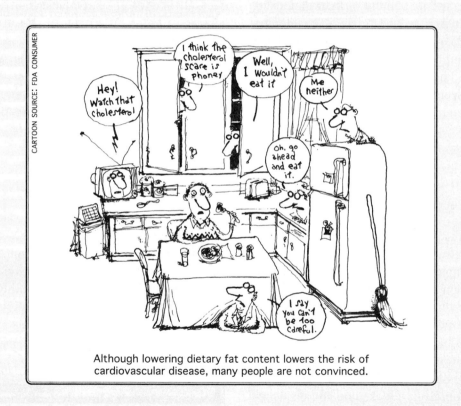

Although lowering dietary fat content lowers the risk of cardiovascular disease, many people are not convinced.

Medical scientists have made tremendous progress in fighting cardiovascular disease. Even so, every 33 seconds an American dies of CVD. . . . In fact, since 1900, the No. 1 killer in the United States has been CVD in every year but one (1918).

AMERICAN HEART ASSOCIATION[1]

Key Concepts
KEEP THESE POINTS IN MIND AS YOU STUDY THIS CHAPTER

- The more risk factors a person has, the greater the risk of developing cardiovascular disease. Heredity, gender, and age cannot be controlled, but the other risk factors can be influenced by the individual's behavior.

- Risk-factor modification can have a significant impact on both the length and the quality of many people's life.

- The prevailing medical view is that all adults should have their blood cholesterol and blood pressure checked and take action if abnormalities are found.

- The cornerstone of a cholesterol reduction program is a balanced, low-fat, high-fiber diet plus regular aerobic exercise.

In recent years few health-related matters have received as much public attention as the relationships between diet, blood cholesterol levels, and heart disease. Consumers are being urged to know their cholesterol numbers, lower the fat content of their diet, exercise, and take other steps to reduce the risk of developing heart disease. The data supporting some of this advice are voluminous, complex, incomplete, and sometimes confusing. Yet, based on these data, individuals are being urged to make decisions that may affect the length and quality of their life. The information in this chapter should help you make intelligent decisions based on the latest available research findings. Most of the research on prevention of heart attacks has been done in men, but there is no reason to believe that the findings do not apply equally to women.

Cardiovascular disease is also an area of explosive technologic development in both diagnostic and treatment procedures. As a result, increasing numbers of people will face complex decisions that can affect both their survival and their pocketbook.

This chapter covers the causes, risk factors, and management of the two most prevalent diseases that affect the heart and blood vessels, with emphasis on strategies for prevention and treatment. The main topic is coronary heart disease, but high blood pressure, which can play a role in both heart attacks and strokes, is included because it involves some of the same considerations. Less common types of heart problems, such as rheumatic heart disease, congenital heart disease, and infections of the heart, are not discussed in this book.

SIGNIFICANCE OF CARDIOVASCULAR DISEASE

Cardiovascular diseases (problems affecting the heart and blood vessels) are the leading cause of illness and death for both men and women in the United States. The American Heart Association estimates that the total cost of treating heart attacks, strokes, and other forms of heart disease in 2000 was \$185.8 billion.[1] About 41% of the deaths in this country are attributable to cardiovascular disease. The majority stem from atherosclerosis.

Before menopause, women tend to have lower blood pressure and fewer heart attacks than do men of equivalent age. (Female hormones exert a protective effect against heart attacks.) After menopause, the rates among women are higher than those of men and increase with advancing age.[2] The American Heart Association[1] estimates that in 1997, 59.7 million Americans had one or more forms of cardiovascular disease. Table 15-1 indicates the prevalence and mortality of the most common types.

RISK FACTORS FOR CORONARY HEART DISEASE

In coronary heart disease (CHD) the arteries to the heart muscle (myocardium) are narrowed. CHD is caused by *atherosclerosis*, a condition in which fibrous tissue infiltrates from the muscular inner layer of the artery due to repeated injury to the delicate lining of the coronary arteries. These fibrous tissue formations, called plaques or atheromas (*-oma* = "tumor"), also incorporate fats,

---

Table 15-1
PREVALENCE OF CARDIOVASCULAR DISEASE (1997 ESTIMATES)

Condition	Prevalence*	# Deaths
High blood pressure	50,000,000	42,565
Coronary heart disease	12,200,000	466,101
Stroke	4,400,000	159,791
Rheumatic heart disease	1,800,000	5,014
Congenital defects	1,000,000	6,800

*Some individuals have more than one of the above conditions.
Source: American Heart Association.[1]

cholesterol, and eventually calcium. These plaques build up on the walls of large and medium-sized arteries. As atherosclerosis progresses, the coronary arteries can narrow and make it difficult for oxygen-rich blood and nutrients to reach the heart muscle. Although atheromas can be reduced by various means, their fibrous structure makes them resistant to anything short of mechanical or surgical intervention—or possibly an intensive cholesterol-lowering program.

Reduced blood supply to the heart can result in chest pain (angina pectoris) or other symptoms, typically triggered by physical exertion. If a narrowed blood vessel is completely blocked by a blood clot, the area of the heart just beyond the blockage is denied oxygen and nourishment, resulting in a heart attack (myocardial infarction). The situation is often complicated by the development of an irregular heart rhythm (arrhythmia) and/or heart failure, in which the heart's ability to pump blood is inadequate to meet the body's needs.

Like other degenerative disease processes, atherosclerosis can take years to develop. Diet is implicated because the deposits on arterial walls contain high levels of fat and cholesterol. Studies of both humans and animals have shown links between dietary habits and atherosclerosis.

At least 10 risk factors can help predict the likelihood of CHD: heredity, being male, advancing age, cigarette smoking, high blood pressure, diabetes, obesity (especially excess abdominal fat), lack of physical activity, and abnormal blood cholesterol and homocysteine levels. The more risk factors a person has, the greater the likelihood of developing heart disease. Heredity, gender, and age cannot be modified, but the others can be influenced by the individual's behavior.

Several of these risk factors are interrelated. Obesity, lack of exercise, and cigarette smoking can raise blood pressure and adversely influence blood cholesterol levels. Several studies suggest that exposure to environmental tobacco smoke ("passive smoking") also increases the risk of developing heart disease.[3] Some authorities believe that emotional stress is a risk factor, but the evidence for this is not clear-cut. A 10-year study of 85,000 women has found that coffee consumption had no effect on the incidence of coronary heart disease in women.[4]

The relationship of blood triglyceride levels to cardiovascular disease is unclear, but recent studies suggest that triglyceride levels of 200 mg/dL or more may be an independent risk factor for coronary heart disease.[5] Regardless, very high levels (over 500 mg/dL) should be treated because this can cause other problems, such as pancreatitis.

The Multiple Risk Factor Intervention Trial (MRFIT), funded by the National Institutes of Health, explored whether an intensive educational program could lower the death rate for heart disease. The study involved 12,866 men, aged 35 to 57 years, whose levels of cigarette smoking, blood cholesterol, blood pressure, or a combination of these factors placed them at high risk for heart disease. After careful evaluation, the men were randomly assigned either to a special intervention program or to their usual sources of health care. After 10 years the intervention group experienced 10.6% fewer heart attacks and had a 7.7% lower overall death rate.[6] Both groups smoked less and had lower blood cholesterol levels, but the improvement was greater in the intervention group.

The age-adjusted death rates due to coronary artery disease and stroke have fallen steadily for more than 20 years. This is due to advances in diagnosis and treatment as well as lifestyle changes that lower the risk for the disease.

Figure 15-1 can help you evaluate your risk of developing coronary heart disease.

BLOOD LIPID AND HOMOCYSTEINE LEVELS

Lipid is the general term for fatty substances, including triglycerides (fats and oils), phospholipids (such as lecithin), and sterols (including cholesterol). In common usage, fats are lipids that are solid at room temperature, whereas oils are lipids that are liquid at room temperature. (See Chapter 11 for discussion of the types of fat found in foods.) *Blood lipids* is a term used to describe the fatty substances circulating within the bloodstream.

Cholesterol is found only in foods of animal origin and is part of every animal cell. It is essential to life, because the body uses cholesterol to make cell membranes, hormones, and bile acids, as well as for other functions. Most of the cholesterol the body uses is manufactured within the body, mainly within the liver. When dietary cholesterol intake is high, the liver tends to compensate by lowering cholesterol production.

Because cholesterol is a fatlike substance and cannot mix with water, the body transports it in protein-containing packages that can flow smoothly throughout the bloodstream. These packages, called lipoproteins, are composed of various amounts of cholesterol, triglycerides (fats), phospholipids, and other special proteins.

Serum lipoproteins are classified according to density. The three main cholesterol-protein combinations are high-density lipoproteins (HDL), low-density lipoproteins (LDL), and very-low-density lipoproteins

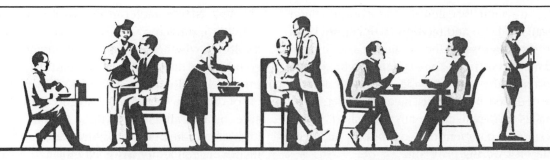

Chart your heart-health status

Good heart health begins with identifying factors that increase your risk for heart disease. In some families, risk factors for heart disease are inherited. If your parents or grandparents suffered from early coronary heart disease (before age 55) or heart attack, your personal risk of developing coronary heart disease may increase.

Other factors that can increase your risk of heart disease include: being male, smoking, having high blood pressure and high cholesterol. Since high cholesterol and high blood pressure may cause no symptoms, only a checkup can show if you have a problem.

Use this chart to record your heart-health status—and actions you need to take.

Checklist for men: Cholesterol _____   Blood pressure _____

☑ **Risk factors** (Check any that apply)
Each risk factor increases your chance of developing heart disease.

☐ High cholesterol   ☐ High blood pressure   ☐ Family history of heart attack before age 55
☐ Male sex   ☐ Smoking   ☐ Obesity (more than 30% over recommended weight)
☐ Diabetes   ☐ Existing blood vessel disease (such as hardening of the arteries)
☐ A level of HDL—"good" cholesterol—under 35, measured by a blood test

☑ **Action** (Check section that applies)

☐ **Total cholesterol under 200—Desirable.** Recheck within five years or sooner if health or diet changes.

☐ **Total cholesterol 200-239—Borderline-high.** (High risk if two other risk factors are present.) Talk to doctor about further evaluation and appropriate management.

☐ **Total cholesterol 240 and over—High risk.** See doctor for further evaluation and appropriate management.

☐ **Blood pressure above 140/90.** See your doctor about treatment steps you may need to take.

Lose weight, if necessary, and **quit smoking** to reduce your risk for heart disease.

Checklist for women: Cholesterol _____   Blood pressure _____

☑ **Risk factors** (Check any that apply)
Each risk factor increases your chance of developing heart disease. This risk increases even more for postmenopausal women who lose the protective benefits of the hormone estrogen.

☐ High cholesterol   ☐ High blood pressure   ☐ Family history of heart attack before age 55
☐ Smoking   ☐ Obesity (more than 30% over recommended weight)
☐ Diabetes   ☐ Existing blood vessel disease (such as hardening of the arteries)
☐ A level of HDL—"good" cholesterol—under 35, measured by a blood test

☑ **Action** (Check section that applies)

☐ **Total cholesterol under 200—Desirable.** Recheck within five years or sooner if health or diet changes.

☐ **Total cholesterol 200-239—Borderline-high.** (High risk if two other risk factors are present.) Talk to doctor about further evaluation and appropriate management.

☐ **Total cholesterol 240 and over—High risk.** See doctor for further evaluation and appropriate management.

☐ **Blood pressure above 140/90.** See your doctor about treatment steps you may need to take.

Lose weight, if necessary, and **quit smoking** to reduce your risk for heart disease.

FIGURE 15-1. Checklist of risk factors and possible corrective steps.

(VLDL). Medical management, however, is based mainly on the levels of total cholesterol, HDL, and LDL.

People with high blood levels of HDL have a low risk of developing coronary heart disease.[7] Although the reason for this is not certain, many scientists believe that HDL serves as a "scavenger" that transports cholesterol from various cells to the liver, from which it can be excreted in the bile. This helps protect blood vessels against atherosclerosis. HDL may also have some ability to remove cholesterol that has already been deposited in atherosclerotic plaque.

Low-density lipoproteins contain about 60% to 70% of the cholesterol carried in the bloodstream. Therefore, when a blood test indicates that total cholesterol is high, this usually means that LDL is undesirably high, but some people (most notably endurance athletes) with high total cholesterol levels have high HDL rather than high LDL. Because the cholesterol from LDL tends to accumulate in the arteries as a component of atherosclerotic plaque, LDL is often called "bad cholesterol," whereas HDL is called "good cholesterol." Since the cholesterol both contain is identical, it would be more accurate to refer to them as good or bad lipoproteins.

Long-range studies of large population groups have shown that the higher the total cholesterol and LDL levels, the greater the risk of a heart attack (Figure 15-2). The most important study began in 1948 in Framingham, Massachusetts, and is still generating valuable information. In 1987 its researchers reported that for people under 50, overall deaths rose 5% and heart-related deaths rose 9% for each 10 mg/dL of total cholesterol.[8] Other studies have shown that lowering the cholesterol level

through dietary and/or drug treatment lowers the incidence of heart attacks.[9,10] For middle-aged men it appears that each 1% reduction in LDL results in a 2% reduction in risk of a heart attack or death from CHD.[11]

A type of LDL called lipoprotein(a), or Lp(a), has been identified as a possible independent risk factor for CHD,[12,13] but the data are conflicting.[14-16] Lp(a) has a strong genetic component and is not influenced by diet or most cholesterol-lowering drugs. Although it may turn out to be an important factor in the development of heart disease for some people, no studies have defined what practical steps can be taken to lower abnormally high levels. One study, however, found that lowering elevated LDL appears to reduce the risk of Lp(a).[17] Another study found no association between Lp(a) concentration and the risk of stroke.[18]

Elevated plasma levels of homocysteine (an amino acid) have been linked to increased risk of premature coronary artery disease and stroke, even among people who have normal cholesterol levels.[19,20] Roughly 10% of cases of coronary heart disease have been linked to elevated homocysteine levels. Both hereditary and dietary factors may be involved. Dietary supplementation with folic acid (typically 1 mg daily) can reduce elevated homocysteine levels in most patients. In cases where it is not effective, high doses of vitamins B_6 and/or B_{12} may be tried. Studies have not yet determined whether lowering blood homocysteine levels reduces the incidence of heart attacks or strokes, but most experts believe that it will prove beneficial.[21] Screening for elevated homocysteine levels is advisable for individuals who manifest coronary artery disease that is out of proportion to their traditional risk factors or who have a family history of premature atherosclerotic disease. Levels above 10 µmol/L warrant treatment.

CHOLESTEROL GUIDELINES

Cholesterol and other blood lipids are measured in milligrams per deciliter (mg/dL—a deciliter is 100 mg, about $^1/_{10}$ of a quart). Total cholesterol, HDL, and triglyceride levels are determined by laboratory tests that measure them directly. LDL can be measured directly or calculated by subtracting HDL plus one fifth of the triglyceride level from total cholesterol. Since triglyceride levels are immediately influenced by eating, a blood specimen for LDL determination must be collected after a fast of 9 to 12 hours, usually overnight. The test to determine total cholesterol, HDL, LDL, and triglyceride levels is called a lipoprotein analysis, or *lipid profile* (see Figure 15-3).

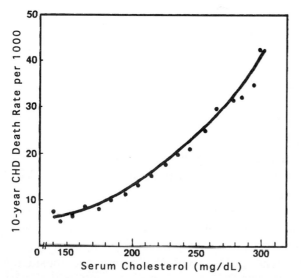

FIGURE 15-2. Relationship between serum total cholesterol level and CHD death rate. (Based on data from 361,662 men screened for MRFIT study.)

TEST	RESULT		UNITS	REFERENCE RANGE
	IN RANGE	OUT OF RANGE		
NAME	**AGE**	**DATE**	**ID #**	
COLLEGE, JOEL	21	2/9/01	987-65-4321	

TEST	IN RANGE	OUT OF RANGE	UNITS	REFERENCE RANGE
LIPID PROFILE				
TRIGLYCERIDES	165		MG/DL	20-190
CHOLESTEROL, TOTAL		210	MG/DL	LESS THAN 200
HDL-CHOLESTEROL	50		MG/DL	GREATER THAN 35
LDL-CHOLESTEROL	127		MG/DL	LESS THAN 130
CHOL/HDL-CHOL RATIO	4.20		(CALC)	< OR = 4.97

FIGURE 15-3. Sample laboratory report of a college student whose total cholesterol value is in the borderline high range. The HDL level is ample. The cholesterol/HDL ratio, a measure of risk, is below average for a male. The student should be counseled about risk factors, lower the fat content of his diet, and be rechecked in a year or two.

In 1987 the National Heart, Lung, and Blood Institute's National Cholesterol Education Program (NCEP) recommended that all Americans aged 20 and over have their total blood cholesterol level measured as part of a routine medical evaluation that also considers other risk factors for heart disease. In 1993 the guidelines were revised to add screening for low HDL levels. Table 15-2 summarizes NCEP's cholesterol-level classification system.

NCEP's current guidelines[22] call for measuring total cholesterol and HDL at least once every 5 years. The most efficient way to do this is to use a lipoprotein analysis as a screening test. If total cholesterol is 240 or more or HDL is less than 35, the test should be repeated. If the first and second LDL levels are similar, the results are averaged. If they are more than 30 mg/dL apart, a third test is done and averaged with the others.

Figure 15-4 summarizes NCEP's recommended actions for adults who do not have heart disease. For those who do, the recommended treatment is based on the individual's average level of LDL and number of risk factors. Regardless, dietary measures should be the cornerstone of any treatment program.

Surveys by the U.S. Centers for Disease Control and Prevention (CDC) indicate that average blood cholesterol levels for adults between the ages of 20 and 74 declined between 1976 and 1991.[23] Based on the 1993 NCEP guidelines, the proportion of Americans with high blood-cholesterol levels fell from 26% in 1976–1980 to 20% in 1988–1991, while the proportion of those with desirable levels rose from 44% to 49%. Based on 1990 population data, about 29% (52 million) would be candidates for dietary therapy and 7% might ultimately be candidates for drug therapy.[24]

In 1991 an NCEP expert panel[25] recommended cholesterol testing for children and adolescents who have a family history of premature cardiovascular disease or at least one parent whose blood cholesterol is over 240 mg/dL. The panel recommended dietary therapy for children whose LDL was 110 or greater and consideration of drug therapy for children over age 10 with persistent LDL levels of 190 or higher (or 160 and other risk factors).

Table 15-2

NCEP CLASSIFICATION OF SERUM CHOLESTEROL LEVELS (mg/dL)*

Total cholesterol

Under 200	Desirable
200-239	Borderline high
240 or more	High

HDL-cholesterol

Under 35	Low HDL-cholesterol

LDL-cholesterol

Under 130	Desirable
130-159	Borderline high-risk
160 or more	High-risk

*Many scientific publications follow the Systeme International, which expresses cholesterol values in millimoles per liter (mmol/L). To convert mg/dL to mmol/L, multiply by 0.02586 and round off to the nearest 0.05. Thus 200 mg/dL would be 5.15 mmol/L, and 130 mg/dL would be 3.35 mmol/L.

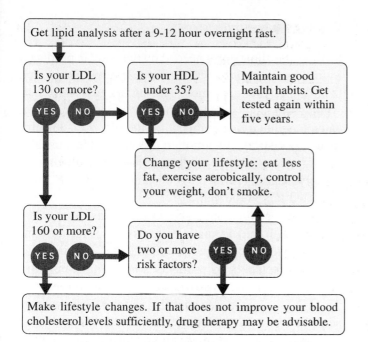

FIGURE 15-4. Simplified version of the NCEP's recommendations for adults with no evidence of heart disease. The positive risk factors are age (male ≥ 45 years, female ≥ 55 years or premature menopause without estrogen therapy); family history of premature coronary heart disease; smoking; high blood pressure; HDL < 35 mg/dL; and diabetes. If HDL ≥ 60, subtract 1 from the total of the others.

Table 15-3 describes the two levels of dietary change recommended for cholesterol reduction. If 3 months on a Step-One diet fail to yield a desirable result, a Step-Two diet should be used. Dietary change must be permanent. Americans currently consume about 37% of their total caloric intake as fat. The Step-One diet would reduce this to 30%, the Step-Two diet to 20%. Dietary cholesterol intake, which typically is 350 to 450 mg/day, would be reduced to 300 mg/day on the Step-One diet and 200 mg/day on the Step-Two diet.

Diets limited to 10% fat are more effective in lowering total blood cholesterol and LDL values,[26] but few people are willing to change their diet that drastically. Mirkin and Rich[27] have noted that for most adults, a 10% fat level will be achieved by limiting daily fat intake to 20 g.

Areas of Controversy

Controversy exists about whether all adults in the United States should aim to improve their blood cholesterol levels or whether efforts should be concentrated on those at highest risk of a heart attack. Some experts believe that NCEP's guidelines are overzealous—particularly for individuals in the 200 to 240 range—and may unduly shift public attention away from other health hazards such as cigarette smoking and high blood pressure.[28]

Expert panels in Canada, England and other European countries have not advocated mass screening for cholesterol but suggest treating individuals on a case-by-case basis. Their guidelines are more conservative, with higher action ranges than those of the NCEP.

The U.S. Preventive Services Task Force[29] recommended periodic screening for all men ages 35 to 65 and women ages 45 to 65. The American College of Physicians (ACP)[30] concurs but advises that only the total cholesterol level should be tested. The American Heart Association Task Force on Risk Reduction called ACP's advice "flawed and misguided" because it would deny young people—particularly those who are at high risk but may not know it—the opportunity to benefit from proven preventive strategies.[31] Task force member John LaRosa, M.D., pointed out:

In approximately 25% of patients with coronary atherosclerosis, sudden death is the first manifestation of disease. Even those who do not die, however, may be crippled by myocardial damage. A catastrophic first event is, of course, a reliable and perhaps even cost-effective way to identify those most susceptible to [high blood-cholesterol levels], but it is hardly a suitable way to practice preventive medicine.[32]

Table 15-3

DIETARY THERAPY OF HIGH CHOLESTEROL

Nutrient	Step-One Diet	Step-Two Diet
Total fat	30% or less of calories	20% or less of calories
Saturated fatty acids	7%–10% of calories	Less than 7% of calories
Polyunsaturated fatty acids	Up to 10% of calories	Up to 10% of calories
Monounsaturated fatty acids	Up to 15% of calories	Up to 15% of calories
Carbohydrates	55% or more of calories	55% or more of calories
Protein	Approximately 15% of calories	Approximately 15% of calories
Cholesterol	Less than 300 mg/day	Less than 200 mg/day
Total calories	To achieve and maintain desirable weight	

Although the risk factors for women appear similar to those of men, little research has been done to determine the appropriateness of using cholesterol-lowering drugs, particularly in premenopausal women.

The female hormone estrogen appears to exert a protective effect against heart disease by lowering LDL levels and raising HDL. After menopause the level of estrogen drops sharply.

The *Harvard Health Letter*[33] states that taking estrogen after menopause may reduce a woman's risk of developing heart disease by almost half. However, there is also some increased risk of cancer of the uterus and possibly of cancer of the breast. This subject is discussed further in Chapter 21. The extent to which cholesterol reduction benefits men and women over age 65 is unknown.[34]

Questions have also been raised about whether lowering cholesterol increases the risk of certain cancers.[35] The prevailing medical view is that it does not.[36]

Problems with Screening Tests

Management of cholesterol levels is complicated by the fact that laboratory tests have considerable potential for error. Test results can vary from sample to sample, and some facilities do not perform the test accurately. Levels vary at different times within the individual.

How the test is done also influences the results. Food intake, changes of position (lying down, sitting, or standing), weight change, alcohol intake, various illnesses, and the technique used to collect the specimen can cause variations.

The CDC recommends using a minimum of two patient specimens to obtain an adequate estimate of cholesterol levels.[37] *Consumer Reports on Health*[38] warns that "finger-stick" tests often used in mass screenings are not as accurate as tests using blood drawn from the arm.

An erroneously high reading can cause needless worry and expense. An erroneously low reading can lead an individual to fail to take appropriate action. Considering the test's relatively low cost and the problems that can result from an inaccurate report, it is wise to obtain the test from a laboratory recommended by one's personal physician.

Although the FDA has approved a home cholesterol test kit, this test is rarely practical because it measures only the total cholesterol level. Current guidelines for screening include HDL testing and a lipid profile for anyone whose total cholesterol is high. Unnecessary expense can be avoided by starting with a lipid profile ordered through a physician's office.

DIETARY MODIFICATION

Most of the cholesterol needed by the body is produced by the body, mainly by the liver. The rest is derived from animal products (meat, fish, milk, eggs) in the diet. Among the dietary factors, the amount and type of fat eaten has the greatest impact on the blood cholesterol level. Decreased consumption of saturated fats usually results in lower blood cholesterol, as does substitution of polyunsaturated or monounsaturated fats for some saturated fats in the diet.

Recent studies have shown that trans-fatty acids, commonly found in margarine, pastries, and fat-containing snack foods, tend to reduce HDL and increase LDL.[39] The labels of products containing trans-fatty acids list "partially hydrogenated oil" as an ingredient. The FDA has proposed that the amount of trans-fatty acids be listed on product labels.[40]

Dietary cholesterol affects the level of blood cholesterol, but to a lesser and more variable extent than does the fat content of the diet. A high intake of soluble fiber (found in oat products, beans, and other complex carbohydrate foods) can help to lower blood cholesterol levels. A recent study found that people who consumed more vegetables, fruits, and cereal fibers had a lower incidence of coronary heart disease.[41] Another study found that fruits and vegetables appear to have a protective effect against strokes in men.[42]

To assist consumers trying to lower their blood cholesterol, the NCEP[43] suggests six general guidelines:

1. Choose foods that are low in saturated fat.
2. Choose foods that are low in total fat.
3. Choose foods high in complex carbohydrates (starch and fiber), such as fruits, vegetables, whole-grain cereals, beans, and other legumes.
4. Choose foods low in cholesterol.
5. Be more physically active.
6. Lose weight, if you are overweight.

In 2000 the American Heart Association issued guidelines containing additional details plus strategies for weight and blood pressure control.[44]

The first practical step toward dietary change is to become more aware of one's diet, especially the amount of food eaten and the brands usually purchased. Toward this end, consumers should get into the habit of checking labels to determine the amount of cholesterol and the amount and type of fat. They should also be aware of the "hidden" fats found in processed foods such as cookies, crackers, and snack cakes, and the kinds of fats and oils used in their own cooking.

The next step is to make substitutions for red meats. For example, leaner beef cuts (select or choice) can be substituted for fatter (prime), and consumption of fish, poultry, fresh fruits and vegetables, beans, and other legumes can be increased. Foods high in complex carbohydrates—such as whole grains, beans, and vegetables—can be made the "main dish," with small amounts of red meats and cheeses becoming the "side dishes." Mixed dishes such as stews, casseroles, and pasta and rice meals can combine small amounts of meat with other foods, such as grains or vegetables.

Finally, consumers should evaluate their progress by having their blood cholesterol tested within a few months and then periodically as recommended by the professional who is guiding them. The goal should be a gradual but steady reduction in the total cholesterol and LDL-cholesterol levels.

Because the major sources of saturated fat in the American diet traditionally have come from beef and dairy products, dietary advice aimed at lowering blood cholesterol often focuses on cutting back on hamburgers and fatty meats, whole milk, and cheeses—and getting into a habit of preparing foods with less fat. Table 15-4 indicates the fatty acid composition of selected fats and oils. The "Dietary Modification" box on page 342 suggests how to reduce the fat and cholesterol content of one's diet.

Food companies have responded to public concern by marketing thousands of products that are fat- and cholesterol-reduced.

Overall Fat Percentage

Following the guidelines in the "Dietary Modification" box will reduce the fat, saturated fat, and cholesterol content of the diet and should come close to the 30%

Table 15-4

FATTY ACID COMPOSITION OF FATS AND OILS

	% Saturated	% Monounsaturated	% Polyunsaturated
Fats and Oils			
Canola (rapeseed) oil	7	58	35
Safflower oil	9	13	78
Walnut oil	10	24	66
Sunflower oil	11	20	69
Corn oil	13	25	62
Olive oil	14	77	9
Soybean oil	15	24	61
Peanut oil	18	48	34
Salmon oil	20	55	25
Wheat germ oil	20	16	64
Cottonseed oil	27	19	54
Tuna fat	30	29	41
Chicken fat	31	47	22
Lard	41	47	12
Mutton (lamb) fat	49	43	8
Palm oil	51	39	10
Beef fat	52	44	4
Palm kernel oil	86	12	2
Coconut oil	92	6	2
Spreads and Shortening			
Mayonnaise (soybean oil)	16	30	54
Mayonnaise (imitation)	18	24	58
Stick margarine (liquid and partially hydrogenated corn oil)	18	51	31
Tub margarine (partially hydrogenated soybean oil)	18	47	35
Shortening (partially hydrogenated soybean and palm oils)	32	53	15
Butter	66	30	4

DIETARY MODIFICATION FOR CHOLESTEROL CONTROL[45]

The following can help you choose and prepare foods lower in saturated fat and cholesterol:

- Trim all visible fat from beef and poultry, and remove the skin from poultry before eating.

- Bake, broil, or roast meat dishes instead of deep-fat-frying them. To prevent drying and add flavor, baste with wine, lemon juice, or a low-fat broth.

- Try experimenting with herbs and spices, such as dill, tarragon, cilantro, and basil.

- Avoid fatty gravies and sauces.

- If pan- or stir-frying, use small amounts of vegetable oils such as canola or safflower oil; also increase your use of olive oil.

- Minimize use of butter.

- Minimize use of products, such as margarines, that contain partially hydrogenated oils (trans-fatty acids).

- To cut down on whole-milk products, switch to 2% or 1% milk, and perhaps eventually to skim milk. Many people find it easy to get accustomed to low-fat milk, and that when they do so, whole milk tastes too rich. Use the low-fat or skim-milk versions of ricotta, cottage, and mozzarella cheese. Low-fat farmer or pot cheeses also are available. All these cheeses should contain no more than 2–6 grams of fat per ounce. For desserts, substitute ice milk, frozen yogurt (especially the nonfat variety), sherbet or sorbet for ice cream. If you do eat ice cream, choose regular rather than super premium types.

- Limit consumption of foods that contain palm, palm kernel, and coconut oils, lard, butter, unidentified shortening, egg-yolk solids, and whole-milk solids. Also, cut down on baked goods made from these ingredients or that are fried, such as doughnuts.

- Use yogurt instead of sour cream in dips and toppings.

- Use only the egg whites or discard every other yolk in recipes requiring eggs (2 whites = 1 whole egg in recipes). Or try commercial cholesterol-free egg substitutes.

- Reduce the amount of fat in recipes by one-third to one-half, and use chiefly polyunsaturated and monounsaturated oils.

- Shrimp, lobster, and other shellfish may be eaten occasionally because they are lower in cholesterol than previously thought, and do not contain too much saturated fat.

- In coffee, use low-fat or skim milk instead of non-dairy creamers containing saturated fats. Skim milk powder also is acceptable.

- Substitute rice and pasta for egg noodles.

- Make your own popcorn for a low-calorie snack, but be sure to omit the melted butter. Beware of high-fat microwave popcorn products.

- Avoid nuts that are high in saturated fats, such as coconuts and macadamia nuts.

- Incorporate oat fiber into your diet, for example, in oat bran muffins or in casseroles. To increase total fiber intake, look for the words "whole wheat" or "whole grain" near the top of the ingredient list when buying breads and cereals.

- Use fresh fruit instead of high-fat desserts.

- Choose lowfat luncheon meats such as turkey breast or pressed turkey instead of salami and bologna. Use frankfurters, other sausages, and bacon sparingly. When eating poultry, remember that white meat has less fat than dark meat.

- Buy or make salad dressings with predominantly unsaturated oils. Olive oil is an especially good choice. Or try a nonfat type or just vinegar or lemon juice.

- Limit use of organ meats that are very high in cholesterol, such as liver, kidneys, brain, and sweetbreads.

- Prepare soups and stews containing meat the day before eating them. After refrigerating, skim off the congealed fat on the surface prior to reheating.

- Be cautious about store-bought baked products such as pies, cakes, croissants, pastries and muffins. Try to find lowfat cookies and crackers. Or bake at home with small amounts of unsaturated oil or with pureed fruit such as applesauce or prune butter substituted for some of the oil. Angel food cake is a good choice because it is low in fat and cholesterol.

- Use some of the many fat-free, cholesterol-free products marketed as substitutes for products that normally are high in fat.

- Make changes gradually to avoid feeling deprived. For most people, enjoying a rich dessert or a prime rib once in a while is not going to significantly affect their cholesterol level as long as the overall cholesterol-lowering diet is followed most of the time. It is better to splurge once in a while than to cheat a little bit each day.

fat and 10% saturated-fat levels recommended in the NCEP Step-One diet. However, the only way to determine how much fat and cholesterol are actually consumed is to add up the amounts contained in the daily diet. While milligrams of cholesterol can be added directly, the percentage of fat must be calculated using information on product labels or from food composition tables. Since there are nine calories per gram of fat, the percentage of calories from fat equals:

$$\frac{\text{grams of fat consumed during the day} \times 9}{\text{total calories eaten}} \times 100$$

Thus someone consuming 2100 calories and 70 g of fat would have a diet that is $[(70 \times 9)/2100] \times 100 = 30\%$ fat. However, precise self-determination of daily fat and cholesterol intake can be difficult. Many foods do not carry complete nutrition labels, and determining the fat and cholesterol content of many restaurant items is difficult or impossible (although many fast food outlets publish information about their products). Table 15-5 compares several popular books that include food composition tables to help consumers plan their diet. More detailed information is available on the USDA Web site.[46]

Computer programs are also available for determining fat and cholesterol intake. Those containing large databases, including nutritional analyses of brand-name products and fast food items, generally provide the most accurate information. Computer programs are accessible to consumers at certain clinics and through nutrition professionals in private practice. Some are also marketed directly to the public for home use.

Kantor[47] states that despite these self-help aids, most consumers wishing to design a diet that is significantly low in fat would be wise to consult a registered dietitian or other professional nutritionist. Chapter 11 describes the training and credentials of nutrition professionals.

Soluble Fiber

It is well established that a diet high in soluble fiber can improve blood cholesterol levels. In 1984, for example, Anderson and colleagues[48] gave 20 men with levels of blood cholesterol above 260 mg/dL diets containing 17 g/day of soluble fiber, derived either from oat bran (100 g/day dry weight) or pinto and navy beans (115 g/day dry weight). Subjects on the "oat diet" consumed one cup of hot oat-bran cereal and five oat-bran muffins each day. Those on the "bean diet" were served cooked beans and bean soup. After 3 weeks, both groups improved their cholesterol levels. Total cholesterol was reduced by about 19%, while LDL levels decreased by approximately 24%. Although the average

---

 Consumer Tip

A Quick Fat-Chemistry Lesson

You need not know the chemical structure of fats to understand a low-fat diet. But for those who want a technical explanation, here it is. Fats are classified by the amount of hydrogen in the fatty acids that make up their basic structure. Fatty acids are composed of chains of carbon atoms tied together:

$$-C-C-C-C-C-C-C-C-C-C-C-C-C-\ldots$$

Each carbon atom has four arms that can attach to other elements:

$$-\overset{|}{\underset{|}{C}}-$$

All the arms must be attached to something else. Fatty acids have hydrogen atoms attached to the carbons:

$$\overset{H}{\underset{H}{-C}}-\overset{H}{\underset{H}{C}}-\overset{H}{\underset{H}{C}}-\ldots$$

All carbons have four binding arms. All hydrogens have one. Some carbons do not have hydrogen attached to them. They have to bind to something else, so they bind twice to the next carbon. This is called a double bond:

$$\overset{H}{\underset{H}{-C}}-\overset{}{\underset{H}{C}}=\overset{}{\underset{H}{C}}-\overset{H}{\underset{H}{C}}-\ldots$$

Fatty acids are classified by the number and location of their double bonds. Those with no double bonds are called saturated:

$$\overset{H}{\underset{H}{-C}}-\overset{H}{\underset{H}{C}}-\overset{H}{\underset{H}{C}}-\overset{H}{\underset{H}{C}}-\overset{H}{\underset{H}{C}}-\overset{H}{\underset{H}{C}}-\overset{H}{\underset{H}{C}}-\ldots$$

Fatty acids that contain several double bonds are called polyunsaturated:

$$\overset{H}{\underset{H}{-C}}-\overset{H}{\underset{H}{C}}-\overset{}{\underset{H}{C}}=\overset{}{\underset{H}{C}}-\overset{}{\underset{H}{C}}=\overset{}{\underset{H}{C}}-\overset{H}{\underset{H}{C}}-\ldots$$

Fatty acids with only a single double bond are called monounsaturated:

$$\overset{H}{\underset{H}{-C}}-\overset{H}{\underset{H}{C}}-\overset{}{\underset{H}{C}}=\overset{}{\underset{H}{C}}-\overset{H}{\underset{H}{C}}-\overset{H}{\underset{H}{C}}-\overset{H}{\underset{H}{C}}-\ldots$$

All fatty acids have a carbon end and an acidic end. Polyunsaturated fats are further classified by where their double bonds are located. Those with the double bond three atoms away from the carbon at the non–acidic end of the chain of carbons are called omega–3's:

$$H-\overset{H}{\underset{H}{C}}-\overset{H}{\underset{H}{C}}-\overset{}{\underset{H}{C}}=\overset{}{\underset{H}{C}}-\overset{H}{\underset{H}{C}}-\overset{H}{\underset{H}{C}}-\overset{H}{\underset{H}{C}}-\ldots$$

Gabe Mirkin, M.D.

Table 15-5

CHOLESTEROL-LOWERING GUIDEBOOKS

Title	Author(s)	Method	Food Analyses	Recipe Analysis	Sample Menus
Beyond Cholesterol: The Johns Hopkins Complete Guide for Avoiding Heart Disease (1989)	Peter Kwiterovich, M.D.	Dietary planning based on selection of foods that are low in saturated fat and/or high in fiber	Calories, total and saturated fat, and cholesterol listed for about 800 foods	Yes	Yes
Controlling Cholesterol (1988)	Kenneth H. Cooper, M.D., Ph.D.	Uses food exchange system to modify sample weekly diet plans	Calories, fat, and cholesterol listed for over 500 food items, with fat composition specified for many	Yes	Yes
Count Out Cholesterol (1989)	Art Ulene, M.D.	Provides system for counting levels of saturated fat and dietary fiber to reach goals based on weight or activity level. Cholesterol is tabulated separately.	Ratings assigned for saturated fat, fiber, and cholesterol for about 300 foods	No	No
Dr. Dean Ornish's Program for Reversing Heart Disease (1990)	Dean Ornish, M.D.	Dietary planning based on counting grams of fat and saturated fat. Advocates a stringent vegetarian "reversal diet" or a less stringent "prevention" diet, plus multivitamin/mineral supplement	Calories, carbohydrate, protein, total and saturated fat, cholesterol, and sodium listed for about 600 foods	Yes	Yes
Eater's Choice (1989)	Ron Goor, Ph.D. Nancy Goor	Dietary planning based mainly on limiting the number of saturated fat calories	Calories and saturated fat listed for about 1500 food items	Yes	Yes
Fat Free, Flavor Full (1995)	Gabe Mirkin, M.D. Diana Rich	Semivegetarian diet that limits fat to 20 g per day in order to achieve a 10% fat diet	All recipes are low in fat	No	No
Good Fat, Bad Fat (1989)	Glen C. Griffin, M.D. William P. Castelli, M.D.	Dietary planning based on limiting the number of grams of saturated fat	Saturated fat and cholesterol listed for about 270 foods	Yes	No
The American Heart Association Low-Fat, Low-Cholesterol Cookbook (1989)	Scott Grundy, M.D., Ph.D.	Primarily a cookbook	Calories, total and saturated fat, cholesterol, and sodium listed for over 500 foods	Yes	Yes
The New American Diet (1989)	William E. Connor, M.D. Sonja L. Connor, M.S., R.D.	Food selection based on "cholesterol-saturated fat index (CSI)," which is the authors' estimate of the foods' overall effect on blood cholesterol levels	Lists calories and CSI for over 100 foods	Yes	Yes

HDL level also decreased slightly in this study, other researchers have found that HDL usually increased modestly or did not change when subjects increased their soluble fiber intake. The addition of psyllium (the soluble fiber in *Metamucil*) to a Step-One diet has been shown to improve cholesterol levels more than the diet alone.[49]

Two large studies have demonstrated that dietary fiber actually protects against cardiovascular disease. One found that among 43,757 male health professionals followed for 6 years, those reporting the highest intake of vegetable, fruit, and cereal fiber had the lowest incidence of coronary heart disease (CHD).[50] The other, which spanned 10 years, compared the incidence of heart attacks and death due to CHD to the amount of dietary fiber consumed by 68,682 women aged 37 to 64 years who had no previously diagnosed angina, heart attack, stroke, diabetes, or high blood cholesterol when the study began. The 20% of women who consumed the most cereal fiber had a 34% lower risk of CHD than the 20% who consumed the least.[51] Two studies support the idea that eating fruits and vegetables may protect against the development of stroke.[52,53]

The foods highest in soluble fiber include oat bran, dry oats, kidney beans, navy beans, pinto beans, lima beans, white beans, Brussels sprouts, kale, broccoli, plums, apples, oranges and grapefruit (including the fibrous partitions). Large amounts of fiber increase the bulk of the stool and can cause bloating, cramps, and diarrhea. However, discomfort can be minimized or prevented if the amount of dietary fiber is increased gradually, so the body can become accustomed to it.

Many studies support the hypothesis that incorporating oat products into the diet causes a modest reduction in blood cholesterol level.[54] A controlled experiment suggests that the water-soluble fiber beta-glucan is responsible for this effect. Six groups of about 20 volunteers following a NCEP Step-One diet were given either oat bran or oat cereal at daily doses of 1, 2, or 3 oz (dry weight) for 6 weeks, while a seventh group received 1 oz per day of farina, which contains no beta-glucan. (A cup of dry oatmeal contains 3 oz.) The groups eating 2 or 3 oz of oat bran or 3 oz of oatmeal had the best results, with total cholesterol falling an average of 7% to 9% and LDL falling an average of 10% to 16%.[55]

Regression of Atherosclerosis

Many studies have shown that improving blood-cholesterol levels can reduce the incidence of and mortality from heart disease.[56,57] Some studies have used angio-graphy or other imaging procedures to determine whether coronary atherosclerosis has increased (progressed), remained the same, or decreased (regressed) during a treatment period. This is done by measuring areas of narrowing and blood flow within the coronary arteries.

Several studies have demonstrated that improving cholesterol levels with drugs can reduce the incidence of heart attacks and strokes in patients with moderately to severely elevated cholesterol levels. In 1994 a study conclusively demonstrated that lowering cholesterol decreases the overall death rate as well as the incidence of heart attacks in people already known to have coronary heart disease. This study involved 4444 patients, all of whom were on a cholesterol-lowering diet. Half were given simvastatin (*Zocor*), and the rest received a placebo. After 5 years, when the groups were compared, the treated group had 42% fewer deaths from coronary disease and a 30% lower overall death rate.[58,59] In 1995 Byington and others reported that the risk can also be decreased in people, both young and old, with *mildly* elevated levels.[60] A subsequent meta-analysis of 35 randomized trials totaling 77,257 patients concluded that every 10% reduction in total cholesterol level reduced the CHD death rate by 13% to 14% and overall mortality by 8% to 10%.[61]

The Lifestyle Heart Trial has demonstrated that regression can occur through changes of lifestyle alone—including a 10% fat vegetarian diet, smoking cessation, stress management techniques, and daily moderate exercise. The only animal products permitted in the treatment group's diet were egg whites and 1 cup a day of nonfat milk or yogurt. Cholesterol intake was 5 mg/day or less. The control group was asked to adhere to a Step-One diet. After 1 year, 18 of the 22 members (82%) of the treatment group showed overall regression of coronary atherosclerosis, while 10 out of the 19 members (53%) of the control group showed substantial progression of their disease.[62,63]

Dean Ornish, M.D., who directed the trial, reported that the degree of regression was related more to compliance with the low-fat diet than it was to the change in blood cholesterol level. After 4 more years, the experimental group continued to do better than the control group, some of whom took cholesterol-lowering drugs.[64,65] Ornish's data have been sufficiently favorable that Medicare and several insurance companies are covering his program as an alternative to bypass surgery or angioplasty. In addition to the full program, Ornish's nonprofit Preventive Medicine Research Institute offers a 1-week residential retreat for learning how to make comprehensive lifestyle changes.

The Pritikin Diet

The Pritikin diet was designed by the late Nathan Pritikin, a successful inventor who had no professional training in medicine or nutrition. Pritikin developed the diet after learning at age 40 that his cholesterol level was high and his coronary arteries were atherosclerotic. It is very low in fat, high in complex carbohydrates, and low in sodium. Its recommended calorie composition is less than 10% fat, 10% to 15% protein, less than 5% simple carbohydrates, and 75% to 80% complex carbohydrates. It allows 3.5 oz of fish, poultry, or lean meat per day, which makes it almost a vegetarian diet. The diet is part of an overall program that includes exercise and prohibits smoking and alcohol intake.[66] In 2000 the residential program, available at Pritikin Longevity Centers in Santa Monica, California, and Aventura, Florida, cost $5435 for 3 weeks, $3695 for 2 weeks, and $1995 for 1 week.

Pritikin claimed that his program helped many people with heart disease, obesity, diabetes, and other health problems. The overall approach is similar to conventional therapy for cardiac patients but uses a more restrictive diet. The Pritikin diet can achieve considerable reduction in blood cholesterol levels. However, its fiber content is quite high (about 30 g per 1000 calories), which may cause abdominal cramps, bloating, and diarrhea. Dr. Ornish's trial suggests that for some patients, the Pritikin diet may protect the heart better than a 20% fat diet. No direct comparative study has been carried out, however, so it is not clear whether the potential benefits of the Pritikin diet justify the radical dietary changes it requires.

Misleading Advertising

Since the public is much more familiar with "cholesterol" than with "saturated fat," many manufacturers have made "no-cholesterol" claims even for foods that are high in fat. Unsuspecting consumers interested in trying to adopt healthier eating habits might actually make things worse by eating these foods. A similar situation exists for some products containing oat bran. Although oat bran can play a valuable cholesterol-lowering role as part of a low-fat diet, some "oat bran" products contain insignificant amounts of oat bran or contain undesirable amounts of fat as well.

In 1991 the New York Department of Consumer Affairs surveyed three supermarket chains in New York City and found 185 products marketed with claims of low or no cholesterol. In some cases the foods were vegetable or grain products that never contained cholesterol to begin with. (Cholesterol is found only in products derived from animal sources.) In other cases the products were free of cholesterol but contained high levels of fat. In some cases a heart symbol was displayed on the package or supermarket shelf for foods that were high in fat. The department's report noted:

Unfortunately, when one product makes a meaningless or deceptive claim, its competitors usually follow suit so they are not competitively disadvantaged. A kind of Gresham's law [the bad driving out the good] of grocery shopping ensues as misleading labels push out honest labels. . . .

Vigorous consumer law enforcement at the federal and local levels is needed to ensure that our supermarket shelves serve—rather than sabotage—our consumer interests.[67]

During 1991 the FDA warned several food companies to stop making health claims that are not backed by scientific evidence. One was Ralston Purina, which was ordered to stop claiming that eating *Oat Chex* "may help reduce cholesterol levels." The company was told that even if scientific evidence eventually supports a link between eating oat bran and reducing the risk of coronary heart disease, *Oat Chex* contained insufficient fiber to support its health claim. The FDA also warned the manufacturers of five corn and canola oils to stop making "no cholesterol" claims and displaying a heart symbol on their product labels.

As noted in Chapter 11, FDA regulations now require that the labels of nearly all packaged foods to disclose the amounts of fat, saturated fat, cholesterol, and fiber per serving size. The regulations also ban "no cholesterol" claims for foods that are high in fat. Presumably accurate information is now displayed in the "Nutrition Facts" boxes on product labels and packages, but misleading slogans still appear on a few products.

LIPID-LOWERING DRUGS

The National Cholesterol Education Program considers dietary treatment the cornerstone of therapy to reduce elevated cholesterol levels. The primary goal of dietary therapy is to maintain an LDL level below 130 mg/dL. It is assumed that this will help prevent heart attacks by inhibiting further buildup of atherosclerotic plaque and perhaps by reducing the amount of plaque already present. If a Step-One diet does not succeed, the more rigorous Step-Two diet should be followed. If all dietary attempts fail to correct elevated LDL levels within about 6 months, drug therapy should be considered in addition to diet.

The choice of drug depends upon the medical condition of the patient, the nature of the patient's blood lipid abnormalities, concern about adverse effects, and

Table 15-6

COMPARISON OF COMMONLY USED CHOLESTEROL-LOWERING DRUGS

Category/Name	⇩LDL	⇧HDL	Cost	Advantages	Adverse Effects
Nicotinic acid (niacin)				Most cost-effective; proven effective for reducing heart attacks; may lower Lp(a)	Flushing and itching of the skin; nausea; abnormal liver function; gout. Sustained-release has fewer side effects but greater incidence of serious complications.
Crystalline niacin	+++	+++	+*		
Sustained-release niacin	+++	+++	+*		
Bile acid sequestrants				Safest; work within the intestine and therefore are not absorbed by the body	Constipation, nausea, bloating, heartburn; can interfere with absorption of fat-soluble vitamins and some drugs.
Cholestipol (Colestid)	++	+	+++		
Cholestyramine (Questran)	++	+	+*		
HMG coA reductase inhibitors ("statins")				Most effective for lowering LDL; proven effective for reducing heart attacks	Side effects are uncommon, but these drugs are too new to have established long-term safety.
Atorvastatin (Lipitor)	+++	+	+++		
Cerivastatin (Baycol)	+++	+	+++		
Fluvastatin (Lescol)	+++	+	++		
Lovastatin (Mevacor)	+++	+	++		
Pravastatin (Pravachol)	+++	+	+++		
Simvastatin (Zocor)	+++	+	++++		
Fibric acid derivatives				Useful against elevated triglyceride levels	GI distress, rash, gallstones.
Fenofibrate (Tricor)	++	++	+++		
Gemfibrozil (Lopid)*	+	++	+*		

*Generic available at much lower cost than brand-name drug.

cost. Niacin and the "statins" reduce cholesterol production. Bile acid sequestrants bind with cholesterol-containing bile acids in the intestines and remove them in bowel movements. Fibric acid derivatives may be used for patients whose problems include high triglyceride levels. Table 15-6 provides an overview of the commonly used drugs. If one drug is not effective, two may be used together. *The Medical Letter* has concluded that, for most patients, statins are the best choice because they are more effective and better tolerated than the rest and have been proven to decrease mortality from coronary heart disease.[68]

Niacin is available in two forms: crystalline (regular) and sustained-release. The usual dosage for cholesterol control is 1 to 3 g daily. Sustained-release products have fewer side effects and may be more potent, but they have a much higher incidence of serious adverse effects. Both varieties are available without a prescription. However, self-medication is extremely unwise. Near-fatal hepatitis has been reported in a previously healthy 32-year-old man who had taken one 500-mg sustained-release niacin tablet daily for 2 months, purchased at a health-food store.[69] Several observers have expressed concern that sustained-released

niacin can be purchased without a prescription.[70-72] Niacin users should have periodic blood tests of liver function to be sure that the niacin is not irritating their liver.

The cost of cholesterol-lowering drugs ranges from about $75 a year for crystalline niacin to more than $1000 a year for simvastatin. Once an appropriate regimen has been found, lipid-lowering therapy should be continued indefinitely because when it is stopped, plasma cholesterol concentrations generally return to their pretreatment levels.

PREVENTIVE USE OF ASPIRIN

Regular use of aspirin appears to have considerable value in preventing heart attacks and strokes.[73] Low doses of aspirin decrease the synthesis of hormone-like substances called *prostaglandins*, which affect blood clotting by causing platelets to cluster where blood vessel walls are injured. Aspirin is believed to prevent heart attacks and strokes by inhibiting the formation of clots that can block the flow of blood in the arteries that nourish the heart and brain. Studies have shown that aspirin (a) reduces the likelihood of a heart attack when taken regularly by apparently healthy men over age 40 and

(b) reduces the risk of heart attacks and strokes among persons who have previously suffered such an event. More research is needed to determine whether apparently healthy people should use it preventively.[74]

The usual recommended daily dosage is from 75 mg (less than a baby aspirin) to 325 mg (an adult-strength tablet). Aspirin's antiplatelet ability will cause some people who use it regularly to develop abnormal bleeding. The American Heart Association recommends that decisions about aspirin use involve consultation with a physician who reviews the patient's risk factors and medical history and other preventive strategies.

QUESTIONABLE PREVENTIVE MEASURES

Many over-the-counter products sold through health-food stores and pharmacies have been touted as useful for preventing cardiovascular disease by lowering blood-cholesterol levels or through another mechanism. Many manufacturers market combinations of such ingredients. Except for crystalline niacin, which should never be taken without medical supervision, no product of this type is rationally formulated.[75] Even if future research demonstrates that any of the substances discussed in this section can exert a protective effect, it is unlikely that any such effect will be significant when compared to the lifestyle modifications and drug therapy already known to be effective.

Garlic extract capsules may lower cholesterol and may also exert an anticoagulant effect. They have not been proven safe or effective for long-term use.[76]

Eating several cloves of garlic daily can also have an impact on cholesterol but will cause the individual to have bad breath and to exude an offensive odor through the skin.

Vitamin E has been touted for its antioxidant effect. Epidemiologic studies have found a relationship between vitamin E intake and the incidence of heart attacks. Other studies have found that vitamin E can have a protective effect by preventing LDL from being oxidized into a more harmful form.

Vitamin E also has an anticoagulant effect, which means that supplementation may increase the risk of stroke. However, no study has demonstrated that vitamin E supplements are safe and effective for long-term use (see Chapter 12). Although aspirin has been proven effective, no study has tested whether combinations of vitamin E, garlic, fish oil, ginkgo, and aspirin—all of which can have anticoagulant effects—are safe for long-term use. A 7-year study of postmenopausal women found: (a) women with an adequate intake of vitamin E in their diet had a lower death rate from coronary heart disease, (b) supplementation with vitamin E had no apparent benefit, and (c) the level of intake of vitamins A and C did not appear to affect the risk of dying from coronary disease.[77] Another study found that high-risk patients age 55 and older who received 400 IU of natural vitamin E for 4.5 years did no better than comparable patients who received a placebo.[78]

Beta-carotene has also been recommended for its antioxidant effect. But long-range studies have found that it is no more effective than a placebo. The most

---

◆ Personal Glimpse ◆

Cholesterol Scam

What could be more timely than a product to reduce blood cholesterol while still allowing you to eat whatever you please? A full-page ad published in 1989 in more than 100 newspapers claimed that Cho Low Tea would do exactly that.

"Don't cut out your favorite foods," the ad advised. "New Tea from China Reduces Cholesterol. Medical studies prove it! Just drinking this refreshing tea every day is as effective as medically prescribed drugs. . . . Cho Low is a rare species of tea grown in China for centuries. Traditionally, the Chinese drink it after every meal as a diet aid. Recently . . . researchers were astonished to discover that besides aiding weight loss, Cho Low Tea has natural cholesterol-reducing properties. . . . And you get none of the possible side effects of . . . cholesterol-reducing drugs." The ad contained endorsements from seven medical sources and the logo of the Better Business Bureau. The tea cost $29.85 for a 30-day supply.

Fortunately for consumers, a newspaper credit bureau executive became suspicious and alerted law enforcement agencies in California, where the promotion was based. It turned out that the claims were false and the endorsements were complete fabrications. In fact, "Cho Low Tea" did not exist. The perpetrators said that they had planned to repackage another tea but were arrested before they could do so. After pleading "no contest" to false and misleading advertising, they were sentenced to brief jail terms followed by 3 years' summary probation. More than 50,000 people had placed orders totalling over $250,000, but the authorities acted so swiftly that none of them lost their money.

notable of these was the Physicians' Health Study[79] in which 22,000 men taking either beta-carotene or a placebo were followed for 12 years.

Fiber pills have no proven value for lowering cholesterol. Although dietary fiber can play a valuable role in a cholesterol-control program, the amount of fiber in these pills is not significant. High-fiber candy bars contain more but cost much more than ordinary foods.

Lecithin has been claimed to lower cholesterol but has not been scientifically demonstrated to do so.[80]

Coenzyme Q_{10} is described in books and pamphlets as a "miracle nutrient" effective against high blood pressure, heart failure, angina pectoris, high blood cholesterol, diabetes, and many other problems. Research with animals has shown that coenzyme Q_{10} can help protect hearts against transient decreases in the amount of oxygen that cells receive. Some researchers hypothesize that coenzyme Q_{10} can function as an antioxidant. Recommending against its use, the *Harvard Heart Letter* states: (a) well-designed placebo-controlled studies that found benefit involved only 10 to 20 patients, (b) larger studies reporting improvement had no controls, (c) no well-designed large-scale study has been reported, and (d) coenzyme Q_{10} is expensive ($8 to $10/week for 100 mg per day in Boston).[81]

Fish-oil capsules that contain omega-3 fatty acids have variable effects on blood lipids (sometimes raising cholesterol levels).[82] Eating fish that provide these fatty acids appears to reduce the risk of death from coronary heart disease. However, the benefit may come from constituents other than the fish oil itself. The fish highest in omega-3s include sardines (in fish oil), pink salmon, albacore tuna, mackerel, lake trout, and halibut. One portion weekly appears sufficient.[83,84] In October 2000, the FDA decided to permit the following claim to be made for fish-oil capsules:

The scientific evidence about whether omega-3 fatty acids may reduce the risk of coronary heart disease (CHD) is suggestive, but not conclusive. Studies in the general population have looked at diets containing fish and it is not known whether diets or omega-3 fatty acids in fish may have a possible effect on a reduced risk of CHD. It is not known what effect omega-3 fatty acids may or may not have on risk of CHD in the general population.

Oil derived from medium-chain triglycerides (MCTs) has been promoted as an alternative to olive or canola oil. It allegedly provide athletes with an energy boost without raising their serum cholesterol level. However, researchers at the University of Texas have demonstrated that the body converts MCTs into long-chain triglycerides, which do raise LDL cholesterol levels.[85]

Alcohol consumption has been studied because it has been shown that drinking alcoholic beverages can raise the level of HDL. Research has also shown that the incidence of coronary artery disease is lower among moderate drinkers than it is among the abstinent.[86] However, it is unclear whether it is advisable to begin using alcohol with the hope of producing a health benefit.[87] "Moderate intake" has been defined as up to two drinks per day for men and one for women, with a drink defined as 1 ounce of hard liquor, 4 ounces of wine, or 12 ounces of beer. Excessive alcohol intake can raise blood pressure; injure the brain, heart, and liver; and cause many other problems.

Sterol-enriched margarines (*Benecol* and *Take Control*) can lower LDL cholesterol by 10% to 15%. They work by decreasing intestinal absorption of cholesterol. However, (a) their effect on the rates of death and illness from coronary heart disease is unknown and (b) the beneficial effects of lowering cholesterol might be offset by increased plasma concentrations of plant sterols, which may foster atherosclerosis.[88]

HIGH BLOOD PRESSURE

Blood pressure is the force created by the heart as it pushes blood throughout the circulatory system. High blood pressure (hypertension) is defined as blood pressure that is persistently higher than normal. Hypertension is sometimes called "the silent disease" because it produces no symptoms until it reaches an advanced state. (Actually, atherosclerosis is equally silent.) High blood pressure often is detected during a routine medical visit or a screening program. However, because the level has some natural variability, the diagnosis cannot be established with a single reading; it should be based on the average of two readings at each of two or more medical visits.[89]

About 50 million Americans age 6 and older have high blood pressure. It tends to rise as people get older and is more common among blacks than among whites. When it is caused by kidney disease, a tumor, or another identifiable condition, curing the cause usually will cure the problem. However, in the vast majority of cases, there is no identifiable cause and the condition is called essential hypertension.[90] When blood pressure is high, the heart must work harder than normal to pump blood throughout the body. The strain often causes the heart to enlarge, promotes atherosclerosis, and can interfere with the blood supply to the kidneys, heart, or brain, leading to kidney failure, heart attack, or stroke. Early treatment is important to reduce the likelihood of these complications.

Table 15-7

CLASSIFICATION OF HIGH BLOOD PRESSURE LEVELS

Category	Systolic Pressure	Diastolic Pressure	Recommended Follow-Up
Normal	Less than 130	Less than 85	Recheck in 2 years
High normal	130–139	85–89	Recheck in 1 year
Stage 1 hypertension	140–159	90–99	Confirm within 2 months
Stage 2 hypertension	160–179	100–109	Evaluate within 1 month
Stage 3 hypertension	180–209	110–119	Evaluate within 1 week
Stage 4 hypertension	210 or more	120 or more	Evaluate within 1 week

From *Fifth Report of the Joint National Committee on Detection, Evaluation, and Treatment of High Blood Pressure.*[91]

Risk Factors for Stroke

A stroke occurs when an artery to the brain bursts or becomes clogged by a blood clot or other particle. Deprived of oxygen, nerve cells in the affected area of the brain cannot function and die within minutes, resulting in loss of function in the parts of the body that are controlled by these cells. The primary risk factors for stroke include hereditary predisposition, high blood pressure, heart disease, cigarette smoking, being male, advancing age, and diabetes. Secondary risk factors, which contribute to the development of heart disease, include lack of exercise, excessive alcohol intake, and abnormal blood cholesterol levels.

A healthy lifestyle can lower the incidence of hypertension. Obesity, high alcohol intake, cigarette smoking, physical inactivity, and high sodium intake can contribute to blood pressure elevation. Stamler and colleagues conducted a 5-year study of 201 people with normal blood pressure, 102 of whom who were counseled about these risk factors. When the trial ended, the incidence of hypertension was 8.8% in the intervention group and 19.2% in the control group.[92] A recent meta-analysis concluded that calcium supplementation may lead to a small reduction in systolic but not diastolic blood pressure. The authors recommended that future research address whether inadequate calcium intake increases the risk of developing high blood pressure.[93]

Diagnosis of Hypertension

Blood pressure varies somewhat during the course of a day. It usually is lowest when resting and higher as activity increases. It also can increase when people are nervous about having it tested, a condition referred to as "white-coat hypertension." For this reason it is important to be relaxed when blood pressure readings are taken. Transient elevations usually do not indicate disease or abnormality.

Blood pressure is expressed as a fraction. Systolic pressure, which is the numerator, reflects the pressure (in millimeters of mercury) when the heart contracts. Diastolic pressure, the denominator, reflects the pressure between beats. Table 15-7 summarizes the current classification[91] of blood pressure levels for adults over age 18 and a timetable for following up initial screening tests.

The optimal pressure with respect to cardiovascular risk is below 120 systolic and 80 diastolic. The goals of treatment are diastolic pressure below 90, systolic pressure below 140, and control of other modifiable cardiovascular risk factors.

Nondrug Therapy

For mild hypertension, nondrug treatment should be tried first. The following measures may help:

- *Weight reduction.* Losing weight usually results in some lowering of blood pressure.
- *Smoking cessation.* Cigarette smoking raises blood pressure because nicotine causes arteries to constrict.
- *Increasing exercise.* As noted in Chapter 14, aerobic exercise can lower blood pressure, help people lose weight, and increase HDL. The American College of Sports Medicine states that endurance exercise training will elicit an average reduction of 10 mm Hg for both systolic and diastolic pressure for individuals in the range of 140–180/90–105 mm Hg.[94]
- *Limiting alcohol intake.* Individuals who consume 6 ounces or more of alcohol per day are twice as likely as nondrinkers to have high blood pressure. Hypertensive individuals should drink no more than 2 ounces daily.
- *Reducing sodium intake.* As noted in Chapter 11, some people with high blood pressure will benefit from lowering their sodium intake. The treating physician should provide dietary instructions and a protocol to test this possibility.[95] The *Harvard Heart Letter* states that "most people can lower their daily sodium intake to about 1.5 g/day of sodium by following a diet of 'no added salt' . . . by avoiding fast foods and keeping the salt shaker out of reach."[96]

- *Reducing caffeine intake.* Since caffeine can temporarily raise blood pressure, reducing or eliminating caffeine could be tried.

Consumer Reports states that nearly all hypertensive people can lower their blood pressure to some extent by improving their lifestyle. The benefit depends on how much they change and how high their pressure was to begin with.[97] About 10 years ago, a study involving people with diastolic pressures between 80 and 89 (high normal) found that weight reduction and sodium restriction were effective and that stress management and supplementation with calcium, magnesium, potassium, or fish oil were ineffective in reducing blood pressure.[98] However, the more recent Dietary Assessment to Stop Hypertension (DASH) study has demonstrated that a diet rich in fruits, vegetables, and low-fat dairy products and with reduced saturated and total fat can achieve reductions comparable to the effects of antihypertensive single-drug therapy seen in many treatment trials. The study involved 459 adults with systolic blood pressures of less than 160 mm Hg and diastolic blood pressures of 80 to 95 mm Hg. Among the hypertensive patients, systolic pressure was reduced by an average of 11.4 mm Hg and diastolic pressure was reduced by an average of 5.5 mg Hg.

Thus the DASH diet may represent an alternative to drug therapy for people with Stage 1 hypertension who are willing to comply with the diet.[99] Additional information about the diet is available on the DASH Web site at http://dash.bwu.harvard.edu.

Drug Therapy

If nondrug measures are unable to normalize blood pressure, drug treatment should be used. The most commonly used antihypertensive drugs fall into four categories:

1. Diuretics increase fluid excretion, which reduces blood volume. They are inexpensive.
2. Beta-blockers slow the heartbeat and decrease the force of the heart. Their cost is moderate.
3. Calcium-channel blockers keep arteries from constricting. They are expensive.
4. ACE inhibitors reduce pressure by keeping arteries from constricting. They have the fewest side effects, but are expensive.[100]

The factors influencing the choice of drug include the doctor's preferences, the extent of the problem, the presence of other health problems, the patient's tolerance of the drugs, side effects, and cost. Side effects can include fatigue, headaches, palpitations, dizziness, loss of sexual desire, and other less common symptoms.

Cost varies according to the drug selected, the dosage and frequency used, the availability of a generic version, and the pharmacist's markup. The cost ranges from a few cents a day for generic diuretics to several dollars per day for brand-name ACE inhibitors or calcium-channel blockers. Some people with mild hypertension are able to discontinue medication safely, but most individuals with moderate or severe hypertension should continue taking it for life. Moderate salt-restriction may enhance the response to some antihypertension medications but can cause difficulty with others.[101]

HEART ATTACKS

The American Heart Association estimated that in 2000, 1.1 million Americans would have a heart attack, and about 40% of them would die as a result.[1] About half of heart attack victims die before they reach a hospital. Heart attacks are typically caused by a blood clot that blocks a segment of coronary artery narrowed by atherosclerosis. The resultant lack of blood can cause damage or death to part of the heart muscle, a condition called myocardial infarction. The typical symptoms are:

- Uncomfortable pressure, fullness, squeezing, or pain in the center of the chest that lasts more than a few minutes.
- Pain spreading to the shoulders, neck, jaw, or arms, particularly the left arm.
- Chest discomfort with lightheadedness, sweating, nausea, and/or shortness of breath.

Not all of these warning signs occur in every heart attack. People who experience them, however, should seek help as soon as possible because early medical intervention can often save a person's life and reduce the amount of damage done to the heart. The American Heart Association advises consumers to know what area hospitals provide 24-hour emergency cardiac care and to call an emergency rescue service if the above symptoms of chest discomfort persist for 10 minutes or longer.

Angina pectoris is a condition in which blood supply to the heart is temporarily inadequate to meet the body's needs. It is typically precipitated by exertion. The discomfort of angina can be similar to that of a heart attack but subsides within a few minutes when the individual rests or takes medication (nitroglycerin) that increases the blood supply to the heart. Recurrent attacks of angina indicate that the risk of a heart attack may be high. Medication that dilates coronary arteries often can prevent or reduce the incidence of angina attacks. In properly selected individuals coronary bypass surgery or angioplasty (discussed later in this chapter) is corrective.

Hospital Care

A myocardial infarction is a medical emergency because it can cause an abnormal heart rhythm that results in sudden death. What takes place within the first few hours may make the difference between life and death, or between recovery and disability.

Hospital care for a heart attack has five basic goals: (1) to prevent sudden death, (2) to determine the location and extent of the problem, (3) to minimize damage to the heart muscle, (4) to prevent and treat complications, and (5) to enable the patient to return to as normal a lifestyle as possible. Upon arrival at the hospital the patient is connected to a device that provides a continuous electrocardiogram on an oscillograph screen that staff members monitor. Anticoagulant therapy may be administered to prevent additional blockage from the blood clot. In some cases it is possible to locate and remove the blockage with clot-dissolving medication and/or surgery. To take advantage of new developments, it is advisable to obtain care from an up-to-date cardiologist who practices in a well-equipped hospital.

DIAGNOSTIC TESTS

The tests used to evaluate the structure and function of the heart and its blood supply vary considerably in complexity and cost. A physical examination is likely to include measurement of the pulse, which provides information about the heart's rate and rhythm; percussion (thumping) of the chest, which may indicate whether the heart is enlarged; and listening to the heart with a stethoscope, which can reveal murmurs that signify abnormalities of the heart valves. A chest x-ray can detect abnormal enlargement of the heart, which can have a variety of causes.

Electrocardiogram

The test that is best known and most widely used to examine heart function is the electrocardiogram, commonly referred to as an ECG or EKG. This test, which usually costs from $35 to $50, detects and measures the flow of tiny electrical currents on the heart's surface. The test is usually performed with the patient lying down, with wires (leads) connected from the patient to the device. The device prints a representation of the electrical activity on graph paper so it can be interpreted by a physician (Figure 15-5).

Electrocardiograms are especially useful for diagnosing disturbances of heart rhythm.[102] Enlargement of the heart and heart muscle damage may also be revealed. A normal ECG report does not ensure that the heart is normal. Following a heart attack, for example, it may

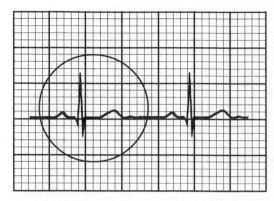

FIGURE 15-5. Normal electrocardiogram. The circled area represents the electrical events related to one heartbeat.

take several hours for abnormal changes to show up on the cardiogram. It is also possible for muscle damage to occur in a part of the heart that a routine ECG procedure does not discern. When a rhythm disturbance is intermittent, a portable device (Holter monitor) that makes a continuous record for at least 24 hours may be needed to demonstrate the abnormality.

Lee and others[103] state: (a) every person with suspected or diagnosed coronary artery disease should have an ECG as part of an initial coronary evaluation, (b) the test is likely to be repeated to determine whether a heart attack occurred between examinations, and (c) how often the test should be done in people without symptoms is controversial. Some physicians worry that routine testing will lead to further testing in people without heart disease, while others argue that a baseline ECG tracing in a person's medical record is useful for comparison if symptoms develop later. Regardless, annual ECGs are not warranted for asymptomatic people.

Stress Testing

A stress test is basically an electrocardiogram performed during gradually escalated exercise. It is useful for detecting unsuspected abnormalities of the heart or to help determine the amount of exercise that can be tolerated by an individual with known heart disease. The exercise usually is performed by walking on a treadmill, although another device such as a stationary bicycle may be used for people who have difficulty walking. Before exercise begins, an ordinary ECG is performed to check for abnormalities and provide a basis for comparison. Blood pressure also is measured beforehand and throughout the procedure.

The strenuousness of the exercise will depend on the individual's health. For those with little or no known impairment, the treadmill speed and elevation will usually be increased until 80% to 90% of the person's maximum heart rate is reached. For individuals with known heart disease, the target rate may be set lower. As exercise increases, the attending physician monitors the subject's blood pressure and electrocardiographic pattern on an oscillograph screen. If chest pain, severe shortness of breath, or certain signs of electrical abnormality appear on the screen, the test is stopped.

A stress test is not appropriate for routine use for people who feel well, because it costs about $300 and can yield false-positive results that trigger even greater expense and intrusive follow-up testing.[28] Testing is likely to be appropriate under the following circumstances:

- Following a heart attack or heart surgery; used to help determine the prognosis and an appropriate heart-strengthening exercise program.
- Sedentary individual aged 40 or more planning to start an exercise program more intense than walking at 50% to 60% of maximum heart rate.[104] However, a gradual and sensible exercise program outlined by a physician is a reasonable alternative.[105] Testing could then be done if symptoms such as chest discomfort or lightheadedness develop.
- People (such as airline pilots) whose health is crucial to the safety of others.
- Coronary occlusion or other evidence of coronary heart disease before the age of 55 in a close blood relative.
- Cigarette smoking, high blood pressure, diabetes, or obesity.
- Chest pain or other symptoms of coronary artery disease during exertion.

Some people who do not develop symptoms but have an abnormal electrocardiogram during a stress test need additional testing to clarify whether they have coronary artery disease. These individuals may be advised to undergo a thallium stress test, a procedure in which radioactive thallium is injected into an arm vein shortly before the end of the exercise period. A scanning procedure is then used to map the distribution of blood to the heart. This test is far more accurate than ordinary stress testing but costs three to five times as much. A thallium stress test may also be used to measure blood flow to the heart following a cardiac rehabilitation program.

A stress test entails slight risk. *The Johns Hopkins Medical Letter*[106] states that the risk of triggering a heart attack is less than 1 in 500, while the risk of dying is less than 1 in 10,000. For this reason, a stress test should be performed in a facility equipped to handle any emergency that may arise, and a physician and at least one technician trained in advanced life support should be present.

Coronary Angiography
Coronary angiography is used to evaluate blood flow to the heart and visualize the location of narrowed or blocked coronary arteries. It is more accurate than a stress test, but it is more expensive and entails a slightly higher risk of provoking a heart attack. The first step, called catheterization, involves passing a small hollow plastic tube (catheter) through the large artery in the groin (femoral artery) or the forearm (brachial artery). The cardiologist anesthetizes the skin over the artery and makes a small incision with a scalpel. Then the catheter is inserted into the artery and threaded through arteries until it reaches the openings of the coronary arteries inside the aorta (the main artery emerging from the heart). The patient may feel some pulling or transient pain when the catheter is inserted into the artery, but the rest of the procedure generally produces no discomfort. When the catheter is in place, an opaque dye is injected into the coronary arteries, enabling the pattern of blood flow to the heart muscle to be visualized. The cardiologist observes the flow with a fluoroscope, and x-ray films are taken throughout the procedure. Coronary angiography typically costs from $2000 to $3500, depending partly on whether it is done on an inpatient or outpatient basis. The American Heart Association estimates that 1,194,000 such procedures were performed in 1997.[1]

Ultrafast Computed Tomography
Ultrafast CT scanning combines electrocardiography with CT scanning so that the heart is imaged only during a particular moment within each cycle of the heartbeat. The resultant images show whether the coronary arteries contain calcium deposits that mark the presence of atherosclerosis.[107] Further testing—usually angiography—might then be performed to pinpoint the extent of disease. If an ultrafast CT scan is negative, the individual has a low probability of having coronary artery disease. However, the test is expensive, not covered by insurance, and produces many false-positive tests that can lead to further unnecessary expense. For this reason the American Heart Association does not recommend routine use in people without heart-related symptoms unless standard cardiac risk assessment is considered insufficient. It may be appropriate for individuals who are anxious to know with a high degree of certainty the state of their coronary arteries and who are willing to undergo a potentially unnecessary catheterization to get that information.[108]

Other Tests
Echocardiography uses ultrasound waves to visualize the heart. It is used to gather information about the functioning of heart valves and the structure and functioning of the heart muscle.[109] Images are observed on a

screen and photographed for later study. Information about the structure and function of the heart valves can also be obtained during coronary angiography.

Echo stress testing combines echocardiography and stress testing in order to detect less-than-normal contraction of heart muscle related to lack of coronary artery circulation to part of the heart. Much research is being done on magnetic resonance imaging (MRI), ultrafast computed tomography, and other imaging procedures for evaluating cardiac function (See Chapter 5 for further information on imaging tests.)

SURGERY TO RESTORE BLOOD FLOW

The heart normally receives its blood supply from the coronary arteries, which connect from the aorta to the heart muscle. If these become clogged near their origin but are open beyond that point, it may be possible to restore the blood supply with a surgical procedure.

Coronary Bypass

In coronary bypass surgery (also referred to as coronary artery bypass graft surgery, or "CABG"), one or more grafts are connected from the aorta to the unblocked portions of the coronary arteries. The grafts are obtained from the patient's mammary artery (which supplies a portion of the chest wall but is not vital to the area) and/or saphenous veins, which serve the lower part of each leg. During the operation, the patient's heart is stopped so the grafts can be sewn in place while circulation is maintained by a heart-lung machine. If no complications occur, most patients will be discharged from the hospital within 1 week and recuperate at home for a few months.

CABG can provide dramatic relief for many people with angina and may also be used to restore blood flow following coronary thrombosis. In 1995, the average cost of a hospital stay that included bypass surgery typically was about $45,000. A 1991 report covering 3055 patients at five medical centers stated that the in-hospital mortality rate for CABG was 3.2% for men and 7.3% for women.[110] Current mortality rates are lower.

In properly selected patients, CABG can prolong life, particularly for those able to reduce their risk factors.[111] Researchers who examined 1974-1991 data on 8221 American bypass patients found that average 5-, 10-, and 15-year survival rates after CABG were 90%, 74%, and 56%, respectively. Of those who underwent bypass surgery at or over 75 years of age, 59% were

---

☑ **Consumer Tip**

Advice to Consumers

Atherosclerosis and high blood pressure develop silently for many years before causing trouble. The difficulty they cause can be prevented or minimized by the following actions:

1. Know the risk factors for atherosclerosis and hypertension and take steps to minimize them. Figure 15-1 provides a convenient summary and checklist for evaluating the status of your risk factors.
2. Do not smoke cigarettes. Smokers develop a much higher incidence of heart disease, stroke, and many cancers.
3. Maintain reasonable weight. Be particularly concerned about developing fatty deposits around the waist (see discussion of waist-hip ratio in Chapter 13).
4. Follow the dietary guidelines in Chapter 11. Eat a balanced diet that is low in fat, particularly saturated fat, adequate in fiber, and moderate in sodium. This will not only help prevent cardiovascular disease but also may help prevent certain cancers.
5. Engage in regular aerobic exercise as outlined in Chapter 14. Exercise can lower total cholesterol and LDL and raise HDL.
6. Have your blood pressure checked at least once a year and take appropriate action if it becomes elevated.
7. Know your "cholesterol number." Have your level checked through a doctor's office and take appropriate action according to the protocols of the National Cholesterol Education Program. If your cholesterol level is high or borderline high, seek expert guidance from a physician who maintains an interest in this subject and pays close attention to recent developments. Usually this can be determined by asking about the physician's level of interest.
8. Do not consume unproven dietary supplements such as fish oil or beta-carotene, but eat fish once or twice a week and have adequate amounts of fruits, vegetables, and whole-grain foods in your diet.
9. If you develop significant cardiovascular disease, seek help from a cardiologist.
10 If you require an invasive diagnostic procedure (such as angiography) or cardiac surgery, select a cardiologist or surgeon who has had adequate experience and works in an up-to-date hospital facility.

still living 10 years after their procedure, while 33% survived for more than 15 years.[112] The researchers concluded that these figures suggest survival exceeding the matched U.S. population. However, there is still controversy over whether the operation is advantageous for people with coronary artery disease who have mild symptoms controllable with drug therapy.[113] Additional studies are needed to answer this question.

Chelation therapy is promoted as an alternative to bypass surgery, although there is no evidence that it is effective (see Chapter 8). Some chelationists even advertise that people advised to undergo bypass surgery should have chelation therapy instead. This advice is extremely dangerous.

Angioplasty

In recent years there has been extraordinary progress in the development of instruments and procedures that can unclog arteries from within. The most widely applicable of these procedures is balloon angioplasty, the medical term for which is percutaneous transluminal coronary angioplasty (PTCA.)[103] In this procedure a very thin wire is placed into the femoral artery in the thigh and threaded into a coronary artery, while the cardiologist watches the wire's progress on an x-ray monitor. Then a guide catheter, a flexible tube whose diameter is about the thickness of a pencil, is passed over the wire and a second catheter tipped with a deflated balloon is threaded through the guide catheter. When the balloon reaches the blockage, it is inflated to compress atherosclerotic plaque against the inner artery walls. The balloon is then deflated and withdrawn together with the guide wire and catheter.

Other angioplasty tools include motorized devices that shave, drill, or pulverize plaque, and laser devices that vaporize it.[114] In some cases a small tube (stent) is left within the artery to maintain the opening. Angioplasty is also used to open arteries in the kidneys, arms, and legs.

In many cases angioplasty provides an alternative to coronary bypass surgery.[113] It costs much less, requires a shorter hospital stay, and has a short recovery period, but it has a much higher likelihood of reclogging. (The restenosis rate for angioplasty is 20% to 45%.) In 1997 a research team reported on 1829 patients with severe coronary artery disease who were randomly assigned to either CABG or PCTA and then followed for about 5 years. The survival rates were similar, but the CABG group tended to have less angina, tended to use less medication, and were much more likely to require another procedure to restore circulation.[115] After 7 years,

CABG provided a much higher survival rate for diabetics but not for patients without diabetes.[116]

The use of bypass surgery and angioplasty has been rising rapidly. About 607,000 bypass operations and 447,000 angioplasties were performed during 1997.[1] Questions have been raised about whether these procedures are performed too often, but there are no simple answers.[117,118] Although several organizations have developed general guidelines, considerably more research is needed to clarify what is most appropriate in individual cases.

REHABILITATION PROGRAMS

After cardiac surgery or recovery from a heart attack, it is important to take steps to restore function and prevent recurrence. Lack of activity, lack of sleep, medication, the surgery itself, and the stress of being ill can leave patients feeling drained, physically and emotionally. Many hospitals and clinics have established programs to help restore the ability to function. These programs provide gradually escalated exercise, dietary counseling, and attention to the individual's risk factors.[119] A cardiologist performs a stress test to determine the individual's exercise tolerance and prescribes an exercise program.[120] Then the exercise is done several times a week while the patient is monitored by a specially trained nurse. The patient wears a device that broadcasts an electrocardiogram to an oscillograph observed by the nurse. If the patient's pulse rises too high or the ECG shows signs that the heart is straining, the patient is advised to slow down or stop. Patients are taught how to monitor their pulse and have the opportunity to use many types of exercise equipment. Most programs involve three sessions a week for 12 weeks. After that, if all goes well, the patient has learned how to perform heart-strengthening aerobic exercise and will continue a home program indefinitely.

SUMMARY

Cardiovascular diseases are the leading cause of illness and death in the United States. The majority of cases stem from atherosclerosis, a condition in which cholesterol, fat, and fibrous tissue build up in the walls of large and medium-sized arteries. The important risk factors for coronary heart disease include hereditary predisposition (a family history of premature heart disease), being male, advancing age, cigarette smoking, high blood pressure, diabetes, obesity, lack of physical activity, and abnormal blood cholesterol and homo-

It's Your Decision

At your doctor's suggestion, you have a lipid analysis, which shows an LDL level of 135 and an HDL of 40. The doctor says that these levels suggest that your risk of a heart attack is above average. What actions should you consider?

cysteine levels. The more risk factors a person has, the greater the risk of developing heart disease. Heredity, gender, and age cannot be controlled, but the other risk factors can be influenced by the individual's behavior.

Medical authorities recommend that all adults have their blood cholesterol and blood pressure checked and take action if abnormal elevations are found. The cornerstone of a cholesterol-reduction program is a balanced, low-fat, high-fiber diet plus regular aerobic exercise. These measures may also be effective in lowering high blood pressure. If nondrug methods are insufficient, drug therapy may be advisable—often on a lifetime basis.

Great progress has been made in both medical and surgical treatment of cardiovascular disease. More research is needed to evaluate newer techniques. If problems arise, expert guidance should be sought from a physician who is well trained and pays close attention to recent developments.

REFERENCES

1. American Heart Association. 2000 Heart and Stroke Statistical Update. Dallas, 1999, The Association.
2. American Heart Association. Silent epidemic: The truth about women and heart disease. Dallas, 1989, The Association.
3. Steenland K. Passive smoking and the risk of heart disease. JAMA 267:94–99, 1992.
4. Willett WC and others. Coffee consumption and coronary heart disease in women: A ten-year follow-up. JAMA 275:458–462, 1996.
5. Triglycerides and heart disease. Harvard Heart Letter 11(1):1–5, 2000.
6. Multiple Risk Factor Intervention Trial Research Group. Mortality rates after 10.5 years for participants in the Multiple Risk Factor Intervention Trial. JAMA 263:1795–1801, 1990.
7. Castelli WP and others. Incidence of coronary heart disease and lipoprotein cholesterol levels—the Framingham Study. JAMA 256:2835–2838, 1986.
8. Anderson KM and others. Cholesterol and mortality: 30 years of follow-up from the Framingham Study. JAMA 257:2176–2180, 1987.
9. Samuelson O and others. Cardiovascular morbidity in relation to change in blood pressure and serum cholesterol levels in treated hypertension. JAMA 258:1768–1776, 1987.
10. Gotto AM Jr and others. The cholesterol facts—a joint statement by the American Heart Association and the National Heart, Lung, and Blood Institute. Dallas, 1990, American Heart Association.
11. Lipid Clinics Research Program. The Lipid Research Clinics Coronary Primary Prevention Trial results. I. Reduction in incidence of coronary artery disease. II. The relationship of reduction in incidence of coronary heart disease to cholesterol lowering. JAMA 251:351–374, 1984.
12. Rader DJ, Brewer HB. Lipoprotein(a): Clinical approach to a unique atherogenic lipoprotein. JAMA 267:1109–1112, 1992.
13. Schaefer EJ. Lipoprotein(a) levels and risk of coronary heart disease in men. JAMA 271:999–1003, 1994.
14. Gurewich V, Mittleman M. Lipoprotein(a) in coronary disease: Is it a risk factor after all? JAMA 271:1025–1026, 1994.
15. Ridker PM and others. A prospective study of lipoprotein(a) and the risk of myocardial infarction. JAMA 270:2195–2199, 1993.
16. Bostom AG and others. Elevated plasma lipoprotein(a) and coronary heart disease in men aged 55 years and younger. JAMA 276:544–548, 1996.
17. Maher VM and others. Effects of lowering elevated LDL cholesterol on the cardiovascular risk of lipoprotein(a). JAMA 274:1771–1774, 1995.
18. Ridker PM and others. Plasma concentration of lipoprotein(a) and the risk of future stroke. JAMA 273:1269–1273, 1995.
19. Boushey CJ and others. A quantitative assessment of plasma homocysteine as a risk factor for vascular disease: Probable benefits of increasing folic acid intakes. JAMA 274:1049–1057, 1995.
20. Morrison HI and others. Serum folate and risk of fatal coronary heart disease. JAMA 275:1983–1896, 1996.
21. Stampfer M, Nalinow MR. Can lowering homocysteine levels reduce cardiovascular risk? New England Journal of Medicine 332:328–329, 1995.
22. Grundy SM and others. Summary of the second report of the National Cholesterol Education Program (NCEP) expert panel on detection, evaluation, and treatment of high blood cholesterol in adults. JAMA 269:3015–3023, 1993.
23. Johnson CL and others. Declining serum cholesterol levels among U.S. adults: The National Health and Nutrition Examination Surveys. JAMA 269:3002–3008, 1993.
24. Sempos CT and others. Prevalence of high blood cholesterol among US adults. JAMA 269:3009–3014, 1993.
25. National Institutes of Health. Report of the expert panel on blood cholesterol levels in children and adolescents. Bethesda, Md., 1991, The Institutes.
26. Barnard RJ. Effects of life-style modification on serum lipids. Archives of Internal Medicine 151:1389–1394, 1991.
27. Mirkin G, Rich D. Fat Free, Flavor Full. Boston, 1995, Little, Brown and Company.
28. Heinz A. Facts and myths about coronary artery disease—a consumer guide. New York, 1989, American Council on Science and Health.
29. U.S Preventive Services Task Force. Guide to Clinical Preventive Services, 2nd edition. Baltimore, 1996, Williams & Wilkins.
30. Garber AM and others. Guidelines for using serum cholesterol, high-density lipoprotein cholesterol, and triglyceride levels as screening tests for preventing coronary heart disease in adults. Annals of Internal Medicine 124:515–517, 1996.
31. Grundy S and others. Cholesterol screening in adults: No cause to change. Circulation 93:1067–1068, 1996.
32. LaRosa JC. Cholesterol agonistics. Annals of Internal Medicine 124:505–508, 1996.

33. A woman's heart. Harvard Heart Letter 17(6):5–7, 1992.

34. Denke MA, Winker MA. Cholesterol and coronary heart disease in older adults: No easy answers. JAMA 274:575–577, 1995.

35. Newman B, Hulley SB. Carcinogenicity of lipid-lowering drugs. JAMA 275:55–60, 1996.

36. Dalen JE, Dalton WS. Does cholesterol lowering cause cancer? JAMA 275:67–68, 1996.

37. Cooper GR and others. Blood lipid measurements: Variations and practical utility. JAMA 267:1652–1660, 1992.

38. What's your cholesterol? You need to understand your cholesterol profile to know what to do about it. Consumer Reports on Health 3:81–83, 1991.

39. Lichtenstein AH. Trans fatty acids, plasma lipid levels, and risk of developing cardiovascular disease: A statement for health professionals. Circulation 95:2588–2590, 1997.

40. Food labeling: Trans fatty acids in nutrition labeling, nutrient content claims, and health claims; Proposed rule. Federal Register 64: 62745–62825, 1999.

41. Rimm EB and others. Vegetable, fruit, and cereal fiber intake and risk of coronary heart disease among men. JAMA 275:447–451, 1996.

42. Gillman MW and others. Protective effects of fruits and vegetables on development of stroke in men. JAMA 273:1113–1117, 1995.

43. Step By Step: Eating to Lower Your High Blood Cholesterol. NIH publication no. 94-2920. Washington, D.C., 1994, Supt. of Documents.

44. Kraus RM and others. AHA dietary guidelines, revision 2000: A statement for healthcare professionals from the Nutrition Committee of the American Heart Association. Circulation 102:2284–2299, 2000.

45. Barrett S, Kantor MA. Tips for lowering your dietary fat content. Quackwatch Web site, March 31, 2000.

46. USDA Food composition data. USDA Nutrient Data Laboratory Web site, accessed Feb 17, 2000.

47. Kantor MA. Nutrition, cholesterol and heart disease. Part V. Dietary modification. Nutrition Forum 6:33–37, 1989.

48. Anderson JW and others. Hypocholesterolemic effects of oat-bran or bean intake for hypercholesterolemic men. American Journal of Clinical Nutrition 40:1146–1155, 1984.

49. Bell LP and others. Cholesterol-lowering effects of psyllium hydrophilic mucilloid—adjunct therapy to a prudent diet for patients with mild to moderate hypercholesterolemia. JAMA 261:3419–3423, 1989.

50. Rimm EB and others. Vegetable, fruit, and cereal fiber intake and risk of coronary heart disease among men. JAMA 273:447–451, 1995.

51. Wolk A and others. Long-term intake of dietary fiber and decreased risk of coronary heart disease among women. JAMA 281:1998–2004, 1999.

52. Gillman MW and others. Protective effect of fruits and vegetables on development of stroke in men. JAMA 273:1113–1117, 1995.

53. Joshipura KJ and others. Fruit and vegetable intake in relation to risk of stroke. JAMA 282:1233–1239, 1999.

54. Ripsin CM. Oat products and lipid lowering: A meta-analysis. JAMA 267:3317–3325, 1992.

55. Davidson MH and others. The hypocholesterolemic effects of β-glucan in oatmeal and oat bran. JAMA 265:1833–1839, 1991.

56. Milani RV, Lavie CJ. Pharmacologic prevention of coronary artery disease. What do clinical trials show? Postgraduate Medicine 99:109–120, 1996.

57. Gotto AM Jr. Lipid lowering, regression, and coronary events: A review of the interdisciplinary Council on Lipids and Cardiovascular Risk Intervention, Seventh Council Meeting. Circulation 92:646–656, 1995.

58. Scandinavian Simvastatin Survival Study Group. Randomised trial of cholesterol lowering in 4444 patients with coronary heart disease: The Scandinavian Simvastatin Survival Study (4). Lancet 344:1383–1389, 1994.

59. Scandinavian Simvastatin Survival Study Group. Baseline serum cholesterol and treatment effect in the Scandinavian Simvastatin Survival Study (4S). Lancet 345:1274–1275, 1995.

60. Byington RP and others. Reduction in cardiovascular events during pravastatin therapy. Pooled analysis of clinical events of the Pravastatin Atherosclerosis Intervention Program. Circulation 92:2419–2925, 1995.

61. Gould AL and others. Cholesterol reduction yields clinical benefit: A new look at old data. Circulation 91:2274–2282, 1995.

62. Ornish D and others. Can lifestyle changes reverse coronary heart disease? Lancet 336:129–133, 1990.

63. Gould KL, Ornish D and others. Improved stenosis geometry by quantitative coronary arteriography after vigorous risk factor modification. American Journal of Cardiology 69:845–853, 1992.

64. Gould KL, Ornish D and others. Changes in myocardial perfusion abnormalities by positron emission tomography after long-term, intense risk factor modification. JAMA 274:894–901, 1995.

65. Ornish D and others. Intensive lifestyle changes for reversal of coronary heart disease. JAMA 280:2001–2007, 1998.

66. Pritikin R. The new Pritikin Program: The easy and delicious way to shed fat, lower your cholesterol, and stay fit. New York, 1990, Simon & Schuster.

67. New York City Department of Consumer Affairs. Supermarket Survey on Misleading Cholesterol Claims. New York, 1991, The Department.

68. Choice of lipid-lowering drugs. The Medical Letter 38:117–122, 1998.

69. Hodes HN. Acute hepatic failure associated with low-dose sustained-release niacin. JAMA 264:181, 1990.

70. Henkin Y. Rechallenge with crystalline niacin after drug-induced hepatitis from sustained-release niacin. JAMA 264:241–243, 1990.

71. Etchason JA and others. Niacin-induced hepatitis: A potential side effect with low-dose time-release niacin. Mayo Clinic Proceedings 66:23–28, 1991.

72. McKenney JM and others. A comparison of the efficacy and toxic effects of sustained- vs immediate-release niacin in hypercholesterolemic patients. JAMA 271:672–677, 1994.

73. Antiplatelet Trialists' Collaboration. Collaborative overview of randomised trials of antiplatelet therapy. British Medical Journal 308:81–106, 159–168, 235–246, 1994.

74. Hennekens CH and others. Aspirin as a therapeutic agent in cardiovascular disease: A statement for healthcare professionals from the American Heart Association. Circulation 96:2751–2753, 1997.

75. A vitamin cocktail for cholesterol? Consumer Reports 55:141, 1990.

76. Goldfinger SE. Good for what ails you? Harvard Health Letter 16(10):1–2, 1991.

77. Kushi LH and others. Dietary antioxidant vitamins and death from coronary heart disease in postmenopausal women. 334:1156–1162, 1996.

78. The Heart Outcomes Prevention Evaluation Study Investigators. Vitamin E supplementation and cardiovascular events in high-risk patients. New England Journal of Medicine 342:145–153, 2000.

79. Hennekens CH and others. Lack of effect of long-term supplementation with beta carotene on the incidence of malignant neoplasms and cardiovascular disease. New England Journal of Medicine 334:1145–1149, 1996.

80. Knuiman A and others. Lecithin intake and serum cholesterol. American Journal of Clinical Nutrition 49:266–268, 1989.

81. Coenzyme Q_{10}: the next aspirin? Harvard Heart Letter 6(6):5–7, 1996.

82. Kwiterovich P. Beyond Cholesterol: The Johns Hopkins Complete Guide for Avoiding Heart Disease. Baltimore, 1989, The Johns Hopkins University Press.

83. Siscovick DS and others. Dietary intake and cell membrane levels of long-chain n-3 polyunsaturated fatty acids and the risk of primary cardiac arrest. JAMA 274:1363–1367, 1995.

84. Ascherio A and others. Dietary intake of marine n–3 fatty acids, fish intake, and the risk of coronary disease among men. New England Journal of Medicine 332:977–982, 1995.

85. Southwestern News, University of Texas Southwestern Medical Center, Jan 2, 1997.

86. Gaziano JM and others. Moderate alcohol intake, increased levels of high-density lipoprotein and its subfractions, and decreased risk of myocardial infarction. New England Journal of Medicine 329:1829–1834, 1993.

87. Friedman GD, Klatsky AL. Is alcohol good for your health? New England Journal of Medicine 329:1882–1883, 1993.

88. Cholesterol-lowering margarines. The Medical Letter 41:56–58, 1999.

89. Reeves RA. Does this patient have hypertension? How to measure blood pressure. JAMA 273:1211–1218, 1995.

90. Farley D. High blood pressure: Controlling the silent killer. FDA Consumer 25(10):28–33, 1991.

91. Gifford RW and others. Fifth Report of the Joint National Committee on Detection, Evaluation, and Treatment of High Blood Pressure. Bethesda, Md., 1993, National Institutes of Health.

92. Stamler R and others. Primary prevention of hypertension by nutritional-hygienic means. Final report of a randomized, controlled trial. JAMA 262:1801–1807, 1989.

93. Bucher HC and others. Effects of dietary calcium supplementation on blood pressure: A meta-analysis of randomized controlled trials. JAMA 275:1016–1022, 1996.

94. American College of Sports Medicine position stand: Physical activity, physical fitness, and hypertension. Medical Science of Sports and Exercise 25(10):i–x, 1993.

95. Weinberger MH and others. Dietary sodium restriction as adjunctive treatment of hypertension. JAMA 259:2561–2565, 1988.

96. Lowering blood pressure without drugs. Harvard Heart Letter 2(9):1–5, 1992.

97. How to lower blood pressure. Consumer Reports 57:300–302, 1992.

98. Hypertension Prevention Collaborative Research Group. The effects of nonpharmacologic interventions on blood pressure of persons with high normal levels. JAMA 267:1213–1220, 1992.

99. Appel LJ and others. A clinical trial of the effects of dietary patterns on blood pressure. DASH Collaborative Research Group. New England Journal of Medicine 336:1117–1124, 1997.

100. ACE inhibitors for hypertension. Harvard Heart Letter 2(6):5–8, 1992.

101. Muntzel M, Drëeke T. A comprehensive review of the salt and blood pressure relationship. American Journal of Hypertension 5:1S–42S, 1992.

102. When the electrocardiogram is abnormal. Harvard Heart Letter 5(3):1–5, 1994.

103. Lee TH and others. Coronary Artery Disease: Diagnosis and Treatment. Boston, 1994, Harvard Publications Group.

104. Fletcher GF and others. Exercise standards: A statement for healthcare professionals from the American Heart Association. Circulation 91:580–615, 1995.

105. Stress tests: Who needs them? Harvard Heart Letter 1(1):1–4, 1990.

106. What is an exercise stress test? The Johns Hopkins Medical Letter 3(10):6–7, 1991.

107. Budoff MJ and others. Ultrafast computed tomography as a diagnostic modality in the detection of coronary artery disease: A multicenter study. Circulation 93:989–904, 1996.

108. O'Rourke RA and others. American College of Cardiology/ American Heart Association expert consensus document on electron-beam computed tomography for the diagnosis and prognosis of coronary artery disease. Circulation 102:126–140, 2000.

109. Feigenbaum H and others. Tracking the advances in echocardiography. Patient Care, pp 14–45, Mar 15, 1991.

110. O'Connor GT and others. A regional prospective study of in-hospital mortality associated with coronary artery bypass grafting. JAMA 266:803–809, 1991.

111. Coronary artery bypass surgery today, Harvard Heart Letter 2(7):1–7, 1992.

112. Myers WO and others. CASS Registry long term surgical survival. Coronary Artery Surgery Study. Journal of the American College of Cardiology 33:488–498, 1999.

113. Bypass surgery. Who really needs it? Consumer Reports on Health 4(7):49–52, 1992.

114. Farley D. Balloons, lasers and scrapers: Help for hearts and blood vessels. FDA Consumer 25(3):22–27, 1991.

115. Writing Group for the Bypass Angioplasty Revascularization Investigation (BARI) Investigators. Five-year clinical and functional outcome comparing bypass surgery and angioplasty in patients with multivessel coronary disease. A multicenter randomized trial. JAMA 277:715–721, 1997.

116. Seven-year outcome in the Bypass Angioplasty Revascularization Investigation (BARI) by treatment and diabetic status. Journal of the American College of Cardiology 35:1122–1129, 2000.

117. Bypass surgery: Making the right choice. The Johns Hopkins Health Letter 3(11):4–5, 1992.

118. Pfeiffer N. The great cardiology debate: Angioplasty. Medical World News, pp 28–30, Jan 1992.

119. Zoler ML. Rehabilitation—a boon of the thrombolytic era. Medical World News, pp 35–44, March 13, 1989.

120. American College of Sports Medicine position stand: Exercise for patients with coronary artery disease. Medical Science of Sports and Exercise 26(3):i–v, 1994.

ARTHRITIS AND RELATED DISORDERS

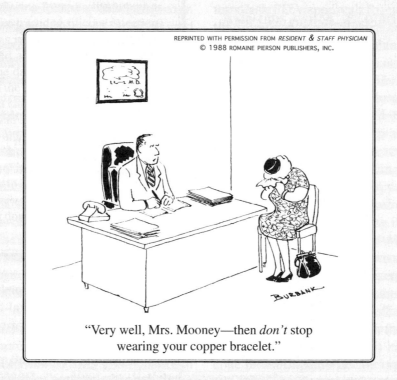

"Very well, Mrs. Mooney—then *don't* stop
wearing your copper bracelet."

*For some curious reason, the idea lingers that "nothing can be
done for arthritis." The very opposite is true. Probably more
progress has been made in the fight against arthritis than in the
struggle against our other major diseases—cancer, heart disease,
and diabetes.*

JAMES F. FRIES, M.D.[1]

*One of the most striking features of most forms of arthritis is
their characteristic flares and periods of lesser disease
activity.... Patients engaging in alternative treatments frequently
do not understand that a "miraculous cure" may simply be a
spontaneous remission.*

FELIX FERNANDEZ-MADRID, M.D., PH.D.[2]

*A*rthritis means "inflammation of a joint." (Joints are the places where bones meet.) "Rheumatic disease," commonly called *rheumatism*, refers to pain and stiffness of joints, muscles, or fibrous tissues. These catch-all terms are used interchangeably for any type of joint disorder, even though some types of rheumatic disease do not affect the joints. There are more than 100 types of arthritis, many of which cause considerable suffering and expense. Regardless of the type, early diagnosis and treatment are likely to produce the most favorable results. Since arthritis is usually a chronic condition, many people with arthritis turn to quackery because of fear, loss of hope, inadequate information, and other psychosocial factors. This chapter focuses on the most common forms of rheumatic disease, how they are treated properly and improperly, and sources of reliable information.

TYPES OF ARTHRITIS

Researchers at the U.S. Centers for Disease Control and Prevention have estimated that nearly 43 million Americans suffered from arthritis in 1998[3] and that this number would grow to nearly 60 million by the year 2020.[4] Some forms are short-lived and curable, whereas others are chronic. The most common forms of chronic arthritis are osteoarthritis, rheumatoid arthritis, ankylosing spondylitis, and gout.[5]

Osteoarthritis, the most widespread type of arthritis, is a degenerative disease of the joints. Although sometimes capable of causing acute inflammation, it is most commonly a "wear-and-tear" disease involving degeneration of joint cartilage and formation of bony spurs within various joints. Trauma to the joints, repetitive occupational usage, and obesity are risk factors. (Pneumatic drill operators and baseball pitchers, for example, are prone to develop osteoarthritis of the shoulder and elbow.) Most people over 60 years of age have this affliction to some extent, with approximately 16 million sufferers requiring medical care. The main goal of treatment is to relieve pain.

Rheumatoid arthritis is an inflammatory disease that involves episodes of pain and swelling, and in some cases deformity and "freezing" of joints, especially the knuckles and middle joints of the fingers. About 2.1 million Americans are afflicted. The disease usually starts between the ages of 20 and 45, affecting about three times as many women as men, but it can occur at any age. Juvenile rheumatoid arthritis, a similar condition, affects about 250,000 children and adolescents. The goals of treatment are to reduce pain and inflammation, maintain joint mobility, and prevent deformity. Figure 16-1 shows the anatomy of a joint and the changes that take place with osteoarthritis and rheumatoid arthritis.

Ankylosing spondylitis, a hereditary condition, is a chronic inflammatory disease of the spine that can also attack the hips and shoulders. About 300,000 Americans have this condition. It affects men considerably more often than women, usually starting in adolescence or the early 20s. As it progresses, calcium is laid down within the joints of the spine, resulting in stiffness, rigidity, and sometimes deformity of the back. The main goals of treatment are maintenance of spinal mobility and retention of muscle strength. Although their most obvious manifestations are on joints, both rheumatoid arthritis and ankylosing spondylitis are systemic diseases and can affect other organs.

Gout is a metabolic disorder that affects about 1 million Americans, the majority of whom are men. The inflammation of acute gout commonly strikes the big toe, causing pain and swelling, but it can also begin in the knee, ankle, or another joint. In chronic gout a buildup of uric acid crystals in various joints can result in disfigurement and disability. Gout's course can vary from a few attacks to a progressive disease that begins at puberty and, if untreated, can be disabling by the age of 40. Effective treatment can relieve or prevent attacks and virtually eliminate the risk of permanent disability.

Fibromyalgia, a form of muscular rheumatism, is discussed in the Personal Glimpse box on the next page.

SCIENTIFIC TREATMENT METHODS

Most patients with chronic forms of arthritis can be helped to lead a productive life if their condition is properly diagnosed and treated before too many irreversible changes occur. In many cases treatment can help relieve the discomfort and maintain or restore joint function. Medications for gout control the abnormal metabolism of uric acid. For the other conditions discussed previously, the treatment can include drugs, rest, exercise, physical therapy, surgery, and various adaptive devices. In obese individuals weight loss is important to reduce further strain on the joints.

Oral Drugs

Medications can be used to relieve pain and counter inflammation. Finding the best one can be a process of trial and error. Generally the safest drugs that are likely to help are tried first. Several drugs may be evaluated in varying doses until the best one is found. The factors to consider are the type of arthritis, stage of the disease, potential benefits and side effects, and cost.

The first lines of pharmacologic defense against inflammation are the nonsteroidal anti-inflammatory drugs (NSAIDs), of which aspirin is the prototype. These drugs can reduce but do not eliminate the signs and symptoms of arthritis. They can relieve pain soon after absorption into the body but have no major effect on the underlying disease process. The other NSAIDs include ibuprofen (*Motrin*), naproxen (*Naprosyn* and *Naprelan*), and about 20 others. In appropriate dosage, they are comparable to aspirin in anti-inflammatory effect. For some patients the side effects seem milder than those from high doses of aspirin—although they can include serious gastrointestinal conditions such as bleeding and stomach perforation. The other NSAIDs are far more expensive than aspirin, and all but ibuprofen (marketed as *Advil* and others), naproxen *(Aleve),* and ketoprofen *(Actron)* require a doctor's prescription. Celecoxib (*Celebrex*) and rofecoxib (*Vioxx*) are newer prescription drugs called cycloxygenase-2 (Cox-2) inhibitors. These work like NSAIDs but have fewer adverse effects and are more expensive.

NSAIDs are considered the safest drugs for long-term treatment of rheumatoid arthritis. In many cases they can control the symptoms while the disease process

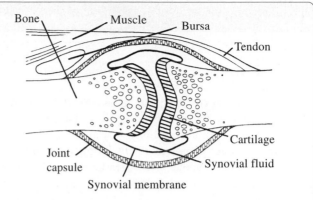

In the normal joint, muscles, bursae and tendons provide support and help bones move. The entire joint is enclosed in a capsule. An inner lining (synovial membrane) releases a slippery fluid into the space between the two bones. The ends of the bones are covered by cartilage, which acts as a shock absorber and keeps bones from rubbing together when the joint moves.

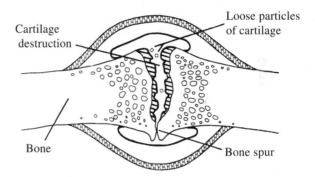

In osteoarthritis, cartilage that cushions the surface of joints breaks down. This causes bones to rub together. The joint loses its shape and alignment. Bone ends thicken and form bony growths called spurs. Bits of cartilage or bone float in the joint space. These changes result in pain and loss of movement.

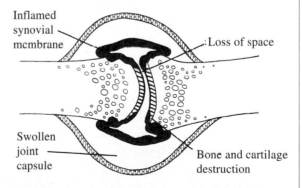

In rheumatoid arthritis a reaction by the body's immune system results in inflammation and thickening of the joint lining (synovial membrane). The whole joint appears swollen. The inflamed joint lining invades and damages bone and cartilage. Inflammatory cells release an enzyme that gradually digests bone and cartilage. The joint loses its shape and alignment. These changes result in pain, loss of movement, and eventually complete destruction of the joint.

FIGURE 16-1. Normal and arthritic joints.
Source: Arthritis Foundation

◆ Personal Glimpse ◆

A Recently Recognized Disease[6-10]

Fibromyalgia is a chronic condition that afflicts an estimated 5 million Americans, most of them women between the ages of 20 and 50. It has three distinguishing characteristics: (1) aching, soreness, or burning pain in muscles throughout the body; (2) an abnormal sleep pattern, often accompanied by fatigue and morning stiffness; and (3) undue muscle tenderness at 11 or more of the 18 "tender points" depicted in the illustration at right. Electroencephalographic (EEG) tracings show a decrease in slow-wave activity, the kind of sleep most restful to the muscles.

Fibromyalgia produces no crippling or deformity but can be extremely painful and frustrating to the patient. The recommended treatments include (a) carefully planned exercise program that includes gentle stretching and gradual progression toward aerobic conditioning and (b) drug therapy, mainly to improve sleep. This is best accomplished with low doses of the antidepressants amitriptyline or *Prozac*. Physical therapy may be helpful and could include techniques such as heat, ice, massage, whirlpool, and electrical stimulation to help control pain.

Fibromyalgia's persistent discomfort, combined with the fact that many physicians know little about it, have made it a fertile field for unsubstantiated treatments. The best professional to consult is a rheumatologist or a physical medicine specialist (physiatrist) who has a special interest in treating fibromyalgia patients.

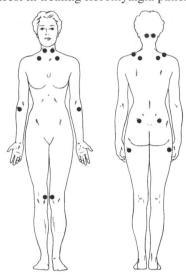

Location of "tender points."
(Drawing courtesy of the Arthritis Foundation.)

---

remits spontaneously. However, if a patient does not respond adequately or if the doctor believes it advisable to attempt to prevent permanent damage to the joints, a disease-modifying antirheumatic drug (DMARD) will be used. These include gold salts; penicillamine; hydroxychloroquine (an anti-malarial drug); methotrexate (a chemotherapeutic agent also used against cancer); sulfasalazine (a drug used for treating inflammatory bowel disease); azathioprine, cyclophosphamide, and cyclosporine (immuno-suppressive drugs); and several others. The newest DMARDs are safer than the rest but far more expensive. Unlike NSAIDs, they do not provide rapid pain relief but may delay progression of the disease. Some must be taken for a few months, whereas others require 1 or 2 years for a beneficial effect. The Arthritis Foundation offers up-to-date information about these drugs.[11]

Corticosteroids such as prednisone are another class of drugs that must be used with caution. Although they can provide dramatic relief of pain and swelling in inflamed joints, their side effects limit their usefulness in prolonged therapy. Unless given in very low dosage, corticosteroids eventually produce serious side effects in all patients during extended therapy. Thus in certain cases when oral corticosteroids are the only alternative,

they are used in the smallest amounts that will improve symptoms, sometimes on an every-other-day basis.

Nonprescription products promoted as "arthritis pain relievers" should be viewed with some skepticism. Most contain either aspirin, acetaminophen, or ibuprofen, which can relieve pain. But the amounts they contain and the cost per dose are usually higher than necessary for this purpose.

Despite the wide use of aspirin to relieve rheumatic symptoms and related muscular discomfort, an FDA expert panel has advised that nonprescription drugs should not be labeled for this purpose. The panel recommended that claims such as "for temporary relief of minor arthritic and rheumatic aches and pains" should be forbidden because salicylates act on two levels, depending on dosage. Up to 4000 mg of aspirin daily can be taken safely for a limited time as self-medication for pain relief and possibly a limited effect on inflammation. But 5300 mg daily (16 5-grain tablets), a more effective anti-inflammatory dosage, should be taken only under close medical supervision.[12] Large amounts can cause stomach irritation and gastrointestinal bleeding, which can be mild or severe. Other common side effects include ringing in the ears and temporary hearing loss. To control such effects, physicians may reduce the dosage, prescribe enteric-coated aspirin (e.g., *Ecotrin*), or try other salicylate drugs similar to aspirin.

For those who take large amounts of aspirin, the Arthritis Foundation has suggested purchasing 5-grain (325 mg) tablets in bottles of 1000. Nonadvertised brands cost the least.

Like aspirin, ibuprofen can be effective against both pain and inflammation. However, the amount contained in the over-the-counter (OTC) products *Nuprin* and *Advil* may be too low for optimal results. For this reason, ibuprofen should not be used for arthritis without instructions from a physician.

For osteoarthritis, which seldom involves inflammation, acetaminophen (*Tylenol, Panadol, Datril*) is considered the best drug to try first.[13] However, newer data suggest that NSAIDs may also be useful. Chapter 19 provides further information about nonprescription pain relievers.

Intra-articular Drugs

When only one or two joints are involved, injection of a steroid drug into the affected joints can provide considerable relief. This should be done sparingly, however, because repeated injections can cause cartilage degeneration, damaging the joint. Some newer injectable drugs can improve joint function and relieve the pain of osteoarthritis but are very expensive.

Physical Treatment Measures

Rest is usually important during acute flare-ups. Exercise is helpful to prevent or relieve pain and to maintain joint flexibility and muscle strength. Splinting of affected joints, particularly the fingers or wrists, can help in some cases of rheumatoid arthritis or tendinitis.

Physical therapy to relieve pain can include external applications of heat by showers, hot or cold packs, whirlpool baths, ultrasound diathermy, or paraffin baths. Range-of-motion exercises may be used to protect against muscle contractures that can lead to permanent disfigurement. Individual joints may be rested in removable, lightweight splints that help lessen inflammation and keep the joint in a normal-use position to protect it against contractures. Splints can also be used to help straighten out a joint that has become fixed in a flexed position. The splints usually are adjusted every few days to move the joint toward the desired position.

Once inflammation and pain subside, more emphasis is placed on exercise. Exercise for arthritis patients should not include activities that are strenuous, involve high impact, or require sudden twisting and turning. It should involve putting joints gently through their full range of motion every day. This helps to maintain normal joint movement and to strengthen muscles weakened by inactivity. As joint function improves, the exercises can be done against slight resistance, provided there is no pain. Low-impact aerobic exercises such as walking, bicycling, swimming, or step aerobics are advisable to foster cardiovascular fitness and help control weight. Each patient may require an individually prescribed program of exercises.

Adaptive devices include braces to relieve strain on painful body parts and various self-help gadgets to enhance restricted function. Some people find that a TENS device can relieve their pain.

Surgery

Various surgical procedures may relieve the pain of severely arthritic joints, particularly hip and knee joints. It is generally best to operate as the need arises rather than wait until the patient has many severely damaged joints and would require long periods of hospitalization and rehabilitation. The operations include:

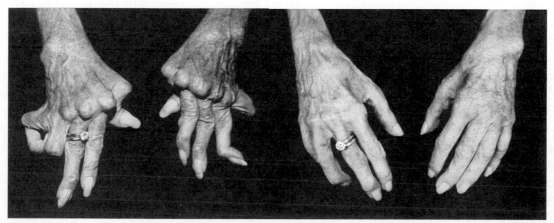

Figure 16-2. Hands of a rheumatoid arthritis patient, in her mid-50s, before and after joint-replacement surgery.
(Photographs provided by the Arthritis Foundation.)

ARTHRODESIS: Fusion of a diseased joint to relieve pain.

JOINT REPLACEMENT: Synthetic materials can be used to replace or rebuild severely afflicted joints. Hip and knee joints are commonly replaced, and operations are sometimes done to replace the joints of the feet, ankles, hands, wrists, and elbows.[14] Figure 16-2 shows a dramatic example of multiple joint replacement.

ARTHROPLASTY: Reconstruction of a diseased joint using a patient's own tissue.

OSTEOTOMY: Separation or cutting of a joint that has become fused or has shifted to an abnormal position.

AUTOLOGOUS CHONDROCYTE TRANSPLANTATION: A small amount of cartilage from a healthy joint is cultivated in a laboratory to obtain tissue that is implanted into a damaged joint. The procedure, which has been used to treat injured joints, is now being tested in osteoarthritic joints.

Competent Help is Essential

Despite medical advances, treatment of arthritis often can frustrate both doctor and patient. Early diagnosis and treatment offer the best results. There are only about 3000 board-certified arthritis specialists (rheumatologists), far fewer than are needed to provide optimal care for the huge number of people with arthritis. Thus most patients must be cared for by their family doctor. Benzaia and Barrett have noted:

Some family doctors provide good care; others are sincere in their wish to help but are not up-to-date in their knowledge of arthritis treatment. . . .
       A . . . common response of the untrained doctor is to sympathize with the patient, shrug his shoulders, indicate that "nothing much can be done," and recommend aspirin to alleviate pain. (Although aspirin can be useful for relieving pain, it must be taken on a regular schedule to reduce inflammation—and not just when pain arises.) You can't call this approach quackery, but it often drives sufferers to go to quacks. People who are discouraged, and have more pain than they think they should, are often willing to try anything that offers hope.[15]

Referral to a rheumatologist can be made by one's personal physician or a local chapter of the Arthritis Foundation. Supervision by a physical medicine specialist (physiatrist) may also be needed.

The Patient's Role

James F. Fries, M.D., professor of medicine at Stanford University, states that successful management of arthritis depends upon the afflicted individual as much as it does on the doctor. He states that people with arthritis must decide how much activity to undertake, whether to see a doctor and when, what kind of doctor to see, when to seek a second opinion, whether to accept medical advice, whether to follow a treatment program carefully, and whether to seek a quack cure or believe a sensational tabloid story. He recommends that a doctor be consulted quickly if joint pain is severe and accompanied by fever or swelling of one or two joints (a possible sign of gout), or if there is inability to use a joint, severe pain from a recent injury, or numbness or tingling related to the joint pain. He also suggests that an appointment should be made for other joint symptoms that have persisted for more than 6 weeks.[1]

External Analgesics

Liniments, rubs, poultices, plasters, and balms—sometimes referred to as external analgesics—are promoted for the relief of aches and pains due to arthritis. Some products of this type have been a part of folk medicine for thousands of years.

External analgesics depend on one or more skin irritants for their effects. They mildly stimulate nerve endings in the skin, producing warmth, coolness, or pain, which can block or distract attention from more bothersome, deep-seated muscular pains. In addition, the rubbing used to apply these products may loosen tight muscles.

Zimmerman[12] has noted that external analgesics were judged with less rigorous standards than were applied to other classes of drugs in the FDA OTC drug-review process (described in Chapters 19 and 26). The expert panel considered popular appeal, indicated by the amounts sold, as one criterion of product effectiveness, and also noted that complaints had been rare and problems mild. The preferred ingredient is methyl salicylate (oil of wintergreen), found in such products as *Ben-Gay Original Ointment* and *Heet Spray*.

Capsaicin, an alkaloid found in hot peppers, can be effective against arthritis pain but may produce an unwanted stinging or burning feeling. In nonprescription dosage, capsaicin is marketed as *Zostrix* and *Zostrix-HP* and costs over $30 per ounce. The *Medical Letter* has expressed skepticism because the supportive studies had very high placebo-response rates. One, for example, had found that applying capsaicin cream over an affected joint decreased pain in about 70% of 34 osteoarthritis patients and 80% of 14 rheumatoid arthritis patients. However, using a cream containing no capsaicin decreased pain in 50% of 30 osteoarthritis patients and 60% of 15 patients with rheumatoid arthritis.[16]

SUSCEPTIBILITY TO QUACKERY

As with many chronic diseases, the major forms of arthritis are subject to periods of spontaneous remission. These conditions may flare up unexpectedly for no apparent reason and then suddenly subside, leaving the individual pain-free for days, weeks, or even months. This can make it difficult for individuals to judge the efficacy of treatment measures—particularly in the short run. If a spontaneous remission takes place after using an unconventional measure (such as wearing a copper bracelet), consuming a particular food, or visiting an unorthodox practitioner, the individual may incorrectly conclude that the measure was effective. The Arthritis Foundation believes that far more money is spent on arthritis quackery than for arthritis research.

The classic 1968 study by the FDA summarizes why people with arthritis are especially susceptible to quackery:

- Arthritis is usually a chronic ailment for which there is no cure.
- Many people do not know how to obtain the best possible help for their condition. Even when they do, treatment may not be effective.
- Arthritis frequently causes great discomfort; afflicted people often fear that their condition will get worse and affect their ability to function.
- Faced with frustration and disappointment, they may lose faith in standard treatment and grasp at any "miracle" they hear about.[17]

A 1986 FDA survey found that 24% of people with arthritis considered their condition serious or very serious, 18% said that they almost always had a significant amount of pain, and 22% said that their condition fre-

quently caused significant pain. About one out of three said they would be willing to try anything for their condition, even if it sounded silly or had a small probability of success. About the same percentage said that they had tried at least one method considered questionable by the survey's designers. The most frequently tried methods were vitamins (17%), vibrators (14%), special diets (12%), chiropractic (12%), alfalfa tablets (9%), copper bracelets (9%), honey/vinegar (8%), and cod liver or fish oil (8%).[19]

QUESTIONABLE TREATMENT METHODS

Questionable arthritis treatments include mechanical devices, environmental methods, fad diets, dietary supplements, acupuncture, and medications. They may be promoted through advertisements, books, newspaper and magazine articles, and word of mouth. Some are available from dubious practitioners and clinics. Some do no direct harm but may cause harmful delay in seeking appropriate treatment. Others, however, can result in severe injury or even death. Quackery tends to keep up with the times by developing methods with supposed actions that are based on current scientific discoveries. For example, after astronauts reached the moon, "moondust" was promoted as an arthritis cure. Gadgets used to be the mainstay of arthritis quackery, but in recent years the emphasis has been on drugs and dietary supplements.[15]

Dubious Devices

Devices cannot cure any form of arthritis. Vibrators and whirlpool baths are commonly sold with exaggerated claims. Vibrators may provide some relief of muscle pain caused by overexertion or fatigue and may have a temporary relaxant effect on some muscle tension, but they can sometimes do serious harm by increasing joint inflammation. Many whirlpool baths for self-use are no more effective than simple hot baths. Therefore, no such device should be purchased without consulting one's physician.[15]

According to modern folklore, copper bracelets worn on both wrists can set up "curative circuits." To avoid prosecution for fraud, such bracelets are usually advertised as costume jewelry (with no health claims), assuming that readers of the ads are sufficiently familiar with the claims that they will try the product.

Magnets worn in clothing and magnetic mattresses are marketed for arthritis pain relief. However, very little research has been done, and there is no reason to believe they are effective.

☑ **Consumer Tip**

"Unproven Remedies"

The Arthritis Foundation[18] has defined unproven remedies as "treatments that have not shown that they work or are safe." You should be wary of any of the following characteristics:

Claimed to work for all types of arthritis
Uses only case histories or testimonials as proof
Only one study is cited as proof that it works
Cited studies have no control group
Contents are not identified
Has no warnings about side effects
Described as harmless or natural
Claimed to be based on a secret formula
Available from only one source
Promoted only through the media, books, or by mail

The following quack gadgets marketed as arthritis cures have been removed from the market by federal enforcement actions:

The *Pulse-A-Rhythm*, a vibrating mattress, was judged by the FDA to be dangerous and ineffective for people in acute phases of rheumatoid arthritis.[20]

The *Micro-Dynameter*, a simple galvanometer made into a complicated-looking box with various dials and wires, was represented as capable of diagnosing and treating virtually all diseases by electronic means.[21] This device was one of many designed by Dr. Albert Abrams, whom the AMA called "the dean of gadget quacks."

The *Vrilium Tube,* promoted with supposed radioactive healing powers, was a brass tube about 2 inches long that contained barium chloride. It cost only a few cents to manufacture but was sold for hundreds of dollars.[15]

The *Solarama Board* (also known as the *Earth Board* or *Vitalator*), when placed under the afflicted person's mattress at night, supposedly released curative "free electrons."

The *Oxypathor* (Figure 16-3), *Oxydonor,* and several similar devices were claimed to cause the body to absorb oxygen and were marketed as cure-alls.[22]

Environmental Approaches

Claims that certain environments offer hope for cure induce many people to spend large sums of money traveling to receive supposedly helpful treatments.

The false claim that radon gas can cure arthritis brought a classic complaint of misrepresentation against the Elkhorn Mining Company, Boulder, Colorado, by the FTC. People with various diseases, especially arthritis, were taken into an abandoned uranium mine for

---

Historical Perspective

A Device that Removed "Poisons" from the Blood (and Money from the Wallet)

The *Oxypathor* was a nickel-plated tube closed at both ends and filled with an inert substance. Flexible wires were attached to the pipe at one end and to small disks at the other. After the disks were fastened to the user's wrist or ankle, the cylinder was placed in cold water, thereby creating a "force" that supposedly caused the body to absorb oxygen from the air and cured a long list of diseases. The manufacturer instructed salespersons that "the less theory you talk the better. . . . It is far better to say, 'Oxygen burns up the wastes and poisons in the blood, leaving it rich and pure' than to undertake to describe these poisons, wastes, and acids. The number of fool questions that you will find hurled your way if you undertake technical presentations will surprise—and disgust you. Side-step as here suggested."

In 1914 the president of the Oxypathor Company was convicted of mail fraud and given a suspended 18-month prison sentence. Records in the case indicate that during the 5 years preceding the trial, 45,541 devices were sold for a minimum of $35 each. At a subsequent proceeding, the administrative law judge stated: "The inherent viciousness of the scheme . . . is apparent when it is remembered that the company sells the treatment for the cure of practically every human ailment, many of which, if allowed to continue without immediate medical treatment, may prove fatal, and that those who, through the false and fraudulent representations of the [seller], buy the machine are lulled into a false sense of security from all disease."[22]

Although device quackery has waned, the notion of ridding the body of unnamed "toxins" is still invoked to market vitamin concoctions, herbs, colonic irrigations, and various diets.

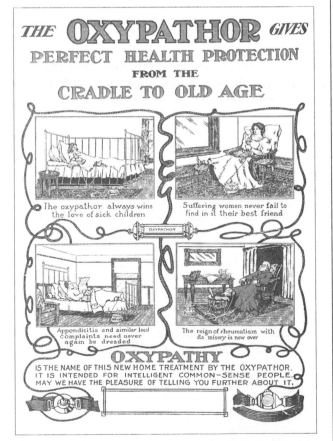

FIGURE 16-3. *Oxypathor* flyer (1911). The reverse side was a letter from a physician who described how a woman had used the device to cure herself of "neurasthenia," "embolism," "atrophy nerves," "weakened mind," and "pains in every limb."
(Courtesy of the Museum of Questionable Devices)

a fee, supposedly to be exposed to helpful radioactive rays. The company also claimed falsely that radon gas stimulated the production of ACTH and hydrocortisone that would help cure arthritis.[23] Benzaia and Barrett have noted: "The radiation level in the mine is so low that it can have no actual effect on the body—which is fortunate—because high radiation levels can increase people's chances of developing cancer."[15]

Real estate promoters sometimes capitalize on the hope that a warm climate will help people afflicted with arthritis. Moving for this reason is not advisable. The majority of scientific studies have found no relationship between weather conditions (temperature, humidity, barometric pressure) and the severity of arthritis symptoms. The most rigorous study followed 18 patients for 15 months, rating the extent of pain (as reported by the patients), joint tenderness (as determined by a doctor), and ability to function (as determined by a standardized test). No relationship was found between weather conditions and the patients' symptoms.[24]

Dietary Methods

The Arthritis Foundation states that no special food, diet, or food supplement can cure arthritis. Gout is partially related to diet, because certain foods increase the blood level of uric acid, but the primary treatment is still medication rather than diet. The Foundation advises people to be wary of claims that any food or food substance can help arthritis. Raw foods, "natural foods," heated milk, honey and vinegar, and alfalfa have been widely promoted as helpful in treating arthritis.

Arthritis Foundation officials believe that improvement following elimination of a food is most likely a placebo effect. The Foundation recommends that rheumatoid arthritis patients who believe their disease is worsened by a food could try avoiding that food under medical supervision to see whether any improvement results. Panush[25] has concluded that a small number (fewer than 5%) of individuals may improve after they stop eating a specific food that appears to aggravate their condition. Jarvis reached a similar conclusion after reviewing double-blind studies conducted before 1989.[26]

In 1991 a Norwegian research team reported that a small group of rheumatoid arthritis patients treated with dietary methods for 13 months had fewer symptoms than a control group who ate normally. During the first 7 to 10 days the treatment group consumed a low-calorie liquid diet with new foods added individually in an attempt to identify foods that might cause arthritis symptoms to worsen. Then these patients followed a vegetarian diet that excluded dairy products, eggs, refined sugar, citrus fruits, and gluten-containing foods (wheat,

oats, rye, and barley) for 1 year. The control group ate as usual. Patients who improved while on the diet relapsed when they resumed their normal eating habits.[27] *Tufts University Diet & Nutrition Letter* cautions that (a) the experimental diet can lead to nutritional shortfalls that require professional monitoring; (b) the results were based on the experience of only 17 individuals; and (c) a much larger sample would be required for confirmation.[28]

Dale Alexander claimed that ingested cod liver oil reduces the pain of arthritis by lubricating the joints.[29] This claim is false because the oil is broken down by digestion into simple substances, before absorption from the intestinal tract, and the oil does not actually reach the joints. Years ago, "immune milk" sold for many times the price of ordinary milk. It was said to produce immunity because the cows producing it had been injected with streptococcus and staphylococcus vaccines.

Nutritional Supplements

Various vitamin and vitamin-mineral supplements are promoted for the treatment of arthritis through articles in "health-food" publications. A number of companies market supplements (for example, *Ar Pak*) whose names suggest effectiveness against arthritis. To avoid legal trouble, product labels make no actual claims.

Green-lipped mussel was promoted by the book *Relief from Arthritis* by John Croft and by articles in health-food magazines and tabloids. The mussel is harvested in New Zealand, made into supplement capsules, and marketed by various American companies. Although in 1976 the FDA banned importation of green-lipped mussel preparations, similar products are still marketed as "mucopolysaccharides." In 1983 the FDA seized a large quantity of products and raw materials from the Aquaculture Corporation of Redwood City, California, manufacturer of *Neptone*. The company contested the seizure on the grounds that their product was a food rather than a drug. However, FDA documents indicated that the company had distributed literature and suggested in advertisements that green-lipped mussel preparations were effective treatment for arthritis.[30]

Superoxide dismutase (SOD) is an enzyme involved in the body's defenses against free radicals. SOD is claimed to reduce inflammation in arthritis, slow the aging process, reverse the effects of radiation, restore damaged tissues after heart attacks, and protect against degenerative diseases. The oral form is digested and has no significant effect on the body. The injectable form (available as *Orgotein* in European countries) has not been proven useful by scientific studies.[31]

Capsules of omega-3 fatty acids, commonly referred to as fish oils, have been marketed with claims that they are effective treatments for several types of arthritis. A few experiments in both animals and humans have had positive results, but it is not known whether there is a dose that is both practical and safe. Fish oil supplements can interfere with blood clotting and increase the risk of stroke, especially when taken with aspirin or other NSAIDs. Fish oils can also cause diarrhea and stomach upset. Responsible medical authorities believe that eating oily fish (mackerel, salmon, sardines, or lake trout) several times a week is preferable to taking fish oil supplements. Eating these fish may help prevent heart attacks as well (see Chapter 15).

Glucosamine and chondroitin sulfate may have some ability to control the pain of osteoarthritis, but the quality of the supporting evidence is not high. In 2000 the *Journal of the American Medical Association* published a meta-analysis whose authors concluded: "Trials of glucosamine and chondroitin preparations for [osteoarthritis] symptoms demonstrate moderate to large effects, but quality issues and likely publication bias suggest that these effects are exaggerated. Nevertheless, some degree of efficacy appears probable for these preparations."[32] An accompanying editorial concluded: "As with many nutraceuticals that currently are widely touted as beneficial for common but difficult-to-treat disorders, the promotional enthusiasm often far surpasses the scientific evidence supporting clinical use. Until high-quality studies, such as the National Institutes of Health study, are completed, work such as [the meta-analysis] is the best hope for providing physicians with information necessary to advise their patients about the risks and benefits of these therapies."[33]

"Research Studies"

Advertisements have solicited people with arthritis for a "research study" that involves buying a product or paying to enroll. The Arthritis Foundation warns that these are marketing ploys that should be ignored. Although advertising is sometimes used to recruit patients for clinical trials, no legitimate study requires those who enroll to pay for the treatment.

Acupuncture

Acupuncture has no known effect on the underlying cause of any form of arthritis. It is alleged that acupuncture provides pain relief in rheumatoid arthritis and osteoarthritis, but controlled experiments suggest that any effect is likely to be temporary. (For details, see the acupuncture discussion in Chapter 8.)

Inappropriate Medications

Medications used inappropriately for arthritis treatment can be classified in two categories: unproven and dangerous.

Clotrimazole, an antifungal drug, was acclaimed by a British physician as a cure for rheumatoid arthritis, which he claims is a protozoan infection. Investigation by the Arthritis Foundation revealed that the doctor was unlicensed in Britain at the time of the report, that he was not an arthritis specialist, that the manufacturers of the drug had no knowledge of any antiprotozoal properties, and that no controlled study had been conducted to investigate its effectiveness.[15]

Injections of the venoms of bees and snakes have been touted for treatment of arthritis. No evidence of their effectiveness exists, and both products are dangerous. Bee venom can produce severe allergic reactions. Snake venom, which has anticoagulant properties, has been implicated in a case of death caused by brain hemorrhage.[34]

Products made from aloe vera, a common houseplant, are promoted with unsubstantiated claims that they are effective treatment for hundreds of ailments, including arthritis. Taken internally, aloe juice is a laxative and can cause gastrointestinal upset (see Chapter 12).

Dimethyl sulfoxide (DMSO) is an industrial solvent that became popular in the 1960s when Stanley Jacob, M.D., University of Oregon Medical School, reported evidence of its use in medical treatment. DMSO has been touted as a "miracle drug," with claims that it relieves pain, decreases swelling, and promotes healing of injured tissue. Its has also been used for sprains, bursitis, scleroderma, rheumatoid arthritis, and other conditions, but there are no controlled studies showing that it is safe and effective for these purposes. Veterinarians have been legally using DMSO on animals. It has been popular among athletes as a treatment for sore muscles and other injuries. When rubbed into the skin, DMSO is quickly absorbed and produces a garlic-like taste and breath odor. If contaminated, it can carry toxic substances into the body. Topical use can also cause a rash, blistering, itching, hives, and skin thickening. Intravenous use can cause kidney damage and many other serious adverse effects.[2]

The news media—most notably CBS-TV's "60 Minutes"—have portrayed DMSO as a medical breakthrough. This claim is premature, however, because adequate evidence is not available and long-term effects are not known. The FDA has approved a drug-grade DMSO drug product for treating interstitial cystitis (a bladder disorder) but not for treating arthritis or

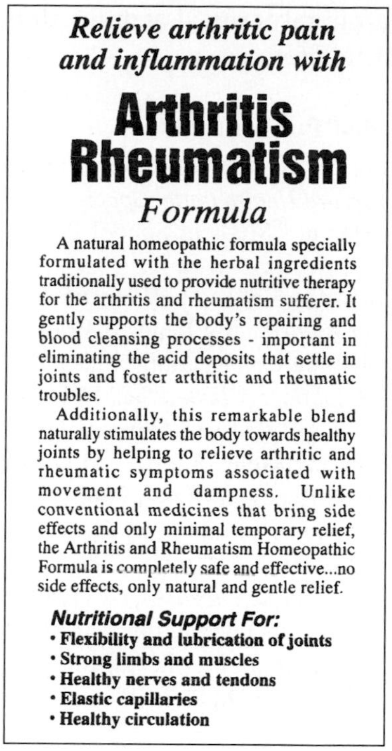

FIGURE 16-4. Recent ad for homeopathic arthritis formula.

any other ailment. A few states have passed laws permitting the manufacture and sale of DMSO as a non-prescription drug, but it cannot be legally marketed in this way in most states. However, it is available in some health-food, surplus, hardware, and other stores, where it is sold as a "solvent" for $5 or more for a small bottle. Industrial-grade DMSO should never be used because contaminants can produce serious reactions.

Dr. Jacob also claims that methylsulfonylmethane (MSM), a DMSO derivative, is effective against arthritis and a long list of other conditions. However, no published research supports his claims.[35]

Since the late 1970s Oriental arthritis remedies said to be "all-natural" herbal products have been illegally marketed in the United States under the names *Chuifong Toukuwan, Black Pearls,* and *Miracle Herb.* Government agencies have found that in addition to herbs, these products contain various potent drugs not listed on their label. The drugs have included antianxiety agents (diazepam [Valium] and chlordiazepoxide [Librium]), anti-inflammatory drugs (indomethacin, phenylbutazone, prednisone, and dexamethasone), pain relievers (mefenamic acid, acetaminophen, and aminopyrine), and the male hormone methyltestosterone. Aminopyrine was banned in the United States in 1938 because it can cause agranulocytosis, a life-threatening condition in which the body stops producing white blood cells. Prednisone and dexamethasone are corticosteroids. Some batches of *Chuifong Toukuwan* have contained amounts of diazepam high enough to cause addiction. In 1975 four users of *Chuifong Toukuwan* were hospitalized with agranulocytosis, and one died. The FDA has banned importation of the product and helped Texas authorities obtain criminal convictions against several marketers.[36]

Homeopathic products are also promoted for arthritis (see Figure 16-4). There is no scientific evidence to support their use (see Chapter 8).

Clinics

Thousands of arthritis sufferers have received improper treatments in unethical clinics in the United States and nearby countries. Some of these are associated with spas where physical therapy and hydrotherapy are available. Some spas feature mineral waters and baths. The National Institute of Arthritis and Metabolic Disease has stated:

Some persons with rheumatic complaints . . . believe that trips to the spas where mineral baths are available were helpful to them, but it has not been shown that it was the mineral content of the waters which accompanied such temporary relief as might have been experienced. In many cases . . . it was simply a matter of rest.[37]

♦ **Personal Glimpse** ♦

Deception in Mexico

After reading about a doctor in Mexico, a 44-year-old woman with rheumatoid arthritis paid him a visit.[38] She did this because she had been in severe pain, could hardly walk, and felt desperate. Cortisone had relieved her symptoms but caused severe adverse effects, including liver and kidney trouble and a stroke that required more than 1 year for full recovery. When she asked the Mexican doctor whether his treatment included any type of steroid drug, he said it did not and it would help her feel better.

Half an hour after receiving an injection, she began to feel dramatically better. She "limbered up," became energetic, and became pain-free for several weeks. However, she then began to experience edema (puffiness) in her face and in other parts of her body and suspected that the injection she had received had contained steroids. The FDA analyzed her medications and confirmed that they contained a combination of steroids. The Mexican doctor had lied to her. She again developed liver and kidney trouble but was able to recover within a few months with appropriate medical treatment.

These events occurred more than 20 years ago, but the problem of Mexican clinics dispensing unidentified and dangerous drugs still exists.

Clinics in Mexico and elsewhere offer other costly treatments not based on scientific principles. Some advertise that the cause of arthritis is constipation caused by "toxemia" and that their treatments are "nonmedical and nonsurgical." Treatment at these clinics may include mud baths, diets, vitamins, salt rubs, pressurized enemas, massages, and the use of electrical devices.

Some clinics dispense steroid drugs such as cortisone or prednisone. Steroid drugs may bring about rapid reduction of pain and inflammation. However, they can have dangerous side effects that make them unsuitable for long-term use in the treatment of arthritis. Steroid drugs should never be used without close medical supervision, yet patients at some foreign clinics are not informed when these drugs are prescribed.[39] As a result, many wind up with stomach ulcers, internal bleeding, weakening of bones, infections, and cataracts.

Dr. Robert E. Liefmann, who fled from the United States to Canada, produced Liefcort, which contained three well-known drugs: prednisone, testosterone (a male hormone), and estradiol (a female hormone). In 1969 he was convicted of violating Canada's Food and Drug Act and was fined $2400. He died in 1972 while the case was being appealed. Hormone/steroid combinations are still prescribed at some clinics in Canada and Mexico. Other potentially dangerous drugs prescribed at these facilities include:

- Dipyrone, which can cause agranulocytosis, a disease in which the white blood count drops and subsequent infection can lead to death
- Aminopyrine (described previously)
- Phenylbutazone, an effective anti-inflammatory drug that requires close medical supervision not offered by the clinics

Some clinics claim to administer DMSO intravenously and dispense DMSO pills to take home. Analysis of the pills has shown that some contain phenylbutazone, diazepam (Valium), and even aminopyrine.

SOURCES OF INFORMATION

Pamphlets and information about reputable treatment facilities are available from the Arthritis Foundation or one of its local offices (listed in the Yellow Pages). The Foundation's bi-monthly magazine *Arthritis Today* provides consumers with a convenient way to keep informed about new developments. However, its coverage of "alternative" topics lacks appropriate criticism and should be considered untrustworthy—as should the Foundation's book on these methods.[40]

Greenwald[41] has observed that the best books are usually written by medical school professors and the worst ones are highly critical of drugs, drug companies, and the medical profession.

Recommended Publications
The following publications are reliable and helpful.

Arthritis: A Harvard Health Letter Special Report, by Daphna W. Gregg. Harvard Medical School Publications Group, Boston, 1995.

Arthritis: A Take Care of Yourself Health Guide for Understanding Your Arthritis, by James F. Fries, M.D. Addison-Wesley Publishing Co., Reading, Mass., 1999.

The Arthritis Helpbook: A Tested Self-Management Program for Coping with Arthritis and Fibromyalgia, by Kate Lorig, R.N., Dr.P.H., and James F. Fries, M.D. Addison-Wesley Publishing Co., Reading, Mass., 2000.

Mayo Clinic on Arthritis, edited by Gene G. Hunder, M.D. Mayo Clinic, Rochester, Minn., 1999.

Primer on the Rheumatic Diseases, ed 11, edited by Cornelia M. Weyand. Arthritis Foundation, Atlanta, 1998.

Treating Arthritis: Medicine, Myth, and Magic, by Felix Fernandez-Madrid, M.D., Ph.D. Plenum Publishing Corp., New York, 1989.

Unproven Remedies Resource Manual, by the Arthritis Foundation, Atlanta, 1991.

Nonrecommended Books
The following books promote unproven methods:

The Arthritic's Cookbook, by Colin M. Dong, M.D., and Jane Banks.

Arthritis and Common Sense #2, by Dale Alexander.

Arthritis and Folk Medicine, by D.C. Jarvis, M.D.

Arthritis Can be Cured: A Layman's Guide, by Bernard Aschner, M.D.

The Arthritis Foundation's Guide to Alternative Therapies, by Judith Horstman.

Arthritis, Nutrition and Natural Therapy, by Carson Wade.

The Arthritis Solution, by Joseph Kandel, M.D., and David Sudderth, M.D.

A Doctor's Proven New Home Cure for Arthritis, by Giraud W. Campbell, D.O., and R. Stone.

Bees Don't Get Arthritis, by Fred Malone.

How To Eat Away Arthritis, by Lauri M. Aesoph, N.D.

Maximizing the Arthritis Cure: A Step-by-Step Program to Faster, Stronger Healing During Any Stage of the Cure, by Jason Theodosakis, M.D., Brenda D. Adderly, M.H.A., and Barry Fox, Ph.D.

The Miraculous Holistic Balanced Treatment for Arthritis Diseases, by Henry B. Rothblatt, J.D., L.L.M., Donna Pinorsky, R.N., and Michael Brodsky.

The New Arthritis Breakthrough, by Henry Scammell.

The Nightshades and Health, by Norman Franklin Childers and Gerard M. Russo.

Pain-Free Arthritis, by Dvera Berson with Sander Roy.

There Is a Cure for Arthritis, by Paavo O. Airola, N.D.

You Can Stay Well and *Let's Get Well,* both by Adelle Davis, M.S.

Tabloid Reports

Tabloid newspapers frequently report so-called arthritis cures—often with front-page headlines. Articles of this type tend to fall into three categories:

1. Sensationalized presentations of useful methods already known to the arthritis community. "New Diet to Ease Pain of Arthritis" (*National Examiner*) was a standard low-fat, high-fiber diet plus vitamin supplements. The method described in "How to Wash Away Arthritis Pain Instantly" (*Examiner*) was a hot bath.
2. One-sided reports touting quack nonsense. "Miracle Caves Cure Thousands of Arthritis" (*Sun*) were tunnels in the mines described earlier in this chapter; "Nature's Miracle Cures for Arthritis and High Blood Pressure" (*Examiner*) were fruits that supposedly rid the body of toxins that cause arthritis.
3. Preliminary reports of research findings. These "breakthroughs" have no practical significance because they are unconfirmed, will not be available for treating people for many years, or might apply to only a tiny percentage of people with arthritis.

GUIDELINES FOR PEOPLE WITH ARTHRITIS

These guidelines can help people with arthritis make intelligent decisions about products and services:

- Leave the diagnosis of ailments to the physician.
- Let the physician prescribe the medications.
- Be wary of testimonials; some are outright lies. Others, sincerely made, are likely to result from spontaneous remission of the disease.
- Ignore anyone who promises a "sure cure" or claims to have a secret formula for arthritis.
- Avoid products claimed to offer more than temporary relief from minor pain of arthritis, unless recommended by your physician.
- Be aware that there is no specific cure for most forms of arthritis.
- Avoid spas or clinics that encourage self-diagnosis by mail or allege therapeutic value of such treatments as mineral salts and baths.
- Understand that just because a product is marketed does not ensure that the claims for it are justified.
- Contact a local Arthritis Foundation chapter for help
- Individuals wishing to use an unproven approach should discuss this with their physician to minimize their chances of deceiving themselves or selecting a dangerous method.

SUMMARY

Arthritis and *rheumatic disease* are general terms applied to about 100 different conditions characterized by aches and pains of joints, muscles, and/or fibrous tissues. Early diagnosis and treatment are likely to produce the most

It's Your Decision

A friend of yours with rheumatoid arthritis has encountered an herbal product sold person-to-person that is claimed to be helpful for arthritis. The friend has been under medical care, with considerable benefit, but would like to "miss no bets." What would you advise? How can the product be investigated? Is there a way to determine whether the product is safe?

favorable results. Most patients with chronic forms of arthritis can be helped to lead a productive life if their condition is properly diagnosed and treated. In many cases treatment can help relieve the discomfort and maintain or restore joint function.

People with arthritis often turn to quackery because of fear, loss of hope, inadequate information, and other psychosocial factors. Because the symptoms of arthritis often vary spontaneously, it may be difficult for people who have arthritis to judge whether an unproven remedy is effective. This chapter describes many types of quackery and tells how to obtain competent professional help.

REFERENCES

1. Fries JF: Arthritis: A Take Care of Yourself Health Guide for Understanding Your Arthritis. Reading, Mass., 1995, Addison-Wesley Publishing Co.
2. Fernandez-Madrid F: Treating Arthritis: Medicine, Myth, and Magic. New York, 1989, Plenum Publishing Corp.
3. National Arthritis Month—May 2000. Morbidity and Mortality Weekly Report 49:365, 2000.
4. Arthritis prevalence and activity limitations—United States, 1990. Morbidity and Mortality Weekly Report 43:433–438, 1994.
5. Lawrence RC and others. Estimates of the prevalence of selected arthritic and musculoskeletal diseases in the United States. Journal of Rheumatology 16:427–441, 1989.
6. Wolfe F and others. The American College of Rheumatology Criteria for the classification of fibromyalgia. Report of the Multicenter Criteria Committee. Arthritis and Rheumatism 33:160–172, 1990.
7. Freundlich B, Levinthal L. The fibromyalgia syndrome. In Schumacher HR Jr., editor. Primer on the Rheumatic Diseases, ed 10. Atlanta, 1993, Arthritis Foundation, pp 247–249.
8. Arthritis information: Fibromyalgia. Atlanta, 1995, Arthritis Foundation.
9. Yunus MB. Fibromyalgia syndrome: Blueprint for a reliable diagnosis. Consultant 36:1260–1274,1996.
10. Yunus MB. Fibromyalgia syndrome: Is there any effective therapy? Consultant 36:1275–1285,1996.
11. Duncan MA. Arthritis Today 2001 Drug Guide. Arthritis Today 15:1:39–60, 2001.

12. Zimmerman DR. Zimmerman's Complete Guide to Non-prescription Drugs. Detroit, 1993, Visible Ink Press.

13. Osteoarthritis: Old scourge, new hope. Consumer Reports on Health 8:3–5, 1996.

14. Lewis R. Arthritis: Modern treatment for that old pain in the joints. FDA Consumer, 25(6):18–25, 1991.

15. Benzaia D, Barrett S. The misery merchants. In Barrett S, Jarvis WT, editors. The Health Robbers: A Close Look at Quackery in America. Amherst, N.Y., 1993, Prometheus Books.

16. Capsaicin—A topical analgesic. The Medical Letter 34:62–63, 1992.

17. Food and Drug Administration: A Study of Health Practices and Opinions. Publ. No. 210978. Springfield, Va., 1972, National Technical Information Service, U.S. Department of Commerce.

18. Arthritis Foundation. Unproven remedies. Atlanta, 1987, The Foundation.

19. Louis Harris and Associates. Health, Information and the Use of Questionable Treatments: A Study of the American Public. Rockville, Md., 1987, U.S. Food and Drug Administration.

20. Janssen WF. The gadgeteers. In Barrett S, Jarvis WT, editors. The Health Robbers: A Close Look at Quackery in America. Amherst, N.Y., 1993, Prometheus Books.

21. Barrett S and others. Health Schemes, Scams, and Frauds. New York 1990, Consumer Reports Books.

22. Propaganda Department of the American Medical Association. Mechanical Nostrums and Quackery of the Drugless Type. Chicago, 1923, American Medical Association.

23. FTC challenges health claims of mine operator, seeks disclosure of material facts. FTC News Summary, No. 14. Washington, D.C., June 28, 1974.

24. Redelmeier DA, Tversky A. On the belief that arthritis pain is related to the weather. Proceedings of the National Academy of Sciences 93:2895–2896, 1996.

25. Panush RS. Nutritional therapy for rheumatic diseases. Annals of Internal Medicine 106:619–621, 1987.

26. Jarvis WT. Arthritis: Folk remedies and quackery. Nutrition Forum 7:1–3, 1990.

27. Kjeldsen-Kragh J and others. Controlled trial of fasting and a 1-year vegetarian diet in rheumatoid arthritis. Lancet 338:899–902, 1991.

28. A ray of dietary hope for arthritis sufferers. Tufts University Diet & Nutrition Letter 9(12):1–2, 1992.

29. Herbert V, Barrett S: The Vitamin Pushers: How the Health Food Industry Is Selling America a Bill of Goods. Amherst, N.Y., 1994, Prometheus Books.

30. USA v Articles of Drug . . . Neptone, Preliminary declarations of Paul J Sage (FDA) and Richard W Dorst (Aquaculture Corporation) in civil case #C-83-0864-EFL, US District Court, Northern District of California, July 22, 1983.

31. Arthritis Foundation. Unproven Remedies Resource Manual. Atlanta, 1991, The Foundation.

32. McAlindon TE and others. Glucosamine and chondroitin for treatment of osteoarthritis: A systematic quality assessment and meta-analysis. JAMA 283:1469–1475, 2000.

33. Tanveer E, Anastassiades TP. Glucosamine and chondroitin for treating symptoms of osteoarthritis: Evidence is widely touted but incomplete. JAMA 283:1483–1484, 2000.

34. HHS News, P80-41, Sept 19, 1980.

35. Lang KL. Methylsulfonylmethane (MSM). Quackwatch Web site, June 9, 2000.

36. McCaleb R, Blumenthal M. Black pearls lose luster. Prescription drugs masquerade as Chinese herbal arthritis formula, HerbalGram No. 22, pp 4–5, 38–39, 1990. The American Botanical Association.

37. Smith RL. The Health Hucksters. New York, 1960, Thomas Y. Crowell Co.

38. Schultz T, Lindeman B. The pain exploiters: A firsthand report on the profiteers who prey on arthritis sufferers. Today's Health, Oct 1973.

39. Diesk A and others. Unconventional arthritis therapies. Arthritis and Rheumatism 25:1145–1147, 1982.

40. Horstman J. The Arthritis Foundation's Guide to Alternative Therapies. Atlanta, 1999, The Foundation.

41. Greenwald RA. Arthritis books: The good, the bad, and the ugly. Priorities for Health 11(1):30–35, 1999.

Chapter Seventeen

CANCER

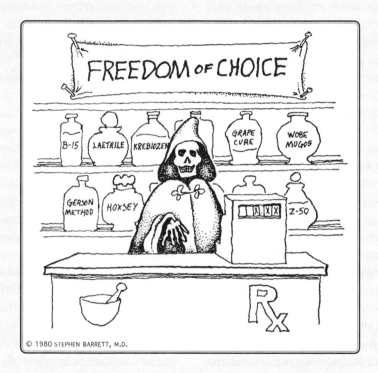

© 1980 STEPHEN BARRETT, M.D.

Suppose someone began marketing automobiles with claims that they can run on water. Most people would want this to be proven and guaranteed or they would pass up the offer. Yet many people who feel desperate about a health problem are vulnerable to promises from individuals who . . . use methods that are unproven according to the criteria of the scientific community. This type of analogy might help patients place dubious cancer treatment in proper perspective.

HELENE BROWN[1]

Key Concepts
KEEP THESE POINTS IN MIND AS YOU STUDY THIS CHAPTER

- The most common direct cause of cancer is tobacco smoking.

- Little evidence exists that food additives increase the risk of cancer in humans.

- Although dietary factors play a role in the development of certain types of cancer, the evidence is weaker than most people realize.

- Antioxidant supplements have not been proven to prevent cancer.

- Cancer treatments promoted with testimonials should be disregarded.

- The National Cancer Institute's computerized database can provide physicians with up-to-date information about cancer treatment. This enables most cancer patients to benefit from current knowledge without having to travel far.

The term *cancer* encompasses more than 100 diseases characterized by abnormal cell growth. The abnormal cells do not function usefully in the body and can destroy normal tissue. No single form of treatment is best for all types of cancer because each type of tumor has its own characteristics. Since cancer cells are quite similar to normal cells, it is not simple to kill the one while preserving the other. These concepts should be useful in understanding why any method proposed as effective against all cancers should be viewed with great skepticism until all the facts are in. Cancer researchers do not expect to find such a "magic bullet" in the foreseeable future.

Cancer ranks as the second leading cause of death in the United States. The American Cancer Society (ACS) estimates that in 2001 about 553,000 Americans will die of cancer and 1,268,000 new cases will be discovered.[2] A similar number will be diagnosed with a superficial form of skin cancer not included in these figures because it is easily detected and cured. Another 100,000 will be diagnosed with cancers of the cervix, female breast, or elsewhere that are so small, localized (in situ), and curable that they are tabulated separately. Except for lung cancer, which has greatly increased, the overall age-adjusted rate of cancer incidence has gradually decreased during the past 35 years. Both cancer prevention activities and improvements in medical care have contributed to this decline.[2]

The American Cancer Society states that one out of four people presently living in the United States will eventually develop cancer, but that half could be saved from cancer death with early diagnosis and current treatment methods.

This chapter discusses the risk factors for cancer, preventive measures, scientific (evidence-based) treatment methods, diet and cancer, susceptibility to quackery, questionable methods, consumer protection laws, and information sources.

RISK FACTORS FOR CANCER

Cancer is the result of a complex interaction of causative agents, both environmental and genetic. The most common direct cause of human cancer is tobacco smoking, which is responsible for 85% to 90% of lung cancer cases as well as cancers of the bladder, mouth, larynx, esophagus, pancreas, and possibly other organs.[3] The ACS estimates that in 2000 about 171,000 cancer deaths resulted from tobacco use. Other risk factors for cancer are related to alcohol, drugs, certain sexual patterns, solar radiation, occupation, and certain infections.[4]

The effect of diet on cancer is not clearly established. However, epidemiologic studies have found an association between low intakes of fruits and vegetables and increased incidence of certain cancers.

Alcohol in large doses increases the risk for cancer of the esophagus, mouth, rectum, and possibly other sites. In combination with cigarettes it acts synergistically to increase oral cancer risk. The ACS estimates that about 19,000 cancer deaths during 2000 were related to alcohol use.

High-dose exposure to ionizing radiation increases the chances of leukemia and skin cancer. Exposure to high indoor levels of radon increases the incidence of lung cancer, particularly among cigarette smokers. The Environmental Protection Agency recommends that homes with average radon levels of 4 picocuries per liter or greater undergo corrective measures. About 6% of homes in the United States have levels that high.[5] Guidance is available from Consumer Federation of America's Radon Fix-It Line (800-644-6999).

In rare cases drugs have increased cancer risk. For example, the use of diethylstilbestrol (DES) during pregnancy has been linked to the subsequent development of a rare form of vaginal cancer in a small number of daughters of exposed women.

Higher risk of cancer of the cervix is associated with human papillomavirus infection (genital warts), intercourse at an early age, and multiple sexual partners.

Ultraviolet rays cause the majority of skin cancers. The principal source is the sun, but indoor tanning devices are another source (see Chapter 20).

High-dose, long-term exposure to a number of occupational chemicals has been shown to increase the risk of cancer. These include benzene, asbestos used for insulating and fireproofing, and vinyl chloride used in the production of plastics.

HIV and hepatitis B are associated with increased incidence of certain cancers.

Despite the presence of carcinogenic substances in the atmosphere, there is no firm evidence that air pollution is a significant cause of cancer. Nor has living or working near electric power lines been shown to increase cancer risk.[6]

There is little evidence that food additives used in the United States increase the risk of any form of human cancer. A 1996 National Research Council report concluded (a) cancer-causing chemicals that occur naturally in foods are far more numerous than synthetic carcinogens, yet both types are consumed at levels so low that they appear to pose little threat to human health; (b) although some chemicals in the diet have the ability to cause cancer, they appear to be a threat only when present in foods that form an unusually large part of the diet; (c) the varied and balanced diet needed for good nutrition seems to provide significant protection from the natural toxicants in our foods; and (d) the human diet contains a mixture of small amounts of thousands of chemicals, some that may cause cancer and some that may help prevent it by acting as anticarcinogens.[7]

PREVENTIVE MEASURES

Cancer prevention can take two forms: primary prevention (before it occurs) and secondary prevention (discovery before symptoms occur). The most important primary preventive measure—probably the most important health decision an individual can make—is to avoid cigarettes and other tobacco products. Other important measures are avoidance of overexposure to the sun and of excessive alcohol intake. The American Cancer Society's dietary recommendations are discussed later in this chapter.

Secondary methods of prevention include self-examination of the breasts, periodic physical examinations, blood tests (to detect leukemia and prostate cancer), Pap smears, sigmoidoscopy, colonoscopy, mammography, and tests to detect blood in the stool. Guidelines for frequency of these examinations are found in Chapter 5. Thermography (a method of measuring heat given off by a part of the body) and transillumination (shining of red and near-infrared light through a body part to illuminate its inner structures)[8] are not valid techniques for breast cancer detection.

DIAGNOSIS

Although cancer is often suspected because of a physical finding, laboratory test, or imaging procedure, standard practice requires confirmation through microscopic examination by a pathologist. Specimens usually are obtained by biopsy of a small piece of tissue suspected of being cancerous. Cancer diagnosis is sometimes difficult. However, although the frequency of diagnostic errors is unknown, it appears low.

Once a cancer is identified, the next step is staging, a method of estimating how far the disease has advanced along its usual course. For most cancers this is based on the size of the primary tumor, the involvement of lymph nodes, and the presence of metastases (tumors that have spread to distant sites through the bloodstream or lymphatic channels). Staging is used to help select appropriate treatment, to estimate prognosis, and to evaluate treatment results.

PROGNOSIS

The National Cancer Institute (NCI)[3] estimates that about 62% of the people diagnosed with cancer are likely

---

✓ **Consumer Tip**

Warning Signals

The American Cancer Society lists the following cancer warning signals as reasons to consult a physician.

- ✔ Change in bowel or bladder habits
- ✔ A sore that does not heal
- ✔ Unusual bleeding or discharge
- ✔ Thickening or lump in breast or elsewhere
- ✔ Indigestion or difficulty in swallowing
- ✔ Obvious change in a wart or mole
- ✔ Nagging cough or hoarseness

to live 5 years or more. Its data from 1989 through 1996 include the following 5-year survival rates by sites: uterus 57% to 86%, larynx 54% to 66%, breast 71% to 86%, cervix 59% to 72%, bladder 64% to 82%, prostate 87% to 94%, colon 52% to 63%, and lung 11% to 14%. (The lower numbers are for African-Americans; the higher ones are for Caucasians.) Treatment with anticancer drugs has caused the overall death rate from cancers that usually occur before age 45 to fall sharply and has resulted in long-term survival for many patients. These cancers include Hodgkin's disease and acute childhood leukemia. The overall survival rate from most other cancers has risen slowly.

The outlook for an individual with cancer depends on the type of tumor, its location, and the extent of its spread. Some tumors grow slowly and remain localized, whereas others grow rapidly and metastasize. Spontaneous remission of certain cancers occurs, although rarely.

Patients with a poor prognosis often face a serious dilemma. In many cases, although surgery, radiation, or chemotherapy might briefly prolong their life, the quality of that life (due to side effects or disability) would be so poor that further treatment is unwarranted. In some cases, measures that have been proven useful against one type of tumor may be inappropriately tried against another type. For these reasons, people with cancer should investigate their options thoroughly.

EVIDENCE-BASED TREATMENT METHODS

The three main types of conventional treatment are surgery, radiation therapy, and chemotherapy. In some cases a combination is more effective than one method alone. Treatment may be done with the hope of curing the patient, or it may be done palliatively, with the hope of relieving discomfort or prolonging life.

Surgery is the primary treatment method for most major forms of cancer, especially in their early stages. Cancer surgery chiefly involves removal of the tumor and nearby tissues that may contain cancer cells.

Radiation therapy, also called radiotherapy, attacks cancers with x-rays or with rays or particles from radioactive substances such as cobalt or radium. Radiotherapy may be administered externally with a machine or internally by inserting radioactive material into a body cavity or organ. The beams do not kill the cancer cells outright but destroy their ability to reproduce so that once they die, they are not replaced.

Chemotherapy (treatment with anticancer drugs) has become increasingly effective. Because these drugs circulate to all parts of the body, they can attack cancer cells that have spread to distant organs. More than 50 anticancer drugs are in use today, and many others are being tested experimentally.[9] The main drug types are alkylating agents (which block cell reproduction), antimetabolites, steroid hormones, and antibiotics. Curative dosages of chemotherapy usually have severe side effects. Lesser doses may be appropriately given for palliation. However, former NCI Director Vincent DeVita has warned that giving lesser dosages to potentially curable patients is "throwing away the cure rate."[10]

Another approach is the use of "biologic response modifiers" that stimulate or use the patient's own immune system to attack cancer cells. These substances, which are quite costly to produce, include interferon and interleukin-2. Interferon is the generic name for a group of hormonelike proteins that can combat many types of viruses. In 1986 it received FDA approval for the treatment of hairy cell leukemia, a rare disease. Monoclonal antibodies are specifically tailored to seek out chosen targets on cancer cells so that they can kill these cells without damaging normal cells.[11] Interleukin-2 (IL-2), produced in the body in tiny amounts, is manufactured by genetic engineering techniques. White blood cells are obtained from the patient, bathed in IL-2 to make them reproduce faster, and reinjected with more IL-2 into the patient's bloodstream. They are attracted to and destroy cancer cells.

Other techniques are used to enhance the effectiveness of current methods. These include "rescue factors" (chemicals used to protect normal cells against otherwise fatal chemotherapy) and use of the patient's own marrow or blood cells to repopulate the bone marrow after chemotherapy.

A limited number of patients for whom no established treatment is available may be eligible to enter a clinical trial of a new approach.[12] Information about clinical trials can be obtained from one's physician or the National Cancer Institute's Cancer Information Service's Web site. Many trials are conducted by cancer specialists in communities throughout the United States.

Scientific treatment facilities maintain a tumor registry in which the details of cases treated at the facility are recorded, with follow-up queries sent annually to patients and/or to their doctors. Data of this type are important in assessing the results of treatment.

DIET AND CANCER

The fact that people with similar hereditary background living in different parts of the world can have different cancer patterns suggests that environmental causes play an important role, but the data are complex and diffi-

Consumer Tip

Diet and Cancer[13]

The public has been bombarded with messages urging everyone to make substantial dietary changes to reduce their risk of cancer. Americans have been led to believe that the link between specific dietary factors and cancer is solid and convincing, and that dietary modification should be top priority in cancer prevention. In actuality:

- Smoking cessation—not diet—is the single most important factor in cancer prevention. There is no dietary change that will counteract the harmful effects of cigarette smoking. People who believe that they can safely continue to smoke as long as they eat healthful diets are dangerously misinformed.

- A substantial body of epidemiologic evidence associates low intakes of fruits and vegetables with increased risks of cancer. It would be wise for all Americans to make an effort to include fruits and vegetables in their daily diets. Current recommendations call for a minimum of five daily servings of fruits and vegetables; this is a reasonable goal.

- The current scientific evidence does not warrant recommendations for widespread supplementation with antioxidant nutrients.

- Reducing dietary fat intake may reduce the risk of colon and prostate cancer but not breast cancer. Evidence for other cancer sites is inconsistent. It is possible that effects attributed to dietary fat may actually be due to related factors such as total caloric intake.

- Dietary fiber has not been convincingly linked with reduced risks of cancer. However, fiber does have other health benefits.

- Reaching and maintaining a desirable body weight is an important health priority. Obesity increases the risk of hypertension, diabetes, and coronary heart disease. It may also increase the risk of some types of cancer, especially in women.

- Previous recommendations that Americans should minimize consumption of cured, smoked, or pickled foods do not have a sound scientific basis.

- "Chemicals" in food—including naturally occurring substances, intentional additives, and contaminants—do not have a significant impact on cancer risk in the United States.

- People who drink alcoholic beverages should do so in moderation. Excessive alcohol intake is linked with many health problems, including risks of some types of cancer. The current evidence does not warrant a recommendation for abstinence from alcohol for the purpose of preventing breast cancer.

---

cult to interpret. Dietary factors may play a role in the development of certain cancers, but the evidence for this is weaker than most people realize.

The idea that dietary strategies might help prevent certain cancers was given impetus by a National Academy of Sciences committee report that included four "interim guidelines":

1. *Include in the daily diet plenty of whole-grain cereals, fruits, and vegetables, especially the fruits and vegetables high in vitamin C and beta-carotene (which the body can convert into vitamin A).* Citrus fruits are rich in vitamin C, and dark-green and deep-yellow vegetables are rich in carotenes. The NAS committee also suggested including members of the family *Cruciferae,* such as cabbage, broccoli, cauliflower, and Brussels sprouts.
2. *Reduce calories from fats from the typical 40% level of the American diet to about 30%.* This was based on a statistical association between fat intake and certain types of cancer. However, a similar association exists between cancer and the intake of proteins and total calories.
3. *Minimize consumption of salt-cured, salt-pickled, and smoked foods.* Epidemiologic studies have found that

people in some parts of the world who frequently consume such foods have a greater incidence of cancer at certain sites, particularly the stomach and esophagus.
4. *Avoid excessive consumption of alcohol, especially in combination with cigarettes.*[14]

Many prominent scientists criticized the NAS report's dietary recommendations as inappropriate, premature, and politically motivated and expressed concern that they might distract people from avoiding the established causes of cancer, most notably cigarette smoking.[15] However, the recommendations have influenced subsequent versions of the *Dietary Guidelines for Americans* and stimulated the American Cancer Society[16] to issue its own guidelines:

1. Maintain a desirable body weight.
2. Eat a varied diet.
3. Include a variety of both vegetables and fruits in the daily diet.
4. Eat more high-fiber foods, such as whole-grain cereals, legumes, vegetables, and fruits.
5. Cut down on total fat intake.

6. Limit consumption of alcoholic beverages, if you drink at all.
7. Limit consumption of salt-cured, smoked, and nitrite-preserved foods.

No scientific data indicate what proportion of cancers may be prevented by following this advice. However, it is unlikely to cause harm and may provide additional benefit such as lowering the incidence of cardiovascular disease (see Chapter 15). A 1993 American Council on Science and Health report[13] concluded that smoking cessation was far more important than all other measures combined (see Consumer Tip box on page 377). Animal studies suggest that the incidence of breast cancer is related to dietary fat intake, but large, long-term studies in humans have found no such relationship.[17]

Questionable Anticancer Supplements

The health-food industry is usually quick to exploit new scientific information to its advantage. The NAS report on diet, nutrition, and cancer specified that since it was not known which dietary factors, if any, might be helpful, supplementation with individual nutrients was not advisable. Within a few months after the report was issued, however, a number of products containing dehydrated vegetables and various nutrients were marketed as though the report had supported their use for cancer prevention. In 1984 the FTC issued complaints against two companies marketing such products: Pharmtech Research, Inc. *(Daily Greens)* and General Nutrition, Inc. *(Healthy Greens)*. The FTC charged that their advertising was misleading because no proof existed that eating a tiny amount of processed vegetables could help prevent cancer. Pharmtech signed a consent order to stop making unproven claims, while General Nutrition was ordered to do so by an FTC administrative law judge. In recent years unsubstantiated cancer-prevention claims have been used to market "antioxidant" supplements (see Chapter 12).

Fiber-containing pills have been marketed with suggestions that they can help prevent certain cancers. However, this idea has no scientific support and has been criticized by many prominent scientific groups and individual scientists. Kritchevsky,[18] for example, has noted that dietary fibers have value beyond their possible role in preventing colon cancer. He emphasized that "a high-fiber diet is not merely a low-fiber diet with fiber added. . . . All components of diets containing fiber-rich foods are important."

Actually, evidence is mounting that no link exists between dietary fiber intake and colon cancer. In 1999 researchers reported that their 16-year prospective study of 88,757 women found no significant relationship between fiber intake and the occurrence of precancerous polyps (colorectal adenomas).[19] In 2000 researchers reported on a clinical trial involving 1429 men and women ages 40 to 80 who had had one or more colorectal adenomas removed within 3 months before the study began. The participants entered a supervised program of dietary supplementation with either high amounts (13.5 grams per day) or low amounts (2 grams per day) of wheat-bran fiber. Of the 1303 subjects who completed the study, 719 had been randomly assigned to the high-fiber group and 584 to the low-fiber group. By the time of the last follow-up colonoscopy, at least one adenoma had been identified in 338 subjects (47%) in the high-fiber group and 299 subjects (51%) in the low-fiber group. The authors concluded that "as used in this study, a dietary supplement of wheat-bran fiber does not protect against recurrent colorectal adenomas.[20]

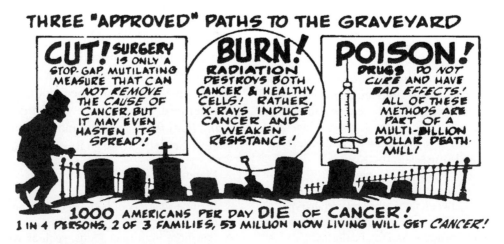

FIGURE 17-1. Message from comic book designed to promote laetrile and undermine public trust in conventional methods of cancer treatment. Condemning accepted methods is a standard practice in medical quackery.

SUSCEPTIBILITY TO CANCER QUACKERY

Cancer is a major field of exploitation of unproven and fraudulent treatments. People use questionable methods mainly because of fears that cancers are incurable and costly to treat, that treatment might be uncomfortable and mutilating, and that they will be socially stigmatized. If treating physicians seem discouraged or state that they can do nothing further, patients often lose hope and feel abandoned. Proponents of "sure cures" cater to these feelings by appearing optimistic and caring while they promote false hopes. Figure 17-1 is an example of literature designed to undermine public trust in proven cancer treatment. Figure 17-2 shows an old ad for a product "guaranteed" to cure any cancer.

People's capacity to be fooled should not be underestimated. During the 1940s, William Koch, M.D., Ph.D., acquired a large following of believers in a remedy that he claimed was 1.32 parts glyoxylide per trillion parts water. More than 3000 assorted practitioners bought it for $25 per ampule and charged patients up to $300 per injection. Analysis of the product could find only distilled water.

Several factors can influence people to believe they have been helped by an unconventional method. Some patients who believe they have been cured of cancer never had it in the first place. Patients who use a questionable treatment along with proven treatment may credit the questionable method for any improvement. Even fatal forms of cancer can have some ups and downs in their course, so that the patient may feel better on some days than others. A period of well-being following use of an unorthodox method can be misinterpreted as "improvement" or even "cure." (See the "Heads I Win, Tails You Lose" box.) Some patients with slow-growing cancers are misrepresented as cured. Doctors sometimes give too pessimistic a prognosis. A patient who tries an unorthodox remedy and lives longer than predicted by a doctor may credit the unorthodox remedy instead of realizing that the doctor's prediction was too pessimistic. Dr. William Jarvis has noted: "Any facility that treats large numbers of cancer patients will encounter some whose survival is much longer than average but still within expected variations. But only the quacks use these people to lure other cancer patients to their facility."

Dr. Malcolm Brigden,[21] a Canadian cancer specialist, believes that unconventional treatments are appealing because their methods are explained in common-sense terms that seem plausible and offer an opportunity to play an active role in fighting the disease: (a) cancer is a symptom, not a disease; (b) symptoms are caused by diet, stress, or environment; (c) proper fitness, nutrition, and mental attitude allow biologic and mental defense against cancer; and (d) conventional therapy treats the symptoms rather than the disease and weakens the body's reserves.

Many "alternative" methods are based on claims that cancer represents a failure of the immune surveillance system to recognize and destroy cancer cells. However, this notion is false, and the claim that cancer can a be cured by strengthening the immune system is unsubstantiated.[22]

Many "alternative" promoters encourage patients to blame themselves for becoming ill. Cassileth and colleagues at the University of Pennsylvania Cancer Center interviewed 304 cancer center inpatients and 356 patients under the care of unconventional practitioners elsewhere. Among those who used "alternative treatment," many believed that their cancer could have been prevented through diet (32% of patients), stress reduction (33%), or environmental changes (26%) and therefore was reversible by the same means. Fifty-three patients had rejected conventional treatment of any kind, while 325 had used both conventional and "alternative" treatments.[23]

In 1987 the American Cancer Society found that 452 (9%) of 5047 cancer patients identified through a

---

◆ **Personal Glimpse** ◆

Heads I Win, Tails You Lose

Quacks capitalize on the natural healing powers of the body by taking credit whenever possible for improvement in a patient's condition. An opposite tack—shifting blame—is used by many cancer quacks. If their treatment does not work, it is because radiation and/or chemotherapy have "knocked out the immune system." Emil J Freireich, M.D., of the M.D. Anderson Hospital and Tumor Institute in Houston, Texas, has combined these ploys into a tongue-in-cheek plan for becoming a successful quack:

1. Pick a "treatment" that is physically harmless.
2. Apply the "treatment" when the patient's disease is getting progressively worse.
3. If the patient's condition improves or stabilizes, take credit. Then stop the treatment or decrease the dosage.
4. If the patient's condition worsens, say that the dosage must be increased or that the treatment was stopped too soon.
5. If the patient dies, say that the treatment was applied too late.

Some Notes on Cancer Quackery

As cancer began to receive considerable attention in the 20th century, many cancer patients became the victims of pseudoscientists and charlatans. Government agencies have driven many from the marketplace, but consumer vigilance remains important.

Members of the Hoque family had no medical training, yet they exploited a cancer-cure salve that contained a corrosive substance. In 1902 and 1908 F.M. Hoque of San Jose, California, was found guilty of practicing medicine without a license. In 1929 W.F. Hoque, a stepson, was found guilty and fined $500 for violation of the Medical Practice Act.

O.A. Johnson of Kansas City, Missouri, sold an alleged treatment called "Mild Combination Treatment for Cancer." In 1910 he was charged with misbranding the product. Later the postal authorities forced him to sign a pledge that he would stop using the mail to sell his product. When two cases concerning women he claimed to have cured were investigated, it was found that both had died of their cancers.

C.R. Chamlee claimed that his mail-order cancer remedy was made from a Pacific island shrub, but chemical analysis found only alcohol and water with small amounts of iron, strychnine, and saccharin (see Figure 17-2). Federal authorities stopped his mail-order business, but for several more years he was able to dispense the product from his offices in Chicago and Los Angeles.

Each decade since 1940 at least one questionable cancer treatment has attracted a large following and become a national issue. The most prominent have been Koch's glyoxylide in the 1940s, the Hoxsey treatment in the 1950s, krebiozen in the 1960s, laetrile in the 1970s, immuno-augmentative therapy in the 1980s, and shark cartilage during the 1990s.

The Hoxsey method of cancer therapy, developed by naturopath Harry M. Hoxsey, has been promoted since the early 1920s. It involved three elements: a liquid for internal use, a corrosive external compound, and supportive treatment. The internal substance contained potassium iodide (an expectorant), licorice, red clover, burdock root, stillingia root, herberis root, poke root, cascara (an herbal laxative), prickly ash bark, and buckthorn bark. The external substance was a yellow powder, a red paste, or a clear solution containing one or more chemicals capable of destroying cancerous tissues on contact. Unfortunately, they destroy healthy tissue as well. The supportive treatment included preparations containing iron, urinary antiseptics, vitamins, laxatives, and antacids.

Three times during the late 1920s, Hoxsey was convicted of practicing medicine without a license. In 1930 he was permanently enjoined for violating the Iowa Medical Practice Act. In 1936, after unsuccessful attempts to practice in other states, he moved to Dallas, Texas, where he maintained a thriving practice until vigorous FDA action drove him to Mexico.

In various trials against Hoxsey, the government presented scientific evidence that his "cured" patients fell into three categories: (1) those who never had cancer, (2) those who had been cured before going to his office, and (3) those who still had their disease or died under the Hoxsey treatment. One case involved a 16-year-old boy who developed cancer of the bone after a football injury. The boy's parents did not wish for the boy's leg to be amputated as recommended by his physician and took the boy to a Hoxsey clinic, where the medical director guaranteed a cure. Four months of tonics were not helpful, and death occurred several months later. The physician who had recommended amputation felt that the boy might have survived had it been performed. Hoxsey, who based his defense on testimonials from 22 patients, won the case. However, the FDA, which suspected that the judge had once been a Hoxsey patient, appealed the case and had the decision reversed. In 1963, after Hoxsey's appeal to the Supreme Court failed, he moved his clinic to Tijuana. He died in 1973, but the clinic is still operated by a nurse who worked with him for many years.

The krebiozen story illustrates how a reputable scientist may become misdirected. In 1949 Dr. Steven Durovic, a physician from Buenos Aires, came to the United States to work with scientists at Northwestern University on a "whitish powder" called kositerin, which he thought was useful in treating hypertension. The substance proved useless, but Durovic met Dr. Andrew C. Ivy, a widely known scientist, physiologist, medical researcher, and vice-president of the University of Illinois. He solicited Ivy's help in testing a compound he called krebiozen, which he claimed was produced by injecting Argentinean horses with *Actinomyces bovis,* the microorganism that causes a disease called "lumpy jaw" in cattle. From the blood of these horses Durovic said he extracted a "whitish powder" that he mixed with mineral oil.

Ivy, who had served as executive director of the National Cancer Advisory Council, was impressed by the results obtained on a number of cancer patients and publicly supported krebiozen. However, in 1952 six prominent physicians reviewed 500 of Dr. Ivy's cases and concluded there was no acceptable evidence that krebiozen had benefited any of them. Dr. Ivy refused to accept these conclusions, and the controversy continued. In 1961 the National Cancer Institute received a small amount of krebiozen along with clinical data from 4200 patients, of which 504 cases were submitted for review. Twenty-four scientists then conducted a study and concluded that krebiozen was ineffective against cancer.

In 1963 the FDA identified krebiozen powder as creatine, an amino acid constituent of meat and normally found in the body. The FDA reported that krebiozen sold before 1960 consisted of mineral oil only, whereas after 1963 it contained creatine monohydrate, which would not dissolve in mineral oil. Meanwhile, the Cancer Advisory Council of the California State Department of Public Health had concluded that krebiozen had no value in the diagnosis or treatment of cancer.

In 1964 Dr. Durovic, his brother Marko, Dr. Ivy, and Dr. William P. Phillips were indicted on 49 counts of violating the Food, Drug and Cosmetic Act, mail fraud, mislabeling, making false statements to the government, and conspiracy. All were acquitted in 1966. The verdict did not alter the fact that krebiozen has no anticancer effect in humans, but it did discourage further criminal prosecutions of this type by the FDA. Since 1966 the agency has initiated few criminal prosecutions against people who market quack products with unproven therapeutic claims.

telephone survey had used questionable treatments. Of these, 49% had used "mind therapies" (mental imagery, hypnosis, or psychic therapy) and 38% had used diets.[24]

QUESTIONABLE METHODS

Cancer quackery is as old as recorded history and almost certainly has existed since cancer was recognized as a disease. Thousands of worthless folk remedies, diets, drugs, devices, and procedures have been promoted for cancer management. The American Cancer Society has defined questionable methods as "diagnostic tests or therapeutic modalities which are promoted for general use in cancer prevention, diagnosis, or treatment and which are, on the basis of careful review by scientists and/or clinicians, not deemed proven nor recommended for current use."[25] The ACS has published detailed critical reports on many questionable methods that have achieved notoriety. In recent years, however, it has softened its approach and issued mostly brief reports on "complementary and alternative methods."

The mere fact that something is unproven does not make it "questionable." For science to advance, researchers and clinicians must be free to try new approaches. Before any cancer treatment is accepted for general use by physicians, it must undergo rigorous scientific scrutiny. When evaluating an unproven method, experts look for:

1. Complete examination of the clinical evidence offered by the proponent, including visits and examinations of treated patients, review of microscopic slides of biopsies, and viewings of x-ray films.
2. Reproducible analysis of laboratory tests on animals and/or tissue culture. No drug that has failed laboratory tests has ever been proven effective against human cancer.
3. Evidence of effectiveness in trials on a sufficient number of patients with biopsy-proven cancers. This must include valid statistical comparison of treated and untreated individuals.
4. Evaluation of autopsy data of treated patients who die.
5. Cooperation with other investigating groups such as the National Cancer Institute, the FDA, and the Sloan-Kettering Memorial Cancer Center.[26]

Questionable methods are broadly classifiable as corrosive agents, plant products, diets and "dietary supplements," drugs, correction of "imbalances," biologic methods, devices, psychologic approaches, and worthless diagnostic tests. Many promoters combine methods to make themselves more marketable.

Corrosive agents. Many salves, poultices, and plasters have been applied directly to tumors with the hope of burning them away. Turpentine is an old favorite. It has been claimed that some corrosive agents "draw out" the cancer. The Hoxsey method (see the Historical Perspective box on page 380) included a product of this type. In recent years scientists have found chemicals that can destroy some superficial skin cancers. Except for these, however, corrosive agents are worthless against cancer.

Plant products. Most folk remedies fall into the plant category. Brews such as a tea from red clover are used as a beverage or for bathing external cancers. *Mucorhicin*, said to be produced by cultivating mold on a nutrient, was composed of yeast, salt, whole wheat, and sterile water. Essiac is an herbal preparation that was prescribed and promoted for about 50 years by Rene M. Caisse, a Canadian nurse who died in 1978. Shortly before her death, she turned over the formula and manufacturing rights to the Resperin Corporation, a Canadian company that has provided it to patients under a special agreement with Canadian health officials. Several reports state that the formula contains burdock, Indian rhubarb, sorrel, and slippery elm, but there may be additional ingredients. Essiac tea claimed to be Caisse's original formulation is also marketed in the United States. Several animal tests using samples of Essiac have shown no antitumor activity.[27] Nor did a review of data on 86 patients performed by the Canadian federal health department during the early 1980s.

Hulda Clark, Ph.D., N.D., claims that (a) all cancers, AIDS, and many other diseases are caused by "parasites, toxins, and pollutants"; (b) cancers can be detected with a blood test for ortho-phospho-tyrosine and a device

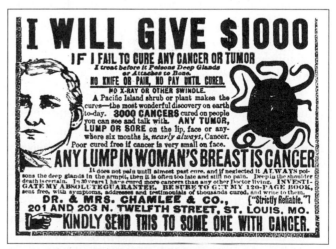

FIGURE 17-2. Ad from the 1920s. C.R. Chamlee claimed that a Pacific island shrub produced his "cures," but chemical analysis revealed that "Chamlee's Cancer Specific" contained only alcohol and water, with small amounts of iron, strychnine, and saccharin.

that identifies diseased organs and toxic substances; (c) cancers can be cured by killing the parasites and ridding the body of environmental chemicals; (d) black walnut hulls, wormwood, and common cloves can rid the body of over 100 types of parasites; and (d) the amino acids ornithine and arginine improve this recipe. Her book *Cure for All Cancers*, contains 103 case histories of her supposed cures. However, judging from her descriptions (a) most did not have cancer, and (b) of those who did, most had received standard medical treatment or their tumors were in early stages.[28]

Pau d'arco tea, sold through health-food stores and by mail, is said to be an ancient Incan remedy prepared from the inner bark of various species of *Tabebuia*, an evergreen tree native to the West Indies and Central and South America. However, stories about its origins contain a variety of geographic and botanical errors. Proponents claim that pau d'arco tea is effective against cancer and many other ailments. *Tabebuia* woods contain lapachol, a chemical that has been shown to have antitumor activity in a few studies on animals. However, human studies have found that as soon as significant blood levels are attained, undesirable effects were severe enough to require that the drug be stopped. Varro E. Tyler, Ph.D., a leading authority on plant medicine, has noted that pau d'arco's "lack of proven effectiveness, potential toxicity, and high cost ($12 to $50 per package) render its use both unwise and extravagant."[29]

Diets and "dietary supplements." Many different dietary approaches have been recommended, including fasting, megadoses of nutrients, consumption of raw foods, and various complicated dietary regimens. The grape cure promoted by Joanna Brandt involves eating large quantities of grapes for 1 or 2 weeks, then adding sour milk, raw vegetables, other fruits, nuts, honey, and olive oil. The macrobiotic diet, discussed in Chapter 12, is a semivegetarian approach claimed to cure cancer and many other health problems.[30]

Powdered shark cartilage is purported to contain a protein that inhibits the growth of new blood vessels needed for cancer to spread. Although a modest effect has been observed in laboratory experiments, it has not been demonstrated that feeding shark cartilage to cancer patients significantly inhibits blood-vessel formation. Even if direct applications were effective, oral administration would not work because the protein would be digested rather than absorbed intact into the body. Nevertheless, in 1993 CBS-TV's "60 Minutes" promoted the claims of biochemist/entrepreneur I. William Lane, Ph.D., co-author of *Sharks Don't Get Cancer*. The program highlighted a Cuban study of 29 "terminal" cancer patients who received shark-cartilage

preparations. Narrator Mike Wallace filmed several doing exercise and reported that most of them felt better several weeks after starting treatment. The fact that "feeling better" does not indicate whether a cancer treatment is effective was not mentioned. Nor was it mentioned that sharks do get cancer, even of their cartilage.[31] National Cancer Institute officials who reviewed the Cuban data called them "incomplete and unimpressive."[32] Figure 17-3 shows how a major health-food-industry book distributor mentioned the "60 Minutes" broadcast in an ad plugging Lane's book.

In 1997, at the American Society of Clinical Oncology's annual meeting, researchers reported a study that found shark cartilage ineffective against advanced cancer in adults with a life expectancy of at least 12 weeks. The study followed 58 people who were prescribed oral doses of shark cartilage as their only form of anti-cancer treatment. After 12 weeks, none achieved a complete or partial response to the shark cartilage treat-

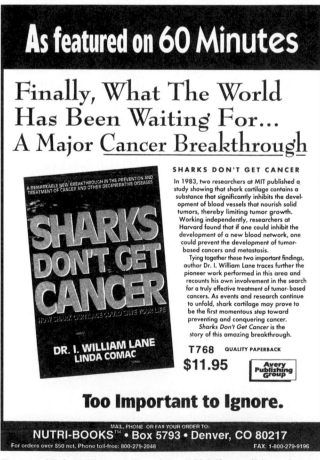

FIGURE 17-3. Within weeks of the "60 Minutes" broadcast, many manufacturers began marketing shark-cartilage products. The false claims in this ad (and the book) would be illegal in marketing products, but freedom of the press protects the authors and the advertiser is merely describing what the book says.

ment. Only 10 showed no progression of their cancer, and only two had a quantifiable improvement in quality of life. (The fact that 10 cancers did not progress is not evidence that the shark cartilage was responsible for this. The progression of cancer is not always rapid.) The researchers concluded: "Shark cartilage was inactive in patients with advanced stages of cancer, specifically in breast, colon, lung, and prostate cancer."[33]

Proponents of the Gerson diet claim to accomplish "detoxification" with frequent coffee enemas and a low-sodium diet that includes more than 1 gallon a day of juices made from fruits, vegetables, and raw calf's liver. Gerson protocols have also included liver-extract injections, ozone enemas, "live cell therapy," thyroid tablets, royal jelly capsules, linseed oil, castor oil enemas, clay packs, Laetrile, and vaccines made from influenza virus and killed *Staphylococcus aureus* bacteria. This approach was developed by Dr. Max Gerson, a German-born physician who emigrated to the United States in 1936. The treatment, available at a clinic in Mexico, is still actively promoted by Gerson's daughter Charlotte through lectures, talk-show appearances, and publications[34] of the Gerson Institute in Bonita, California. Although Ms. Gerson claims high cure rates, these claims are not based on systematic monitoring of patients after they leave the clinic.[35] Three naturopaths who visited the Gerson Clinic in 1983 were able to track 18 patients over a 5-year period (or until death) through annual letters or phone calls. At the 5-year mark, only one was still alive (but not cancer-free); the rest had succumbed to their cancer.[36] Green has concluded that the Gerson rationale is unfounded because (a) the "poisons" Gerson claimed to be present in processed foods have never been identified, (b) frequent coffee enemas have never been shown to mobilize and remove poisons from the liver and intestines of cancer patients, (c) there is no evidence that any such poisons are related to the onset of cancer, and (d) there is no evidence that a "healing" inflammatory reaction exists that can seek out and kill cancer cells.[37]

The American Cancer Society advises that although dietary measures may help prevent certain cancers, there is no scientific evidence that any nutrition-related regimen is appropriate as a primary *treatment* for cancer.[38]

Drugs. Iscador, an extract of mistletoe, was proposed for the treatment of cancer in 1920 by Rudolf Steiner, a Swiss physician who espoused occult beliefs. Steiner founded the Society for Cancer Research to promote mistletoe extracts and occult practices he called anthroposophical medicine. A 1962 report by the society claimed that the time of picking the plants was important because they react to the influences of the sun,

moon, and planets. Various mistletoe juice preparations have been studied with the hope of finding an effective anticancer agent. However, in 1984, the expert working group of the Swiss Society for Oncology concluded that there was no evidence that Iscador was effective against human cancers.[39]

During the past decade, oxygen-rich substances (germanium sesquioxide, hydrogen peroxide, and ozone gas) have been utilized by many promoters of questionable cancer regimens. Their use is based on the erroneous notion that cancer is caused by oxygen deficiency and can be cured by exposing cancer cells to more oxygen than they can tolerate. Although these compounds have been the subject of legitimate research, there is little or no evidence that they are effective for the treatment of any serious disease, and each has demonstrated potential for harm.[40,41] Germanium products, for example, have caused irreversible kidney damage and death. The FDA has banned their importation and seized products from several American manufacturers.

CanCell, originally called *Entelev*, is a liquid claimed to cure cancer by "lowering the voltage of the cell structure by about 20%," causing cancer cells to "digest" and be replaced with normal cells. Accompanying directions have warned that bottles of *CanCell* should not be allowed to touch each other or be placed near any electrical appliance or outlet. *CanCell* has also been promoted for the treatment of AIDS, amyotrophic lateral sclerosis, multiple sclerosis, Alzheimer's disease, "extreme cases of emphysema and diabetes," and several other diseases. In 1989 the FDA reported that *CanCell* contained inositol, nitric acid, sodium sulfite, potassium hydroxide, sulfuric acid, and catechol.[42] Subsequently, its promoters claimed to be modifying the formulation to make it more effective. They have also claimed that *CanCell* cannot be analyzed because it varies with atmospheric vibrations and keeps changing its energy. Laboratory tests conducted between 1978 and 1991 by the NCI found no evidence that *CanCell* was effective against cancer. The FDA has obtained an injunction forbidding its distribution to patients.[43]

In the mid-1970s hydrazine sulfate was proposed for treating the progressive weight loss and body deterioration characteristic of advanced cancer. Based on animal data and preliminary human studies, it has also been claimed to cause tumor regression and subjective improvement in patients. However, three recent trials sponsored by the National Cancer Institute found that hydrazine sulfate was no better than a placebo.[44] The trials involved a total of 636 patients with three types of cancer. In one study nerve damage occurred more often and the quality of life was significantly worse in the hydrazine sulfate group. Beginning in 1995, Kathy Keeton, wife of *Penthouse* magazine publisher Bob Guccione, achieved widespread publicity with claims that hydrazine sulfate had enabled her to recover from stage IV metastatic cancer after doctors gave her only 6 weeks to live. However, she died of her disease in 1997. The 5-year survival rate with such a cancer is 12% to 20%. A 2-year survival is certainly not unusual.[45]

"Antineoplastons" is the name given by Stanislaw R. Burzynski, M.D., to substances that he claims can "normalize" cancer cells. He has published many papers in which he claims that antineoplastons extracted from urine or synthesized in his laboratory have proven effective against cancer in laboratory experiments. He also claims to have helped many people with cancer get well.

In 1982 two Canadian experts visited Burzynski's clinic and asked for information on the patients he felt best demonstrated that his treatment was effective. After reviewing the status of about a dozen cases, they concluded that all who were still alive had either had slowly growing tumors or had received effective treatment before seeing Burzynski. In a report to the Canadian Ministry of Health they stated:

We were surprised that Dr. Burzynski would show us such questionable cases. We were left with the impression that either he knows very little about cancer and the response of different tumors to radiation and hormonal measures, or else he thinks that we are very stupid, and he has tried to hoodwink us.[46]

In 1988 talk-show hostess Sally Jesse Raphael featured four patients of Burzynski whom she described as "miracles." The patients stated that Burzynski had cured them when conventional methods had failed. In 1992 the television program "Inside Edition" reported that two of the four patients had died and a third was having a recurrence of her cancer. (The fourth patient had bladder cancer, which has a good prognosis.) The widow of one of Raphael's guests stated that her husband and five others from the same city had sought treatment after learning about Burzynski from a television broadcast—and that all had died of their disease.

Saul Green, Ph.D.,[47] a biochemist who worked for many years at Memorial Sloan-Kettering Hospital investigating the mechanisms and treatment of cancer, has found no evidence that any of the substances Burzynski calls "antineoplastons" have been proven to "normalize" tumor cells. In 1998, the Texas Attorney General secured a consent agreement stating that Burzynski (a) cannot distribute unapproved drugs in Texas; (b) can distribute "antineoplastons" only to

patients enrolled in FDA-approved clinical trials, unless the FDA approves his drugs for sale; (c) cannot advertise "antineoplastons" for the treatment of cancer; and (d) his Web site and promotional material and ads must include a disclaimer that the safety and effectiveness of "antineoplastons" have not been established. The agreement also called for Burzynski to pay $50,000 to reimburse the Attorney General's office and the Texas Health Department for the cost of their investigation.[48] The *Cancer Letter* subsequently noted that although Burzynski has set up many "clinical trials," they do not conform to usual standards.[49]

714X is a chemical solution produced in Quebec by Gaston Naessens, who also operates the International Academy of Somatidian Orthobiology. He claims that 714X can "fluidify the lymph" and "direct nitrogen into the cancerous cells in order to stop their toxic secretions which block the organism's defense system." 714X has been analyzed by the Canadian Health Protection Branch and found to contain a mixture of camphor, ammonium chloride and nitrate, sodium chloride, ethyl alcohol, and water. The Health Protection Branch has received no scientific data to support claims that 714X can cure cancer or AIDS. Its Expert Advisory Committee has deplored its use for these purposes and warned that there could be adverse side effects.[50] In 1956, in connection with alleged cancer remedy called GN-24, Naessens was convicted of illegal medical practice and ordered by a French court to pay the maximum applicable fine. He was prosecuted again in 1964 after another alleged cancer remedy he administered in Corsica was proven not to work.

Laetrile, which achieved great notoriety during the 1970s and early 1980s, is discussed later in this chapter.

Correction of "imbalances." Revici Cancer Control (also called lipid therapy) is based on the belief that cancer is caused by an imbalance between constructive (anabolic) and destructive (catabolic) body processes. This approach was developed by Emmanuel Revici, M.D. (1896–1998), who practiced in New York City. To treat the patient, Revici prescribed lipid alcohols, zinc, iron, and caffeine—which he said were "anabolic"—and fatty acids, sulfur, selenium and magnesium—which he classified as "catabolic." His formulations, which varied from visit to visit, were based on his measurements of the specific gravity, pH (acidity), and surface tension of single samples of the patient's urine. Revici also claimed success against AIDS.

Scientists offering to evaluate Revici's methods were never able to agree with him on procedures to ensure a valid test. However, his method of urinary interpretation is not valid. The specific gravity of urine reflects the concentration of dissolved substances and varies with the amount of fluid a person consumes. The acidity depends mainly on diet and varies considerably throughout the day. Thus, even when these values are useful for a metabolic evaluation, information from a single urine sample would be meaningless. The surface tension of urine has no medically recognized diagnostic value.[51]

In 1983 Revici's medical license was suspended for 60 days while the New York Board of Medical Conduct reviewed charges that he had promised to cure three cancer patients. One was a 49-year-old woman whom other doctors had advised to have a marble-sized lump removed from her left breast. Revici persuaded her to undergo treatment with him instead. After 14 months, the tumor had filled one breast and spread to the opposite breast and to many lymph nodes—requiring removal of both breasts and treatment with radiation and chemotherapy. State licensing authorities placed Revici on probation in 1988 and revoked his license in 1993 after concluding that he had violated the terms of his probation.

Biologic methods. "Vaccines" and similar products have been prepared from various substances including pooled cancers, the patient's own blood and/or urine, animal blood and/or urine, and cultures of germs. Virginia Livingston, M.D., who died in 1990, postulated that cancer is caused by a bacterium that invades the body when resistance is low.[52] To combat the cancer, she allegedly strengthened the body's immune system with various vaccines (including one made from bacteria taken from the patient's urine); a vegetarian diet that avoids chicken, eggs, and sugar; vitamin and mineral supplements; visualization; and stress reduction. She claimed to have a very high recovery rate but published no clinical data to support this. Scientists who attempted to isolate the organism she postulated found that it was a common skin bacterium. Researchers at the University of Pennsylvania Cancer Center compared 78 patients with advanced cancer treated at the center with 78 similar patients given various vaccines, a vegetarian diet, and coffee enemas at the Livingston-Wheeler Clinic. The study found no difference between average survival time of the two groups. However, the Livingston-Wheeler patients reported more problems with appetite and pain.[53]

Fresh cell therapy, also called live cell therapy and cellular therapy, involves injections of fresh embryonic animal cells taken from the organ or tissue that corresponds to the unhealthy organ or tissue in the patient. Proponents claim that the recipient's body automatically transports the injected cells to the target organ where they repair and rejuvenate the ailing cells. The originator of this approach was Paul Niehans, a Swiss physician who died in 1971. The American Cancer Society[54] states that fresh cell therapy has no proven benefit and has caused serious side effects (infections and immunologic reactions to the injected protein) and death.

Hariton Alivizatos, a Greek physician who died in 1991, claimed to have developed a blood test that can determine the type, location, and severity of any cancer. He also claimed to have developed a "serum" that enabled the patient's immune system to destroy cancer cells and helped the body rejuvenate parts destroyed by cancer.[55] Knowledgeable observers believe the principal ingredient of the so-called Greek Cancer Cure was niacin.

Immuno-augmentative therapy, another biologic method, is discussed later in this chapter.

Devices. Numerous gadgets have been falsely claimed to diagnose and/or treat cancer.[56] One of the most notorious was the Orgone Energy Accumulator, which was claimed by Wilhelm Reich, M.D., to treat disease by absorbing "blue bions" or "Cosmic Orgone Energy." In 1956 Reich and an associate were sentenced to prison for violating an earlier injunction against distributing his devices. Devices used or marketed by others have included equipment that passes low-voltage electrical current through tumors or the body; "electroacupuncture" devices purported to measure the electrical resistance of so-called "acupuncture points" for diagnosis and prescription; colonic irrigation machines claimed to "detoxify the system"; electrical devices claimed to "charge" blood samples taken from patients and later returned; negative ion generators claimed to have an effect against tumors; radionics devices claimed to diagnose and cure cancer by analyzing and emitting radio waves at the correct frequencies; magnets claimed to cure cancers by "improving circulation" or by intracellular effects; crystals alleged to have curative powers; pendulums used to diagnose or locate tumors in a manner similar to that of divining rods; pyramidal objects alleged to focus occult energies for healing purposes; and a brassiere claimed to prevent breast cancer and either increase or decrease the size of the bosom. Neither quacks nor their victims seem to have any limit to the scope of their imagination.

Psychologic approaches. Various psychologic methods are promoted to cancer patients as cures or as adjuncts to other treatment. The techniques include imagery, visualization, meditation, progressive muscle relaxation, and various forms of psychotherapy. These techniques may reduce stress, alleviate depression, help control pain, and enhance patients' feelings of mastery and control. Individual and group support can have a positive impact on quality of life and overall attitude. A positive attitude may increase a patient's chance of surviving cancer by increasing compliance with proven treatment. However, it has not been demonstrated that emotions directly influence the course of the disease.

Bernie Siegel, M.D., author of *Love, Medicine & Miracles* and *Peace, Love & Healing*, is a surgeon who claims that "happy people generally don't get sick" and that "one's attitude toward oneself is the single most important factor in healing or staying well." He also states that "a vigorous immune system can overcome cancer if it is not interfered with, and emotional growth toward greater self-acceptance and fulfillment helps keep the immune system strong." No scientific study supports these claims. Siegel co-authored a report of a 10-year study which found that 34 breast cancer patients participating in his Exceptional Cancer Patients program lived no longer after diagnosis than comparable non-participants.[57] The program consisted of weekly peer support and family therapy, individual counseling, and the use of positive imagery.

O. Carl Simonton, M.D., claims that cancers can be affected by relaxation and visualization techniques. He asserts that this approach can lessen fears and tension, strengthen the patient's will to live, increase optimism, and alter the course of a malignancy by strengthening the immune system. However, he has not published the results of any well-designed study testing his ideas. Simonton theorizes that the brain can stimulate endocrine glands to inspire the immune system to attack cancer cells. He and his wife Stephanie (a psychotherapist) taught cancer patients to imagine their cancer being destroyed by their white blood cells. However, there is no evidence that white cells actually attack cancer cells in this manner or that "immune suppression" is a factor in the development of common cancers. Friedlander[58] has noted:

When the Simontons developed this technique, many people thought that the white blood cells of the immune system were the body's major defense against cancer. Cancerous cells supposedly are produced on a steady basis but destroyed by the body's white cells; and malignancies that become evident are the ones that "got away." Unfortunately for the "immune surveillance" theory, we now know that people who are given immunosuppressant drugs . . . or who are immunodeficient because of hereditary disease or AIDS, are not prone to develop any of the common cancers. Rather, they tend to develop unusual cancers—such as Kaposi's sarcoma in AIDS—that arise from cells made abnormal by the underlying diseases. Nevertheless, imagers still meditate about white cells making their cancers go away.

Simonton's book *Getting Well Again* included reports on patients who got better after using his methods. However, Friedlander[59] analyzed five of the reports he thought might impress laypersons most and noted that two of the patients had undergone standard treatment, one had a slow-growing tumor, and one probably did not have cancer. The fifth patient's tumor was treatable by standard means.

Some people suggest Simonton's program may have positive psychologic effects because it may help people relax and give them a feeling that they are doing something positive. However, hundreds of scientific studies have found no clear-cut relationship between emotions, personality factors, stresses, and cancer. Simonton has done some studies, but the American Cancer Society and others have questioned their design.[59] Although his method is physically harmless, it may encourage some patients to abandon effective care.

Worthless diagnostic tests. H.H. Beard, a biochemist, claimed that his Beard Anthrone Test could detect cancer in the body within 2 or 3 weeks after it started by measuring a sex hormone in the urine. He was indicted for mail fraud in 1967 and subsequently received a 6-month suspended prison sentence. The Arthur (or Automated) Immunostatus Differential Test (also called the AID Test), which Beard claimed could detect cancer before it developed, involved computerized microscopic examination of blood from the earlobe.

Two tests were used by William Kelley, D.D.S., the dentist whose methods were used unsuccessfully to treat actor Steve McQueen. Kelley's Protein Metabolism Evaluation Index was based on the premise that cancer is a foreign protein. His Kelley Malignancy Index was claimed to be " the most accurate and extensive cancer detection system ever developed." It was supposed to determine "the presence or absence of cancer, the growth rate of the tumor, the location of the tumor mass, prognosis of the treatment, age of the tumor, and the regulation of medication for treatment."[60] A booklet by Kelley claimed "at least 86% of all cancer conditions can be treated by diet alone" and that "cancer is nothing more than a pancreatic enzyme deficiency" caused by eating too much of the wrong kind of protein. "If people would not eat protein after 1:00 PM," the booklet stated, "83% of cancer in the United States could be eliminated."

In 1970 Kelley was convicted of practicing medicine without a license after witnesses testified that he had diagnosed lung cancer on the basis of blood from a patient's finger and prescribed dietary supplements, enzymes, and a diet as treatment.[61] In 1976, following court appeals, his dental license was suspended for 5 years for unprofessional conduct. However, he continued to promote his methods until the mid-1980s through his Dallas-based International Health Institute.[62] Under the institute's umbrella, licensed professionals and "certified metabolic technicians" throughout the United States would administer a 3200-item questionnaire and send the answers to Dallas. The resultant computer printout provided a lengthy report on "metabolic status" plus detailed instructions covering foods, supplements (typically 100 to 200 pills per day), "detoxification" techniques, and lifestyle changes.[27]

Treatment said to be similar is still provided today by Nicholas Gonzalez, M.D., of New York City, who claims to have analyzed Kelley's records and drafted a book about his findings. The manuscript was never published, but experts who evaluated its chapter on 50 cases found no evidence of benefit.[27]

In 1994, after investigating six of Gonzalez's cases, New York State licensing authorities had concluded (a) his "alternative protocol" did not entitle him to an alternative standard of care, (b) he had failed to correctly interpret signs and symptoms of disease progression, (c) he had treated the patients incompetently, and (d) his record-keeping was inadequate. He was placed on probation for 3 years with stipulations that he undergo retraining and his work be supervised by the Office of Professional Conduct.

In 1997 a jury in New York City awarded $2.5 million in actual damages and $150,000 in punitive damages to a former Gonzalez patient. The woman testified that she had been diagnosed with an early stage of uterine cancer in 1991 and underwent a hysterectomy. Instead of following through with medically recommended radiation and chemotherapy, she consulted Gonzalez who discouraged her from following her cancer specialist's advice. Gonzalez prescribed up to 150 dietary supplement pills a day plus frequent coffee enemas. Later he claimed that the cancer was cured even though it was progressing. It eventually damaged her spine and left her blind. An appeals court upheld the $2.5 million verdict but dismissed the punitive damage award. In April 2000, a jury awarded $282,000 in damages to the husband of a 40-year-old college professor who had died of Hodgkin's disease in 1995. According to an article in the *New York Daily News*, the jury found Gonzalez negligent because he failed to arrange "appropriate testing" to track the cancer, relying instead on an unproven method of hair analysis.[63]

Immuno-Augmentative Therapy

Immuno-augmentative therapy (IAT) was developed by Lawrence Burton, Ph.D., a zoologist who claimed that IAT could control all forms of cancer by restoring natural immune defenses. He claimed to accomplish this by injecting blood serum proteins isolated with processes he had patented. However, experts have shown that the substances he claims to use cannot be produced by these procedures and do not exist in the human body.[64] Burton did not publish detailed clinical reports, divulge the details of his methods, publish meaningful statistics, conduct a controlled trial, or provide independent investigators with specimens of his treatment materials for analysis. During the mid-1980s, several of Burton's patients were reported to have developed serious infections following IAT.

In 1974 Burton declined an offer from the National Cancer Institute to help test his methods. Shortly afterward, after failing to complete a satisfactory application to the FDA to test humans in the United States, he established a clinic on Grand Bahama Island, where patients paid more than $5000 for a few weeks of treatment. In 1979 Burton received an enormous boost when CBS-TV's "60 Minutes" gave him favorable publicity. A prominent physician stated that one of his patients treated by Burton appeared to have miraculously recovered. The patient died within 2 weeks after the program was shown, but "60 Minutes" never informed viewers of this fact.

William A. Nolen, M.D., who visited Burton's clinic in 1982, reviewed many records and had follow-up conversations with at least 10 patients and some of their doctors. Nolen concluded that most of the patients had never had cancer or had tumors that typically grow slowly, while some had undergone conventional treatment that was probably responsible for any positive results.[65]

Burton's literature included a booklet summarizing the experiences of 35 IAT patients and their status as of February 1988. However, Dr. Wallace Sampson, a cancer specialist who examined the data, concluded:

The sampling of cases is not meaningful. To estimate prognosis accurately, the stage and grade of a tumor are needed. Only a few of these vignettes provide both of these. Any facility that treats large numbers of cancer patients will have some patients who survive a long time—with or without treatment. It would not be possible to determine IAT's effectiveness without knowing how these outcomes compare with the rest of Burton's patients who had similar cancers. Moreover, 30 of the 35 received standard or near-standard treatment before undergoing IAT. All of these had a significant probability of living as long as was recorded in the booklet.[66]

In 1985 public health officials found antibodies to the AIDS virus in vials of serum obtained from several patients and were able to culture the virus from one specimen—suggesting that blood infected with the virus had been used to prepare IAT treatment materials.[67]

In 1986, in response to Congressional action, the Congressional Office of Technology Assessment (OTA) appointed a group of technical experts and representatives of Dr. Burton to design a clinical trial to evaluate IAT. However, communication broke down after Burton insisted on having a "pre-test" conducted at his clinic. The OTA report concluded that "no reliable data are available on which to base a determination of IAT's efficacy."[27] Burton died in 1993, but his former medical director is still operating the clinic.

The Personal Glimpse box below describes how trickery may have been used to make patients think they had been helped by IAT.

Laetrile

Laetrile, which achieved great notoriety during the 1970s and early 1980s, is the trade name for a synthetic relative of amygdalin, a chemical in the kernels of apricot pits, apple seeds, bitter almonds, and some other stone fruits and nuts. Many Laetrile promoters have called it "vitamin B_{17}" and falsely claimed that cancer is a vitamin deficiency disease that Laetrile can cure.

Claims for Laetrile's efficacy have varied considerably.[68–70] First it was claimed to prevent and cure cancer. Then it was claimed not to cure, but to "control" cancer while increasing feelings of well-being. Then it was claimed to be effective, not by itself but as a component of "metabolic therapy" (described on the opposite page).

Laetrile was first used to treat cancer patients in the 1950s. Proponents claim that it kills tumor cells selectively while leaving normal cells alone. Although Laetrile has been promoted as safe and effective, clinical evidence indicates that it is neither.[72] When subjected to enzymatic breakdown in the body, it forms glucose, benzaldehyde, and hydrogen cyanide.

Some patients treated with Laetrile have suffered nausea, vomiting, headache, and dizziness, and a few have died from cyanide poisoning. Laetrile has been tested in at least 20 animal tumor models and found to have no benefit either alone or together with other substances. Studies of human case reports have also been uniformly negative. During the 1970s, for example, Dr. Ernesto Contreras, a Mexican physician who claimed to have treated more than 16,000 cancer patients with Laetrile, submitted 12 cases to illustrate his successes. However, the FDA found that six had died of their disease, one still had cancer, and three could not be located. Two others had been treated with conventional therapy, which made it impossible to tell whether Laetrile had helped them.[73]

In 1982, in response to political pressure, the Mayo Clinic and three other cancer centers began a clinical

---

◆ **Personal Glimpse** ◆

A Victim's Experience

In 1982 my father-in-law was diagnosed as having unresectable, incurable, widely disseminated cancer of the lung, and advised that essentially his condition was terminal. As could be expected, the family was distraught, and we began to grasp at straws and looking into alternative modes of treatment. . . . Some of the local press carried stories about . . . so-called immuno-augmentative therapy. . . . Soon thereafter he went to the Bahamas to get the treatment.

His main symptom had been pain from the tumor. It had metastasized to the bones. When he went down there, he was told to go off pain medication and to begin the serum injections, and that . . . the serum injections, if they work and dissolve the tumor, will cause pain. So he went down there knowing he had a tumor growing in him and causing him pain, and through a pretty good ploy he came back convinced that the pain he was having was a cure. In addition, he was told the tumor was shrinking. The x-ray film they took was overexposed, which has the technical problem of making masses look smaller than they really are.

Upon his return I encouraged him to go to Fox Army Hospital and have another chest x-ray made. Several radiologists corroborated that they could see no evidence of any shrinkage in the tumor. I was then faced with the unpleasant task of telling my father-in-law for the second time he was dying.

It was interesting that both he and his wife came back with total euphoria—that he was cured. They told everyone they saw he was cured. When they realized that they had been fooled, it was really a shock, and, of course one doesn't usually go around telling people you have been fooled.

He died approximately 2 months after he returned. In addition to the emotional turmoil and being away from the rest of the family for essentially half the remaining life he had, this cost them approximately $10,000, including travel and lodging, for this phony cancer cure.

Carl Barnes, M.D.[71]

trial sponsored by the National Cancer Institute. Laetrile and "metabolic therapy" were administered as recommended by their promoters. The patients had advanced cancer for which no proven treatment was known. Of 178 patients, not one was cured or stabilized or had any lessening of any cancer-related symptoms. The median survival rate was about 5 months from the start of therapy. Several patients experienced symptoms of cyanide toxicity or had blood levels of cyanide approaching the lethal range.[74] Dr. Arnold S. Relman, editor of the *New England Journal of Medicine*, commented on these results:

Laetrile, I believe, has had its day in court. The evidence, beyond reasonable doubt, is that it doesn't benefit patients with advanced cancer, and there is no reason to believe that it would be any more effective in the earlier stages of the disease. Some undoubtedly will remain unconvinced, but no sensible person will want to advocate its further use and no state legislature should sanction it any longer. The time has come to close the books on Laetrile and get on with our efforts to understand the riddle of cancer and improve its prevention and treatment.[75]

In 1975 a class action suit was filed to stop the FDA from interfering with the sale and distribution of Laetrile. Early in the case, a federal district court judge in Oklahoma issued orders allowing cancer patients to import a 6-month supply of Laetrile for personal use if they could obtain a physician's affidavit that they were "terminal." In 1979 the U.S. Supreme Court ruled that it is not possible to be certain who is terminal and that even if it were possible, both terminally ill patients and the general public deserve protection from fraudulent cures. In 1987, after further appeals were denied, the district judge (a strong proponent of Laetrile) finally yielded to the higher courts and terminated the affidavit system. Today few sources of Laetrile are available within the United States, but it still is utilized at Mexican clinics.[76]

"Metabolic Therapy"

"Metabolic therapy" is based on the idea that cancer and other chronic illnesses result from a disturbance of the body's ability to protect itself. Its most visible proponent was Harold Manner, Ph.D., a former biology professor who left his academic position to market his treatment ideas. Manner defined metabolic therapy as "the use of natural food products and vitamins to prevent and treat disease by building a strong immune system." He theorized that chemicals in food, water, and air cause large numbers of primitive cells to become cancerous. He said that when the immune system is functioning normally, the cancer cells are destroyed. But if

it is weakened by poor nutrition, environmental pollutants, or debilitating stress, cancer cells are uninhibited and multiply rapidly. Therefore, the way to treat cancer is by revitalizing the body's immune system with diet, dietary supplements, and "detoxification." In 1982 Manner became affiliated with a clinic in Tijuana, Mexico, that was later renamed the Manner Clinic.

During 1988 the clinic charged $7500 for its 21-day program of vegetable juices; "natural foods"; intravenous Laetrile; coffee enemas; and large amounts of vitamins, minerals, enzymes, glandular extracts, other products, and inspirational messages. Although Manner claimed a 74% success rate against cancers, there is no evidence that he kept track of how patients fared once they left his clinic.[77] Manner died in 1988, but the clinic is still operating.

The components of metabolic therapy vary from practitioner to practitioner. No controlled study has shown that any of its components has any value against cancer or any other chronic disease. However, many people find its concepts appealing because they do not seem far removed from scientific medicine's concerns with diet, lifestyle, and the relationship between emotions and bodily responses.

Insurance Fraud

In 1988 a reporter who attended a Manner seminar for doctors (mostly chiropractors and naturopaths) uncovered a scheme to defraud insurance companies. The scheme was carried out by North American Health Insurance Coordinators (NAHIC), a company that filed claims on behalf of patients at "alternative" treatment facilities. Instead of indicating what actually took place, it would enter code numbers for standard treatment on the claim forms.[77] In 1994, after a lengthy FBI investigation, three NAHIC officials were indicted when a federal grand jury concluded that the company's "principal business was the filing of false and fraudulent claims" for health-insurance benefits. The indictment charged that fraudulent claims inflated the fees for services rendered, billed for services never provided, utilized false dates of service, falsified diagnoses, and pretended that services provided at Mexican clinics had been administered within the United States. The FBI estimated that claims submitted by NAHIC had caused insurance companies to pay out more than $43 million during the previous 7 years, mostly for treatment at Mexican clinics. The indictment papers identified six clinics whose services were fraudulently described on claims submitted by NAHIC. Figure 17-4 illustrates a misleading "credential" the reporter acquired at the Manner Seminar.

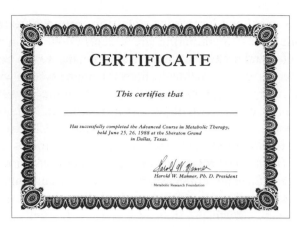

FIGURE 17-4. This certificate was obtained by a reporter who gained admission to Harold Manner's "Advanced Course in Metabolic Therapy" by pretending to be a chiropractor. Attendees who joined the Manner Metabolic Foundation were promised a $200 "referral fee" for each patient they referred to Manner's Mexican clinic.

PROMOTION OF QUESTIONABLE METHODS

Promoters of cancer quackery run the gamut from ignorant individuals to highly educated scientists with advanced degrees. A few even hold medical degrees. Such individuals typically (a) discount biopsy verification, (b) fail to keep adequate records, (c) spread claims through the media rather than through scientifically acceptable channels subject to peer review, (d) tend to be isolated from established scientific facilities or associates, and (e) claim persecution by the medical establishment.

Many promoters claim that cancer is the result of adverse environmental influences, excess protein intake, self-pollution by bad habits, and incorrect spiritual attitudes. The methods promoted by proponents of these ideas include meatless diets; "cleansing" of the body by special diets, enemas, and antioxidants; megadoses of vitamins and trace minerals; and various spiritual approaches. Cassileth has noted:

Most [such programs] are within the control of the patient, who can choose which part . . . to accept, which part to cheat on, and which part to amplify. There is no FDA regulation of most of these programs since the FDA has no jurisdiction over dietary theories, personal vitamin consumption or spiritual improvement. What's more, no action can be taken against the proponents for claiming that orthodox approaches are unnatural and bad.[78]

Dubious Information Sources

Cancer patients can obtain information about questionable methods in many ways:

1. *Personal contacts.* Referrals may be made by friends, neighbors, or other individuals who know someone supposedly improved or cured by an unconventional treatment. In some communities, traffic in questionable methods is so well organized that proponents infiltrate hospitals to tout their methods during "chance meetings" in waiting rooms.

2. *Magazines and books.* Articles promoting questionable treatments appear frequently in magazines that cater to the health-food industry and sporadically in other magazines. The promotional books include:

Vitamin B-17: Forbidden Weapon against Cancer, by Michael L. Culbert, 1974
World without Cancer, by G. Edward Griffen, 1974
Laetrile Case Histories, by John A. Richardson, M.D., 1977
Recalled by Life: The Story of My Recovery from Cancer, by Anthony Satillaro, M.D., 1982
The Cancer Industry, by Ralph Moss, 1989
A Cancer Therapy, Results of Fifty Cases, by Max Gerson, M.D., revised 1990
The Macrobiotic Approach to Cancer, by Michio Kushi, 1991
How I Conquered Cancer Naturally, by Eydie Mae, 1992
Third Opinion, by John M. Fink, 1992
Options: The Alternative Cancer Therapy Book, by Richard Walters, 1993
Beating Cancer with Nutrition, by Patrick Quillen, Ph.D., R.D., 1994
Nutrition: The Cancer Answer II, by Maureen Salaman, 1995
Definitive Guide to Cancer, by W. John Diamond, M.D., and W. Lee Cowden, M.D., 1997

These books are skillfully written and can cause the average reader to conclude that they provide enough information to make a valid judgment. In some cases,

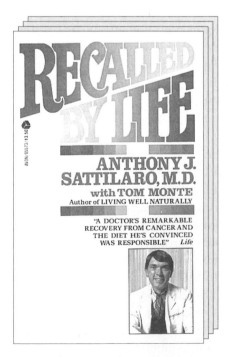

FIGURE 17-5. The author of this 1982 book had conventional treatment for prostate cancer but credited macrobiotics for placing him in "permanent remission." He died of his disease in 1989.

readers are given the impression that the author is impartial and factual, even though the book strongly advocates "alternative" methods. Figure 17-5 depicts a popular book whose author died after claiming that his prostate cancer had been cured by macrobiotic eating.

3. *Proponent organizations.* The International Association of Cancer Victors and Friends (IACVF)[79] was founded by Cecile Hoffman, a cancer patient who believed her life had been saved by the use of Laetrile. Mrs. Hoffman died in 1969 of metastatic cancer. Other groups that promote questionable methods include the Cancer Control Society, which offers tours of the Mexican clinics, the National Health Federation (see Chapter 12),[80] the Committee for Freedom of Choice in Medicine (CFCM),[81] People Against Cancer,[82] the Foundation for Alternative Cancer Therapy, Ltd, and the Center for Advancement in Cancer Education. Their activities may include (a) publishing a magazine or newsletter, (b) selling books and tapes, (c) orchestrating letter-writing campaigns, (d) referring patients to "alternative" treatment facilities, and (e) sponsoring conventions that attract large numbers of participants. Another organization, Project Cure, promotes questionable treatments through the media and distributes promotional literature. Figure 17-6 illustrates CFCM's aggressive language.

4. *Commercial information services.* Several proponents of questionable methods provide individual clients with reports on cancer treatment based on computer searches and other sources. Some reports include some information about conventional treatment but are slanted toward unconventional treatment. In 1991 investigative reporter David Zimmerman probed a report from one such service, CANHELP, operated by Pat McGrady, Jr. The report, which had cost $400, said that no effective conventional treatment was available and recommended a restricted diet plus 100 to 150 supplement pills each day. McGrady apparently was unaware of a new treatment that appeared to have extremely good results. The results had not yet been published in a scientific journal but were readily available to physicians and the public from the National Cancer Institute's information services. Zimmerman indicated that McGrady's advice, if followed, would have led to an unnecessary death.[83] People against Cancer offers advice through its "Alternative Therapy Program," which is available after joining as a sustaining member.[82] In 1995 the group's executive director, Frank Wiewel, advised an undercover investigator to use organic foods, an air purifier, and a water filter to help reduce the odds that her breast cancer would recur.

5. *Radio and television programs.* Proponents of controversial remedies are frequently interviewed on talk shows. A few talk show hosts, most notably Gary Null (syndicated from a station in New York City), give a great deal of favorable publicity to questionable cancer treatments. A few individuals, such as Harry M. Hoxsey, have had their own radio stations.

6. *Internet channels.* Claims for various methods are promoted through Web sites, news and patient support groups, and unsolicited e-mail messages.

7. *Sponsorship by prominent individuals.* Entertainers, socially prominent persons, celebrities, congressional representatives, and others may be persuaded to promote various questionable methods of cancer management. These individuals often are sincere but lack the scientific background to judge the merit of the approach and may not be aware of the strict criteria necessary for scientific investigation before a drug or method is acceptable for medical use.

FIGURE 17-6. This passage from a newsletter of the Committee for Freedom of Choice in Medicine implies that organized medicine, drug companies, government agencies, and various consumer groups are conspiring against the public interest. In 1977 the committee's founder, Robert Bradford, and its vice-president, Frank Salaman, were convicted of conspiracy to smuggle Laetrile into the United States. Bradford now operates American Biologics, a Mexican clinic offering a broad spectrum of unorthodox and unproven treatments for cancer, cardiovascular disease, arthritis, multiple sclerosis, and other conditions. Bruce Halstead, M.D., CFCM's vice president for more than 10 years, was convicted in 1986 of cancer fraud and had his license revoked in 1992.

Fedstapo targeting our medical freedom

U.S. medical orthodoxy and government regulatory agencies have joined forces in an all-out attack on the burgeoning alternative health movement.

To date, the campaign . . . has meant stepped-up prosecution of alternative medical practitioners, assembling of "hit lists" of suspect doctors and professional propagandizing in favor of allopathic, drug-industry medicine.

Joined in the alliance against what they choose to call "health fraud" are such governmental agencies as the Food and Drug Administration (FDA), Postal Service, and Federal Trade Commission (FTC), as well as such nongovernmental but establishment-lining propaganda groups such as the National Council Against Health Fraud, Inc. (NCAHF), the U.S. Council of Better Business Bureaus, national groups of state and federal health officials and other quasi-official organizations.

Institutions that provide standard treatment may also add questionable treatments or exaggerate the quality of their offerings. In recent years, many otherwise reputable facilities have added "alternative" and/or "complementary" services that have little or no value.

Cancer Treatment Centers of America (CTCA), which manages hospitals in Zion, Illinois, and Tulsa, Oklahoma, advertises frequently on television and in health-related magazines and chiropractic journals. Many of its ads have featured testimonials from patients who said CTCA had helped them after other doctors had given up. The ads claimed that CTCA's facilities offer innovative treatment and "specialize in treating cases other hospitals call hopeless." However, no statistics comparing their survival rates with those of other facilities have been published in a scientific journal. Critics have charged that in addition to standard approaches, CTCA patients have been subjected to questionable treatments, expensive and unnecessary tests, and hospital treatment in situations where less expensive outpatient treatment is standard practice.[84] In 1996 CTCA settled FTC charges that it had falsely represented that (a) survival rates for its cancer patients were among the highest recorded and (b) the consumer testimonials in its ads reflected the typical experience of its patients.[85]

RELIABLE INFORMATION SOURCES

The American Cancer Society (ACS), the National Cancer Institute (NCI), and the University of Pennsylvania Cancer Center maintain comprehensive Web sites. The ACS and the NCI also answer telephone queries and distribute printed materials.

Information on treatment protocols, results, and clinical trials is available through NCI's Physician Data Query (PDQ), a computerized database maintained and updated monthly. This enables most cancer patients to benefit from the latest scientific knowledge without having to travel far.

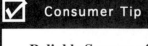 Consumer Tip

Reliable Sources of Advice about Cancer

ACS: http://www.cancer.org   (800) 227-2345
NCI: http://cis.nci.nih.gov   (800) 226-4237
           http://cancernet.nci.nih.gov
           http://cancertrials.nci.nih.gov
Oncolink: http://oncolink.upenn.edu
Quackwatch: http://www.quackwatch.com

The Quackwatch Web site has comprehensive information about questionable methods. The American Cancer Society has published a well reasoned book about "alternative methods,"[86] but many of its Web site articles on this subject are either misleading or written so blandly that they provides little guidance. The Consumer Tip box tells how to access these sources.

TREATMENT GUIDELINES

FDA historian Wallace Janssen has suggested the following treatment guidelines for people with cancer:

- Don't bet your life on any method that has not been FDA-approved for marketing or research.
- Go after the best possible treatment offered by known cancer experts.
- Avoid any "fad" treatment promoted by a crusading group of laypersons.
- Don't trust testimonials from laypersons who think they have been cured by unrecognized treatments. Such people mean well but are not qualified to diagnose or to determine what cured them.
- Stick with a prescribed treatment even if results are not immediately apparent.
- Have faith in experts who are devoting their careers to cancer research and treatment.
- If a specialist "gives up," look for another. A good physician does not abandon a patient to hopelessness.[87]

CONSUMER PROTECTION LAWS

The FDA, which has jurisdiction over drugs and devices marketed in interstate commerce, has been able to drive many fraudulent cancer treatments out of the American marketplace. Regulation of health professionals is handled primarily by state licensing agencies. State attorneys general and local district attorneys can take action against anyone—licensed or not—who violates laws involving fraud and deception. California has a special law to control the sale of worthless cancer remedies. This law has established precise procedures to test and investigate cancer treatment products, with the seller bearing the burden of proving that the method is safe and effective. Approval of the State Department of Public Health is required to sell, prescribe, or administer any drug or device for diagnosing or treating cancer.

The vigor with which government officials work to protect the public against cancer frauds varies considerably from agency to agency and depends in part on the extent of other matters competing for their attention. It also depends upon the extent to which fraud victims (or their survivors) complain and press for action.

SUMMARY

Cancer is a general term applied to more than 100 diseases characterized by cell growth. Early diagnosis and treatment are likely to produce the most favorable results. Victims may turn to quackery because of fear, loss of hope, inadequate information, and other psychosocial factors. This chapter describes many types of quackery and tells how to obtain competent professional help.

REFERENCES

1. Brown HG. A final challenge. In Barrett S, Cassileth BR, editors. Dubious Cancer Treatment. Tampa, 1990, American Cancer Society, Florida Division.
2. Cancer Facts &Figures 2001. Atlanta, 2001, American Cancer Society.
3. American Council on Science and Health. Cigarettes: What the Warning Label Doesn't Tell You. Amherst, N.Y., 1996, Prometheus Books.
4. Greenlee RT and others. Cancer Statistics, 2000. CA 50:7–33, 2000.
5. Radon: Worth learning about. Consumer Reports (60):464–465, 1995.
6. Health CW. Electromagnetic field exposure and cancer: A review of epidemiologic evidence. CA—A Cancer Journal for Clinicians 46:29–44, 1996.
7. Estabrook RW and others. Carcinogens and Anticarcinogens in the Human Diet. Washington, D.C., 1996, National Academy Press.
8. Unreliable breast cancer screening halted. FDA Consumer 25(9):42–43, 1991.
9. Krakoff III. Systemic treatment of cancer. CA—A Cancer Journal for Clinicians 46:134–141, 1996.
10. Shaving chemotherapy: Killing patients with kindness. Medical World News, pp 24–25, Apr 28, 1986.
11. Monoclonal antibodies: What's their role in cancer? Cancer Smart 2(1):6–9, 1996.
12. National Cancer Institute. What are clinical trials all about? NIH Publication No. 90–2706, Washington, D.C., 1989, U.S. Government Printing Office.
13. Meister KM and others. Diet and cancer, 2nd edition. New York, 1993, American Council on Science and Health.
14. NAS Committee on Diet, Nutrition, and Cancer. Diet, Nutrition, and Cancer. Washington, D.C., 1982, National Academy Press.
15. Whelan EM. Dietary recommendations for cancer prevention. ACSH News & Views 3:4, Nov/Dec 1982.
16. American Cancer Society guidelines on diet, nutrition, and cancer. CA—A Cancer Journal for Clinicians 41:334–338, 1991.
17. Hunter DJ and others. Cohort studies of fat intake and the risk of breast cancer: A pooled analysis. New England Journal of Medicine 334:356–361, 1996.
18. Kritchevsky D. Diet and cancer. CA—A Cancer Journal for Clinicians 41:328–333, 1991.
19. Fuchs CS and others. Dietary fiber and the risk of colorectal cancer and adenoma in women. New England Journal of Medicine 340:169–176, 1999.
20. Alberts DS and others. Lack of effect of a high-fiber cereal supplement on the recurrence of colorectal adenomas. New England Journal of Medicine 342:1156–1162, 2000.
21. Brigden ML. Unorthodox therapy and your cancer patient. Postgraduate Medicine 81:271–280, 1987.
22. Green S. Can alternative treatments induce immune surveillance over cancer in humans? Scientific Review of Alternative Medicine 4(1):6–9, 2000.
23. Cassileth BR. Contemporary unorthodox treatments in cancer medicine. Annals of Internal Medicine 101:105–112, 1984.
24. Lerner IJ, Kennedy BJ. The prevalence of questionable methods of cancer treatment in the United States. CA—A Cancer Journal for Clinicians 42:181–191, 1992.
25. American Cancer Society. Questionable methods of cancer management. New York, 1992, The Society.
26. American Cancer Society. Unproven methods of cancer management. New York, 1982, The Society.
27. Congress, Office of Technology Assessment. Unconventional Cancer Treatments, OTA-H-405. Washington, D.C., 1990, U.S. Government Printing Office.
28. Barrett S. The bizarre claims of Hulda Clark. Quackwatch Web site, Oct 13, 2000.
29. Tyler VE. Pau d'arco. Nutrition Forum 2:8, 1985.
30. American Cancer Society. Unproven methods of cancer management: Macrobiotic diets for the treatment of cancer. CA—A Cancer Journal for Clinicians 39:248–251,1989.
31. Barrett S, Herbert V. The Vitamin Pushers: How the "Health Food" Industry Is Selling America a Bill of Goods. Amherst, N.Y., 1994, Prometheus Books, pp. 370–375.
32. Mathews J. Media feeds frenzy over shark cartilage as cancer treatment. Journal of the National Cancer Institute 85:1190–1191, 1993.
33. Miller DR and others. Phase I/II trial of the safety and efficacy of shark cartilage in the treatment of advanced cancer. Journal of Clinical Oncology 16:3649-3655, 1998.
34. Healing, Journal of the Gerson Institute and the Gerson Therapy, vol 1, Fall 1981.
35. Lowell J. The Gerson clinic. Nutrition Forum 3:9–12, 1986.
36. Austin S, Dale EB, DeKadt S. Long-term follow-up of cancer patients using Contreras, Hoxsey and Gerson therapies. Journal of Naturopathic Medicine 5(1):74–76, 1994.
37. Green S. A critique of the rationale for cancer treatment with coffee enemas and diet. JAMA 268:3224–3227, 1992.
38. American Cancer Society. Questionable methods of cancer management: Questionable "nutritional" therapies in the treatment of cancer. CA—A Cancer Journal for Clinicians 43:309–319, 1993.
39. Working group on unproven methods in oncology. Iscador. File No. 10E, Bern, 1994, Swiss Cancer League, 1984.
40. American Cancer Society. Questionable methods of cancer management: Hydrogen peroxide and other "hyperoxy-

genation" therapies. CA—A Cancer Journal for Clinicians 43:47–55, 1993.

41. Green S. Oxygenation Therapy: Unproven treatments for cancer and AIDS. Scientific Review of Alternative Medicine 2(1):6–12, 1998.

42. Gelb L. Unproven cancer treatments: Help or hoax? FDA Consumer 26(2):10–15, 1992.

43. Segal M. Court says cancel the CanCell. FDA Consumer 27(4)–40–41, 1995.

44. National Cancer Institute studies of hydrazine sulfate. NIH news release, Aug 19, 1997.

45. London WM. The Penthouse politics of cancer: The promotion of hydrazine sulfate and a medical conspiracy theory. Priorities for Health 10(4):7–13, 34–35, 1998.

46. Blackstein ME, Sergsagel DE. Report to the Ontario Ministry of Health on the treatment of cancer patients with antineoplastons and the Burzynski clinic in Houston, Texas. Undated, circa 1983.

47. Green S. "Antineoplastons": An unproved cancer therapy. JAMA 267:2924–2928, 1992.

48. Texas Attorney General's Office. Morales halts use of unapproved cancer treatment. News release, Feb 10, 1998.

49. The antineoplaston anomaly: How a drug was used for decades in thousands of patients, with no safety, efficacy data. Cancer Letter, Sept 25, 1998.

50. Canadian Health Protection Branch. 714X: An unproven product. Issues, Jan 24, 1990.

51. Cancer "cure" challenged. Consumer Reports on Health 2:21–22, 1990.

52. American Cancer Society. Unproven methods of cancer management: Livingston-Wheeler therapy. CA—A Cancer Journal for Clinicians 40:103–107, 1990.

53. Cassileth BR and others. Survival and quality of life among patients receiving unproven as compared with conventional cancer therapy. New England Journal of Medicine 324:1180–1185, 1991.

54. American Cancer Society. Unproven methods of cancer management: Fresh cell therapy. CA—A Cancer Journal for Clinicians 41:126–128, 1991.

55. American Cancer Society. Unproven methods of cancer management: Greek cancer cure. CA—A Cancer Journal for Clinicians 40:368–371, 1990.

56. American Cancer Society. Questionable methods of cancer management: Electronic devices. CA—A Cancer Journal for Clinicians 44:115–127, 1994.

57. Gellert G, Maxwell RM, Siegel BS. Survival of breast cancer patients receiving adjunctive psychosocial support therapy: A 10-year follow-up study. Journal of Clinical Oncology 11:66–69, 1993.

58. Friedlander ER. Mental imagery. In Barrett S, Cassileth BR, editors. Dubious Cancer Treatment. Tampa, 1990, American Cancer Society, Florida Division.

59. American Cancer Society. Unproven methods of cancer management: O Carl Simonton, MD. CA—A Cancer Journal for Clinicians 32:59, 1982.

60. American Cancer Society. Kelley malignancy index and ecology therapy. In Unproven Methods of Cancer Management. New York, 1971, The Society.

61. Dentist directed McQueen therapy. ADA News, Nov 17, 1980.

62. Herbert V, Barrett S. Vitamins and "Health" Foods: The Great American Hustle. Philadelphia, 1981, George F. Stickley Co.

63. Arena S. Doctor liable in death of patient. New York Daily News, April 20, 2000.

64. Green S. Immunoaugmentative therapy: An unproven cancer treatment. JAMA 270:1719–1723, 1993.

65. Nolen, WA. Dr. William Nolen challenges unorthodox healers. 50 Plus, pp 43–45, 70–71, Nov 1983.

66. Questionable methods of cancer management: Immuno-augmentative therapy (IAT). CA—A Cancer Journal for Clinicians 41:357–363, 1991.

67. Centers for Disease Control and Prevention. Isolation of human T-lymphotropic virus type III/lymphadenopathy-associated virus from serum proteins given to cancer patients—Bahamas. Morbidity and Mortality Weekly Report 34:490–491, 1985.

68. Young, JH. Laetrile in historical perspective. In Merkle GE, Petersen JC, editors. Politics, Science, and Cancer: The Laetrile Phenomenon. Boulder, Colo., 1980, Westview Press.

69. Wilson B. The rise and fall of Laetrile. Quackwatch Web site, September 9, 2000.

70. American Cancer Society. Laetrile background information. New York, 1977, The Society.

71. Barnes C. Testimony before the Subcommittee on Health and Long-Term Care of the U.S. House of Representatives Select Committee on Aging. In Pepper C and others. Quackery: A $10 Billion Scandal. Washington, D.C., 1984, U.S. Government Printing Office.

72. American Cancer Society. Unproven methods of cancer management: Laetrile. CA—A Cancer Journal for Clinicians 1:187–192, 1991.

73. Laetrile: The political success of a scientific failure. Consumer Reports 42:444–447, 1977.

74. Moertel C and others. A clinical trial of amygdalin (Laetrile) in the treatment of human cancer. New England Journal of Medicine 306:201–206, 1982.

75. Relman A. Closing the books on Laetrile. New England Journal of Medicine 306:236, 1982.

76. American Cancer Society. Questionable methods of cancer management: Questionable cancer practices in Tijuana and other Mexican border clinics. CA—A Cancer Journal for Clinicians 41:310–319, 1991.

77. South J. The Manner clinic. Nutrition Forum 5:61–67, 1988.

78. Nourse AE. Quack cancer cures. Good Housekeeping, pp 58–69, Sept 1983.

79. Unproven methods of cancer management: International Association of Cancer Victors and Friends. CA—A Cancer Journal for Clinicians 39:58–59, 1991.

80. American Cancer Society. Unproven methods of cancer management: National Health Federation. CA—A Cancer Journal for Clinicians 41:61–64, 1991.

81. Barrett S. Some notes on Robert W. Bradford and his Committee for Freedom of Choice in Medicine. Quackwatch, Web site, Dec 2, 1999.

82. Barrett S. People against Cancer. Quackwatch Web site, Feb 14, 2000.

83. Zimmerman D. A case report: How Pat McGrady's 'CAN-HELP' helps patients with cancer. Probe 1(2):4–7, 1991.

84. Weiss J. Critics say cancer ads deceptive. Dallas Morning News, June 21, 1992, pp 1A, 26A.

85. Companies that purport to successfully treat cancer agree to settle FTC charges over their claims. FTC News, Mar 13, 1996.

86. Bruss K and others. American Cancer Society's Guide to Complementary and Alternative Cancer Methods. Atlanta, 2000, American Cancer Society.

87. Janssen WF. Cancer quackery: Past and present. FDA Consumer 11(6):27–32, 1977.

Chapter Eighteen

AIDS

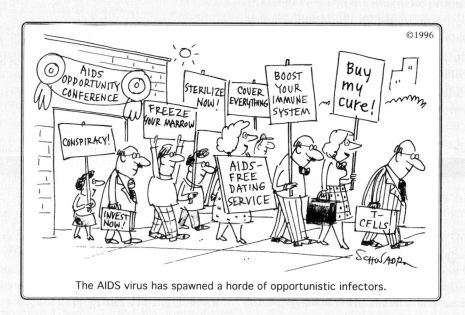

The AIDS virus has spawned a horde of opportunistic infectors.

*AIDS has rightly been called the greatest health threat of the 20th
century. AIDS has also been called a quack's dream come true.*

FRANK E. YOUNG, M.D., PH.D.
FDA COMMISSIONER
JAMES H. MCILHENNY, PRESIDENT
COUNCIL OF BETTER BUSINESS BUREAUS[1]

*In addition to illness, disability, and death, AIDS has brought fear
to the hearts of most Americans—fear of disease and fear of the
unknown.*

C. EVERETT KOOP, M.D., SC.D.[2]
SURGEON GENERAL

*HIV disease, a social and medical disaster, has produced oppor-
tunities for fraud and fraud watchers. As opportunists make small
fortunes, we have the opportunity to observe the natural history
of pseudoscience and society's responses.*

WALLACE I. SAMPSON, M.D.[3]

Acquired immunodeficiency syndrome (AIDS) is a fatal disease caused by the human immunodeficiency virus (HIV). This organism can remain in a person's body for years before symptoms appear and the individual is considered to have AIDS. The virus disrupts the functioning of the body's immune system, rendering the infected individual progressively unable to resist microorganisms that would normally be harmless. The Joint United Nations Program on HIV/AIDS has estimated that at the end of 1999, 34.3 million people were living with HIV/AIDS and 18.8 million had died from AIDS.[4]

From June 1981 to the end of 1999, a total of 733,374 cases of AIDS were reported to the U.S. Centers for Disease Control and Prevention (CDC), with 430,441 deaths.[5] AIDS is the fifth leading cause of death among all adults aged 25 to 44 in the United States. Among African-Americans in the 25 to 44 age group, AIDS is the leading cause of death for men and the second leading cause of death for women. Among women, African-Americans and Hispanics account for about 77% of cases; among men, they account for about 59%. The seriousness of HIV disease and the high cost of treating infected persons is having great impact on our health-care system as well as our society as a whole.

This chapter discusses the course of the disease, HIV testing procedures, preventive measures, treatment approaches, economic factors, and AIDS-related quackery and frauds.

COURSE OF THE DISEASE

Most people infected with HIV are adults in their 20s, 30s, and 40s, but the disease can occur at any age. The initial stage of the disease is a brief illness that typically includes fever, sore throat, skin rash, swollen lymph glands, headache, and malaise. This phase, termed acute HIV syndrome, usually lasts 1 to 2 weeks and is followed by a period in which the virus keeps multiplying but causes no symptoms. The median length of the symptom-free period in untreated individuals is about 10 years, but the disease progresses much faster in some people and may remain quiescent indefinitely in a small percentage of others. Thus, at any given time, most individuals who carry the AIDS virus exhibit no signs of illness. However, regardless of the stage of the disease, an infected person can transmit the virus to others.

Once clinical symptoms appear, the course of the disease can vary considerably, depending in part on the extent of immune damage and the treatment received by the patient. Eventually most people with AIDS become thin, easily fatigued, and prone to diarrhea, swollen lymph glands, and multiple infections. *Pneumocystis carinii* pneumonia, other opportunistic infections, and a skin cancer called Kaposi's sarcoma are life-threatening complications. In addition, some patients suffer from dementia. Opportunistic infections are caused by organisms that normally are harmless but can thrive when immunity is impaired.

In 1981 the diagnosis of AIDS was reserved for patients with severe symptoms. In 1985[6] and 1987[7] the definition was modified to include certain HIV test results and additional AIDS-related diseases. As medical understanding increased, authorities concluded that it was better to classify the later stages of HIV disease by measuring the number or functioning of CD4 cells (part of the body's immune system) rather than by considering only the patient's symptoms. These cells—also called T-lymphocytes, helper cells, or T4 cells—are HIV's primary target. CD4 counts are used as markers to estimate the health of the immune system of people infected with HIV and to determine when to start treatment to prevent the common opportunistic infections. CD4 counts are also used to measure the effectiveness of different treatments, even though they can vary by as much as 20% to 40% from test to test from the same patient at the same laboratory. Viral load tests, which measure the concentration of viral particles in the blood or other body tissues, may be more accurate and can also be used.

The CDC's current definition of AIDS, which took effect in 1993, raised the number of reported cases per year but gives a more accurate count of the number of infected individuals.[8] It requires laboratory confirmation of HIV infection and a CD4 cell count below 200 per cubic microliter of blood or below 14% of the total number of lymphocytes. In healthy people the CD4 cell count is usually 800 to 1200 per cubic microliter. (A microliter is one millionth of a liter.)

TESTING PROCEDURES

In 1985 the FDA approved a test for use in commercial blood banks and public health clinics to screen blood for HIV infection. The test, called ELISA (enzyme-linked immunosorbent assay), does not diagnose AIDS but indicates whether an individual has developed antibodies to the AIDS virus. This test, which is highly sensitive but can yield false-positive results, is also used to screen individuals. If it is positive, more specific tests, such as the Western blot or an immunofluorescence assay, are used to test for AIDS antigens, which indicate that the disease is present. AIDS testing is not foolproof, however. HIV antibody is detectable in at least 95% of patients within 6 months after infection. False-negative results occur when an infected individual has not yet developed antibodies to the AIDS virus.

Testing is most likely to be accurate if done several months after the potentially risky behavior has taken place. Testing can be performed on either a blood sample or a saliva sample[9] obtained by swabbing the mouth. Although most people test positive within 4r months of becoming infected, the virus can take 1 year to show up in some people. Because a positive test report (even if falsely positive) can have serious consequences, it is important that HIV testing be preceded by appropriate counseling and that strict confidentiality be maintained.

Some dating services require HIV testing for prospective clients. Although a negative test might reduce the chance of contact with an infected individual, it would not guarantee that the person is free of HIV. Antibodies to HIV are not present during the first few weeks or months of infection. Moreover, a negative test cannot ensure that an individual will remain uninfected.

Consumers worried about whether they have AIDS should seek testing from a reliable source. In most parts of the country, reliable testing can be obtained anonymously and free of charge through a local health department. Testing can also be done through one's personal physician. The cost of private testing depends on the number of tests required and the fee charged by the physician for counseling. A single negative test would cost at least $60, but the tests needed to evaluate an initial positive result can cost hundreds of dollars.

Only one home sample collection system has FDA approval: the *Home Access Express HIV-1 Test System* manufactured by Home Access Health Corporation and marketed directly to consumers. The user performs a finger-stick to obtain a dried-blood spot specimen on a special filter paper. The dried blood spots are mailed to a laboratory with a confidential and anonymous personal identification number (PIN) and analyzed at a certified laboratory. The results are obtained by the purchaser through a toll-free telephone number using the PIN; and post-test counseling is provided by telephone when results are obtained. Clinical studies have shown that the test system is able to correctly identify 100% of known positive blood samples, and 99.5% of HIV negative blood samples.[10]

People who have shared drug needles or who have had sexual contact with a man or woman who could be infected with HIV should consider being tested, even if no symptoms have appeared. Testing can be particularly important for people thinking about entering a new sexual relationship or having children.

PREVENTION

AIDS is not acquired through casual contact, such as sharing meals, kissing, shaking hands, or being near an infected person who coughs or sneezes. Intimate contact with human body fluids (blood, semen, vaginal secretions, or possibly breast milk) is required. Thus the disease is spread through having sexual intercourse (especially anal intercourse) with an infected person, sharing contaminated needles and syringes, or being born to an infected mother. Transmission through oral-genital contact appears to be possible but rare.[11] Blood transfusions are another potential source of infection, but this problem has decreased greatly since a method of identifying infected blood has been developed. All donated blood is now routinely tested for HIV and hepatitis and discarded if antibodies to either are found.[12] The estimated risk of AIDS transmission through donated blood is 1 per 677,000 units.[13] In 1994 the CDC issued guidelines for preventing the transmission of HIV through organ and tissue transplants.[14]

At the end of 1999, an estimated 800,000 to 900,000 U.S. residents were living with HIV infection, but one third of them were unaware of their infection.[15] Of new infections among men in the United States, about 60% were acquired through homosexual sex, 25% through injection drug use, and 15% through heterosexual sex. Of new infections among women in the United States, about 75% were acquired through heterosexual sex and 25% through injection drug use.[16] In many other parts of the world, the primary mode of transmission is heterosexual contact.[17]

Consumers Union[18] and the American Council on Science and Health[19] recommend the following protective measures:

- Abstain from sex outside a mutually faithful relationship with a partner who you know is not infected with the AIDS virus.
- If you choose to have sexual relations with someone who may be infected with the AIDS virus or whose history is unknown, avoid exchange of body fluids. A latex (rubber) condom should be used during each sexual act, from start to finish. Use of a spermicide provides additional protection.
- Never use a nonsterile needle or syringe for injections of any kind.

Hearst concurred with these recommendations but stressed that avoiding high-risk partners is far more important than anything else.[20] Today's high-risk groups include anyone who, within the past 10 years has engaged in male homosexuality or intravenous drug use, has resided in Haiti or central Africa, or has had a regular partner who fits any of these descriptions.

Studies have demonstrated that the incidence of HIV transmission among intravenous drug users is much lower if sterile syringes are readily available.[21] In 1995 a joint panel of the National Research Council and the Institute of Medicine concluded that needle-exchange programs (in which new needles are exchanged for used ones) will reduce the spread of HIV without increasing either the injection of illegal drugs among participants or the number of new users. The panel also recommended repealing all laws barring the sale and possession of injection paraphernalia and requiring a prescription to purchase needles and syringes.[22] As of 1997, about 100 needle-exchange programs were operating in the United States,[23] but only a few states permit both nonprescription purchase and possession of drug paraphernalia.

Because transmission of HIV to the fetus can be prevented, the American College of Obstetricians and Gynecologists advises pregnant women to undergo HIV screening.[24]

Much effort is being given to developing vaccines that can decrease the spread of HIV infections.

Provider/Patient Contact

Many people have wondered whether health-care workers who have AIDS or who have contact with AIDS patients are likely to become infected or to transmit HIV infection to their patients. The evidence so far suggests that few health-care workers acquire HIV infections from their patients. A study of 2500 health workers who cared for very ill AIDS patients found that only three of 750 who had stuck themselves with a needle had a positive antibody test for exposure to HIV.[2] Another study involving 5425 health workers with AIDS concluded that most had acquired their disease through nonoccupational exposure.[25] Fraser and Powderly estimated that the overall risk of HIV infection in health-care personnel through contact with HIV-infected blood is about 0.3% per incident and can be reduced by paying close attention to infection-control procedures and minimizing risky procedures.[26]

The likelihood of provider-to-patient HIV transmission is much smaller. The only documented transmission is the case of David Acer, a Florida dentist who appears to have infected seven of his 1100 patients.[27,28] The evidence against transmission during dental procedures is bolstered by a study of 1279 patients of a dentist with AIDS who, during a 5-year period, had treated at least 28 patients with HIV infection. Although the dentist admitted that he did not always follow recommended infection-control procedures, no evidence of dentist-to-patient or patient-to-patient transmission was found. Genetic testing showed that the viruses harbored by the dentist and these patients were different strains.[29]

In 1995 CDC investigators published the results of a survey of investigators from health departments, hospitals, and other agencies who had elected to notify patients who had received care from health-care workers infected with HIV. Test results were available for about 22,171 patients of 51 such workers. For 37 of the 51, no positive findings were reported among 13,063 patients tested for HIV. For the remaining 14 health-care workers, 113 positive tests were reported among 9108 patients, but epidemiologic and laboratory follow-up did not show that any health-care worker was the source of their infections.[30] CDC still advises that precautions be taken to prevent the transmission of HIV (and other blood-borne infections):

- All health-care workers should use special care when handling blood specimens or disposing of needles and other sharp instruments.
- Those who do exposure-prone procedures should know their HIV status.

- Those who know they are infected with AIDS should not perform exposure-prone procedures unless they have sought counsel from an expert review panel and been advised under what circumstances, if any, they may continue to perform these procedures.
- Mandatory testing of workers is not advisable.[31]

The American Public Health Association, the National Commission on AIDS, and most health-care leaders do not believe that mandatory testing of health-care workers would be cost-effective. Philips and others[32] estimated that the cost per case averted would depend on several factors and would range from $29.8 million in low-risk scenarios to $81,000 in high-risk scenarios. The AMA House of Delegates has called for voluntary testing of physicians who do invasive procedures that risk transmission of HIV and for supervision of doctors who know they are infected with the virus. Invasive procedures are those in which the doctor's hands or instruments enter the patient's body or touch mucous membranes, as in abdominal, heart, or dental surgery.

TREATMENT

Finding a cure for AIDS will be difficult because HIV infects several types of cells and inserts a copy of itself into their genetic material (DNA). This "tricks" the cells into treating the virus's genes as their own. The virus is then safe from attack by the body's immune system and is reproduced each time the host cells reproduce. The *Harvard Health Letter*[33] has noted that it is difficult to envision a drug that could eradicate the virus from multiple sites without doing extensive harm to vital body tissues. In addition, drug resistance occurs readily because the virus constantly evolves into new forms by mutating its own genes. AIDS develops when something triggers rapid reproduction and spillage of the virus into the blood stream, where it destroys CD4 lymphocytes and weakens the patient's immune system.

Although no cure for AIDS has been found, significant progress has been made. Early treatment of HIV-infected individuals can delay the onset of AIDS and increase survival time. The treatment goal should be to achieve maximum suppression of HIV replication in order to avoid the emergence of resistant organisms. The most effective approach is to combine antiretroviral drugs with which the patient has not been previously treated. More than 20 drugs are now available. Combinations that include a protease inhibitor have produced remarkable improvements in some patients.[34] Progress has also been made in preventing or fighting *P. carinii* pneumonia and several other AIDS-related infections.

The seriousness of AIDS, the growing worldwide epidemic, and political pressure from AIDS activists have led the FDA to streamline its procedures for approving new drugs for treating HIV infections. Under new regulations, developers of drugs for AIDS and other serious illnesses can make promising drugs available before clinical testing is complete.[35]

People with AIDS have difficulty maintaining adequate nutritional status. This results from a combination of lack of appetite, poor nutrient absorption, and high nutrient losses. Infection of the mouth and throat can make chewing and swallowing painful. Malnourished people are more susceptible to infection than are well-nourished people. Because their resistance is low, people with AIDS should be especially careful to avoid food-borne infections such as dysentery caused by salmonella bacteria. The Task Force on Nutrition Support in AIDS[36] recommends that all HIV patients have a complete nutritional assessment and dietary counseling with a health professional.

TREATMENT COSTS

The cost of treating people with HIV or AIDS is estimated to range from about $1000 to $4000 per month, depending on the stage of the disease. Total lifetime costs have been estimated to be about $155,000 to $195,000 per infected person, but statisticians have warned that as survival times increase, lifetime costs will also increase.[37] The Health Insurance Association of America estimates that health insurance companies paid $474 million in AIDS-related claims in 1997.[38]

Many insurance companies and self-insured employers have taken steps to minimize or avoid these costs. Some companies, for example, have established lifetime limits on HIV-related claims. Some insurers have denied coverage to single men living in certain zip code areas or working as hairdressers. Some insurers require HIV testing of applicants and deny coverage to those who test positive. Critics of these practices claim that they are unfairly discriminatory, and some have filed lawsuits attacking these practices. The American Association of Retired Persons (AARP) has expressed concern about attempts by insurers to limit or exclude by disease category. An AARP official has said, "Once you start with one disease, like AIDS, the next step could be Alzheimer's or other chronic conditions. I think that would be a disaster for the people who need help the most."[39]

When people with AIDS are seriously ill, home care is often an alternative to hospitalization. However, in 1991 the New York City Department of Consumer

Affairs[40] concluded that some private high-tech home care suppliers were committing "bedside robbery." The biggest problem was the provision of total parenteral nutrition (TPN), a liquid protein and fat supplement fed intravenously through a surgically implanted catheter to patients whose digestive systems no longer function normally. The Department's report cited instances in which insurance companies and government agencies have been billed more than $15,000 per month for treatment that costs much less to deliver. Only three of 12 companies responded to the Department's questionnaire about prices for their services. Several patients reported that buying supplies through a pharmacy and administering TPN themselves could more than halve their home care costs. Hospice care is another alternative that can be more compassionate and is less expensive than hospitalization. Many hospice providers have developed innovative programs for people with AIDS.[41]

Some manufacturers have programs through which needy patients with HIV or AIDS can obtain free medication for up to 90 days until they can secure financial assistance from other sources such as state or federal programs.[42]

AIDS-RELATED QUACKERY AND FRAUD

The fact that AIDS causes great suffering and is deadly has encouraged the marketing of hundreds of unproven remedies to AIDS victims. In addition, many companies in the "health-food" industry have produced vitamin concoctions claimed to "strengthen the immune system" of healthy individuals.[43] John Renner, M.D., president of the Consumer Health Information Research Institute, who attended meetings of groups promoting unorthodox methods, has commented that "many of the expert quacks in arthritis, cancer, and heart disease have now shifted into AIDS" and that "every quack remedy seems to have been converted into an AIDS treatment." The "cures" he observed have included processed blue-green algae (pond scum), hydrogen peroxide, BHT (an antioxidant used as a food preservative), pills derived from mice given the AIDS virus, herbal capsules, bottles of "T cells," and thumping on the thymus gland.[44] Young and McIlhenny[1] have noted that some firms have offered to freeze and store bone marrow, claiming that it could be used to restore an AIDS victim's marrow when AIDS began to deplete the body's supply of bone marrow (which manufactures blood cells).

Many Mexican cancer clinics offer their unproven treatments to AIDS victims, and a black market has developed in drugs that have shown promise but lack FDA approval because the agency is not convinced they are

safe and effective. Several drugs available without a prescription in Mexico are being smuggled into the United States. Drugs are also imported through "buyers' clubs," which obtain the drugs from other countries where they are legally prescribed or used in clinical trials. "Legitimate" buyers' clubs require a prescription written by an American physician who supervises the patient's care. However, some buyers' clubs obtain drugs for people who are not under medical care. Some also supply drugs to victims of cancer, Alzheimer's disease, chronic fatigue syndrome, and other diseases. Braun and others[45] have observed that the FDA appears willing to permit buyers' clubs to operate, even though technically illegal, provided: (a) patrons are purchasing drugs for their own use under medical supervision, (b) the club does not commercialize or promote its product, and (c) the products do not present "unreasonable" safety risks

Some entrepreneurs have attempted to exploit public fear of acquiring AIDS. Covers for public toilets and telephone receivers are worthless because AIDS is not transmitted in this manner. Figure 18-2 shows how a disinfectant product was claimed to offer protection against the AIDS virus. Rubber dental dams to prevent direct contact during oral-genital sex have been marketed despite the minuscule likelihood of HIV transmission by this route.

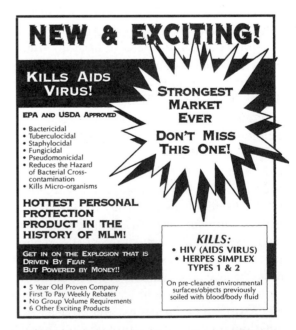

FIGURE 18-1. Ad seeking distributors for a multilevel company that marketed a disinfectant. The ad suggested that the product could be sold by capitalizing on the fear of AIDS. However, HIV is not transmitted through contact with countertops or other "environmental surfaces."

A few people have marketed shares of companies falsely claimed to have developed an effective method of diagnosing or treating HIV infections.[3,47,48] Several individuals and groups have claimed that the U.S. Army, the Central Intelligence Agency, the World Health Organization, and Russian agents have conspired in various ways to eliminate African-Americans or gays by introducing HIV into vaccines for smallpox, polio, and/or hepatitis.[3] A few skeptics have even claimed that HIV is not the cause of AIDS.[49] The National Institute of Allergy and Infectious Diseases has published a detailed rebuttal.[50]

Several studies have shown that a significant percentage of people with AIDS use questionable treatment. A study of patients hospitalized in Illinois found that 18 out of 50 with AIDS and two of 30 patients with cancer had used "alternative" treatments.[51] Acupuncture was used by 15 of the AIDS patients, mental imagery by 12 of them, massage therapy by 11, megavitamins by 10, acupressure by 8, unapproved medications by 7, and a high-cereal diet by 1 patient.

A study of 79 patients attending the St. Louis AIDS Clinical Trials Unit found that 44 (56%) had tried an "alternative" remedy. The most commonly used were vitamins (46% of patients), herbal therapy (16%), imagery or meditation (14%), and nonapproved drugs (14%).[52] Most patients using these methods thought they had improved their general well-being but readily admitted that the benefit was largely psychologic. The average yearly cost was $356, but 14 of the patients spent between $500 and $2700, and two patients spent more than $9000 each.

Interviews with 114 patients attending the AIDS Clinic of the University of California San Francisco Medical Center indicated that 25 (22%) had taken one or more herbal products during the 3 months before the survey.[53] The study's authors expressed concern that herbal extracts can produce diarrhea, liver toxicity, and other symptoms common in AIDS itself.

Dutch sociologists who interviewed people who used alternative treatments reported that 46% assumed that the treatment was effective, 66% thought it would strengthen their resistance, and 34% said they felt better because they had the feeling of being actively involved in their treatment.[54]

A telephone survey of 180 patients who had attended a general medicine practice at a university-based teaching hospital in Boston found that 122 (68%) used herbs, vitamins, or dietary supplements and that 81 (45%) visited an "alternative" provider during the previous year.[55]

A recent study of 68 HIV-infected adults assessed the effect of a 35-ingredient Chinese herbal preparation on disease progression, viral loads, CD4 and CD8 cell counts and scores on standard questionnaires for quality of life, depression, anxiety, and coping. The researchers found no difference between those who received the herbs and those who received a placebo over a 6-month period.[56]

The widespread use of herbal products has aroused concerns about their potential to interfere with the action of prescribed drugs. In 2000, following a report in *Lancet*,[57] the FDA warned that the herb St. John's wort can interfere with the AIDS drug indinavir and certain other types of drugs.[58]

Government Regulatory Actions

In 1993 the New York City Department of Consumer Affairs charged four supplement companies with deceptively promoting products characterized as "immune boosters." The action was taken under a city consumer protection law, passed in 1990, which regulates advertising of products and services claimed or implied to "boost, enhance, stimulate, assist, cure, strengthen or improve the body's immune system." Under this law, no such effect can be claimed without

Internet Fraud Stopped[59]

In April 1996 the Massachusetts Attorney General obtained a restraining order against Marjorie Phillips of Brockton, Massachusetts, after charging that she had engaged in consumer fraud on the Internet. Her "New Discoveries" Web page advertised information on the cause and cure of HIV infection. One version of the ad proclaimed that customers could be "HIV Negative in Six Weeks!" Phillips further advertised that HIV infection was caused by a flatworm that could be eliminated by using herbs or administering a *SyncroZap*, a 9-volt battery-powered device that would eliminate the flatworms in 7 minutes.

an accurate statement about whether the product or service is effective in preventing HIV infection or improving the health of an infected individual. The cited products were *Immune Protectors* (Twin Laboratories, Inc.), *Immunizer Pak Program* and *Immune Nectar* (Nature's Plus), *Pro-Immune Anti-Oxidant* (Nutritional Life Support Systems), and *Ecomer (*a shark liver oil capsule marketed by Scandinavian Natural Health & Beauty Products, Inc.).

The FDA has issued more than 60 warning letters, conducted more than 20 seizures, and obtained a few injunctions against AIDS-remedy purveyors, many of whom marketed products with "immune" or "immu-" in their name. Despite these actions, many products are still marketed with "immune-boosting" claims.

In 1993 postal inspectors arrested a California couple for conducting a phony charity scheme using the name American Society for AIDS Prevention (ASAP). Documents in the case charged that brochures mailed to potential donors contained numerous misrepresentations about ASAP's track record in helping AIDS victims as well as about the manner in which solicited funds would be used. Many of the services that had been claimed had not been performed, and money collected had been used to perpetrate the scheme even further.

Several companies have marketed bogus home-use test products. In 1997, the FDA warned pharmacists and consumers about "Lei-Home Access HIV Test," which was being illegally marketed by Lei-Home Access Care, a division of Jin-Greene Biotechnology, Inc. in Sunnyvale, California.[60]

In 1999, the FTC announced that it had tested several kits advertised on the Internet and found that they didn't work. In every case, the kits showed a negative result when used on a known HIV-positive sample that

should have shown a positive result. These kits can give people who might be infected the false impression that they are not.[61] In February 1999, a federal judge sentenced Larry Greene, 51, of Los Banos, California, to 63 months in prison for marketing unapproved kits and furnishing bogus test results to several purchasers.[62,63] The FDA also has issued a public warning about one of these products, the EZ MedTest distributed by Cyberlinx Marketing, Inc., of Las Vegas, Nevada.[64]

Although ads for home-use kits may say they are for sale outside the United States only, consumers in the United States have been able to purchase them. Some ads state or imply that the kits have been approved by the World Health Organization (WHO) or a similarly well-known health organization, or that the home-use test kits have FDA approval. WHO does not approve or license HIV test kits. The FDA has approved the Home Access Express HIV-1 Test System, in which the user collects the sample at home but sends it to a laboratory for analysis. However, it has not and will not approve any HIV test kit in which the test itself is done by the user.

In July 1999, Donald L. MacNay, M.D., and two others were indicted on criminal charges of conspiring to commit violations of federal drug laws in connection with the promotion, sale, and distribution of "T-UP," an aloe vera concentrate they claimed was effective against

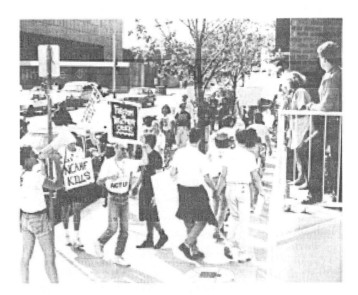

FIGURE 18-2. AIDS activists picketing for "freedom of choice" at the 1990 National Health Fraud Conference. The pickets alleged that the conference represented efforts by the AMA and big drug companies to suppress competition, and by the insurance industry to reduce coverage. What do you think their activity illustrates about the emotions of desperately ill people?

Photograph courtesy of Lauren Chapman, Kansas City, Mo.

It's Your Decision

Which of the following would you do if you contemplated having sex with someone? What is your reasoning?

_____ Have partner use a condom

_____ Ask whether partner is HIV-infected

_____ Ask whether partner uses intravenous drugs

_____ All of the above

_____ None of the above

---

cancer, AIDS, herpes, and other auto-immune disorders.[65] The indictment stated that intravenous administration of the T-UP cost the patients or their family members approximately $12,000 for a 2-week course of treatment and was also sold for $75 per 2-ounce bottle to cancer patients. MacNay, who had practiced orthopedic surgery in Manassas, Virginia, had his license revoked in February 1998 by the Virginia Board of Medicine, which cited fraud, unprofessional conduct, and gross malpractice. Four patients he had treated in 1997 had died shortly after receiving his aloe therapy.

Since no cure for AIDS is known, people with AIDS should be wary of anyone who claims to have one. Up-to-date information can be obtained through the National STD Hotline or the U.S. Public Health Service AIDS Hotline [800 342-AIDS] and through several reliable sites on the Internet.

SUMMARY

AIDS is a disease of the immune system that is incurable but largely preventable. It is caused by the human immunodeficiency virus, which escapes the body's immune defenses by inserting its genes into the genetic material of the body's cells.

This organism can remain in a person's body for years before symptoms appear and the person is considered to have AIDS. By disrupting the functioning of the body's immune system, it renders the infected individual progressively unable to resist organisms that would normally be harmless.

Regardless of the stage of the disease, an infected individual can transmit the virus to others. The best way to minimize AIDS transmitted through sexual contact is to (a) use a latex condom and (b) abstain from sex outside a mutually faithful relationship with a partner who is unlikely to be infected with the AIDS virus. Easy access to sterile needles and syringes can greatly reduce the spread of AIDS by intravenous drug abusers.

In most parts of the country, reliable testing can be obtained anonymously and free of charge through a local health department. It can also be ordered through one's personal physician.

Considerable progress has been made in identifying drugs that can delay the onset of AIDS and control some of its complications. However, the fact that AIDS causes great suffering and is deadly has created a market for many unproven remedies.

REFERENCES

1. Young FE, McIlhenny JH. AIDS: False hope from fraudulent treatment. Letter to consumer reporter, May 22, 1989.
2. Koop CE. Surgeon General's Report on AIDS. Rockville, Md., 1990, U.S. Department of Health and Human Services.
3. Sampson WI. AIDS fraud, finances, and fringes. New York State Medical Journal of Medicine 99:92–95, 1993.
4. Report on the global HIV/AIDS epidemic. Joint United Nations Program on HIV/AIDS, June 2000.
5. HIV/AIDS Surveillance Report, Vol 11, No 2, 1999.
6. Revision of the case definition of acquired immunodeficiency syndrome for national reporting—United States. Morbidity and Mortality Weekly Report 34:373–375, 1985.
7. Revision of the CDC surveillance case definition for acquired immunodeficiency syndrome. Morbidity and Mortality Weekly Report 36 Suppl 1S:1S–15S, 1987.
8. 1993 revised classification system for HIV infection and expanded surveillance case definition for AIDS among adolescents and adults. Morbidity and Mortality Weekly Report 41 RR-17:1–19, 1992.
9. Gallo D and others. Evaluation of a system using oral mucosal transudate for HIV-1 antibody screening and confirmatory testing. JAMA 277:254–258, 1997.
10. Testing yourself for HIV-1, the virus that causes AIDS—Home test system is available. FDA Web site, May 6, 1999.
11. Cohen J. HIV data raise concern of oral-sex risk. Science 272:1421–1422, 1996.
12. Sloan EM and others. Safety of the blood supply. JAMA 274:1368–1373, 1995.
13. Kleinman S and others. The incidence/window period model and its use to assess the risk of transfusion-transmitted human immunodeficiency virus and hepatitis C virus infection. Transfusion Medicine Review 11:155–172, 1997.
14. Guidelines for preventing transmission of human immunodeficiency virus through transplantation of human tissue and organs. Morbidity and Mortality Weekly Report 43(RR-8):1–17, 1994.
15. Centers for Disease Control and Prevention (CDC). Guidelines for national human immunodeficiency virus case surveillance, including monitoring for human immunodeficiency virus infection and acquired immunodeficiency syndrome. Morbidity and Mortality Weekly Report 48 (RR-13):1–27, 29–31, 1999.
16. HIV/AIDS Statistics. National Institute of Allergy and Infectious Diseases Fact Sheet, Nov 8, 2000.
17. World Health Organization. Current and future dimensions of the HIV-AIDS pandemic. Geneva, Switzerland, 1992, World Health Organization.
18. Hein K and others. AIDS: Trading Fears for Facts. Yonkers, N.Y., 1991, Consumer Reports Books.

19. Popescu CB. Answers about AIDS. New York, 1988, American Council on Science and Health.
20. Hearst N. Preventing the heterosexual transmission of AIDS. JAMA 259:2428–2432, 1988.
21. Watters JK and others. Syringe and needle exchange as HIV/AIDS prevention for injection drug users. JAMA 271:115–120, 1994.
22. Moses LE and others. Preventing HIV Transmission: The Role of Sterile Needles and Bleach. Washington, D.C., 1995, National Academy Press.
23. Interventions to prevent HIV risk behaviors. NIH Consensus Statement 11-13;15(2):1–41, Feb 1997.
24. American College of Obstetricians and Gynecologists. HIV tests urged for all pregnant women: Ob-gyns launch campaign for universal HIV screening. News release, May 23, 2000.
25. Chamberland ME and others. Health care workers with AIDS—national surveillance update. JAMA 266:3459–3462, 1991.
26. Fraser VJ, Powderly WG. Risks of HIV infection in the health care setting. Annual Review of Medicine 46:203–211, 1995.
27. Update: investigations of persons treated by HIV-infected health-care workers—United States. Morbidity and Mortality Weekly Report 42(17):329–331, 337, 1993.
28. Risk of HIV transmission in dental offices 'very low'. AIDS Alert 10(1):10–11, 1995.
29. Jaffe HW and others. Lack of HIV transmission in the practice of a dentist with AIDS. Annals of Internal Medicine 121:855–859, 1994.
30. Robert LM and others. Investigations of patients of health care workers infected with HIV. The Centers for Disease Control and Prevention database. Annals of Internal Medicine 122:653–657, 1995
31. Polder JA and others. Recommendation for preventing transmission of human immunodeficiency virus and hepatitis B virus to patients during exposure-prone invasive procedures. Atlanta, 1991, U.S. Department of Health and Human Services.
32. Phillips KA and others. The cost-effectiveness of HIV testing of physicians and dentists in the United States. JAMA 271:851–858, 1994.
33. Combating HIV in the nineties. Harvard Health Letter 16(11):1–4, 1991.
34. Waldholz M. Strong medicine: New drug cocktails make exciting turn in the war on AIDS. Wall Street Journal, June 14, 1996, pp A1, A6.
35. Stone B. How AIDS has changed FDA. FDA Consumer 24(1):14–17, 1990.
36. Task Force on Nutrition in AIDS. Guidelines for nutrition support in AIDS. Nutrition Today 24(4):27–33, 1991.
37. Holtgrave DR, Pinkerton SD. Updates of cost of illness and quality of life estimates for use in economic evaluations of HIV prevention programs. Journal of Acquired Immune Deficiency Syndromes and Human Retrovirology 16:54–62, 1997.
38. Source Book of Health Insurance Data, 1999–2000. Washington, D.C., 1999., Health Insurance Association of America.
39. Henry S. Health insurance caps—redlining people with AIDS. The Nation, Nov 11, 1991.
40. DeStefano G. Making a Killing on AIDS: Home Health Care and Pentamidine. New York, 1991, New York City Department of Consumer Affairs.
41. Buckingham RW. Among Friends: Hospice Care for the Person with AIDS. Buffalo, N.Y., 1992, Prometheus Books.
42. Directory of Prescription Drug Patient Assistance Programs, 1999–2000. Washington, D.C., 1999, Pharmaceutical Research and Manufacturers Association.
43. Barrett S. Strengthening the immune system—a growing fad. Nutrition Forum 3:24, 1986.
44. Segal M. Defrauding the desperate. FDA Consumer 21(8):17–19, 1987.
45. Braun JF and others. A guide to underground AIDS therapies. Patient Care 27(12):53–70, 1993.
46. Martin N. AIDS fraud rampant in Houston. Nutrition Forum 7:16, 1990.
47. Abraham L. Slick marketing tactics used to push new class of phony treatments for AIDS. American Medical News, April 1, 1988.
48. Barrett S. Some notes on ImmuStim and the credentials of its proponent. Quackwatch Web site, Aug 25, 2000.
49. Harris SB. The AIDS heresies: A case study in skepticism taken too far. Skeptic 3(3):42–79, 1995.
50. The evidence that HIV causes AIDS. National Institute of Allergy and Infectious Diseases Fact Sheet, Oct 10, 2000.
51. Hand R. Alternative therapies used by patients with AIDS. New England Journal of Medicine 320:672–673, 1989.
52. Rowlands C, Powderly WG. The use of alternative therapies by HIV-positive patients attending the St. Louis AIDS Clinical Trials Unit. Missouri Medicine 88:807–810, 1991.
53. Kassler WJ and others. The use of medicinal herbs by human immunodeficiency virus-infected patients. Archives of Internal Medicine 151:2281–2288, 1991.
54. Wolffers I, de Moree S. Alternative treatment as contribution to care of pwHIV/AIDS. International Conference on AIDS 10(2):66 (abstract no. 540B), 1994.
55. Fairfield KM, Eisenberg DM, and others. Patterns of use, expenditures, and perceived efficacy of complementary and alternative therapies in HIV-infected patients. Archives of Internal Medicine 158:2257–2264, 1998.
56. Weber R and others. Randomized, placebo-controlled trial of Chinese herb therapy for HIV-1-infected individuals. Journal of Acquired Immune Deficiency Syndrome 22:56–64, 1999.
57. Jobst KA and others. Safety of St. John's wort. Lancet 355:576, 2000.
58. Lumpkin MM, Alpert S. Risk of drug interactions with St. John's wort and indinavir and other drugs. FDA Health Advisory, Feb 10, 2000.
59. Massachusetts Attorney General news release, April 3, 1996.
60. FDA. FDA warns consumers about two unapproved home-use test kits. News release, Sept 26, 1997.
61. Federal Trade Commission. Home use tests for HIV can be inaccurate, FTC warns. FTC Consumer Alert, June 1999.
62. U.S. Department of Justice. Businessman sentenced to over five years: Selling bogus HIV-testing kits. News release, Feb 17, 1999.
63. Kurzweil P. Internet sales of bogus HIV test kits result in first-of-kind wire fraud conviction. FDA Consumer 33(4):34–35, 1999.
64. Michaels DM. Warning: HIV Rapid Home-Use test kits distributed by Cyberlinx Marketing, Inc. cannot be trusted. Do not use them! FDA Web site, July 6, 1999.
65. U.S. Department of Justice. Indictments in "T-Up" Case. News release, July 7, 1999.

PART V

OTHER PRODUCTS AND SERVICES

DRUG PRODUCTS

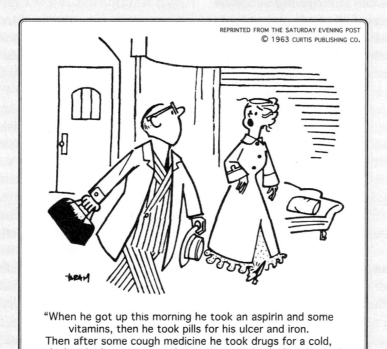

"When he got up this morning he took an aspirin and some vitamins, then he took pills for his ulcer and iron. Then after some cough medicine he took drugs for a cold, and when he lit a cigarette there was some kind of explosion."

No drug is perfectly safe. Any drug powerful enough to do good is powerful enough to do harm.

MORTON MINTZ
THE THERAPEUTIC NIGHTMARE

This chapter focuses on common drug products and strategies for using them wisely. It explains the differences between prescription and over-the-counter products, describes the training and professional activities of pharmacists, states why generic drugs usually provide good value, describes how government regulation has improved the quality of nonprescription drugs, and recommends sources of comprehensive information about individual drugs.

MEDICATION TYPES

Two basic types of medications can be legally purchased in the United States: *prescription* (**Rx**) drugs and *over-the-counter* (OTC) drugs. Including different packages sizes, dose strengths, and forms, about 65,000 prescription products[1] and 100,000 OTC[2] products are marketed in the United States.

Prescription drugs can be prescribed by a physician or other designated health professional, such as a dentist or podiatrist, and most commonly are dispensed by registered pharmacists. They are sometimes referred to as ethical or legend drugs. They require professional supervision because (a) they are generally stronger than OTC drugs, (b) they pose a greater risk of adverse side effects, and (c) the conditions for which they are prescribed are generally unsuitable for self-treatment because expert knowledge is required for their diagnosis and management. By law, a pharmacist cannot fill or refill a prescription without an order written or telephoned by an authorized provider. Under the Food, Drug, and Cosmetic Act, manufacturers may not label or market drugs for uses that lack FDA approval. However, federal law does not limit how physicians may use approved drugs.

OTC products can be purchased without a prescription from pharmacies, supermarkets, convenience stores, and mass merchandisers—a total of about 750,000

outlets. They generally are weaker than prescription drugs and have less severe side effects. Most are intended for relieving the symptoms of relatively benign, self-limiting conditions rather than for curing or controlling diseases. They include common remedies such as pain relievers, antacids, laxatives, and cough and cold remedies. Their labeling must contain all the information consumers need for appropriate use. New regulations, which will take effect within the next few years, call for a "Drug Facts" panel in which a product's active ingredients will be listed first, along with their purposes, followed by uses, warnings, directions, and inactive ingredients.[3]

Drugs can be marketed under a brand name or simplified chemical name. New prescription drugs, which are marketed under brand names, are protected by patents. After the protection period ends, other manufacturers can copy and market a drug under its chemical name or another brand name. Originally the patents were good for 17 years from the early stages of the drug's development. The federal Drug Price Competition and Patent Term Restoration Act (1984) extended the protection for up to 5 more years to compensate for the time required to get FDA approval. The General Agreement on Tariffs and Trade (GATT) Act, which took effect in 1995, extended patent protection to 20 years from the time the manufacturer files for a patent. A federal court has ruled that 94 drugs can qualify for both extensions, which will cover them for up to 25 years.

Drugs sold under their chemical name are called *generic drugs*. FDA regulations require them to undergo limited testing to demonstrate equivalence to their brand-name counterparts. Generic drugs cost less—often considerably less—but some controversy exists over whether they actually are equivalent. Although their active ingredients are identical, their inert ingredients (binders) may affect their absorption and other characteristics of bioavailability.

PHARMACISTS

Pharmacy is concerned with safety and efficacy in procuring, storing, dispensing, and using medications, related substances, and appliances. Pharmacists are also trained in methods of compounding and manufacturing drugs and testing them for purity and potency, although most of the items they dispense are compounded by drug manufacturers.

The American Council on Pharmaceutical Education accredits 82 schools and colleges of pharmacy in the United States. Two years of prepharmacy college work are required for admission. In 1992 the American Association of Colleges of Pharmacy recommended that pharmacy schools offer a doctoral curriculum for their entry degree. Eighty-one of the schools now offer the doctor of pharmacy degree (Pharm.D.) as the first professional degree, nine still offer a bachelor of pharmacy (B.Pharm.) degree, and 60 offer a Pharm.D. degree as a postgraduate degree. The Pharm.D. program includes clinical practice under faculty supervision.

Pharmacists practice in community pharmacies, hospitals, clinics, extended care facilities, and nursing homes. All states require a license to practice. Licensure requires graduation from an accredited college of pharmacy, a prescribed period of internship (in most states), and passage of an examination given by the state board of pharmacy. Pharmacists with a doctoral degree, referred to as "clinical pharmacists," can teach in schools of pharmacy or medicine, provide patient care services in teaching hospitals, and engage in clinical research.[4] There are about 250,000 pharmacists in the United States. In 1986 Florida passed a law that permits pharmacists to prescribe fluorides and a limited number of drugs. About 20 other states have granted limited power to prescribe. However, the majority of pharmacists have chosen not to do this.

Problem Areas

Most pharmacists who work in retail pharmacies have a serious potential conflict of interest. On the one hand, they are professionals, expected to be knowledgeable about drugs and to dispense them in a responsible and ethical manner. On the other hand, their income depends on selling products. Before the FDA's OTC Drug Review drove most of the ineffective ingredients out of OTC drug products, few pharmacists protested or attempted to protect their customers from wasting money on products that did not work. Today nearly all pharmacies carry irrationally formulated dietary supplements and many stock dubious herbal, homeopathic, and dietary supplement products in addition to standard drugs.

Pharmacists are also the only recognized health professionals who sell tobacco products, which cause more death and years of lost life than any other consumer product. Although some pharmacists have stopped (see Figure 19-1), the majority do not consider tobacco sales unethical. The American Pharmaceutical Association's code of ethics does not state that pharmacists have a duty to prevent dubious products from lining their shelves. A few states have laws against pharmacists selling ineffective products, but these laws have never been applied to the sale of OTC products.

If asked directly whether an ineffective product is worthwhile, most pharmacists will answer to the best of their ability. However, many are poorly informed. In 1987 two pharmacy school professors sent a questionnaire to 1000 pharmacists in the Detroit metropolitan

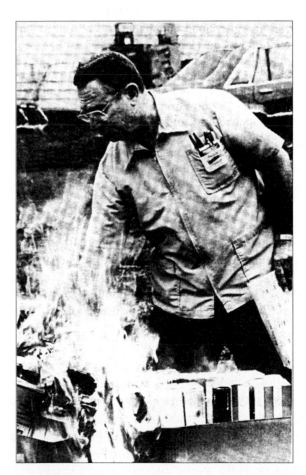

FIGURE 19-1. Pharmacist strikes a blow for public health. Adrian Thomas, owner of the Thomas Pharmacy in Meyersville, Pennsylvania, decided it was hypocritical to give health advice in one part of his store and sell health-destroying products in another. In 1992 he burned his entire tobacco inventory, along with his license to sell tobacco products. He told reporters he was tired of seeing his customers die of cancer and heart disease.

Photo courtesy of *Johnstown Tribune-Democrat.*

area and received 197 responses. Among the 116 who identified their five most-common reasons for recommending vitamins or minerals, 66 (56%) listed fatigue and 57 (49%) listed stress.[5] (Neither reason is valid.) In response to a question about homeopathy, 27.4% said it was "useful," 18.3% judged it "useless," and 54.3% "didn't know."[6]

Pharmacy trade publications, such as *Natural Pharmacist*, suggest that "natural products" offer opportunities to make up for prescription drug revenues lost as a result of managed care and other cost-containment programs. Barrett[7] has noted that at least two companies are marketing elaborate systems in which pharmacists advise customers to buy supplements products to replace nutrients that their prescription drugs are supposedly depleting. These companies also encourage pharmacists to prescribe supplements, herbs, and homeopathic products for many diseases.

Bouts[8] has expressed concern about inappropriate compounding of drugs. Compounding (creation of a drug product by mixing ingredients) has legitimate uses and is most often done honestly at physician request. However, some compounding pharmacists are networked with "alternative" practitioners to provide products that lack scientific substantiation, and some compounders are marketing such products independently. Quality control is also a significant problem. Bouts advises consumers to avoid compounded products that are sustained-release, administered by injection or inhalation, or available in brand-name or generic form.

PRESCRIPTION DRUGS

In 1961 there were 656 different prescription medicines on the market. Today there are more than 2500. In 1999 retail expenditures for prescription drugs totaled about $111 billion and the average prescription cost about $39.

The National Council on Patient Information and Education[9] states that half of prescriptions are used incorrectly by the patient, and many hospital admissions and deaths can be traced to drug-induced problems. Many people fail to fill prescriptions they receive, take doses that are too small or too large, take their medication at the wrong intervals, forget to take one or more doses, or discontinue medication too soon.

Cramer and others[10] studied the compliance of 26 epileptic patients who used special bottles equipped with a microprocessor that recorded when the bottles were opened and closed. Even though the patients had a serious disease and were closely monitored, they took an average of only 76% of their medication doses as prescribed.

It is useful to know how to read a physician's prescription. Figure 19-2 illustrates the typical format for prescriptions, and Table 19-1 provides the common abbreviations used by doctors. It is also helpful to be familiar with prescription labels and to understand them. Labels should state:

- Patient's name
- Physician's name
- Pharmacy name, address, and telephone number
- Name of the medication
- The number of units (tablets, capsules, ounces, etc.)
- The amount of each active ingredient in each unit
- How often and when to take the medication
- How much to take each time
- Any special instructions for use
- Pertinent warnings regarding sedation or allergy
- Number of refills permitted

When dispensing a generic drug, some pharmacists indicate which brand-name drug is equivalent. In December 2000 the FDA proposed that package inserts use a new format intended to reduce medical errors.[11]

Table 19-1		
COMMON PRESCRIPTION ABBREVIATIONS*		
Latin	**Abbreviation**	**Meaning**
ad libitum	ad lib	freely, as needed
ante cibos	ac	before meals
bis in die	bid	twice a day
capsule	cap	capsule
gutta	gt	drop
hora somni	hs	at bedtime
per os	po	orally
post cibum	pc	after meals
pro re nata	prn	as needed
quaque 4 hora	q4h	every 4 hours
quaque die	qd	daily
quater in die	qid	four times a day
ter in die	tid	three times a day
ut dictum	ut dict	as directed
Metric units:	cc	cubic centimeter
	mg	milligram
	ml	milliliter
	g	gram (1000 mg)
Quantity:	ī, īī, īīī	1, 2, 3

*The R in the symbol ℞ is an abbreviation of the Latin verb *recipte,* meaning "take thou." The *thou* refers to the pharmacist. The "tail" on the R is a contraction of the sign of Jupiter. Thus the symbol is an order to the pharmacist to "take in the name of Jupiter," with the physician invoking the name of Jupiter to ensure that the pharmacist does not make a mistake in carrying out the instructions.

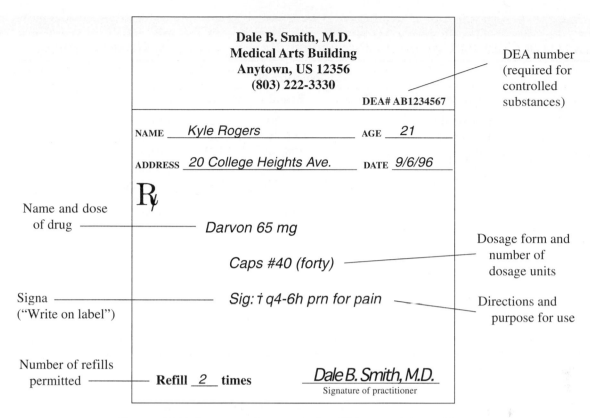

FIGURE 19-2. Anatomy of a prescription. This one advises taking one tablet of *Darvon* every 4 to 6 hours when needed for pain.

GENERIC VS. BRAND-NAME DRUGS

Drugs may be identified by generic or brand name. The term *generic* refers to the name of the active chemical or chemicals in a drug. Generic names are written in lowercase letters. The brand name (trade name) is the manufacturer's exclusive property, usually by reason of trademark rights. The first letter of a brand name is capitalized.

Some drugs are marketed under only one brand name, while others are marketed under more than one. Brand-name manufacturers market about 80% of the generic drugs, while a few hundred smaller companies make the rest. The fact that identical drugs are marketed under different names is a potential source of confusion for consumers and possibly even for physicians.

All drug products must meet FDA requirements for form, strength, route of administration, safety, purity, and effectiveness. The official standards of identity, strength, and purity are set forth in the *United States Pharmacopeia and the National Formulary (USP-NF)*, which is continuously revised by experts. The compendium is published by the United States Pharmacopeial Convention, an independent organization that establishes officially recognized standards for medicines and related products. The 2001 update of

USP24-NF19 contains more than 4000 monographs on drug substances and dosage forms for medicines and dietary supplements.

Product labels sometimes contain the term USP or NF to indicate that the active ingredient meets USP or NF standards. Therapeutic equivalence is established by demonstrating bioequivalence. If the rate of absorption and the blood levels achieved are allowably close to those of a brand-name drug in the same dosage, a generic substance is considered bioequivalent.

The Drug Price Competition and Patent Term Restoration Act requires the FDA to expedite approval of generic drugs. To approve a generic for marketing, the FDA does not have to judge the safety and effectiveness of its active ingredient(s), since the same chemical substance(s) have already been approved for use in the drug's brand-name counterpart. However, the FDA must test for and approve the bioequivalence of generic drugs.

FDA officials state that properly evaluated generic drugs are therapeutically equivalent to their brand-name counterparts.[12] More than 400 different generic drugs are available. All states let pharmacists substitute a generic product if authorized by a physician. Some states require that when a generic version of a prescribed drug is available, it *must* be dispensed unless the physician forbids substitution.

Table 19-2

COMPARATIVE COST OF COMMONLY PRESCRIBED BRAND-NAME AND GENERIC DRUGS

Brand Name	Generic Name	Price per 90			Drug Type or Purpose
		Dosage	Brand	Generic	
Amoxil	amoxicillin	250 mg	19.20	19.20	Antibiotic
Ativan	lorazepam	1 mg	96.05	34.24	Antianxiety agent
Calan SR	verapamil	120 mg	104.34	14.85	Calcium-channel blocker (for high blood pressure)
Deltasone	prednisone	5 mg	6.74	6.40	Antiinflammatory drug
Elavil	amitriptyline	25 mg	42.17	8.43	Antidepressant
Flexeril	cyclobenzaprine	10 mg	103.53	11.70	Muscle relaxant
HydroDIURIL	hydrochlorthiazide	25 mg	14.44	5.49	Diuretic
Inderal*	propranolol	10 mg	37.83	7.57	Beta blocker (for high blood pressure, migraine headaches)
Lasix	furosemide	40 mg	24.48	5.63	Diuretic
Motrin	ibuprofen	400 mg	21.39	8.56	Antiinflammatory drug
Valium	diazepam	5 mg	73.12	10.97	Antianxiety agent, muscle relaxant
Zantac	ranitidine	300 mg	276.16	24.98	H_2 blocker (for ulcers and acid reflux)

*Inderal prices are for 100 tablets. Source: Drugstore.com Web site, December 2000.

Generic drugs are usually less expensive than brand-name drugs. Table 19-2 compares the prices of several commonly prescribed products. For consumers to realize savings it is necessary for doctors and pharmacists to make generic drugs available. Pharmacies pay less for generics than for brand-name prescription drugs, but they do not always pass these savings to the consumer; in some stores consumers have paid higher prices for generics. Because prices vary from store to store, it is advisable to shop for drugs. Many pharmacists are willing to quote prices over the telephone.

Some manufacturers try to frighten consumers away from generics because brand-name drugs generally are priced higher and yield larger profits. These companies claim that generics are not as safe, that they don't do the job as well and take longer to act, and that patients may suffer side effects. The *FDA Consumer*[13] has reported that all of these claims are myths, and *Consumer Reports*[14] has also criticized this tactic, in an article titled "The Big Lie About Generic Drugs." However, authorities generally agree that if a generic drug is used over a long period and appears to be working, it is best to not switch brands when refilling the prescription. Using a single brand will avoid any problem of brand-to-brand variation.

In 1989 it was revealed that several FDA employees had accepted payoffs from generic drug firms and that seven companies had substituted brand-name drugs in tests needed for approval of 57 generic versions. Sub-

sequent investigation disclosed that the bribes had not affected the approval process. The FDA banned the 57 products but stated that no evidence of product ineffectiveness had been uncovered. The agency then analyzed about 3000 samples of 54 different generic drugs obtained from pharmacies and wholesale distributors. It found that only about 1% did not comply with FDA standards. *Consumer Reports*[15] again expressed confidence in the safety and effectiveness of generic drugs.

DRUG INTERACTIONS

Two or more drugs taken at the same time may interfere with each other's absorption, distribution, metabolism, or excretion. For example, taking an anticoagulant (which helps prevent blood clots) with an antacid may slow the absorption of the anticoagulant so that it is not effective. Aspirin increases the clot-preventing ability of oral anticoagulants and can cause someone on anticoagulant therapy to have a hemorrhage. Thousands of people who combine alcohol with other drugs are treated in hospital emergency rooms yearly, and some die. Alcohol is a central nervous system depressant, as are narcotics, barbiturates, tranquilizers, sedatives, and certain prescription painkillers. Alcohol causes drowsiness and, depending on the amount consumed, can affect walking, talking, and driving. When mixed with another depressant drug, the combined effect may be greater than the sum of the two drug actions.[16]

The "Evolution" of Patent Medicines

Patent medicines were also known as nostrums and proprietary medicines. Nostrums are remedies recommended by their preparers, usually without scientific proof of effectiveness. Strictly speaking, patent medicines are those for which patents have been obtained from the U.S. Patent Office to deter other manufacturers from copying them. (A patent permits a monopoly for at least 17 years.) However, many products referred to as "patent remedies" were actually not patented. A proprietary medicine is one whose name, composition, or manufacturing process is protected from use by competitors.

Thousands of patent medicines were produced and distributed in the United States, with sales reaching their peak during the 19th century and part of the 20th century. The 19th century has been called the "patent medicine era" because of the extensive variety of materials sold to the public. Toxic substances could be legally marketed.

Some products were said to be for specific ailments, while others were supposedly cure-alls. They were claimed to affect afflictions such as "female weakness," "worn-out kidneys," yellow fever, goiter, cancer, paralysis, and "piles" (hemorrhoids). Tonics, bitters, and other substances were widely used, but their ingredients were kept secret. The worse a product tasted, the greater its curative powers were assumed to be. Many of the products were neither helpful nor toxic, but some were as hazardous as the ministrations of the doctors practicing "heroic" medicine of the period.

Whiskey was considered the all-purpose remedy on the frontier. It was used as an antiseptic, painkiller, and courage builder. Tonics and cough medicines were popular because of their alcoholic content, as illustrated by these products: *Hood's Sarsaparilla* (18%), *Hotstetter's Bitters* (44%), and *Parker's Tonics* (42%). Most hard liquors today are about 40% to 45% alcohol.

The home-remedy books of this era promoted patent medicines as well. These volumes included *Indian Doctor's Dispensatory, Dr. John Williams' Last Legacy, A Useful Family Herbal, Dr. Chase's Recipes, Gunn's Domestic Medicine,* and *Poor Man's Friend in Pain and Sickness.* Most patent remedies had ingredients derived from the leaves, flowers, seeds, bark, and roots of plants.

Notable Promoters and Remedies

In 1796 Samuel H.P. Lee, a doctor from Windham, Connecticut, became the first American to prepare a patent medicine, which he called *Bilious Pills.* The ingredients were gamboge, aloe, soap, and nitrate of potassium. The pills supposedly would cure biliousness, yellow fever, jaundice, dysentery, dropsy (edema), worms, and female complaints.

The patent medicine business was very lucrative. Thomas W. Dyott, king of America's nostrum makers, marketed products that contained large amounts of alcohol. He assumed the title of M.D. and fabricated experience as a doctor. By 1830 his income was $25,000 per year; when he died, his estate was valued at $250,000.

During the early 1800s Samuel Thomson, a New Hampshire farmer, devised a treatment system intended to make people their own physicians. He believed that the diminished "power of heat" and water caused an imbalance of body elements. The cure was to restore heat with a 30-minute steam bath, which was followed by washing the body with cold water, taking a powerful vomitive containing herbs mixed in brandy, drinking warm water until vomiting occurred, taking another bath, resting in bed, and taking two herbal enemas.[17] This treatment was repeated for several days. Thomson was labeled "the sweating and steaming doctor." The idea of cleaning out the patient's system and strengthening the patient with tonics was common to both orthodox and folk medicine at that time and is still common among nonscientific practitioners and products today.

Lydia E. Pinkham's Vegetable Compound was advertised in 1873 for female weaknesses, irregular menstruation, inflammation, and ulceration of the womb. The Bureau of Investigation of the American Medical Association could find no medical evidence to support these claims. The compound originally contained 18% alcohol. Eventually vitamins and minerals were added and the alcohol content was reduced. The company appealed to women disenchanted with their doctors by suggesting that the grandmotherly Mrs. Pinkham was compassionate and understood their needs. The *Pinkham Guide for Women*, a publication important to the product's success, had over 1 million copies distributed.

In 1890 Dr. Samuel Brubaker Hartman produced *Peruna,* which he claimed could cure catarrh of the lungs; disorders of the stomach, head, kidneys, bladder, and pelvis; and other conditions. *Peruna* contained 25% alcohol. For 25 years no other patent medicine in the United States devoted as much newspaper space to testimonials.

Rampant Narcotic Use

Brecher[18] described 19th-century America as a "dope fiend's paradise." Opium was sold legally at low prices. Morphine was commonly used, and heroin was marketed toward the end of the century. These opiate (narcotic) drugs could be purchased as easily as aspirin is today. Physicians dispensed them in prescriptions, drugstores sold them over the counter, grocery and general stores made them available, and they could be ordered by mail.

More than 600 patent medicines and other products contained opium. They were widely advertised in

Continued . . .

Historical Perspective

The "Evolution" of Patent Medicines — *Cont'd.*

newspapers and on billboards as effective against pain, cough, and other problems. Physicians prescribed them for pain, cough, diarrhea, and other illnesses for which they actually were effective. Opiates were also used as a substitute for alcohol. They apparently helped to calm rather than excite the baser passions and hence were considered less conducive to violent or criminal behavior. Many physicians converted alcoholics into narcotic addicts because morphine addiction was thought to be far less damaging than chronic alcoholism.

During the Civil War, men who had been injured in battle were given large doses of opium to ease their pain. Soldiers often left hospitals cured of their wounds but addicted to opiates. This affliction acquired the name "soldier's sickness." However, addiction was more widespread among civilians. Federal narcotics laws passed after the turn of the century ended the inclusion of opiates in nonprescription remedies (see Chapter 26).

Marketing Strategies

Advertising played an important role in the patent medicine business. By 1860 there were 4000 newspapers, including 400 dailies. By 1900 there were 100 magazines in production. In 1804 about 100 patent medicines were marketed. By 1858 over 1500 were advertised, not only in newspapers and magazines but also on handbills, buildings, steamboat decks, and the surfaces of rocks.

During the 19th century no laws controlled advertising, and product claims by manufacturers were never modest. The main advertising techniques included:

- Making the product's name memorable: *Burdock's Blood Bitters, Swift's Sure Specific.*
- Distributing books and pamphlets giving medical advice.
- Using cures from afar (e.g., China, Turkey).
- Stating that a product was a powerful remedy used by the American Indians.
- Invoking mythology (*Hygeia*, the Minerva pill for syphilis).
- Indicating that diseases may cause pain and death.
- Using biblical quotations and testimonials from ministers.
- Using testimonials from supposedly satisfied customers. Some of these people later died from the disease the medicine was supposed to have cured.
- Using a doctor's name or picture on the label.
- Distributing free items such as an almanac or booklet; offering a money-back "guarantee."

During this period, patent medicine promoters often met their customers face-to-face. They went to towns and villages, especially during fairs, setting up platforms, putting on shows, delivering spiels, selling their wares, and then moving on. The performances evolved into full evenings of drama, vaudeville, musical comedy, bands, parades, and other spectacles. This was all considered respectable, as were the sidewalk exhibits in store windows that lured young men to "free exhibits" inside, where they were terrified into believing they suffered from some strange disease. The men were then spirited into examining rooms, where "doctors" asked a few hasty questions and pressured them into buying secret remedies. Often the cost was the exact amount of money found in their wallets.

Perhaps the greatest spectacle of the day was produced by John A. Healy and Charles Bigelow and their Kickapoo Indian Medicine Company.[19] The entertainment consisted of Indians and Wild West performers who were professional actors. Healy's "liver pads" supposedly contained a mixture of roots, bark, gum, leaves, oils, and berries prepared by the Kickapoo Indians. Actually they contained sawdust, red pepper, and glue.

Dudley J. LeBlanc, a Louisiana state senator, introduced *Hadacol* to the public in 1943. It was an elixir containing 12% alcohol, B-vitamins, iron, calcium and phosphorus, diluted hydrochloric acid, and honey. An 8-ounce bottle sold for $1.25, and a 24-ounce bottle cost $3.50. A pamphlet entitled "Good Health—Life's Greatest Blessing," produced by LeBlanc in 1948, contained testimonials by people supposedly cured of conditions such as anemia, arthritis, asthma, diabetes, epilepsy, heart trouble, and high and low blood pressure. It was claimed that a 13-year-old boy who lacked the energy to ride his bicycle took *Hadacol* and became a center on his football team.

LeBlanc revived the old-time medicine show. In 1950 a caravan of 130 vehicles, including steam calliopes, toured 3800 miles through the South. LeBlanc's medicine troupe played one-night stands in 18 cities with an average of 10,000 people attending. *Hadacol* boxtops were accepted as admission to hear a Dixieland band play "Hadacol Boogie" and "Who Put the Pep in Grandma?" In August 1951, shortly after LeBlanc claimed sales of $75 million, he sold his business for $8 million plus a $100,000-a-year salary as sales manager. The new owners, however, soon filed for bankruptcy, charging that LeBlanc had concealed $2 million in unpaid debts and grossly inflated the amount owed from previous sales.

The broad reach of medicine shows has given way to the even broader reach of radio and television. The spectacular productions have given way to talk shows and infomercials, and the products have been replaced by a myriad of questionable vitamin products, herbs, homeopathics, and exotic "dietary supplements."

Many OTC cough, cold, and allergy medicines contain antihistamines, and some also contain alcohol. When these products are taken with alcoholic beverages, they can increase drowsiness and be dangerous to someone driving an automobile or operating machinery.

Foods can interact with drugs, making them work faster or slower or preventing them from working at all. For example, the calcium in dairy products interferes with the absorption of tetracycline (an antibiotic), and carbonated beverages and fruit juices with a high acid content can cause some drugs to dissolve in the stomach rather than in the intestine.

Consumers can minimize the likelihood of taking an adverse combination of drugs by telling their physician when they are taking drugs from another source and by carefully following the directions when using any nonprescription product.

DRUG RECALLS

Since 1997, the FDA has banned or restricted distribution of eleven popular drugs:

DURACT (ANTI-INFLAMMATORY): liver damage
HISMANAL (ANTIHISTAMINE): interactions with other drugs
LOTRINEX (FOR IRRITABLE BOWEL): intestinal problems
POSICOR (BLOOD PRESSURE DRUG): interactions with other drugs
PROPULSID (FOR HEARTBURN): distribution restricted to patients who have failed to benefit from other therapies
RAXAR (ANTIBIOTIC): irregular heartbeat
REDUX (DIET DRUG): heart damage
RESULIN (DIABETES DRUG): liver failure
ROTASHIELD (ROTAVIRUS VACCINE): bowel obstruction suspected
SELDANE (ANTIHISTAMINE): interactions with other drugs
TROVAN (ANTIBIOTIC): liver failure (may still be used for some patients in hospitals or nursing homes)

FDA officials have stated that many problems with these drugs arose because doctors ignored safety warnings and prescribed them for patients who did not meet appropriate criteria. In a recent interview, FDA Commissioner Jane Henney, M.D., advised consumers that if a doctor wishes to switch them to a brand-new drug, they should ask how it is different and indicate that just being new is not sufficient reason.[20]

INTERNET PHARMACY SALES

Many Web sites sell prescription products directly to the lay public. Although these outlets may enable consumers to save money, it should not be assumed that prices are actually lower. In 1999 Bloom and Iannacone[21] located 46 Web sites, 37 of which required a prescription or online physician consultation and nine (located outside of the United States) that did not. The investigation also found that the two most commonly offered medications, *Viagra* (for impotence) and *Propecia* (for hair growth) cost 10% more than they did at five Philadelphia pharmacies.

Doing business with sites outside of the United States may be risky because the quality of the medications may not meet U.S. manufacturing standards. FDA officials advise against buying from Web sites that offer to prescribe a drug for the first time without a physical examination, sell prescription drugs without a prescription, sell drugs not approved by the FDA, or require going to another site to purchase the drug.[22]

The National Association of Boards of Pharmacy has developed a voluntary Verified Internet Pharmacy Practice Sites (VIPPS) program. To earn the right to display the VIPPS logo, companies must have appropriate licensure and written policies and procedures for drug utilization review, patient counseling, patient confidentiality, and quality improvement programs.[23]

INNOVATIONS IN DRUG DELIVERY

Increasing numbers of drugs are becoming available in delivery systems that deliver the drug at a slow rate for a long time rather than immediately releasing them into the body.[24]

Medicine-impregnated skin patches permit absorption through the skin at a steady rate. This maintains blood levels high enough to be effective but low enough to prevent toxicity. This controlled release reduces the frequency with which the drug must be taken and makes it easier for the patient to follow the physician's orders. *Transderm-Nitro*, for example, is a disk that contains a one-day supply of nitroglycerin and is placed on the chest to prevent angina pectoris (heart-related chest pain). Several brands of patches that release nicotine are available to help people stop smoking cigarettes (see section on smoking deterrents). *Estroderm* and *Climara* are patches that deliver estrogen to the body for about half a week.

Pumps have also been developed to deliver drugs at a controlled rate. Infusion pumps can be programmed to deliver drugs at precise dosages and delivery rates. To date, pumps have been approved for the delivery of insulin, a cancer drug, and morphine (for severe chronic pain). The *Norplant* system (see Chapter 21), implanted under the skin, protects against pregnancy for about 5 years. It consists of flexible silicon tubes filled with a hormone that is released gradually.

OVER-THE-COUNTER DRUGS

OTC drugs are those obtainable without a prescription. They frequently provide temporary relief from simple discomforts. They can relieve minor complaints when used properly but can cause many problems when used improperly. They include acne products, antacid products, antimicrobials, antiperspirants, analgesics, corn and callus removers, cough and cold remedies, menstrual products, laxatives, ophthalmics, skin protectants, antismoking products, and sunscreen products.

The Consumer Healthcare Products Association (CHPA), formerly called the Nonprescription Drug Manufacturers Association (NDMA), estimates that in

1999 Americans spent $18 billion for OTC products. The average cost of an OTC product is about $5. A 1989 survey published in the pharmacy news publication *Drug Topics* found that nearly all consumers said they practice self-medication at some time, and nearly 75% said they do so frequently.[25] A 1992 NDMA survey of 1500 households found that 38% of the problems experienced during a 2-week period were treated with an OTC product. The most frequent of these problems were headache, athlete's foot, lip problems, the common cold, chronic dandruff, premenstrual symptoms, menstrual symptoms, upset stomach, painful dry skin, and sinus problems.[26]

For many people the chief source of information about OTC drugs is television advertising. Advertise-

---

Table 19-3

OTC CATEGORIES FOR WHICH NO PRODUCT HAS BEEN FOUND SAFE AND/OR EFFECTIVE

Category	Ingredients/Comments
Anticholinergics in cough-cold products	Atropine sulfate, belladonna alkaloids, to "relieve excessive secretions of the nose and eyes"
Antifungal diaper rash products	Antifungals should be used only under a doctor's supervision
Antifungal nail products	Camphorated metacresol, chloroxylenol, nystatin
Aphrodisiacs	Cantharides, ginseng, yohimbine
Boil treatments	Ichthammol, juniper tar, calomel
Digestive aids	Cellulase, garlic, ox bile extract, pancreatin
Hair growers and hair loss prevention remedies	(Minoxidil subsequently approved for OTC use)
Ingrown toenail relief	Chlorbutanol, chloroxylenol, sodium sulfide
Nailbiting or thumbsucking deterrents	Denatonium benzoate, sucrose octaacetate
Ophthalmic antiinfectives	Yellow mercuric oxide, boric acid, for eyelid infections
Oral treatment of fever blisters and cold sores	Lysine, *Lactobacillus acidophilus*
Oral wound healing agents	Allantoin, carbamide peroxide in anhydrous glycerin, for "minor oral injury"
Products for oral use as insect repellents	Thiamine hydrochloride
Products to relieve the symptoms of benign prostatic hypertrophy	Amino acids "to relieve symptoms of urinary urgency and frequency"
Products marketed as daytime sedatives	Antihistamines, bromides, for claims such as "simple nervous tension, helps you relax"
Products to treat and/or prevent nocturnal leg cramps	Quinine sulfate
Products to prevent swimmer's ear	(None listed)
Smoking deterrents	Silver acetate, lobelia alkaloids, ginger
Stomach acidifiers	Betaine hydrochloride, diluted hydrochloric acid, pepsin, to treat lack of acid production
Theophylline-containing products to treat symptoms of asthma	People with asthma require individualized dosing by a doctor
Topical hormone products	Estrogens, progestins, androgens, for claims such as "removing wrinkles"
Sweet spirits of nitre	Benefits insignificant in view of risks
Camphorated oil drug products	Often mistaken for castor oil, resulting in a large number of accidental ingestions

Source: FDA Medical Bulletin 26(1):4, 1996.

ments generally are poor sources of drug information. Their message is often deliberately unclear and misleading (see Chapter 4). Their primary purpose is to increase usage of the product, even if this involves inappropriate or unnecessary use.

Federal law requires the following information on all OTC labels:

- Name or statement of identity of the product
- Net quantity of the contents and the number of tablets or ounces
- Active ingredients and strength
- Name and address of the manufacturer, distributor, or packer
- Directions for the safe use by the consumer, including the following:
  - Individual dose or unit dose
  - Frequency of use
  - Maximum dose for one day
  - Maximum number of days product should be used
  - Cautions or warnings such as, "If symptoms persist more than 24 hours, see your doctor," or "Should not be taken by persons with high blood pressure or heart disease unless directed by a doctor"
  - Side effects, such as drowsiness
  - Date of expiration of use when drug is no longer effective
  - Drug interaction precautions
  - Warning about serious allergic reactions if the product contains sulfites.

Many manufacturers voluntarily list inactive ingredients on their labels. These substances include flavors, colors, binders, emulsifiers, and preservatives.

FDA's OTC Review

In 1972 the FDA began an extensive evaluation to ensure the effectiveness and safety of over-the-counter drugs. Rather than attempting to evaluate each of the huge number of products, it divided the ingredients into categories and appointed expert advisory panels to evaluate the categories.[27]

The following sequence of events was planned: As each panel report was completed, the FDA would publish a proposed monograph in the *Federal Register* for public comment. After comments were received and revisions made, a tentative final monograph would be published to provide manufacturers with an additional opportunity to comment. After this period, a final monograph would be issued, and ingredients that had not been judged both safe and effective would be banned. When the FDA determines that no ingredient meets the criteria for a particular use, a "nonmonograph" is published and the entire category is banned for OTC use.

The panel phase of the review spanned about 10 years and covered 722 ingredients, some of which fell into more than one category.[28] The advisory panels concluded that only one third of these ingredients were safe and effective. As a result, manufacturers reformulated many products by removing unsafe and ineffective ingredients or by adding others. Many other unapproved ingredients were banned by the FDA. So far, about 80% of the proposed monographs and nonmonographs have been promulgated as final rules,[29] but most of the remaining OTC products are safe and effective for their intended purposes.

The advisory panels recommended shifting a number of active ingredients from prescription to OTC status. Today, more than 700 OTC products use ingredients and dosages available only by prescription less than 30 years ago.[2] These include certain antihistamines and nasal decongestants for colds and allergies, sleep aids, pain relievers, cough medicines, antimicrobial products, and anti-itch medicines. Examples are sodium and stannous fluoride rinse (anticaries), chlorpheniramine maleate (antihistamine), hydrocortisone (topical anti-inflammatory drug), ibuprofen (pain reliever), oxymetazoline hydrochloride (topical nasal decongestant), and the antifungal drugs clotrimazole and miconazole nitrate (for vaginal yeast infections).

The regulations resulting from the OTC Review prevent further interstate shipment of products with unacceptable ingredients. The FDA did not require that these products be recalled from the marketplace unless they pose a safety risk. As a result, some can still be found on retail shelves. To warn consumers, the FDA has published a summary of the categories for which no OTC product was found to be safe and/or effective.[30] Table 19-3 lists most of these categories. A 1995 investigation by *U.S. News & World Report* found products from a dozen categories, most of which had been "banned" for at least 1 year. The investigators noted that drugs with banned ingredients often were shelved next to FDA-approved formulations with nearly identical packaging.[31]

Despite these problems, today's OTC marketplace differs remarkably from that of a century or two ago—or even 10 years ago! Except for homeopathics, the vast majority of OTC drugs are backed by scientific evidence that they are safe and effective for their intended purposes. Ironically, as this transformation took place, the United States Congress *weakened* the laws governing the sale of herbs, vitamins, minerals, amino acids, and other substances marketed as "dietary supplements" (see Chapters 12 and 26). As a result, the marketplace has been flooded with dubious non-drug products.

Suggestions for Using OTC Medicines

Before purchasing an OTC drug, be certain that you have a rational use in mind, and consider whether a physician should be seen instead. If your goal is temporary relief, a pharmacist may offer sound advice. The best way to choose OTC drugs is to identify the chemical names of the ingredients useful for the condition in question and check product labels to obtain what you need. A pharmacist can help select a suitable compound. Before using any OTC drug, learn about its purposes, side effects, recommended dosage, precautions for use, and limitations. Directions for use will be found on the product label or an accompanying instruction sheet. Generally these directions are accurate and conservative. Medicines should not be taken in higher dosage or more frequently than indicated unless specified by a physician.

Many OTC products contain more than one active ingredient. Some contain one ingredient that is effective when taken alone plus others that are questionable or ineffective. The combination is then potentially less safe and at best no more effective than the single ingredient. The AMA Council on Drugs and the National Academy of Sciences have criticized OTC combination drugs and noted that a mixture can be irrational, even though one or more ingredients in the mixture is effective. Moreover, it may be advisable to adjust the dosage of one ingredient more than another. This can be done only if the ingredients are available separately. Thus it is generally best to select single-ingredient products. Zimmerman has noted:

Single-ingredient products are safer because they carry the risk of only one set of side effects. They are also safer because they help consumers identify the lowest effective dose of one drug that is capable of relieving the distress they feel.[32]

ALLERGY PRODUCTS

Allergy is the hypersensitivity to a specific substance (called an antigen or allergen) that results in a condition such as hay fever, asthma, urticaria (hives) or other skin eruption, itching of the eyes, and certain types of headaches. About 50 million people in the United States suffer from allergic reactions, the most common of which is seasonal allergic rhinitis (hay fever). The common substances that may trigger allergic reactions include the following:

INHALED SUBSTANCES: Pollens from weeds, grasses, trees, and plants; dusts in the home and in industry; mold spores; animal skin (dander) and hair; feathers; cosmetics; hair lotions; tobacco smoke; insecticide sprays; and many other chemicals.

FOODS: Lobster, crab, other shellfish, fish, cocoa, peanuts, spices, eggs, milk, wheat, soy products, some fruits and vegetables.

SUBSTANCES THAT CONTACT THE SKIN: Plastics, metal, rubber, fabrics, dyes, cosmetics, resins, drugs, pesticides, plants such as poison ivy.

MEDICATIONS: Aspirin, various antibiotics, and other drugs.

Common Allergic Conditions

Eczema is a skin eruption characterized by itching, swelling, blisters, oozing, and scaling. It has many causes, and often there is a family history of allergy.

Bronchial asthma is marked by difficulty in breathing accompanied by wheezing, a sense of constriction in the chest, coughing, and expectoration. It afflicts several million people in the United States. Many asthmatics are allergic to dust mites, microscopic insects that inhabit furniture, bedding, and carpets.

Contact dermatitis is a skin eruption that occurs after contact with various industrial chemicals, metals (hairpins, curlers, bobby pins, thimbles, needles, scissors, coins, items with nickel in them), plastics, cosmetics, deodorants, mouthwashes, dyes (bleaching peroxides, shampoos, rinses), certain textiles, adhesive tape, rubber (garments, swim suits, surgical bandages, support hose, dress shields), medicines, resins, pesticides, and plants (poison ivy, poison oak, poison sumac).

Drug allergies may occur in the form of skin rashes, fever, and other reactions.

Food allergies usually result in digestive disturbances, but hay fever, asthma, eczema, hives, and anaphylaxis can also occur.

Seasonal allergic rhinitis (hay fever) is characterized by nasal congestion and discharge, sneezing, and redness and itching of the eyes in response to allergens. The most common allergens are dust mites, mold, ragweed pollen, and grasses.

Insect stings can cause allergic reactions. Both immediate and delayed reactions can result from the stings of bees, wasps, hornets, and yellow jackets. Desensitization injections may be recommended for persons who experience a severe reaction.

Urticaria is characterized by itching welts (hives) on the face, lips, tongue, eyelids, ears, or other parts of the body. Infections, emotional stress, foods, drugs, and inhalants may be causative factors.

Management of Allergies

Medical treatment of an allergy may entail more than the mere prescription of a drug. It may require a

Table 19-4

COMPARISON OF SELECTED ANTIHISTAMINES

Chemical Name	Brand Names	Generic Available	Antihistamine Effect	Sedative Effect	Drying Effect
Prescription					
Fexofenadine	Allegra		+ + +	–	–
Loratadine	Claritin		+ + +	–	–
Nonprescription					
Brompheniramine	Dimetane Aller-Chlor	✔	+ + + + +	+	+ + +
Chlorpheniramine	Chlorate Chlor-Trimeton	✔	+ + +	+	+ + +
Dexbrompheniramine	*Drixoral Polaramine	✔	+ + + +	+	+ + +
Dexchlorpheniramine	Benadryl 25	✔	+ + + + +	+	+ + +
Diphenhydramine	Nytol Sleep-Eze-3	✔	+ +	+ + + + +	+ + + + +
Doxylamine	Sominex 2 Unisom Nighttime Sleep Aid		+ +	+ + + + +	+ + + + +
Phenindamine	Nolahist		+ + +	–	+ + +
Pyrilamine	Dormarex	✔	+	+	–
Triprolidine	Actidil *Actifed *Alleract	✔	+ + + +	+	+ + +

*Combined with pseudoephedrine to counteract sedation.
+ + + + + = High   + + + + = Moderate to high   + + + = Moderate   + + = Low to moderate   + = Low   – = Low to zero

thorough review of the patient's life situation for clues to the causes. Consultation with an allergy specialist may be advisable, particularly when the cause is not readily apparent. Skin tests or blood tests may be performed. However, although these can identify suspected allergens, they must be interpreted in light of the patient's history. Substances that test "positive" do not necessarily cause the patient to develop symptoms. Once an offending substance is identified, it may be possible to avoid it or desensitize the individual with a series of injections. In many cases of asthma, steps to reduce contacts with household dust (and dust mites) can be important.

Allergy shots may be effective against some allergens that are inhaled, such as the pollens that cause hay fever or aggravate asthma, and against insect stings.[33] But they are not effective against food allergies.[34]

Although self-treatment with OTC medications is suitable for mild allergies, it is probably advisable to have at least one consultation with a physician to confirm the diagnosis and discuss the various treatment options.

Unsupervised self-treatment is not suitable for severe or chronic allergies. However, well-informed patients can play a major role in managing their treatment.

Drugs
Many products are available to relieve the symptoms of allergies. Antihistamines may provide temporary relief, especially for hay fever and itching skin. Table 19-4 compares the effectiveness and side effects of several such products. Most OTC antihistamines can cause drowsiness; the extent depends on the ingredient, the dosage, and the individual's susceptibility. Drowsiness is rarely a problem with *Allegra* or *Claritin*, but they require a prescription and cost considerably more than the others. Several products also contain the decongestant pseudoephedrine, which can counteract the sedative effect of the antihistamine. However, it may be best to purchase the ingredients separately so that their dosages can be adjusted separately.

The response to antihistamines varies from one person to another. Therefore it is best to experiment with different ones to find one that works without causing oversedation. It may be prudent to take a nonsedating product during the day and a sedating one at bedtime.[35] *Consumer Reports on Health*[36] states that antihistamines are most effective when allergy symptoms are mild or when used before symptoms become severe. It also suggests that sustained-release products be avoided because their rate of absorption into the bloodstream and onset of action are unpredictable.

When using antihistamines, it is best to avoid alcohol and psychiatric drugs that cause sedation, because they may multiply each other's sedative effect. Pregnant and breast-feeding women, men with prostate problems, and people with glaucoma should not use antihistamines without consulting a physician. It is inadvisable for someone using a potentially sedative antihistamine to drive a car or operate industrial equipment without knowing from experience that a drug will not interfere with performance.

Corticosteroid hormones (cortisone, hydrocortisone, and prednisone) may be prescribed for short periods to treat severe allergic reactions. However, for most conditions, the risk of side effects is too great for long-term use. Steroid drugs can also be very helpful when used in ointments (for skin problems), inhalants, and nasal sprays. Topical products are available without a prescription. Steroid nasal products are sprayed into each nostril once a day and take about a week to reach full effectiveness.

Nasalcrom (cromolyn) is a prescription nasal spray that can prevent allergy symptoms. It has no side effects, but must be used for 2 to 4 weeks before it takes effect.

Topical nasal decongestants, available as OTC products, are sprayed into the nose to shrink nasal blood vessels and membranes. Since frequent use can cause rebound congestion, they are not appropriate for the treatment of hay fever or other chronic conditions.

Epinephrine (adrenaline) is a prescription drug that may be injected for the treatment of acute allergic attacks. It is a powerful drug that takes effect quickly. Other useful measures for asthma include aerosols to be inhaled to dilate the air passageways, antibiotics for acute infection, cough-controlling agents, expectorants for loosening bronchial secretions, and steroid inhalants.

Emergency Medical Identification

Individuals with severe or life-threatening allergies should carry some form of emergency medical identification. This can be a health card to be carried in the person's pocket, purse, or wallet or a plastic card or metal tag worn around the neck or wrist. These items should specify any major allergies or sensitivities and the drugs (such as penicillin) likely to produce an adverse reaction. If someone is found unconscious or is seriously injured and unable to communicate, the information may be important.

Poison Ivy, Poison Oak, Poison Sumac

Each year millions suffer from contact dermatitis caused by poison ivy, poison oak, or poison sumac. It may be acute or chronic, depending on the intensity of the exposure and the degree of sensitivity to the allergens. It can develop as a result of direct contact with plants or indirectly from contaminated clothing, pets, or other sources. About 70% of adults are sensitive to the oily resin produced by these plants. A thorough washing with soap and water within 10 to 20 minutes after exposure may remove the resin from the skin before it causes trouble. Clothing is decontaminated by machine washing with laundry detergent.

Severe dermatitis caused by poison ivy, oak, or sumac can be dangerous and painful. The eyelids may be swollen shut; there may be swollen lymph nodes, flulike symptoms, or kidney damage; even blood changes are possible. Extreme cases may require hospitalization. However, most cases clear up within 1 to 3 weeks.

The itching of the rash may be relieved by applying cold compresses, a paste made of baking soda and water, calamine lotion (without phenol), or a nonprescription hydrocortisone cream. Nonprescription products containing a local anesthetic or antihistamine should be avoided. Although these measures may be helpful for mild cases, a prescription product containing higher dosage of a topical steroid is likely to be far more effective. The medical treatment of severe cases may include an antihistamine and a few days of oral steroid medication.

Some physicians inject or orally administer extracts of the offending plant to try to desensitize (build up an immunity) to dermatitis. Desensitization is at best temporary, expensive, and relatively inconvenient.

EXTERNAL ANALGESICS

External analgesics are topically applied lotions, creams, liniments, and gels that have analgesic, anesthetic, antipruritic, or counterirritant effects. The analgesic, anesthetic, and antipruritic substances depress skin receptors for pain, itching, and burning and act directly to reduce or obliterate symptoms resulting from burns, cuts, abrasions, insect bites, and other lesions. Topical counterirritants are applied to the intact skin for the relief of pain. They differ from the other agents because their effect results from irritation of the skin that draws attention away from deeper-seated sources of discomfort. (By stimulating blood flow, they may also speed removal of lactic acid and other substances that contribute to local discomfort.) Equally effective relief may be obtainable by applying heat with a warm compress, hot water bottle, hot shower, or other means.

Counterirritants produce a mild inflammatory reaction. Some products bring extra blood to the surface of the skin by dilating the small blood vessels, thus warming the area; the heat supposedly provides pain relief. The use of counterirritants has a strong psychologic component and may exert a placebo effect. However, they can cause contact dermatitis in individuals with sensitive skin. The most common active ingredients are methyl salicylate (the active substance in oil of wintergreen), menthol, camphor, and capsaicin (a red pepper derivative).[37]

Several precautions should be considered in using these counterirritants: (a) do not use when there is severely restricted blood circulation in the legs; (b) do not bandage the area, since the skin may blister; (c) to prevent irritations, do not bring the preparations in contact with the eyes; (d) do not apply to wounds or broken skin; (e) do not apply to large parts of the body; (f) do not use to mask the discomfort of a serious injury; and (g) discontinue use if an adverse reaction occurs.

INTERNAL ANALGESICS

Internal analgesics are used for pain relief but have other uses as well. Americans spend about $3 billion a year for them. The most significant ingredients are aspirin, acetaminophen, ibuprofen, ketoprofen, and naproxen sodium. These substances are generally safe when used as directed but cause adverse reactions in some people. Table 19-5 summarizes their potential benefits, dosage, adverse effects, and cost.

Most pain-relief products contain an appropriate amount of one of these ingredients. A few contain both aspirin and acetaminophen, even though such combinations have no proven advantage. Several products contain caffeine, which may enhance the effect of aspirin or acetaminophen on certain types of pain but can produce nervousness as a side effect.[38] Some include an antacid ingredient that may lessen the incidence of stomach upset from an occasional dose. However, taking a full glass of water or other liquid with each dose can accomplish this also.[39]

Aspirin

Aspirin (acetylsalicylic acid) is effective against pain, fever, and inflammation. The adult dose of two 5-grain tablets (325 mg each) provides substantial relief from mild to moderate pain. Enteric-coated tablets are slow to dissolve and cause less stomach irritation. They may benefit those who are arthritic and take aspirin regularly, but the onset of relief is not as prompt. Aspirin risks include the following.

Hypersensitivity: Allergic reactions include asthma, hives, eczema, other rashes, and, rarely, anaphylactic shock.

Gastrointestinal disturbances with internal bleeding: Approximately 5% of the individuals who take one dose complain of heartburn and dyspepsia. The incidence of gastroduodenal bleeding is high. Of those who take two tablets three times daily, 70% lose 2 to 6 ml ($^1/_2$ to 1 tsp) of blood daily, and 10% lose as much as 10 ml (2 tsp) per day. This level of blood loss is usually not clinically significant.

Ototoxicity: Large doses of aspirin (9 to 25 tablets, 325 mg each) can cause tinnitus (ringing in ears), vertigo (dizziness), and bilateral hearing loss. The conditions generally disappear within a few days after use of the drug is stopped.

Prothrombin depression: In large doses, salicylates reduce plasma prothrombin (involved in blood coagulation) levels, and in some cases increase the time it takes blood to clot. This condition may be significant in patients with fever, rheumatoid arthritis patients taking large doses, people with liver damage, people with vitamin K deficiency, and surgical patients. No one taking anticoagulants should take aspirin without close medical supervision.

Overdose: A dose of 25 to 35 "baby aspirins" (81 mg each) can kill a child 1 to 5 years of age. Signs of overdose include bloody urine, diarrhea, dizziness, severe drowsiness, and ringing and buzzing in the ears.

Reye's syndrome: Aspirin taken by children who have chickenpox or flu can cause Reye's syndrome, a disease that is very rare but can be fatal. Therefore, children with chickenpox, flu, or an undiagnosed viral illness should be given only acetaminophen for fever. Although small children have mistaken flavored aspirin for candy, childproof packaging has almost eliminated aspirin poisoning in this age group.

Pregnancy: Large amounts during the latter months of pregnancy may cause adverse effects for both mother and fetus. Over 3250 mg/day (10 adult tablets) can delay or prolong labor, cause greater blood loss at delivery, increase perinatal mortality, and decrease neonatal birth weight.

During the last few years it has been found that taking low doses of aspirin (a) can help prevent heart attacks and strokes among individuals who have previously suffered such events, (b) may save the life of heart attack victims if started within hours after the onset of an attack, (c) may prevent an initial heart attack if taken by apparently healthy people with no history of heart disease, (d) may prevent serious complications from high blood pressure during pregnancy, (e) may lessen the frequency of migraine headaches, and (f) may reduce the risk of developing colon cancer.[40] However, none of these uses should be attempted without discussion with a physician.

The FDA expert panel that reviewed internal analgesics concluded that the addition of alkaline buffers makes aspirin dissolve more quickly, speeding its absorption into the system. This reduces but does not eliminate the effect of aspirin on the stomach. However, the panel indicated there had been no well-controlled clinical studies proving that buffered aspirin works faster or is more effective than plain aspirin. Also, some brands of buffered aspirin dissolve at different rates, and not all dissolve faster than plain aspirin.

Acetaminophen

Acetaminophen—the ingredient found in *Tylenol*—is as effective as aspirin in relieving pain and reducing fever. However, it has little antiinflammatory effect.

Table 19-5

COMPARISON OF OTC PAIN RELIEVERS

	Acetaminophen	Aspirin	NSAIDs
Common brand names	Anacin-3 Datril Tylenol	Bayer Bufferin Empirin Norwich	Ibuprofen: Advil, Medipren, Motrin IB, Nuprin, Pamprin-IB Ketoprofen: Actron, Orudis-KT Naproxen sodium: Aleve

Therapeutic uses	Pain relief
	Fever reduction
		Pain relief
		Fever reduction
		Antiinflammatory effect in
		  higher doses (requires medical
		  supervision)
		Heart attack prevention with
		  small doses (requires medical
		  supervision)
			Pain relief
			Fever reduction
			Menstrual pain
			Dental pain
			Soft tissue injuries
			Antiinflammatory effect in higher
			  doses (requires medical supervision)

Appropriate amount per tablet	325 mg	325 mg	Ibuprofen: 200 mg Ketoprofen: 12.5 mg Naproxen: 220 mg
Usual adult dosage*	2 every 4–6 hours	2 every 4–6 hours	Ibuprofen: 1 or 2 every 4–6 hours Ketoprofen: 1 or 2 every 4–6 hours Naproxen: 1 or 2 every 8–12 hours
Cost per 100*	3¢ to 6¢ per tablet	1¢ to 4¢ per tablet	Ibuprofen: 3¢ to 9¢ per tablet Ketoprofen: 9¢ per tablet Naproxen: 9¢ per tablet
Advantages	Fewer side effects than aspirin	Lowest cost	Fewer side effects than aspirin; anti-inflammatory doses better tolerated
Adverse effects	Stomach upset, but less than aspirin Some risk of kidney disease with prolonged daily use	Stomach irritation Interferes with blood clotting Allergic reactions, ranging from itching to asthma Ringing in ears (very high doses) Should never be given to children under 16 with viral illness, because of risk of Reye's syndrome	Stomach upset (ibuprofen inbetween aspirin and acetaminophen; naproxen and ketoprofen have higher incidence) High doses can cause bleeding and perforation of the stomach

*The NSAID dosages are based on general medical knowledge. The upper range of frequency is slightly higher than product labels suggest for initial use. The prices are based on a mid-1996 survey at a major chain drugstore. Where a range of prices is stated, the lower numbers are for generic brands.

Therefore it should not be relied upon for treating inflammatory arthritis or other types of inflammation. Acetaminophen has three advantages over aspirin: (1) it can be used by people allergic to aspirin, (2) it does not cause gastric mucosal damage and bleeding, and (3) it is less apt to affect anticoagulant therapy. Its disadvantages resulting from excessive ingestion are kidney damage and liver toxicity, primarily in heavy drinkers.

Ibuprofen, Naproxen, and Ketoprofen

Ibuprofen, naproxen, and ketoprofen are nonsteroidal antiinflammatory drugs (NSAIDs) that are available in higher dosage as prescription drugs. Like aspirin, all offer pain relief and fever reduction in addition to antiinflammatory action. Ibuprofen (now marketed as *Advil, Medipren, Nuprin*, and *Motrin IB*) was approved for over-the-counter sale by the FDA in 1984. Naproxen (marketed as *Aleve*) was approved in 1994, and ketoprofen (*Actron, Orudis KT)* was approved in 1995.

Ibuprofen is the active ingredient in *Motrin*, a prescription drug used for the treatment of arthritis (see Chapter 16) and menstrual pain. The prescription versions of naproxen and ketoprofen include *Naprosyn* and *Orudis,* respectively.

NSAIDs can cause troublesome and potentially serious side effects if taken in high doses or for prolonged periods. The most frequent is gastrointestinal irritation, including heartburn, nausea, constipation, or diarrhea. Taking them with food reduces the chance of stomach irritation. The serious side effects include perforation of the stomach lining, but this is unlikely to occur with OTC dosage. Chapter 16 discusses newer prescription drugs used for arthritis that are safer but more expensive.

Some advertisements for *Actron* and *Orudis-KT* suggest that they are more powerful than the other OTC pain relievers on a milligram-for-milligram basis. An article in *Consumer Reports on Health* called this comparison meaningless because "People take pills, not milligrams. So what if one active ingredient requires fewer milligrams to have the same effect as another?"[41] The article also stated that naproxen and ketoprofen are not more effective than ibuprofen and should be considered only as a fallback to ibuprofen.

The Medical Letter has noted that alcohol ingestion may increase the risk of liver damage or gastrointestinal bleeding caused by NSAIDs or acetaminophen, but the risk with small amounts of alcohol is unknown. It recommends that people who drink regularly should use analgesics infrequently and at the lowest possible doses.[42]

Costs

An effective dose of an OTC pain reliever can cost anywhere from 1¢ up to about 20¢. Generic products are generally less expensive than brand-name products. The cheapest pain reliever will usually do the job. Brands with similar amounts of the same ingredients should do the job equally well. Higher-than-usual doses are usually unnecessary unless pain is intense, but intense pain is probably reason to consult a physician. Extra-strength products, which contain higher doses per tablet, are more expensive than regular-strength products and are unnecessary. An individual wishing to take more than the regular dose can easily use regular-strength tablets to do so. For example, someone wishing to take 1000 mg of acetaminophen can save money by using three 325-mg tablets instead of two 500-mg tablets.

Antacids and H₂ Blockers

Overeating, eating quickly, or eating certain foods may lead to feelings of fullness, nausea, heartburn, or other symptoms identified as "sour stomach," "upset stomach," or indigestion. Individuals seeking relief may reach for an antacid or an H$_2$ blocker. Antacids function by neutralizing the hydrochloric acid present in gastric juice. Heartburn is usually caused by a backup of stomach acid into the esophagus. H$_2$ blockers can prevent symptoms by reducing the production of stomach acid. Antacids provide rapid relief, whereas H$_2$ blockers take about 45 minutes.[43]

All antacids are safe when used occasionally by healthy individuals. However, if taken on a regular basis they may cause bowel irregularities, aggravate kidney disorders, or mask a serious problem such as a peptic ulcer. Regular use requires medical diagnosis and supervision. Table 19-6 compares the major antacid ingredients.

Simethicone, which is approved by the FDA as an antigas ingredient, is said to relieve gas symptoms by breaking up gas bubbles, making them easier to eliminate from the body. Simethicone is found in several antacid products. However, Consumers Union's medical consultants believe that it does not help relieve heartburn and is "effective only in increasing the price of those antacids that contain it."[44]

Some antacid products combine calcium and magnesium compounds in an attempt to balance the tendency of some ingredients to cause diarrhea while others cause constipation. Consumers Union's medical consultants say that aluminum/calcium/magnesium combinations are more sensible than calcium/magnesium combinations but are far more expensive. Products that combine antacids and other drugs are not advisable unless each ingredient is needed to provide the relief that is sought.

Prescription-strength H_2 blockers are used to treat severe problems, such as stomach inflammation (gastritis), ulcer, or gastroesophageal reflux disease (GERD). GERD is a chronic form of heartburn that, if untreated, can lead to esophageal bleeding and other serious complications.[45] In 1995 three lower-dose products became available for OTC purchase for the treatment of heartburn: *Pepcid AC Acid Controller* (famotidine), *Tagamet HB* (cimetidine), and *Zantac 75* (ranitidine).

Consumers who use or contemplate use of an antacid or an H_2 blocker may find these suggestions helpful:

- Instead of habitually using these products, reduce or eliminate the causes of frequent heartburn or upset stomach, such as excess fatty food, alcohol, or stress.
- Use these products only occasionally. Don't exceed the maximum dosage or frequency without consulting a physician.
- Liquid or powdered antacids neutralize acid more effectively than tablets. Chew tablets thoroughly to help them dissolve or disperse quickly in the stomach. To increase effectiveness, take antacids 30 minutes to 2 hours after a meal.
- Antacids may interfere with the absorption of tetracyclines, digitalis, anticoagulants, and many other categories of drugs. Consult your pharmacist or doctor before combining medications.
- People on a sodium-restricted diet should avoid antacids that contain sodium.
- Seek medical help immediately if your heartburn is severe and accompanied by chest pain, weakness, breathlessness, or sweating.

- Pregnant women and people with ulcers or kidney problems should consult a physician before using any antacid.
- If using an antacid (such as *Tums*) as a calcium supplement, avoid aluminum-based products, which can actually deplete calcium.[66]
- Remember that symptoms similar to "indigestion" or heartburn can be caused by other conditions such as heart attacks, gallstones, and peptic ulcers. It is not necessary to see a doctor for occasional heartburn or indigestion. However, if symptoms are severe or recur over a week or two, a doctor should be consulted (see Box on ulcer treatment).

ANTIBIOTICS

Antibiotics (also called antimicrobial drugs) are substances used to fight infections caused by disease-producing microorganisms. They are prescription items (except for a few topical products) and should not be used without the advice of a physician. They can be harmful if misused. More than 100 antibiotics have been developed. The physician may conduct culture and sensitivity tests to help determine the appropriate drug to prescribe for a patient's illness.

Penicillin is effective against common types of blood poisoning, boils, scarlet fever, ear and bone infections, and many types of nonviral pneumonia. It is widely used and is among the safest of antibiotics. It can, however, cause allergic reactions in some people, and bacteria may develop a resistance to it. The allergic reactions include hives, skin rash, and edema; a small percentage involve anaphylactic shock, an extreme form of sensitivity that can be fatal.

Amoxicillin is similar to penicillin but is effective against a broader spectrum of bacteria.

Table 19-6

COMPARISON OF ANTACID INGREDIENTS

Ingredient/Brand	Relative potency	Disadvantages
Sodium bicarbonate Alka Seltzer Bromo-Seltzer	Fast-acting, high potency	Can cause belching and flatulence; high sodium content makes it unsuitable for individuals on low-sodium diet
Calcium carbonate Alka-2, Titrilac, Tums	Fast-acting, high potency, and lasts long	Frequent or heavy use can cause constipation, kidney damage, kidney stones; can cause "acid rebound" (increased acid production) when stopped
Magnesium compounds Gelusil, Maalox, Mylanta, Riopan, WinGel	Fast-acting, medium potency	Can cause diarrhea, kidney stones, drop in blood pressure
Aluminum compounds AlternaGEL AmphoGel, Rolaids	Relatively weak and slow-acting, but lasts long	Heavy use can weaken bones of people with kidney disease

Historical Perspective

Revolutionary Treatment for Peptic Ulcers

Everybody "knows" that peptic ulcers are caused by excess stomach acid that erodes the lining of the stomach or upper part of the small intestine (duodenum). In the early 1980s two Australian physicians theorized that the underlying cause is a bacterium able to live within the layer of mucus that normally protects the stomach wall.[47] The organism was later named *Helicobacter pylori*.

The conventional treatment of ulcers has been guided by findings made during the 1960s, when it was assumed that surplus stomach acid was the cause. The conventional treatment uses drugs to suppress acid secretion or antacids to render the acid harmless. Although these cause most ulcers to heal, they do not prevent recurrences. Today most cases can be *cured* by antibiotics or antibiotics plus bismuth (the active ingredient in *Pepto Bismol*). The new discovery makes it more important than ever that patients with persistent symptoms of pain, burning, or related symptoms seek a medical diagnosis rather than merely trying to suppress their symptoms with antacids.

The American College of Gastroenterology (ACG) has issued guidelines for the medical treatment of peptic ulcer disease.[48] ACG's recommendations include (a) antibiotic therapy for all ulcer patients infected with *H. pylori*; (b) temporary conventional therapy to provide relief of symptoms; (c) continued conventional therapy only for refractory cases; and (d) stopping any use of nonsteroidal antiinflammatory drugs (NSAIDs), which are another possible cause of peptic ulcers. The presence of *H. pylori* can be determined with a blood test, a breath test, or tests on a specimen obtained by endoscopy (a procedure in which a diagnostic instrument is inserted through the mouth into the patient's stomach). Because these tests are negative 5% to 15% of the time there is actually an infection, a therapeutic trial of antibiotics may be appropriate even if the tests are negative. ACG also advised endoscopic examination and biopsy to be sure that the ulcers are not caused by a stomach cancer.

The drugs used to treat *H. pylori* should be taken for at least 2 weeks, even though they can cause diarrhea and other unpleasant side effects. Stopping treatment too soon can leave behind resistant bacteria that can cause further trouble.[49]

Cephalosporins resemble penicillin chemically. They are used to combat a broad spectrum of infections, including staphylococcal infections that are resistant to penicillin. They are often considered to be safe substitutes for patients with minor allergy to penicillin. Diarrhea is a possible side effect.

Erythromycin is one of the safer, more effective agents against certain strains of streptococci and staphylococci in pneumonia, infections of the heart lining, and carbuncles. However, many strains of staphylococci are resistant to the drug.

Fluoroquinolones are useful for treating bronchitis and urinary tract infections. Newer versions have a broader spectrum.

Chloramphenicol, because it can cause aplastic anemia, is used only for treating typhoid fever, certain types of meningitis, and a few other severe infections.

Tetracyclines, including chlortetracycline and oxytetracycline, are used to treat urinary tract infection, gonorrhea, chlamydia, cholera, brucellosis, trachoma, and infections caused by Rickettsia (organisms transmitted by ticks, lice, and mites). Side effects may include vomiting, diarrhea, sore tongue, and rectal itching.

Antibiotics are also used in nonprescription products for the treatment of cuts, abrasions, and burns (see "OTC First-Aid Antimicrobials" later in this chapter).

Antibiotics have been called miracle drugs. They have dramatically reduced death rates and prevented much suffering among people. However, as a result of the vast increase in the use of these substances, the incidence of adverse reactions has increased. Certain organisms have grown more resistant to certain antibiotics, rendering these drugs less useful. There are also indications that the drugs are being misused and overused.

Antibiotics are useless against the viruses that cause colds. They may be appropriate, however, if a secondary bacterial infection occurs.

Acyclovir for Genital Herpes

Infection with the herpes simplex virus can cause clusters of small red lumps that turn into painful blisters. Type 1 (HSV-1) is usually responsible for cold sores (fever blisters) on or near the lips. Type 2 (HSV-2), a venereal disease that affects millions of Americans, usually causes blisters on the genitalia and sometimes on the buttocks and thighs. Following the first outbreak the HSV virus remains latent in the cranial nerves or spinal cord until some stimulus triggers migration down a nerve to where it produces the characteristic skin eruptions. Type 2 infections occur far more commonly and more frequently than those of Type 1 and are potentially more serious.

A Difficult Germ

Clostridium difficile can produce toxins that damage the large intestine (colon). The bacterium is carried harmlessly by about one person in 50 but is more common among patients in hospitals and nursing homes. It is usually held in check by friendly bacteria that inhabit the colon, but when the normal balance is disturbed, it may overgrow. This can happen when any antibiotic is administered but most often occurs with clindamycin, ampicillin, or the cephalosporins.

Clostridium difficile overgrowth can result in a mild, self-limiting diarrhea, a more severe diarrheal illness (colitis), or a life-threatening disease called pseudomembraneous colitis. The symptoms can range from simple loosening of the stools to relentless bloody diarrhea with fever and severe abdominal pain. They can begin during the period of antibiotic therapy, a few days afterward, or even as long as 6 weeks later.

These infections can be expensive and sometimes difficult to diagnose and treat. Hospitalization may be required. Relapses occur in 20% to 40% of cases.

The point of this story is that antibiotics are a two-edged sword and should not be taken promiscuously. Intelligent consumers should adhere to four strategies:

- Don't take antibiotics unless they are prescribed for you.
- Don't press a doctor to prescribe antibiotics for colds or for other viral infections for which there is no proven benefit.
- If you develop diarrhea while taking an antibiotic, stop taking it and notify your doctor quickly. Failing to do so could result in serious worsening of the diarrhea.
- If you have taken an antibiotic within 6 weeks before contracting a diarrheal illness, mention this fact when you consult your doctor.

Acyclovir (*Zovirax*) is used to treat genital herpes. It speeds the healing of herpetic sores and reduces the multiplication of the causative virus. It helps prevent recurrences and can reduce the duration of outbreaks. Acyclovir works by preventing the herpes virus from spreading to uninfected cells,[50] but it does not cure the infection or eradicate the virus from the body. The drug is usually administered by mouth but may be used intravenously in immunosuppressed individuals (such as people with AIDS). An ointment is also available. No other drug or diet, vaccine, or other product has been proven effective in preventing, curing, or alleviating genital herpes.

Individuals with genital herpes may need to decide with their doctor whether to use acyclovir to minimize recurrences or to take it only when outbreaks occur. Kaplowitz and others[51] completed a 3-year study of acyclovir in 525 patients who had had more than six recurrences per year. Daily dosage of acyclovir reduced the overall recurrence rate about 90% and enabled 61% of patients who completed the study to be recurrence-free during the third year. About 10% of the patients experienced side effects, which included weakness, headache, abdominal pain, nausea, and diarrhea. Whether steady use of *Zovirax* is practical depends on the frequency and severity of recurrences; the individual's tolerance for the drug; and the ability to afford the drug's cost, which is several dollars per day. Similar new drugs offer convenient once-a-day dosage but are also expensive.

OTC First-Aid Antimicrobials

First-aid antimicrobials are products applied to the skin to help prevent infection in minor cuts, scrapes, and burns. These products should not be used for longer than 1 week or to treat existing infections, animal bites, sunburn, punctures, or cuts that are deep or contain imbedded particles that can not be flushed away. The FDA approved seven topical antibiotics in 1987 and is evaluating topical antiseptics under a proposed rule issued in 1991. The antiseptics tentatively considered safe and effective are ethyl alcohol (48% to 95%), isopropyl alcohol, benzalkonium chloride, camphorated metacresol, camphorated phenol, hexylresorcinol, hydrogen peroxide solution, iodine tincture, iodine topical solution, methylbenzethonium, and povidone-iodine. However, the National Safety Council advises against using hydrogen peroxide, and an American Pharmaceutical Association handbook advises against using ethyl alcohol.[52]

"Aphrodisiacs" (Alleged Sex Enhancers)

In 1990 the FDA banned the sale of nonprescription aphrodisiac drug products. An FDA advisory panel had examined various ingredients, including gotu kola, ginseng, licorice, sarsaparilla, cantharides (Spanish fly), Pega Palo, strychnine, and yohimbine, as well as the hormones testosterone and methyltestosterone. They concluded that there was no scientific evidence to support claims that these products can increase sexual arousal or desire or improve sexual performance.[53] Herbal products, if taken in quantity, can cause high blood pressure and sleeplessness. Spanish fly can irritate the urinary tract. The FDA states that individuals with sexual problems should seek professional medical help.

"Poppers" sold under the trade names of *Rush, Thrush, Hardware, Locker Room,* and *Bolt* are used as inhalant drugs to enhance sexual pleasure but are sold as room odorizers or liquid incense; thus they have avoided FDA jurisdiction. The products are readily available in bars, discos, and some bookstores. They contain either amyl nitrite or butyl nitrite, which cause dilation of blood vessels in the hands, feet, and face. Some people find the increased blood flow pleasurable. Little is known about their long-term effects, but they can cause bronchitis and burns around the nose.[54] Amyl nitrite is a prescription drug used to relieve heart pain.

Harvey and Beckman[55] report that a study of sexually active women between the ages of 18 and 34 failed to show any significant effects of alcohol on sexual arousal, pleasure, or orgasm. Large amounts of alcohol can cause temporary impotence in men.

REMEDIES FOR COMMON FOOT PROBLEMS

This section discusses the management of athlete's foot, corns, calluses, and warts.

Athlete's foot (*tinea pedis*) is the most prevalent superficial infection in humans. It is classified symptomatically as acute (weeping and inflammatory lesions) or subacute/chronic (dry, scaly skin). In both cases itching, burning, and stinging are the primary complaints. The fungus is probably acquired most often by people walking barefoot on infected floors. Treatment preparations are available in creams, ointments, liquids, powders, and sprays.

The FDA expert advisory panel judged the following ingredients in OTC antifungal medications as safe and effective: clioquinol, tolnaftate, and undecylenic acid and its salts, haloprogin, miconazole nitrate, and nystatin. Tolnaftate can be used to prevent as well as to treat athlete's foot.

Effective therapy for athlete's foot involves proper hygiene that includes (a) cleaning and thoroughly drying the feet daily, (b) reducing heat and perspiration by wearing light shoes and cotton socks for ventilation, (c) changing clothing and towels frequently, (d) using a drying powder between toes, and (e) wearing protective footwear in public and home shower and bathing areas. A medical doctor or podiatrist should be consulted if the eruptions are oozing, the space between the toes has a foul odor, the foot looks inflamed or swollen, or the patient has diabetes or eczema.

Calluses and corns are protective responses to friction or pressure, usually caused by ill-fitting shoes, improperly fitted hosiery, or orthopedic problems. Calluses are skin thickenings with no central core, usually found on the palms of the hands and soles of the feet. Corns are skin thickenings with central cores that press on nerve ends, causing pain. The types include (a) hard corns, most commonly found on joint surfaces; (b) soft corns, resulting in a whitish thickening of the skin between the fourth and fifth toes; (c) intermediate corns, which are hard rimmed, soft in the center, and painful; and (d) neurovascular corns, which contain a large amount of blood and occasionally rupture. Most OTC products for treating corns and calluses contain salicylic acid, which softens and destroys the outer layer of the skin. The product is applied once or twice daily for up to 2 weeks. If no improvement occurs within 2 weeks, a medical doctor or podiatrist should be consulted.

Warts are caused by a viral infection of the epidermis (outer layer of the skin). They are contagious, and scratching can spread them. They can occur on any part of the body but most often appear on the hands, fingers, and soles of the feet. They typically are rough, scaly areas of the skin that have a cauliflower-like appearance. Those occurring on the feet (plantar warts) can resemble calluses but tend to be painful because of the pressure and irritation of weight-bearing. (Calluses are usually not tender.) Many warts disappear eventually without treatment.

The best strategy for managing a wart is early medical treatment. The treatments include freezing with liquid nitrogen or dry ice, burning with an electric cautery, surgical excision, and destruction with chemicals. Small warts of the hands or feet are also self-treatable with an OTC salicylic acid product, which is applied once or twice daily as needed for up to 12 weeks. Warts in other parts of the body should be treated only by a physician.

When using a salicylic acid product, it is important to follow the directions carefully so the surrounding skin does not get burned. The product should not be used on skin that looks irritated, infected, or reddened; nor should it be used by anyone with diabetes or poor circulation.

COUGH AND COLD REMEDIES

Almost any congestion in the nose may be labeled a cold, even though the congestion may be caused by pollutants or allergens rather than by one of the 120 or so viruses that cause cold symptoms. Colds can be classified as abortive (symptoms subside in 24 hours), mild, moderate, and severe. Medical science cannot cure a cold, but several types of medicines can help to control the symptoms.

Most coughs are caused by acute respiratory tract infections, such as the common cold. Coughs are usually mild and self-limiting. The cough reflex, controlled by a cough center in the brain, helps the lower respiratory tract rid itself of secretions and foreign matter. Dry, hacking coughs, which are usually caused by irritation rather than secretions that need to be cleared, often can be controlled by an OTC medication that suppresses the cough reflex. Productive coughs reflect the body's need to clear the respiratory passageways of secretions. Coughs that are productive or last for more than 1 week indicate a need for medical attention.

OTC Ingredients

Americans spend over $3.5 billion annually for OTC cough, cold, and allergy remedies that contain one or more of the following ingredients.

Antihistamines: Table 19-4 lists the characteristics of commonly used antihistamines. They are most useful for controlling seasonal allergic rhinitis. They have no ability to prevent or abort the common cold. They are found in almost all cold remedies. Many of them have a drying effect on mucus secretion in the nose. Some can cause drowsiness. *Consumer Reports*[56] believes that antihistamines have not been proven more effective than a placebo in stopping a runny nose and should be removed from OTC cold remedies.

Topical decongestants: Various sympathomimetic amines are available in nosedrops or inhalants to provide temporary relief from nasal stuffiness. These products produce physiologic effects resembling those caused by the activity or stimulation of the sympathetic nervous system. They work by constricting dilated blood vessels and opening the nasal passages. The substances include phenylephrine, oxymetazoline, and xylometazoline. Although topical decongestants are more effective than oral decongestants, frequent use can cause rebound nasal stuffiness that is worse than the original stuffiness.

Oral decongestants: Sympathomimetic amines ingested orally last longer but cause less intense vasoconstriction than topical sprays or drops. They do not produce rebound congestion but can produce insomnia and irritability. The most commonly used ingredients identified as safe and effective by the FDA[57] are phenylephrine and pseudoephedrine. Phenylpropanolamine (PPA) has been marketed as a single-ingredient decongestant in cold remedies and in appetite suppressants

(see Chapter 13). Consumer's Union's medical consultants recommend that PPA be avoided because it can cause dangerous blood pressure elevation.[58] The FDA is proposing to ban it.

Expectorants: Expectorants are administered orally to stimulate the flow of respiratory tract secretions to help with dry coughs. The only currently approved substance is guaifenesin, which has been shown to loosen phlegm but not to help relieve a cough.[59]

Oral cough suppressants: Cough suppressants are used for dry, hacking coughs. The FDA has approved two ingredients as safe and effective OTC use: dextromethorphan and codeine (in combination products only).[60] These ingredients work by inhibiting the brain's cough reflex. However, many states prohibit the inclusion of codeine in OTC cough suppressants because of the potential for abuse. Codeine as the sole active ingredient is available by prescription.

Topical cough suppressants: Camphor and menthol may be sold for use in hot steam vaporizers and in ointments rubbed on the chest. Their label must read: "For steam inhalation only. Do not take by mouth." They can quiet coughs by acting locally on the throat.

Fever-reducing pain relievers: In adults 325 to 650 mg (5 to 10 grains: 1 to 2 tablets) of aspirin or acetaminophen or 200 mg of ibuprofen, every 4 to 6 hours should help relieve discomfort and fever. Ketoprofen and naproxen have similar properties (see Table 19-5).

There is no evidence that vitamin C supplements can prevent the common cold. At best they may *slightly* reduce symptoms (see Chapter 12). Vitamin C is not an approved ingredient in OTC products for colds but is promoted as a cold remedy by the health-food industry.

Suggestions for Treatment

It has been said, "You can cure a cold with treatment in 1 week and without treatment in 7 days." The best a person can do about a cold is to get symptomatic relief. These suggestions are worth considering when cold symptoms appear.

- Rest in bed for a day or so, especially if the symptoms are severe.
- Take aspirin for aches and pains, or take acetaminophen or ibuprofen if allergic to aspirin.
- Decongestant nose drops can provide temporary relief from a stuffy nose, but symptoms may worsen if they are used too frequently.
- The use of antihistamines to stop a running nose is controversial. Some authorities believe that antihistamines are effective, while other authorities are skeptical.
- A vaporizer can help relieve a cough by putting moisture into the air and loosening secretions.

- Sucking cough drops or lozenges, increasing fluid intake, and drinking hot beverages may be beneficial. Lozenges and cough drops offer no advantages over less expensive hard candies.
- A cough suppressant is appropriate for a dry, hacking cough but not for a productive one. The best choice is single-ingredient dextromethorphan. A physician should be consulted if a cough lasts longer than 1 week.

SORE-THROAT PRODUCTS

Most sore throats are caused by an infection; more throat infections are viral than bacterial in origin. Use of an antiseptic gargle or medicated lozenges can do nothing to cure a cold or throat infection. The offending organisms are deep in the throat tissues and cannot be eliminated by gargling. Lozenges promoted for relief of pain from sore throats usually contain a topical anesthetic such as benzocaine. At best, the pain relief obtained may be short-lived.

OTC mouthwashes are dilute solutions of aromatic substances that may be sweetened with saccharin and colored. They may contain ethanol, astringents (zinc salts), surface-active agents (for foam), and quaternary ammonium halides (antiseptic agents). The halides have no significant ability to kill germs during a gargle. Comparable relief could be obtained from salt water ($^1/_2$ tsp of salt to an 8-oz glass of warm water). The FDA does not permit mouthwash manufacturers to claim their products have medicinal value or can stop bad breath. An oral pain reliever might help to relieve general discomfort.

Untreated throat infections caused by streptococci may lead to rheumatic fever or kidney disease. If a sore throat lasts more than a day or two or is accompanied by fever or severe malaise, a physician should be consulted to assess the likelihood of a streptococcal infection.

DIARRHEA REMEDIES

Most attacks of diarrhea are self-limiting; the symptoms are relieved within a day or two, with or without treatment. However, if the symptoms do not subside after a brief time, or if they are accompanied by fever, severe abdominal pain, severe malaise, or bloody stools, a physician should be consulted.

Two main types of ingredients are used in diarrhea remedies: adsorbents and antiperistaltic agents. Adsorbents attract and hold fluid so that the bowel movements become less watery. Antiperistaltic agents help stop diarrhea by slowing down the motility of the intestine. The adsorbents approved for OTC use for mild to moderate acute diarrhea are activated attapulgite (in *Kaopectate*), kaolin, pectin, bismuth salts (in *Pepto-Bismol*), and polycarbophil. The antiperistaltic ingredient in OTC products is loperamide, which is available in *Imodium A-D*, *Kaopectate II,* and *Pepto Diarrhea Control Liquid.*

In mild and moderate diarrhea, if the patient is not vomiting, the replacement of lost fluid is important. To help maintain fluid and electrolyte balance, ingest fruit juices, caffeine-free soft drinks, and salted crackers. Avoid alcohol and caffeine-containing beverages.

Traveler's diarrhea occurs as a result of consuming food or water that contains unfriendly bacteria. It can often be prevented if these simple rules are followed while traveling abroad: do not eat anything that is not cooked, except for fruit that you peel yourself; do not eat salads; do not drink beverages with ice in them; do not brush your teeth with water that you would not consider safe to drink; and drink only bottled water, soft drinks, beer, or wine. The basic rule is "boil it, cook it, peel it, or forget it."

Bismuth subsalicylate (*Pepto-Bismol*) is somewhat effective for preventing and treating traveler's diarrhea. The prophylactic dose is 30 to 60 ml or 2 tablets four times each day during the first 2 weeks of travel. For acute illness, 30 to 60 ml can be taken every 30 minutes for a total of eight doses. The salicylate content can be a problem for people who are taking other salicylate-containing drugs (if the combined total is too high) or who are allergic to aspirin.

OPHTHALMIC PRODUCTS

Nonprescription ophthalmic products are basically safe and effective only to relieve minor symptoms such as itching, tearing, tired eyes, dry eyes, or eyestrain caused by minor irritation and redness of the eyes. These problems are usually self-limiting. OTC products may cause allergic reactions due to the active ingredients or to preservatives. The FDA requires that OTC products to relieve symptoms carry the warning: "If you experience eye pain, changes in vision, continued redness or irritation of the eye, or if the condition worsens or persists for more than 72 hours, discontinue use and consult a doctor." Eyewashes must carry the same warning but without the 72-hour limit on use.

Smarting, burning, itching, conjunctivitis, and blepharitis (inflammation of the eyelid) are often caused by infection by bacteria or viruses, or by allergic sensitivity to dust, pollens, and molds. These generally can be cured fairly quickly with appropriate antibiotic drops or ointments prescribed by a physician.

Eye fatigue may result from errors of refraction (nearsightedness, farsightedness, and astigmatism), or it may be associated with general fatigue caused by a sleepless night, for example. There are also some systemic conditions that affect eye muscles and lids and cause fatigue. However, these conditions are not suitable for OTC treatment but require medical aid.

Should a simple eye irritation occur from smog, strong light, sea bathing, or swimming in chlorinated water, placing one or two drops of cold tap water on the lower lid with a clean eye dropper is generally helpful. The application of iced, wet compresses for about 15 minutes safely relieves tired but otherwise healthy eyes. Boric solutions have not been demonstrated to be more effective than plain water for the relief of eye discomfort.

A stye is an eyelid infection caused by the staphylococcus bacterium. The symptoms are a red, swollen, tender area and some pain. The condition is usually self-limiting, but if it persists or worsens, a physician should be consulted. Warm compresses can provide temporary relief and speed up the healing process. An ophthalmic antibacterial ointment may be useful.

ALLEGED HANGOVER PRODUCTS

The FDA's advisory panel[61] could not identify any product or single ingredient that would relieve the symptoms of a hangover (unpleasant physical effects that follow the heavy use of alcohol) or any ingredient that could entirely prevent drunkenness. To relieve hangovers, the panel recommended the use of pain relievers for headaches, antacid for gastric distress, and caffeine for fatigue and dullness. The panel concluded that activated charcoal was safe to use in the doses found in products for reducing and minimizing hangover symptoms, but its effectiveness had not been demonstrated. Some evidence indicates that the use of fructose prevents and reduces inebriation, but the panel stated that the evidence was not clinically significant and recommended further research.

HEMORRHOIDALS

Hemorrhoids are clusters of dilated (varicose) veins in the lower rectum and anus; they generally occur between 30 and 50 years of age. They may be internal or may protrude outward. Internal hemorrhoids are rarely painful, but external hemorrhoids can be painful.

Hemorrhoids are frequently self-treatable. They may be related to lack of sufficient dietary fiber, drinking few liquids, the overuse of laxatives, chronic constipation, pregnancy, and lifting heavy objects. Some symptoms that lead people to believe they have hemorrhoids may be caused by a different problem. Itching can be the result of poor anal hygiene, perianal warts, intestinal worms, medication allergies, psoriasis, or nervous scratching.

These suggestions can help individuals to minimize the symptoms of hemorrhoids:

- Increase the amount of fiber in the diet. This helps to soften the stool and reduce constipation. Eat fruits, vegetables, whole-grain breads, and whole-grain cereals.
- Practice good anal hygiene to control irritation and itching by keeping the skin around the anus clean and dry. Avoid vigorous wiping with dry toilet paper; use cotton or a rag moistened with warm water and pat dry. Completely remove soap residue after showering or bathing. Use sitz baths in warm water two to three times daily for 10 to 15 minutes at a time. Wear loose cotton underwear, and lightly sprinkle the anus with talcum powder.
- If hemorrhoid symptoms persist despite self-treatment, professional help may be needed.

Consumer Reports[62] has expressed reservations about the use of OTC products containing anesthetics, astringents, counterirritants, and skin protectants. Some of the ingredients can cause allergic reactions and make irritations worse. Hemorrhoidal products are marketed in three basic forms: cleansers, suppositories, and creams or ointments.

Cleansers: The best products keep the anal area clean; for example, *Tucks* and *Preparation H* pads.

Suppositories: They can lubricate the rectum and make hard bowel movements less painful, but they have minimal effect.

Creams and ointments: These may soothe irritation. Creams are preferable because ointments are greasier, retain moisture, and encourage itching and irritation. Hydrocortisone in some products is an effective anti-itch ingredient, but its overuse may lead to dependency and cause thinning of the skin.

Consumer Reports states: "There is no acceptable evidence that the heavily promoted *Preparation H* . . . can shrink hemorrhoids, reduce inflammation, or heal injured tissue."[62] *Preparation H* contains live yeast cell derivative and shark liver oil in addition to petroleum jelly. The *Public Citizen Health Research Group Health Letter*[63] stated that yeast cell derivative has not been proven beneficial, and that the product contains too little shark liver oil to protect the skin around the anus.

Historical Perspective

Autointoxication Theorists

Many faddists have claimed that the "bowels" (intestines) are a major source of health problems. One unfounded theory ("autointoxication") suggests that intestinal sluggishness leads to the absorption of poisons; another suggests that fecal material collects on the lining of the intestine and causes trouble unless removed by laxatives or enemas. Many chiropractors and naturopaths still espouse this theory.

The concept of enemas may have originated from observations of the ibis, a bird that supposedly uses its curved beak to give itself a rectal infusion of Nile water. The Egyptians gave enemas with beer, oil, or other fluids, adding such ingredients as honey, herbs, hemp, or ox brain. Enemas were used to "resist poison," to nourish weak and consumptive patients (wine), to prevail against dropsy (urine), and to exorcise devils from possessed nuns (holy water). In 18th-century England tobacco enemas were used to attempt to resuscitate drowned persons. In the United States in the 1930s children were often subjected to colonic irrigation for all sorts of complaints. Today various fringe practitioners still use colonics to "detoxify" the body.

Elie Metchnikoff, a Russian chemist who won the 1908 Nobel Prize for his contributions to immunology, was a strong proponent of yogurt. His 1907 book, *The Prolongation of Life,* described his search for the elixir of life and his discovery of Bulgarians who supposedly lived to the age of 100. He concluded that the sour milk (yogurt) they consumed was the cause of this extended life. Metchnikoff claimed that putrefaction of proteins in the intestines released poisons that caused disease. He called this "auto-intoxic action" and said that yogurt drove out the poisons by supplying microorganisms that were gentle, friendly, and happy.

Dr. John Harvey Kellogg, who had advocated an immaculate bowel, capitalized on Metchnikoff's theory and changed his treatment at Battle Creek. He did not permit putrescible foods and "disinfected" all fruit with chemicals. Patients would have the "poisons" flushed out of the alimentary canal by taking half a pint of whey culture by mouth and injecting another half pint into the colon by enema. Kellogg was probably more responsible than anyone else for the common belief that a daily bowel movement is necessary.

IRON-CONTAINING PRODUCTS

A well-balanced diet usually supplies enough iron, even for most women with heavy menstrual periods. The body normally absorbs the correct amount of iron that it needs. However, some people are prone to iron overload (hemochromatosis), which can cause serious damage to body organs. It is inadvisable to take iron-containing supplements without first determining whether they are needed.

Government action has put an end to the once-commonplace pitches "for people with tired blood" (see Historical Perspective box on page 57). However, advertisements that exaggerate the difficulty of getting enough dietary iron still occur.

Although severe anemia can cause fatigue, only a small percentage of people with fatigue or lack of energy have anemia. Moreover, if someone is anemic, iron tablets by themselves may not help. Anemia is a condition in which there are not enough red blood cells. The causes include iron deficiency, abnormal absorption of vitamin B_{12}, liver and thyroid diseases, hidden infections, and internal bleeding. Blood tests are necessary to make an accurate diagnosis, and the treatment should attempt to correct the cause. Supplementary iron may be appropriate for a short period when anemia is caused by a dietary deficiency, but dietary iron intake should be increased to prevent future difficulty. *Consumer Reports*[64] estimates that only 6% of women between 18 and 44 are iron-deficient due to heavy menstrual-blood losses.

Iron-containing products should be stored carefully if there are children in the home, because an overdose can be fatal.[65,66]

LAXATIVES

Constipation (hard stools) is a functional impairment of the colon, which normally produces properly formed stools at regular intervals. Constipation is related to an individual's habits and can occur when the customary pattern of bowel action is disrupted. The most common cause is too little fiber in the diet. Various medications have constipation among their side effects.

Some people believe that the colon is like an unsanitary sewer and requires vigorous, periodic cleaning. Many quacks have thrived by promoting this notion (see Historical Perspective box on "Autointoxication Theorists"). There is no scientific support for this idea. Nor is it necessary to have a daily bowel movement. Some people normally have a bowel movement only once every two or three days. Others do so only once per week, although this is not common

Table 19-7

COMPARISON OF OTC LAXATIVE INGREDIENTS

Type	Examples	Products	Mechanism of Action	Comments
Bulk-forming agents	Bran, cellulose, methylcellulose psyllium, polycarbophil	FiberCon, Metamucil, Serutan	Absorb water in the intestine and swell the stool into an easily passed soft mass.	Safe to take indefinitely
Lubricant	Mineral oil	Agoral Plain, Fleet Mineral Oil Enema	"Grease" stools to facilitate excretion.	Should be used only sparingly and for short periods; can interfere with absorption of fat-soluble vitamins, and can leak from rectum
Stool softeners	Docusate	Colace, Dialose, Regutol, Surfak	Merge with feces to soften their consistency. Useful for people who are temporarily bedridden, have hard, dry stools, or must avoid straining. Not effective for chronic constipation.	Should be used only sparingly and for short periods
Saline laxatives	Magnesium salts, sorbitol, sulfate salts	Citrate of Magnesia, Epsom Salts, Milk of Magnesia	Promote secretion of water into the intestine.	Safe with prolonged use, but promote dependency
Chemical stimulants	Bisacodyl, casanthranol, cascara, senna, castor oil	Carter's Little Pills, Castor Oil, Dulcolax, Ex-Lax, Feen-A-Mint, Fletcher's Castoria, Modane	Promote secretion of water into the intestine; some stimulate more vigorous contractions of the colon. Should be considered a last resort.	Can lead to dependency and can damage the bowel with daily use for months or years

and need not be encouraged. After limited irregularity, bowel rhythm usually returns to regular action with no treatment; there should be no ill effects except a slight feeling of discomfort. If it fails to return after 1 week, a physician could be consulted.

Temporary bowel changes can result from travel, change of diet, emotional tension, or a side effect of medication. In such cases, if consumption of additional fruits, vegetables, fluids, and high-fiber foods is not successful, a prepackaged saline enema or glycerin suppository is generally the quickest and safest approach. Properly administered, an enema cleans only the distal colon and most nearly approximates a normal bowel movement. Increasing exercise can also help.

Consumer Reports on Health[67] recommends that if these measures don't work, use of a bulk-forming laxative or stool softener should be the next step. If that does not work, a saline laxative for a day or two may be advisable. However, overdependence on laxatives can be harmful; they should not be used on a regular basis.

Americans spend about $870 million per year on laxatives. Table 19-7 compares various types.

Pain in the abdomen can be caused by a variety of conditions. Some of them, including an inflamed appendix, a bowel obstruction, or certain cancers, are serious and require skilled medical assistance. The use of laxatives in such cases is dangerous. A laxative should not be used when nausea or vomiting is present or for longer than 1 week. Overuse suppresses the normal urge to defecate and leads to dependency. Rectal bleeding or failure to have a bowel movement after the use of a laxative may indicate a serious condition and is reason to consult a physician.

The following measures may help prevent constipation:

- Eat a well-balanced diet that includes whole-grain breads or cereals, prunes and prune juice, fresh fruits, and vegetables.
- Drink adequate amounts of liquids.
- Exercise regularly.

- Set aside time after breakfast or dinner to allow for an undisturbed visit to the toilet.
- When possible, defecate fairly soon after feeling the urge to do so.

MOTION SICKNESS REMEDIES

The FDA has approved four OTC ingredients for use in OTC motion sickness drugs: cyclizine, meclizine, dimenhydrinate, and diphenhydramine.[68] The most common is dimenhydrinate, which is used in *Dramamine* and most other products. These drugs are antihistamines that can cause drowsiness and should not be combined with alcoholic beverages.

Transderm Scop, a prescription product for adults, can prevent motion sickness without causing sedation. The product is a patch that is placed behind the ear of the user at least 4 hours before its effect is desired. The patch releases small amounts of scopolamine over a 3-day period.

SLEEP AIDS

Nonprescription sleep aids rely on an antihistamine for their sedative effects. Sedation effects vary from individual to individual. An FDA advisory panel stated that occasional use of a sleep aid is not harmful, but a person with a chronic sleep problem should consult a physician. Their investigation revealed that many sleep-aid products contained ingredients that were ineffective (for example, aspirin, vitamins, and passionflower extract) or unsafe (for example, bromides and scopolamine). The experts believed that an antihistamine could be safe and effective if given in proper dosage. As a result of their findings, OTC sleep aids were reformulated to include an antihistamine, either diphenhydramine (used in *Compoz, Nytol, Sleep-eze 3, Sleepinal, Sominex,* and *Sominex 2*) or doxylamine succinate (used in *Unisom, Doxysom,* and *Ultra Sleep*), as their sole active ingredient.

Prescription sleep aids are far more potent than nonprescription products and can have more significant side effects. These, too, should not be used for long periods of time.

Alcohol has sedative qualities, but if used on a regular basis the quantity may have to be continually increased to induce sleep. In addition, the user may awaken in the middle of the night when the sedative effect wears off. A warm glass of milk is safer and might work.

A common but frequently unsuspected cause of insomnia is the consumption of caffeine-containing beverages such as coffee, tea, and cola drinks. Caffeine can interfere with sleep even when it is ingested during the early part of the day. A National Institutes of Health Consensus Conference concluded that insomnia for

---

☑ **Consumer Tip**

Self-Help for Sleepless Nights

Self-help and traditional remedies may be sufficient to cope with occasional bouts of insomnia. Before reaching for drugs, insomniacs may want to try one or more of these measures:

- Cut back on caffeine consumption, particularly in late afternoon or evening.
- Don't drink alcohol before bedtime. Although alcohol may help people fall asleep, it tends to wake them up a few hours later when its sedative effects wear off.
- Before bedtime, take a warm shower or, better yet, a warm bath.
- Retire to an environment conducive to sleep; use bedding that's clean and comfortable, and be sure the bedroom is quiet and dark.
- Stick to a regular sleep schedule throughout the week and avoid daytime napping or oversleeping on weekends.
- When anxiety is a problem, set aside a time during the day as a regular worry period; meanwhile, be mentally armed with a list of pleasant, relaxing subjects to crowd out anxieties at bedtime—and try not to worry about going to sleep.

- Regular exercise can help, but avoid exercising within a couple of hours of bedtime.
- Avoid excitement before retiring. Relax with light reading, restful music, or television.
- Don't eat large meals before bedtime. Instead, eat a light snack high in carbohydrates.
- Try sleep restriction, a strategy based on the finding that many insomniacs spend too much time in bed, hoping to make up for lost sleep: Go to bed later than usual, and get up at the same time each morning. Stay in bed only as long as you actually sleep, even if it is only for a few hours. When you sleep at least 90% of your allotted time in bed for 5 days in a row, go to bed 15 minutes earlier. After a week or two you should be sleeping better and, after a few months, as long as you want. The American Sleep Disorders Association says that this method is generally easier when under medical supervision.[69]

more than 3 weeks may warrant an extensive diagnostic evaluation.[70]

L-Tryptophan, an amino acid that was available for many years as a food supplement, was promoted as a sleep aid, although it had never been proven safe and effective for this purpose. The FDA banned it in 1989, after it was implicated in an outbreak of eosinophilia-myalgia syndrome, a rare but serious disorder characterized by severe muscle and joint pain. More than 1500 cases and 38 deaths were reported. The difficulty was due to a contaminant introduced during the manufacturing of L-tryptophan by a Japanese supplier.[71]

Scientific studies may eventually show that melatonin can promote sleep safely, but the appropriate dosage and the potential for adverse effects are currently unknown (see Chapter 12).

The box on "Self-Help for Sleepless Nights" suggests measures that can help restore a normal sleep pattern.

SMOKING DETERRENTS

Much of the difficulty people have in quitting smoking is caused by nicotine withdrawal symptoms. Within 24 hours of stopping, about 80% of smokers experience withdrawal symptoms that can include a craving for nicotine, irritability, anxiety, difficulty in concentrating, restlessness, and difficulty with appetite (either too much or too little). Nicotine-replacement therapy is intended to make the transition from smoker to nonsmoker easier.

In 1984 nicotine gum (*Nicorette*) was approved for use under a physician's prescription. Chewing the gum can produce blood nicotine levels similar to those obtained with cigarette smoking. Any nicotine that is swallowed has little effect on the body. The gum provides a substitute for oral activity and can prevent nicotine withdrawal symptoms, allowing the smoker to break the behavioral habits of smoking without suffering the discomforts of nicotine withdrawal at the same time. After a few months, use is tapered off.

In 1996 the FDA switched *Nicorette* to nonprescription status, permitting it to be sold as a 12-week smoking-cessation program that includes a user's guide and audiotape.

Since 1992 several companies have begun marketing prescription products (*Nicoderm, Habitrol, Nicotrol, Prostep*) that deliver nicotine through the skin. The products are small patches that release nicotine slowly and steadily when placed on the upper body or upper outer part of the arm. These products are appropriate for people who (a) smoke 1 pack or more per day and are unable to quit with willpower alone or (b) smoke about 15 cigarettes per day but developed

tobacco withdrawal symptoms during their last attempt to quit.[72] The recommended period of use is 6 to 8 weeks, with dosage decreased as the user becomes more accustomed to not smoking. The side effects, which usually are dose-related, include diarrhea, nausea, dry mouth, joint pains, abnormal dreams, insomnia, nervousness, and headache. *Zyban* (bupropion), a prescription drug that works differently from nicotine-replacement products, is also effective. None of these products has been proven more effective or better tolerated than the others.[73] The results are best if the prescribing physician is familiar with smoking-cessation techniques and provides appropriate counseling.[73,74] In 1996 the FDA approved OTC sale of *Nicotrol* and *NicoDerm CQ* patches and prescription sale of *Nicotrol NS* nasal spray.

STIMULANTS FOR FATIGUE

Fatigue is a normal physiologic result of physical exertion. It disappears after adequate rest has been obtained. However, students who want to avoid fatigue and stay awake while cramming for exams, truck drivers taking long trips, and others seeking greater alertness for another reason may resort to OTC drugs or illegally

Table 19-8
CAFFEINE CONTENT OF SELECTED SOURCES

Source	Caffeine (typical amount)
Beverages	
Brewed coffee*	100 to 150 mg/cup
Instant coffee*	90 mg/cup
Tea*	50 to 70 mg/cup
Decaffeinated coffee	2 to 4 mg/cup
Cola drinks/many soft drinks	30 to 55 mg/12 oz
Cocoa	25 mg/cup
Milk chocolate	3 to 6 mg/oz
OTC products	
Caffedrine capsules	200 mg
Nodoz Extra Strength	200 mg
Vivarin	200 mg
Quick-Pep tablets	150 mg
Nodoz tablets	100 mg
Excedrin Extra Strength	65 mg
Anacin, Cope	32 mg

*The amount of caffeine in coffee and tea varies with the brand, the size of the cup, and the strength of the brew. A cup is 6 fluid ounces.

obtained prescription drugs that contain a stimulating substance.

The ingredient in the OTC products is caffeine. It can help to reduce drowsiness and fatigue and stimulate muscular function. An FDA advisory panel said, "In cases where mental alertness or motor performance is necessary, such drugs (caffeine) can modify fatigue states to allow successful completion of a required task."[75] The FDA panel stated that caffeine in doses of 100 to 200 mg every 3 to 4 hours is safe and effective in OTC products. Table 19-8 illustrates the caffeine contents of selected sources.

Too much caffeine can cause several problems. It can mask fatigue to the point where a person may suddenly collapse from exhaustion. It may make a person excessively nervous and irritable, cause palpitations and heart irregularity, and stimulate excess stomach acid-

ity. Tolerance and physical dependence can occur with habitual ingestion of caffeine; some individuals will experience withdrawal symptoms (headache, irritability, restlessness, and fatigue) if they suddenly stop a daily regimen of coffee consumption.

Caffeine is not advisable for people with high blood pressure. It may cause palpitations and tachycardia. It should also be avoided by ulcer patients because it can increase gastric secretion.

Some OTC pain relievers contain as much as 64 mg of caffeine per dose, the amount in half a cup of coffee. The inclusion of caffeine in product mixtures for relief of headache is questionable.

Consumers should also be wary of products claimed to improve one's personality, marriage, sex life, or other farfetched benefits. The main ingredient may be caffeine.

Table 19-9

HOME MEDICINE CABINET

First-Aid and Medical Supplies

Band-aids of various sizes	Hydrogen peroxide (for cleansing wounds)*
Absorbent cotton	Sterile gauze pads
Ace bandage	Adhesive tape
Tongue depressors	Cotton-tipped applicators
Ice bag	Hot water bottle or heating pad
Sunscreen product	Safety pins
Flashlight	Small, blunt-edged scissors
Dosage spoon	Oral and rectal thermometers
Fine-point tweezers and sewing needle (for removing splinters)	Petroleum jelly
	First-aid manual

Drug Items / For Treatment of:

Drug Items	For Treatment of:
Aspirin, acetaminophen, and/or ibuprofen	Fever, headache, other aches and pains
Antacid	Heartburn and upset stomach
Hydrocortisone ointment or cream	Minor skin irritations and allergies
Antibiotic ointment or cream	Minor skin infections
Antidiarrhetic	Diarrhea
Antihistamine (chlorpheniramine)	Allergic reactions and colds
Cough syrup (suppressant)	To reduce the intensity of a cough
Decongestant (pseudoephedrine)	Stuffy nose
Antinausea (dimenhydrinate)	Nausea (including motion sickness)
Mild laxative (Milk of Magnesia)	Occasional constipation
Glycerine suppositories or prepackaged enemas	Occasional constipation
Calamine lotion	Contact dermatitis (e.g., poison ivy)

Additional Products for Children

Pediatric acetaminophen	Fever
Syrup of ipecac	Poisoning (to induce vomiting only if use is advised by a physician or poison control center)

HOME MEDICINE CABINET

It is prudent to have medical supplies and drug products available for self-treatment of certain illnesses, injuries, and emergency situations. Select from Table 19-9 on page 435 according to the anticipated needs of your household. Drugs should be stored where they will not be exposed to excess humidity.

Keep drug items out of reach of children. Discard medications that have reached their expiration date or have changed in color, odor, or consistency. The telephone numbers of your doctor, hospital, poison control center, ambulance or rescue squad, and police and fire emergency switchboards should be kept handy.

PRUDENT USE OF MEDICATION

Safe, effective drug use depends upon the patient's understanding of the drug regimen, its risks and benefits, and the necessary precautions associated with each medication. In many cases, the key to safe and effective use of medication is open communication with the prescriber.[76] Prudent use of medication requires knowledge of the following:

- *The name of the drug.* Knowing the name will not only enable you to look up information about the drug, it will also enable you to discuss it with your doctor (or another doctor) should this be necessary.
- *The drug's purpose.* This information will help you understand your treatment and whether or not it is working.
- *How and when should it be taken?* This basic information will be on the product's label. Some medications are best taken on an empty stomach (before meals) for maximum absorption. Some are best taken on a full stomach to prevent the medications from irritating the stomach. Some

are inactivated by food and must be taken on an empty stomach. Some have to be taken on an exact schedule, while others do not. It may be helpful to keep a written record of what you are doing—particularly when several medications are being taken on different schedules.

- *Are there any special instructions?* Sometimes specific foods, alcoholic beverages, or other medicines will react unfavorably with the medicine just prescribed.
- *What side effects might occur?* All drugs have possible side effects. If they occur, in some cases nothing needs to be done and the medication can be continued. In others, a change of dosage or medication will be advised. The occurrence of certain side effects would be a reason to stop using the drug. It can help to know the common side effects and what to do if they occur. One of the most important side effects is drowsiness—which is common with antihistamines, sedatives, and drugs for mental and emotional problems. People taking any of these drugs should not drive a car until they have determined that the drugs will not interfere with their ability to do so safely. Information about side effects can be obtained by asking your physician or pharmacist or consulting a reliable reference.
- *How long should the drug be taken?* Some drugs need to be taken only until symptoms stop, while others should be taken for a period specified in advance. For example, pain relievers can be stopped when your pain goes away, but antibiotics are typically prescribed for 7 to 14 days to eradicate germs that remain even though symptoms of the infection have disappeared.
- *What should I do if I miss a dose?* In some cases it will be advisable to make up the dose to maintain an adequate blood level of a medication. In other cases it will not matter, and doubling the dose will increase the likelihood of side effects.
- *Is written information about the drug available?* Some doctors provide instruction sheets on common prescription drugs. A package insert may be available from the

---

Table 19-10

RELIABLE DRUG REFERENCES

Title	Price	Description
Complete Drug Reference, 2001 (updated annually)	$44	Detailed compilation of the purposes and side effects of more than 9000 brand-name prescription and OTC drug products.
The Essential Guide to Prescription Drugs, 2001 (updated annually)	$22	Detailed compilation of the uses, benefits, risks, and date of introduction of more than 300 drugs of major importance.
PDR Family Guide to Prescription Drugs (1999)	$23	Explains why each drug is prescribed and how it works. Less detail than the *Complete Drug Reference.* Comes with CD-ROM.
Physician's Desk Reference, 2001 (updated annually)	$84	Written for physicians. Impractical for laypersons because it provides little perspective on the frequency of side effects and what to do if they occur.
MEDLINEplus Drug Information from U.S. Pharmacopeial Convention	Free	Excellent database of 9000 prescription and OTC drugs at http://www.nlm.nih.gov/medlineplus/druginformation.html.

pharmacist who fills the prescription, but these tend to be overly technical. Table 19-10 describes several excellent information sources for consumers.

- *Is a generic form available?* Generic drugs usually cost less and are just as potent as name brands. Some doctors routinely prescribe them, but others either think they are inferior or simply do not bother. With a few medicines for serious diseases there may be a medical reason to avoid a generic drug. But in most cases there is no reason they cannot be used.

It should not be necessary to ask all the aforementioned questions each time you visit a doctor and receive a prescription. A good doctor will communicate most of this information when the medicine is prescribed. But do not expect or demand a lengthy discussion on the uncommon side effects and complications of common drugs. If you think your doctor is not communicating enough, a tactful question may lead to clarification.

Various types of aids can help people take their medications properly. These include medication calendars, individual instruction sheets, color-coded bottles, blister cards, calendar trays, self-sealing plastic bags on which the dates and times for medicating are written, special bottlecaps that record when bottles are opened, and bottlecaps and boxes that beep or buzz when it is time to take a dose.

When traveling, try to take along enough medicine to meet your needs. Carrying an extra prescription may be wise in case your luggage is lost or your supply runs out. If a childproof container is hard to handle, ask the pharmacist for one that is easy to open.

Safety Precautions

The following suggestions may help you use medications safely.

- If you go to more than one doctor, tell each about any prescription and OTC medications you are taking. It is a good idea to keep a record with you. Also tell the doctor about any adverse drug reaction you have had.
- Stick to the dosage the doctor prescribes. Taking extra may increase the chances of adverse reactions without increasing the chances of benefit. And don't stop a medicine because you don't think it is working. Some drugs have to be taken for several days or even weeks before their effect is apparent. Instead, contact your doctor for instructions. Keep a daily record of all drugs being taken, especially if treatment schedules are complicated.
- Remember that alcohol and sedatives can multiply each other's effect on the brain. Don't mix alcohol and sleeping pills, antianxiety agents, or any other drugs that have sedative effects. If you drink regularly, make sure your doctor knows about it.

- Keep your drugs in their original containers so no mix-up occurs about which drug is which.
- Clean out your medicine cabinet periodically. Throw away any drugs that have reached their expiration date or changed in color, odor, or texture. Drugs prescribed for a previous illness or for another person should not be taken without first checking with the physician. The drug may have lost its strength or changed its composition, or a more appropriate drug may be available for the illness.
- Call the doctor promptly if an unusual drug reaction occurs.
- Consider purchasing all of your prescription products at a pharmacy with a computer that tracks them and alerts the pharmacist to possible adverse drug interactions. This might have protective value if your physician overlooks a significant interaction. However, this potential benefit should be weighed against the advantage of comparison shopping to save money.
- Remember that it may be risky to share medicines with others. When prescribing medications, doctors take into account the patient's age, weight, sex, other medications being taken, and other factors. What is good for one person may not be good for someone else.

Cost-Saving Strategies

Although the total amount Americans spend on drug products is only a small percentage of total health-care costs, the proportion spent out of pocket is high (see Chapter 25). Several strategies can lead to savings.

Many people can save significant sums by asking their doctors to consider cost when choosing which drugs to prescribe and to give preference to generic drugs when possible. Higher-priced drugs are not necessarily better than low-priced drugs. If a product seems especially expensive, ask whether a less costly alternative is available. This is often the case with antibiotics. Some of the newer antibiotics are very expensive. Although they may be important for certain infections, most infections can be managed with older, less expensive antibiotics.

For nonprescription drugs it is wise to learn the names, dosages, and purposes of common active ingredients and list those that seem useful for the self-treatment of minor ailments. This information will make it possible to choose the least expensive products that contain the desired ingredients. As with prescription drugs, prices vary from product to product and from store to store. Information about ingredients in specific products can be obtained from product labels, package inserts, a pharmacist, or the American Pharmaceutical Association's *Handbook of Nonprescription Drugs.*

People who require prescribed medication for a long-term illness may find it economical to purchase pills in large quantities. Consumers who can wait 1 week

---

It's Your Decision

Your doctor has prescribed an antibiotic for a respiratory tract infection. On the second day you took the drug, you develop nausea and diarrhea. Which of the following actions would you take?

Reason

☐ Consult the *Physician's Desk Reference* to see whether this is a common side effect.

☐ Telephone your doctor to report the new symptom.

☐ Wait 24 hours to see what happens.

☐ Stop taking the drug.

☐ Telephone the pharmacist.

☐ Other (specify) _____

---

or longer to obtain a drug may find that discount mail-order services can save them money. Some of these are open only to members, whereas others are available to anyone. Members of the American Association of Retired Persons (AARP), for example, can purchase both prescription and nonprescription drugs from the AARP Pharmacy Service. AARP membership is open to people age 50 and older and costs about $5 a year.

Many pharmacies give 10% discounts to senior citizens, and several states have passed laws that reduce prescription drug costs for low-income elderly. Price should not be the sole reason for selecting one's pharmacy, however. Convenience, courtesy, and service may be worth the extra price paid for a product. A pharmacist may be able to help you assess the quality of products and should be willing to answer questions readily.

Summary

The two basic types of medicines that can be purchased in the United States are prescription and over-the-counter (OTC) drugs. Prescription drugs generally are more powerful and have more side effects. Prudent consumers learn the name, purpose, dosage, side effects, and other significant characteristics of drugs that are prescribed for them. This information can be obtained from one's physician, a pharmacist, product labels, package inserts, and drug reference books.

OTC drugs are intended mainly for self-treatment of minor illnesses and injuries. Since 1972, expert advisory panels have reviewed the ingredients in these products to determine their safety and efficacy. As a result, most ingredients that were hazardous or ineffective have been removed from the marketplace. In addition, many potent ingredients that were available only by prescription 20 years ago are now available over the counter.

The commonly used OTC products include pain relievers, antacids, antihistamines, cough and cold remedies, laxatives, and remedies for diarrhea and motion sickness. The best way to choose most OTC remedies is to determine what ingredients are desirable and select products that contain them. In most cases, single-ingredient products are best. It is also prudent to have medical supplies and drug products available at home for the self-treatment of minor illnesses and injuries and for first aid. Generic drugs usually are equivalent to brand-name drugs and usually are less expensive.

References

1. Physicians' Desk Reference for Nonprescription Drugs. Montvale, N.J., 1996, Medical Economics.
2. OTC facts & figures. Consumer Health Products Association Web site, accessed Dec 17, 2000.
3. Over-the-counter human drugs; labeling requirements; Final rule. Federal Register 64:13253–13303, 1999.
4. Blies JA. The doctor of pharmacy. JAMA 249:1157–1160, 1983.
5. Nelson MV and others. A survey of pharmacists' recommendations for food supplements in the U.S.A. and the U.K. Journal of Clinical Pharmacy and Therapeutics 15:131–139, 1990.
6. Nelson MV, Bailie GR. Pharmacists' perceptions of alternative health approaches—a comparison between U.S. and British pharmacists. Journal of Clinical Pharmacy and Therapeutics 15:141–146, 1990.
7. Barrett S. Unethical behavior of pharmacists. Quackwatch Web site, Dec 8, 1999.
8. Bouts BA. The misuse of compounding by pharmacists. Quackwatch Web site, Dec 5, 1999.
9. Talk about prescriptions. Washington, D.C., 2000, National Council on Patient Information and Education.
10. Cramer JA and others. How often is medication taken as prescribed? A novel assessment technique. JAMA 261:3273–3277, 1989.
11. Food and Drug Administration. Requirements on content and format of labeling for human prescription drugs and biologics; Requirements for Prescription Drug Product Labels; Proposed Rule. Federal Register: 65:81081–81131, 2000.

12. Nightingale SL, Morrison JC. Generic drugs and the prescribing physician. JAMA 258:1200–1204, 1987.

13. Myths and facts of generic drugs. FDA Consumer 21(7):13–14, 1987.

14. The big lie about generic drugs. Consumer Reports 52:480–485, 1987.

15. Generic drugs: still safe? Consumer Reports 55:310–311, 1990.

16. Alcohol, caffeine, and tobacco are drugs, too. Consumer Reports on Health 3:12, 1991.

17. Whorton JC. Traditions of folk medicine in America. JAMA 257:1632–1635, 1987.

18. Brecher EM and the editors of Consumer Reports. Licit and Illicit Drugs. Boston, 1972, Little, Brown & Co.

19. McNamara B. Step Right Up. Garden City, N.J., 1976, Doubleday & Co.

20. Neergaard L. Drug bans blamed on doctors who ignored safety warnings: FDA says death resulted from patients using new medicines. Associated Press, Dec 12, 2000.

21. Bloom BS, Iannacone RC. Internet availability of prescription pharmaceuticals to the public. Annals of Internal Medicine 131:830–833, 1999.

22. Henney JE and others. Internet purchase of prescription drugs: Buyer beware. Annals of Internal Medicine 131:861–862, 1999.

23. Barrett S. Internet drug sales attacked by Kansas Attorney General. Quackwatch Web site, Dec 19, 2000.

24. Segal M. Patches, pumps, and timed release: New ways to deliver drugs. FDA Consumer 25(8):15–17, 1991.

25. Gannon K. Exclusive consumer OTC survey. Drug Topics, Jan 8, 1990.

26. Heller Research Group: Self-Medication in the '90s: Practices and Perceptions. Washington, D.C., 1992, Nonprescription Drug Manufacturer's Association.

27. Young JH. Self-Dosage Medicines: An Historical Perspective. Lawrence, Kan., 1974, Coronado Press.

28. Gilbertson WE. FDA's review of OTC drugs. In Handbook of Nonprescription Drugs, ed 10. Washington, D.C., 1993, American Pharmaceutical Association.

29. Bradley WW. OTC Review summary. Washington, D.C., June 28, 2000, Consumer Healthcare Products Association.

30. Unapproved over-the-counter (OTC) drugs still marketed? FDA Medical Bulletin 26(1):4, 1996.

31. Podolsky D. Questionable medicine: Many FDA-banned pills and potions are still sold—legally. U.S. News & World Report, May 15, 1995, pp 101–105.

32. Zimmerman D. Zimmerman's Complete Guide to Non-prescription Drugs. Detroit, 1993, Visible Ink Press.

33. Stehlin IB. Taking a shot at allergy relief. FDA Consumer 30(4):6–11, 1996.

34. Barrett S and the editors of Consumer Reports. Health Schemes, Scams, and Frauds. Mount Vernon, N.Y., 1990, Consumer Reports Books.

35. How to relieve allergy symptoms—and stay awake. Consumer Reports on Health 4:37, 1992.

36. Antihistamines. Consumer Reports on Health 1:12–13, 1989.

37. Jacknowitz AI. External analgesic products. In Handbook of Nonprescription Drugs, ed 10. Washington, D.C., 1993, American Pharmaceutical Association.

38. Migliardi JR and others. Caffeine as an analgesic adjuvant in tension headache. Clinical and Pharmacological Therapeutics 56(5):576–586, 1994.

39. What's the best pain reliever? Depends on your pain. Consumer Reports 61:62–63, 1996.

40. Jonas M, Hennekens CH. Aspirin and health: Impressive new benefits of a very old remedy. New York, 1993, American Council on Science and Health.

41. How to pick a pain reliever. Consumer Reports on Health 8:30–32, 1996.

42. Acetaminophen, NSAIDs, and alcohol. The Medical Letter 38:55–56, 1996.

43. Over-the-counter H_2-receptor antagonists for heartburn. The Medical Letter 37:95–96, 1995.

44. Antacids. Consumer Reports on Health 2:12–13, 1990.

45. When heartburn goes from "nuisance" to "dangerous." Tufts University Diet & Nutrition Letter 14(6):4–5, 1996.

46. How to use antacids safely and effectively. University of California at Berkeley Wellness Letter 2(6):3, 1986.

47. Lewis R. Surprise cause of gastritis revolutionizes ulcer treatment. FDA Consumer 28(10):15, 1994.

48. Soll AH and others. Medical treatment of peptic ulcer disease: Practice guidelines. JAMA 275:622–629, 1996.

49. New treatment for ulcers—and other stomach pains. Consumer Reports 60:552–553, 1995.

50. The pill for herpes—for whom? Harvard Medical School Health Letter 10(2):6, 1985.

51. Kaplowitz LG and others. Prolonged continuous acyclovir treatment with normal adults with frequently recurring genital herpes simplex virus infection. JAMA 265:747–551, 1991.

52. Farley D. Help for cuts, scrapes, and burns. FDA Consumer 30(4):13–15, 1996.

53. Hecht A. Of hangovers and love potions. FDA Consumer 16(10):10–11, 1982.

54. Hse E. Warning on gay enhancers. San Francisco Chronicle, March 24, 1983.

55. Harvey SM, Beckman ZD. Alcohol consumption, female sexual behavior, and contraceptive use. Journal of Studies of Alcohol 47:327–332, 1986.

56. Cold remedies. Which ones work best? Consumer Reports 54:8–11, 1989.

57. Hecht A. More yesses, no's and maybes for OTC drugs. FDA Consumer 19(3):16–19, 1985.

58. Cold comfort: Which remedies should you choose? Consumer Reports on Health 9:133–137, 1997.

59. Cough remedies. Consumer Reports on Health 1:30–31, 1989.

60. Final rule issued on OTC cough medicines. FDA Consumer 21(9):3, 1987.

61. Herndon ML. Guaranteed hangover remedy revealed! FDA Consumer 17(10):16–17, 1983.

62. Help for hemorrhoids. Consumer Reports 51:578–580, 1986.

63. Hemorrhoids. Public Citizen Health Research Group Health Letter 7(3):1–6, 1992.

64. Iron in the diet: Do you need supplements? Consumer Reports 61(3):6–7, 1996.

65. Litovitz T, Manoguerra A. Comparison of pediatric poisoning hazards: An analysis of 3.8 million exposure incidents. Pediatrics 89:999–1006, 1992.

66. Hinglet AT. Preventing childhood poisoning. FDA Consumer 30(2):7–11, 1996.

67. Laxatives. Consumer Reports on Health 2:85, 1990.

68. Farley D. Taming tummy turmoil. FDA Consumer 29(5):21–23, 1995.

69. Segal M. OTC options: Help for the sleepless. FDA Consumer 28(7):14–17, 1994.

70. Freedman DX. Drugs and insomnia. Consensus Development Conference Summary, 4:1, Bethesda, Md., 1984, National Institutes of Health.

71. Barrett S. Notes on the tryptophan disaster. Skeptical Inquirer 19(4):6–9, 1995.

72. Rennard SI, Daughton DM. The transdermal nicotine experience: Safety, efficacy, and tips for smoking cessation. Modern Medicine 62 Supp 1:28–33, 1994.

73. Fiore MC and others. Treating Tobacco Use and Dependence. Clinical Practice Guideline. Rockville, Md., 2000, U.S. Department of Health and Human Services.

74. Fiore MC and others. Tobacco dependence and the nicotine patch: Clinical guidelines for effective use. JAMA 268:2687–2694, 1992.

75. Hecht A. Panel reports on sleep aids. FDA Consumer 10(1):10–13, 1976.

76. Tips on prescription drugs and pharmacies. Arlington, Va., 1990, Council on Better Business Bureaus.

Chapter Twenty

SKIN CARE AND BEAUTY AIDS

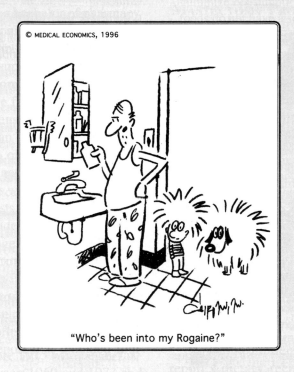

© MEDICAL ECONOMICS, 1996

"Who's been into my Rogaine?"

Man can be cured of every folly but vanity.
ROUSSEAU

*Beauty is a conspiracy of pain forced upon women.
. . . In the boardroom and in the bedroom, women
are entrapped by a cult that is the equivalent of the
iron maiden.*
NAOMI WOLF[1]

*To think that a moisturizer with herbs, vitamins,
botanicals, or some other skin care ingredient can
feed the skin, is like thinking that you can put a bologna sandwich on your face and have lunch.*
PAULA BEGOUN[2]

Key Concepts

KEEP THESE POINTS IN MIND AS YOU STUDY THIS CHAPTER

- Many ingredients in cosmetic products are included for marketing purposes and serve no useful purpose. Price is not a reliable measure of quality.

- Antiperspirants and deodorants have been oversold. Bathing is by far the most important body-odor control measure.

- By masking tiny lines, some moisturizing agents may help the skin look and feel better for a few hours.

- Tretinoin may slightly reduce fine wrinkles and age spots, but no cosmetic product can prevent or eliminate wrinkles, repair sun-damaged skin, or retard or reverse the aging process of the skin.

- The most important causes of premature aging of the skin are exposure to ultraviolet light and smoking cigarettes.

- Effective over-the-counter and prescription products are available to treat acne.

- People contemplating cosmetic surgery should think carefully about why they want it, thoroughly investigate the credentials of a prospective surgeon, and gather realistic information about the limitations and possible adverse effects of the procedure.

Americans spend more than $30 billion each year on cosmetic products they hope will make them more attractive. The American Academy of Dermatology states that the average adult uses at least seven skin-care products a day.[3] Americans also spend several billion dollars a year on cosmetic surgery. This chapter focuses on products and services that are intended to improve the way people look.

COSMETIC REGULATION

The federal Food, Drug, and Cosmetic Act defines cosmetics as "articles (other than soap) intended to be applied to the human body for cleansing, beautifying, promoting attractiveness, or altering the appearance without affecting the body's structure or functions." The FDA has classified cosmetics into 13 categories: skin-care products (creams, lotions, powders, and sprays); fragrances; eye makeup; other makeup (lipstick, foundation, and blush); manicure products; hair coloring preparations; deodorants; shaving products; baby products (shampoos, lotions, and powders); bath oils and bubble baths; mouthwashes; sunscreens; and shampoos, permanent waves, and other hair products.[4]

Cosmetic product labels must list all ingredients that compose more than 1% of a product (by weight), in the order of predominance, with the ingredient present in the largest amount first. This enables allergic individuals to avoid known irritants and can help people compare differently priced products. More than 5000 ingredients are used in cosmetic products. Information about the most widely used ingredients can be obtained from the *International Cosmetic Ingredient Dictionary*, which is available at many public libraries. This book provides both definitions and trade names.

Cosmetics marketed with claims that they can affect structure or function must meet the labeling standards for drugs in addition to those of cosmetics. Such products include dandruff shampoos, fluoride toothpastes to prevent dental decay, and sunscreen and sunblocking cosmetics. Dual-classification products must be proven safe and effective for their therapeutic claims before marketing. Color additives also require FDA approval.

Under the FDA's good manufacturing practice guidelines, even cosmetic products that are not regulated as drugs should be tested for safety and subject to quality control during manufacture. FDA review of the tests is not necessary, but safety warnings are required if problems become apparent. The products that currently require warnings include products in pressurized containers (potentially dangerous to children), detergent bubble bath products (may irritate the skin or urinary tract), genital deodorant sprays (may cause irritation or allergic reaction), hair-dye products that contain coal-tar dyes (can irritate skin), depilatories and hair straighteners (alkaline ingredients can cause burns), shampoos and conditioners (can irritate eyes), and nail builders (can irritate skin).[5]

SOAPS

Soap cleans the skin more effectively than any other product. It is the best cleanser for most people. Soaps are traditionally made of natural ingredients: fatty acids from animal fat or vegetable oils, alkalis, scent, and coloring materials. Solid soaps are made from sodium alkalis, such as lye, whereas liquid soaps are based on potassium alkalis. Dishwashing liquids, which are not soaps, are detergents made from synthetic, often petroleum-based, chemicals. Most bar soaps are inexpensive, but some marketed for their scent or other aesthetic feature are priced quite high. Low-priced bar soaps usually cost less than low-priced liquid soaps.

A small percentage of people react adversely to alkaline soap. A soap's pH indicates the extent of its acidity or alkalinity. A pH of 7 is neutral; a higher number means the product is alkaline; and a lower number means it is acidic. High-alkaline soaps can cause the skin to become rough, red, and dry. Individuals with dry skin may find that a superfatted soap (containing additional fats or oils such as moisturizing cream, lanolin, or cocoa butter) will leave the skin feeling more comfortable. However, a moisturizing lotion used after bathing is likely to be more effective.

Deodorant soaps include an antibacterial agent. Perspiration has no odor; body odor is caused by bacteria that thrive on perspiration. However, all soaps provide some protection from unwanted odors by washing off bacteria along with dirt, bacterial products, grease, and skin debris.

In 1995 *Consumer Reports* rated *Dove* and *Caress Original Peach* highest among 28 bar soaps and *Ivory Dishwashing Liquid* best among 14 liquid detergents. The editors commented that, "Boutique soaps come in nice colors, but their fancy prices won't buy you more cleanliness than what you'll get with a soap from the supermarket."[6]

MOISTURIZERS

Moisturizing lotions, creams, and gels can help the skin feel smoother by increasing the amount of water retained in the outermost layer of the skin. The skin constantly renews itself through multiplication of cells beneath the surface. Dead cells are gradually pushed toward the surface, where they lose their moisture and eventually slough off. If the skin loses moisture too quickly, its outer layer dries out and may even crack. Glands within the skin produce oil that retards evaporation of the skin's water. If the glands become less active (as usually happens when people age) or too much oil is removed by washing, the skin will become too dry.

Moisturizers contain ingredients that can penetrate the outer layer of the skin but not the living cells underneath. Emollient ingredients block moisture from leaving the skin by coating it with a thin layer of oil. The most common ones are petrolatum, lanolin, mineral

Consumer Tip

Cosmetics Safety Precautions

- Read the labels carefully and follow directions exactly. This is especially important when using antiperspirants, depilatory (hair-removing) preparations, hair dyes, home permanents, and skin packs.
- Apply a small amount on the inside of your forearm and leave it for 24 hours to determine if you are allergic to the cosmetic.
- Stop using the cosmetic immediately if it causes an adverse effect such as burning, breaking out, stinging, or itching. See your physician if the condition appears serious.
- To prevent contamination, wash your hands before applying a cosmetic.
- Close containers after each use to prevent contamination.
- Do not borrow cosmetics from others.
- Do not buy cosmetics without preservatives, which help prevent contamination.
- Avoid scented soaps; fragrance chemicals may be responsible for allergy and irritation.
- Be cautious when using cosmetics around the eyes.
- Report adverse effects of cosmetics to the manufacturer and the FDA as a public service.
- Use aerosol products in well-ventilated rooms.

oil, propylene glycol, and dimethicone. Humectant ingredients slow down the rate of water loss by attracting water from the skin and surrounding air. The most commonly used humectants are glycerine, propylene glycol, and phospholipids. Most moisturizers contain both types of ingredients, but products intended for dry skin have more oil, whereas products for oily skin contain only humectants. The best time to apply a moisturizer is after washing, while the skin is still damp, so that the moisturizer traps some of the water.

In 1999 *Consumer Reports*[7] tested 28 moisturizing lotions and creams and concluded that some low-cost products worked better than expensive ones. The top-rated products included *L'Oréal Penituse Active Daily Moisture SPF 15* ($1.32 per ounce), *Pond's Nourishing Moisturizer SPF 15* ($1.40 per ounce), *Curél Soothing Hands Moisturizing with Chamomile* ($1.05 per ounce), and *Vaseline Intensive Care Advanced Healing with Skin Protection Complex* (29¢ per ounce). All the products increased the skin's moisture during the first 2 hours after they were applied; then the moisture level usually decreased. The most effective products caused large, long-lasting increases in the moisture level; the least effective products boosted moisture very little. In a previous report[8] the editors concluded that people with oily skin or who live in a humid climate may only need regular cleaning and a sunscreen to keep their face looking its best, whereas people with dry skin may benefit from a moisturizer. They recommended the following test for determining your skin type.

A few hours after washing with a nonmoisturizing soap hold pieces of eyeglass lens-cleaning paper for 10 seconds against your forehead, nose, chin, and a cheek. If the paper from all areas is oily, your skin is oily. If the paper from all areas is dry, your skin is dry. For normal skin, the paper held to the cheek will be less oily than the paper held to the forehead, nose, and chin.

QUESTIONABLE CLAIMS

A certain amount of wrinkling is inevitable as people get older. Both cigarette smoking[9] and excess sun exposure can cause facial wrinkling to become apparent in middle age. When both occur, the effects are multiplied.[10]

Many cosmetic manufacturers suggest that their moisturizers and other products can help people look more youthful. Moisturizers may help the skin look and feel better for a few hours. By preventing water loss from the skin, they can fill in fine lines to make the skin look smoother. Alpha hydroxy acids can facilitate removal of dead skin cells, making the skin smoother and enabling the moisturizer to work more effectively.[11] But no cosmetic can prevent or eliminate wrinkles, repair sun-damaged skin, or retard or reverse the aging process of the skin. Specific statements to that effect would be *drug* claims because they would indicate that the product is intended to affect a bodily function or the body's structure. Such claims are illegal because no product has been proven safe and effective for these purposes. Table 20-1 comments on several questionable cosmetic ingredients.

In 1988 the FDA[12] ordered Alfin Fragrances, Inc., Estée Lauder, Inc., Christian Dior Perfumes, Inc., Avon Products, Inc., and 18 other manufacturers to stop

Table 20-1

QUESTIONABLE COSMETIC INGREDIENTS

Substance	Description	Comment
Aloe vera	Plant with anti-irritant properties	Most skin lotions listing aloe vera as an ingredient do not contain enough (5% to 10%) to work as an anti-irritant; those that do are expensive
Amniotic fluid	Fluid that surrounds the developing fetus (from cow or ox) to protect it from injury	Does not promote tissue growth or remove wrinkles
Bovine albumin	Protein from a cow	Federal court ordered manufacturer to stop claiming it can give a "face lift without surgery"
Cerebrosides and ceramides	Phospholipids similar to compounds formed in the skin that help the skin retain its moisture	The claim that they "help fortify and replenish the skin's moisture barrier" is merely a fancy description of what all emollient ingredients in moisturizers do
Collagen and elastin	Proteins under the top layer of skin; tend to deteriorate with age or sun damage	Skin proteins cannot be "replenished" by a cosmetic product
Liposomes	Microscopic capsules made from phospholipids and other fatty substances, some of which occur naturally in the skin	Does not "work beneath the skin's surface" or carry useful ingredients to underlying skin layers, because moisturizers do not penetrate living cells
Nayad	Trade name of a yeast extract	Use claimed to result in "smoothing of lines and wrinkles." FDA has no data to substantiate or refute this claim
Vitamin E	Fat-soluble vitamin that can preserve the fatty components in cosmetic creams and lotions	Prevents products from discoloration and rancidity, but has no proven value for skin preservation or "rejuvenation"
Other vitamins	Vitamins included in various cosmetic formulations	Vitamins applied to the skin do not nourish the skin

Sources: Modified from data in *Consumer Reports*[6] and *FDA Consumer*.[13]

☑ **Consumer Tip**

Healthy Perspectives on Makeup

- The information you get at the cosmetics counter is rarely accurate when it comes to skin care.
- There are no antiaging products available besides sunscreens.
- No one needs more than a daytime moisturizer with an SPF of 15 or greater and a nightime moisturizer without a sunscreen.
- Spending more money doesn't mean you will look more beautiful. Knowing how to apply makeup is the key to looking good.
- All the makeup and skin care products in the world can't cover up an unhealthy lifestyle of no exercise, smoking, and/or a high-fat diet.
- Find ways to feel good about yourself that don't come from your appearance.

Paula Begoun[2]

making antiaging claims for their skin-care products. One product was *Glycel*, which had been promoted by Dr. Christiaan Barnard, the South African surgeon who performed the first successful heart transplant. *Glycel* was said to contain a "rejuvenating" agent called glycosphingolipid (GSL), and advertisements claimed that lack of GSL causes wrinkles. *Glycel* sold for $75 a jar. Dr. Vincent DeLeo,[14] a dermatologist at Columbia Presbyterian Medical Center in New York, said it was merely a moisturizer that smoothes out lines and wrinkles temporarily.

Despite the FDA's action, misleading claims are still common. In mid-1996, for example, Lancôme's *Primordiale Visibly Revitalizing Solution* was said to "help insulate the skin from premature aging factors," Estée Lauder's *Advanced Night Repair* was claimed to "help prevent environmental damage that can cause up to 80% of premature aging," and its *Lipton Anti-Feathering Complex* was touted to "boost the skin's natural ability to produce new elastin and collagen."

Paula Begoun, author of *Don't Go to the Cosmetics Counter Without Me*, advises her readers to be wary of phrases like "appears to," "leaves the skin looking smoother," "changes the appearance of," "lessens the signs of," "reduces the chances of," "reduces the temporary signs of aging," and "reverses the visible damage of aging." She states that because they refer to the skin's appearance, rather than its structure, they are cosmetic claims and do not have to be truthful.[2] Her book discusses the ingredients in more than 10,000 cosmetic products and states what she and people who responded to her surveys have concluded about the products.

Alpha hydroxy acids (AHA) are claimed to reduce wrinkles, spots, and other signs of aging, sun-damaged skin. Although some evidence suggests that they may work, the FDA has received reports of adverse reactions such as severe redness, swelling (especially in the area of the eyes), burning, blistering, bleeding, rash, itching, and skin discoloration. Since they have been available only since 1992, their long-term effects are unknown. An industry-sponsored study found that people who use AHA products have greater sensitivity to sun, which may mean that they increase the risk of photoaging and skin cancer.[15]

Many products are sold with false claims that rubbing them on the skin will eliminate "cellulite." This subject is discussed in Chapter 13.

The Federal Trade Commission, which has jurisdiction over advertising claims, could attack the deceptions that are common in cosmetic advertising, but it has not done so.

OTC TRETINOIN

In 1996 the FDA approved the marketing of Renova, an over-the-counter (OTC) tretinoin product capable of slightly reducing fine wrinkles and age spots. The product is similar to the prescription acne remedy *Retin-A* but has an oilier formulation. Renova is labeled as "an adjunctive agent for use in the mitigation (palliation) of fine wrinkles, mottled hyperpigmentation, and tactile roughness of facial skin in patients who do not achieve such palliation using comprehensive skin care and sun avoidance programs alone." The label must also state: "Renova does not eliminate wrinkles, repair sun damaged skin, reverse photoaging, or restore more youthful or younger skin."

The FDA's action was based on evidence from two clinical trials in which patients treated with *Renova* for 24 weeks were compared with patients who used an emollient cream, with both groups following a comprehensive skin care and sun avoidance program.[16] Although about 65% of the *Renova* group showed some improvement of wrinkling and mottling, *Consumer Reports on Health* has noted: (a) 40% to 50% of the people who used the emollient cream reported seeing similar improvement; (b) nearly all users experienced redness, dryness, itching, and peeling of the skin; (c) any benefit should be apparent within 6 months; and (d) the benefit will disappear if use of the drug is stopped.[17] OTC tretinoin, marketed as *Renova*, costs about $60 for a tube that should last 4 to 6 months. No study has determined how safe it is to use *Renova* for longer than 48 weeks.

FADE CREAMS

Skin bleaches (fade creams) are used to lighten skin discoloration (hyperpigmentation) caused by freckles, flat moles, and age spots. However, they make the skin especially sensitive to the sun. An FDA expert panel reported that the only safe and effective ingredient for OTC use is hydroquinone in concentrations from 1.56% to 2%. Nonprescription products containing 2% hydroquinone include *Esoterica*, *Porcelana*, and *Artra*. More concentrated products are available by prescription.

Hydroquinone does not actually bleach the skin but inhibits the cells that produce melanin. Since these cells are deep within the skin, lightening products work slowly, if at all. Results may not be apparent for 3 months. Users (including those who do not sunbathe) should apply a sunscreen because fade creams increase sensitivity to the sun. *Consumer Reports*[18] has offered these additional comments:

• When fade creams work, they work only against freckles and age spots.
• They will not cause blemishes to completely disappear.
• Apply them only to the pigmented areas and not the surrounding skin.
• If no results are obtained after three months, consider professional treatment.
• Protect hands and face from excessive exposure to the sun to prevent pigment production.
• Foundation creams can cover skin blemishes and serve as an alternative to fade creams.

ANTIPERSPIRANTS AND DEODORANTS

Sweating is a natural body function that helps regulate body temperature and protect the skin against dryness. Normal skin secretions do not have an objectionable odor. However, when skin bacteria interact with sweat, the result may be unpleasant.

There are two types of sweat glands: eccrine and apocrine. Eccrine glands, the main source of perspiration, are located near all body surfaces except the margins of the lips and certain parts of the sex organs. They secrete watery or water-soluble substances. The apocrine glands are located in the armpits, around the nipples, on the abdomen, and in the genital area. They do not function in body temperature regulation but respond to hormonal stimulation. After puberty they produce a milky secretion that emits a strong odor when metabolized by local bacteria. Perspiration from these glands can be triggered by heat and emotional stress.

Antiperspirants reduce secretions from the eccrine glands by astringent action, which contracts the skin to prevent the flow of perspiration. Deodorants either reduce the number of odor-causing bacteria in the underarm area or cover up the odor. Combination products are also available. Antiperspirants are regulated as OTC drugs because they affect a bodily function. Deodorants are regulated as cosmetics. More powerful antiperspirant drugs are available by prescription. However, no product can stop sweating completely.

The *University of California at Berkeley Wellness Letter* states: (a) bathing is by far the best way to control body odor; (b) antiperspirants and deodorants have been oversold; (c) many people use more of them than they need; (d) people who use these products daily should try using them two or three times a week to see whether this works just as well; (e) sticks, roll-ons, and creams tend to provide more protection than aerosols; and (f) inhaling aerosol mist may pose a safety hazard.[19]

Some ingredients in antiperspirants and deodorants can cause allergic reactions. People who are unable to tolerate these products may be helped by washing more frequently or by using an antibacterial soap.

ACNE CARE

Acne is a skin condition characterized by whiteheads, blackheads, pimples, and sometimes cysts, all of which result from the clogging of sebaceous glands. About 80% of teenagers are afflicted, and it remains a problem for many people into their 20s and sometimes beyond. At puberty the sebaceous glands increase in size and activity and secrete more sebum (a mixture of fats and waxes), which normally exits from the pores and lubricates the skin and hair.

Figure 20-1 shows the anatomic relationship between a hair follicle and its nearby sebaceous glands, which secrete sebum into the follicle. In acne, follicles become plugged with comedos composed of sebum and dead cells. If bacteria invade, the surrounding skin can become inflamed, and pimples or pustules may form. Most people with acne have a mild (noninflammatory) form and get occasional whiteheads or blackheads. Severe (inflammatory) acne involves a constant outbreak covering the face and sometimes also the neck, back, chest, and groin. Pimples and pus-filled cysts occur and can result in pitting and scarring of the skin.

Heredity is often a factor in acne. In adult women, cosmetics (especially greasy, heavy creams) may be the cause. In some, acne can be triggered by hormone fluctuations. Jobs that involve exposure to grease or oil may also be a factor. There is little evidence that acne is related to diet. However, if self-experimentation suggests that a specific food aggravates acne, avoiding the food may be reasonable.

Acne cannot be prevented or cured, but it can be controlled and minimized. Only about 10% of cases need medical supervision. Most cases respond to self-treatment with nonprescription products, although physician-directed treatment might produce quicker and better results. The first step is to keep the skin as free of oil as possible by washing twice a day, shampooing as needed, keeping oily hair off the face, and avoiding cosmetic products that contain oil or grease.

If this is insufficient, the next step should be treatment with a topical product containing benzoyl peroxide. Benzoyl peroxide produces irritation that speeds up the turnover of cells lining the follicle. This increases the sloughing of these cells and promotes resolution of the comedos. Benzoyl peroxide often stings and burns the skin and sometimes causes redness and scaling. Self-treatment can be done with an OTC product, but a medical consultation would be more prudent. A doctor can determine which type of product would be best, provide instructions about comedo removal, and advise whether anything else is needed. Kligman[20] states that 2.5%, 5% and 10% benzoyl peroxide solutions are equally effective, but the lowest concentration is the least irritating.

If treatment with benzoyl peroxide is not effective, a doctor may prescribe a topical retinoid such as tretinoin (*Retin-A*), which is stronger but more irritating to the skin. When severe infection exists, an antibiotic will also be prescribed. Because tretinoin increases susceptibility to sunburn, prolonged exposure to the sun should be avoided, and an effective sunscreen should be used.

Accutane, a prescription drug taken orally, can be prescribed for severe acne that does not respond to other forms of therapy. Treatment takes several months and is expensive. Women who are pregnant or might become pregnant should not use *Accutane* because it can cause severe birth defects.

Ultraviolet light from sunlight or a sunlamp can be effective for some people with acne but will aggravate the condition of others. However, it is no longer recommended, because it increases the risk of skin cancer.

Dermatologists and plastic surgeons can improve the appearance of people with severe acne scars. The procedures they use include dermabrasion (facial planing), cryosurgery, and injections of silicone or collagen.

HAIR AND SCALP CARE

The hair shaft, which is the visible part of the hair, is a complex, nonliving structure made of protein. The shaft is produced by the bulb-shaped hair root, at the bottom end of the shaft, deep in the scalp (see Figure 20-1). The shaft and root are encased together in a cellular

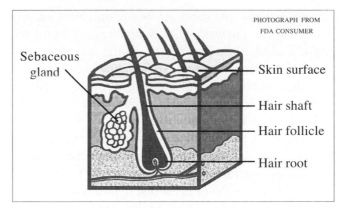

FIGURE 20-1. Cross-section of skin. If the openings of sebaceous glands are blocked by sebum, cells and sebum accumulate to form plugs (comedos).

structure called the follicle, which supplies nourishment and support. Hairs go through three stages.

During the growth stage, which lasts 2 to 6 years, each individual hair is formed by rapidly dividing cells pushing up the follicle from the root. During this stage they grow about half an inch per month. As the cells multiply, those near the surface of the skin die and harden into what we perceive as hair.

During the resting stage, which lasts about 3 months, the hair cells stop reproducing and the entire hair gradually moves up to the skin's surface.

During the dormant stage, which lasts a few weeks, the hair becomes completely separated and a new hair usually begins to grow at the base of the follicle. The hair eventually is pulled out, falls out, or is pushed out by the hair growing from below. Hairs that are growing do not come out unless they are pulled vigorously enough to cause pain.

The healthy scalp of a young adult normally has about 100,000 hairs and loses 50 to 100 each day. In most people, the loss is not significant because the replacement rate is about the same as the rate of loss. As people age, however, the rate of loss increases, and a permanent thinning may be inevitable. Hair can be split or otherwise damaged by rough handling or excessive use of bleach, hair dye, or certain other hair-care products. This section focuses on hair-related problems that may require the use of a medication or the services of a health-care provider.

Shampoos and Conditioners

Some oiliness and flaking of the scalp are normal. Sebaceous glands located just beneath the skin secrete an oil that lubricates the hair follicle and the scalp, keeping the hair glossy and the scalp comfortable. Washing the hair once or twice weekly is usually sufficient to control oiliness and dandruff, but people with an oily scalp may have to wash daily. Soaps remove the oil and leave a residue of mineral salts on the hair shafts that can make the hair look dull. So it is better to use a shampoo that enables some of the natural oil to remain or that contains lanolin as a replacement. That way the hair remains shiny and manageable.

The main function of shampoo is to clean the hair by removing dirt, dead skin scales, and excess sebum. Shampoos generally contain (a) water, (b) a synthetic detergent, (c) a sudsing agent that makes rinsing easier, (d) antistatic and detangling agents, (e) a moisturizing agent, (f) a thickener to give the shampoo a pleasing consistency, and (g) a fragrance. Many shampoos contain a conditioner such as collagen, protein, amino acids, or panthenol. Conditioners are intended to counteract the depletion of natural hair oils, but most are washed away. People who want maximum benefit from a conditioner should apply a separate product after shampooing. Dry shampoos are useful for people who are ill or incapacitated and unable to wash their hair. These are left on the hair for a specified time and then are brushed or combed out.

Begoun[21] states that shampoos are 70% to 90% water, that most cost less than 50¢ a bottle to manufacture, and that most sell for $3 to $20 per item. She states that exotic ingredients such as tea tree oil and awapuhi have no effect on the hair. She also notes that people can tell immediately after use if their hair feels clean, soft, defrizzed, and easy to style, and whether or not it stays put. Most people who wash their hair frequently do not need a medicated shampoo.

Consumer Reports[22] adds that the "workhorse" ingredients in shampoos are (a) detergents (or surfactants), such as ammonium lauryl sulfate, which clean the hair; (b) cationic polymers that can attach to the hair shaft to add smoothness and volume; and (c) silicones such as dimethicone, that can coat the hair, making it feel soft, pliable, and easy to comb. The magazine has also noted that other ingredients such as herbs, vitamins, proteins, AHA, and moisturizers do nothing to improve the condition of the hair. Its recent tests found that expensive brands performed no beter than inexpensive brands.

Dandruff

The skin at the top of the head renews itself once a month. Dead scalp cells are constantly being pushed from the skin's deepest layer to its surface, where they gradually die. Usually this process is not apparent. Dandruff occurs when the dead cells are shed in clumps or flakes. It is a problem with the scalp, not the hair. Nearly everyone has dandruff to some extent.

Dandruff is usually treatable with an OTC product and causes no general health problem or permanent damage. But care should be taken not to confuse simple dandruff with other conditions that cause flaking of the scalp, such as seborrheic dermatitis or psoriasis.

Seborrheic dermatitis is characterized by redness, inflammation, itching, and flaking of the skin. It most commonly affects the scalp and face but can also occur on the ears, chest, and other parts of the body. Hormones, heredity, diet, emotions, medications, cosmetics, and climate can be factors in seborrhea, but often the cause is an infection with a yeast (fungus) called *Pityrosporum ovale*. Mild cases are treatable with OTC products, but severe cases should be treated by a physician. Some cases respond well to treatment with a shampoo containing ketoconazole, which kills the fungus.

Psoriasis is an inflammatory skin disease in which cells reproduce about 10 times faster than normal, but the rate of shedding is unchanged.[23] Live cells then accumulate and form thick patches covered with flaking skin. The scales can occur in many areas of the body, most commonly the knees, elbows, back, and buttocks. Although coal tar and salicylic acid preparations are approved for OTC use against psoriasis, more effective drugs are available by prescription. Because coal tar can make skin overly sensitive to sunlight, people using a coal-tar product should be cautious about exposing their skin to sunlight.

In 1990 the FDA banned 27 ingredients in dandruff shampoos because they had not been proven safe and effective.[24] Five ingredients were approved for use in shampoos, rinses, or products consumers apply to the scalp: salicylic acid, pyrithione zinc, sulfur, selenium sulfide, and coal tar.

Hair Removal

Many people wish to remove hair they consider excessive or unsightly. Excess hair (hirsutism) results from an overabundance of androgens produced in the adrenal glands and ovaries. About one third of women of reproductive age have at least a few long, coarse facial hairs.

Except for electrolysis, all methods of hair removal are temporary. The reappearance time depends on the location of the hair and how much of the hair is removed. Shaving is the fastest method but results in the quickest regrowth. Tweezing is also quick and, because it removes a portion of the hair below the skin, tends to have a longer-lasting effect than shaving. Small amounts of hair can be removed with a pumice stone or other abrasive. However, this can irritate the skin.

Waxing, which is similar in effect to tweezing, is done by applying melted wax to a hairy area. When the wax cools, it can be stripped off in the direction of hair growth, carrying hairs with it. Waxing can irritate the skin and can cause infection of the hair follicles.

Depilatory creams and lotions contain a chemical agent (most commonly thioglycolate) that breaks down the protein in the hair, turning it into a soft mass that is easily wiped off the skin. The root of the hair is left intact. The products are applied to the skin and removed after 5 to 15 minutes. Since the chemicals can irritate or burn the skin, depilatories should not be used without testing them on a small area of the skin. The test is carried out by applying the product to a small area of skin and inspecting the area 24 hours later.

Electrolysis is the only way to remove unwanted hair permanently. It is performed by inserting a fine needle into the hair follicle and delivering an electric current to destroy the hair root. Its safety and effectiveness depend on the expertise of the operator. The competence of nonmedical electrolysis operators varies widely. Thirty-one states license electrologists. Two professional organizations offer certification based on a written examination. Electrolysis devices are also available for self-treatment.

Electrolysis can be tedious, time-consuming, expensive, and uncomfortable, depending on the areas involved and the amount of hair to be removed. In addition, excessive exposure to electric current can damage the skin and cause scarring or infection. A fresh needle should be used for each patient to prevent the spread of hepatitis or AIDS.

People considering electrolysis should consult a dermatologist to determine whether it is advisable and to obtain the name of a suitable practitioner. Growths that contain hair, such as moles, should be diagnosed and evaluated by a physician.

In 1995 the FDA approved medical use of the ThermoLase Softlight laser for hair removal, based on a clinical trial showing that 60% to 70% of people treated had at least a 30% temporary reduction of hair in treated areas. The manufacturer is permitted to state that the procedure can cause hair reduction for up to 3 months after treatment.[25]

Some women may need medical treatment for hirsutism. A physician may advise the use of drugs to inhibit androgen production or block its effect on hair follicles. These substances can have undesirable side effects, and none is uniformly effective. The limitations of the therapy and the extent of the side effects should be discussed thoroughly before making a decision about treatment.

HAIR LOSS

Temporary hair loss may be associated with hormonal imbalance and can occur after surgery, childbirth, radiation, cancer chemotherapy, or certain diseases that are accompanied by a high fever. Other causes of temporary hair loss include reactions to hair products and procedures (permanent waving, drying, and weaving); iron deficiency, toxic intake of vitamin A or mercury; and medications such as heparin and warfarin (anticoagulants), amphetamines, L-dopa, and propranolol (*Inderal*). In such instances, regrowth usually occurs within a few months.

There is no specific therapy for temporary hair loss. To minimize it, one should brush hair only moderately with a soft brush, shampoo regularly and gently with a mild shampoo, dry hair by letting the towel soak up moisture rather than by vigorous rubbing, and avoid hair styles that require pulling the hair excessively.

Alopecia areata, a condition in which hair falls out in patches, occurs with equal frequency in men and women. The cause is unknown, but it may be related to heredity or to the body's immune system. About 90% of people with this condition regrow their hair spontaneously.

The so-called normal or common baldness is male-pattern baldness (androgenic alopecia), which is responsible for 95% of all hair loss in men and also occurs in women. Although a specific cause cannot be identified, it is probably related to hereditary factors (especially among Caucasians), an excess of male hormones (androgens) such as testosterone, and possibly attacks on scalp hair follicles by the body's immune system. Nutritional deficiencies are not a factor.

Minoxidil, marketed as *Rogaine*, has some ability to retard male-pattern baldness. Minoxidil was originally approved by the FDA for the treatment of high blood pressure. However, in certain concentrations it was found to spur the growth of body hair. In 1988 the FDA approved minoxidil as a prescription drug for the treatment of hair loss. Studies indicated that applying minoxidil to the scalp would restore hair growth in some men with thinning hair. In 1996 the FDA switched minoxidil to nonprescription status, enabling it to be marketed as *Rogaine Topical Solution*.

Most of the evidence supporting the use of *Rogaine* is based on a study that began with 2300 men between the ages of 18 and 49 with male-pattern baldness. The study, carried out at 27 research centers, was sponsored by the manufacturer and is summarized in the package insert. After 4 months, 57.7% of the treatment group and 41.4% of the control group reported some hair growth. After 8 more months, 8% of the treatment group reported dense hair growth, 40% reported moderate growth, 36% reported minimal growth, and 16% reported no growth. "Moderate growth" meant that new hairs covered some or all thinning areas, but not as closely together as hair on the rest of the head. "Minimal growth" meant that new hairs were seen, but not enough to cover thinning areas. The second phase of this study had no placebo group. A 32-week study of 600 women with diffuse hair thinning had slightly better results. Two controlled studies of women with alopecia areata found no benefit.[26]

The FDA states that about 25% of men and 20% of women who use *Rogaine* appropriately will attain meaningful (at least moderate) hair growth.[27] Whiting[28] states that the people who respond best are usually younger than 40 years of age, have a history of hair loss for less than 10 years, and have a bald area less than 4 inches in diameter near the top of the skull.

In 1997 the FDA approved *Propecia* for hair loss in men, making it the first such treatment in pill form. The active ingredient in *Propecia* is finasteride, which was approved initially in 1992 as *Proscar*, a treatment for prostate enlargement. It was observed that some patients being treated for prostate enlargement had some regrowth of hair in areas of male-pattern hair loss. Subsequent studies found that 1 mg of finasteride produced hair growth in men with male-pattern hair loss. (*Proscar* contains 5 mg of finasteride; *Propecia* contains 1 mg. Both are prescription drugs.)

The Medical Letter states (a) both *Rogaine* and *Propecia* can produce a modest increase in hair on the scalps of young men with mild-to-moderate hair loss, (b) both must be taken daily and continued indefinitely to maintain the effect, (c) the long-term safety of both drugs has not been determined, and (d) the slight advantage of 5% minoxidil (*Rogaine Extra Strength*) over 2% minoxidil does not justify the higher cost and possible risk of the higher concentration.[29]

No other products are legally marketable as hair-growth stimulants. In 1991 the FDA banned the OTC sale of all other externally applied products said to grow hair or prevent baldness.[30] In announcing the ban, the agency noted that nothing done to a hair shaft once it emerges from the surface of the scalp will influence hair growth.

Hair Implant Surgery

Hair implantation is a form of cosmetic surgery in which patches of skin containing healthy hair follicles are transplanted into areas that are bald or becoming bald. The procedures include punch grafting, strip grafting, scalp reduction, scalp expansion, and various types of flap grafting.[31]

In *punch grafting*, a punch is used to remove small areas of bald scalp and replace them with plugs of healthy scalp.

Minigrafting and *micrografting* involve transferring only a few hairs at a time.[32] In some cases they are used to make the hairline created by punch grafting look more natural.

In *strip grafting*, strips of bald skin are cut from the top of the head and replaced by strips of healthy scalp.

In *scalp reduction* a portion of bald scalp is removed and the wound is closed by pulling surrounding areas of the scalp toward the bare spot. The remaining bald spot can be filled with transplanted hair plugs.

In *scalp expansion*, a balloon-like device is inserted under part of the scalp and gradually filled with dilute salt water, causing the skin to stretch and grow so that a subsequent scalp reduction can cover a larger area.[33]

Flap grafting is done by removing bald areas and replacing them with surrounding areas of hairy skin that have been lifted and swiveled into position. The swiveled portion is left attached to its original location until a new blood supply is established.

These procedures cost thousands of dollars and are often unsuccessful. Sometimes the areas from which the grafts are taken fail to regrow hair properly. Even successful transplants do not last indefinitely, because the transplanted hair lasts only as long as it would have at its original location. A hairpiece, wig, hair weaving, or simply accepting one's baldness may be a better choice.

Hair-Growth Frauds

Hundreds of bogus baldness products have been marketed by mail and through health-food stores, beauty salons, barber shops, and department stores. Most include vitamin combinations said to provide the nutrients needed to nourish the hair. Although severe malnutrition can result in hair loss, there is no evidence that dietary supplements will increase hair growth for anyone who is eating normally. Since the hair shaft is dead tissue, no product can make it healthier or faster-growing by "feeding" it.

Some entrepreneurs have claimed that scalp massage and heat treatments can stimulate hair growth by increasing circulation of the scalp. Aldhizer[34] and others have noted out that this claim is readily refuted by the fact that bald scalps do not lack adequate circulation; they bleed readily when cut and can sustain transplanted hair.

The following cases illustrate government action against bogus hair products.

In 1983, to settle charges by the FTC, Braswell, Inc., and its president, A. Glenn Braswell, agreed to pay $610,000 in civil penalties and to stop claiming that any product or service could cure or prevent hereditary baldness. Braswell was also convicted of mail fraud and perjury and served a brief prison sentence. The mail-fraud charges involved the faking of "before-and-after" photographs for ads for bust-developer, hair-growth, and cosmetic products. Evidence indicated that Braswell had received over $2 million for a worthless baldness cure in one 6-month period.[35]

In 1989, in response to action by the Pennsylvania Department of Health, General Nutrition Corporation agreed to stop marketing a "Helsinki Formula" hair treatment. The product, which included a shampoo, a conditioner, and a vitamin tablet, had been marketed with false claims that it was a proven treatment for thinning hair and that the vitamin supplement contained "those special nutrients that have been proven helpful in an overall hair-care regimen."[36] Two other companies selling bogus hair-growth products through infomercials were sued in civil court by the manufacturer of *Rogaine*.[37]

In 1991 the FTC ordered a California manufacturer to pay $2 million plus court costs for falsely and deceptively claiming that "New Generation" products prevent baldness and stimulate hair growth in those with male-pattern baldness.[38] The products included shampoos and cleanser/conditioners, one of which contained polysorbate 60 in a formula allegedly developed and tested at the University of Helsinki.

In 1994, General Nutrition, Inc., agreed to pay a $2.4 million penalty in an FTC case that included false claims for hair-loss products that contained biotin.[39]

In 1995, Nature's Bounty, of Bohemia, New York, settled FTC charges that it was making deceptive claims for weight-loss, body-building, disease-treatment, or other health-related claims for 26 nutrient supplements it marketed. The company agreed to pay $250,000 and to stop making unsubstantiated claims. The prohibited claims included (a) the amino acid L-cysteine promotes hair growth and (b) the amino acid L-methionine prevents premature hair loss.[40]

SUN PROTECTION

The sun emits several types of radiation. The two that consumers should be concerned about are ultraviolet B (UVB) and ultraviolet A (UVA). UVB is the most active radiation wavelength for producing both sunburn and skin cancer. Its greatest intensity occurs from late morning to early afternoon. UVA penetrates the skin more deeply. It speeds up skin aging by causing changes in the skin's collagen, the protein in its connective tissue. This effect is most noticeable in people, such as farmers and fishermen, who work long hours outside. UVA rays may also cause changes in the eyes that lead to cataracts. The intensity of UVA is relatively constant throughout the day. Most people get about half of their lifetime sun exposure by the age of 18. DeSimone states that an apt warning is "fry now, pay later."[41]

When the skin is exposed to ultraviolet radiation the body responds by producing melanin, a dark pigment that provides some protection against sunburn. A "base tan" is equivalent to an SPF (sun protection factor) of 2 or 3. The darker a person's skin, the more melanin and natural protection it has. However, even the darkest-skinned people can burn when sufficiently exposed to the sun, and melanin is not completely protective against skin cancer. Skin does not have to be burned to develop cancer. Damage also accumulates from everyday exposure.

Skin cancers are most common among fair-skinned (lightly pigmented) people. There are three main types of skin cancer:

BASAL CELL CARCINOMAS: These usually appear on the face, ears, or scalp as pale, waxlike, pearly nodules. They do not metastasize (spread through the body) but if untreated can harm surrounding tissues.

SQUAMOUS CELL CARCINOMAS: These appear as red, scaly, sharply outlined patches. If untreated, they can metastasize.

MELANOMAS: These typically start as a molelike growth that increases in size and darkness. They metastasize early and are highly malignant.

More than 95% of basal and squamous carcinomas are easy to cure when detected early. About 1.3 million cases are diagnosed annually. The American Cancer Society[42] estimates that in 2001 about 51,400 new cases of melanoma of the skin will be diagnosed and about 7800 people will die from the disease.

Sunscreen products help absorb, block, or scatter UVB radiation. They are used primarily to prevent sunburn but can also help people tan without burning. The products are available as lotions, creams, gels, oils, alcohol solutions, and wax substances for lips. Their potency is expressed by the letters "SPF" and a number that follows. The higher the number, the greater the protection.

SPF 15 products permit sun exposure for a few hours with no tan or burn. The product should be applied 15 to 30 minutes before sun exposure begins. The FDA recommends that the product be applied liberally, using about an ounce for an average-size person. Since some sunscreens can irritate the skin, it may be prudent to test for this by applying a small amount to the inside of the upper arm one day before exposure to the sun is planned. In 1998 *Consumer Reports* tested 25 products labeled SPF 15 or 30 and found that all but two provided the amount of designated protection. It also found that an "SPF 50" product tested about 41 and an "SPF 45" product scored only 33.[43]

The American Academy of Dermatology[44] recommends using a broad-spectrum sunscreen that is SPF 15 or higher and applying it every two hours. "Broad spectrum" refers to the ability to block UVA as well as UVB. *Consumer Reports* found that all of the SPF 30 products and a few of the SPF 15 products provided excellent UVA blockage. However, it is not known whether UVA blockage prevents skin cancer.

Since 1994 the National Weather Service has issued daily forecasts of the intensity of ultraviolet light expected the next day in about 60 cities. The *UV index* is based on the sun's position, cloud movements, altitude, ozone, and other factors. It is expressed as minimal (0–2), low (3–4), moderate (5–6), high (7–8), and very high (10–15). The higher the number, the more important it is to take protective measures such as wearing tightly woven clothing and a broad-brimmed hat, using sunglasses, or avoiding the sun altogether. About 80% of ultraviolet radiation can pass through clouds, so the fact that it is cloudy may not protect people.

Tanning Devices

Tanning at a salon or using a home tanning device is no safer than tanning in the sun. FDA regulations require that sunlamp products have a warning label, an accurate timer, and an emergency stop control and that they include an exposure schedule and protective eyewear. Although the FDA permits tanning beds to be marketed, it advises that they be completely avoided.[45]

Spencer and Amonette[46] state that the indoor tanning industry is a billion-dollar-a-year industry. After reviewing 118 studies on skin damage and indoor tanning they concluded that tanning lamps can deliver two or three times the dose of UVA found in outdoor sunlight. They also noted that increasing numbers of melanomas are turning up in people under age 40 who have used indoor tanning machines. Investigators have found that high percentages of tanning-parlor operators tell their patrons that they cannot burn or develop skin cancer as a result of using their device.[47]

FDA scientists have concluded that people who use sunlamps about 100 times a year may be increasing their exposure to "melanoma-inducing" radiation by up to 24 times the amount they would receive from sun exposure. (The amount would depend on the type of lamp used and whether sunscreen is used regularly.)[48]

Tanning Accelerators

The cosmetic industry has marketed "tan accelerator" creams claimed to stimulate faster and deeper tans. Tyrosine, the major ingredient, is naturally present in the skin's cells and is needed for melanin production. The companies claim that the tyrosine causes more melanin to form and that tanning therefore results. Skepticism is warranted because Jaworsky and others[49] studied two brands of tanning accelerators in 18 volunteers and found no augmentation of tanning.

Tanning Pills and Lotions

Some "tanning pills" do not provide a tan but dye the skin orange or yellow by coloring the fat cells under the skin's outer layer. The pills contain a food-coloring agent in doses much higher than the amount consumed in the normal diet. The skin color fades when the pills are no longer taken. One ingredient is beta-carotene, which is found naturally in many foods and is permitted as a color additive in foods and drugs. Another ingredient is canthaxanthin, a fat-soluble carotenoid that the human body cannot convert to vitamin A.

Canthaxanthin is legal to use as a food-coloring agent. Despite a warning by the FDA, it has been illegally sold in tanning parlors and by mail as a tablet for skin tanning under such names as *Orobronze, Darker Tan, French Bronze,* and *BronzGlo*. Ads for *Darker Tan* promised "a rich dark bronze glowing tan without risking skin cancer." A case has been reported of a 20-year-old woman who took high doses and developed aplastic anemia, a serious condition in which the production of blood cells is impaired. Previous reports have linked canthaxanthin use to hepatitis, generalized itching, hives, and eye problems.[50]

Two other types of "tanning" products are legally marketable as cosmetics. Bronzers, made from color additives, stain the skin but can be washed off with soap and water. Bronzers may produce different shades in different areas of the body. Extenders, when applied to the skin, interact with a surface protein to produce color that tends to wash off after a few days. The only color additive approved for extenders is dihydroxyacetone. Although they give the skin a golden color, these products offer no sunscreen protection.

COSMETIC SURGERY

The term "plastic surgery" refers to the repair or remodeling of injured or defective body parts. The terms "cosmetic surgery" and "aesthetic surgery" refer to reshaping or remodeling of otherwise normal body features to improve a person's appearance. The term "reconstructive surgery" means restoration of an injured, congenitally absent, or abnormal body feature. More than 4000 physicians specialize in plastic and reconstructive surgery. Otolaryngologists, ophthalmologists, dermatologists, and general surgeons perform some plastic surgical procedures in the areas of the body within their scope.

The cosmetic procedures done by plastic and reconstructive surgeons include breast augmentations, eyelid surgery, face lifts, nose reshaping, liposuction, and about 20 other cosmetic procedures. Some ophthalmologists perform eyelid tucks. The procedures done by dermatologists include hair transplants, dermabrasion, chemical peeling, laser procedures (to remove birthmarks, age spots, freckles, unwanted tattoos, and other types of blemishes[51]), soft-tissue augmentation (to correct wrinkles and scars), and sclerotherapy (injection of a solution that will remove unwanted small veins near the skin's surface). Most of the plastic surgery done by otolaryngologists is reconstructive.

Table 20-2 describes the purpose, cost, side effects, risks, and duration of the results of 10 procedures that plastic surgeons commonly perform. The cost of cosmetic surgery is not covered by most insurance policies and is not tax-deductible for federal income tax purposes.

Choosing a Plastic Surgeon

The best choice for cosmetic surgery is a physician who has had special training in plastic surgery, has been certified by an appropriate specialty board, and has staff privileges at an accredited hospital. The American Board of Plastic Surgery (ABPS) requires at least 3 years of postgraduate training in surgery (or its equivalent), 2 years of postgraduate training in plastic surgery, 2 more years of experience, and passage of written and oral examinations. The American Board of Dermatology and the American Board of Ophthalmology do not offer subspecialty certification in plastic surgery. Information about the relevant training and experience of dermatologists or ophthalmologists can be obtained by contacting their offices.

The American Society of Plastic Surgeons (ASPS) represents 97% of ABPS-certified surgeons. Its Web site (http://www.plasticsurgery.org) maintains a directory of its members and the procedures they do. The certification status of other types of doctors is available from the American Board of Medical Specialties Web site.

Hospital privileges can be verified by contacting the hospital. Other sources are primary-care physicians, operating room nurses, local hospital referral services, and individuals who have had satisfactory surgery. Flamboyant advertising is not a favorable sign.

Once names have been gathered, you might want to visit two or three surgeons for an initial consultation. That way you can compare their personalities, their opinions on the type of surgery you should have, their fees, and the way they answer your questions about the likely results and the risks. You can also ask how often the doctor has performed the procedure you are considering. Some doctors have photographs of their patients before and after surgery. Even if the surgeon would like to do a contemplated procedure on an outpatient basis, it would be prudent to check whether the physician has been approved for performing that procedure at the hospital. The FTC advises consumers to be wary of physicians who suggest "fixing" a feature that does not bother you, use a hard sell to obtain your business, or brush aside your concerns about safety.[52]

Breast Implants

Since the early 1960s more than 2 million American women have had implant surgery to increase the size of their breasts or to reconstruct a breast after breast-cancer surgery. Until 1992 most of the implants were filled with silicone, and about 10% contained saline (salt water). Silicone was generally preferred because it gives the breast a more natural look and feel. (Silicone implants differ from silicone injections, which enable the liquid silicone to spread to the surrounding tissues.)

In 1992, after receiving many thousands of reports of adverse reactions, the FDA banned the use of silicone-filled implants except for reconstructive breast surgery and certain medical conditions—provided that the patient is enrolled in a clinical study. Women who wanted silicone-gel implants for breast augmentation were not eligible for enrollment.[53] In 1993 the AMA Council on Scientific Affairs agreed that more data should be obtained but felt that silicone-gel implants should remain available for augmentation procedures as long as the results are properly monitored.[54] FDA Commissioner David A. Kessler, M.D., J.D., responded that the FDA was required to uphold the law that devices be proven safe before marketing.[55]

The risks of implant surgery include hardening of the breast caused by scar-tissue formation; leakage or rupture of the implant; temporary or permanent loss of sensation in the nipple or breast tissue; pain caused by calcium deposits; shifting of the implant; and interfer-

Table 20-2

Purposes, Risks, and 1999 Fees of Selected Cosmetic Surgical Procedures

Procedure and Average Fee*	Purpose/Description	Side Effects/Risks	Duration
Abdominoplasty (tummy tuck) $4198	Flatten abdomen by removing excess fat and skin and tightening muscles	Temporary discomfort; blood clots, infection, conspicuous scarring	Permanent
Breast enlargement $2984	Enhance size and shape of breast using artificial implants	Temporary swelling and discomfort; infection; asymmetry; hardening of scar tissue around implant; rupture of implant; change in sensitivity of nipples or breast skin	Variable; implants may require removal or replacement
Breast lift $3735	Raise and reshape sagging breasts by removing excess skin and repositioning remaining tissue and nipples	Temporary swelling and discomfort; thick, wide scars; infection; permanent loss of feeling in nipples or breast	Variable; new sagging may occur; results may last longer if combined with implants
Chemical peel Regional $760 Full face $1271	Restore wrinkled, blemished, unevenly pigmented, or sun-damaged facial skin using a chemical solution to peel away skin's top layers	Temporary swelling and discomfort; tiny whiteheads, infection, scarring	Permanent if phenol is used; variable with trichloroacetic acid
Collagen injections $302/cc	Plump up creased, furrowed, or sunken facial skin; add fullness to lips and backs of hands	Temporary discomfort; allergic reactions, contour irregularities	A few months to 1 year
Dermabrasion $1755	Mechanical scraping of outer skin layers using a high-speed rotary wheel; lessens surface irregularities from acne, other scars, and fine wrinkles	Temporary swelling and discomfort; abnormal permanent color changes	Permanent, although new wrinkles may form as skin ages
Eyelid surgery $3030	Correct drooping upper eyelids and puffy bags below the eyes	Temporary swelling and discomfort; temporary blurred vision	Several years; sometimes permanent
Facelift $4956	Improve sagging facial skin, jowls, and loose neck skin by removing excess fat, tightening muscles, and redraping skin	Temporary swelling and discomfort; injury to nerves that control facial muscles and feeling; infection, scarring, asymmetry	Usually 5 to 10 years
Fat injection $951-$1064	Fat extracted from the patient's abdomen, thighs, buttocks, or elsewhere is reinjected into the skin beneath the face	Temporary swelling or puffiness; rare instances of infection	Effect usually is halved in 3-6 months but may persist for 1 year or longer
Liposuction $1923	Reshape parts of body using tube and vacuum device to remove unwanted fat deposits that don't respond to dieting and exercise	Temporary swelling and discomfort; infection, bagginess of skin, pigmentation changes	Permanent if person does not regain weight
Rhinoplasty Open $3573 Closed $3360	Reshape nose by reducing or increasing size, removing bump, narrowing span of nostrils, or changing angle between nose and upper lip	Temporary swelling and discomfort; infection; small burst blood vessels resulting in tiny but permanant red spots; incomplete improvement requiring additional surgery	Permanent
Sclerotherapy n/a	Lighten or shrink small superficial veins by injecting sclerosing material	Rare occurrence of blood clots in the veins, severe inflammation, allergy to the solution, scarring	Vein obliteration is permanent, but new veins may emerge

*Fees do not include the costs of anesthesia, operating room facilities, or other related expenses. The averages are based on a survey of members of the American Society of Plastic Surgeons.[56] The cost of sclerotherapy depends on the area involved and the number of sessions required.

Historical Perspective

Silicone Injections

In the 1960s many women underwent breast augmentation in which liquid silicone was injected into their breasts. However, the initial enthusiasm for this operation cooled quickly as reports of serious and sometimes fatal complications poured in. These included swelling; discoloration; cyst formation; and migration of silicone particles to the brain, lungs, or heart. During the 1970s silicone injections of the face underwent a similar surge of popularity until serious complications became apparent.[57]

In 1974 the *San Francisco Chronicle* reported that silicone injections were available in Mexico for $800 for a series of injections plus the use of plastic molds to reshape the breasts. During the previous 7 years, surgeons in the San Diego area had treated nearly 400 women suffering from mutilated breasts and infections that were traced to silicone injections by Mexican physicians in border cities. About 20% of the women required amputation of both breasts because of the extreme damage.[58]

The FDA banned the use of medical silicone for cosmetic purposes, but clandestine use has continued in the United States, and silicone injections can still be obtained in many other parts of the world from both licensed and unlicensed practitioners. The reported complications include 20 cases of severe pneumonia subsequent to injections of the breasts[59,60] and five cases of severe problems following injections of the penis done to enlarge the penis or to treat impotence.[61]

ence with the ability to detect cancer through mammography. Breast implants last for many years in some women, whereas in others frequent replacement seems necessary.[62]

Saline-filled implants remain freely available. The FDA considers these less risky because, although they have the same silicone rubber envelope as gel-filled implants, leakage or rupture would release only salt water, not silicone gel, into the tissues. However, the frequency of rupture is far from clear. In 1995 Commissioner Kessler informed a congressional subcommittee that published studies had reported rates from 5% to 51%, but the size of this range indicated that the real rupture rate was unknown. The FDA then established protocols for clinical studies to study the safety of both silicone and saline implants, and thousands of women enrolled. Further information on this subject is available from the FDA's consumer information hotline at (800) 532-4440.

In 1994 Mayo Clinic researchers reported on a study that compared 749 women who had had implants and 1498 who had not. The women were followed for an average of about eight years. The researchers found no association between silicone implants and the incidence of 12 types of connective tissue diseases.[63] In 1995 the *New England Journal of Medicine* reported on a study of 87,501 nurses who had been followed for other research purposes from 1976 through the middle of 1990, when there were widespread media reports of a possible association between breast implants and connective tissue disease. The study found no relationship between the two.[64] Another large study concluded that a small association may exist, but a large one does not.[65]

A few laboratories offer to detect the levels of antibodies to silicone alleged to indicate that an implant is ruptured or leaking. FDA officials have warned (a) such tests lack FDA approval; (b) neither the existence nor the significance of "silicone antibodies" has been established; (c) since small amounts of silicone "bleed" from intact implants, tests can not tell whether an implant has ruptured; (d) even if silicone is detectable, the source could be a commonly used medication or cosmetic; and (e) diseases are defined by their signs and symptoms, not by the mere presence of antibodies. An FDA official stated that the tests cost $500 to $1000 and that "a lot of them are being done for litigation purposes rather than to help the patient medically."[66,67] In 1994 the FDA ordered a company called Structural Biologicals to stop marketing its *Detectsil* test.

In 1999, the Institute of Medicine concluded that no association existed between silicone gel implants and cancer, immunologic disease, or other systemic diseases. They also reported that implants pose no risk for breast-feeding or to unborn infants.[68]

Scientists affiliated with the American Council on Science and Health (ACSH) have concluded that silicone breast implants do not increase the risk of developing breast cancer, other cancers, or any immune or neurologic disease. ACSH believes that the controversy has been fueled by irresponsible media reports and sustained by unfounded product-liability lawsuits.[69]

Penile Enlargement (Phalloplasty)

In 1996 *The Wall Street Journal*[70] reported that 20 to 30 surgeons were performing large numbers of operations purported to enlarge the penis permanently. About half of these surgeons were located in Southern California. The operation is done by cutting an internal attachment of the penis to the pubic bone, which causes more of the organ to protrude. Fatty tissue injections and grafts have been used to enlarge penile girth. The American

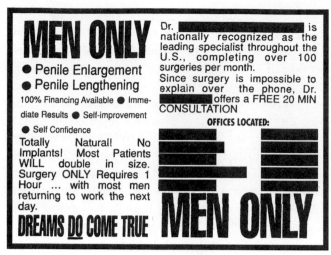

FIGURE 20-2. Ad for dubious penile surgery, 1994.

Urological Association states that these procedures have not been proven safe or effective.

Figure 20-2 shows an advertisement that offered a "free 20-minute consultation" for penis surgery. In January 1994, after spotting the ad, Dr. William M. London posed as a prospective patient. The "consultation" was performed by the surgeon's stepson, who had had no medical training. The stepson said that the lengthening procedure usually added 2 to 2.75 inches and had no health risks except "minor infections at the area worked on." London also noted that no attempt was made to explore whether it was sensible for him to have the operation. The *Wall Street Journal*'s report stated (a) the doctor had performed 6 to 14 operations a day and had grossed $7.4 million during the first 6 months of 1994 and (b) more than 50 malpractice suits had been filed against him by patients who said they had suffered great pain, been disfigured, been rendered impotent, or had other serious complications. Charged with unprofessional conduct, the doctor permanently surrendered his medical license in 1996. Payments in the malpractice suits exceeded $6 million.

LASER PHOTOTHERAPY

PhotoDerm®VL delivers very brief bursts of pulsed light to remove vascular birthmarks, spider veins on the legs and face, and other vascular conditions. Treatment is applied by placing a hand-held treatment unit on the patient's skin. Usually four to six treatments are required. The light coagulates the small blood vessels, which are sealed off and gradually fade away. There may be slight reddening or local swelling for a few days. Other temporary side effects, which are rare, include blistering, burning, or changes in skin color.

CAMOUFLAGE COSMETICS

Corrective cosmetics offer an alternative to surgery for the correction of various blemishes. They can be used to conceal birthmarks, broken capillaries, dark circles under the eyes, abnormal pigmentation, cleft lip deformities, varicose veins, stretch marks, scars, and other blemishes. They are also used to conceal bruising and other temporary after-effects of surgery. Concealers have an opaque foundation that makes them more effective than ordinary cosmetics for masking scars and other imperfections of the skin. Color correctors can be used to disguise discolored areas. Contouring products can be used to disguise swollen areas. Corrective cosmetics are waterproof and smudgeless and can adhere longer to the skin than ordinary cosmetics. However, they should be removed at night. The American Society of Plastic and Reconstructive Surgeons recommends that removal be done with a cleansing cream, followed by alcohol-free toner applied with a cotton ball, followed by application of a moisturizer.[71]

SUMMARY

Consumers spend over $30 billion yearly on skin care and beauty aids that may help their appearance but will not perform miracles. Much of this expense occurs

---

It's Your Decision

Suppose you are dissatisfied with your appearance and think it may hamper your social success. Check which of the following actions you would take.

Reason

☐ Discuss the situation with a friend   _____
☐ Discuss the situation with a parent   _____
☐ Consult your family doctor or a student health physician   _____
☐ Consult a professional who counsels people about their appearance _____
☐ Consult a dermatologist or plastic surgeon   _____
☐ Other (specify) _____   _____

because our youth-oriented culture prods people to try to look younger. For cosmetic products, price is generally not a reliable indicator of quality.

Soaps and various cosmetic products can help keep the skin clean, moist, and soft. But no cosmetic can eliminate wrinkles, repair sun-damaged skin, or retard or reverse the aging process of the skin. Mild cases of acne can be improved through hygienic practices and generally can be treated with OTC products. Severe conditions should have professional assistance.

The three most important things you can do for your skin are (1) keep it clean, (2) protect it from the sun, and (3) don't smoke cigarettes.

Cosmetic surgery can improve many people's appearance. Consumers contemplating cosmetic surgery should investigate thoroughly to determine the potential benefits, the risks, and the surgeon's credentials.

REFERENCES

1. Wolf N: The Beauty Myth. New York, 1991, William Morrow.
2. Begoun P. Don't Go to the Cosmetics Counter Without Me: An Eye Opening Guide to Brand Name Cosmetics, ed 2. Seattle, 1994, Beginning Press.
3. Cosmetics & skin care products. Schaumburg, Ill., 1994, American Academy of Dermatology.
4. Stehlin D. Cosmetic safety: More complex than at first blush. FDA Consumer 25(9):18–23, 1991.
5. Foulke JE. Decoding the cosmetic label. FDA Consumer 28(4):20–23, 1994.
6. Can soaps do more than clean? Consumer Reports 61:730–733, 1995.
7. The skin game. Radiant? Refined? Forget the claims. Here's the latest on which products moisturize best. Consumer Reports 65(1):38–41, 2000.
8. Moisturizers. Consumer Reports 59:577–581, 1994.
9. Smith JB, Fenske NA. Cutaneous manifestations and consequences of smoking. Journal of the American Academy of Dermatology 34:717–732, 1996.
10. Kadunce DP and others. Cigarette smoking: Risk factor for premature facial wrinkling. Annals of Internal Medicine 114:840–844, 1991.
11. Winter R. Do antiaging creams really work? Consumers Digest 33(4):61–64, 1994.
12. Antiaging creams challenged, FDA Talk Paper, May 14, 1987.
13. Foulke JE. Cosmetic ingredients: Understanding the puffery. FDA Consumer 26(4):11–14, 1992.
14. Fisher AA. Cosmetic warning: this product may be detrimental to your purse. Cutis 39:23–24, 1987.
15. Kurtzweil P. Alpha hydroxy acids for skin care. Smooth sailing or rough seas? FDA Consumer 32(2):30–35, 1998.
16. Ortho Renova to be launched in February at $10–$15/month retail; anti-wrinkle agent shows moderate improvement in 24% of patients treated at 24 weeks. F-D-C Reports Jan 8, 1996, pp 4–5.
17. Renova: Wrinkle cream or skin game? Consumer Reports on Health 8:62, 1996.
18. Fade creams. Consumer Reports 50:12, 1985.
19. Buying guide: Antiperspirants and deodorants. University of California at Berkeley Wellness Letter 2(7):3, 1986.
20. Kligman AM. Acne vulgaris: Tricks and treatments. Part II: The benzoyl peroxide saga. Cutis 56:260–261, 1995.
21. Begoun P. Don't Go Shopping for Hair Care Products Without Me. Seattle, Wash., 1995, Beginning Press.
22. Shampoos: Head games are a lot of lather. Consumer Reports 65:18–23, 2000.
23. Mayfield E. Psoriasis treatments: Relieving that terrible itch. FDA Consumer 29(3):12–15, 1995.
24. Hingley AT. Controlling dandruff. FDA Consumer 28(8):25–27, 1994.
25. Segal M. Hair today, gone tomorrow. FDA Consumer 30(7):21–24, 1996.
26. Topical minoxidil for baldness: A reappraisal. The Medical Letter 36:9–10, 1994.
27. FDA approves Rogaine for OTC marketing. FDA Talk Paper T96–9, Feb 12, 1996.
28. Whiting DA. Hair disorders. In Rakel RE. Conn's Current Therapy. Philadelphia, 1995, W.B. Saunders Co.
29. Propecia and Rogaine Extra Strength for alopecia. The Medical Letter 40:25–27, 1998.
30. FDA. Federal Register, Aug 1, 1991.
31. Cosmetic plastic surgery: Procedures at a glance. Arlington Heights, Ill., 1993, American College of Surgeons.
32. Berland T. Baldness 'cures': Does anything really work? Consumers Digest 32(4):68–70, 1993.
33. General reconstructive plastic surgery (brochure). Arlington Heights, Ill., 1996, American Society of Plastic Surgeons.
34. Aldhizer TG and others. The Doctor's Book on Hair Loss. Englewood Cliffs, N.J., 1983, Prentice-Hall.
35. Nelson CP. Testimony before the Subcommittee on Health and Long-Term Care of the U.S. House of Representatives Select Committee on Aging. In Pepper C and others. Quackery: A $10 Billion Scandal. Washington, D.C., 1984, U.S. Government Printing Office.
36. Helsinki Hair Formula. Nutrition Forum 6:30, 1989.
37. Companies sued for false hair-growth claims. NCAHF Newsletter 11(6):3, 1988.
38. FTC wins $2 million judgment in "New Generation" baldness remedy case. Judge also halts sale of products. FTC news release, Sept 10, 1991.
39. General Nutrition Inc. agrees to pay $2.4 million civil penalty to settle charges it violated two previous FTC orders. FTC news release, April 28, 1994.
40. Nature's Bounty to pay $250,000 redress as part of settlement with FTC over nutrient supplement claims. FTC news release, April 27, 1995.
41. DeSimone EM II. Sunscreen and suntan products. In Handbook of Nonprescription Drugs, ed 10. Washington, D.C., 1993, American Pharmaceutical Association.
42. Cancer Facts & Figures, 2001. Atlanta, 2001, American Cancer Society.
43. A spectrum of sun protection: We tested lotions, moisturizers and clothing. Consumer Reports 63(5):20–23, 1998.
44. Ultraviolet index. Schaumburg, Ill., 1996, American Academy of Dermatology.
45. Strange CJ. Thwarting skin cancer with sun sense. FDA Consumer 29(6):10–14, 1995.
46. Spencer JM, Amonette RA. Indoor tanning: Risks, benefits, and future trends. Journal of the International Academy of Dermatology 33:288–298, 1995.

47. Kahn J. Tanning salons do not provide a 'safer tan.' Emerging body of evidence suggests UVA radiation causes long-term damage to skin. Medical Tribune, Aug 24, 1995, p 12.

48. Kurzweil P. Seven steps to safer sunning. FDA Consumer 30(5):6–11, 1996.

49. Jaworsky C and others. Efficacy of tan accelerators. Journal of the American Academy of Dermatology 16:769–771, 1987.

50. Bluhm R and others. Aplastic anemia associated with canthaxanthin ingested for 'tanning purposes.' JAMA 264:1141–1142, 1990.

51. Arndt KA, Thomas P. Laser resurfacing slows the hands of time. Harvard Health Letter 21(1):4–5, 1996.

52. Cosmetic surgery. Washington, D.C., 1990, FTC Bureau of Consumer Protection.

53. Breast Implants: An information update. Rockville, Md., 1996, Food and Drug Administration.

54. AMA Council on Scientific Affairs. Silicone gel breast implants. JAMA 270:2602–2606, 1993.

55. Kessler DA and others. A call for higher standards for breast implants. JAMA 270:2606–2608, 1993.

56. 1999 Plastic surgery statistics. Arlington Heights, Ill., 2000, American Society of Plastic Surgeons.

57. Klevan P. New face lift not all smiles. FDA Consumer 13(2):15, 1979.

58. Tijuana silicone rot. San Francisco Chronicle, Aug 16, 1974.

59. Lai YF and others. Acute pneumonitis after subcutaneous injections of silicone for augmentation mammoplasty. Chest 106(4):1152–1155, 1994.

60. Chastre J and others. Acute and latent pneumonitis after subcutaneous injections of silicone in transsexual men. American Review of Respiratory Disease 135(1):236–240, 1987.

61. Wassermann RJ, Greenwald DP. Debilitating silicone granuloma of the penis and scrotum. Annals of Plastic Surgery 35(5):505–510, 1995.

62. Breast implants: An information update. FDA Center for Devices and Radiologic Health, Aug 22, 2000.

63. Gabriel SE and others. Risk of connective-tissue diseases and other disorders after breast implantation. New England Journal of Medicine 330:1697–1702, 1994.

64. Sanchez-Guerrero J and others. Silicone breast implants and the risk of connective-tissue diseases and symptoms. New England Journal of Medicine 332(25):1666–1701,1995.

65. Hennekens CH and others. Self-reported breast implants and connective-tissue diseases in female health professionals. A retrospective cohort study. JAMA 275:616–621, 1996.

66. Segal M. Silicone breast implants: Available under tight controls. In Current Issues in Women's Health, ed 2. DHSS Publication no. (FDA)94-1181, pp 76–79, 1994.

67. Segal M. A status report on breast implant safety. FDA Consumer 29(9):11–16, 1995.

68. Institute of Medicine. Safety of Silicone Breast Implants. Washington, D.C., 1999, National Academy Press.

69. Rohrich RJ, Muzaffar AR. Silicone gel breast implants: Health and regulatory update 2000. New York, 2000, American Council on Science and Health.

70. Growth industry: How a risky surgery became a profit center for some L.A. doctors. The Wall Street Journal, Jun 6, 1996, pp A1, A8.

71. Camouflage techniques. Arlington Heights, Ill., 1992, American Society of Plastic Surgeons.

Chapter Twenty-One

ESPECIALLY FOR WOMEN

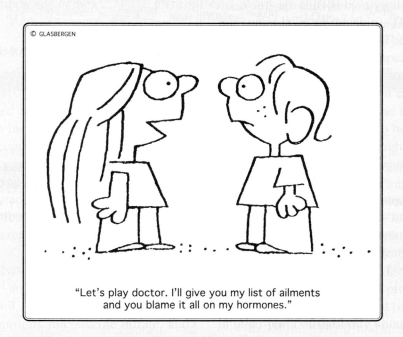

"Let's play doctor. I'll give you my list of ailments and you blame it all on my hormones."

© GLASBERGEN

One need spend only a day in a women's clinic or hospital emergency room to appreciate the difficulties that can visit the female reproductive system when women are not educated to be vigilant in self-protection.

SADJA GOLDSMITH GREENWOOD, M.D.[1]
UNIVERSITY OF CALIFORNIA MEDICAL CENTER
SAN FRANCISCO

Think of your bones as a retirement account: They're where you stash calcium when you're young, so you'll have enough to last through old age.

CONSUMER REPORTS[2]

Key Concepts

KEEP THESE POINTS IN MIND AS YOU STUDY THIS CHAPTER

- People who wish to use contraception should consider effectiveness, convenience, safety, protection against sexually transmitted diseases (STDs), and personal and partner preferences.

- Prenatal care that includes sensible eating, regular exercise, screening examinations, and childbirth can greatly benefit both mother and child.

- Osteoporosis is a serious but largely preventable condition. Women should take preventive measures throughout adulthood.

- For most postmenopausal women the potential benefits of hormone-replacement therapy far outweigh the risks.

Women face a variety of health concerns related to the anatomy and physiology of their reproductive organs. This chapter discusses feminine hygiene, menstrual discomfort, vaginitis, and contraception (including the methods used by men). Information is also provided about hormone-replacement therapy, osteoporosis, pregnancy testing, infertility services, prenatal care, birthing and delivery options, and mastectomy prostheses.

MENSTRUAL PRODUCTS

Menstruation takes place approximately once a month as the uterus sheds the vascular lining it has prepared in response to the woman's hormones. The debris exits through the vagina over several days. Most women use tampons to dispose of the menstrual fluids. Sanitary napkins and reusable sponges are other options.

An effective tampon is absorbent enough to protect against leaks, but not so absorbent that it dries out the delicate vaginal tissues. It should also be easy to insert, comfortable to wear, and easy to remove. It may help to use a more absorbent one when menstrual flow is heavy and a less absorbent one when flow is light. Using a highly absorbent tampon when flow is light may result in excess absorption of natural vaginal lubrication.

Excessive drying of the vaginal tissue can render a woman susceptible to toxic shock syndrome (TSS), a rare but potentially fatal infection caused by staphylococcus bacteria. TSS is characterized by high fever, vomiting, diarrhea, sunburnlike rash, liver or kidney failure, and a rapid blood pressure drop that can cause shock. In 1989 the FDA ordered manufacturers to standardize tampon labeling so that "junior," "regular," "super," and "super plus" means the same thing regardless of a manufacturer's brand. Packages now must explain the basis for the rating and advise on choosing the lowest appropriate absorbency.[3] A 1994 study by *Consumer Reports* found that most tampons absorbed amounts within their labeled range.[4]

MENSTRUAL PROBLEMS

Many women who menstruate experience significant symptoms before or during their monthly periods. Symptoms fall into three general categories: dysmenorrhea (painful menstruation), premenstrual syndrome (PMS), and menstrual irregularities.

Dysmenorrhea

Dysmenorrhea is typically experienced as cramplike lower abdominal discomfort that may come and go in waves. There may also be dull lower backache and, in some women, nausea and vomiting. These symptoms begin shortly before the onset of menstrual flow and

---

 Consumer Tip

The following measures can help prevent toxic shock syndrome:

- Wash hands with soap and water before and after inserting or removing a tampon. Use care to avoid carrying bacteria from the skin or rectum into the vagina.
- Choose the lowest absorbency product that is effective.
- Do not use a plastic applicator that may be more likely to scratch the vagina. Cardboard applicators tend to be gentler. On days when secretions in the vagina are scanty, use a water-soluble lubricating jelly on the tampon applicator to avoid nicking the vaginal surface.
- Change tampons often—at least as frequently as every 6 to 8 hours.
- Alternate tampon use with pads during a given menstrual period. Do not use a tampon on days when bleeding is light.
- If symptoms of high fever (102.7° F or higher), vomiting, diarrhea, or sunburnlike rash occur, discontinue tampon use and immediately consult a physician.

usually last 2 or 3 days. A small percentage of women have symptoms severe enough to interfere with their usual activities.

Dysmenorrhea may be primary or secondary. Primary dysmenorrhea, by far the more common type, begins during the first year or two after the onset of menstruation, usually lasts only a few years, and is dramatically relieved after childbirth. Self treatment with a nonprescription pain reliever may be effective when started the day before a menstrual period. (See Chapter 19 for dosage information.)

Primary dysmenorrhea does not usually require consultation with a physician unless symptoms are severe and do not respond to self-treatment. The prescribed drugs fall into two categories: (1) nonsteroidal anti-inflammatory drugs (NSAIDs) such as naproxen and mefenamic acid *(Ponstel)* and (2) oral contraceptives, particularly for women who also want contraceptive protection.

Secondary dysmenorrhea refers to menstrual pain that develops in women who previously had little or no cramping with their periods. It is usually associated with some type of abnormality of the reproductive organs such as a benign uterine tumor (polyp or fibroid), a pelvic infection, or endometriosis. It can also be caused by an intrauterine device (IUD) used for contraception. A physician should be consulted in all cases of secondary dysmenorrhea to determine the presence of any underlying disease that requires treatment. In most cases of secondary dysmenorrhea, treatment by a physician is more effective than self-treatment.

Premenstrual Syndrome

Premenstrual syndrome (PMS; also called premenstrual tension) is a combination of physical and/or emotional symptoms that occur a week or two before menstruation and disappear or become minimal during periods. PMS is said to be very common, but estimates of its incidence are clouded by lack of a precise definition. The symptoms vary from person to person, but are usually consistent for each individual; they include tension, depression, irritability, fatigue, difficulty concentrating, crying spells, aggression, headaches, abdominal bloating, swelling of the hands and feet, breast tenderness, constipation, acne, abnormal thirst, and cravings for sweets and/or salty foods. Usually relief occurs when the menstrual period begins. In contrast to dysmenorrhea, PMS usually starts during the late 20s or 30s and worsens with age and after childbearing. When symptoms include depression and are severe enough to interfere with occupational and social functioning, the con-

dition is called premenstrual dysphoric disorder (PMDD).

Most women with PMS do not need treatment by a physician. Only symptoms that disrupt their life need medical intervention. Understanding what occurs in the body when symptoms are present often provides significant relief. The following suggestions may also help:

- For premenstrual water retention (abdominal bloating and swelling of the hands and feet), refrain from adding salt to meals and restrict sodium-containing foods for a few days before the time of the menstrual cycle when the symptoms typically occur. Diuretic drugs may be helpful.
- For symptoms of anxiety, avoid or limit coffee, tea, cocoa, cola, and other foods and medications that contain caffeine or related compounds. Although this may not help, it is harmless and relatively easy to do.[5]
- Try to identify and deal with psychosocial stresses.
- If eating sweets appears to produce symptoms, try to satisfy cravings with complex carbohydrates, such as fruits, rather than simple sugars, which tend to produce greater variability of blood sugar levels.[6]

Over-the-counter (OTC) products for premenstrual discomfort contain one or more of up to four main ingredients: a pain reliever, a diuretic, an antihistamine, and caffeine. OTC diuretic ingredients are weak compared to those available by prescription, but they may alleviate the symptoms of premenstrual tension by helping the body shed water.

Some doctors recommend pyridoxine (vitamin B_6) for PMS. The FDA Advisory Review Panel on OTC Miscellaneous Internal Drug Products concluded that pyridoxine had not been proven effective.[7] Subsequent reports of nervous system toxicity indicate that pyridoxine supplementation is unsafe (see Chapter 12). Other supplementary vitamins were summarily disapproved by the expert panel.

Some studies suggest that the antidepressant drug fluoxetine and other serotonin reuptake inhibitors can be effective against PMS and PMDD.[8] These products are prescription drugs that raise the level of serotonin in the brain. Serotonin is an organic compound involved in the transmission of impulses between nerve cells and in the regulation of cyclic body processes. Fluoxetine is marketed as *Prozac* for depression and *Sarafem* for PMDD. A generic version is expected soon.

PMS Escape, a powdered drink mix that costs $10 for a 5-serving box, is claimed to be "the first clinically tested nutritional product to effectively manage disturbances in mood, appetite and memory associated with premenstrual syndrome." The product is alleged to work by raising the level of serotonin in the brain. However, the *Tufts University Diet & Nutrition Letter* has noted: (a) the "test" involved only 24 patients, which is far too small to evaluate a PMS treatment; (b) the theory that PMS occurs when serotonin levels fall has not been proven; and (c) the researchers did not measure the serotonin levels of the participants in the test.[9]

Menstrual Irregularities

During the first few years of menstruation, irregularity is common and may be related to ovarian dysfunction. The treatment of abnormal uterine bleeding depends on the cause, the woman's age, and her plans regarding pregnancy. Persistent irregularity at any age or excessive bleeding after age 35 are reasons to consult a physician. Bleeding for longer than 7 days is considered excessive and warrants evaluation by a physician. Bleeding that occurs 1 year or more after menstrual periods cease (postmenopausal bleeding) should be evaluated promptly, because it may be a sign of cancer.

Women normally lose 1 to 4 tablespoons of blood during a menstrual period, with a daily iron loss of up to 1.4 mg. This amount of iron can be provided by a sensible diet. Individuals with a heavy blood flow (which may result in clots) should be sure that their iron intake is adequate. This can be accomplished by eating iron-rich foods (e.g., liver, veal, other meats, fish, soybeans), cooking in an iron pot, or using iron supplements. However, self-medication with supplementary iron is unwise unless a deficiency is medically diagnosed with a blood test (see Chapter 19). Even if an individual is iron-deficient, the cause should be established before treatment is begun.

VAGINAL HYGIENE

Under normal circumstances the healthy vagina cleans itself. Like the eyes, nose, and mouth, it is lined with epithelial cells that produce secretions that flush surface debris toward the outside. At the same time, bacteria normally present maintain the normal acidity of the vagina, which discourages the growth of other microorganisms

Douching

Douching consists of forcing water or other fluids into the vagina for "cleansing" purposes. Except for douches prescribed for treating medical problems, douching is unnecessary and may be harmful. Many preparations cause drying of the vaginal tissues and disturb the normal bacteria that help to keep the vagina healthy. Some products contain local anesthetics (e.g., phenol, menthol)

that can mask symptoms of infection. Reusable douching materials carry added dangers. Douching within 3 days before a pelvic examination or Pap smear can interfere with the accuracy of these procedures. Douching should never be done during pregnancy or within 6 weeks after giving birth or having a miscarriage.

The FDA, which once considered douches to be cosmetics, requires that they be labeled: "For cleansing purposes only. Do not use more than twice weekly unless directed by a physician," or "For cleansing purposes only, after menstruation and after marital relations." However, it should be noted that postcoital douching is not an effective contraceptive.

External Hygiene

Vaginal secretions and perspiration can collect on the external surfaces of the vaginal folds, where they can break down and become odorous if allowed to accumulate. This is more likely to happen with the use of pantyhose and nylon panties, which increase the accumulation of perspiration. These garments should be washed after each use in mild, nonperfumed soaps. If pantyhose are used, those with a cotton crotch are less apt to allow the buildup of heat and moisture

Washing the skin of the vulva is all that is needed for adequate hygiene. Care should be taken to avoid getting soap on the delicate tissue at the entrance of the vagina and the urethra (where the urine exits the bladder). So-called feminine deodorant sprays are not necessary and can cause trouble not only for women but also for their sexual partners. Some women who have used these products have experienced infections, irritations, burns, and rashes.[10] Women who decide to use a spray despite these facts should follow the manufacturer's directions carefully. The FDA requires the following label warning:

Caution: For external use only. Spray at least eight inches from skin. Use sparingly and not more than once daily to avoid irritation. Do not use this product with a sanitary napkin. Do not apply to broken, irritated, or itching skin. Persistent or unusual odor may indicate the presence of a condition for which a physician should be consulted. If a rash, irritation, unusual vaginal discharge, or discomfort develops, discontinue use immediately and consult a physician.

VAGINITIS

Vaginitis means inflammation of the vagina. It is often accompanied by vulvitis, an inflammation of the outer tissues of a woman's genital area, in which case the problem is called vulvovaginitis. Most women have vaginitis at some time during their life. The symptoms are vaginal discharge with or without itching, burning, odor, or burning with urination.

The most common causes of vaginitis and vulvitis are chronic irritation by bacteria or yeast (*Candida albicans* and sometimes other species). These microorganisms are normally present in small numbers but are kept in check by the normal bacteria that dominate the vagina (lactobacilli). Anything that disturbs the normal lactobacilli or reduces their numbers can provide the opportunity for such infections. This includes douching, sprays, heat and moisture buildup from clothing, irritants in spermicides and some condoms, soaps, tissues, swimming pool water, antibiotics, lost tampons, and even high fevers from other illnesses. Women with diabetes are more vulnerable to vaginitis, especially vaginal yeast infections. The introduction of fecal bacteria into the vulvar and vaginal areas by sexual practices or poor hygiene can cause infections. Vaginitis and vulvitis are also caused by sexually transmitted organisms such as trichomonas vaginalis and the herpes virus. Rarely, overgrowth of the normal lactobacilli causes similar symptoms. Some of the aforementioned agents can also irritate the vaginal tissues without causing an infection.

The treatment of vaginitis and vulvitis depends on the cause. Nonprescription remedies that are effective against yeast contain the drugs clotrimazole or miconazole. Those that contain benzocaine (a local anesthetic) may be helpful for the temporary relief of symptoms of burning and itching until a physician can be consulted. Homeopathic products, which contain no actual antifungal agent, are worthless for treating yeast infections.

Theoretically, treatment with the right strains of lactobacilli could be helpful, and scientists continue to study this. One small study suggested, for example, that women who regularly eat yogurt (which contains a lactobacillus) are less prone to vaginal yeast infections.[11] But "acidophilus" preparations have not been shown to help, and many such products do not contain the proper variety of lactobacilli.[12] Nor is there any scientific evidence that dietary factors such as coffee, alcohol, sugar, or carbohydrates play any role in the cause or treatment of vaginitis.

Because vaginitis and vulvitis have many causes, some of which are serious, a doctor should be consulted unless a woman is certain that she has a recurrence of a previously medically diagnosed problem that is suitable for self-treatment. In some cases, treatment of a woman's sexual partner(s) is also necessary.

CONTRACEPTION

Throughout history, both men and women have sought effective ways to control their fertility. Many of these treatments were not effective, and many caused infections and burns. As far back as 1850 BCE in ancient Egypt, recipes for barrier contraceptive methods were buried with the dead to prevent pregnancy in the afterlife. They advised using honey, carbonate of soda, and crocodile dung as spermicides.

Five major types of contraception are used today in the United States: fertility awareness (rhythm) methods, barrier methods, intrauterine devices (IUDs), hormonal methods (oral contraceptives, subdermal implants, injections), and surgical sterilization.

Despite recent medical advances, a completely safe, effective, and nonpermanent method has yet to be developed. Nearly 60% of all pregnancies in the United States are unintended, and slightly fewer than half of these occur after contraception has failed or was used improperly.[13] Planned Parenthood Federation of America[14] suggests five considerations when selecting a method:

1. *Personal preference*: Choose a method with which you are physically and emotionally comfortable and can use consistently.
2. *Safety:* Be aware of any health risks involved, including the risk of sexually transmitted diseases.
3. *Effectiveness:* Choose a method that provides the amount of protection you need to feel secure. For maximum effectiveness, the method must be understood and used carefully and consistently.
4. *Convenience:* Choose a method that is available and affordable.
5. *Partner preference:* You may also want to consider this when deciding which method is most appropriate.

Table 21-1 compares the failure rates, risks, side effects, and other noteworthy features of the various methods. Additional information and services can be obtained from physicians, women's centers, or Planned Parenthood clinics.

Fertility Awareness Methods

Fertility awareness (rhythm) methods depend on abstaining from intercourse or using other forms of contraception during the fertile days of the menstrual cycle. The fertile days are the few days leading up to and including the day of ovulation. Ovulation can be determined by counting days (calendar method), noting changes in body temperature taken each morning, noting changes in the character of cervical mucus, or a combination of these methods. Rhythm methods are economical, free

Table 21-1

COMPARISON OF CONTRACEPTIVE METHODS

Method	Typical Yearly Pregnancy Rate per 100 Women*	Typical Cost†	Risks and Side Effects	Comments
Subdermal implant (Norplant)	0.05	$600 to $800 including removal	Menstrual irregularities, weight gain, headaches	Usually removed after 5 years No STD protection
Male sterilization	0.1	$300 to $1000	Pain, swelling, bleeding	Success must be confirmed by a negative sperm count after 15–20 ejaculations
Female sterilization	0.5	$1000 to $2500	Risks associated with surgery	No STD protection
Depo-Provera	0.3	$60/3 months plus costs of doctor's exams	Irregular bleeding and spotting Weight gain, headaches, acne	No STD protection
Pill	5.0*	Cost of doctor's exam plus $20 to $35 per month for the pills	Minor problems include tender breasts, nausea, gain or loss of weight Mild high blood pressure Slight increase in incidence of gallbladder disease Thromboembolic phenomena: blood clots in legs (1 in 2000 yearly), less commonly in lungs, heart, or brain; heart attack incidence is significantly increased in smokers	Must be taken daily to be effective Reduces menstrual bleeding and cramping Reduces risk of several cancers and heart disease No STD protection
Intrauterine device Mirena® ParaGard® Progestasert®	 0.4 0.8 2.0	$300 to $750 for device, exam, insertion, and follow-up	Pelvic infection Perforation of uterine wall (rare) Less protection against ectopic pregnancy (pregnancy outside uterus); infection or miscarriage can result if pregnancy occurs	Mirena is approved for up to 5 years, Progestasert for 1 year, and ParaGard for up to 10 years No STD protection

*More conscientious use will greatly decrease the failure rates for these methods, but relative effectiveness remains approximately the same.
†Clinics offer some of these services at lower cost.
Source: Based on data from *The Medical Letter*[15]; Knowles J. Facts about birth control[16]; and product literature and price information on the Internet.

of side effects, and practiced successfully by many women, but these methods are among the least effective. They work best in women whose menstrual cycles are regular.

Test kits that attempt to predict ovulation are available for home use, but they are not reliable for contraceptive purposes (see Chapter 9). Since sperm can live in the female reproductive tract for a few days, pregnancy can result from having unprotected intercourse a few days before the test shows that ovulation has occurred.

Barrier Methods

Barrier methods work in one of two ways: the sperm is either immobilized by a chemical (cream, jelly, foam, or suppository) or mechanically blocked (diaphragm, cervical cap, or condom) from entering the uterus. Effectiveness depends upon how conscientiously the method is used. Combinations of a mechanical and a chemical method are far more effective than either type used alone. Barrier products include the following:

Diaphragm: The diaphragm is a flexible rubber barrier that covers the cervix. It must be fitted by a doctor. Learning to use it may take time and patience. It should be used with contraceptive jelly and left in place for at least 6 hours after intercourse.

Condom, male: The male condom is a sheath of thin latex or animal tissue that fits over the penis; it offers good protection against sexually transmitted diseases, though this protection is not absolute. Simultaneous use of a spermicide provides additional protection and also can kill sperm if the condom breaks. Some condoms contain spermicide, but the extra protection is likely to be greater with the other large amounts of spermicide used in the vagina. *Consumer Reports* states that skin condoms (made from part of the intestine of a lamb) are less likely to break than latex condoms but do not prevent transmission of the viruses that cause AIDS,

Table 21-1

COMPARISON OF CONTRACEPTIVE METHODS - *CONT'D.*

Method	Typical Yearly Pregnancy Rate per 100 Women*	Typical Cost†	Risks and Side Effects	Comments
Condom (female)	21*	$2.75 each	Allergic reaction (rare)	Significant protection against STDs, especially when used with spermicide; skin condoms may not protect as well as latex condoms
Condom (male)	14*	50¢ to $3 each	Rough handling may tear	
Cervical cap		Doctor's visit plus $13 to $25 for cap	Abnormal Pap smears	Some protection against certain STDs
Have given birth	40*		Cervical irritation	
Never given birth	20*			
Diaphragm	20*	Doctor's visit plus $13 to $25 for diaphragm	Bladder infections Allergic reaction (rare)	Should be checked for weak spots or holes before insertion
Coitus interruptus (withdrawal)	19	No cost	No physical risk	May make satisfaction less likely Pregnancy can result from sperm in pre-ejaculatory fluid No STD protection
Vaginal sponge	18*	–	Allergic reactions	Not available in United States
Fertility awareness methods ("rhythm")	20*	Charts and kits are inexpensive	No physical risk	The frequency of unwanted pregnancy varies with the type of method used No STD protection
Vaginal foam, cream, jelly, film, or suppository	26*	70¢ to $1 per use –	Active ingredient (nonoxynol-9) may irritate vagina or provoke a vaginal infection	Some protection against certain STDs
No method used	85		Very high risk of unwanted pregnancy	No STD protection

genital herpes, or hepatitis.[17] Marketing surveys show that 40% to 50% of condoms are purchased by women.

Condom, female ("vaginal pouch"): The female condom is a soft, loose-fitting polyurethane sheath and two diaphragm-like, flexible polyurethane rings. One ring, which lies inside the sheath, fits internally like a diaphragm and anchors the sheath inside the vagina. The other ring forms the outer edge of the sheath and remains outside the vagina. The female condom is easy to use and does not require fitting by a health professional. It is thicker and covers more of the genital area than the male condom, which means it may offer more protection against sexually transmitted diseases.

Cervical cap: The cervical cap is a flexible cup-like device about 1½ inches in diameter that fits snugly over the cervix. It can be inserted many hours before sexual activity and left in place for up to 48 hours. A pelvic examination by a physician is needed to determine the correct size. The cap is recommended only for women with a normal Pap smear, and another Pap smear should be obtained after 3 months of use to be sure that abnormal changes have not occurred in the cervical tis-

sue. (They occur in about 4% of users.) It is also recommended that users apply spermicide with each use and leave the device in for 6 to 8 hours after intercourse.

Foam, cream, jelly, film, suppositories: These products contain nonoxynol-9, a chemical that kills sperm on contact. To be effective, the product must cover the cervix. Combining them with a condom, diaphragm, or cervical cap greatly enhances their effectiveness. Used alone, aerosol foams are the most effective of these products. Contraceptive suppositories tend to lose their effectiveness within 30 minutes after insertion.

Vaginal contraceptive sponge: The vaginal sponge is a soft, round sponge, approximately 2 inches in diameter, made of polyurethane, and impregnated with a spermicide that is activated by moistening the sponge with water. When properly inserted, it covers the cervix. The sponge is considered effective for 24 hours after insertion. During this period it continuously releases a spermicide and acts as a barrier to block spermatozoa from entering the cervix. A polyester loop attached across the bottom of the sponge permits easy removal. In 1995 the only American manufacturer suspended production, stating that FDA manufacturing requirements would force it to raise prices beyond what many consumers would be willing to pay. Another manufacturer expects to market it again in the near future.

Intrauterine Devices (IUDs)

IUDs are the world's most often used method of temporary contraception for women. They involve the insertion by a doctor of a small piece of shaped plastic or other object into the uterus, where it can block the transport of sperm through the uterus. When the IUD is in place, an attached string hangs through the opening of the cervix so the position of the IUD can be checked. Protection is increased with use of a condom and/or spermicide during the woman's most fertile period (usually the week beginning 19 days before the next period is due).

IUDs offer convenience and a high rate of effectiveness as long as they stay in place. In some women they have major side effects: bleeding, menstrual cramping, and infections. If a sexually transmitted infection occurs, the presence of an IUD may make it more serious.

◆ Personal Glimpse ◆

Sample Script for Safer Sex[18]

If your partner says: What's that?
You can say: A condom, sweetheart.

If your partner says: What for?
You can say: To use when we're making love.

If your partner says: Rubbers are gross.
You can say: Being pregnant when I don't want to be is more gross. Getting AIDS is totally gross.

If your partner says: Rubbers aren't romantic.
You can say: What's more romantic than making love and protecting each other's health at the same time?

If your partner says: Let's face it. Making love with a rubber on is like taking a shower with a raincoat on.
You can say: You face it. Doing it without a rubber isn't making love; it's playing Russian roulette.

If your partner says: But I love you.
You can say: That won't protect me against disease or pregnancy.

If your partner says: I guess you don't love me.
You can say: I do, but I'm not risking my future to prove it.

If your partner says: We're not using a rubber and that's it.
You can say: O.K. You know how to play checkers?

Three types of IUDs have FDA approval in the United States: *Progestasert*, a progestin-releasing IUD that must be replaced annually; *ParaGard*, which is approved for up to 10 years of use; and *Mirena*, another progestin-releasing device that was approved in 2000 for up to 5 years. IUDs are not recommended for women with multiple partners (because the risk of sexually transmitted disease is higher) or those who have had a recent or recurrent pelvic infection, tubal pregnancy, very heavy periods, or previous trouble with an IUD.

Hormonal Methods

Three types of contraceptives prevent pregnancy through the effects of female hormones: oral contraceptives ("the pill"), *Norplant* (an implant), and the long-acting injectable drugs *Depo-Provera* and *Lunelle*. These hormones suppress ovulation, thicken the cervical mucus, interfere with the transport of sperm through the tubes, and make the tissue lining the uterus thinner and less receptive to implantation of an early embryo.

Oral contraceptives (OCs), available only by prescription, contain one or two hormones similar to those that naturally regulate menstruation. Pills that contain estrogen and progestin (a synthetic progesterone) are more effective than those that contain only progestin (called minipills). OCs provide the best reversible protection, but only if they are taken properly with no missed doses. Most women also experience lighter and less painful periods, a reduction in breast tenderness and lumps, and, with some OCs, reduced acne. The FDA has approved one of these (*Ortho-Tricylcen*) for treating acne, but no studies show that this pill is superior to the others.

Extensive studies have not established that long-term use of oral contraceptives increases the incidence of breast cancer.[19] Those containing both estrogen and progestin offer some protection against ovarian and uterine (endometrial) cancer.[20] Both kinds of pills reduce the risk of serious pelvic infections of the uterus and tubes. Although cervical cancer is more common among OC users, this appears to be due to sexual factors (multiple partners) rather than the pill itself.

The list of possible side effects is long, but serious problems are rare. Mild side effects, such as nausea, weight gain, fluid retention, spotting between periods, and breast tenderness, usually subside within a few months. Moderately troublesome side effects include headaches and depression. The incidence of side effects is less with the minipill, but its effectiveness is a bit lower. For this reason, use with a spermicide or condom is advantageous. Most women who take either type of pill have no side effects or complications.

OCs pose a significant risk for smokers and for individuals with a history of blood clots in the legs or elsewhere. The smoking-related risk increases with age. Smokers over 35 should not take them. OCs are also unsuitable for women who are pregnant or who have active liver disease, cancer of the breast or internal sexual organs, or abnormal vaginal bleeding.

In 1990 the FDA approved use of the contraceptive implant *Norplant,* which consists of six silicone tubes that are about the size of matchsticks.[21] The tubes are implanted in the underside of a woman's upper arm in a fanlike arrangement that can be felt but not easily seen. Once in place, the tubes steadily release a low dose of progestin into the bloodstream. The implant procedure takes 10 to 15 minutes. *Norplant* is highly effective for up to 6 years but often causes menstrual irregularities. *Norplant* usually costs $500 to $600 for the insertion and an additional $100 to $200 for eventual removal.

In 1992 the FDA approved use of depot medroxyprogesterone acetate (DMPA), a synthetic drug that is nearly 100% effective when injected every 12 weeks. Marketed as *Depo-Provera,* it takes effect within 24 hours and halts ovulation for at least 14 weeks, which provides a 2-week grace period before the next injection. The most common side effects are menstrual changes: irregular bleeding and spotting, particularly in the first few months. After 1 year about half of the users do not get their periods, a situation that poses no medical risk.

In 2000, the FDA approved *Lunelle,* a once-a-month injection that combines progestin and estrogen to inhibit ovulation. Several clinical trials have reported failure rates of less than 1%. The injections are given by a health-care provider every 28 to 30 days, and no longer than 33 days apart. *Lunelle* should not be used by women known or suspected to be pregnant; smokers who are over the age of 35; or women with severe high blood pressure. Most women who receive it experience changes in their menstrual cycle. Ovulation resumes 2 to 4 months after stopping the injections. To ensure that *Lunelle* or *Depo-Provera* are not accidentally given to a pregnant woman, the first injection should be given during the first 5 days of the menstrual period.

All of the hormonal methods tend to promote weight gain by increasing appetite. However, weight gain can be avoided by eating and exercising sensibly.

Emergency Contraception

Emergency contraception pills (ECPs) are hormonal products that, if taken within 72 hours following intercourse, can prevent ovulation or, if that has already occurred, can block implantation of a fertilized egg in the uterus. They have minimal side effects and are about 75% effective after unprotected intercourse.[22,23] ECPs are commonly referred to as "the morning-after pill." This term is incorrect, however, because treatment involves more than one pill and does not need to occur on the "morning after." Two ECP products have received FDA approval since 1998. The American Medical Association has asked the FDA to make them available without a prescription, because some women might not be able to obtain ECP soon enough through a physician.

Surgical Sterilization

Close to half the married couples who intend to avoid pregnancy include one partner who has been sterilized. Sterilization has the advantage of being permanent, although it occasionally can be surgically reversed. Because of this, however, a decision to undergo sterilization should be made only after careful consideration and discussion with one's physician. Although sterilization procedures can sometimes be reversed, it is important to be certain that no more pregnancies are desired.

Sterilization in women (tubal ligation) destroys a portion of the fallopian tubes by placing clips or bands, burning them with an electric current, or cutting them directly. Most of these procedures are performed by laparoscopy through a small incision just inside the navel. In most cases, a second incision just inside the pubic hairline is also used.

Tubal ligation is also performed through a larger incision at the time of a cesarean delivery or through an incision in the vagina. These procedures are usually performed as outpatient operations in the hospital or a surgery center.[24] After tubal ligation, sperm can no longer reach the eggs released by the ovaries, which die and are resorbed just as they are during any other cycle in which pregnancy does not occur.

Male sterilization (vasectomy) is accomplished by cutting and sealing off the tube (vas deferens) from each testicle through which spermatazoa travel before they are stored for ejaculation. In the traditional method, a local anesthetic is injected into the area, an incision is made on each side of the scrotum, and the tubes are located and blocked. Minor complications (swelling, tenderness, blood clots, infections, and sperm leakage under the skin) occur in a small percentage of cases.[25] With the no-scalpel method (microvasectomy), the scrotal skin is opened by puncture to reach the vas deferens. Microvasectomy decreases the possibility of complications. The procedures take about 20 minutes and are done on an outpatient basis. A number of ejaculations must take place (typically 15 to 20) before all stored spermatozoa are expelled, and success of the operation can be confirmed by laboratory examination of semen specimens (sperm counts).

Voluntary Abortions

A 1973 Supreme Court decision prohibits the states from banning voluntary abortions during the first and second trimesters of pregnancy. About 1.5 million voluntary abortions are performed each year.

The surgical technique used depends on the stage of pregnancy and the preference of the physician.[26] During the first 12 weeks of pregnancy, uterine contents are evacuated by a suction procedure (vacuum curettage) usually performed on an outpatient basis using local anesthesia. From 13 to 16 weeks the cervix requires additional stretching before the uterine contents can be sucked out; a dilation and evacuation procedure (D&E) is commonly performed under general anesthesia. From 17 to 24 weeks a D&E may still be performed or a solution of saline (salt), prostaglandin, and/or urea is injected into the uterus. Prostaglandin can also be administered by vaginal suppository. These substances cause the uterus to become irritable and to contract, expelling its contents in a procedure that resembles labor. The complication rate of induced abortion is less than 1% during the first trimester, but rises gradually (to 2% to 3%) the later the procedure is performed. About 95% of voluntary abortions take place during the first 13 weeks. Many of the rest are done because of fetal abnormality detected with screening tests.

Abortion is a highly controversial subject.[27] "Pro-choice" advocates believe that women should have the freedom to choose whether to have a child or terminate unwanted pregnancies. "Pro-life" advocates state that abortion is morally wrong because it involves the destruction of human life. The opposition comes primarily from Roman Catholic, fundamentalist, and evangelical churches. Much of the controversy involves debate about when personhood begins.

Since the 1973 Supreme Court decision, opponents of abortion have lobbied for passage of state and federal laws that make it more difficult for women to obtain abortions. Federal funding through Medicaid has been restricted to cases in which an abortion is deemed necessary to protect the woman's life or when the pregnancy resulted from incest or rape. Laws requiring a waiting period, parental or spousal consent, or another procedural delay have been enacted, but some have been overturned by the courts.[28,29] Opponents hope for passage of a constitutional amendment that would nullify the Supreme Court decision, but so far this seems unlikely.

Women who need help in deciding whether to terminate a pregnancy can obtain counseling from some physicians, clergy, local family planning clinics, women's centers, and Planned Parenthood offices. In 1991 the U.S. Supreme Court upheld a law that forbids federally funded facilities from discussing abortion with their clients. The "pro-life" viewpoint is available from some physicians and clergy, as well as from Birthright USA, Alternatives to Abortion, and similar groups that maintain offices in many American cities.

Many antiabortion information centers have been listed in the Yellow Pages under abortion services, alternatives to abortion, birth-control information centers, or family planning information centers, despite the fact that their only service was antiabortion advice.[30] In 1991 Representative Ron Wyden (D–OR) held a Congressional hearing in which he charged that as many as 2000 clinics were operating in this matter.[31] After the hearing, some Yellow Pages directory publishers announced that they would segregate such ads and clearly indicate that facilities listed under "abortion alternatives" do not provide abortions or abortion referrals.[32] Court rulings have forced several antiabortion counseling centers to change their name, but some are still deceptively advertised.

In recent years some opponents have campaigned to intimidate abortion providers and their patients. Their activities have included picketing, blockades, and invasions of facilities where abortions are performed; stalking of staff members; bombings; arson; death threats; assaults; and other personal attacks.[33] Several physicians and other staff members have been murdered by antiabortion extremists. The 1994 federal Freedom of Access to Clinic Entrances Act makes it a federal crime to use or attempt to use force, the threat of force, or physical obstruction to injure, intimidate, or interfere with providers of reproductive health-care services or their patients. It also outlaws damaging or destroying the property of a reproductive health-care facility. By 1998, at least 15 individuals had been convicted under this law.[34] These cases and civil lawsuits have reduced some types of harassment, but pro-choice leaders believe their facilities are still under siege.

Mifepristone, commonly called RU-486, is an antiprogesterone drug that can prevent pregnancy if taken within 72 hours after unprotected intercourse and can induce abortion if taken within the first 6 weeks of pregnancy. When prescribed with prostaglandin, it is more than 95% effective in ending the pregnancy and has a low incidence of side effects. However, blood loss is greater than with a D&E, and about half of the users require a D&E to complete the process. Mifepristone is given only very early in pregnancy; D&E is used to abort pregnancies that are much further along.

RU-486 was approved by the FDA in 2000. Advocates predict that its availability will greatly reduce the incidence of surgical abortions,[35,36] but that remains to be seen. The FDA's terms of approval require that a woman make three visits to a physician, first to receive the mifepristone, then 2 days later for a dose of misoprostol, and again on day 14 for follow-up. Information from the FDA is posted at http://www.fda.gov/cder/drug/infopage/mifepristone.

INFERTILITY

About one out of every 12 American couples trying to achieve pregnancy despite one year of regular sexual intercourse without contraception. The problem is attributable to the man in about one third of couples, and to the woman in about another third. In some couples, both are impaired; and in others, no problem can be identified. With specialized help, about half the infertile couples achieve pregnancy. Certain procedures increase the likelihood of multiple births.

Evaluation of the man begins with a sperm count. Evaluation of the woman is more complex and involves checking for problems with structure and function of the ovaries, fallopian tubes, and uterus. This usually begins with blood and x-ray tests that are the simplest and least expensive. For men, the best doctor may be a board-certified urologist who has 2 years of special training in andrology. For women, the best doctor is a board-certified obstetrician-gynecologist who has had 2 years of further training in reproductive endocrinology. Resolve, a nonprofit group, maintains a list of specialists and provides comprehensive information about infertility. It advises using an infertility specialist if (a) the woman is age 35 or older, (b) microsurgery is needed, (c) there have been three or more miscarriages, (d) the menstrual cycle and ovulation have not responded to clomiphene citrate (*Serophene*), (e) the semen is seriously defective, (f) the woman has a history of pelvic infection, (g) the couple has been unable to conceive for 2 years despite "normal" basic tests, or (h) the couple is considering in vitro fertilization or other assisted reproductive technology.[37]

The FTC[38] suggests that couples seeking infertility services check the doctor's qualifications carefully, rather than relying on advertisements.

Some infertility procedures are very expensive and often are not covered by insurance policies. *Kiplinger's Personal Finance Magazine* recommends checking one's insurance policy carefully and obtaining written confirmation that any contemplated procedure is covered.[39]

GENETIC TESTING AND PRENATAL COUNSELING

Most of the body's cells have a nucleus containing 23 pairs of chromosomes, one originally contributed by the mother and one by the father. Each chromosome is a tightly coiled strand of DNA (deoxyribonucleic acid), which, in turn, is composed of two ribbon-like strands of polynucleotides. A gene is a tiny segment of DNA capable of reproducing itself exactly at each cell division and directing the formation of an enzyme or other protein. About 4000 diseases are known to be caused by defective chromosomes or genes.[40]

Until recently, hereditary tendencies were determined mainly by examining the family history of the individuals involved. Within the past decade, however, genes have been identified that cause or contribute to Alzheimer's disease, amyotrophic lateral sclerosis (Lou Gehrig's disease), cystic fibrosis, neurofibromatosis, familial colon cancer, Huntington's disease, myotonic dystrophy, and several other conditions.[40] About 500 laboratories, most affiliated with hospitals, provide genetic testing services. Research in this field is progressing very rapidly.

Genetic counseling can help prospective parents review the facts in light of their personal beliefs. It is commonly recommended for all women over 35 and for others at risk for bearing a child with hemophilia, sickle cell anemia, thalassemia (a severe type of anemia), cystic fibrosis, the hereditary form of Down syndrome, and Tay-Sachs disease (a degenerative disease that results in considerable suffering and death by the age of 4).

The Harvard Guide to Women's Health[41] states that genetic counseling has become a routine part of prenatal care for many women at increased risk of carrying a congenitally abnormal fetus. Some abnormalities are life-threatening or will result in disabilities so severe that the offspring will suffer greatly or be incapable of becoming self-sufficient. Other abnormalities will result in only minor dysfunction. Detection of certain conditions may lead to a decision to terminate the pregnancy or can facilitate planning for the special needs of a physically or mentally handicapped child.

The counseling process usually starts with the woman's primary care physician or obstetrician but may require the services of a specialist. The American Board of Medical Genetics offers certification in clinical genetics and related fields to physicians and others with doctoral degrees. The American Board of Genetic

Counseling offers certification in genetic counseling, for which at least a master's degree is required.

Pregnant women who are at risk giving birth to a child with genetic abnormalities may be candidates for screening procedures in which fetal chromosomes are examined. In chorionic villus sampling, which can be done between the 8th and 12th week of pregnancy, a long needle is inserted through the abdomen or vagina to remove a tiny specimen of placental tissue for examination. In amniocentesis, which is performed between weeks 16 and 20, about 1 ounce of the fluid surrounding the fetus is removed from the uterus. The findings may lead to a decision to terminate the pregnancy.

Alpha-fetoprotein screening is recommended for all pregnant women. This test can be performed on a blood sample or directly on the amnionic fluid. A positive test indicates that a neural tube defect is likely and that further testing should be done to clarify the situation.

Pregnancy and Delivery

This section covers some of the decisions that must be made about self-care, professional services, and birthing options.

Pregnancy Testing

When a woman is pregnant, human chorionic gonadotropin (HCG) becomes present in her urine and blood. This hormone, which is produced by the chorion (the membrane surrounding the embryo in the uterus), is the substance tested for in pregnancy tests performed on urine. The most accurate tests (radioreceptor assay or radioimmunoassay) are performed by laboratories on blood samples.

Do-it-yourself test kits are available (see Chapter 9). If done carefully, the tests are usually accurate when positive, but they may be a needless purchase. If the result is positive, indicating that pregnancy is probable, a visit to a physician is advisable. If the physician believes it is important to confirm the diagnosis, the woman will wind up paying for two pregnancy tests.

Prenatal Care

The vast majority of women receive their prenatal care from a physician and deliver their child in a hospital. Prenatal care is best begun when pregnancy is suspected and will involve evaluation of the woman's medical history, a physical examination, and discussion of any special concerns. Current medications should be discussed to determine whether they pose any risk to the developing baby. Diet should be discussed to be certain that the mother-to-be has an adequate nutrient intake, particularly of calcium, iron, and folic acid. (Chapter 11 discusses the importance of adequate folic acid intake to prevent certain birth defects.) Although an appropriate diet will supply what most women need, a prenatal supplement is usually recommended. Appropriate formulas, which contain the essential vitamins and minerals in no more than the RDA amounts, can be purchased for less than 10¢ per day.

Most obstetricians recommend that prenatal visits take place monthly until the seventh month of pregnancy and then increasing visits to weekly as the due date approaches.

Table 21-2 summarizes the screening tests and other medical interventions that the U.S. Preventive Services Task Force recommends for pregnant women.

The U.S. Centers for Disease Control and Prevention recommends testing all pregnant women during the seventh or eighth month of pregnancy to see whether they are carrying *Streptococcus B*.[42] This bacterium is the most common cause of life-threatening infections in newborns. Detecting it and treating the mother can greatly reduce the risk of the infant becoming infected. The test is performed by culturing bacteria found in the vagina and rectum.

Ultrasound screening is popular but has not been demonstrated to improve outcome without a definite medical reason to use it.[43]

Consumer Reports recommends that women who are selecting an obstetrician should ask about the doctor's attitude toward cesarean deliveries.[44] Inquiries also should be made about the doctor's practice style, fees, hospital policies regarding labor and delivery, and the likelihood that the doctor will be the person who actually does the delivery.[45] The best choice is likely to be an obstetrician/gynecolgist who (a) trained at a university-affiliated program; (b) is board-certified, (c) is a Fellow of the American College of Obstetricians and Gynecologists (F.A.C.O.G.), (d) is easy to talk to, and (e) answers questions adequately.

Childbirth education classes can help prepare the woman (and usually her partner) for labor and delivery. They typically teach how breathing and relaxation exercises can lessen the fear of labor and may reduce the amount of anesthesia required. Women who are pregnant for the first time are likely to benefit considerably from knowing what to expect.

Delivery Options

An out-of-hospital childbirth movement began in the mid-1970s in response to feelings that hospital care was too cold and impersonal and did not pay sufficient

Table 21-2

INTERVENTIONS RECOMMENDED FOR PREGNANT WOMEN

Initial Evaluation	Subsequent Screening	Counseling
Blood pressure	Blood pressure (each visit)	Multivitamin with folic acid
Hemoglobin/hematocrit	Urinalysis (each visit)	Tobacco cessation; effects of
Hepatitis B surface antigen	Diabetes screen (blood sugar test	passive smoking
RPR/VDRL (for syphilis)	following glucose administration)	Alcohol and other drug use
Chlamydia and gonorrhea screen	Urine culture (12–16 weeks)	Nutrition, including adequate
Rubella antibody test	Multiple marker testing: serum	calcium intake
Rh incompatibility	alpha-fetoprotein, HCG, and	Encourage breastfeeding
Assess for problem or risk drinking	estriol (15–18 weeks)	Lap/shoulder belts
HIV screening for high-risk patients	Amniocentesis and/or other genetic	Regular physical activity
or if required by state law	tests as desired (15–18 weeks)	Infant car seats
Discuss genetic counseling and testing	Culture for Group B *Streptococcus*	STD prevention

Source: Updated from the 1996 U.S. Preventive Services Task Force Report[46] with help from Timothy N. Gorski, M.D., F.A.C.O.G.

attention to emotional needs. Since then, however, most hospital programs have integrated the concept of family-centered childbirth. The improvements include permitting the woman's partner to stay with her during labor and delivery and permitting mother and child to share a room after delivery. Freestanding childbirth centers are less expensive but can pose additional risk for the 10% to 15% of women in labor who develop a problem that needs urgent medical attention. Women considering this option should carefully inquire about the qualifications of the person performing the delivery and the availability of emergency care. Home birth is suitable only for normal deliveries and runs an additional risk of infection. Timothy N. Gorski, M.D., F.A.C.O.G., of Arlington, Texas, likens home birth to skiing under conditions where medical help is not readily available. He warns that, "In most instances everything works out fine, but the consequences can be catastrophic when an unexpected complication arises."

INFANT FEEDING

Although formula feeding can adequately meet the physical and emotional needs of the newborn infant, many studies have shown that breastfeeding is advantageous.[47] Human milk and breastfeeding of infants are better for general health, growth, and development and significantly decrease the risk for many diseases. Lactating women have an earlier return to prepregnant weight, reduction in hip fractures in the postmenopausal period, and reduced risk of ovarian cancer and premenopausal breast cancer. The success of breastfeeding is facilitated by guidance from a knowledgeable relative or

health professional.[48] Chapter 11 contains additional information on infant nutrition.

OSTEOPOROSIS

Osteoporosis is a condition, occurring mostly in women, in which bones lose calcium and become less dense (more porous) and more brittle. It occurs most commonly in postmenopausal women, whose ovaries no longer produce the estrogen needed to help maintain bone mass. Caucasian women who are fair, small-boned, and thin-skinned are especially vulnerable. Other risk factors are long-term use of thyroid hormones and cortisone, cigarette smoking, lack of weight-bearing exercise, insufficient calcium and vitamin D intake, alcohol abuse, and early menopause. Regardless of risk factors, the incidence and severity of osteoporosis can be greatly reduced by estrogen-replacement therapy (discussed later in this chapter).

The early stages of osteoporosis produce no symptoms. Often the first sign is a fracture of the hip or wrist after a minor fall. Some women lose height or develop a hunched back ("dowager's hump") caused by collapse of spinal vertebrae. Lost bone tissue cannot easily be replaced, but further bone loss can be minimized by preventive measures. About half the untreated women who reach age 75 suffer at least one fracture due to osteoporosis.

The key to bone health late in life is prevention. Bone density progressively increases until age 30 to 35 and gradually decreases after that. Adequate calcium intake is necessary to maximize bone density and slow down the rate of loss. The current (1997) Dietary

Reference Intake values for calcium are 1300 mg/day for ages 9–18, 1000 mg per day for ages 19–50, and 1200 mg/day for age 51 and older.[49] These values are higher than the 1989 RDAs, which ranged from 800 to 1200. Surveys indicate that many do not consume the amount of calcium recommended in the report. Calcium intake can be increased by consuming more lowfat or nonfat dairy products or fortified food products or by taking supplements. The report states that supplements may be appropriate for those at high risk of health problems due to low calcium intake.

In 1995 *Consumer Reports* tested 21 brands of calcium supplements and found that all contained the amount of calcium stated on their label, and all would dissolve properly after swallowing. The editors recommended using the cheapest brand of calcium carbonate available, which should cost less than $3 per month.[2] Absorbability can be tested by placing a tablet in vinegar. One that does not disintegrate within 30 minutes is unlikely to be well absorbed. This problem can be overcome by chewing the tablet or letting it dissolve in the mouth before swallowing it or by switching to a better brand.

X-ray examination (densitometry) can be used to measure bone mass in the spine, hip, and/or wrist, the most common sites of fractures due to osteoporosis. Density can also be measured in the middle finger and the heel or shinbone. Spine and hip tests are the most accurate and should be the ones used for definitive diagnosis; the others are mostly appropriate for screening. The test findings are compared to two standards, or norms, known as "age matched" and "young normal." The age-matched reading compares bone density to what is expected in someone of the same age and gender. The young normal reading compares density to the optimal peak bone density of a healthy young adult of the same gender. The information enables a doctor to identify where a patient stands within ranges of normal and to determine whether the patient is at risk for fracture.

In general, the lower the bone density, the higher the risk for fracture. Test results will help determine the best course of action for bone health.

Regardless of what a bone scan might show, women should minimize their chance of developing osteoporosis by heeding its risk factors throughout their adult life. They should consume adequate amounts of calcium, engage in weight-bearing exercise,[50] and not smoke cigarettes or abuse alcohol. Before menopause, there is little reason to screen women who have no risk factors for bone loss.

Certain blood and urine tests can measure the rate of bone turnover, which may reflect the rate bone loss. However, these tests provide no indication of bone mass and thus are not useful for diagnosing osteoporosis. A urine test showing whether bone turnover has slowed after treatment has begun may be useful in checking a patient's response to treatment. But these biochemical tests should not be regarded as a cheaper, more convenient alternative to bone mass measurements.[51]

HORMONE-REPLACEMENT THERAPY

Menopause is the complete disappearance of a woman's monthly cycles for 6 to 12 months and is caused by declining production of estrogen and progesterone hormones by the ovaries. When the ovaries are removed, this is referred to as "surgical menopause." Hormone-replacement therapy (HRT) provides a postmenopausal woman with the absent hormone(s), although not in the amounts once produced by the ovaries. About 10 million women take HRT, making these drugs among the most prescribed in the United States

HRT is often prescribed to relieve menopausal symptoms such as "hot flashes," night sweats, and vaginal dryness. In recent years it has become clear that HRT can provide important health benefits as well. Estrogen reduces (a) cardiovascular risk factors after the age of 50,[52,53] (b) the lifetime risk that a woman will develop

---

It's Your Decision

You have encountered unusual difficulty with premenstrual syndrome.
Which of the following actions would you take?   Reason

☐ Take a pain reliever   _____
☐ Attempt to reduce tension and stress   _____
☐ Increase vitamin intake   _____
☐ Increase intake of herbal tea   _____
☐ Get more rest by going to bed earlier   _____
☐ See a doctor   _____
☐ Other (specify) _____   _____

osteoporosis, and (c) the risk of vertebral fractures up to 50% and hip fractures, 25%, if treatment begins at menopause. Several studies suggest that estrogen also helps to protect against colon cancer[54] and that the overall death rate is lower among women taking HRT.[55] Estrogen's protective effect against heart disease is partially related to its ability to raise the blood level of HDL-cholesterol and lower the blood level of LDL-cholesterol.[56] Estrogen may also improve mental function and help prevent Alzheimer's disease. Consumers Union's medical consultants believe that women at high risk for osteoporosis or heart disease should consider HRT if they have no medical reason not to do so.[57]

Recent studies suggest that HRT may not prevent further heart attacks or death among postmenopausal women whose arteries are already partly blocked by atherosclerosis.[58,59] A 4-year study in such women actually showed increased risk in the first year and only a slight trend toward protection over longer periods.[59] Another study found that women who started HRT after an attack did worse during the next year than women who had never taken it.[60] It is still considered appropriate for women without heart disease and those with heart disease who have used it for 1 year without difficulty.[58,61]

Women with a uterus have a higher risk of uterine cancer if they take estrogen alone. This risk is eliminated by the standard practice of taking a progesterone as well. Women who no longer have a uterus can take estrogen alone. Some women, particularly those who have undergone surgical menopause, may benefit from very small doses of androgens (male hormones).

Many studies have examined whether HRT increases the risk of breast cancer. The prevailing view is that it may pose a slight risk, but for most women, the risk is far outweighed by the proven reduction of heart disease and osteoporosis. This view is supported by a study of 232 women born before 1915 who began taking daily estrogen tablets between 1969 and 1973 and continued for an average of 17.1 years. These women had 46% fewer deaths than 222 similarly aged women who had never taken estrogen or took it for 1 year or less. The difference was attributable mainly to less cardiovascular disease. The overall cancer mortality rate of the two groups was similar.[62] Another recent study found no association between breast cancer and the use of combined estrogen/progestin therapy.[63]

The American Council on Science and Health[64] has concluded (a) for most women, the benefits of HRT far outweigh the risks; (b) dietary supplements sold as "alternatives" have not been shown to be safe or effective; and (c) the amounts of active constituents in some of these products may vary from batch to batch. Gorski[65]

warns that although wild yam cream and other "natural" progesterone-containing skin creams may provide some relief from hot flashes and other menopausal symptoms, they have not been proven to help prevent osteoporosis or provide HRT's other benefits. The American Cancer Society states that HRT cannot be safely recommended for patients who have had breast or endometrial cancer,[66] but recent data suggest that it could be used for some women in this situation. For most women, the question is whether an uncertain small risk for cancer is an acceptable tradeoff for HRT's well-documented benefits. Other drugs are available to help maintain or rebuild the bones of women who are unable or unwilling to use HRT or who need additional help in coping with osteoporosis.

Mastectomy Prostheses

Women who undergo breast removal surgery for cancer or other conditions may wish to retain a normal breast contour as much as possible. Sometimes plastic surgery can be performed to reconstruct the breast. If the surgery is not too radical, reconstructive surgery may be relatively simple. At other times, the plastic surgery may involve using skin grafts from other parts of the body.

An alternative approach is use of an artificial breast form that is worn inside the woman's brassiere. Ready-made devices, which cost $100 or more, may be filled with silicone gel, air, liquid, weighted or unweighted foam rubber, or polyester. The liquid or silicone gel forms are generally heavier and more expensive, but are usually preferable because they assume a natural breastlike contour and do not slip out of position.[67] Custom-made forms, made from molds, cost $300 or more. Comparison shopping is advisable. One should not buy a product until completely satisfied with both appearance and comfort. Particular attention should be paid to fit; one should be sure that both breasts appear matched from the side, top, and bottom. Breast prostheses are often covered by medical insurance, but many insurers only pay for the initial one after the surgery.

Advice and emotional support after mastectomy can be obtained from the American Cancer Society program called Reach to Recovery, a network of local support groups composed of women who have undergone mastectomy.

Summary

Women are faced with many health problems related to the anatomy and physiology of their reproductive organs. Menstrual cramps that begin during the first year after the onset of menstruation are usually mild and self-treatable. Premenstrual syndrome will usually respond to self-help measures. Persistent menstrual irregularity is a reason to consult a physician.

Many choices are available to sexually active individuals who wish to prevent pregnancy. Contraceptive methods should be judged by considering effectiveness, safety, convenience, reversibility, and personal acceptability.

Genetic testing, counseling, or other procedures may be advisable when there is a significant risk of producing an abnormal fetus. Childbirth education and appropriate provider choice can reduce the stress and risks of delivery.

All women should attempt to prevent osteoporosis by avoiding or correcting the lifestyle factors that tend to increase the risk of it developing. After menopause, estrogen-replacement therapy should be considered.

References

1. Shephard BD and Shephard CA. The Complete Guide to Women's Health. Tampa, Fla., 1983, Mariner Publishing Co.
2. Calcium: How to get enough. Consumer Reports 60:510–513, 1995.
3. Farley D. Preventing TSS: Tampon labeling lets women compare absorbencies. In FDA Consumer's Current Issues in Women's Health, 2nd edition. Rockville, Md., 1994, Food and Drug Administration.
4. Tampons and pads: Should you use what Mom used? Consumer Reports 60:51–55, 1995.
5. Rossignol A, Bonnlander H. Caffeine-containing beverages, total fluid consumption, and premenstrual syndrome. American Journal of Public Health 80:1106–1110, 1990.
6. Beaudette T. Premenstrual syndrome: Is it nutrition-related? Nutrition Forum, Aug 1987.
7. Zimmerman DR. Zimmerman's Complete Guide to Nonprescription Drugs. Detroit, 1993, Visible Ink Press.
8. Endicott J and others. PMS: New treatments that really work. Patient Care 30(7):88–123, 1996.
9. 'PMS Escape' escapes scientific rigor. Tufts University Diet & Nutrition Letter 14(3):2–3, 1996.
10. Holt LH, Weber M. The American Medical Association Book of Womancare. New York, 1984, Random House Inc.
11. Hilton E and others. Ingestion of yogurt containing *Lactobacillus acidophilus* as prophylaxis for candidal vaginitis. Annals of Internal Medicine 116:353–357, 1992.
12. Hughes VL, Hillier SL. Microbiologic characteristics of *Lactobacillus* products used for colonization of the vagina. Obstetrics and Gynecology 75:244–248, 1990.
13. Rosenfield A and others. Contraceptive Research and Development: Looking to the Future. Washington, D.C., 1996, National Academy Press.
14. Over the counter birth control for women. New York, 1988, Planned Parenthood Federation of America.
15. Choice of contraceptives. The Medical Letter 37:9–12, 1995.
16. Knowles J. Facts about birth control. New York, 1995, Planned Parenthood.
17. Condoms get better: Tests of 30 models show far fewer failures than in past years. Consumer Reports 64:46–49, 1999.
18. Knowles J. The condom. New York, 1995, Planned Parenthood Federation of America.
19. Romieu J and others. Oral contraceptives and breast cancer: Review and meta-analysis. Cancer 66:2253–2263, 1990.
20. Snider S. The pill: 30 years of safety concerns. FDA Consumer 24(10):8–11, 1990.
21. Segal M. Norplant: Birth control at arm's reach. FDA Consumer 25(4):8–11, 1991.
22. Fact sheet: A brief history of emergency hormonal contraception. Planned Parenthood Federation of America, July 2000.
23. Trussel J, Rodrigues R, Ellerson C. New estimates of the effectiveness of the Yuzpe regimen of emergency contraception. Contraception 57:363–369, 1998.
24. Knowles J. All about tubal sterilization. New York, 1991, Planned Parenthood Federation of America.
25. Knowles J. All about vasectomy. New York, 1995, Planned Parenthood Federation of America.
26. Dudley S. Fact sheet: What is surgical abortion? Washington, D.C., 1996, National Abortion Federation.
27. Baird RM, Rosenbaum SE. The Ethics of Abortion: Pro-Life vs. Pro-Choice, revised edition. Amherst, N.Y., 1993, Prometheus Books.
28. Fact sheet: Abortion & waiting period/mandatory information laws. New York, 1994, Planned Parenthood Federation of America.
29. Fact sheet: Laws requiring parental consent or notification for minors' abortions. New York, 2000, Planned Parenthood Federation of America.
30. Anti-abortion counseling centers: A consumer's alert to deception, harassment & medical malpractice. New York, 1989, Planned Parenthood Federation of America and the National Abortion Federation.
31. Consumer Protection and Patient Safety Issues Involving Bogus Abortion Clinics. Hearing before the Small Business Subcommittee on Regulation, Business Opportunities, and Energy, Committee on Small Business, U.S. House of Representatives, Washington, D.C., Sept 20, 1991.
32. Abortion clinics. Associated Press news release, Nov 7, 1991.
33. Fact sheet: Protecting women and their health care providers from violence and harassment. New York, 1995, Planned Parenthood Federation of America.
34. Abortion Clinics: Information on the Effectiveness of the Freedom of Access to Clinic Entrances Act. Washington, D.C., 1998, General Accounting Office.
35. Fact Sheet: Mifepristone. New York, 1994, Planned Parenthood Federation of America.
36. Lader L. A Private Matter: RU 486. Amherst, N.Y., 1995, Prometheus Books.
37. Clapp DN. Selecting an infertility physician. Resolve Web site, accessed June 2000.
38. Infertility services. Washington, D.C., 1993, Federal Trade Commission.
39. Davis K. The agonizing price of infertility. Kiplinger's Personal Finance Magazine 50(5):50–54, 1996.
40. Genetic testing and preventive medicine: A new approach to health care. (A backgrounder for journalists.) Collegeville, Pa., 1995, SmithKline Beecham Laboratories.
41. Carlson KJ and others. The Harvard Guide to Women's Health. Cambridge, Mass., 1996, Harvard University Press.
42. Prevention of perinatal Group B streptococcal disease: A public health perspective. Morbidity and Mortality Weekly Report 45(RR-7):1–24, 1996.
43. LeFevre ML and others. A randomized trial of prenatal ultrasonographic screening: Impact on maternal management

and outcome. American Journal of Obstetrics and Gynecology 169:483–489, 1993.

44. Too many cesareans. Consumer Reports 56:120–126, 1991.

45. Planning Your Pregnancy and Birth. Washington, D.C., 2000, American College of Obstetricians and Gynecologists.

46. U.S. Preventive Services Task Force. Guide to Clinical Preventive Services, 2nd edition. Baltimore, 1996, Williams & Wilkins.

47. American Academy of Pediatrics Work Group on Breast-feeding. Breastfeeding and the use of human milk. Pediatrics 100:1035–1039, 1997.

48. Lawrence RA. A 35-year-old woman experiencing difficulty with breast feeding. JAMA 285:73–80, 2001.

49. Standing Committee on the Scientific Evaluation of Dietary Reference Intakes, Food and Nutrition Board, Institute of Medicine. Dietary Reference Intakes for Calcium, Phosphorus, Magnesium, Vitamin D, and Fluoride. Washington, D.C., 1997, National Academy Press.

50. American College of Sports Medicine position stand on osteoporosis and exercise. Medical Science of Sports and Exercise 27(4):i–vii, 1995.

51. Osteoporosis. Boston, 1997, Harvard Women's Health Watch.

52. The Writing Group for the PEPI Trial. Effects of estrogen or estrogen/progestin regimens on heart disease risk factors in postmenopausal women. The Postmenopausal Estrogen/Progestin Interventions (PEPI) Trial. JAMA 273:199–208, 1995.

53. Healy B. PEPI in perspective: Good answers spawn pressing questions. JAMA 273:240–241, 1995.

54. Newcomb PA, Storer BE. Postmenopausal hormone use and risk of large-bowel cancer. Journal of the National Cancer Institute 87:1067–1071, 1995.

55. Sturgeon SR and others. Evidence of a healthy estrogen user survivor effect. Epidemiology 6:227–231, 1995.

56. Facts about hormone replacement therapy and heart disease: The PEPI Trial. NIH Publication No. 95-3277. Bethesda, Md., 1995, National Heart, Lung, and Blood Institute.

57. Estrogen replacement: More important than ever. Consumer Reports on Health 7:121–124, 1995.

58. Hulley S and others. Randomized trial of estrogen plus progestin for secondary prevention of coronary heart disease in postmenopausal women. JAMA 280:605–613, 1998.

59. Herrington DM and others. Effects of estrogen replacement on the progression of coronary-artery atherosclerosis. New England Journal of Medicine 343:522–529, 2000.

60. Josephson WD. Women with heart disease cautioned about HRT. British Medical Journal 318:753, 1999.

61. Petitti DB. Hormone replacement therapy and heart disease prevention: Experimentation trumps observation. JAMA 280:650–652, 1998.

62. Ettinger B and others. Reduced mortality associated with long-term postmenopausal estrogen therapy. Obstetrics and Gynecology 87:6–12, 1996.

63. Stanford JL and others. Combined estrogen and progestin hormone replacement therapy in relation to risk of breast cancer in middle-aged women. JAMA 274:137–142, 1995.

64. Meister KM. Postmenopausal hormone replacement therapy: Benefits, risks, and options. New York, 2000, American Council on Science and Health.

65. Gorski T. "Wild yam cream" threatens women's health. Quackwatch Web site, June 16, 1997.

66. Hormone replacement therapy and cancer. American Cancer Society Newsletter 5(1):1–2, 1996.

67. Kushner R. Why Me? Philadelphia, 1982, WB Saunders.

Chapter Twenty-Two

HEALTH DEVICES

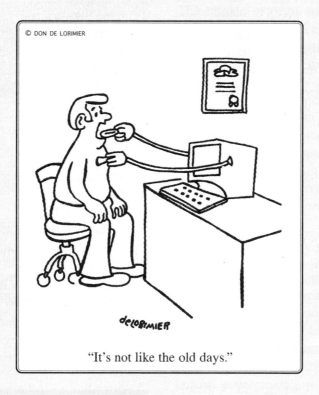

© DON DE LORIMIER

deLORIMIER

"It's not like the old days."

QUESTION: *What [device] can reduce bothersome background noise, magnify nearby conversation, allow you to focus on sounds you want to hear, overcome nerve deafness, and improve speech clarity?*
ANSWER: *Nothing.*

AARP SENIOR CONSUMER ALERT[1]

Medical devices include several thousand types of health products, from simple articles such as thermometers, heating pads, contact lenses, and hearing aids to complex medical equipment such as heart pacemakers, kidney dialysis machines, and lasers used for surgery. Federal laws define "medical device" as any health-care product that does not achieve any of its principal intended purposes by chemical action in or on the body or by being metabolized.[2] (Products that work by chemical or metabolic action are defined and regulated as drugs.) The term "devices" also includes laboratory equipment; diagnostic test kits; and components, parts, and accessories of medical devices. The Advanced Medical Technology Association estimates that 1999 sales in the United States totaled $62.1 billion for medical devices and $11.4 billion for diagnostic products.[3] More than 10,000 medical-device manufacturers have registered with the U.S. Food and Drug Administration (FDA).[4]

In most cases where consumers encounter a device used by or prescribed by a physician, they have little need or opportunity to make a choice. It would be pointless, for example, for a patient whose blood pressure is being checked to attempt to determine whether the instrument is designed well and calibrated properly. Nor would it be appropriate or even possible for someone undergoing general anesthesia to evaluate the quality or reliability of the anesthetist's equipment. The only practical way for consumers to protect themselves is to choose competent practitioners who presumably select and maintain their equipment properly.

This chapter emphasizes devices (and related services) about which consumers frequently make decisions: eyeglasses, contact lenses, sunglasses, hearing aids, water purifiers, humidifiers, and personal response systems. It also calls attention to the little-publicized problems of latex allergy and quack devices.

MEDICAL-DEVICE REGULATION

The FDA is responsible for device regulation. It has the extremely difficult task of trying to keep unsafe or ineffective products off the market while ensuring timely access to new ones.

FDA jurisdiction over devices began with passage in 1938 of the Food, Drug, and Cosmetic Act (FD&C Act), which required that devices be safe and labeled with adequate directions for use. Premarket approval from the FDA was not required. The burden of proving that a device was dangerous or ineffective fell upon the FDA. To stop the marketing of a dubious device, the agency often had to expend much time, effort, and expense for research and court procedures. As legitimate devices became more sophisticated and more numerous, it became clear that the 1938 law did not adequately protect the public.

The 1976 Congress amended the law to require that all devices be safe and effective, that new devices have premarket clearance, and that manufacturers bear the burden of proof. The Medical Device Amendments divided medical devices into three classes (I, II, and III) based on the principle that the greater the potential hazard, the more rigorous the regulatory requirements and the higher the class.[5] The first products banned under the 1976 law were prosthetic hair implants used to treat baldness (see Historical Perspective on page 479).

The Medical Device Reporting Act (1984) required for the first time that adverse reactions and significant malfunctions be reported to the FDA. Within the first 3 years after it took effect, 1554 device-related deaths and 21,176 nonfatal injuries were reported.[6] In 1989 the General Accounting Office reported that only about 25% of the expected number of device manufacturers had filed problem reports. FDA inspectors found that many firms were unaware of the reporting requirement, and some had records of deaths and serious injuries that had not been reported to the FDA.

After it became apparent that the 1976 law needed further reform, Congress passed the Safe Medical Devices Act of 1990. This extends the reporting requirement to hospitals, nursing homes, and outpatient facilities (except physicians' offices), and also requires notification of the manufacturer. The 1990 law also enables the FDA to order an immediate recall of any device it deems unsafe and to initiate large civil penalties for violations of the act (see Chapter 26). While underreporting of device-associated problems has decreased, the result is not entirely positive. In fiscal year (FY) 1999, the FDA received over 90,000 reports of problems associated with medical devices, far more than it can usefully manage.

The current classification system considers (a) the extent to which use of the device involves matters of life or death or serious injury and (b) whether the device is entirely new or is similar to a previously approved device. Most Class I products are subject only to the general controls that apply to all devices. These include registration of manufacturers, recordkeeping requirements, labeling requirements, and good manufacturing practice regulations. Most of the devices in this category are simple products such as bandages, tongue depressors, bedpans, dentures, orthopedic shoes, and other items in which failure is unlikely to cause serious harm. Most Class I products do not require permission from the FDA before they can be legally marketed.

Class II products are required to meet performance standards established by the FDA. However, no standards have been written. To market a new Class II

Historical Perspective

The First Banned "Device"

The first device banned under the 1976 device law was prosthetic hair fibers. Before the ban, which took effect in 1983, plastic fibers or processed human hair from another person were used as implants. The procedure consisted of implanting hundreds to thousands of fibers, cost thousands of dollars, and was usually performed by someone who was not a physician. It was unrelated to legitimate operations (described in Chapter 20) in which a person's own natural hair and surrounding tissue are grafted onto another part of the scalp.

Contrary to advertising claims, the fibers were not effective either in stimulating natural hair growth or concealing baldness. Within a short time after the operation, the fibers usually fell out, broke off, or were rejected by the body. Hundreds of people complained to federal agencies that the procedure had caused them to experience infections, facial swelling, severe pain, scarring, scalp disfigurement, or permanent loss of their remaining real hair.

The FDA had issued a public warning about the implants in 1979, but it took multiple regulatory actions by federal and state agencies to drive the procedure from the marketplace.[7]

device, a manufacturer usually must go through an approval process called "premarket notification," commonly referred to as a "510k," which is the section number of the relevant regulation. This regulatory pathway can be used for devices "substantially equivalent" to others already approved. The amount of substantiation is much less than would be required for a device that is entirely new. In FY 1999 the average time for the premarket notification approval process was 102 days. (In 1988 the average time was about 2 months.) Over 98% of the devices marketed today have gone this route.

Class III products are usually devices that are entirely new and involve life support and other critical functions. Cardiac pacemakers and heart valves are examples. Most Class III products require premarket FDA approval based on substantial evidence that they are safe and effective for their intended uses. The evidence must include human clinical trials as well as physical, scientific, biologic, and engineering tests. The average elapsed time for a premarket approval increased from about 11 months in FY 1988 to about 27 months in FY 1993, but it dropped to 7 months in the first half of FY 1999. The length, complexity, and cost of the approval process is discouraging the development of "breakthrough" products, particularly by smaller companies.

Many observers contended that the FDA's approach was too conservative, that the approval process was too slow, and that the agency lacked the resources to speed it up.[8] In 1996, to deal with its backlog, the FDA initiated a pilot program in which manufacturers of certain low- to moderate-risk devices can choose to have one of seven FDA-approved private agencies evaluate their submission. Although the FDA must still make the final decision, the agency has promised swift action on devices approved by a designated agency.

The 1997 FDA Modernization Act requires the agency to adopt the least burdensome method of getting new medical devices to market. Among other things, it requires expansion of the third-party 510(k) review program. Currently there are 12 accredited organizations, many of them overseas. While this program requires paying an independent laboratory for a something that the FDA would provide at no cost, it enables products to be marketed many months sooner.

The act also reduces the number of reported medical device problems to a manageable level. Rather than requiring that every serious incident be reported, FDA is testing a Medical Device Surveillance Network in which a small-but-representative number of user facilities would be contracted to report serious problems. The Consumer Product Safety Commission has been using such a system for many years.

While reducing regulations that affect hospitals, nursing homes, and other professional users, the FDA has increased attention to the reuse of disposable devices labeled for single use. As government and insurance reimbursement have been cut, many facilities have begun to reprocess certain single-use devices. Certain devices can be reprocessed safely. However, not all products are suitable (for example, some crevices cannot be cleaned properly), and some facilities simply don't do the job well. The FDA plans to issue regulations for devices labeled for single use.

Criticism by Congress and others of the FDA's medical-device regulation has suggested that the public is not adequately protected. Robert Mosenkis, president of CITECH (one of the FDA-designated review agencies), says this perception is not valid. Mosenkis served for many years as editor of *Health Devices,* a magazine similar to *Consumer Reports* but written for large purchasers of medical devices. He states that the quality of medical devices generally is high and that "the device industry is, overwhelmingly, very effective at policing itself, if only because of the large awards being made in liability suits." Manufacturers are also trying harder to design equipment so that health-care professionals make fewer errors when using it.[9] FDA has also placed increased emphasis on human factors, by requiring manufacturers of new devices to include and document that they have tried to design their devices so that user errors are minimized.

VISION PRODUCTS AND SERVICES

The ability to see well depends mainly on the shape of the cornea and eyeball (Figure 22-1), the status of the lens of the eye, and the condition of the retina. The common visual problems include:

NEARSIGHTEDNESS (MYOPIA) is a condition in which close objects can be seen clearly, but distant ones cannot.
FARSIGHTEDNESS (HYPEROPIA) is a condition in which distant objects are usually seen clearly, but close ones are not brought into proper focus.
ASTIGMATISM is an irregularity of the front surface (cornea) of the eye, which causes vision to be blurred at all distances.
PRESBYOPIA occurs when the lens of the eye loses its elasticity and becomes unable to focus sharply on close objects. This happens gradually as people get older and is usually noticeable in the early- to mid-40s. The change in the lens enables people with a certain amount of nearsightedness to read without glasses, but they will still need glasses for distance vision. Everyone else will need corrective lenses for reading.
CATARACTS are a clouding of the lens that distorts entering light, causing blurred or hazy vision. Cataracts usually develop slowly.
GLAUCOMA is a buildup of excess fluid within the eye, which causes pressure that can damage the optic nerve. Untreated glaucoma can cause blindness.
AGE-RELATED MACULAR DEGENERATION is an irreversible disorder in which the light-sensing cells in the macula (central zone of the retina) deteriorate, leading to loss of central and detailed vision.

The degree of sharpness of *visual acuity* is expressed as a fraction. The normal value, 20/20, means that the person can see clearly at 20 feet what the average person can see at 20 feet. Someone with 20/100 vision would have to be as close as 20 feet to see what someone with normal vision could see at 100 feet. The legal definition of blindness is vision that cannot be corrected to better than 20/200. About half the people in America and about 95% of those over the age of 45 wear glasses or contact lenses.

Friedlander and Donev[10] note that corrective lenses do not "strengthen" or "weaken" the eyes and do not make the wearer "addicted" to wearing glasses. They also note that people rarely develop headaches because they need glasses, and that the few who do usually are farsighted and went for prolonged periods without wearing glasses.

Eye-Care Professionals

The three main types of professionals involved in vision care are ophthalmologists, optometrists, and opticians.

Ophthalmologists are physicians who have completed several years of postgraduate residency training. Unlike optometrists, they can perform surgery and have full prescribing privileges. Some ophthalmologists restrict their practice to the medical and surgical

---

Historical Perspective

A Deluded Physician

William Horatio Bates received his M.D. degree from Cornell University in 1885. He was an attending physician at the New York Eye Infirmary and taught ophthalmology at the New York Postgraduate School from 1886 to 1891. In 1920 Dr. Bates wrote *Cure of Imperfect Eyesight by Treatment without Glasses.* He stated (incorrectly) that the lens of the eye was not a factor in accommodation, and that refractive errors were simply "strain due to an abnormal condition of the mind" that could be helped through various prescribed eye exercises. He also advocated looking directly at the sun for short moments to "strengthen" the eyes. Although his methods have no validity, they are still advocated by a few practitioners today. Staring directly into the sun can seriously damage the retina.

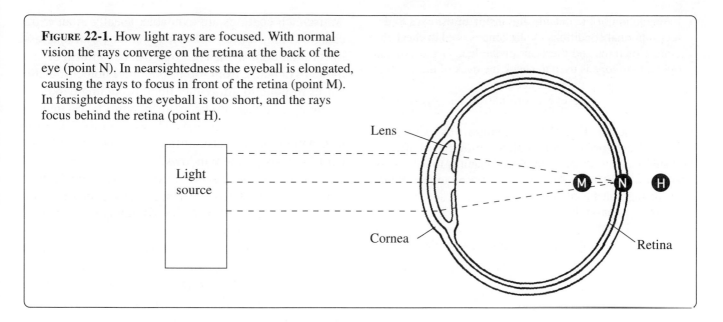

FIGURE 22-1. How light rays are focused. With normal vision the rays converge on the retina at the back of the eye (point N). In nearsightedness the eyeball is elongated, causing the rays to focus in front of the retina (point M). In farsightedness the eyeball is too short, and the rays focus behind the retina (point H).

treatment of the eye. Increasing numbers, however, are refracting eyes and selling eyeglasses and contact lenses.

Optometrists (O.D.s) are trained to examine the eyes and related structures to detect vision problems, eye disease, and other abnormalities. They principally perform vision examinations for the purpose of prescribing glasses and contact lenses. Optometrists do not perform surgery but can use diagnostic drugs as part of the eye examination. In 46 states they are also permitted to use drugs to treat certain eye diseases. Most optometrists are graduates of one of the 16 accredited colleges of optometry in the United States. Admission to these schools requires a minimum of 3 years of undergraduate work, although, as in medicine, few matriculants have less than a baccalaureate degree. This is followed by 4 years of optometry school. Two states require a 6-month internship. In all states, passage of a state board examination is required. Currently there are about 29,000 practicing optometrists in the United States, nearly 70% of whom belong to the American Optometric Association.

Opticians are technicians who make and fit eyeglasses and contact lenses as prescribed by optometrists and ophthalmologists. Opticians do not examine eyes and are not legally authorized to prescribe lenses. They may be trained through apprenticeship or a 2-year community college or vocational school program and are licensed in about half the states. The American Board of Opticianry/National Contact Lens Examiners offers certification in dispensing opticianry and contact lens–fitting. Licensing and board certification may indicate that an optician has had appropriate training, but they do not guarantee this.

Professional Evaluation

The American Optometric Association (AOA) recommends a yearly examination for everyone from preschool to age 25, exams every 2 years between ages 25 and 35, and annual exams for those 35 and older. This timetable will enable detection of some changes that have not become apparent to the individual, such as the early stages of presbyopia. However, people with no known eye problems can have their vision checked less often.

The U.S. Preventive Services Task Force (USPSTF)[11] has concluded: (a) there is insufficient evidence to support or discourage routine screening of children and young adults for visual impairment; (b) recommendations against such screening can be made on grounds such as cost, inconvenience, and the fact that refractive errors are readily correctable when they produce symptoms; (c) routine screening is recommended for elderly patients; and (d) the optimal frequency for visual acuity screening is unknown and should be left to clinical discretion. The USPSTF also recommends that people at high risk for developing glaucoma undergo periodic screening. This recommendation applies to African-Americans over 40, all people over 65, people with diabetes or severe nearsightedness, and people with a family history of glaucoma.

A complete eye examination usually takes 30 to 45 minutes, costs $40 to $60, and includes:

• A review of the patient's general health and eye history. The presence of diabetes or high blood pressure is significant because they can damage retinal blood vessels if not controlled.

- Examination of the outside and inside of the eyes to detect abnormal conditions. A slit lamp is used to check the outer structures and the front of the lens of the eye. An ophthalmoscope is used to check the back of the eye (the retina and part of the optic nerve).
- Tests to determine eye coordination and eye-muscle function.
- Measurement of the eye's fluid pressure to check for glaucoma. This is usually done with an air-puff machine.
- Visual acuity testing to determine the ability to see clearly at various distances. An eye chart is used to test distant vision; a printed card is used to test near vision (the ability to read small print).
- Visual field testing to check peripheral vision. The doctor may do this by asking whether you can see the doctor's fingers as they move to various locations near your head. Mechanized testing is also available.
- Refraction to determine which lenses can correct your vision problem. This is usually done with a Phoropter, a device that you look through while the doctor switches lenses to determine which ones enable you to see the best.

Selection of Eyeglasses

When eyes have been examined and glasses are indicated, the doctor prepares a prescription for the appropriate type of lenses. Glasses may be purchased from an ophthalmologist, optometrist, or optician. The cost of ordinary glasses depends on the nature of the lenses, the type of frame, and the vendor's markup. The most variable factor in the price of eyeglasses is the frame. These often are sold for twice their wholesale cost and can cost $200 or more, while the lenses often cost $100 or more, depending on the features desired. Some chains have discount outlets that offer complete glasses for considerably less.

Lenses are made of plastic, glass, or a laminated combination of plastic and glass. Most lenses today are plastic. The FDA requires that all lenses be resistant to shattering on impact. Plastic lenses are more easily scratched but weigh less and are break-resistant.

 Consumer Tip

Shopping for Eyeglasses

- Obtain a thorough examination by a competent ophthalmologist or optometrist.
- The FTC Eyeglass Rule requires that consumers receive a copy of the prescription. This makes it possible to shop to compare prices.
- Wear the glasses for a few days, and have them checked if they do not feel right.
- If the glasses seem defective, do not hesitate to ask the vendor to rectify the problem.

Antiscratch coatings are available, usually at an extra charge. Tinting is available in many colors, with sunglass tints for outdoor wear. The color can be uniform or can lighten gradually from top to bottom. Photochromatic lenses respond to ultraviolet light, becoming darker in sunlight and lighter in shade. Such lenses take a minute or two to make their changes. They do not work as well in an automobile because sufficient ultraviolet light may not filter through the windows.

About half the lenses sold yearly are bifocals (two lenses in one), trifocals (three lenses in one), or progressives (multifocal with no dividing line between different portions of the lens). These lenses enable people to focus sharply at more than one distance. It is important that glasses be checked by the doctor or office staff after they have been received from the dispenser to be certain that the prescription has been accurately filled.

Ready-to-wear reading glasses are available in many stores for $10 to $15. These come in different strengths and can be tried out in the store. They may be adequate (though not optimal) for people who are nearsighted or presbyopic and have no astigmatism. They should not be used as a substitute for periodic professional examinations.

In 1997 *Consumer Reports*[12] published the results of a survey of about 55,000 of its subscribers who had purchased prescription glasses within the previous 2 years. The survey showed (a) readers were slightly more satisfied when they bought their glasses from independent opticians, private optometrists, and ophthalmologists rather than from large optical chain stores; (b) examinations by ophthalmologists and private optometrists generally were more thorough; (c) nearly one third paid more than expected; (d) the average cost at big chains ($160) was lower than the average at private offices ($171); (e) the three chains rating highest in customer satisfaction (Costco Wholesale, For Eyes, and Shopko Optical), also had the lowest prices; and (f) about 12% of those who used a big chain store had to return at least once because of a problem such as an improperly fitting frame or a loose lens.

Prescription glasses can be purchased by mail. This is unwise, however. Frames often need an adjustment to fit properly. This and other problems are much more easily handled at a local source.

Contact Lenses

Contact lenses are plastic or glass discs worn in front of the pupil and in contact with the cornea. They adhere to the cornea by capillary action on the normal layer of tear fluids. Not everyone can wear them, and they do

Refractive Surgery

It is possible to permanently alter the refractive state of the eye by making appropriate incisions in the cornea. These incisions change the shape of the cornea and enable light rays to converge properly on the retina. Various operations can reduce or correct nearsightedness, farsightedness, and astigmatism.

Modern refractive surgery became popular in the United States through radial keratotomy (RK), which was introduced from Russia in the early 1980s. In this operation, incisions made in the outer part of the cornea cause the central part of the cornea to flatten, which can correct a mild degree of nearsightedness.

Initially, even though the procedure looked promising, many eye surgeons cautioned that there were no long-term data showing that the procedure was safe and likely to improve vision permanently. Many authorities also objected to the idea of surgery being performed on healthy eyes when the use of eyeglasses or contact lenses could enable them to see adequately.

In 1990 the *Journal of the American Medical Association* published the Prospective Evaluation of Radial Keratotomy (PERK) study of about 400 patients, most of whom had been followed for 4 years.[13] About two thirds of the patients achieved their goal of eliminating glasses or contact lenses, and nearly all of the others improved considerably.[14] No severe complications occurred. Many patients reported seeing radiating light (glare) around light sources such as headlights or street lights at night. In most cases this diminished as time went on. Most patients reported that it did not interfere with their normal activities, but some said it interfered severely with night driving. A 10-year follow-up study of 374 of the patients found that 70% said they did not use corrective lenses for distance vision and 53% had 20/20 vision without glasses.[15]

We now know that the accuracy of the operation can be increased by varying the incisions according to the patient's age. In 1993 the American Academy of Ophthalmology noted that about 10% of ophthalmologists were doing RK, that hundreds of thousands of procedures had been performed, and that the operation usually improved the vision of patients with non-progressive low and moderate amounts of near-sightedness.[16] Today RK is used mostly for refractive errors of 4.00 diopters or less. The required incisions are small and far enough from the center of the cornea that postoperative glare is uncommon.

Newer techniques involving computerized assessment, precisely calculated cutting patterns, and lasers have made refractive keratotomy more predictable. Computerized topography can be used preoperatively

to determine the best procedure and postoperatively to determine whether additional correction might be indicated. The newer operations include the following.

Photorefractive keratotomy (PRK): An excimer laser is used to correct up to 6.00 diopters of nearsightedness. The correction is fairly precise, but not completely predictable. The recovery period varies, and the final refractive state may not be known for 3 to 6 months. During the procedure, the corneal surface is removed, which means that the eye will be very painful for a few days until the cornea regrows. Haziness of the cornea (with cloudy vision) is common after a few months, but goes away eventually in most cases.

Automated lamellar keratoplasty (ALK): The cornea is reshaped by a precise mechanical instrument that peels an outer flap and then removes a calculated amount of material from underneath. The flap is then put back into place. This operation can correct high degrees of nearsightedness (up to 20.00 or more diopters) and works well in most cases. Since the corneal surface is not removed, there is little if any postoperative discomfort, and postoperative glare is uncommon.

Laser in-situ keratomileusis (LASIK): The first corneal flap is made as in ALK, and an extremely precise underlying cut is made with an excimer laser. LASIK techniques can be used to correct astigmatism and farsightedness as well as myopia. The results are nearly always predictable, there is no postoperative discomfort, and glare is uncommon. The operations is preferred by eye surgeons throughout the world who have sufficient experience and have access to the necessary equipment. Several eye-surgery centers in the United States have FDA approval to perform LASIK, and some individual ophthalmologists have acquired unapproved but high-quality devices through foreign channels.

For people who are severely nearsighted, an alternative approach is replacement of their natural lens with an artificial lens which is more appropriately shaped.

People contemplating refractive surgery should discuss the potential benefits and risks with an ophthalmologist who is well regarded by the medical and optometric communities. Although the procedures have a low incidence of complications, the risk involved may not justify their use if adequate vision can be achieved with eyeglasses or contact lenses. Individuals who wish to have laser surgery should seek someone who is well trained and thoroughly experienced.

Herbert J. Nevyas, M.D.
Clinical Professor of Ophthalmology
Medical College of Pennsylvania

not correct all vision problems. Except for extreme near-sightedness, vision is no better with contacts than with regular glasses. Many individuals use them for cosmetic reasons, and they also serve a useful purpose in athletics.

Friedlander and Donev describe the history of contact lens development in their book *20/20: A Guide to Improving Your Vision and Preventing Eye Disease*.[1] Modern contact lenses developed after it was understood that the outer covering of the eye (cornea) required a steady supply of oxygen from the air. This led to development of lightweight glass lenses small enough to permit oxygen dissolved in the tears to reach the underlying cornea. In the late 1950s a soft plastic lens was created that was flexible, absorbed water, and permitted the cornea to breathe more normally. Extended-wear lenses introduced in the 1970s were more convenient but turned out to cause potentially serious infections if not properly cleaned. The more recently developed gas-permeable lenses permit more oxygen to reach the cornea and are less prone to cause infections. Disposable extended-wear contacts offer the same advantages plus additional convenience.

The prices charged for contact lenses include the cost of the lenses, the amount of time spent to fit them and to provide follow-up care, the nature of the warranty, and the value of the services as determined by the practitioner. Prices may or may not include the initial examination, the fitting, follow-up care, a good lens-care kit, or a good warranty. Many sellers guarantee to issue a refund or furnish a pair of glasses if the buyer is unable to adapt to the use of contacts.

Hard lenses and gas-permeable lenses are the most economical and durable. Soft lenses are most comfortable and can be worn longer but their care is more difficult. Table 22-1 summarizes the advantages and disadvantages of currently marketed contact lenses.

Examinations for prescribing contact lenses are conducted by optometrists and ophthalmologists. They include tests for corneal sensitivity and lacrimal (tear) secretion, a refraction to determine the strength of the lenses, and measurement of the eye's curvature to determine the type of lens needed. The FTC's "Eyeglass Rule" requires the eye specialist to give a copy of the prescription to the patient when requested after the examination.

Once contact lenses have been purchased, the directions for use, maintenance, storage, and cleaning should be followed scrupulously. Serious infections and

Table 22-1

COMPARISON OF CONTACT LENSES

Lens Type	Advantages	Disadvantages
Rigid gas-permeable (RGP) Made of slightly flexible plastics that allow oxygen to pass through to the eyes.	Excellent vision; short adaptation period; comfortable to wear; correct most vision problems; easy to put on and to care for; durable with a relatively long life; available in tints (for handling purpose) and bifocals.	Require consistent wear to maintain adaptation; can slip off center of eye more easily than other types.
Daily wear soft Made of soft flexible plastics that allow oxygen to pass through to the eyes.	Very short adaptation period; more comfortable and more difficult to dislodge than RGP lenses; available in tints and bifocals; great for active lifestyles.	Do not correct all vision problems; vision may not be as sharp as with RGP lenses; require careful cleaning and care; need replacement at least annually.
Extended-wear Available for overnight wear in soft or RGP lenses.	Can usually be worn up to 7 days without removal.	Do not correct all vision problems; require regular office visits for follow-up care; must be replaced at least annually.
Disposable soft Soft lenses worn for 1 to 2 weeks, and then discarded.	Require little or no cleaning; minimal risk of eye infection if wearing instructions are followed; available in tints and bifocals; spare lenses available.	Vision may not be as sharp as RGP lenses; do not correct all vision problems; handling may be more difficult.
Planned replacement soft Soft daily wear lenses that are replaced on a planned schedule, most often either every 2 weeks, monthly, or quarterly.	Require simplified cleaning and disinfection; good for eye health; available in most prescriptions.	Vision may not be as sharp as RGP lenses; do not correct all vision problems; handling may be more difficult.

Source: American Optometric Association.[17,18]

damage to the eye can result from improper maintenance and from wearing lenses for longer periods than recommended.

Sunglasses

Many studies have shown that prolonged exposure to the sun's rays increases the chances of developing cataracts, retinal degeneration, cancer of the eyelids, and photokeratitis, a temporary but painful burn of the eye's surface (sometimes called snow blindness or welder's flash).[19] The sun's glare can also interfere with comfort and the ability to see clearly. Reducing glare can make driving and outdoor recreational and occupational activities safer.

The American Optometric Association (AOA) says that sunglasses have gone from a fashion accessory to a necessity. There are three main types. *Polaroid* lenses cut glare and are especially useful when driving or boating. *Photochromatic* lenses change color with varying light intensity. *Mirrored* lenses reflect rather than absorb light and are primarily useful when there is intense glare from snow or water. However, they show dirt and are hard to clean.

The AOA advises consumers to insist that sunglasses block out at least 99% of ultraviolet radiation; screen out at least 75% of visible light; be perfectly matched in color and free of distortion; and have lenses that are gray (the preferable color), green, or brown.[20] Prescription lenses may be advisable for people with vision problems, but clip-on or overfitting sunglasses may be an acceptable substitute.

Color can be checked by looking at the glasses against a white background. Distortion can be observed by holding them at arm's length and looking through them with one eye at something with a rectangular pattern. Any distortion will be apparent as the glasses are moved back and forth or rotated. To be sure the lenses block enough light, try them on in front of a mirror. If your eyes are clearly visible through the lenses, the lenses are probably are not dark enough for glare reduction and comfort. This test does not apply to photochromatic lenses.

In 1988 *Consumer Reports* tested more than 180 pairs of nonprescription sunglasses with prices that ranged from $2 to nearly $200. The investigators found little relation between price and quality.[21]

Pinhole Glasses

Many entrepreneurs have marketed "pyramid" or "pinhole" glasses consisting of opaque material with multiple slits or perforations. The mechanism involved has been known for centuries and was used before glass lenses were invented. Light passing through a small hole (or holes) is restricted to rays coming straight from the viewed object; these rays do not need focusing to bring them to a point. Modern promoters claim their products are better than conventional lenses. Worrall[22] states that although both reduce the focus effort needed to read, pinhole glasses are much less useful because they restrict contrast, brightness, and the field of view. Worn as sunglasses, they can even be harmful because the holes allow damaging ultraviolet rays to reach the eye.

In 1992 the Missouri Attorney General obtained a consent injunction and penalties totaling $20,000 against a New York company that sold "aerobic glasses." These glasses, which sold for $19.95 plus postage and handling, had black plastic lenses with tiny holes. The company's ads had falsely claimed that its "Aerobic Training Eyeglass System exercises and relaxes the eye muscles through use of scientifically designed and spaced 'pin dot' openings that change the way light enters the eye." The ads claimed that the glasses would help nearsightedness, farsightedness, astigmatism, and presbyopia, and that wearing them and doing eye exercises would enable users to change to weaker prescription lenses and possibly eliminate the need to wear glasses.

Cataract Surgery

A cataract is an opacity of the lens of the eye that impairs vision. The cause is unknown, but diabetes and exposure to ultraviolet light are important factors. Low dietary intake of antioxidant vitamins may also be a factor.[23,24] Cataracts can cause double or blurred vision, sensitivity to light and glare, less vivid perception of color, and frequent changes in eyeglass prescription. Cataracts develop in about 400,000 Americans each year, but most remain small and never need treatment.

Cataract surgery is the most frequently performed operation on people age 65 or older. More than 1 million cataract extractions are performed each year. During the operation, the lens is removed from its supporting capsule either by pushing it out or by phacoemulsification (shattering it with ultrasound and sucking out the remnants). A plastic intraocular lens is then placed inside. The procedure takes 20 to 30 minutes and does not require hospitalization. About 95% of patients emerge with better than 20/40 vision with eyeglasses (the minimum required for a driver's license). Eyeglasses are still needed for reading because the inflexible lens focuses at only one point, usually in the distance.

The operations are not risk-free. A small percentage of patients develop swelling or detachment of the retina, glaucoma, infection, or displacement of the intraocular lens. About one third of patients develop clouding of the lens capsule, which can be remedied by cutting a hole through the capsule with a laser. *Consumer Reports on Health* cautions against having the operation unless a cataract hampers daily activities. This usually does not occur unless a person's visual acuity drops to 20/50 with glasses.[25]

HEARING AIDS

Hearing loss affects about 28 million Americans, about half of whom are over the age of 50. In 1995 the International Hearing Society estimated that about 6 million Americans use a hearing aid, but many more people who could benefit do not do so. The reasons for not using a hearing aid include (a) lack of awareness of problem, (b) cost, (c) not wishing to call attention to disability, (d) dealer practices, (e) sounds when amplified are still not clear, (f) difficulty in manipulating controls, and (g) not knowing where to go for help.[26,27]

Hearing loss is most common among the elderly. One person in four over 65 years and one in three over 75 years experience this problem. Noise-induced hearing loss is common among young and middle-aged people exposed to high levels of noise from sources such as motorcycles, snowmobiles, powerboats, radios with headphones, poorly designed telephones, live rock band music, and other types of occupational exposure.[28]

Types of Hearing Loss

There are two types of hearing loss: sensorineural and conductive. Sensorineural deafness, also called perceptive or nerve deafness, is caused by damage to the auditory nerve, which connects the inner part of the ear to the brain. Nerve deafness can result from birth defects, illnesses that produce a high fever, overexposure to high noise levels, use of certain medications, head injuries, vascular problems, and tumors. Nerve deafness often is related to aging and is the most common reason for using a hearing aid.

In conductive deafness, which is less common, sound waves cannot be transmitted to the auditory nerve. Conductive deafness is related to the outer and middle portions of the ear and can be caused by (a) impacted wax in the external ear; (b) injury to the eardrum by an explosion, blow to the ear, infection, or sharp implement; or (c) arthritic disease, middle ear infection (otitis media), and other condition that prevents the three tiny bones of the inner ear from vibrating.

Some individuals have "mixed" hearing loss—both conductive and sensorineural. Elderly individuals with a hearing loss often have damage to the auditory nerve as well as a defect in the ear mechanism that relays sound to that nerve. Some impairments can be medically or surgically treated. If there is partial hearing, a hearing aid may be effective.

People with a hearing loss may find that words are difficult to distinguish; sounds seem muffled or subdued; and high-pitched sounds, such as the ticking of a watch, dripping of a faucet, or high tones of a musical instrument, are difficult or impossible to hear. Other signs of possible impairment include asking people to repeat themselves, turning up the volume of a radio or television set, favoring one ear, or straining to hear. Many people with a hearing loss also have tinnitus (continual hissing or ringing of their ears). If a hearing loss is suspected, a physician should be consulted. In most cases an evaluation by an otolaryngologist is advisable.

Professional Evaluation

An evaluation for suspected hearing loss should include (a) a review of the symptoms and past medical history, (b) examination of the ears and throat, (c) an audiometric test, and (d) other special tests as needed. Audiometry is performed in a soundproof room, usually by an audiologist. Some otolaryngologists employ one in their office, whereas others refer the patient elsewhere. During the test, various tones and levels of sound are transmitted to the patient through an earphone. The patient signals to the tester which sounds are heard, and the tester records the information on a graph (audiogram). The information is analyzed and the hearing level, measured in decibels (dB), is established. When all tests are completed, the otolaryngologist informs the patient of the nature and extent of the problem, if any, and whether a hearing aid might be helpful.

Some common sounds and their decibel values include: rustling leaves (20 dB), whisper at 5 feet (30 dB), conversational speech at 3 feet (60 dB), loud radio music (65 dB), shouted speech (90 dB), a loud amplified rock band (110 dB), and a jet engine at 100 feet (140 dB). Hearing loss is also expressed in decibels. Someone with a 30 dB loss, for example, could not hear someone 5 feet away who is whispering. Table 22-2 indicates how the levels of dB loss relate to the possible usefulness of a hearing aid.

Types of Hearing Aids

A hearing aid is a miniature, battery-powered, amplifier system with a microphone that picks up sound waves and a speaker that sends them to the ear canal.

Table 22-2

SIGNIFICANCE OF HEARING LOSS LEVELS

Level of Loss	Description	Effect	Need for Hearing Aid
25 to 40 decibels	Mild	Difficulty understanding normal speech	Needed in some situations
41 to 55 decibels	Moderate	Difficulty understanding loud speech	Frequently needed
56 to 80 decibels	Severe	Can understand only amplified speech	Needed for all communication
81 or more decibels	Profound	Difficulty understanding amplified speech	May need to supplement hearing aid with lip-reading, aural rehabilitation, or sign language.

Source: American Association of Retired Persons.[29]

Monaural systems serve one ear, while binaural systems serve both. To benefit from a hearing aid it is necessary to have some degree of hearing. Most hearing aids work similarly, although their designs differ somewhat. Because hearing losses vary in pattern and severity, no single hearing aid is right for everyone. There are four commonly used types: (1) behind the ear, (2) in the ear, (3) in the canal, and (4) completely in the canal. Behind-the-ear models, which are the largest type, are best for people with limited dexterity who would have difficulty adjusting the controls, cleaning the device, or changing the batteries on smaller models.

Hearing aids range from about $700 to several thousand dollars. Hundreds of models are available. The price depends mainly on the sophistication of the electronic circuitry. Multichannel adaptive models can be set to amplify certain frequencies and lower the volume of others. Digital programmable models can be adjusted through a computer hookup. Digital sound models use a microprocessor to provide the "cleanest" sound possible.

Rezen and Hausman[30] have noted that some dealers charge twice as much for two hearing aids as they do for one. If the price for one includes compensation for the dealer's time, doubling it is unfair because it takes no more time to provide instruction for two than it does to provide instruction for one. They suggest asking the dealer how much each component of the sales package costs.

Selecting a Hearing Aid
Hearing aid dealers sell, lease, or rent equipment. They conduct hearing tests for selection and fitting, encourage prospective users to try amplification, make impressions for ear models, counsel the hearing-impaired on

ways to adapt to the aid, and repair malfunctioning hearing aids. The best way to select a dealer is probably through a physician's recommendation. Your family doctor or an otolaryngologist may be able to make a suitable recommendation. Some otolaryngologists employ a qualified person in their office who fits hearing aids.

All states require that hearing aid sellers be licensed. Dealers certified by the National Board of Hearing Instrument Specialists can use the letters BC-HIS after their name. The International Hearing Society also has a certification program (National Board for Certification in Hearing Instrument Sciences) and can provide the names of local dealers. Information can also be obtained from American Speech-Language-Hearing Association. Although hearing aids have been marketed door-to-door and by telephone (sometimes with a survey or prize offer), accepting such a solicitation is senseless because reputable dealers do not solicit this way.

Before visiting a dealer, it may be helpful to visit a local noncommercial hearing aid center. Such centers are usually connected with a hospital and are staffed by qualified personnel who help to determine the proper type of hearing aid. They do not sell hearing aids, but they recommend specific brands and models and will also check what a consumer purchases to be sure it is appropriate. *Consumer Reports* recommends avoiding dealers who sell only one brand of hearing aid.[31]

Obtaining a proper fit may require several visits to the dealer. Adjusting to the device may take weeks or months. Before purchasing, it is prudent to rent it for a trial period. Many manufacturers offer a trial rental or purchase-option plan, usually for 30 days.

Buyers should not be influenced solely by the price or appearance of a hearing aid, but should obtain answers to these questions:

- What is the quality of the sound?
- Does the aid help you to understand speech in quiet places? In noisy places?
- Is the aid comfortable to wear?
- Are the tone and volume controls easy enough to operate?
- Does the price include the initial testing, the device itself, the fitting, and follow-up costs? If a device proves unsatisfactory, what costs will be involved if it is returned?
- Who will provide maintenance and repair services? What will they cost?
- What are the warranty terms?
- Does the dealer offer an aural rehabilitation program (a program that teaches how to use facial expression and other visual cues to help interpret what people say)?

Government Regulation

The hearing aid industry has a long history of making deceptive claims for its products. Between 1934 and 1976 the Federal Trade Commission secured orders, consent decrees, or voluntary compliance agreements against manufacturers or sellers in 66 cases.

Since 1977 FDA regulations have imposed certain conditions for the sale of hearing aids. The hearing aid dispenser must obtain a written physician's statement that the patient has been medically evaluated and that the patient is considered a candidate for a hearing aid. The evaluation must have occurred no longer than 6 months before the date of sale. The dispenser must give the patient written instructions for the hearing aid selected and make sure that the patient understands them. Patients over 18 may waive the medical evaluation requirement, but the dispenser is required to warn them beforehand that it is not in their best interest to do so. Patients under the age of 18 must be medically evaluated before a sale can be legally made.

Patients must also be advised to consult a physician or ear specialist if any of the following conditions are discovered: visible congenital deformity of the ear; history of active drainage from the ear within the previous 90 days; acute or chronic dizziness; one-sided hearing loss within the previous 90 days; evidence of wax accumulation or the presence of a foreign body in the ear canal; pain or discomfort in the ear; or an audiometric airborne gap equal to or greater than 15 dB at tonal frequencies of 500 Hz, 1000 Hz, and 2000 Hz.

In 1993 an official of the American Academy of Otolaryngology–Head and Neck Surgery testified at a Senate hearing that the waiver requirement had questionable value because 85% of first-time hearing aid purchasers had signed a waiver.[32]

In 1993 the FDA told eight major hearing aid manufacturers and distributors to stop making misleading claims about their products.[33] The companies included Dahlberg, Inc., Electone, Inc., Siemens Hearing Instruments, Omni Hearing Systems,, Starkey Laboratories, Inc., and Beltone Electronics Corp. All had advertised that their hearing aids would help users discriminate between background noise and speech and would improve the user's ability to hear words in noisy places. During the same year, the FTC obtained consent decrees barring seven hearing aid retailers from continuing to falsely imply in advertisements that Medicare would cover the cost of hearing aids.

In 1994 the FTC and 36 state attorneys general sued Dahlberg, Inc., in a Minnesota court. The FTC case was resolved by a consent decree that involved a $2.75 million penalty. The state cases were resolved by an agreement in which Dahlberg paid $700,000; promised to stop making unsubstantiated claims; and pledged to disclose that the benefit of hearing aids may depend on proper fit, degree of hearing loss, and accuracy of patient evaluation. The company had advertised that the Miracle-Ear *Clarifier* (a) contained a filter system that reduced low-frequency noise to make conversations easier to hear, even in noisy situations, and (b) adjusted automatically so that the user could go from a quiet conversation in one room into a noisy room without having to adjust the amplification.

◆ Personal Glimpse ◆

Negative Ion Therapy

Ions are atoms or groups of atoms bearing electrical charges. Positive ions lack one or more electrons; negative ones possess a surplus of electrons. Polluted air may be lower in negative ions and higher in positive ions. Weather conditions can also affect ion concentrations. According to folklore, an excess of positive ions can cause a variety of physical and emotional problems.

Proponents of negative ion therapy (aeroionotherapy) claim that illness can be prevented by neutralizing positive ions with negative ones produced by small generators. But negative ion generators cannot actually produce enough ions to change the air in a room effectively. Ions have a short half-life; their energy dissipates rapidly as they leave the generators. Scientific studies carried out during the past 20 years have failed to support the claims of negative ion proponents. Moreover, the generators may produce toxic amounts of ozone.

Wallace I. Sampson, M.D.[34]

DUBIOUS WATER PURIFIER PROMOTIONS

Water treatment devices may be useful for removing contaminant or improving the water's taste.[35] However, the water treatment business has been rife with fraud. Companies that offer free testing of home water supplies for "contamination" are interested in selling water-treatment devices whether needed or not. *Consumer Reports*[36] has noted that some in-home demonstrators add chemicals to a prospective customer's tap water to change its color or to form particles that supposedly indicate contamination.

Some entrepreneurs try to sell devices without having the water tested. Multilevel marketers typically cite a few localized problems to suggest that water pollution is widespread. Other entrepreneurs notify large numbers of people by mail or telephone that they have been selected to win a prize. To "qualify," they are required to purchase a water treatment device or other products costing hundreds of dollars. The price is invariably more than similar merchandise would cost if obtained from a legitimate firm. In many cases no device is delivered. Regardless, it is never a good idea to reveal your credit card number to an unfamiliar solicitor.

A 1999 federal law now requires water utilities serving more than 10,000 people to explain what is in the water exiting their water-treatment plant and whether it is within government safety limits. People with further concerns can call the Environmental Protection Agency (EPA)'s Safe Drinking Water Hotline [800 426-4791] or consult their local or state health department or a state-certified laboratory. A free booklet, "Is Your Drinking Water Safe," is available from the EPA. The FTC[37] and others have offered the following additional tips:

- If your tap water meets current federal standards, there is no need to consider drinking bottled water. The *University of California at Berkeley Wellness Letter*[38] stated that many people drink bottled water because they think it is "healthier" and "purer." About 25% of the bottled water in the United States comes from tap water and municipal systems.
- *If you have reason to be concerned, obtain an independent opinion.* Ask the local water authority for the latest test of your community's water supply. If you have your own supply, ask the local or state health department whether free testing is available; most will test for bacterial contents. A consumer can also engage a private laboratory that is certified by the state health department or the state environmental agency. Tests for bacteria are inexpensive, but tests for chemicals can cost hundreds or even thousands of dollars, depending on the depth of the analysis. *Consumer Reports* has identified two mail-order laboratories it considers reliable: National Testing Laboratories [800 458-3330] and Suburban Water Testing Laboratories [800 433-6595].
- *If a problem is found, carefully decide what you need.* There are many water purifiers, ranging from simple filter devices for a kitchen faucet to expensive sophisticated systems. No device can solve every problem. Ask the testing firm or a local government official what system would be best for your problem.
- *Avoid "free" home water tests.* Checking for acidity/alkalinity, iron, manganese, or color is meaningless because none of these is harmful. Home testing cannot provide the in-depth analysis required to determine whether water actually needs treatment or what type of system would be best.
- *Comparison shop.* See "Home Water Treatment Units,"[39] a brochure the FTC developed with cooperation with the Environmental Agency.
- *Be wary of claims of government approval.* The government does not endorse water tests, water treatment, or purification systems. An EPA registration number merely indicates the product has been registered with the EPA.

All bottled waters are now strictly regulated by the EPA and the FDA for purity and safety. Genuine spring water is always identified as such.

HUMIDIFIERS

A humidifier may help relieve a dry, hacking cough or discomfort from an acute respiratory infection or dry air, especially in the winter heating season. However, harmful bacteria and molds can multiply in the water tank of a humidifier and be blown into the air. For this reason humidifiers should be cleaned daily and disinfected weekly.

Consumer Reports notes that each type of humidifier has some drawbacks. Ultrasonic models, now rare, can spew an annoying white dust. Cool-mist models can do the same unless the water is demineralized. Steam-mist models (vaporizers) can scald people who get too close to them. Steam- and warm-mist models use a large amount of electricity. Evaporative models can breed bacteria.[40]

Tabletop models can handle one or two rooms. Console models can raise humidity throughout a whole house. In-duct models require less maintenance but are considerably more expensive. The best models have a humidistat that controls the moisture level. The top-rated tabletop was Duracraft DH-904, a warm-mist model that cost $60 to $70.

Several years ago a hand-held humidifying device called the *Viralizer* was marketed with claims that it could relieve the symptoms of a cold or allergy. The device delivered a steady flow of heated air saturated with water. *Consumer Reports* investigated the evidence claimed to substantiate its use and concluded that the device was ineffective and could cause undesirable dryness and increased congestion of the nose.[41] A subsequently published double-blind study of 66 patients found that using a similar device was no more effective than inhaling ordinary room-temperature air.[42] In 1992 the manufacturer signed an FTC order prohibiting unsubstantiated claims that the *Viralizer* can eliminate, relieve, or temporarily reduce symptoms of a cold or allergy. In the future, any such claim must either be supported by at least one well-controlled, double-blind study or be approved by the FDA.

PERSONAL EMERGENCY RESPONSE SYSTEMS

A personal emergency response system (PERS) is an electronic device designed to let the user summon help in an emergency. It has three components: a small, battery-powered radio transmitter with a help button; a console connected to the user's telephone; and an emergency response center that monitors calls. When the button is pressed, it signals the console, which automatically dials one or more preprogrammed numbers. Most systems can dial out even if the telephone is off the hook. When its button is pressed, a radio signal prompts a machine connected to the telephone to call the monitoring center for help. The monitoring center usually tries to call back to find out what is wrong. If the center is unable to reach the person or help is needed, the center will try to reach a designated person (friend, family member) to follow up the call. If a medical emergency appears evident, an ambulance or other emergency provider will be dispatched

There are two types of emergency response centers. Provider-based centers usually are located in the user's local area and are operated by hospitals or social service agencies. Manufacturer-based operations usually have one national center.

The device can be purchased, rented, or leased. The purchase prices normally range from $200 to more than $1500. However, some consumers have paid several thousand dollars. There is also a small installation fee, and a monthly monitoring charge of $10 to $30. Monthly rental fees range from $15 to $50 and usually include the monitoring service. Lease agreements can be long term or can include an option to buy. Some contracts have a cancellation charge.

A local social agency might be the best source of referral to prospective vendors. The Federal Trade Commission[43] recommends the following precautions:

- Check out several systems before making a decision.
- Ask about the pricing, features, and servicing of each system, and compare costs.
- Make sure that the system is easy to use. Buttons should be easy to operate and batteries easy to change.
- Ask whether the monitoring center is available 24 hours a day, what kind of training its operators receive, and what the average response time is.
- Test to be sure that the system works from every point in and around your home. Make sure nothing interferes with transmissions.
- If unsure of a company's reputation, check with the Better Business Bureau.
- Read the written agreement carefully before signing it.

THE LATEX ALLERGY EPIDEMIC

During the past 15 years allergic reactions to latex have become a significant public health problem, particularly among health-care workers. When exposed to latex or latex dust, sensitized persons can develop hives; nasal and eye irritation; asthma; and anaphylaxis, a life-threatening condition in which the breathing passageways swell closed. About 1% of the general public and 5% to 15% of health-care workers and others exposed to latex on their jobs have become sensitized.[44-47] Some have even been forced to terminate their careers for this reason. Medical and dental procedures on sensitized individuals may be complicated by anaphylactic events, as may the use of latex pacifiers by infants. By 1997 the FDA received more than 1700 reports of severe allergic reactions and 16 reports of death associated with latex allergy.[44] Since 1998, latex-containing devices that can come in contact with humans must be labeled: "Caution: This Product Contains Natural Rubber Latex Which May Cause Allergic Reactions."[44]

Latex is a common component of disposable gloves, intravenous tubing, syringes, stethoscopes, catheters, condoms, dressings, bandages, and other medical supplies. Gloves are the most significant source because they are frequently used, and the powder used to line some of them can absorb latex proteins and become airborne. Asthmatic reactions have occurred among people who did not use gloves but merely inhaled latex-containing dust.

The increased prevalence of latex allergy has been attributed primarily to the increased use of disposable gloves to prevent the spread of AIDS and hepatitis B. Increased demand and cost pressures for gloves has led some manufacturers to shorten the manufacturing time by reducing the number of washing and purifying steps, which reduces the amount of sensitizing protein that the gloves will transmit.

Latex allergy can be suspected from the patient's history and confirmed by a skin test. People with frequent latex exposure should also be tested, even though the test entails some risk.[18] The FDA approved a test system for marketing in 1995.[44] The American Academy of Allergy, Asthma & Immunology has published guidelines and recommends that people who have been diagnosed as allergic wear an identification card (or bracelet) and a self-injectable adrenalin device.[49]

QUACK DEVICES

The FDA[50] has grouped quack devices into nine general categories. The following devices can be considered complete fakes:

- Figure enhancers, such as bust developers and spot reducers.
- Arthritis and pain relievers claimed to relieve all types of pain.
- Sleep aids claimed to produce electrical impulses that cause natural sleep.

- Mail-order sex aids claimed to cure impotence or frigidity.
- Hair and scalp devices claimed to eliminate baldness or remove unwanted hair painlessly and permanently.
- Youth prolongers claimed to eliminate wrinkles and restore youthful facial contours.
- Air purifiers claimed to destroy bacteria and TB germs and reduce the aging process.
- Disease diagnosers claimed to be capable of diagnosing all diseases or a wide variety of diseases.
- Cure-all devices claimed to be effective for diagnosing or treating a wide variety of illness.

The Historical Perspective box provides a brief account of quack devices used many years ago.

Magnetic Products

In recent years, many magnetic products have been marketed with claims that they are effective against pain and a wide variety of medical problems. Pulsed electromagnetic fields—which induce measurable electric fields—have been demonstrated effective for treating slow-healing fractures and have shown promise for a few other conditions. However, few studies have been

---

Historical Perspective

Electrical Fakery

Elisha Perkins, a practicing physician from Connecticut, announced the invention of his Perkins Metallic Tractors in 1796. These were two rods of brass and iron about 3 inches long, rounded at one end and pointed at the other. At that time, electricity was considered a powerful force despite little knowledge of its properties. Having observed during surgery that muscles may contract when touched by a metallic instrument, Perkins concluded that metallic substances influenced nerves and muscles. He announced that his tractors could draw diseases from the body and could help against inflammation; rheumatism; and pains in the head, face, and breast. Although the state medical society expressed skepticism, the Chief Justice of the Supreme Court bought a pair and President Washington was a customer and wrote letters recommending the treatment.

In 1799, after spending several weeks combating a yellow fever outbreak in New York City, Perkins caught the disease and died. His son Benjamin continued selling the device in England until a physician discovered that rubbing patients with wooden rods was equally effective and concluded that the curative agent was the patient's imagination.[51]

Dr. Albert Abrams became professor of pathology at Cooper Medical College in San Francisco and in 1889 was appointed vice president of the California State Medical Society. His 1910 book, *Spondylotherapy,* theorized that the reflex center in the spinal cord could be stimulated by rapid percussion (tapping). He said that every disease had a vibratory rate and could be diagnosed by tapping the spine and abdomen to discover the patient's disease frequency. He claimed he could determine the severity and exact location of any ailment.

Abrams also claimed he could determine a person's age, sex, and even religion from a drop of blood and could diagnose ailments from a handwriting sample. Later he introduced the reflexophone and said he could diagnose a person's condition by telephone. Another of his devices was the oscilloclast, a sealed box with a rheostat, condenser, ohmmeter, and various wires. He claimed that the device would cure by sending into the body electrical waves that duplicated the rate of disease vibrations. Actually it was a galvanometer that reflected the amount of perspiration on the patient's skin. Traveling around the country, Abrams taught courses that enabled several thousand chiropractors, naturopaths, and others to become electronic practitioners."[52] Abrams got little attention until an attack in the *Journal of the American Medical Association* made him a cause célèbre and spurred unorthodox practitioners to clamor for his devices.[51]

A blue-ribbon committee created by *Scientific American* magazine investigated Abrams and concluded

Historical Perspective

Electrical Fakery – *Cont'd.*

that his methods were "at best an illusion, at worst a colossal fraud." When he died in 1924, Abrams left several million dollars to his Electronic Medical Foundation to perpetuate the devices. Some continued to be used into the 1980s.

Dr. Ruth B. Drown, a chiropractor, developed and sold similar instruments and conducted business with her daughter in the Los Angeles area for about 40 years.[53] One of her patients was a woman with a lump in her breast whose doctor had advised her to go to a hospital for treatment. Instead she visited Drown, who "diagnosed" her condition by placing a drop of her blood on a blotter, which was then inserted into a small black box as Drown ran a finger across a rubber plate. The lady was informed that she did not have cancer but a fungus had spread through her digestive system and liver. Drown also concluded that the woman had gallstones, a non-functioning kidney, and a deficiency of hydrochloric acid. The victim was told that her conditions could be cured if she would visit a practitioner near her home in Chicago. Despite treatment by this practitioner (at $50 per visit) and further reassurance from Drown, the woman died of breast cancer.

In 1949 Drown demonstrated her machine to scientists at the University of Chicago. Blood was drawn from 10 patients whose health status had been medically determined. Drown provided diagnoses for three of them. She said the first had cancer of the left breast that had spread to the ovaries and pancreas; actually the patient had tuberculosis of the right lung. Drown said that the second patient had an improperly functioning uterus, but the actual condition was high blood pressure. The third patient, said by Drown to have prostate cancer, was a healthy young physician on the hospital staff.

Drown was brought to trial in 1950. Her device was shown to be a simple electrical circuit with a variety of wires. The galvanic instrument generated small voltages that registered on a dial. However, the values were apparently irrelevant to treatment, and the dried blood on the blotter was not linked to the galvanic circuit. Yet 19 patients testified to marvelous benefits from her therapy. Drown was found guilty, fined $1000, and given a 1-year suspended sentence with 5 years' probation. The case cost $50,000 to prosecute.

Drown stopped distributing her devices in interstate commerce but continued to practice in California, eventually treating a total of 35,000 individuals. In 1963 she was indicted for grand theft. As part of the investigation, an undercover agent from the district attorney's office had submitted samples of blood that were supposedly from her three children but actually came from a healthy turkey. At $50 per test, reports were returned claiming the children suffered from chickenpox and mumps. The agent was told how to use a Drown-supplied device to treat these conditions. Drown died at age 74 while awaiting trial.

Although the devices marketed by Abrams are no longer marketed, dozens of similar ones have taken their place. Some have their galvanometers connected to dials that provide a numerical readout; others are computerized. Used by a few hundred chiropractors, homeopaths, naturopaths, acupuncturists, bogus nutrition counselors, and "holistic" physicians and dentists, the devices are variously claimed to detect allergies, vitamin deficiencies, "imbalances in the flow of electromagnetic energy," and other alleged dysfunctions of bodily organs. Chapter 8 describes these further.

published on the effect on pain of small, static magnets marketed to consumers. Explanations that magnetic fields "increase circulation," "reduce inflammation," or "speed recovery from injuries" are simplistic and are not supported by the weight of experimental evidence.

The claims that magnets relieve pain are based primarily on testimonials from athletes. The marketing was given impetus by a study comparing the effects of magnets and sham magnets on the knee pain of 50 adult patients who had had poliomyelitis during childhood. The 29 who received an active magnet reported a significantly greater reduction in pain than the 21 treated with a sham magnet.[54] However, this finding was based on completion of a questionnaire following a single 45-

minute exposure, with no follow-up study to determine whether any alleged effect persisted. No published study of other painful conditions has found any benefit. Some products are too weak to provide a magnetic field that penetrates the skin or are complete fakes that exert no magnetic force whatsoever.

In 1998, Magnetherapy, Inc., of West Palm Beach, Florida, agreed to pay the State of Texas $30,000 and to stop claiming that wearing its magnetic device near areas of pain and inflammation will relieve pain due to arthritis, migraine headaches, sciatica or heel spurs. Magnetherapy was also required to stop making claims that its magnets can cure or mitigate any disease or can affect any change in the human body, unless its devices are FDA-approved for those purposes. The company had provided retailers with display packages that included testimonials and posters of sports stars.[55]

In 1999, the FTC obtained a consent agreement barring Magnetic Therapeutic Technologies, of Irving, Texas, from claiming that its magnetic sleep pads or other products (a) are effective against cancers, diabetic ulcers, arthritis, degenerative joint conditions, or high blood pressure; (b) could stabilize or increase the T-cell count of HIV patients; (c) could reduce muscle spasms in persons with multiple sclerosis; (d) could increase bone density, immunity, or circulation; or (e) are comparable or superior to prescription pain medicine. In another FTC case, Pain Stops Here! Inc., of Baiting Hollow, N.Y., agreed to stop claiming that its "magnetized water" or other products are useful against cancer and many other diseases and could stimulate the growth of plants.[55]

In 2000, Florsheim, Inc., began advertising on its Web site that the magnetic insoles in its *MagneForce* shoes "generate a deep-penetrating magnetic field which increases circulation; reduces foot, leg and back fatigue; provides natural pain relief and improved energy level." The site also claimed that some people might suffer from "magnetic deficiency." After Quackwatch[56] posted an analysis of these claims, the Consumer Justice Center, of Laguna Niguel, California, sued Florsheim for false advertising. The offending claims quickly vanished from Florsheim's site.

EMF Protectors

Many individuals and organizations are marketing low-magnetic-field electric blankets, clocks, and computer terminals for "electrically hypersensitive" people"; measuring devices; and various "protective" devices said to protect against electromagnetic fields. For example, an ad for a $39.95 *Cell Censor Cellular Phone/EMF Detection Meter* has stated:

It's Your Decision

1. You are nearsighted and dislike wearing glasses. You have tried contact lenses and consider them a nuisance. What information should you seek to make an intelligent decision about refractive surgery?

2. Your friend appears to have difficulty hearing clearly. You have detected this problem because the person frequently asks you to repeat yourself. What should you suggest? Would a visit to a local hearing aid dealer be a suitable first step?

Learn to detect and measure: cellular phone RF radiation, electromagnetic fields generated by power lines, computer monitors, TVs, appliances, home wiring, and other unsuspected sources. . . . It lets you instantly measure the levels in your environment, and helps you make informed purchasing decisions regarding appliances.

Contrary to what the ad implies, there is no scientific evidence that proximity to electric power lines or electric appliances causes any health problem or that "electrical hypersensitivity" exists.[57] A National Research Council committee has thoroughly evaluated published studies related to electric and magnetic fields and found no evidence of a human-health hazard.[58]

SUMMARY

Medical devices include several thousand types of health products, from simple articles to complex medical equipment. Federal laws define "medical device" as any health-care product that does not achieve any of its principal intended purposes by chemical action in or on the body or by being metabolized. The general quality of professionally used medical devices is high.

The devices commonly used by consumers include eyeglasses, contact lenses, and hearing aids. Purchase of these products should be preceded by a thorough professional examination. Since prices vary considerably, comparison shopping may also be wise.

Some devices have been marketed with misleading claims. Some hearing aid manufacturers and salespeople have exaggerated what hearing aids can do. Scare tactics are often used to sell water-treatment devices that are unnecessary or overpriced. Quack devices are still a significant problem—especially the "electrodiagnostic" devices used by certain "alternative" practitioners.

REFERENCES

1. Hearing aid claims—Just a lot of noise? AARP Senior Consumer Alert, Spring 1995.
2. Food and Drug Administration. Federal Food, Drug, and Cosmetic Act, as Amended, and Related Laws. HHS Publication No. (FDA) 93-1051. Washington, D.C., 1993, U.S. Government Printing Office.
3. U.S. Medical Technology Industry Fact Sheet, 1999. Washington, D.C., 2000, Health Industry Manufacturers Association.
4. Strongin RJ. The Dialog of Device Innovation: An Overview of the Medical Technology Innovation Process. Alexandria, Va., 1993, Health Care Technology Institute.
5. Kessler DA and others. The federal regulation of medical devices. New England Journal of Medicine 317:357–366, 1987.
6. GAO finds FDA drags feet in medical device safety. Public Citizen Health Research Group Health Letter 5(6):10–11, 1989.

7. FDA news release P83-11, June 3, 1983.
8. Briones MN. 1995 Reference Guide for the Health Care Technology Industry. Arlington, Va., 1995, Health Care Technology Institute.
9. Mosenkis R. Human factors design—Do's and don'ts. Medical Design & Diagnostics Industry 12(9):58–61, 1990.
10. Friedlander MH, Donev S. 20/20: A Total Guide to Improving Your Vision and Preventing Eye Disease. New York, 1994, Wings Books.
11. U.S Preventive Services Task Force. Guide to Clinical Preventive Services, ed 2. Baltimore, 1996, Williams & Wilkins, pp 373–391.
12. The specs on specs. Consumer Reports 62(7):10–15, 1997.
13. Waring GO III and others. Results of the Prospective Evaluation of Radial Keratotomy (PERK) Study 4 years after surgery for myopia. JAMA 263:1083–1091, 1990.
14. Waring GO III and others. Results of the Prospective Evaluation of radial keratotomy (PERK) study 10 years after surgery. Archives of Ophthalmology 112:1298–1308, 1994.
15. Bender P. Radial keratotomy in the 1990s and the PERK Study. JAMA 263:1127, 1990.
16. American Academy of Ophthalmology. Radial keratotomy for myopia. Ophthalmology 100(7):1103–1115, 1993.
17. So you want to wear contact lenses. St. Louis, 1995, American Optometric Association.
18. Consumer guide to contact lenses. St. Louis, 1997, American Optometric Association.
19. Sunglasses are more than shades. St. Louis, 1994, American Optometric Association.
20. Consumer guide to sunglasses. St. Louis, 1997, American Optometric Association.
21. Sunglasses. Consumer Reports 53:504–509, 1988.
22. Worrall RS. The eye exorcisors. In Barrett S, Jarvis WT. The Health Robbers: A Close Look at Quackery in America. Amherst, N.Y., 1993, Prometheus Books.
23. Taylor A and others. Relations among aging, antioxidant status, and cataract. American Journal of Clinical Nutrition 62(6 Suppl):1439S–1447S, 1995.
24. Christen WG Jr. Antioxidants and eye disease. American Journal of Medicine 97(3A):14S–17S, 1994.
25. Cataract surgery: Beware the traps. Consumer Reports on Health 5(5):48–50, 1993.
26. Franks JR, Beckman NJ. Rejection of hearing aids: Attitudes of geriatric sample. Ear and Hearing 6:161–166, 1985.
27. Hearing loss and you. Livonia, Mich., 1995, International Hearing Society.
28. NIH Consensus Conference: Noise and hearing loss. JAMA 263:3185–3190, 1990.
29. AARP Product report: Hearing aids. Washington, D.C., Dec 1989, American Association of Retired Persons.
30. Rezen SV, Hausman C. Coping with Hearing Loss: A Guide for Adults and Their Families. New York, 1985, Dembner Books.
31. How to buy a hearing aid. Consumer Reports 57:716–722, 1992.
32. Goldstein J. Testimony reported in The Hearing Aid Marketplace: Is the Consumer Adequately Protected? Hearing Before the Senate Special Committee on Aging, 1993, pp 85–89.
33. Misleading claims about hearing aids must end, FDA warns. FDA Medical Bulletin, June 1993, p 8.
34. Sampson WI. The holistic hodgepodge. In Barrett S, Jarvis WT. The Health Robbers: A Close Look at Quackery in America. Amherst, N.Y., 1993, Prometheus Books.
35. Fit to drink: Devices that help keep water in good taste and you in good health. Consumer Reports 66(10):52–55, 1999.
36. The selling of water safety. Consumer Reports 55:27–43, 1990.
37. Water testing scams. Washington, D.C., 1993, Federal Trade Commission.
38. Bottled water. University of California at Berkeley Wellness Letter 7(9):5, 1991.
39. Home water treatment units. Washington, D.C., 1994, Federal Trade Commission.
40. Humidifiers: Relief for winter dryness. Consumer Reports 59:659–664, 1994.
41. Hot air for sale. Consumer Reports 54:12, 1989.
42. Macknin ML and others. Effect of inhaling heated vapor on symptoms of common cold. JAMA 264:989–991, 1990.
43. Personal emergency response systems. Washington, D.C., 1993, Federal Trade Commission.
44. Latex labeling required for medical devices. FDA talk paper T97-50, Sept 30, 1997.
45. Nightingale SL. Latex allergy test cleared for marketing. JAMA 273:1564, 1995.
46. ACAAI Latex Hypersensitivity Committee. Latex allergy—an emerging healthcare problem. Annals of Allergy, Asthma & Immunology 75:19–20, 1995.
47. Slater JE. Latex allergy. Journal of Allergy and Clinical Immunology 94(2Pt1):139–149, 1994.
48. Weido AJ, Sim TC. The burgeoning problem of latex sensitivity: Surgical gloves are only the beginning. Postgraduate Medicine 98(3):173–184, 1995.
49. Task Force on Allergic Reactions to Latex. American Academy of Allergy and Immunology: Committee report. Journal of Allergy and Clinical Immunology 92(1Pt1):16–18, 1993.
50. FDA. The big quack attack: Medical devices. HHS publication No (FDA) 80-442, Washington, D.C., 1980, US Government Printing Office.
51. Gevitz N. Three perspectives on unorthodox medicine. In Gevitz N, editor. Other Healers: Unorthodox Medicine in America. Baltimore, 1988, Johns Hopkins University Press.
52. Smith RL. The strange world of mechanical quackery. Today's Health 42:42–47, 1964.
53. Smith RL. The incredible Drown case. Today's Health 46:46, 1968.
54. Vallbona C and others. Response of pain to static magnetic fields in postpolio patients: A double-blind pilot study. Archives of Physical Medicine and Rehabilitative Medicine 78:1200–1203, 1997.
55. Barrett S. Magnetic therapy. Quackwatch Web site, May 18, 2000.
56. Barrett S. Florsheim's MagneForce shoes: Should we worry about "magnetic deficiency? Quackwatch Web site, Aug 8, 2000.
57. Farley JW. Power lines and cancer: Nothing to fear. Quackwatch Web site, Sept 24, 2000.
58. National Research Council Committee on the Possible Effects of Electromagnetic Fields on Biologic Systems. Possible Health Effects of Exposure to Residential Electric and Magnetic Fields. Washington, D.C., 1997, National Academy Press.

Chapter Twenty-Three

COPING WITH DEATH

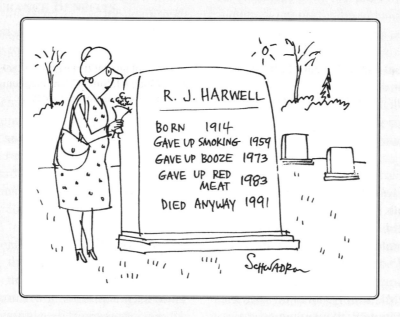

It is a myth to think that death is only for the old. Death is there from the very beginning.

HERMAN FEIFEL[1]

Most Americans have difficulty accepting death as a normal physiological process. In the current system of care many dying persons suffer needlessly, burden their families, and die isolated from family and community.

AMA COUNCIL ON SCIENTIFIC AFFAIRS[2]

The burden of death can be eased by understanding the emotions involved and planning ahead to deal with various issues that pertain to dying. This chapter can help you make intelligent decisions about preparing an advance medical directive, donating body parts, hospice care, euthanasia, body disposition arrangements, dealing with grief, and quackery related to life extension. Preparation for the inevitable should also include consideration of life insurance, estate planning (including a will), and other financial matters beyond the scope of this textbook.

ADVANCE DIRECTIVES

Consumer Reports on Health states that the need to prepare for death is pressing because machines often can keep a seriously ill or permanently unconscious patient alive, sometimes indefinitely, with no hope of recovery. However, people do have certain rights to refuse treatment.[3] Anyone 18 years or older who wishes to invoke the right to refuse medical treatment should prepare an advance medical directive, which may be a living will, a durable power of attorney for health care (DPAHC), or a combination of the two.

A living will is a document in which a patient states whether artificial life-support procedures such as a respirator or intravenous feeding should be used. This document is activated if the patient becomes terminally ill (as defined by state law) or is too sick (e.g., in a coma) to communicate treatment preferences.[4] A durable power of attorney designates another individual (proxy), usually a family member or intimate friend, to make treatment decisions when the patient cannot.

Living wills are advantageous because they enable people to specify what they want done. However, a very specific document may not provide guidance for situations that were not anticipated, and a broadly written document may not be clear about actual situations. The DPAHC enables the signer's agent to make decisions not covered by a living will and to discuss the situation with the patient's doctor. Its major disadvantage is that there may not be anyone with whom the signer feels comfortable as an agent. Experts advise preparing both documents and making sure that one's family and physician are aware of them. Many states provide model forms, and a few states require their use. The American Medical Association (AMA)[5] advises that if a state form seems too restrictive, an alternative form can be followed. However, it is advisable to be sure that the form and witnessing procedure comply with state law. Figure 23-1 illustrates a wallet card for indicating where your advance directive can be located. Figure 23-2 illustrates a simply worded living will and DPAHC combination.

A study of more than 9000 patients found that "do not resuscitate" (DNR) orders were not written promptly, many patients still died in pain in intensive care surroundings, and most of the doctors seemed to misunderstand their patient's wishes to forego futile medical

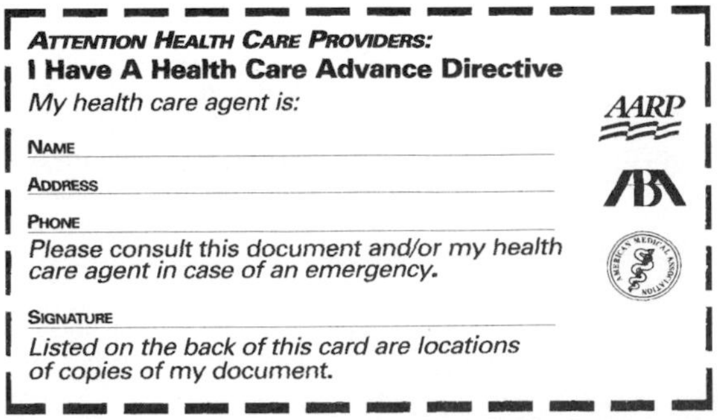

ATTENTION HEALTH CARE PROVIDERS:
I Have A Health Care Advance Directive
My health care agent is:

AARP

NAME

ADDRESS

/B\

PHONE
Please consult this document and/or my health care agent in case of an emergency.

SIGNATURE
Listed on the back of this card are locations of copies of my document.

FIGURE 23-1. Wallet card for advance directive. The name and address of the signer's physician and location of the advance directive are noted on the reverse side.

DECLARATION

I, _____, being of sound mind, willfully and voluntarily make this declaration to be followed if I become incompetent. This declaration reflects my firm and settled commitment to refuse life-sustaining treatment under the circumstances indicated below.

I direct my attending physician to withhold or withdraw life-sustaining treatment that serves only to prolong the process of my dying, if I should be in a terminal condition or in a state of permanent unconsciousness.

I direct that treatment be limited to measures to keep me comfortable and to relieve pain, including any pain that might occur by withholding or withdrawing life-sustaining treatment.

In addition, if I am in the condition described above, I feel especially strongly about the following forms of treatment:

I ( ) do I ( ) do not want cardiac resuscitation.

I ( ) do I ( ) do not want mechanical respiration.

I ( ) do I ( ) do not want tube feeding or any other artificial or invasive form of nutrition (food) or hydration (water).

I ( ) do I ( ) do not want blood or blood products.

I ( ) do I ( ) do not want any form of surgery or invasive diagnostic tests.

I ( ) do I ( ) do not want kidney dialysis.

I ( ) do I ( ) do not want antibiotics.

I realize that if I do not specifically indicate my preference regarding any of the forms of treatment listed above, I may receive that form of treatment.

Other instructions: _____

_____

I ( ) do I ( ) do not want to designate another person as my surrogate to make medical treatment decisions for me if I should be incompetent and in a terminal condition or in a state of permanent unconsciousness.

Name and address of surrogate (if applicable): _____

_____

Name and address of substitute surrogate (if surrogate designated above is unable to serve):

I made this declaration on the _____ day of _____, 200__.

Declarant's signature: _____

Declarant's address: _____

The declarant or the person on behalf of and at the direction of the declarant knowingly and voluntarily signed this writing by signature or mark in my presence.

Witness' signature: _____

Witness' address: _____

Witness' signature: _____

Witness' address: _____

FIGURE 23-2. Sample form for advance medical directive and living will combination.

procedures.[6] DNR orders can be written by the attending physician in accord with the wishes of the patient or—if the patient is incompetent—those of the patient's next-of-kin. (An incompetent patient is one who is too ill to communicate or to comprehend the situation.)

Federal Law

Sections 4206 and 4751 of the Omnibus Budget Reconciliation Act of 1990 apply to hospitals, nursing homes, hospices, health maintenance organizations, and home health-care agencies that receive Medicare or Medicaid funding. The law provides that when a person is admitted to a health facility, the medical staff must:

- Provide all adults with written information about their rights under state law to accept or refuse treatment and to execute advance directives.
- Inform the individual of the facility's policy on implementing advance directives.
- Make the person's living will or advance directive part of the person's medical record.
- Take no discriminatory action because of any decision regarding life-sustaining medical treatment.[7]

Guidelines for Physicians

The AMA Council on Ethical and Judicial Affairs states that it is ethical to stop or withhold life-support treatment to let a terminally ill patient die, but that a physician should not intentionally cause death. The Council also has ruled that when the duty to prolong life conflicts with the duty to relieve suffering, the physician, the patient, and/or a surrogate decision-maker (usually a family member) have discretion to resolve the conflict.[8]

Participants in an international conference have proposed guidelines to help physicians deal ethically with issues related to foregoing treatment. They concluded that all people should (a) feel morally obligated not to inflict harm or risk harming others; (b) respect patients' choices selected according to their own conscience, values, and religious convictions; and (c) act fairly and justly in allocating scarce resources. The other guidelines included:

FOR PATIENTS WITH AN ADVANCE DIRECTIVE WHO BECOME INCOMPETENT: Should patients refuse treatment: (a) the physician should not impose treatment even if potentially life-prolonging and (b) the physician should not be obligated to provide physiologically futile treatments.

FOR PATIENTS WITHOUT AN ADVANCE DIRECTIVE WHO BECOME INCOMPETENT: The physician: (a) should ensure patients' preferences as far as possible, (b) has a duty to discuss all alternatives with the family or significant others and seek an acceptable plan of action, (c) should consult with other professionals if the patient has no family or friends, and (d) if requested, should not provide futile treatment.

FOR PATIENTS WHO HAVE NEVER BEEN COMPETENT: The physician: (a) does not have an absolute duty to order life-prolonging treatment; (b) should weigh benefits and burdens of treatment in terms of quality of life; (c) should involve family, surrogates, physicians, and other caregivers in decisions; (d) should act in a trustworthy manner; and (e) may withhold life-prolonging treatment if its burdens outweigh potential benefits.

◆ Personal Glimpse ◆

The Naturalness of Dying

Dying, which was once viewed as natural and expected, has become medicalized into an unwelcome part of medical care. It has been distorted from a natural event of great social and cultural significance into the end point of untreatable or inadequately treated disease or injury. Worse, death has become medicine's enemy—a reminder of our limitations of medical diagnosis and management. After an anticipated death from a known terminal illness, for example, medical colleagues would be expected to make humane efforts to help family and caregivers understand this natural event and assuage their feelings of loss and sadness. Instead, the medical decisions leading up to the death may be defensively reviewed with the family, then scrutinized for mistakes by peers at clinicopathologic conferences, reported to risk management to be certain that liability issues are addressed, or critiqued in mandated quality assurance reviews. It is little wonder that physicians engage in inappropriately heroic battles against dying and death, even when it may be apparent to physician, patient, and family that a rapid, good death is the best outcome.

Viewing dying and death as merely a failure of medical diagnosis and therapy . . . trivializes the final event of our lives, stripping it of important nonmedical meaning for patients, family, and society. This narrow view of dying may be a particular concern for the very elderly, for whom death is an expected and sometimes desired event.

Respect for the wholeness of life requires that we not debase its final stage; art, literature, and the social sciences teach us that a good death can be a natural, courageous, and thoughtful end to life.

Jack D. McCue, M.D.[9]

© 1995 American Medical Association

SCARCITY OF RESOURCES: (a) Society must establish limits and priorities, (b) processes used to establish limits should be open and fair, (c) established policies that are restrictive must be publicized in advance of patient admission, and (d) the patient has no right to any treatment that has no reasonable expectation of benefit.[10]

Drafting an Advance Directive

The *Johns Hopkins Medical Letter*[11] suggests following these procedures when preparing an advance directive:

- Contact your lawyer or state attorney general's office to get information on living will and DPAHC legislation in your state, as well as appropriate forms.
- Sign your advance directive and designation of DPAHC before two witnesses (other than the person designated to carry out your wishes, a potential heir, or any health-care professional who is caring for you) and, if required by your state, a notary. A lawyer is not required, although you might want to consult one.
- Give a copy to your family, your doctor, your lawyer, and your cleric. Do not store your living will only in a safe deposit box, where it may be inaccessible to anyone but you.
- To keep the living will current (and more likely to be upheld should it ever go to court), re-examine the document every 2 years or so, and sign and date it again. Every 5 years, sign again in front of witnesses and a notary.

Forms and instructions specific for each state can be downloaded free from the Choice in Dying/Partnership in Caring Web site (http://www.choices.org).

Viatical Settlements

Faced with the financial burden of a terminal illness, some people choose to sell their life-insurance policy for an immediate lump sum. The viatical settlement company (or a third-party investor who purchases the policy) pays any subsequent premiums and collects the face value when death occurs. The Federal Trade Commission has warned that decisions about insurance benefits can have a profound financial and emotional impact on dependents, friends, and caregivers. The 1996 Health Insurance Portability and Accountability Act permits people with a life expectancy of less than 2 years to receive the distribution tax-free. However, the sale may hinder eligibility for Medicaid coverage.

Some agents fraudulently recruit terminally ill people to apply for multiple policies.[12] They misrepresent the truth and answer "no" to all of the medical questions. Healthy impostors then undergo the medical evaluation. In many cases, the insurance agent who issues the policy is a party to the scheme. The agent or one applicant may even submit the same application to many insurance companies. Viatical settlement

◆ Personal Glimpse ◆

Who Should Determine When Someone Has the Right to Die?

In 1990 the U.S. Supreme Court affirmed that competent people have a right to refuse life-sustaining treatment, including artificially given food and fluids. But when patients are incompetent, the court said, they are unable to make informed and voluntary choices. States are therefore justified in requiring "clear and convincing evidence" of the patient's wishes before allowing withdrawal of such support measures. The ruling was applied to the case of 32-year-old Nancy Cruzan, who had been in a coma as a result of irreversible brain damage since a 1983 car accident. By a 5-4 vote the Supreme Court upheld a Missouri Supreme Court ruling that Ms. Cruzan's guardian could not terminate her treatment because there was not sufficient evidence of her wishes. The verdict stimulated many hospitals to become more aggressive about having patients sign a living will or other "advance directive" to be used if they become irreversibly ill and are unable to speak for themselves.

What is your reaction to the court's decision?

companies then purchase the policies and sell them to unsuspecting third-party investors. The insurance industry is the biggest victim of this fraud and could incur huge losses (conservatively estimated at more than $1 billion) within the next few years. Some investors receive nothing in return for their "guaranteed" investment. People considering a viatical settlement should read the FTC's brochure[13] and consult a professional adviser.

DONATIONS OF ORGANS AND TISSUES

Transplantation is usually thought of in terms of major organs such as the heart, kidney, or lung. However, many body tissues can also be used to help the living. Corneal transplants can restore sight. Skin grafts can help burn victims. Heart valves can aid those with congenital heart disease. Ligaments can help people with athletic injuries. Bones are also suitable for grafting. Bone marrow from a live donor can be used to save certain patients with leukemia and several other disorders. However, this discussion focuses on the organs whose use is related to whether the recipient lives or dies.

The best opportunities for organ donation occur when death results from a head injury or stroke that results in brain death. However, if death results from heart

Table 23-1
SELECTED ORGAN TRANSPLANT DATA, 1997–1998

Transplanted Organ(s)	Number 1997-98	Patient Survival[*] 1-Year	Patient Survival[*] 5-Year	Longest Pt. Survival (1997)	Cost (1996)[†] 1st Yr.	Cost (1996)[†] Follow-Up	Median Waiting Time (1998)	Waiting List Death Rate (1999)
Heart	4,012	85.7%	69.5%	23 years	$228,000	$19,600	217 days	19.2%
Liver	3,652	87.5%	73.9%	28 years	290,000	20,800	496 days	12.8%
Kidney, live donor	3,007	97.8%	91.0% }	35 years	94,000	15,600	n.a	6.3%
Kidney, cadaveric	8,384	94.4%	81.6% }					
Pancreas	842	96.6%	82.7%	17 years	110,000	9,800	210 days	2.1%
Heart-lung	70	63.3%	44.3%	15 years	n.a	n.a	n.a	18.0%
Lung	722	75.1%	44.1%	9 years	241,600	14,200	n.a	17.3%

[*]Median survival time: 1-year figures based on 1996–1997 data; 5-year figures based on 1989–1997 data; "n.a." means not available.

[†]Estimated total for surgeon, operating room personnel, anesthesia, hospital stay, and extensive laboratory tests. Organs average $24,000 more.

Source: UNOS Web site (http://www.unos.org)

disease, donation may be limited to eyes and certain tissues. The National Transplant Act of 1984 initiated development of a national system to ensure equitable allocation. The Department of Health and Human Services then contracted with the United Network for Organ Sharing (UNOS) to implement this.

UNOS now operates a patient waiting list and an organ matching system; coordinates the logistics of matching the organs; collects, analyzes, and publishes transplant data; and educates health professionals about the donation process. Its centralized computer network links all organ procurement organizations and transplant centers and is accessible 24 hours a day, 7 days a week, with specialists available to answer calls. The waiting list on the last day of 2000 had about 73,400 registrants.

When a donor becomes available, the transplant center or organ procurement organization will access the computer, which generates a list of patients ranked according to the UNOS policies. The transplant coordinator then asks the transplant team to select a patient for further evaluation. The factors that affect ranking include tissue match, blood type, urgency of need, length of time on the waiting list, immune status, and distance from the available organ. The identities of the donor and recipient are confidential, although some basic information may be shared.

UNOS[14] reports that in 1999, 21,612 organs were transplanted from living donors and 4690 organs were transplanted from 5848 cadaveric (posthumous) donors. About 98% of the living donors were kidney donors between the ages of 18 and 64. Most of the posthumous donors were killed by a motor vehicle accident, another source of head injury, or a stroke. Table 23-1 provides data on the costs and waiting and survival times for the major types of organ transplant operations.

Although Americans generally feel favorably toward organ donation, fears and misconceptions still influence whether people become donors.[15] The positive factors include humanitarian feelings and pride experienced by the donor. The negative factors include fears of body mutilation and of receiving inadequate medical treatment when one's life is at risk.[16]

In some parts of the world the selling of body organs is a commercial enterprise. However, because of the shortage of donors and the large number of patients awaiting body parts, proposals have been made to provide financial aid or material incentives to the heirs of posthumous donors. This might come in several ways: (a) burial expenses, (b) rebates or deferral of state and federal income taxes, (c) a fixed grant for the surviving spouse and/or dependent children, (d) a government-sponsored or paid-for insurance policy payable to a designated beneficiary. Most religious groups support organ donation.

How to Donate

Every state has adopted some form of the Uniform Anatomical Gift Act, which recognizes the right of all Americans to donate their organs and tissues. These laws provide that when the individual's intent is not known, the next-of-kin can make this decision. The simplest way to make donation possible is to fill out an organ donor card that can be carried in one's wallet or other easily locatable place. The decision should also be discussed with family and friends. In some states permission to use tissues after death may be indicated on one's driver's license or an attached card. A Uniform Donor Card is available from UNOS and several other organizations (Figure 23-3). Identification bracelets indicating a wish to donate are available from Medic

Alert Foundation. The Living Bank maintains an unofficial national registry and publishes a free newsletter . Family wishes take precedence over donor card wishes. However, several studies suggest that both medical professionals and family members are more likely to favor donation when the deceased carries a donor card.[17]

Hospice Care

Hospice care is a way of helping people who are expected to live 6 months or less and their family members. It is provided mostly in the home by family and friends with the support of health professionals and volunteers. Beresford[18] describes it as "an alternative to conventional, cure-oriented medical treatment aimed at fighting the disease by any means possible, at the time when that approach has become counterproductive." This includes situations where continued treatment could delay death a bit longer but would have severe side effects.

The modern hospice movement began in 1967 with the founding of St. Christopher's Hospice in England.[19] The first American program began in 1974 in Connecticut. In 1999 there were about 3100 hospices in the United States, 75% of which were Medicare-certified or pending certification.[20] To achieve certification, a hospice must providc 24-hour availability; medical and nursing care; home care services; access to inpatient care; social work services; medications, medical supplies, and durable medical equipment related to the illness; and physical, occupational, and speech therapy as appropriate. At least 5% of the hours required must be contributed by unpaid volunteers.

ORGAN DONOR CARD

____
Print or Type Name of Donor

In the hope that I may help others, I hereby make this anatomical gift, if medically acceptable, to take effect upon my death. The words and marks below indicate my desires.

I give: (a)______ any needed organs or parts
(b)______ only the following organs or parts

____
Specify the Organ(s) or Part(s)

for the purposes of transplantation, therapy, medical research or education;
(c)______ my body for anatomical study if needed.

Limitations or special wishes, if any:______________

Figure 23-3. Uniform Organ Donor card. The back of the card states that it is a legal document under the Uniform Anatomical Gift Act or similar laws. It also asks for the donor's date of birth, the signature of the donor and two witnesses, and the date signed.

Most hospices are independently based community organizations (44%) or divisions of hospitals (33%) or home health agencies (17%). A few are divisions of hospice corporations or nursing homes. About 80% of hospice programs belong to the National Hospice and Palliative Care Organization (NHPCO), a nonprofit advocacy group founded in 1978. The NHPCO estimates that in 1999, hospices served about 700,000 patients (about 29 % of all Americans who died that year). About 78% had cancer, 10% had heart disease, and 4% had AIDS.

Hospices provide palliative (symptom-relieving) care to patients and families in both home and hospital settings. This includes physical (personal care), psychologic (fear, anxiety, grief), social (individual and family support), and spiritual (religious) aid by a medically supervised, interdisciplinary team of professionals and volunteers. Specialists in death awareness are available. Medications are generally given not to prolong life but to relieve distressing symptoms such as pain. Emotional support is also offered during the bereavement phase of care.

Hospice care was originally designed to help terminally ill individuals (particularly cancer patients) who wished to die at home and be as pain-free and alert as possible. This has been broadened so that programs now cover general care for anyone who may be dying. The emphasis is on quality of life rather than quantity.[21]

In 1983 Medicare began offering an option to cover hospice care for physician fees, nursing care, counseling, medical social services, short-term inpatient care, medical supplies, and the services of home health aides and homemakers. To qualify, the patient must (a) be medically certified as terminally ill with a life expectancy of 6 months or less and (b) sign a statement choosing hospice care instead of standard Medicare.

A Medicare beneficiary may elect to receive hospice care for two 90-day periods, followed by a 30-day period, and, when necessary, an extension period of indefinite duration. In 2000 the daily Medicare rates were about $101.84 for routine home care and $453.04 for general inpatient care. More than 90% of hospice-care hours are provided in the patient's home, thus substituting for more expensive multiple hospitalizations. In 1999 the average length of enrollment for patients admitted to hospice care was 48 days and the median length of service was 25 days. A 1995 study found that for every dollar Medicare spent on hospice during 1991 and 1992, it saved $1.52 in Medicare expense and that, during their last year of life, people who used hospice services incurred $2737 less cost than those who did not.[22]

Locating and Selecting a Hospice

The names and addresses of hospice care organizations and agencies may be obtained from the National Hospice Organization; the National Cancer Institute (telephone [800 4-CANCER]; a discharge planner, community relations person, or social worker at a local hospital; or a local religious institution, health department, social service office, bureau of aging, or American Cancer Society office. The following questions may be useful[23]:

About the Hospice

What nurses, doctors, volunteers, or others will
    provide services? What services will they provide?
What will the physician's role be, and will the hospice
    be communicating with the physician?
What services will be available 24 hours a day?
Will someone help with the insurance forms?
How often will the nurse, doctor, or other staff
    member visit the home or provide services?
Will bereavement counseling be available after the
    patient dies?
How are middle-of-the-night crises handled?
What follow-up services are provided if the patient
    must return to the hospital?

About Costs

What are the fees? Are they charged by the hour, day,
    or visit?
Will the hospice accept fee payments by private
    insurance, Medicare, or other payee? Will there be
    additional charges not covered by these providers?
Will the hospice handle billing with Medicare or a
    private insurance carrier? Will the hospice negotiate
    with the insurance carrier should charges be denied?

About the Program

Does the hospice mainly involve home or inpatient
    institutional care? How does it arrange for hospital
    care if necessary?
Does the program provide services to nursing home
    residents?
Is the hospice Medicare/Medicaid certified?
What kind of accreditation does the hospice have?
Does the program adhere to National Hospice Organi-
    zation standards?
Are any nurses certified in hospice care?

Other organizations that can provide information are the National Homecaring Council, National Consumers League, and Joint Commission on Accreditation of Healthcare Organizations.

EUTHANASIA AND ASSISTED SUICIDE

This section does not discuss the philosophical or moral issues involved in euthanasia. Rather, it presents information about its nature, related laws, and the ethics of physician responsibilities.

Euthanasia is derived from Greek words that mean "a good death." The term is used to describe situations in which a compassionate decision is made to terminate a person's life by applying a lethal treatment (active, or direct, euthanasia) or by withholding life-sustaining treatment (passive, or indirect, euthanasia).

If the patient asks for and gives competent consent to euthanasia, the euthanasia is called *voluntary*. If the patient cannot give consent or has not issued an advance directive, the euthanasia is called *nonvoluntary*. If action were taken against the will of a patient, it would be termed *involuntary* and would be illegal.[24] Voluntary active euthanasia is legal in the Northern Territory, Australia, and is government-sanctioned in The Netherlands, where physicians can administer a drug to someone who is suffering from an incurable disease or condition. However, it is illegal in the United States.

Many hospitals have an ethics committee to help hospital staff members deal with ethical issues related to patient care. Its activities include education of staff members; formulation of hospital policies, particularly about death and dying; and advising providers and possibly families. Garrett and others[25] have stressed that ethics committee opinions are most valuable if they reflect independent judgments rather than those of the institution or its dominant figures.

With physician-assisted suicide, doctors provide or prescribe lethal doses of drugs to suffering patients who intend to end their lives. This practice is illegal in almost all states. Jack Kevorkian, M.D., a retired pathologist and author of *Prescription Medicide*,[26] is a controversial crusader for the legalization of physician assistance to help certain terminally ill patients commit suicide. Since 1990 he has attended the deaths of more than 100 people who had requested suicide assistance.

In 1998, Kevorkian provided voluntary euthanasia by injecting a patient with a lethal dose of drugs and provided CBS-TV's "60 Minutes" with a videotape of the procedure. Following broadcast of the event, he was convicted of second-degree murder and sentenced to 10 to 25 years in prison. He is appealing this conviction.

Kevorkian has proposed that clinics called obitoriums be made available where terminal patients could receive pain treatment or help from "obitiatrists" in ending their life.[27] Derek Humphrey, president of the

Euthanasia Research and Guidance Organization (ERGO), states that, "Assistance in suicide should be voluntary, legal and rare and arranged by a team of health professionals, not one acting alone and covertly as now."[28] However, the AMA thinks it should remain illegal.[29]

In 1994 voters in Oregon narrowly passed a state law allowing physicians to prescribe lethal drugs to adults who are mentally competent and who request the drugs so that they can self-administer them.[30] In 2000 voters in Maine defeated a referendum that asked, "Should a terminally ill adult, who is of sound mind, be allowed to ask for and receive a doctor's help to die?"

In 1996 the United States Court of Appeals for the Ninth Circuit struck down a Washington state law against physician-assisted suicide, ruling that the law was contrary to a constitutional "right to die."[31]

Infant Euthanasia

With dramatic advances in the technology available in neonatal intensive care units (NICUs), survival of premature and congenitally deformed newborns has dramatically improved since the early 1960s. NICUs have enabled many infants to survive and live a productive life. For some, however, the expensive NICU treatment can only prolong suffering.

For example, infants with meningomyelocele are born with a malformed and exposed spinal cord and typically die within days or weeks. Some infants with Down syndrome can live satisfactorily despite mental retardation. But others have such serious defects that, even with the best medical and surgical treatment, there is little hope for significant autonomy or personal development.

Decisions about the appropriate way to care for hopelessly imperiled infants can be complicated. Physicians and hospital ethics committees may provide helpful input.[32] The courts generally recognize that parents have the primary responsibility for deciding whether to withhold or withdraw care. However, in 1992 the Florida Supreme Court upheld a lower court ruling that prevented an anencephalic infant from being declared dead so her organs could be used for transplants as requested by her parents.

In 1994 the U.S. Supreme Court turned down an appeal by a Virginia hospital to discontinue life-sustaining treatment after 2 years for "Baby K," an anencephalic infant. Anencephaly is a rare neural tube defect in which all or part of the brain is absent, thereby precluding the possibility of consciousness or feelings.[33] Most anencephalic infants survive only a few days. Baby K's

anencephaly had been diagnosed during pregnancy, but the mother completed the pregnancy and asked for maximal care for the infant, who was placed on a respirator. The hospital ethics committee was unable to convince the mother that such care was futile. A district court ruled that the hospital was obligated to provide full medical care under both the federal Emergency Medical Treatment and Labor Act and the Federal Rehabilitation Act of 1973. By 1994 the total cost to the state of Virginia exceeded $800,000.[34]

REASONS FOR AN AUTOPSY

When there is a sudden, violent, or unexpected death, the coroner or medical examiner may be called to investigate. A coroner is an elected official who may have no medical background or training. A medical examiner is an appointed public official who is a qualified physician, generally with special training in forensic medicine. If it appears that foul play is involved, the coroner or medical examiner will order an autopsy.

An autopsy is a comprehensive postmortem examination done for the purpose of determining the cause of death. Unless ordered by a government official, consent of the next-of-kin is required. The county or state pays for autopsies requested by the coroner or medical examiner. If a hospital physician requests the autopsy, the hospital is legally obliged to bear the cost. If the next-of-kin makes the request, that person would be responsible for the cost. Such a request might be made if the cause of death is uncertain or if medical malpractice, a hereditary disease, or a serious contagious disease is suspected but not confirmed.

BODY DISPOSITION

Each year Americans arrange more than 2 million funerals for family and friends. When someone dies, the bereaved must consider two things: disposal of the body and a ceremony acknowledging the person's death. Funerals and memorial services provide opportunities for expressing and validating grief, celebrating the life of the deceased, reaffirming religious or community ties, and expressing sympathy for the bereaved. The body of the deceased is present at a funeral, but not at a memorial service. Death certificates state the cause of death and are necessary to settle the financial affairs of the deceased.

The business that provides help to bereaved persons is called a mortuary or funeral home. Morticians (funeral directors) can arrange funerals, notify friends and relatives, obtain permits and death certificates, handle arrangements for the body, place obituary and funeral notices in the newspaper, assist with cremation and cemetery arrangements, provide transportation to and from the funeral, and attend to various other details. Some also provide a modest amount of counseling. Nearly all states license funeral directors, and all states license embalmers. (Embalming replaces the blood and other body fluids with disinfecting chemicals that retard the decomposition of the corpse.) The schools at which they train include courses in anatomy, microbiology, pathology, communicable diseases, business practices, and the psychology of grief. There are about 22,000 funeral homes and 100,000 cemeteries in the United States.

Funeral services are among the biggest expenditures that many Americans make during their lifetime. The average cost of funeral and burial arrangements in the United States is about $5800,[35] a figure that does not include the cost of a cemetery plot or opening, closing, or perpetually caring for the grave. However, alternative arrangements to the traditional funeral can be dignified without being costly. Funerals are much more expensive than simple burial, cremation, or cremation plus a separate memorial service.

Methods

Three general options for body disposal are available: burial, cremation, and donation. The corpse can be buried below ground in a grave or above ground in a mausoleum. Direct burial, usually within 1 day, is the least expensive burial option because (a) mortuary services are minimal; (b) refrigeration or embalming are not needed to preserve the body; and (c) burial can be done in a container of unfinished wood, pressboard, cardboard, or canvas, rather than an expensive casket.

The casket is frequently the most expensive funeral item, but prices vary widely.[36] Caskets are usually made of metal or wood, although some are constructed of fiberglass or plastic. Most metal caskets are made from rolled steel; the lower the gauge, the thicker the steel. Wooden caskets come in hardwood, softwood, and plywood. Some metallic caskets have a rubber gasket or other feature that delays the penetration of water and retards rust formation. Some also come with a warranty for durability. Protective features add to their cost. Wooden caskets are usually not gasketed and do not carry a warranty for durability. However, both types are usually warranted for workmanship and materials.

Burial requires a cemetery plot and involves the cost of opening and closing the grave, a grave marker, and cemetery upkeep. For below-ground burials, cemeter-

ies typically require that the casket be placed in a grave liner or burial vault to prevent the ground above the casket from caving in. A grave liner, also called a "rough box," is made of reinforced concrete and lowered into the grave before burial. A burial vault, which is more substantial and expensive than a grave liner, is typically sold for its visual appeal and is usually gasketed. Most vaults are constructed of steel-reinforced concrete and lined with other materials, including plastic. Like some caskets, the vault may be sold with a warranty of protective strength.

Cremation reduces the corpse to coarse, sandlike pieces of bone by heating it at 2000° F to 2500° F for a few hours. The remains can be kept at home (typically in an urn) or scattered at sea or over land in accordance with state and local laws. There are added costs if the remains are buried in a cemetery plot or placed in a columbarium (an above-ground vault containing niches into which urns are placed). The Cremation Association of North America states that there were 1100 crematories and over 470,000 cremations in 1994 and that cremation follows about 21% of deaths in the United States. Some religions forbid the practice.

A 1995 *Consumers Digest* survey found that burial containers cost $26 to $33,000, concrete burial vaults cost $100 to $5000, cremation urns cost $100 to $1500, and burial spaces cost $500 to $250,000. In 12 large cities, the lowest prices found ranged from $400 to $1122 for direct burial and from $375 to $695 for cremation.[37] In some situations it may be practical to purchase a casket from a local discounter or through the Internet. However, in some states a funeral director or funeral establishment license is required in order to sell burial containers.

The spouse or dependent children under 18 of someone whose work was covered by Social Security are entitled to a $255 payment for funeral expenses. Some veterans are entitled to free burial at a national cemetery and a grave marker at any cemetery.

The least expensive method of body disposal is donation to a medical school that, when notified, will provide free pick-up and eventual cremation. However, the donation must be arranged before death occurs, and some schools do not have a shortage of bodies.

Memorial Societies

A memorial society is a nonprofit cooperative that provides consumer education and information about the funeral industry and alternatives to traditional funerals. There are more than 100 local and regional memorial societies in the United States. Consumers can join one by paying a small one-time fee.

Memorial societies typically have formal contracts with one or more local funeral directors to provide members with a simple dignified burial or cremation at a cost much lower than normally offered to mortuary clients. Most memorial societies are affiliated with the Continental Association of Funeral and Memorial Societies (CAFMS), a consumer organization that encourages advanced planning and cost efficiency. If a member of a local society affiliated with CAFMS moves, discounted services can still be made available if there is another local CAFMS affiliate society in the area.

FTC Funeral Rule

The FTC Funeral Rule, which went into effect in 1984 and was revised in 1994, bans several types of deceptive practices.[38,39] The rule is intended to help people select what they want and to pay only for what they select. It requires providers to disclose prices and give truthful and complete information in person or if requested by telephone. The General Price List should include the cost of direct cremation; immediate burial; basic services (overhead); transfer of remains to funeral home; forwarding or receiving the remains; embalming and other preparation; use of facilities or staff for viewing or a ceremony; use of staff or equipment for a graveside service; a hearse or limousine; and caskets, liners, and vaults.

Providers must also (a) truthfully disclose whether state law requires embalming, (b) state that a casket is not required for direct cremation, (c) make an unfinished wood box or alternative container available for cremation, and (d) provide a Statement of Funeral Goods and Services listing the prices of individual items as well as the total price. The rule prohibits (a) charging a "handling fee" for receiving a casket or other goods or (b) stating that embalming, a specially sealed casket, or any other item or service can indefinitely preserve the body of the deceased in the grave. The rule does not cover pre-need funding or direct sales by cemeteries.

Consumer Problems

Most decisions about purchasing funeral goods and services are made by people when they are grieving and under time constraints. Most customers will not engage in comparison shopping, and many are vulnerable to sales pressure. Former funeral director Gregory W. Young[40] states that "the biggest moneymaker for the funeral director is consumer ignorance." His book *The High Cost of Dying* describes three main types of deceptive practices:

SUBSTITUTION OF MERCHANDISE: The casket or burial vault used is a less expensive model than the one for which the consumer is charged, or floral arrangements contain fewer or less expensive flowers than were promised.

CHARGING FOR SERVICES NOT NEEDED: The prime example is embalming, which is seldom needed unless there is a viewing of the body. It is never needed if the casket is kept closed or the body is directly cremated.

SUBTLE PERSUASION: Some funeral directors try to mobilize guilt to induce the family to order a more expensive casket and a higher-priced funeral. This can be done with phrases like "You have only one chance to do it right for Mom" or claims that a higher-priced casket will last longer.

Some people choose to make these arrangements for themselves before they die. Traditionally this has been done through a funeral home (mortuary) that offers several types of products and services. In 1995 *Consumers Digest* stated that the death-care industry is being transformed from simple agreements with local funeral homes and cemeteries to aggressively marketed plans sold by multinational corporations. Funeral arrangements are now being sold over the phone, through the mail, and door-to-door. The magazine reported that during the previous 5 years at least $50 million ij advance payments had been stolen or reported missing nationwide. Its 6-month investigation found that only half of the states regulated "pre-need" plans but there was little or no funding for auditing and enforcement to stop future theft.[37]

In 1995 ABC's "20/20" visited 26 funeral homes with a hidden camera and found that about half of the salespeople lied, broke the law, or gave misleading advice. For example, one funeral director offered a $1600 casket as the cheapest, and another offered an "inexpensive" funeral package with a $2385 casket and a total cost of $7208. The television moderator stated that prepayment is unwise because the money might be lost.

In 1996, the FTC launched the Funeral Rule Offenders Program ("FROP") to boost compliance with the Funeral Rule. Under the program, funeral homes that fail to give test shoppers the itemized price lists required by the Rule can enter the FROP program rather than face possible formal legal action. If they choose FROP, they make a voluntary payment and enroll in a compliance program, administered by the National Funeral Directors Association (NFDA), which includes a review of price lists, training on compliance, and follow-up testing and certification. Since that time, compliance has been substantially increased.[41]

The best strategy for people concerned about funeral costs is probably to join a memorial society, which will enable them to locate and use a low-cost provider if the need arises. Those wishing to make complete preneed arrangements should carefully investigate the reputation of any provider under consideration. (The local Better Business Bureau or state consumer protection office may have information.) The contract should be revocable, refundable, and portable (usable in any state). The price should be guaranteed, and the deposit placed in a revocable bank trust with interest payable to the purchaser or the purchaser's estate.

Sources of Information or Other Help

The National Research and Information Center, an independent, nonprofit organization, offers information on death, grief, and funeral services and handles disputes. The Conference of Funeral Service Examining Boards, which represents licensing boards in the United States and Canada, provides information on laws and responds to consumer inquiries or complaints about funeral providers. The NFDA offers consumer information and operates an arbitration program. The American Association of Retired Persons offers two free publications: "Cemetery Goods and Services" and "Pre-Paying Your Funeral." Information is also available online from the Federal Trade Commission.

GRIEF AND MOURNING

Grief is the sadness, pain, and suffering that occur when a family member or friend is terminally ill or dies. The intensity and duration of these emotions depend on the nature of the relationship to the dying person and the emotional makeup of the grieving persons.

The *Mayo Clinic Health Letter*[42] states that adult grief predominantly involves four reactions:

1. *Shock, numbness, and disbelief.* Bereaved persons may appear to be holding up well even though they feel terrible.
2. *Pining, yearning, and sadness.* Usually numbness turns to intense feelings of separation and mental pain in the months after the death.
3. *Acceptance of loss.* When death occurs, complete failure to mourn is a sign that something may be wrong.
4. *Resolution of grief.* As the individual "lets go," it becomes possible to reinvest in continuing life—for example, resuming former behavior patterns, seeking new relationships.

Loss of a loved one can cause guilt, shame, sadness, and a fear of dying. Bereaved persons must learn to cope with reality. This process involves gradual acceptance of the fact that a loved one has died, followed by gradual reinvolvement in day-to-day activities. Mourners typically must cope with a feeling of emptiness related to the fact that a part of their emotional investment has been lost. When mourning is successful, the emotions are "reinvested" as the individual becomes reinvolved in activities.

Many people believe that crying and other expressions of sadness are abnormal and a sign of emotional weakness. Displays of emotions may be painful to other people. However, expressions of grief are normal and healthy. Cassem[43] has noted:

Allowing the bereaved to express feelings is essential. The most important part of this process is to avoid the maneuvers that nullify grieving. Clichés ("It's God's will"), self-evident but irrelevant reassurances ("After all, you've got three other children"), and outright exhortations to stop grieving ("Life must go on") should be avoided.

Bereaved individuals can best deal with grief by recognizing that the sadness they feel is normal and resuming activity when they are able to do so. Friends often can help simply by expressing their sympathy and acknowledging the upset of the bereaved. Religious involvement may also be helpful.

Physicians often see people who feel that it is wrong to feel upset. Usually all such people need in order to proceed with mourning is reassurance that it is all right to grieve. An opportunity to ventilate both positive and negative feelings toward the ill or deceased individual may be helpful. Antidepressant drugs usually are not appropriate in the treatment of uncomplicated grief. The act of giving a drug to a grieving person may convey the message that grief is abnormal. Some communities have support groups for those who need help.

Normal vs Abnormal Grief

The length of the grieving or mourning process varies among individuals. When a loved one has passed on, most people take 6 to 12 months to recover, but some take less and some take considerably more. Horowitz[44] has noted:

In normal grief . . . the person passes through such states of mind with a sense of progressing along a mourning process. However, in pathological [abnormal] grief, the person may become frozen in one or more of these states, without progress over weeks or even months. There may be additional signs of inertia, hypochondriasis, numbness, unaccountable irritability, feelings of gross worthlessness, and apathy.

The *Johns Hopkins Medical Letter*[45] states that the "success" of the grieving process should not be measured by a predetermined timetable but by the griever's acceptance of the loss. The signs of unresolved grief include suicidal thoughts, chronic sleep difficulty, overuse of alcohol or drugs, persistent depression, failure to carry out normal daily routines, and persistent symptoms resembling those of the deceased. A shift to positive and realistic plans for the future is a sign that mourning is nearing completion.[46] Professional help is unlikely to be needed unless severe depression or social isolation persists for 6 to 12 months.

LIFE-EXTENSION QUACKERY

The wish to delay aging and prolong life is almost universal. Many entrepreneurs have capitalized on these wishes and proposed modern equivalents of the "fountain of youth." Chapter 20 describes how cosmetics manufacturers have made unproven claims that their products can rejuvenate the skin and/or remove wrinkles. Some product lines include vitamin supplements in addition to skin creams. Other manufacturers have marketed products claimed to prevent or delay aging, boost immunity, cure chronic disease, and/or improve memory.

Some spas offer therapeutic baths (in mineral water or seawater), mud packs, seaweed wraps, and a variety of other services claimed to promote rejuvenation or healing. Van Italie and Hadley[47] note that whereas most American spas offer fitness activities, European facilities are more likely to feature "cures," stress reduction, or various forms of pampering. Rejuvenation claims are also made by physicians engaged in unfounded practices here and abroad. Fresh cell therapy, which is claimed to rejuvenate body organs, is described in Chapter 17.

Antiaging and Life-Extension Claims

The limit of the human lifespan is probably not much more than 120 years. Many dietary methods, nutritional supplements, and drugs have been claimed to delay aging and/or extend life. During the early 1980s books by Saul Kent,[48] Durk Pearson and Sandy Shaw,[49] and Roy Walford, M.D.,[50] called considerable public attention to this matter. The books were based mainly on misinterpretations or inappropriate extrapolations of animal experiments.

Kent's *The Life Extension Revolution* summarized and commented on a large number of studies he believed were related to aging. Although the book gave little direct advice, it magnified the potential value of many of the strategies it discussed. Pearson and Shaw's 900-page *Life Extension—A Practical Scientific Approach* outlined an extensive program of supplements and drugs, combined with laboratory testing to look for signs of improvement or toxicity. The authors claimed that their program might extend an average individual's

Consumer Tip

Quackery and Terminal Illness

The notion that terminal patients have nothing to lose by turning to quackery is dead wrong. Most people faced with a life-threatening disease can make a reasonable psychological adjustment. . . . Those who accept their fate are in the best position to use their remaining time wisely. . . . Quacks discourage people from making the difficult adjustment by reinforcing their denial. Such people usually die unprepared because preparation for death is an admission of failure.

William T. Jarvis, Ph.D.[46]

lifespan by several decades and improve quality of life as well. Yetiv,[51] however, who published a detailed review of the book, found it to be "extremely inaccurate." He said that some of its recommendations were potentially life-threatening, many of the references cited did not support the book's claims, and some directly contradicted the book's claims. Walford's *Maximum Life Span* suggested that the human lifespan could be extended by eating fewer than 1500 calories a day and taking certain supplements. Walford's theories are based on experiments in which laboratory animals fed a highnutrient, low-calorie diet lived longer than normal.

Each of the three books was followed by a sequel providing detailed advice on following the programs they recommended. The resultant publicity inspired many manufacturers to market products claimed to influence some aspect of aging. The FDA has driven some products of this type from the marketplace, but many others are still sold.

In 1980, the year his first book was published, Kent launched the Life Extension Foundation in Hollywood, Florida. The foundation's stated purpose was to "mobilize support for life extension, provide the public with products and services, and raise money for life extension research." Regular membership now costs $75 a year and entitles members to product discounts, a directory of "life extension" doctors, a directory of "innovative medical clinics," a copy of "The Physician's Guide to Life Extension Drugs," and two monthly newsletters. In 1987 FDA officials and U.S. marshals seized large quantities of products marketed by the Life Extension Foundation, including *BHT* (promoted for herpes and AIDS), *Coenzyme Q*$_{10}$ (for cardiovascular disorders and increased longevity), *DMSO* (for arthritis and bursitis), and *Cognitex* (to enhance mental function). In 1991 Kent and the foundation's vice president were charged with 28 criminal counts related to importing and selling unapproved new drugs and misbranded prescription drugs. However, the case did not proceed to trial.

Substances claimed to retard aging include Gerovital H3 (GH3), human growth hormone, dehydroepiandrosterone (DHEA), and melatonin.

GH3 was developed by Dr. Anna Aslan, a Rumanian physician. It has been promoted by the Rumanian National Tourist Office and a few American physicians as an antiaging substance—"the secret of eternal vigor and youth." Claims have been made that GH3 can prevent or relieve a wide variety of disorders, including arthritis, arteriosclerosis, angina pectoris and other heart conditions, neuritis, deafness, Parkinson's disease, depression, senile psychosis, and impotence. It is also claimed to stimulate hair growth, restore pigmentation to gray hair, and tighten and smoothen skin. The main ingredient in GH3 is procaine, a substance used for local anesthesia. Although many uncontrolled studies describe great benefits from the use of GH3, controlled trials using procaine have failed to demonstrate any. Low blood pressure, breathing difficulty, and convulsions have been reported among users. Noting that para-aminobenzoic acid (PABA) appears in the urine of people receiving procaine injections, a few American manufacturers have been selling procaine tablets containing PABA with false claims similar to those made for GH3. The FDA has taken regulatory action against several "GH3" marketers, but other brands still are marketed.

Human growth hormone has been shown to increase muscle mass and skin thickness when injected into elderly men who produce little or no hormone of their own. However, no study has demonstrated that it is safe and effective for long-term use for any such purpose. It is very expensive, and long-term use can cause joint inflammation and diabetes-like symptoms. At present, the only proven indication for human growth hormone is to treat children with short stature caused by growth-hormone deficiency.[52]

DHEA is a hormone that peaks around age 25 and gradually declines after that. Scientists have speculated that declining levels of this adrenal hormone play a role in aging. On the basis of animal experiments, DHEA has been claimed to cure cancer and heart disease and to delay aging. However, significant dosages in humans can cause unwanted hair growth, liver enlargement, and other adverse effects that make its use impractical. "DHEA pills" have been also promoted with false claims that they can cause effortless weight loss (see Chapter 13).

Melatonin, a hormone secreted by the pineal gland, peaks during childhood and gradually declines. Experiments with small numbers of people have found that melatonin influences the "body clock" and may be useful against "jet lag" and as a sleep aid. However, the fact that melatonin declines with age does not mean that the body needs larger amounts. Claims that melatonin can protect against heart disease, cancer, and cataracts and may help people with AIDS, Alzheimer's disease, asthma, and Parkinson's disease should be considered speculative.

Health professionals interested in "anti-aging" strategies have formed the American Association for Anti-Aging Medicine (A$_4$M), which holds conferences and has a certifying board that is not recognized by the American Board of Medical Specialties. An affiliated organization, the American Board of Anti-Aging Health Professionals (ABAAHP), was established in 1999 to provide "advanced education, representation, and specialty recognition of healthcare professionals," including chiropractors, PhDs, registered nurses, podiatrists, naturopaths, and pharmacists. Eligible individuals who pass a 1-day examination are certified as an "Anti-Aging Health Professional." These certifications are not recognized by the American Board of Medical Specialties or other mainstream groups.

Scientific Responses

Schneider and Reed[53] and Yetiv[54] have summarized and evaluated life extension strategies proposed in both popular books and the scientific literature. Their findings include:

- Several studies in animals have shown that cutting calories 50% to 60% can significantly increase maximum lifespan. However, the restriction also retards their growth and development and thus is not suitable for humans.
- Many types of immunologic manipulation have been proposed, including the transplantation of immune cells from young animals. However, no such approach has been demonstrated safe or effective in humans.
- Antioxidant nutrients such as selenium, vitamins C and E, and BHT are claimed to delay aging by soaking up "free radicals" that have escaped the body's own "free radical patrols." Although antioxidants can deactivate free radicals in the test tube, they have not been proved to do so in humans.
- Superoxide dismutase (SOD) is an enzyme whose tissue levels in various animal species appears related to their lifespan. However, consumption of SOD supplements has no effect in humans because SOD (a protein) is digested into its component amino acids and does not reach the tissues as intact SOD.

Much research is being done to see whether anti-oxidant supplements can protect against heart disease, cancer, and other diseases. In 1992, after reviewing current research data, *Consumer Reports* concluded:

No one has yet proven the theory that antioxidants slow aging and fight disease by protecting the body from free radicals, although evidence is accumulating. Very few studies so far have examined the effect of supplements directly, and more prospective clinical trials are still essential.[55]

So far, studies of antioxidant vitamin supplements have demonstrated no life-prolonging benefit (see Chapter 12).

No controlled clinical trial has tested whether taking high-dose multivitamin/multimineral preparations can prolong life. However, a study of the death rates of elderly readers of *Prevention* magazine, most of whom took high doses of supplements, found no evidence of this.[56] Another epidemiologic study[57] found that people who consumed 300 to 400 mg of vitamin C daily (with roughly half from food) tended to live longer and have less heart disease than those who averaged 50 mg/day. (The current RDA is 90 mg/day for men and 75 mg/day for women.) The study did not prove that supplementation is beneficial, however, because the people with higher vitamin C intake had generally healthier lifestyles, which could explain why they lived longer.

Cryonics

Cryonics is defined by its proponents as "the freezing of humans as shortly as possible after death with the hope of eventual return to life."[58] Proponents claim that it is possible to preserve "with reasonable fidelity" the basic biologic components of the brain and that future technology will be able to repair brain damage caused by "imperfect preservation, premortal disease, and postmortem changes." In 2000 the cost for whole-body freezing and permanent maintenance ranged from about $28,000 to $135,000. "Brain only" suspension, which is less expensive, is also available.

Cryonic technology has not been demonstrated to work in laboratory animals. Even if the rest of a person's body could be revived after hundreds of years, the brain could not. Brain cells deteriorate within minutes after death, and any still viable when the body is frozen would be burst by the freezing process. Cryonics might be a suitable subject for scientific research, but marketing an unproven method to the public is quackery.[59] National Council Against Health Fraud founder William T. Jarvis, Ph.D., calls cryonics "quackery's last shot at you."

SUMMARY

The burden of death may be eased by understanding the emotions involved and planning ahead to deal with various issues that pertain to dying. The need to prepare for death has become more pressing because machines often can keep a dying, permanently unconscious patient alive, sometimes indefinitely. An advance directive can help people control what care they receive if terminally ill. Hospice care provides another way to reduce suffering for patients with a terminal illness.

The technology and success rates of organ transplantation have improved greatly during recent years, but the cost is high and there is a serious shortage of available organs.

The intensity and duration of grief and mourning depend on the nature of the relationship to the dying person and emotional makeup of the survivors.

Most decisions about body disposition are made by people who are grieving and under time constraints, leaving them vulnerable to price-gouging and fraud.

Many entrepreneurs have capitalized on people's wishes to prolong life and delay aging.

It's Your Decision

One of your parents is in the hospital with a terminal illness from which there is no hope of recovery. How can you resolve the following questions?

- Should a discussion be made with the physician to clarify what medical interventions might be used or withheld?
- Should your parent be encouraged to prepare—or should you prepare—a living will, durable power of attorney, or other type of advance medical directive?
- Which friends or family members, if any, should participate in helping to resolve these questions?

REFERENCES

1. The New York Times, July 21, 1974.
2. AMA Council on Scientific Affairs. Good care of the dying patient. JAMA 275:474–478, 1996.
3. Avoiding prolonged death. Consumer Reports on Health 2(8):1–2, 1990.
4. Lieberson AD. The Living Will Handbook. Mamaroneck, N.Y., 1991, Hastings House.
5. Orentlicher D and others. Advance medical directives: A guide to living wills and powers of attorney for health care. Chicago, 1992, American Medical Association.
6. The SUPPORT Investigators. A controlled trial to improve care for seriously ill hospitalized patients. The study to understand prognoses and preferences for outcomes and risks of treatments (SUPPORT). JAMA 274(20):1591–1598, 1995.

7. HCFA fact sheet: A summary of Federal statute concerning advance directives. Washington, D.C., 1991, Health Care Financing Administration.

8. AMA Council on Ethical and Judicial Affairs. Code of Medical Ethics, 1994 Edition. Chicago, 1994, American Medical Association.

9. McCue JD. The naturalness of dying. JAMA 273:1039–1043, 1995.

10. Stanley JM. The Appleton Consensus: Suggested international guidelines for decisions to forego medical treatment. Journal of Medical Ethics 15:129–136, 1989.

11. Living wills: Limitations and alternatives. The Johns Hopkins Medical Letter, Health After 50 2(8):4–5, 1990.

12. Betting on death: Insurance settlements intended to help the dying have short-changed them and fleeced many investors. Consumer Reports 66:3739, 2001.

13. Viatical settlements: A guide for people with terminal illness. Washington, D.C., 1998, Federal Trade Commission.

14. Critical data: U.S. facts about transplantation. United Network for Organ Sharing Web site, accessed Dec 31, 2000.

15. Horton RL, Horton PJ. Knowledge regarding organ donation: Identifying and overcoming barriers to organ donation. Social Science and Medicine 31:791–800, 1990.

16. Parisi N, Katz I. Attitudes toward posthumous organ donation and commitment to donate. Social Science and Medicine 5:565–580, 1986.

17. Ford LA, Smith SW. Memorability and persuasiveness of organ donation message strategies. American Behavioral Science 34:695–711, 1991.

18. Beresford L. The Hospice Handbook: A Complete Guide. Boston, 1993, Little, Brown & Co.

19. Rymes J. Hospice care in America. JAMA 264:369–372, 1990.

20. Facts and figures about hospice care in America. Alexandria, Va., Sept 2000, National Hospice and Palliative Care Organization,

21. Dying with dignity: A guide to hospice care. Harvard Health Letter, Special supplement, April 1993.

22. Lewin-VHI, Inc. An analysis of the cost savings of the Medicare hospice benefit. Arlington, Va., 1995, National Hospice Organization.

23. Coleman B. A consumer guide to hospice selection. Washington, D.C., 1990, National Consumers League.

24. Zucker A. Rights and the dying. In Wass H, Niemeyer RA, editors. Dying: Facing the Facts, ed 3. Washington, D.C., 1995, Taylor & Francis.

25. Garrett TM and others. Health Care Ethics: Principles & Problems. Englewood Cliffs, N.J., 1989, Prentice Hall.

26. Kevorkian J. Prescription Medicide. Amherst, N.Y., 1991, Prometheus Books.

27. Dr. Kevorkian mulls California suicide clinic. American Medical News, Feb 5, 1996.

28. Statement from ERGO Web site, June 1996.

29. Gianelli DM. Association stands firm in opposition of suicide. American Medical News, July 8/15, 1996.

30. Doctor-assisted suicide law spurs care improvements. American Medical News, Feb 5, 1996.

31. Court voids a law barring help in suicide. New York Times, March 7, 1996.

32. Stokely J. Withdrawing or withholding medical care from premature infants: Who should decide, and how? North Dakota Law Review 70(1), 1994.

33. In the matter of baby K. 16F3d 590 (4th Circuit, 1994).

34. Zimmerman D. Supreme Court will not allow brainless 'Baby Girl K' to die. Probe 3(11):1,4, 1994.

35. Funeral Price Information (1999). National Funeral Directors Association Web site, accessed Dec 17, 2000.

36. Caskets and Burial Vaults. Washington, D.C., 1992, Federal Trade Commission.

37. Wasik JF. Fraud in the funeral industry. Consumers Digest 34(5):53–59, 1995.

38. Funerals: A consumer guide. Washington, D.C., June 2000, Federal Trade Commission.

39. Federal Trade Commission. Funeral industry practices; final amended trade regulation rule. Federal Register 59:1592–1614, 1994.

40. Young GW. The High Cost of Dying: A Guide to Funeral Planning. Amherst, N.Y., 1994, Prometheus Books.

41. FTC announces results of compliance testing of over 300 funeral homes in the second year of the Funeral Rule Offenders Program. News release, Feb 25, 1998.

42. Grief—time can be the greatest healer of all. Mayo Clinic Health Letter 8(3):3–4, 1990.

43. Cassem NH. The person confronting death. In Nicholi AM Jr, editor. New Harvard Guide to Psychiatry. Cambridge, Mass, 1988, Harvard University Press.

44. Horowitz MJ. Posttraumatic stress disorders. In American Psychiatric Association Task Force on Treatments of Psychiatric Disorders, vol 3. Washington, D.C., 1989, American Psychiatric Association, pp 2069–2070.

45. Charting a course through grief. The Johns Hopkins Medical Letter, Health After 50 3(12):6–7, 1992.

46. Jarvis WT. How quackery harms. In Barrett S, Cassileth BR, editors. Dubious Cancer Treatment. Tampa, Fla., 1991, American Cancer Society Florida Division.

47. Van Italie TB, Hadley L. The Best Spas. New York, 1989, Harper & Row.

48. Kent S. The Life Extension Revolution: the Source Book for Optimum Health and Maximum Life-Span. New York, 1980, William Morrow and Company.

49. Pearson D, Shaw S. Life Extension: A Practical Scientific Approach. New York, 1982, Warner Books.

50. Walford RL. Maximum Life Span. New York, 1983, W.W. Norton & Co.

51. Yetiv JZ. Popular Nutritional Practices: A Scientific Appraisal. New York, 1988, Dell Publishing.

52. "Fountains of Youth." Lahey Hitchcock Health Letter 7(2):1–3, 1996.

53. Schneider EL, Reed JD. Life extension. New England Journal of Medicine 312:1159–1168, 1985.

54. Yetiv J. Life extension, part I: Theories of aging. Nutrition Forum, Oct 1986.

55. Can you live longer? What works and what doesn't. Consumer Reports 57:7–15, 1992.

56. Enstrom JE, Pauling L. Mortality among health-conscious elderly Californians. Proceedings of the National Academy of Sciences 79:6023–6027, 1982.

57. Enstrom JE, Kanin LE, Klein, MA. Vitamin C intake and mortality among a sample of the United States population. Epidemiology 3:194–200, 1992.

58. The cryobiological case for cryonics. Undated paper distributed in 1989 by Alcor Life Extension Corporation, Riverside, Calif.

59. Jarvis WT. Quotation in Butler K. A Consumer's Guide to "Alternative" Medicine. Amherst, N.Y., 1992, Prometheus Books.

PART VI

PROTECTION OF THE CONSUMER

Chapter Twenty-Four

HEALTH INSURANCE

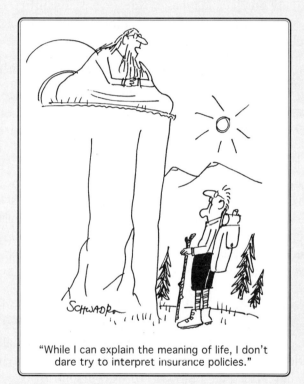

"While I can explain the meaning of life, I don't dare try to interpret insurance policies."

Shopping for health insurance ranks somewhere between grouting the tub and giving blood. A good thing, a necessary thing, but, at best, a chore.

PAUL COHEN[1]

Health insurance policies contain hidden benefits that you can't tap into because you aren't told about them. It's like you're being mugged without even knowing it.

KATHLEEN HOGUE[2]

Bring together any group of citizens and the dimensions of the health care crisis emerge from their stories. Stories about insurance coverage lost, policies cancelled, fear of financial ruin, better jobs not taken, endless forms filled out. They are stories of frustration and insecurity—and, too often, pain and fear.

HILLARY RODHAM CLINTON[3]

Health insurance can help people budget by paying in advance for relatively predictable types of health-care expenses. It can also protect against costs that are less predictable and can be ruinously high. This is important because hospital care costs about $1000 a day and surgical procedures can cost thousands apiece.

Modern health insurance in the United States began as hospital insurance in 1929, when a Dallas hospital administrator told a group of local schoolteachers that for 50¢ a month per teacher his hospital would provide up to 20 days of care. In the 1930s and through World War II health insurance expanded to cover hospital, surgical, and medical services, and employers began to include it in collective bargaining contracts. In the early 1950s insurers began offering major medical policies that covered the cost of illnesses requiring long hospital stays or other extensive treatment. Protection grew rapidly and, by the mid-1950s, 77 million people had coverage for hospital expenses.

During the next few years, insurance companies began offering high-benefit major medical plans and comprehensive coverage with limits placed on out-of-pocket expenses (100% of costs beyond set limits were covered by most insurance plans). Medicare (primarily for people over 65) and Medicaid (for certain low-income populations) became available in 1966.

In the 1970s escalating health-care costs stimulated rapid growth of health maintenance organizations (HMOs), preferred provider organizations (PPOs), and other types of managed-care plans. By 1997 approximately 226 million Americans (84% of the total U.S. population) were covered to some extent by private and/or public insurance. Of these, about 195 million were under 65 years of age, and 31 million were over 65 years old.[4]

This chapter discusses the types of benefits and plans, gives guidelines for selecting coverage, explains the procedures used to collect benefits, and briefly describes disability insurance. Chapter 25 covers national health insurance and insurance fraud.

BASIC HEALTH INSURANCE

Basic health insurance includes benefits for hospital, surgical, and medical expenses. The extent of these benefits differs from contract to contract.

Hospital benefits may pay specified amounts for a specified number of days, which may or may not pay all the costs. Many policies cover the full charges for daily room (usually semiprivate), board, routine nursing services, and intensive care up to a maximum number of days. The insured individual may be responsible for payment of a specific amount (deductible) before coverage begins or may be required to pay a percentage of costs (co-insurance). Additional benefits may be provided up to a fixed dollar amount or for the full cost of other inpatient or outpatient hospital services (other than physicians' fees). Inpatient services are services during hospital confinement and can include laboratory tests, drugs, diagnostic x-ray procedures, operating room, anesthesia, surgical dressings, and physical therapy.

Surgical benefits after any deductible generally pay a surgeon's fee up to a specific limit set forth in the contract (commonly 80% of charges), or the insurer may agree to pay the full amount up to but not exceeding the surgeon's "usual, customary, and reasonable" (UCR) fee. (See Table 24-1 for definitions of these terms.)

Medical benefits provide for payment of nonsurgical physician's fees. They may cover UCR charges or a stated amount for each hospital visit by the attending physician. They generally pay 80% of the bills, including prescription drugs, laboratory tests, private nurses, and other out-of-hospital care. They may also include the maximum number of visits or dollar amounts to be paid for office and home calls plus other professional

Table 24-1

GLOSSARY OF COMMON INSURANCE TERMS

ASSIGNMENT OF BENEFITS: By signing a form (usually the insurance claim form), you authorize the insurance company to pay the physician directly. Otherwise payment must be made directly to you. Most physicians will ask you to sign the form if you don't want to pay your bill before the insurance company pays its share.

CAPITATION: Payment to health providers according to the number of patients they agree to serve rather than the amount of service rendered.

CLAIM FORM: Form stating what information an insurance company needs to make payment. Many providers submit this information electronically rather than on paper.

CO-INSURANCE: Arrangement whereby the patient and the insurance company share costs. The insurer typically pays 75% to 80% of covered costs beyond any deductible amount, and the patient pays the rest. Some policies set an upper limit to co-insurance expense, after which the company pays all additional charges.

CONVERSION PRIVILEGE: Provision that enables those insured by group contracts to obtain an individual policy under various circumstances, such as leaving the job that provided the group coverage.

COORDINATION OF BENEFITS: Provision that prohibits collecting identical benefits from two or more policies, thereby profiting when you are ill. After the primary company pays, other companies calculate their coverage of the remainder. All group policies contain a coordination clause, but some individual policies do not.

COPAYMENT: Fixed dollar amount paid whenever an insured person receives specified health-care services.

DEDUCTIBLE: The amount you must pay before the insurance company starts paying.

ENDORSEMENT OR RIDER: Attachment to the basic insurance policy that changes its coverage.

EXCLUSIONS: Specified conditions or circumstances for which the policy does not provide benefits.

GATEKEEPER: Health-care provider, usually a primary care specialist, who supervises all aspects of a patient's care and must authorize care (except in emergencies) from other providers before the plan will pay for it.

GRACE PERIOD: Number of days that you may delay payment of your premium without losing your insurance.

GUARANTEED RENEWABILITY: Policy where the company agrees to continue insuring you up to a certain age (or for life) as long as you pay the premium. Under this provision, the premium structure cannot be raised unless it is raised for all members of a group or class of insured, such as all people living in your state with the same kind of policy.

INDEMNITY CARRIER: Insurance company or other organization offering specified coverage within a framework of fee schedules, limitations, and exclusions.

INPATIENT SERVICES: Services received while hospitalized.

MANAGED CARE: Health-care system (such as an HMO or PPO) that integrates the financing and delivery of services by using selected providers, utilization review, and financial incentives for members who use the providers and procedures authorized by the plan.

OPEN ENROLLMENT: Period during which insurance plan must accept eligible people regardless of their health status.

OUTPATIENT SERVICES: Services obtained at a hospital by people who are not confined to the hospital.

PARTICIPATING PHYSICIAN: Physician who agrees to abide by the rules of a plan in return for direct payment by the insurance company. The agreement includes acceptance of a fixed fee schedule, a monthly fee per eligible patient, or other fee limitation.

PRE-EXISTING CONDITION: Health problem a person had before becoming insured. Some policies exclude these conditions, while others do not.

PARTICIPATING PROVIDER: Someone who has contracted with an insurance company to provide services to insured individuals under specified conditions. The conditions may include fee limits, utilization review, continuing education requirements, availability during specified hours, and several other factors.

PORTABILITY: The legal right, after employment terminates, to transfer from a group insurance plan to another group or individual plan.

QUALITY ASSURANCE: Internal peer-review process that audits the quality of care delivered. The process should include a mechanism to identify and prevent discrepancies in care.

PROVIDER: Any source of health-care services, such as a hospital, physician, pharmacist, or laboratory.

REASONABLE CHARGE: The amount a company will pay for a given service based on what most providers charge for it.

SUBSCRIBER: Individual who contracts for health insurance coverage.

UTILIZATION REVIEW: Case review to determine whether the care rendered was necessary and appropriate.

WAITING PERIOD: Specified time between issuance of a policy and coverage of certain conditions. Typically there are waiting periods for maternity benefits and pre-existing conditions. Also called elimination period.

WAIVER OF PREMIUM: Policy provision that, under certain conditions, a insurance policy will remain in force without further payments by the policyholder. It is used most often in cases of permanent and total disability.

services. These medical benefits are usually available only with other basic coverages such as hospital and surgical insurance.

Maternity care may be considered a medical benefit, but some policies treat it as a separate category. Hospital care for childbirth may be paid in full, or a maximum amount may be specified. Physicians' fees are usually covered according to a schedule of benefits, with higher amounts permitted for complicated procedures. When available, major medical contracts often cover complications of pregnancy (for example, cesarean section) if expenses exceed maximum benefits of the basic health insurance plan.

Skilled nursing care benefits provide a fixed daily allowance or full charges for a certain type of room for a maximum number of days, usually within a limited number of days after discharge from a hospital. Payment is provided only for medically necessary services, not for mere residential or custodial care. Skilled nursing is much more likely to be covered in major medical policies than in basic insurance.

Benefits for mental or emotional disorders are often treated as a separate category. Some policies have a deductible or co-insurance provision that applies to psychiatric treatment. Other contracts exclude or limit coverage. Some policies provide coverage for vision care, dental care, and prescribed drugs.

MAJOR MEDICAL COVERAGE

Major medical contracts (also called comprehensive coverage) are designed to offset large medical expenses resulting from prolonged illness or serious injury. They take over where basic insurance plans leave off. Major medical policies usually contain deductible and co-insurance provisions. The deductible amount may vary from $50 to $1000 or more. Co-insurance is usually 20%.

Many policies have a "stop-loss" feature that limits out-of-pocket expenses in any year. For example, the insurer may pay 100% of all expenses over $1500 for one person or $3000 for a family within a 1-year period. Maximum lifetime benefits can range from $50,000 to $1 million or can be unlimited. Because most health insurance claims fall within basic coverage, it is possible to buy high maximum benefits under major medical policies for a relatively small increase in premium. It is also possible to purchase an *excess major medical policy* with a very high maximum lifetime benefit and a deductible of $15,000 or more.

Major medical insurance generally covers every type of medically necessary care prescribed by a physician both in and out of the hospital. It can include office visits, nursing care (including special duty nurses), physical therapy, accident-related dental services, durable medical equipment (such as a respirator or feeding device), emergency ambulance service, prescription drugs, prosthetic appliances, pediatric immunizations, and psychiatric care or rehabilitation. The following are desirable components.

CONVERTIBILITY: Ensures conversion to an individual policy if a person changes jobs or divorces.
RENEWABILITY: Guarantees renewability to age 65 and conversion to Medicare.
MAXIMUM BENEFITS: Covers expenses of $1 million or more for each family member.
DEDUCTIBLE: Should not exceed $750 to $1000; policy should start to pay for services when deductible has been met within a 12-month period.
CO-INSURANCE: Should pay 20% to 25% up to a cutoff point of $1500 to $3000, after which the insurer should pay 100%.
CHANGES IN COVERAGE: Insurer may not reduce benefits or coverage.
HOSPITAL EXPENSE LIMIT: Should be at least as high as the daily semiprivate room charges in one's area.
INTENSIVE AND CARDIAC CARE: Should be fully covered.
PRIVATE NURSING: Provision should include care both in and out of the hospital when specified by physician, usually with a limit.
PSYCHIATRIC: At least 50% of the psychiatric bills in and out of the hospital; should have a $10,000 or higher benefit limit.
CONVALESCENT HOME CARE: Coverage should include 60 to 120 days; benefits usually are about half of the daily hospital limits.
BLOOD, PLASMA, AND PROSTHETICS: Should be fully covered.

CONTRACT PROVISIONS

A health insurance policy is a business agreement formalized by a written contract that details both benefits and obligations. When selecting insurance it is useful to understand the significance of the following terms.

Waiting periods. When medical examinations are not required, coverage generally does not become effective until a probationary period, usually 2 weeks to 1 month, has elapsed. Maternity benefits may not be granted until 10 to 12 months after a policy has been issued. There may also be waiting periods for surgery involving the tonsils, adenoids, and appendix, as well as for hemorrhoid surgery and hernia repair. Specific waiting periods may be imposed if an illness or disorder is identified in a subscriber's health history.

Pre-existing illness. An illness or a condition due to injury that is present prior to the contract's date is often excluded from coverage for a specific time, often

1 year. Some contracts deny coverage for illnesses that were present when the policy was taken out, even if an individual was unaware of them.

Conversion privileges. Many group contracts contain a clause that allows an employee, when leaving a job or in the case of marriage, death, divorce, having a child, or reaching maximum age, to convert all or part of the contract to an individual or family plan. There is usually a limit of 15 to 30 days for converting.

Coverage in other countries. Many contracts cover medical care wherever received.

Exclusions. Most contracts exclude coverage for care in hospitals owned and operated by the federal government and for injuries or diseases covered by worker's compensation laws. In addition, conditions resulting from acts of war, riot, and military duty are excluded. Most basic policies do not pay for dental services, hearing aids, or vision aids.

Dependent coverage. Dependents can be protected under a family plan. Coverage for infants may begin at birth or several weeks afterward. Others are usually covered until age 19 years (sometimes longer if full-time students). Coverage is usually dropped automatically when children reach the maximum age listed in the contract, marry, or enter the armed forces, but some policies continue coverage for totally disabled or handicapped children as long as they are dependent. Dependents often have the option of converting their terminating coverage to policies of their own, regardless of medical history. Because the premiums for such individual coverage are higher, it is best to keep dependents under family coverage for as long as the policy allows. Some policies provide fewer benefits to family members than to the principal insured person.

Coordination of benefits. When someone is eligible for benefits under more than one contract or policy, a coordination of benefits provision may apply. This limits payment so the total amount paid under all contracts does not exceed the medical expenses incurred.

Cancellation and renewal provisions. Some policies permit the company to cancel the policy when it wishes to do so. A guaranteed renewable clause prevents the company from canceling the policy, changing the provisions, or charging more to people who incur high expenses. (Rates can be raised, however, for everyone having the same kind of coverage). Conditionally renewable plans are guaranteed renewable as long as the company continues to insure people in your state with the same kind of policy. An optional renewal clause permits changes when the policy comes up for renewal, although any current claims must be paid.

Portability

People covered by a group plan at work have certain rights if their employment is terminated. The 1986 Consolidated Omnibus Budget Reconciliation Act (COBRA) gives an employee who quits or has been laid off the right to remain in the company's plan for 18 months (or 36 months for the family if the person dies or gets divorced). This law applies to most employers of 20 or more people. The cost of the new policy is slightly higher than the cost of coverage under the group policy. A 1989 amendment provides additional help for disabled employees who leave their job. The 1996 Health Insurance Portability and Accountability Act guarantees additional portability to individuals who have group coverage for at least 18 months before leaving a job.

TYPES OF PLANS

Insurance plans can be classified into two main types: indemnity and managed care. (The word *indemnity* means "compensation for damage, loss, or injury.") Indemnity insurance provides monetary benefits rather than services. It includes traditional fee-for-service plans and plans that pay fixed amounts per service, per day, or per week. Managed-care programs are responsible for delivering services in addition to funding them. They include HMOs, PPOs, and point of service (POS) plans. They are based on networks of providers who have contracted to provide services.[5] Managed-care companies try to recruit providers who they believe will furnish cost-effective care. The distinction between indemnity and managed-care plans is not clear-cut, however, because some plans contain features of both.

The term "managed care" is also used to describe various procedures intended to reduce costs while preserving quality of care. These include requirements that nonemergency hospitalization, elective surgery, and various other services be specially authorized in order to be covered. Managed-care companies may also inspect the offices of providers, audit patient charts, issue guidelines, and provide financial incentives to providers that meet certain standards. The economics of managed care is discussed further in Chapter 25.

Health insurance is available through groups and to individuals. *Group insurance* is offered through employers, labor unions, professional organizations, and other benevolent associations. Group health insurance has several advantages. Group policies usually offer greater benefits at lower premiums because economies of scale make administration less expensive. Group insurance seldom requires evidence that individuals are insurable (have no serious pre-existing health problem) if they enroll when they become eligible for coverage.

As an employee benefit, much of the cost of group insurance may be borne by an employer, although there is a trend toward sharing those costs with employees. Employers who have more than 25 employees and offer health insurance may be required by federal law to offer membership in an HMO as an option. Some large groups offer employees a choice of fee-for-service and managed-care plans, either at initial enrollment or once a year. Some group plans offer dental insurance as well as medical. Some also offer long-term care coverage, as an employee-paid option, for employees and their relatives.

Fee-for-Service Plans

In fee-for-service plans, physicians, hospitals, and other providers bill the patient or insurance carrier for each service rendered. Fee-for-service policies include both group and individual plans, with premiums usually billed monthly or quarterly. The benefits received depend on (a) the deductible amount and whether it has been met; (b) the policy's co-insurance provision, which typically is 20% of the covered amount until a specified amount has been reached; and (c) whether the policy pays UCR fees or follows a specific fee schedule. For benefits to be paid, claims must be filed by the insured individual or the provider.

Fixed Dollar Plans

Hospital indemnity plans pay fixed amounts of dollars during hospital confinement. Some policies specify coverage for such items as hospital room, surgery, or prescription drugs. For example, a hospital indemnity policy may pay $50, $75, $100, or more for each day a patient is hospitalized. Because the average length of hospital stay is about 5 days, and the average daily cost is more than $1000, such amounts will only cover a small percentage of the total cost. People who wish to increase their insurance coverage would be wiser to purchase a higher-limit policy or disability insurance.

"Dread disease" policies cover treatment for cancer or other specified serious diseases. Although promoted as a way to supplement basic or major medical coverage, they are a very poor investment. Some of the benefits offered would duplicate existing coverage and thus are unnecessary. Other benefits typically are so narrowly defined that even if the dreaded illness occurs, the policy will cover only a small part of the cost. Moreover, the odds of developing a specific dread disease are small compared to the odds of becoming seriously ill from all causes added together. Therefore someone who wishes greater protection should purchase a high-limit comprehensive policy that covers all illnesses rather than one or a few. A few states have banned or restricted the sale of policies limited to specific diseases. Consumers Union would like all hospital indemnity and dread disease policies banned by federal law.[6]

Health Maintenance Organizations

HMOs are health-care systems in which enrollees (or their employers) pay monthly or quarterly premiums that entitle them to treatment from designated providers. In most cases, providers receive capitated payments or have another incentive to hold down costs. HMOs began operating in the 1930s, but they did not become a major factor in the marketplace until the 1973 Health Maintenance Organization Act allocated $375 million in seed money to start new ones. This law was passed with the hope that managed care would reduce national health expenditures. The law requires all employers with 25 or more employees to offer workers an opportunity to join a qualified HMO if one exists in the area.

HMOs can be classified according to the way in which they are organized. There are five basic types:

INDEPENDENT PRACTICE ASSOCIATION (IPA): An HMO contracts with an association (group) of physicians in various settings and specialties. These doctors include solo and group practitioners. Physicians are paid on a fee-for-service basis. These fees may be 15% or 20% less than the usual and customary fees. Patients see physicians in their individual offices. This model has the largest enrollment and number of plans.

GROUP MODEL: An HMO contracts with a single multispecialty group of physicians to provide health services to its members. A capitation payment is made to the group for each HMO member services regardless of the number of office visits made by members.

NETWORK MODEL: An HMO contracts with two or more independent physician group practices to provide services to its members.

STAFF MODEL: This is the original model (used by Kaiser Permanente), in which physicians are employed directly by the HMO and practice in a central office facility with the necessary administrative support. Doctors receive a salary and bonuses based on the HMO's profits, costs of operation, physician performance, and other factors. Patients can select a primary care physician who can direct them to staff specialists as needed.

DIRECT CONTRACT: An HMO contracts directly with individual physicians.

Mixed-model plans use various combinations of these arrangements.[7]

Table 24-2

HMO Enrollment, 1998

Model	Number of Plans	Enrollment
IPA	606	62.8 million
Network	175	20.1 million
Group	91	19.8 million
Staff	30	2.7 million
Totals	902	105.3 million

Source: Hoechst Marion Roussel, Inc.[8]

HMO enrollment has been growing about 10% per year. Table 24-2 gives the number of plans and their enrollments in 1998.

Preferred Provider Organizations

PPOs combine features of HMOs and fee-for-service indemnity plans. PPOs contract with networks or panels of providers who agree to a negotiated fee schedule that usually is 15% to 20% lower than their standard fees. Subscribers can obtain services from any provider they wish but must pay a higher percentage of the cost if they use a nonparticipant. An exclusive provider organization (EPO) is a less expensive form of PPO that does not reimburse for the services of nonparticipating providers. In 1998 there were 1127 operating PPOs covering 98.3 million eligible persons in the United States.[8]

Point of Service Plans

POS plans are HMO/PPO hybrids. Subscribers choose a primary physician who provides basic care and can authorize referrals to specialists. As in HMOs, subscribers pay only their copayments and deductibles for services rendered from participating providers, and they do not have to file claims. Subscribers who elect to see nonparticipating providers are reimbursed, but their out-of-pocket costs are significantly higher.

Medicare

Medicare is a federal insurance program created by amendments to the Social Security Act. It provides benefits for persons 65 years or older and for certain disabled persons younger than 65. It is administered by the Health Care Financing Administration (HCFA), an agency of the U.S. Department of Health and Human Services. Various commercial insurance companies are under contract with HCFA to process and pay Medicare claims, and groups of doctors and other health-care professionals have contracts to monitor the quality of care given to Medicare beneficiaries.

Medicare has two parts. Part A helps pay for inpatient hospital care, inpatient care in a skilled nursing facility, and hospice care. Part A is financed by Social Security taxes. Employers and employees now pay 1.45%, and the self-employed pay 2.9% on all earnings. Part B helps pay for doctors' services, outpatient hospital services, laboratory services, ambulance service, durable medical equipment, and various other medical services and supplies. Part B subscribers pay monthly premiums that cover about 25% of the government's cost of running the program. The premium is either billed quarterly or deducted from the insured person's Social Security check.

Most people over 65 are eligible for Part A. There is no monthly charge, but eligible individuals must request coverage. When signing up, they are automatically enrolled in Part B. Enrollment in Part B is voluntary, however. Those who decline can enroll during the first quarter of the following year at a higher premium. People planning to begin Medicare coverage at age 65

Managed Care Consumers' Bill of Rights

The Public Policy and Education Fund of New York, in cooperation with the Citizens Fund, has published a report stating that managed-care consumers should have the right to:

1. Timely access to appropriate health care.
2. Affordable choice of qualified health-care professionals.
3. Comprehensive health care benefits that meet consumers' health-care needs.
4. Receive health care that is affordable and free of financial barriers that impede access to health care.
5. High-quality health care.
6. Challenge decisions a plan makes about any practices or services that impact access to and quality of health care.
7. Accurate, current, and understandable information about a managed care plan.
8. Have medical information remain confidential and not to be discriminated against in managed care.
9. Be represented in decision making and in the organization and regulation of managed care.
10. Vigorous enforcement of the Managed Care Consumers' Bill of Rights.[9]

Table 24-3

SUMMARY OF 2001 MEDICARE PART A BENEFITS*[10]

Services	Benefit	Medicare Pays
Hospitalization	First 60 days	All but $792
Semiprivate room and board, general nursing	61st to 90th day	All but $198 a day
and other hospital services and supplies	91st to 150th day (once in a lifetime)	All but $396 a day
	Beyond 150 days	Nothing
Skilled nursing facility care	First 20 days	100% of approved amount
Semiprivate room and board, skilled nursing	Next 80 days	All but $99 a day
and rehabilitative services, and other services and supplies	Beyond 100 days	Nothing
Home health care	Unlimited if patient is	100% of approved amount; 80%
Part-time or intermittent skilled care, home	homebound and meets	of approved amount for durable
health aide services, durable medical equip-	other Medicare	medical equipment
ment and supplies, and other services	conditions	
Hospice care	For as long as doctor	All but $5 for outpatient drugs
Pain relief, symptom management, and support	certifies need	and 5% of the approved amount
services for the terminally ill		for inpatient respite care
Blood	Unlimited if medically	All but first 3 pints per calendar
When furnished by a hospital or skilled nursing	necessary	year; no obligation if replaced
facility during a covered stay		or paid for under Part B

*Most people do not have to pay a premium for Part A.

should contact their local Social Security office 3 months beforehand to obtain the enrollment forms.

The 1989 federal Physicians Payment Reform Act limits the amount that doctors who do not accept Medicare's assigned fees are permitted to charge patients over the age of 65. The current limit is 15% above what Medicare pays. The law requires physicians to file claims for all reimbursable services. The law also states that if Medicare denies payment for services (as not reasonable or necessary), the physician may not collect from the patient unless the patient was notified in advance or should have known that the services were not reimbursable. (In many cases the patient will be asked to sign an advance notice.) In 1996 a federal court ruled that the 1989 law does not limit hospital outpatient charges. This means that Medicare patients who are responsible for 20% of the charges, can have sizable out-of-pocket expenses for hospital outpatient services.[11]

Tables 24-3 and 24-4 summarize the coverage under Medicare. Noncovered services include long-term nursing home stays, custodial care in a nursing home, private-duty nurses at home, homemaker services, routine dental services and dentures, routine physicals, preventive care (except for influenza and pneumococcal pneumonia vaccines), vision examinations and eyeglasses, hearing tests and hearing aids, routine foot care,

physician charges above the approved amount, care received outside the United States, and items or services not considered medically reasonable or necessary.[10] People who believe that a Medicare payment is less than it should be have the right to appeal for reconsideration. Additional details about Medicare coverage are published in a handbook that is updated annually and is available online at http://www.medicare.gov or from the Medicare Hotline [800 638-6833].

Supplemental Insurance
Medicare supplement insurance (commonly called "Medigap" insurance) is commercial insurance tailored to cover some of the gaps in Medicare coverage. In 1990 Congress ordered the National Association of Insurance Commissioners to develop 10 standard packages of Medicare supplement benefits. States were given until mid-1992 to choose which of these policies can be sold within their borders. All 10 packages must fill the gaps in Part A so that the beneficiary is covered for hospital co-insurance and 365 additional lifetime hospital days after the Medicare hospital benefit is exhausted. The price of the policy reflects the number of additional benefits (such as skilled nursing co-insurance, prescription drugs, Part B deductible, and certain preventive care) that are included.

Table 24-4

SUMMARY OF 2001 MEDICARE PART B BENEFITS*[10]

Services	Benefit	Medicare Pays
Medical expenses Doctors' services, inpatient and outpatient medical and surgical services and supplies, physical and speech therapy, diagnostic tests, durable medical equipment, and other services	Unlimited if medically necessary	80% of approved amount (after $100 deductible) 50% for most outpatient mental health services
Clinical laboratory services Blood tests, urinalyses, and other tests	Unlimited if medically necessary	Generally 100% of approved amount
Home health care Part-time or intermittent skilled care, home health aide services, durable medical equipment and supplies, and other services	Unlimited if medically necessary	100% of approved amount; 80% of approved amount for durable medical equipment
Outpatient hospital treatment Services for the diagnosis or treatment of illness or injury	Unlimited if medically necessary	Medicare payment to hospital based on hospital cost
Blood	Unlimited if medically necessary	80% of approved amount (after $100 deductible and starting with 4th pint)
Ambulatory surgical services	Unlimited if medically necessary	80% of predetermined amount (after $100 deductible)

*The 2001 Part B monthly premium for most people is $50.

The best time to purchase a Medigap policy is during the open enrollment period, which is 6 months from the date of Medicare Part B enrollment (after age 65). During this period, no applicant can be refused. After it ends, companies have the right to restrict which policy they sell. State insurance commissioners can provide information on the types of policies approved for sale within their state.

Another way to decrease out-of-pocket expenses is to enroll in an HMO or other managed-care plan. They provide all of Medicare's benefits with little or no paperwork but with limited choice of providers. These plans entail a copayment whenever various services are used. About 65% of HMOs charge no premium (but the insured must be enrolled in Medicare Part B), and 30% charge less than $40 a month.[12] All plans that contract with Medicare must have an enrollment period of at least 30 days per year, during which no applicant can be rejected because of poor health.

The standardization of Medigap policies was ordered to protect the elderly from widespread, unscrupulous sales practices. In 1994, after a 7-month investigation, *Consumer Reports* concluded that many insurance companies and agents were thwarting the law's intent. The investigation found: (a) companies and agents were steering consumers to only one or two of

the plans, while strongly disparaging the others; (b) agents failed to give their prospects the price information required by law; (c) agents were still urging consumers to buy benefits they did not need; and (d) in many cities there was a wide range of prices for policies offering the same benefits.[13]

The Health Research Group (HRG) has reported that some capitated HMOs did not provide adequate service to their Medicare enrollees. This conclusion was based on its analysis of a survey by the Office of the Inspector General of about 4000 enrollees from 45 HMOs. Nineteen percent had complained that their doctors' phone lines were busy "all or most of the time," and 11% had reported giving up trying to make appointments.[14]

Diagnosis-Related Groups (DRGs)

Since 1983 Medicare has paid for hospital services according to a predetermined schedule for about 500 diagnosis-related groups (DRGs). The DRG system replaced the system whereby hospitals in various parts of the United States received widely divergent fees for the same services. It was instituted in an effort to control medical costs. Hospitals able to provide services for less than the government rate can retain the difference. Thus a hospital that keeps a patient for 2 days receives as much as one that keeps a similar patient for 6 days. To ensure that the quality of care is not affected, hospitals treating Medicare patients must conduct strict peer review.

DRG procedures have helped spur hospitals to reduce the average number of days that patients spend per hospital admission. Concerns have been raised that some hospitals discharge patients who still need treatment. Patients who believe they are being prematurely discharged can: (a) ask for a written notice, which will be needed for appeal, (b) seek help from their doctor, and (c) appeal to the hospital peer review organization (PRO).

MEDICAID

Medicaid is a federal grant-in-aid program under which the states may contract with the Secretary of Health and Human Services to finance health-care services for public assistance recipients. It provides comprehensive care and nursing home coverage for certain categories of indigent and medically indigent persons. There are about 29 million eligible persons, including the aged, blind, disabled, and members of single-parent families with dependent children.[4] The proportion of state-to-federal funding of the program is determined by a formula based on each state's per capita income. Eligibility requirements differ from state to state but generally require a low income and few assets. Some people establish eligibility by incurring medical expenses until their assets are depleted and their net income after medical expenses is low enough to qualify. Of those eligible for Medicaid, nearly half are eligible to receive Medicare.

LONG-TERM CARE INSURANCE

Long-term care refers to the nursing, medical, and social services provided to an individual over a prolonged period (see Chapter 10). The most common settings are nursing homes and individual homes.

The levels of service provided in nursing homes are classified as skilled nursing care (intensive medical and rehabilitative care by trained personnel), intermediate nursing care (less intensive care by trained personnel), and custodial care (daily activities such as meals, bathing, and dressing). In home care, patients may receive skilled nursing care (also occupational and physical therapy), home health aide services (personal and custodial care), and homemaker services (cleaning, cooking, and running errands).

In 1991 Kemper and Murtaugh[15] estimated that 43% of Americans who were 65 in 1990 would enter a nursing home some time before they die, that half of these would spend at least 1 year there, and that 21% would spend at least 5 years there.

Nursing homes typically cost $3000 to $6000 per month. Home care averages about $75 per visit and can easily total over $1000 per month for just three visits per week. These costs have encouraged the elderly to seek protection and have stimulated insurance companies to offer policies to offset some of the expenditures for long-term care.

The premiums for long-term care insurance depend on the age of the person, daily benefit levels, and length of elimination period (number of days or home visits before coverage begins). Most policies require passage of a period of time before covering care needed because of pre-existing conditions. The cost can be reduced by selecting a policy with a long waiting period (such as 100 days) or a shorter benefit period (3 or 4 years rather than lifetime benefits). Policies with benefits that increase with inflation cost 30% to 90% more than those that provide a fixed monthly amount. Eligibility for benefits is based on the severity of impairment and the inability to perform a certain number of activities of daily living.

In 1997, a policy offering a $100 per day nursing home benefit for 4 years, with a 20-day deductible, cost about $364 per year when purchased at age 50, $980 when purchased at age 65, and $3907 for a 79-year-old. The same policy with an inflation feature cost $802 at age 50, $1829 at age 65, and $5592 at age 79.[16] The Health Insurance Association of America (HIAA)[4] estimates that more than 4.9 million long-term care policies were purchased between 1987 and 1996. The 1996 Health Coverage and Affordability Act made premiums for long-term care insurance deductible a medical expense for income tax purposes.

Oshiro and Snyder[17] advise that people whose income and assets are low enough or nearly low enough to qualify for Medicaid cannot afford to purchase long-term care insurance. Those with modest assets who do not qualify immediately for Medicaid will quickly have their assets depleted to the point that they do qualify. Financial planners consulted by *Kiplinger's Personal Finance Magazine* said (a) prime candidates for long-term care insurance are couples with over $100,000 in assets or single individuals with at least $40,000 in assets, not including the value of their home, and (b) premiums should not exceed 5% to 6% of the buyer's income.[18]

Consumers investigating long-term care insurance policies should obtain answers to these questions:

- Does the policy cover skilled nursing, intermediate care, and custodial care, at a nursing home, other assisted living facilities, and at home? What services are covered?
- What is the daily benefit? It should pay half to two thirds of the cost. Will benefits increase with inflation?
- How long will the benefits last?
- When do benefits begin? (The longer the elimination period, the less costly the policy.)
- Under what circumstances can the premiums be increased?
- Is payment of further premiums waived if the insured person stays in a nursing home?
- Are policies guaranteed renewable?
- Do benefits hinge on prior hospitalization? (Nearly two thirds of the patients who enter a nursing home have not been hospitalized beforehand.)
- Is Alzheimer's disease covered? To what extent? Is any other illness or injury excluded from coverage?
- What are the restrictions on pre-existing conditions? Waiting periods? Deductible?
- Are there any other limitations or exclusions?
- May I have an outline of the coverage and sample copy of the policy?
- Is the company's loss ratio 80% or more?
- Can I receive a 30-day free look at the policy with refund of the premium if requested?
- Is the company rated "B" or better by *Weiss Ratings' Guide to HMOs and Health Insurers*? This can be checked by asking the agent or consulting the guide at a library.

A consumer's guide to long-term care insurance is available on the Health Insurance Association of America Web site (http://www.hiaa.org).

DENTAL INSURANCE

Dental insurance programs were started by nonprofit dental service corporations sponsored by local dental societies. Currently almost all private plans are group plans sponsored by employers or labor unions. Medicaid also provides coverage in some states.

The American Dental Association (ADA)[19] states that the most common plans can be grouped into five categories:

DIRECT REIMBURSEMENT PROGRAMS reimburse a percentage of the dollar amount spent and provides free choice of dentist.

USUAL, CUSTOMARY, AND REASONABLE (UCR) programs pay a set percentage of the dentist's fee or the plan administrator's UCR limit, whichever is lower. The limits are set by a contract between the insurer and the plan purchaser (usually the employer).

TABLE or SCHEDULE OF ALLOWANCE programs assign dollar amounts to a list of covered services. Most often the fees are below the dentist's full fee, and the patient pays the difference.

PREFERRED PROVIDER ORGANIZATION (PPO) programs are plans in which contracting dentists agree to discount their fees

as a financial incentive for patients to select their practices. Patients who choose a nonparticipating dentist will have benefits reduced or lost completely.

CAPITATION PLANS (HMOS) pay contracting dentists a fixed amount (usually monthly) per enrolled family or patient. In return, the dentist agrees to provide specific types of treatment at no charge or with a copayment.

The most recent survey by the National Center for Health Statistics found that in 1995, about 55% of Americans over the age of 2 had private dental insurance.[20] Dental insurance usually covers examinations, fillings, x-ray films, extractions, cleaning, and dentures. Orthodontic and endodontic care, bridgework, oral surgery, and periodontics are often limited or excluded unless a higher premium is paid. Other common exclusions or limitations apply to pre-existing conditions, replacement of lost dentures, dentures and bridgework to replace teeth lost prior to coverage, and expenses covered by other insurance. Monthly premiums typically range from $20 to $30 for individuals and $40 to $60 per family. Individual plans, purchasable directly from an insurance company, have higher premiums, more limited coverage, and larger out-of-pocket expenses.

Dental costs that can be covered by insurance are much more predictable than medical costs and can fit within most budgets. People whose teeth and gums are healthy do not need dental insurance because the annual cost of dental checkups and cleaning will be less than the cost of dental insurance. People who expect to need more care should compare their anticipated expenses with the cost of insurance premiums.

LOSS RATIOS

The amount of money a company pays out in claims can be expressed as the benefit-cost ratio or loss ratio. This is calculated by dividing the amount paid in benefits by the amount received in premiums. It is one way that consumers can assess the value of health insurance policies. A high loss ratio is a favorable sign. A low loss ratio indicates that a company is either inefficient or is making excess profits. According to the A.M. Best Company, the average loss ratio for all 1995 accident and health policies was 81.2%, which means that for every $100 premium dollars, $81.20 was paid in benefits. The average for all group plans was 82.2%.[21] Nonprofit plans and most HMOs tend to have higher loss ratios.

Data on individual companies are compiled by state insurance departments and are also published by A.M. Best in manuals available at most public libraries. However, loss ratios vary not only from company to company but from one type of policy to another within a company. Data on specific policies may be available from company representatives or agents.

INDEMNITY VS MANAGED CARE

Traditional (fee-for-service) indemnity plans tend to cost most, HMOs least, and PPOs and POS in between. *Managed Care* magazine has reported, for example, that in 1998 the average monthly premiums for individual coverage offered to the employees of "Fortune 500" companies were $200 for indemnity plans, $161 for HMOs, $171 for PPOs, and $178 for POS plans.[22] (Family plans tend to cost about three times as much.) However, the pattern is not consistent. Some indemnity and PPO plans are less expensive than HMOs. Surveys have found that higher-priced plans tend to be rated higher by their subscribers, but some lower-priced plans also have been rated highly.

Among more than 20,000 *Consumer Reports* readers who responded to a 1995 survey, about 10% said they didn't get treatment they felt they needed because their HMOs discouraged it, whereas only 2% with traditional plans described that problem. About 18% of managed-care subscribers went outside their plan to get what they believed they needed. The respondents also tended to be more satisfied with the nonprofit plans.[23] A 1999 survey of *Consumer Reports* readers found that

34% of managed-care participants reported getting inappropriate care and that those who were sick were more satisfied in less-restrictive plans.[24]

A Group Health Association of America survey found generally greater satisfaction with HMOs, but senior citizens in fair or poor health were more satisfied with fee-for-service coverage.[25] A Robert Wood Johnson Foundation survey of 473 significantly ill people ages 18 to 64 found that those in managed-care plans spent less out-of-pocket but were somewhat less likely to get the services they or their doctors thought were necessary.[26] A Commonwealth Fund survey found that dissatisfaction was higher among managed-care enrollees than among fee-for-service enrollees. This study involved 3000 people with employer- or union-sponsored plans. Those who did not have a choice of plan were less likely to be satisfied with managed care.[27]

It has been hoped that accreditation might provide a valuable guideline for judging the quality of a managed-care plan. The National Committee on Quality Assurance (NCQA) is an independent, nonprofit organization that evaluates managed care. Its more than 60 standards cover access and service, provider qualifications, health maintenance strategies, and quality of care. NCQA also operates the Health Employer Data Information System (HEDIS), a "report card" intended to enable employers and consumers to compare plans.

Table 24-5

COMPARISON OF INSURANCE PLANS

Characteristic	Fee-for-Service	PPO	POS	HMO
Are consumers free to choose providers?	Yes	PPO providers can be seen at discounted fees. Out-of plan providers can be seen but cost more.	Coverage provided for providers in plan. Other providers paid according to fee schedule; consumer must pay any additional cost.	Coverage provided only for providers in plan. Some providers use physician assistants for screening.
Are providers free to prescribe treatment?	Yes, if medically necessary and appropriate	Yes, if medically necessary and appropriate	Some restrictions	Many services must be preapproved in order to be covered.
Does insurer bear financial risk?	Yes	Yes	Yes	Yes
Do providers share financial risk with insurer?	No	Rare	Sometimes	Yes; penalties or incentives discourage use of "unnecessary" services.
Is insurer obliged to provide health-care services?	No	Yes, within provider network	Yes, within provider network	Fully responsible for necessary and appropriate services
Must consumer file claim forms?	Yes, unless provider does	Only for out-of-network services	Only for out-of-network services	No
Relative cost of premiums	Tends to be highest	Between fee-for-service and HMO	Between fee-for-service and HMO	Tends to be lowest
Relative out-of-pocket expense	Lower cost policies have highest out-of-pocket expense	Low if out-of-network services are not used	Low if out-of-network services are not used	Tends to be lowest

By October 31, 2000, 265 commercial plans, 141 Medicare plans, and 63 Medicaid plans had completed NCQA's accreditation process (19 of these were denied), and 13 others were waiting to be evaluated.[28] A 1998 survey of *Consumer Reports* readers found that their assessments closely matched the data reported by NCQA participants and that NCQA nonparticipants were rated significantly worse than participants.[29] An analysis of HEDIS data gathered in 1996 has concluded that nonprofit HMOs scored higher than investor-owned programs.[30] The Center for the Study of Services[31] has concluded:

Given the possible advantages and disadvantages of different plan types, no type is a clear winner for all. Some consumers will be more concerned than others about the restrictiveness of HMOs, and some may weigh HMOs' cost advantages or care management potential most heavily. Even if you prefer one plan type in theory, you might choose another type because that specific plan is extraordinary.

Managed-care plans tend to have lower premiums and result in fewer out-of-pocket costs, particularly for young adults and families with young children. Traditional indemnity policies tend to cost more and involve more paperwork (in filing claims) but provide greater choice of providers, which may be important for people who are chronically or seriously ill. Table 24-5 provides additional comparative data. People inclined toward managed care should carefully investigate whether a suitable primary physician is available to them in any plan they consider. Other favorable signs are affiliation with an accredited teaching hospital, access to enough specialists, and a high percentage of board certification among its physicians. Some HMOs provide data on subscriber satisfaction with their primary care physicians. *Consumer Reports*[29] and *U.S. News & World Report*[32] have published ratings of several hundred plans. The NCQA publishes an accreditation status list and summaries of its findings for individual plans.

MEDICAL SAVINGS ACCOUNTS

The 1996 Health Coverage and Affordability Act set up a trial program for up to 750,000 Americans who open medical savings accounts (MSAs). Eligibility requires that an individual (a) be self-employed or employed by a firm with 50 or fewer employees and (b) be covered by an insurance policy with an annual deductible between $1500 and $2250 for an individual or $3000 to $5000 for a family. Each year the individual (or employer) can contribute up to 65% of the deductible for an individual or 75% of the deductible for a family.

The contribution is nontaxable if paid by the employer, and tax-deductible if paid by the individual. The money can be invested with no tax due as the investment grows. Distributions to pay medical expenses will be tax-free. Other distributions would be taxable, with an additional 15% penalty unless made after age 65, death, or disability. MSAs combine insurance coverage with an opportunity for tax-free investing and an incentive for keeping medical costs as low as possible. Participants whose expenses are small can accumulate a substantial sum by age 65.

MSAs are most suitable for young adults with a healthy lifestyle that makes them less likely than most people to have high medical expenses. MSAs may also help reduce overall health-care costs by lowering the demand for health-care services. (When people have to pay directly for health-care services, they tend to use fewer of them.) However, Keeler and others[33] state that this is unlikely unless the required insurance policies have high deductibles and are purchased by individuals. Critics have also pointed out that MSAs might drive up costs for traditional plans if healthy people, who stand to accumulate considerable savings with MSAs, leave the insurance pool, while those with chronic ill health remain.[34]

CHOOSING A POLICY

Choosing health insurance can be complicated. There are many types of plans, and contracts can vary greatly from company to company and even within the same company.

Colleges typically provide outpatient health services through a student health service, usually at a low fee that is paid along with tuition. Some also require students to purchase additional insurance to cover hospitalization or other outside services. Students covered under their family's policy may not be required to purchase additional insurance. It is usually most economical to remain covered under a family policy as long as possible rather than obtaining a separate policy.

After college it is usually best to see whether group coverage is available through work or membership in an organization. If you work for a large company, several plans may be available. If no group coverage is available, contact Blue Cross/Blue Shield and agents for several other insurance companies, including some that provide managed-care plans. If you find it difficult to obtain insurance because of a pre-existing health problem, find out from your state insurance department or a broker whether your state has a risk pool similar to the assigned-risk pools for automobile insurance.

Table 24-6

QUESTIONS TO ASK WHEN COMPARING HEALTH INSURANCE POLICIES

When choosing health insurance, become familiar with all the literature provided. It is best to obtain a copy of the policy and read it carefully. If the language appears conflicting or difficult to understand, ask the company representative for clarification. Be sure the coverage is suitable, and don't hesitate to shop around. Coverage and costs vary greatly from plan to plan. The following questions can help you to compare plans.

Type of policy
- Is the policy a group or individual one?
- Is the insurance comprehensive, providing basic health insurance that includes hospital, surgical, medical, and (if needed) maternity benefits? Does it also include major medical provisions, or is such insurance available?

Hospital coverage
- How many days are covered for each illness? What is the per diem rate? Is the allowance sufficient to cover the entire daily rate? Is there coverage for intensive care?
- What services are covered?
- Is there a deductible clause?
- Is the choice of hospitals limited?
- Are in-hospital physicians' services covered?
- Is consultation permissible? Under what conditions?
- Are the covered days limited to one period of hospitalization, or is there more than one period covered up to a maximum number of days?
- Are there limitations on readmission to a hospital for the same illness?

Surgical coverage
- What surgical procedures are covered, and to what extent? What is the surgical fee schedule?
- Are there provisions for consultant services?
- Are second opinions required?
- Are there limits in the choice of surgeons or where they may conduct the surgery?
- How do the fees allowed compare to what local surgeons charge?

Medical coverage
- Which services are covered? Excluded? Limited?
- Are home and office visits covered? Are there any limitations?
- Is there a deductible clause?
- Does it include service for accidents?
- Is the choice of physicians limited?
- Are periodic well-person physical examinations, preventive immunizations, Pap tests, and other preventive measures covered?
- Are prescription drugs covered?
- Is treatment for mental and emotional problems and drug and alcohol abuse covered? To what extent?
- Are there provisions for concurrent services of more than one physician when medically necessary?

Maternity care
- What expenses are covered? What are the limitations?
- What complications are covered?
- What is the waiting period?

Major medical insurance
- What services are covered?
- What is the maximum coverage? The minimum recommended is $1 million. What is the stop-loss limit (the amount over which the company pays $100%)?
- Is there a deductible? How much?
- Is co-insurance required? Limits?
- Can maximum limits be restored after illness?
- What percentage above the deductible is paid by the company?

Nursing home or home care
- What services are covered? For how many days? At what daily rate?
- Is prior hospitalization required for coverage?
- Are services of RNs, LVNs, LPNs, or other allied health professionals covered?
- Are medications and medical supplies covered?

Contract provisions
- Are all family members covered? To what ages?
- Are there waiting periods? What is the effective policy date?
- What are the conditions and limitations for pre-existing conditions? Do they apply for more than 1 year?
- Can the policy be converted to an individual plan? To a family plan if an individual marries? Is it convertible after retirement?
- What are the conditions regarding cancellation and renewal of policy? By whom? Is renewal guaranteed?
- What are the exclusions? Are they more restrictive than the usual ones, such as dental, vision, hearing?
- Does coverage include out-of-area services, and services in foreign countries?
- Can rates be changed? What are the conditions under which rates may be changed?

Selecting an insuring organization
- Is the company licensed in your state?
- Is the company or agent a reliable and reputable one?
- Is it rated at least C by *Weiss Ratings' Guide*?
- Does the company have a reputation for paying promptly and without hassles?
- What is the loss ratio? Is it at least 80%?

After discussing your needs, obtain both a summary and a copy of each policy that sounds suitable, read them carefully, and be sure you understand what they say. If you want both basic and major medical coverage, they should be obtained from the same company to avoid gaps in coverage. However, your aim should be to insure mainly against the most serious types of losses. In the long run, it is more economical to absorb the cost of minor medical expenses as part of your overall budget. Policies that pay a daily amount and other types of overlapping policies should be avoided.

Table 24-6 can help you compare policies. Some state insurance departments can provide information on complaints made against health insurance companies. The *Weiss Ratings' Guide to HMOs and Health Insurers* provides data on the financial stability of hundreds of plans.[35]

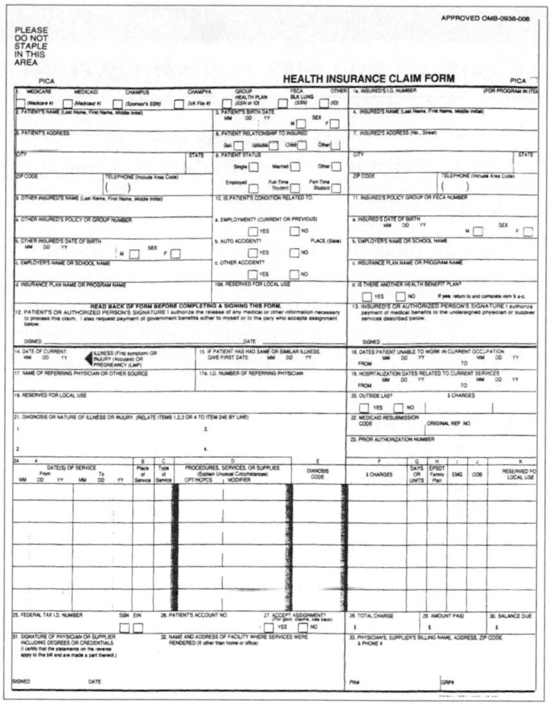
APPROVED OMB-0938-008

PLEASE DO NOT STAPLE IN THIS AREA

PICA HEALTH INSURANCE CLAIM FORM PICA

1. MEDICARE (Medicare #) MEDICAID (Medicaid #) CHAMPUS (Sponsor's SSN) CHAMPVA (VA File #) GROUP HEALTH PLAN (SSN or ID) FECA BLK LUNG (SSN) OTHER (ID)
1a. INSURED'S I.D. NUMBER (FOR PROGRAM IN ITEM 1)
2. PATIENT'S NAME (Last Name, First Name, Middle Initial)
3. PATIENT'S BIRTH DATE MM DD YY SEX M F
4. INSURED'S NAME (Last Name, First Name, Middle Initial)
5. PATIENT'S ADDRESS
6. PATIENT RELATIONSHIP TO INSURED Self Spouse Child Other
7. INSURED'S ADDRESS (No., Street)
CITY STATE
8. PATIENT STATUS Single Married Other
CITY STATE
ZIP CODE TELEPHONE (Include Area Code) ( )
Employed Full-Time Student Part-Time Student
ZIP CODE TELEPHONE (Include Area Code) ( )
9. OTHER INSURED'S NAME (Last Name, First Name, Middle Initial)
10. IS PATIENT'S CONDITION RELATED TO:
11. INSURED'S POLICY GROUP OR FECA NUMBER
a. OTHER INSURED'S POLICY OR GROUP NUMBER
a. EMPLOYMENT? (CURRENT OR PREVIOUS) YES NO
a. INSURED'S DATE OF BIRTH MM DD YY SEX M F
b. OTHER INSURED'S DATE OF BIRTH MM DD YY SEX M F
b. AUTO ACCIDENT? PLACE (State) YES NO
b. EMPLOYER'S NAME OR SCHOOL NAME
c. EMPLOYER'S NAME OR SCHOOL NAME
c. OTHER ACCIDENT? YES NO
c. INSURANCE PLAN NAME OR PROGRAM NAME
d. INSURANCE PLAN NAME OR PROGRAM NAME
10d. RESERVED FOR LOCAL USE
d. IS THERE ANOTHER HEALTH BENEFIT PLAN? YES NO If yes, return to and complete item 9 a-d.
READ BACK OF FORM BEFORE COMPLETING & SIGNING THIS FORM.
12. PATIENT'S OR AUTHORIZED PERSON'S SIGNATURE I authorize the release of any medical or other information necessary to process this claim. I also request payment of government benefits either to myself or to the pary who accepts assignment below.
SIGNED DATE
13. INSURED'S OR AUTHORIZED PERSON'S SIGNATURE I authorize payment of medical benefits to the undersigned physician or supplier for services described below.
SIGNED
14. DATE OF CURRENT: MM DD YY ILLNESS (First symptom) OR INJURY (Accident) OR PREGNANCY (LMP)
15. IF PATIENT HAS HAD SAME OR SIMILAR ILLNESS. GIVE FIRST DATE MM DD YY
16. DATES PATIENT UNABLE TO WORK IN CURRENT OCCUPATION FROM MM DD YY TO MM DD YY
17. NAME OF REFERRING PHYSICIAN OR OTHER SOURCE
17a. I.D. NUMBER OF REFERRING PHYSICIAN
18. HOSPITALIZATION DATES RELATED TO CURRENT SERVICES FROM MM DD YY TO MM DD YY
19. RESERVED FOR LOCAL USE
20. OUTSIDE LAB? YES NO $ CHARGES
21. DIAGNOSIS OR NATURE OF ILLNESS OR INJURY. (RELATE ITEMS 1,2,3 OR 4 TO ITEM 24E BY LINE)
1. 3.
2. 4.
22. MEDICAID RESUBMISSION CODE ORIGINAL REF. NO.
23. PRIOR AUTHORIZATION NUMBER
24. A DATE(S) OF SERVICE From MM DD YY To MM DD YY | B Place of Service | C Type of Service | D PROCEDURES, SERVICES, OR SUPPLIES (Explain Unusual Circumstances) CPT/HCPCS MODIFIER | E DIAGNOSIS CODE | F $ CHARGES | G DAYS OR UNITS | H EPSDT Family Plan | I EMG | J COB | K RESERVED FOR LOCAL USE
25. FEDERAL TAX I.D. NUMBER SSN EIN
26. PATIENT'S ACCOUNT NO.
27. ACCEPT ASSIGNMENT? (For govt. claims, see back) YES NO
28. TOTAL CHARGE $
29. AMOUNT PAID $
30. BALANCE DUE $
31. SIGNATURE OF PHYSICIAN OR SUPPLIER INCLUDING DEGREES OR CREDENTIALS (I certify that the statements on the reverse apply to this bill and are made a part thereof.)
SIGNED DATE
32. NAME AND ADDRESS OF FACILITY WHERE SERVICES WERE RENDERED (If other than home or office)
33. PHYSICIAN'S, SUPPLIER'S BILLING NAME, ADDRESS, ZIP CODE & PHONE #
PIN# GRP#

FIGURE 24-1. HCFA 1500 insurance claim form.

COLLECTION OF INSURANCE BENEFITS

When a policy is issued, covered individuals will be issued a card indicating the name of the company, the policy number, and the type of plan.

Providers generally ask new patients to complete a registration form that includes basic information (name, address, and age), current problem, past medical history, medications taken, and insurance information. The insurance card will also be requested and a copy made. For HMOs, a plastic card may be used to fill out encounter and referral forms.

After the service is completed, the patient will be given a bill, a receipt for payment, or a computer printout, or the provider will submit the bill for the patient. (For Medicare, the provider must submit the bill). Figure 24-1 shows the HCFA 1500 form required by Medicare but used by many other companies. Forms completed with a computer or typewriter can be processed by scanning, which may result in earlier payment. Many providers submit the data electronically, which makes processing even more efficient.

The patient (or other responsible party) will usually be asked to sign the claim form. If payment is not made at the time of the visit, the patient will usually be asked to *assign* payment to the doctor, either by indicating this on the claim form or by signing a separate statement. When this is done, payment is made directly to the provider. Hospitals and most other providers routinely file claims for basic insurance coverage either electronically or by filling out forms. If not, the patient is responsible for the filing. For reimbursement under major medical policies, the insured files the claims.

Physicians often elect to accept what insurance pays in return for a guarantee that payment will be made directly to them rather than to the patient. This procedure is known as *accepting assignment*. When a physician accepts assignment, the patient may not be billed for the difference between the provider's charge fee and the amount paid by the insurance company (except for amounts that involve deductibles or co-insurance). Providers are likely to accept assignment when patients have financial difficulties or when the physicians think that a patient might pocket a direct insurance payment without paying the medical bill. If the provider does not belong to a fixed-fee plan and has not accepted assignment, the patient will be liable for the difference between the physician's fee and the policy allowance. Patients who belong to an HMO are responsible only for copayment (usually $5 to $20 per visit) for covered services, plus any fees for noncovered services.

Since 1989 physicians have been required to submit appropriate codes when billing for services to Medicare recipients. The diagnosis codes are listed in the *International Classification of Diseases, Ninth Edition, Clinical Modification (ICD-9-CM),* which is available from several publishers. Most insurance companies have the same requirement. Procedure codes have been standardized in *Current Procedural Terminology*, which is updated annually by the American Medical Association and incorporated into manuals published by the AMA, insurance companies, and commercial publishers. These codes are usually referred to as "CPT codes." The codes for medical evaluation and management are based on the complexity of the service and whether the patient has been seen previously. Some insurance companies

Table 24-7

CPT CODE GUIDELINES FOR OUTPATIENT MEDICAL CARE OF NEW AND ESTABLISHED PATIENTS

CPT Code	Key Components*			Typical Severity	Typical Time with Patient	Typical Examples of Problems or Professional Services
	Extent of History	Examination	Complexity			
First visit (new patient)						
99201	Problem-focused	Focused on one problem	Straight-forward	Self-limited	10 minutes	Baby with diaper rash / Skin bump requiring no treatment
99202	Expanded	Expanded problem-focused	Straight-forward	Low to moderate	20 minutes	Adolescent with acne / College student with seasonal allergies
99203	Detailed	Detailed	Low	Moderate	30 minutes	Vasectomy counseling / Knee injured during football game
99204	Comprehensive	Comprehensive	Moderate	Moderate to high	45 minutes	Chest pain on exertion, 63-year-old man / Multiple joint pains, 70-year-old woman
99205	Comprehensive	Comprehensive	High	Moderate to high	60 minutes	Unexplained 15-pound weight loss / Evaluation and counseling, suicidal patient
Subsequent visits (established patient)						
99211	Problem-focused	Minimal, if any	Low	Minimal	5 minutes; doctor not required	Blood pressure check / Changing a dressing
99212	Expanded	Expanded problem-focused	Straight-forward	Self-limited or minor	10 minutes	Student with sore throat, fever, and fatigue / Child with sore throat and headache
99213	Detailed	Detailed	Low	Low to moderate	15 minutes	Diabetic needing to change insulin dosage / Quarterly follow-up visit for asthmatic
99214	Comprehensive	Comprehensive	Moderate	Moderate to high	25 minutes	Recent heart attack patient with intolerable side effects from a medication
99215	Comprehensive	Comprehensive	High	Moderate to high	40 minutes	Elderly patient with recent onset of fainting / Discussion of treatment options with patient recently proven to have colon cancer

*All three of these components are required for the first visit. For subsequent visits, only two are required.
Source: Pennsylvania Blue Shield 1996 Procedure Terminology Manual.

EXPLANATION OF BENEFITS STATEMENT

COLLEGE, JOEL
200 CAMPUS DRIVE
ANYTOWN, US 90000

DATE 1/29/01
CLAIM NO. 123454321

MEMBER COLLEGE, JOEL
S.S. NO. 999-99-0001
PATIENT COLLEGE, JOEL

Date(s) of Service	Description of Service		Provider's Charge	Excluded Amount	Code	Covered Charge	Deductible	%	Benefit Amount
11/18/00	VISIT	99213	43.00	.00		43.00	5.00	80	30.40
11/18/00	ECG	93000	40.00	5.00	A1	35.00	0.00	100	35.00
11/29/00	SURG	11200	30.00	30.00	D7	0.00	0.00	0	0.00
	TOTALS		113.00	35.00		78.00	5.00		65.40

FIGURE 24-2. Portion of sample explanation-of-benefits statement. The insurance policy covered 80% of medically necessary office visits and 100% of procedures but had a copay of $5 per visit. On November 18th the insured had an office visit and an electrocardiogram (ECG). Nothing was excluded from the office visit fee because it was in line with the company's usual, customary, and reasonable (UCR) fee allowance. After deducting the $5 copayment, the company paid 80% of what was left. The doctor charged $5 more than the company paid for ECGs. ("Code A1" indicated that the provider's fee exceeded the company's UCR fee.) Since the doctor had agreed to accept the company's allowable fees, the patient did not have to pay the $5. The operation on November 29 was removal of two skin tags (little outgrowths of skin) of the neck, which the patient wanted removed because they interfered with shaving. ("Code D7" indicated that the procedure was not covered because it was not medically necessary.)

ask providers to submit a descriptive phrase in addition to the CPT code.

In 1992 Medicare implemented the resource-based relative value system, a method of payment quite different from the UCR method. The system is intended to help control costs and to provide more equitable reimbursement for services rendered. Under this system:

- Payment is made according to the resource-based relative value scale (RBRVS), a nationwide fee scale that takes into account (a) the extent of history taking and physician examination, (b) the complexity of medical decision making, (c) the time spent counseling the patient, (d) the severity of the patient's health problem, and (e) the time spent with the patient.
- Fees that Medicare patients can be charged by doctors who do not accept assignment cannot exceed Medicare-approved fees by more than 15%. Several states have established a similar limitation.
- Doctors are prohibited from offsetting fee reductions by ordering more tests, doing more procedures, or submitting a higher proportion of claims for higher-priced services.
- Restrictions were placed on referral of patients to clinical laboratories or other health-care facilities in which the referring physician has a financial interest.

Table 24-7 illustrates how the severity and complexity of the problem are related to the level of care for which physicians are permitted to bill Medicare. Virtually all health insurance companies now use the RBRVS coding system.

After the insurer receives the claim, it determines what the provider and patient should be paid. Payment is accompanied by an "explanation of benefits" report that itemizes the services, indicates what is covered, and explains whatever amounts are not paid. Figure 24-2 illustrates a sample report.

Health insurance companies process billions of claims each year, and errors and delays do occur. These suggestions may help you collect the benefits to which you are entitled:

- Keep careful and complete records of all health-related bills.
- Be sure that claim forms are filled out accurately and completely. Keep a photocopy for reference.
- If asked for documentation, send photocopies. *Never* send your only copy of a bill to an insurance company.
- If a problem arises, contact the company for an explanation or to register a complaint. The contact can be by telephone or mail. If you phone and the person to whom you speak cannot resolve the problem, ask to speak with a supervisor.
- If that does not resolve the problem, write to the company president or the state insurance department.

DISABILITY INSURANCE

Disability insurance provides income when sickness or injury interferes with ability to earn a living. It is available through employer-paid and government-sponsored programs. Individuals can also purchase private policies, but these tend to be much more expensive. Policies vary in terms of eligibility requirements, premiums charged, how disability is defined, extent of benefits, waiting periods before benefits begin, length of coverage, protection against inflation, coverage of office overhead, and other features. Employees are also

It's Your Decision

You will soon have the opportunity to select a health insurance plan for yourself or your family from several offered by your employer. Which of the following actions would you take?

Reason

☐ Ask a friend, neighbor, or relative for advice
☐ Select an HMO or PPO policy
☐ Select a fee-for-service policy
☐ Try to determine your health insurance needs
☐ Obtain sample policies for review
☐ Compare sample policies using a list of guidelines
☐ Ask your family doctor for assistance
☐ Other: (specify) _____

In considering policies, which things are most important to you?

☐ The amount of the premium
☐ The freedom to choose whichever doctors you want
☐ The size of the deductible or copayments
☐ The company's reputation
☐ Other factors (specify)_____

covered in every state through a workers' compensation program for job-related injury and (when they have worked long enough) through Social Security for long-term disability from any cause. Before buying a disability policy it is wise to assess whether coverage already exists, what additional coverage would be needed to meet expenses, and how soon benefits would be needed.

SUMMARY

Health insurance enables people to budget in advance for health care and is important for nearly everyone. A health insurance policy is a business agreement formalized by a written contract that details both benefits and obligations. Basic health insurance includes benefits for hospital, surgical, and medical expenses. The extent of these benefits differs from contract to contract. Major medical contracts take over where basic insurance plans leave off. Managed-care policies combine insurance with health-delivery systems.

Group policies generally offer more coverage and cost less than individual policies. Most people are insured through a group policy obtained through their place of employment. Because the extent and type of covered services vary widely from contract to contract, policies should be read carefully to understand what protection they provide.

Managed-care plans tend to have lower premiums and result in fewer out-of-pocket costs. Traditional indemnity policies tend to cost more and involve more paperwork (in filing claims) but provide greater choice of providers. To get the full benefit of their health plan, consumers should understand the extent of their coverage and any procedures (such as preauthorization) required when seeking care.

REFERENCES

1. Cohen P. Health plan roulette. In Health 4(4):78-82, 1990.
2. Hogue K and others. Complete Guide to Health Insurance: How to Beat the High Cost of Being Sick. New York, 1990, Avon Books.
3. Clinton HR. Foreword to White House Domestic Policy Council. Health Security: The President's Report on the American People. Washington, D.C., 1993, U.S. Government Printing Office.
4. Source Book of Health Insurance Data, 1999–2000. Washington, D.C., 1999, Health Insurance Association of America.
5. Miller RH, Luft HS. Managed care plan performance since 1980: A literature analysis. JAMA 271:1512–1519, 1994.
6. The Clinton Health Care Act: What Will It Mean for Consumers? Washington, D.C., 1993, Consumers Union.
7. Gold MR and others. A national survey of the arrangements managed-care plans make with physicians. New England Journal of Medicine 333:1678–1683, 1995.
8. HMO-PPO/Medicare-Medicaid Digest. Kansas City, Mo., 1999, Hoechst Marion Roussel.
9. Finkelstein R, Hurwit C, Kirsch R. The Managed Care Consumers' Bill of Rights. New York, 1995, Public Policy and Education Fund of New York.
10. Medicare & You 2001. Baltimore, 2000, Health Care Financing Administration.
11. McLeod D. Medicare outpatient debacle: Hospitals allowed to charge more for outpatient care. AARP 37(8):4, 1996.
12. Choosing a Medicare HMO. Kiplinger's Personal Finance Magazine 50(8):73–77, 1996.
13. Filling the gaps in Medicare. Consumer Reports 60:523–532, 1994.
14. Serious Problems for Older Americans in Health Maintenance Organizations. Washington, D.C., 1995, Public Citizen Health Research Group.
15. Kemper P, Murtaugh CM. Lifetime use of nursing home care. New England Journal of Medicine 324:595–600, 1991.
16. Guide to long-term healthcare. Washington, D.C., 1999, Health Insurance Association of America.
17. Oshiro C, Snyder H and the editors of Consumer Reports. Medicare/Medigap. Mount Vernon, N.Y., 1994, Consumer Reports Books.
18. Stover S. Considering long-term care insurance. Kiplinger's Personal Finance Magazine 50(3):111–114, 1996.
19. A Guide for patients. Managed care: Understanding your dental benefits plan. Chicago, 1995, American Dental Association.
20. Dental service use and dental insurance coverage—United States, Behavioral Risk Factor Surveillance System, 1995. Weekly Mortality and Morbidity Report 46:1199–1203, 1997.
21. Best's Aggregates and Averages–Life-Health. Olwick, N.J., 1996, A.M. Best Co.
22. Concern about premium hikes rises as plans' ability to cut costs questioned. Managed Care, March 1999.
23. How good is your health plan? Consumer Reports 61:28–42, 1996.
24. Is an HMO for you? Consumer Reports 65(7):38–41, 2000.
25. Regardless of health status–HMO and FFS patients report similar levels of satisfaction. GHAA News, July 18, 1995.
26. Sick people in managed care have difficulty getting services and treatment. News release, Robert Wood Johnson Foundation, June 28, 1995.
27. Davis K and others. Choice matters: Enrollees' views of their health plans. Health Affairs, Summer 1995.
28. NCQA's health plan report card. NCQA Web site, accessed, Oct 31, 2000.
29. How does your HMO stack up? 19,000 readers help us judge 54 health plans. Consumer Reports 64(8):23–29, 1999.
30. Himmelstein DU and others. Quality of care in investor-owned vs not-for-profit HMOs. JAMA 282:159–163, 1999.
31. Consumers' Guide to Health Plans, ed 2. Washington, D.C., 1996, Center for the Study of Services.
32. Shapiro JP. America's Top HMOs. There when you need it. U.S. News & World Report, Oct 5, 1998, pp 65–91.
33. Keeler EBB and others. Can medical savings accounts for the nonelderly reduce health care costs? JAMA 275:1666–1671, 1996.
34. Editorial: Unacceptable solution to US health-care costs. Lancet 347:69, 1996.
35. Weiss Ratings' Guide to HMOs and Health Insurers. Palm Beach, Fla., Weiss Ratings., Inc., updated quarterly.

Chapter Twenty-Five

HEALTH CARE ECONOMICS

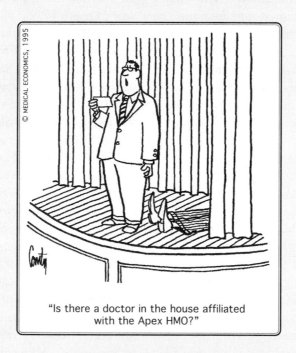

© MEDICAL ECONOMICS, 1995

"Is there a doctor in the house affiliated with the Apex HMO?"

The American health care system, and especially its cost, is out of control, inhibiting access to care for many, lessening quality of care for some, and creating an almost palpable angst among physicians and others concerned with this enormous national problem.

NICHOLAS E. DAVIES, M.D.[1]
LOUIS H. FELDER, M.D.

The nation's health care system is in a historic transformation driven by rising prices, pressures on public and private budgets, and scientific and technological change.

COMMITTEE ON THE ADEQUACY OF NURSE
STAFFING IN HOSPITALS AND NURSING HOMES[2]
INSTITUTE OF MEDICINE

Stripped to its simplest form, managed care is an attempt to lower the nation's medical bill by putting an end to the American way of health care—a costly approach that has included unlimited tests, treatments on demand, multiple visits to specialists, emphasis on expensive high-tech procedures, long hospital stays, and unrestricted choice of doctors.

CONSUMER REPORTS[3]

The term "health-care system" refers to the network of individuals and organizations involved in providing health services. The participants include independent practitioners, allied health-care providers, hospitals, outpatient clinics, nursing homes, voluntary agencies, and public and private insurance programs.

America is said to be undergoing a "health-care crisis" due to skyrocketing costs and inequalities in the distribution of services. Part of the problem is due to the high cost of new technology. But many critics of our health-care system describe it as choked by paperwork, strangled by bureaucracy, and riddled with waste and inefficiency. Corrective legislation has been stymied by the complexity of the problems and the competing demands of special-interest groups.

The National Coalition on Health Care concluded that most Americans had little confidence in the health-care system. Its 1997 poll found that 8 out of 10 said that medical care quality was being compromised in the interest of profit.[4] The Center for Health Economics Research has concluded that the major source of public dissatisfaction is not quality but out-of-pocket costs, and that these costs fall with better insurance coverage.[5] Other polls have found that the primary concern is with public access and that satisfaction with the system is far greater among those who are wealthy rather than poor, white rather than nonwhite, and healthy rather than disabled.[6,7]

This chapter examines health-care costs, cost-control strategies, insurance fraud, and proposals for health-care reform.

HEALTH-CARE COSTS

National health-care expenditures have risen steadily. The Health Care Financing Administration (HCFA) states that the total spent rose an average of 10.5% per year between 1960 and 1970, 13% between 1970 and 1980, 10.3% between 1980 and 1990, about 8% from 1991 through 1993, and about 5% from 1994 through 1998.[8,9] The rate of increase has outpaced the inflation rate and the overall Consumer Price Index throughout most of this period. Health-care expense amounted to 5.7% of disposable income in 1960 and rose nearly every year to reach 17.5% of disposable income in 1994.[10]

In 1998 expenditures for health care in the United States totaled $1149 billion ($4094 per person).[11] As shown in Table 25-1, $1019 billion of this was spent for personal health care, and the rest was spent for administration, research, construction, and public health activities. HCFA actuaries have estimated that the total will continue to rise about 6.5% per year and reach $2200 billion (16.2% of the Gross Domestic Product) by 2008.[9]

In 1998, 80% ($819.8 billion) of personal health expenses were paid by third parties (private health insurers and public agencies) and 20% ($199.5 billion) were paid by individuals. U.S. Department of Commerce data indicate that in 1997 personal-consumption expenditures for medical care totaled $957.3 billion. (The Commerce Department's medical-care total differs from that of HCFA because it does not include moneys from Medicare, worker's compensation, or temporary disability insurance.) This amount exceeded expenditures for food and tobacco ($832.3 billion); housing ($829.8 billion); transportation ($636.4 billion); household operation ($620.7 billion); recreation ($462.9 billion); personal business ($459.1 billion); clothing, accessories, and jewelry ($353.3 billion); religious and welfare activities ($157.6 billion); and private education and research ($129.4 billion).[12] Figure 25-1 summarizes how America's health-care costs were financed and how the money was spent.

The reasons for the rise have included (a) increasing use of costly high-tech equipment,[13] (b) the high cost of treating such illnesses as AIDS and cancer, (c) aging of the population, (d) fraudulent practices by some providers, (e) the large number and high cost of malpractice suits, (f) the administrative costs of complying with government regulations,[14] and (g) the practice of defensive medicine—testing that is medically

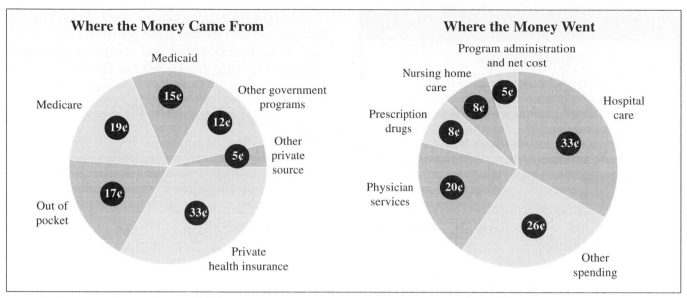

FIGURE 25-1. How America's health-care dollars were spent in 1998.[11]

Table 25-1

SOURCES OF FUNDS FOR HEALTH-CARE EXPENDITURES, 1998 (BILLIONS OF DOLLARS)

Expense Category	Category Total	Out-of-Pocket Payments	Private Insurance	Other Private	Government Programs
Personal health care (89%)					
Hospital care	$382.8 (37.6%)	$ 12.8	$118.0	$19.1	$232.9
Physician services	229.5 (22.5%)	35.7	116.0	4.5	73.3
Dental services	53.8 (5.3%)	25.8	25.5	0.2	2.3
Other professional services	66.6 (6.5%)	27.2	20.2	5.0	14.2
Home health care	29.3 (2.9%)	6.0	4.0	3.7	15.5
Drugs and other nondurable products	121.9 (12.0%)	55.4	47.8	–	8.1
Vision products and other medical durables	15.5 (1.5%)	8.2	0.8	–	6.5
Nursing home care	87.8 (8.6%)	28.5	4.7	1.6	53.0
Other personal health care	32.1 (2.6%)	–		3.8	28.3
Total, personal health care	1019.3 (100%)	199.5	337.0	37.9	444.9
Other expenditures (12%)					
Program administration and net cost of private insurance	57.7	–	38.0	0.9	18.8
Govt. public health activities	36.6	–	–	–	36.6
Research	19.9	–	–	1.6	18.3
Construction	15.5	–	–	11.5	4.0
Total, all expenditures	1149.1	199.5	375.0	51.8	522.7

Source: Health Care Financing Administration.[11] Some numbers do not add to totals because of rounding.

unnecessary but is ordered to protect the physician against the danger of a malpractice suit—which adds tens of billions of dollars yearly to the cost of medical care.[15] Another factor is that greater insurance coverage (more people insured and greater coverage per person)

has led consumers to demand more and better services and doctors to recommend more services.[16] The Health Care Technology Institute[17] has pointed out that Americans have mixed feelings about cost-control (see "Conflicting Attitudes" Personal Glimpse box).

Costly Problems

What else could anyone expect in America but rapidly rising health-care costs, with 3 million desperate drug abusers at large on our streets, 18 million alcohol abusers loose on our highways, 55 million tobacco abusers causing 1000 costly, painful deaths every day, and nearly 1 million new cases of venereal disease adding to our society's existing burden every year. . . .

Waiting in the wings are growing crises involving long-term care, homelessness, Alzheimer's disease, and the uninsured and underinsured working poor, not to mention the burgeoning tragedy of a million or more men, women, and children infected with the AIDS virus.

Timothy B. Norbeck[15]
Executive Director
Connecticut Medical Society

Personal health expenditures are very unevenly distributed. Consumers Union[18] has concluded that (a) the sickest 10% of the population accounts for 68% of health care expenditures; (b) for households with head younger than 65, the percent of family income spent on premiums and out-of-pocket payments ranged from a high of 17% for families with income under $10,000 to 3% for families with income of $100,000 or more; (c) one in six households with a head younger than 65 spends 10% or more of its income on out-of-pocket costs plus directly paid premiums; and (d) half of households headed by a person 65 or older pays more than 10% of its income on such costs, mainly because Medicare does not cover prescription drugs.

Hospital and Nursing Home Charges

In 1998 the average hospital cost per inpatient day was slightly over $1000, and the average length of stay was about 5 days. This is what it cost the hospitals to deliver their services, not what patients or insurance companies paid, which probably averaged about $300 more per day. These figures do not include medical and surgical fees.

Consumers may be able to reduce hospital and surgery costs by (a) getting a second opinion when elective surgery is advised; (b) not extending hospital stays for the sake of convenience, (c) comparing prices when hospitalization is needed (some areas have developed consumer guides that provide information about charges, services, and other matters); and (d) monitoring hospital bills carefully to be certain all charges are valid. Billing errors, which are common, can include charges for unreceived services, as well as overcharges.

The cost per day at a nursing home depends on the nature of the care rendered, the type of facility, the region of the United States, and several other factors. Typical costs range from $3000 to $6000 per month. For many people, nursing home expenses are by far the largest health-related out-of-pocket expense.

Reducing nursing home expenses may be difficult, but it may help to investigate Medicare and Medicaid coverage, purchase long-term insurance (see Chapter 24), or explore less expensive alternatives to nursing home care (see Chapter 10). Some people qualify for Medicaid by incurring medical expenses until their net income after medical expenses is low enough to qualify. This method is called "spending down."[19] Some people transfer assets to someone other than their spouse so these assets will not have to be spent to establish Medicaid eligibility. Since recently transferred assets are considered part of the applicant's net worth, the transfer must take place several years before applying. This method is controversial but legal.

Medical Fees

Physicians generally base their fees on (a) the nature, extent, and complexity of the service; (b) the time involved; (c) the office overhead—rent, heat, lighting, equipment and supplies, salaries of personnel; (d) the experience and expertise of the practitioner; (e) the area in which the physician practices; (f) the fees customarily charged by others in the community; and (g) in some circumstances, the economic status of the patient. Medical fees are also influenced by the forces of supply and demand. Table 25-2 shows the average fees physicians charged in 2000 for typical office and hospital visits.

Conflicting Attitudes

Since 1980, Americans often expressed, simultaneously, two contradictory attitudes on medicine and its costs—they repeatedly wanted unrestricted access to the best medical care and related technology, and, at the same time, they wanted lower medical costs and cited expense as a major shortcoming of the U.S. health care system. During the same period, respondents who were asked to consider cost-stabilizing health insurance plans were unwilling to give up complete access to the latest—even if it was the costliest—medical technology. Respondents were willing to exclude only purely elective care (i.e., cosmetic surgery) from national health care plans for cost control purposes.

Health Care Technology Institute[17]

Table 25-2

MEAN PHYSICIAN FEES FOR LEVEL-3 OFFICE VISITS AND ALL HOSPITAL VISITS (2000)

Type of Physician	Level-3 Office Visits*		Hospital Visits	
	New Patient	Established Patient	First Day	Subsequent Days
All physicians	$ 95	$ 55	–	–
Family practioners	90	60	$ 100 to 175	$ 50 to 100
Internal medicine specialists	99	60	100 to 150	58 to 100
Pediatricians	80	55	–	60 to 110
Surgeons	100	60	Usually included in surgical fee	
Obstetricians/gynecologists	100	65	Usually included in surgical or obstetric fee	

*Level-3 office visits for new patients (code #99203) typically last 30 minutes. Level-3 office visits for established patients (code #99213) typically last 15 minutes. Table 24–7 explains the coding system further. Source: Medical Economics.[20]

Insurance plans pay for medical services in three ways. In the fee-for-service method, providers are compensated for each service they render. Another arrangement is a salary from a hospital, group health insurance plan, or governmental or private organization or agency. Some members of group or managed-care plans may also receive a share of the profits at the end of each year, based upon the amount of service rendered. The third method is capitation, a fixed monthly amount paid for each patient (per capita) regardless of the amount of services used.

Insurance companies generally base fee-for-service payments on what they consider usual, customary, and reasonable (UCR). "Usual" refers to a physician's own charges for the previous year or years. "Customary" refers to the range of fees charged by all physicians in a given region. "Reasonable" refers to a fee within a given region or area that falls below the 90th percentile of the customary charges. Medicare uses the 75th percentile and pays 80% of this amount. Except for deductibles and co-insurance, physicians who accept assignment are not permitted to bill the patient for the difference between what they bill and what they collect from third-party payers. Federal regulations prohibit medical organizations from establishing fee guidelines or fee schedules, which are considered anticompetitive.

Many attempts have been made to control escalating medical and hospital costs without affecting the quality of care. They have included (a) reduction of the time patients stay in hospitals; (b) the use of second opinions to reduce unnecessary surgery; (c) the Medicare DRG (diagnosis-related group) program, whereby hospitals are paid a set fee per admission based on the patient's diagnosis; (d) emphasis on preventive care; (e) development of HMOs, PPOs, and other managed-care programs; and (f) a switch to outpatient surgery

for the repair of hernias, removal of tonsils, breast biopsies, and many other procedures.

Another practice intended to influence medical costs has been the publishing of physician directories that include fee information. These publications are not very useful because they quickly become outdated, many physicians refuse to provide the information, and fees do not reflect the quality of care, which is generally much more important.

Dental Fees

Table 25-3 lists the average and 95th percentile fees charged for common procedures by general dentists and specialists in the United States in January 2000. This information may be helpful when preparing a budget for dental care or considering the purchase of dental insurance (see Chapter 24).

Considerable evidence indicates that self-care and preventive dentistry can save consumers money. More important, however, are the benefits of freedom from pain and discomfort, retention of teeth, and less time spent obtaining dental care. The incidence of dental caries and periodontal disease can be substantially and cost-effectively reduced through the fluoridation of water supplies, topical application of fluorides, and plaque-control measures (see Chapter 7).

Budgeting Considerations

When budgeting for health care, consumers should consider that (a) out-of-pocket expenses are likely to occur each year; (b) the 1998 average was $711 per person; (c) health-care costs tend to increase as people grow older; and (d) the appropriate amount to allocate should depend on the number of people in the family unit, how old they are, and the extent of insurance coverage. Table 25-4 lists per capita health-care expenses for 1998.

Table 25-3

FEES FOR COMMON DENTAL SERVICES, 2000

Services	Average Fee	95th Percentile
Diagnostic		
Complete intraoral x-ray series	$ 77	$ 110
Bitewings, four films	35	55
Preventive		
Prophylaxis (cleaning)—adult	54	84
Prophylaxis (cleaning)—child	38	62
Topical fluoride plus prophylaxis—child	32	43
Sealant, per tooth	27	43
Restorative		
Amalgam—one surface, permanent teeth	79	107
Inlay, composite, one surface	332	418
Crown, porcelain	643	911
Oral surgery		
Extraction, single tooth	80	145
Implant placement	1531	3250
Periodontics		
Gum resection or reshaping, per quadrant	477	670
Endodontics		
Therapeutic pulpotomy (without final restoration)	79	118
Root canal, molar (without final restoration)	593	970
Prosthodontics		
Complete denture, upper or lower	874 or 900	1500
Orthodontics		
Comprehensive treatment (cost depends on age)	3876–4438	5314–6251

Source: The Orthodontic Page (http://www.bracesinfo.com), Jan 12, 2000. Specialists tend to charge more than general dentists for similar services.

COST-CONTROL METHODS

Traditional insurance companies can use several measures to reduce costs. They can raise deductibles and copayment amounts, limit what they pay for each service, limit or exclude certain services, limit maximum total benefits, and exclude people with pre-existing illness. They can use utilization management to limit payment to medically necessary services. (For example, they can require that confirmatory second opinions be obtained before a person can undergo certain types of elective surgery.)

Managed-care plans limit their subscribers' choice of providers to those who have agreed to accept lower fees (or capitation) or have exhibited a pattern of providing lower-cost care. These plans also deny coverage of diagnostic tests and the services of specialists unless the primary physician authorizes them.

Managed-care plans use additional measures that influence physician behavior. They may require preauthorization from the plan before hospitalizing a patient or ordering certain expensive tests. They may exclude certain drugs from coverage and require that generic drugs be prescribed when available. They use aggressive utilization review programs to detect what they consider medically unnecessary or inappropriate care. They can also reduce costs by creating economies of scale, reducing duplication of services, issuing treatment guidelines, and using financial incentives to encourage cost-conscious decisions.

Managed-care plans usually compensate physicians with capitation fees or a salary. In addition, they typically use incentives to limit use of diagnostic tests, referrals to other physicians, hospital care, or other ancillary services. Many plans pay bonuses that depend on how little the plan has to spend for these services. Some plans withhold a percentage of the physician's compensation until the end of the year to cover any shortfalls in the amounts budgeted for patient-care expenditures. If there is no shortfall, or if the shortfall can be covered by part of the withheld fees, the remainder of the withheld amount is distributed to the physicians.

Many authorities have expressed concern that financial considerations may undermine patient care. Wenger and Shapiro,[21] for example, suggest that utilization review programs should explore possible underuse of care in addition to overuse. The AMA Council on Ethical and Judicial Affairs has stated:

> While efforts to contain costs are critical and while many of the approaches of managed care have an impact, managed care can compromise the quality and integrity of the physician-patient relationship and reduce the quality of care received by patients. In particular, by creating conflicting loyalties for the physician, some of the techniques of managed care can undermine the physician's fundamental obligation to serve as patient advocate. Moreover, in their zeal to control utilization, managed care plans may withhold appropriate diagnostic procedures or treatment. . . .
>
> Efforts to contain health care costs should not place patient welfare at risk. Thus, financial incentives are permissible only if they promote the cost-effective delivery of health care and not the withholding of medically necessary care.[22]

Many state legislators have expressed concerns that HMO cost-cutting measures have been too stringent.[23,24] Many states have passed laws requiring HMOs to permit women to remain in the hospital at least 48 hours (or a time recommended by the American College of Obstetricians and Gynecologists) after giving birth. At least 12 states have made it harder for HMOs to deny payments for emergency-department visits that turn out not to be emergencies. A few states have enacted laws that require prospective enrollees to be told how HMO

physicians are compensated. Many states have banned "gag clauses" (HMO rules that prevent doctors from telling patients about treatment options the HMO does not pay for), even though HMO industry leaders maintain that no such clauses exist.

Provider Strategies

Escalating costs and the prospect of greater government intervention have stimulated rapid and sweeping changes in the way in which the health marketplace is organized. There is widespread concern that small organizations will be unable to compete effectively with large ones because large ones can achieve economies of scale. Hospitals have been merging with other hospitals, forming purchasing alliances, hiring large numbers of physicians, and developing integrated managed care systems that include the full gamut of medical services. Profit-making organizations have been buying hospitals and physician practices. Physicians have been forming independent practice associations and other networks so that they can bargain more effectively with managed-care organizations. Group practices are becoming larger.[25] Some Blue Cross/Blue Shield organizations have converted from nonprofit to commercial status, and more are expected to do the same.[26]

Employer Strategies

In 1998 about 155 million people (more than 90% of insured individuals) obtained their health insurance through their employers. As health-care costs have escalated, it has become increasingly difficult for businesses to absorb the expense while still remaining profitable. As a result, many have reduced health-care benefits, switched to managed-care plans, cut retiree benefits, or are requiring employees and retirees to pay part of the premium costs. About half of employers now self-insure (assuming the financial risk) but hire an insurance company or other third party to administer their program.[27] Today the vast majority of those who obtained health services through an employer are in some form of managed care.

Consumer Strategies

Health-care costs and benefits can be defined both in terms of dollars and in terms of the presence or absence of disease. The National Health Council's "Principles of Patients' Rights and Responsibilities" box and the Consumer Tip box on pages suggest 538 and 539 how to protect your health and avoid unnecessary expense. Some of the suggestions are simple to carry out, whereas others require diligent effort.

Table 25-4
PER CAPITA OUT-OF-POCKET PERSONAL HEALTH-CARE EXPENDITURES, 1998

Category	Amount
Hospital care	$ 46
Physician services	127
Dental services	92
Other professional services	97
Home health care	21
Drugs and other nondurable products	197
Vision products and other medical durables	29
Nursing home care	102
Total	711

Source: Health Care Finance Administration, 2000.[9]

NATIONAL HEALTH COUNCIL'S PRINCIPLES OF PATIENTS' RIGHTS AND RESPONSIBILITIES

- *All patients have the right to informed consent in treatment decisions, timely access to specialty care, and confidentiality protections.* Patients should be treated courteously with dignity and respect. Before consenting to specific care choices, they should receive complete and easily understood information about their condition and treatment options. Patients should be entitled to: coverage for qualified second opinions; timely referral and access to needed specialty care and other services; confidentiality of their medical records and communications with providers; and, respect for their legal advanced directives or living wills.

- *All patients have the right to concise and easily understood information about their coverage.* This information should include the range of covered benefits, required authorizations, and service restrictions or limitations (such as on the use of certain health care providers, prescription drugs, and "experimental" treatments). Plans should also be encouraged to provide information assistance through patient ombudsmen knowledgeable about coverage provisions and processes.

- *All patients have the right to know how coverage payment decisions are made and how they can be fairly and openly appealed.* Patients are entitled to information about how coverage decisions are made, i.e., how "medically necessary" treatment is determined, and how quality assurance is conducted. Patients and their caregivers should have access to an open, simple and timely process to appeal negative coverage decisions on tests and treatments they believe are necessary.

- *All patients have the right to complete and easily understood information about the costs of their coverage and care.* This information should include the premium costs for their benefits package, the amount of any patient out-of-pocket cost obligations (e.g., deductibles, copayments, and additional premiums), and any catastrophic cost limits. Upon request, patients should be informed of the costs of services they've been rendered and treatment options proposed.

- *All patients have the right to a reasonable choice of providers and useful information about provider options.* Patients are entitled to a reasonable choice of health care providers and the ability to change providers if dissatisfied with their care. Information should be available on provider credentials and facility accreditation reports, provider expertise relative to specific diseases and disorders, and the criteria used by provider networks to select and retain caregivers. The latter should include information about whether and how a patient can remain with a caregiver who leaves or is not part of a plan network.

- *All patients have the right to know what provider incentives or restrictions might influence practice patterns.* Patients also have the right to know the basis for provider payments, any potential conflicts of interest that may exist, and any financial incentives and clinical rules (e.g., quality assurance procedures, treatment protocols or practice guidelines, and utilization review requirements) which could affect provider practice patterns.

- *All patients, to the extent capable, have the responsibility to pursue a healthy lifestyle.* Patients should pursue lifestyle factors known to promote positive health results, such as proper diet and nutrition, adequate rest, and regular exercise. Simultaneously, they should avoid behaviors known to be detrimental to one's health, such as smoking, excessive alcohol consumption and drug abuse.

- *All patients, to the extent capable, have the responsibility to become knowledgeable about their health plans.* Patients should read and become familiar with the terms, coverage provisions, rules and restrictions of their health plans. They should not be hesitant to inquire with appropriate sources when additional information or clarification is needed about these matters.

- *All patients, to the extent capable, have the responsibility to actively participate in decisions about their health care.* Patients should seek, when recommended for their age group, an annual medical examination and be present at all other scheduled health care appointments. They should provide accurate information to caregivers regarding their medical and personal histories and current symptoms and conditions. They should ask questions of providers to determine the potential risks, benefits and costs of treatment alternatives. Where appropriate, this should include information about the availability and accessibility of experimental treatments and clinical trials. Additionally, patients should also seek and read literature about their conditions and weigh all pertinent factors in making informed decisions about their care.

- *All patients, to the extent capable, have the responsibility to cooperate fully on mutually accepted courses of treatment.* Patients should cooperate fully with providers in complying with mutually accepted treatment regimens and regularly reporting on treatment progress. If serious side effects, complications, or worsening of the condition occur, they should notify their providers promptly. They should also inform providers of other medications and treatments they are pursuing simultaneously.

Endorsed by the National Health Council, March 22, 1995.

☑ **Consumer Tip**

Guidelines for Reducing Personal Health-Care Costs

- Acquire a primary physician, preferably before you are ill. Chapter 5 will help you find one. Check fees in advance, and learn to communicate efficiently. The *Healthwise Handbook* described in Chapter 9 provides many useful tips on patient-doctor communication. Don't attempt to seek care from one specialist after another without a primary physician as a coordinator.
- Use the preventive measures described in Chapter 9. Do not smoke, eat sensibly, maintain optimum weight, exercise sufficiently, avoid excessive intake of alcohol, keep immunizations up-to-date, wear a safety belt in automobiles, and have a smoke detector and possibly a carbon monoxide detector in your home.
- Have periodic health examinations as recommended in Chapter 5.
- Find out in advance about fees and payment policies. If you have insurance, ask whether the doctor will accept assignment. If paying for particular services may be a problem, discuss it with your doctor or the doctor's office staff. Some fees are negotiable, and most doctors will permit payment in installments.
- Use the telephone discriminately to obtain needed information from your personal physician. However, do not expect this procedure always to be a substitute for an office visit. Remember that the physician's time is valuable; have your thoughts well organized before telephoning.
- A local health department clinic may provide certain tests without cost and will inform your physician of the results. Keep in mind, however, that isolated tests are not a substitute for an overall diagnostic evaluation. The local health department may also provide immunizations and other health services without charge.
- Take advantage of outpatient services, including surgery, whenever possible, since these are much less costly than inpatient services.
- Visit your doctor during regular office hours except in emergencies. Avoid unnecessary use of hospital emergency rooms, which are far more costly than physicians' offices or ambulatory care centers.
- Do not press to remain in a hospital longer than necessary. Avoid entering the hospital on a weekend if tests or procedures you need will not begin until Monday. Check your hospital bill carefully.
- Become familiar with local health facilities and organizations. (For example, the American Cancer Society and the American Lung Association have brochures and programs for people who want to stop smoking.) Know ahead of time what to do and whom to call in case of emergency.
- A dental school clinic may be able to provide dental services at lower cost.

- When elective surgery is recommended, seek a reasonable explanation of what it entails, why it is recommended, and what the risks are. Ask if a medical alternative is available and consider getting a second opinion (see Chapter 5). Your primary physician's opinion may be as valuable as that of a second surgeon, or even more valuable.
- Mental health care may be less expensive through group therapy, self-help groups, or clinics.
- Appropriate home-care services, where available, are generally less expensive than hospital and nursing home care. Medicare, Medicaid, and insurance companies are often willing to pay for these services.
- Attempt to purchase prescription drugs by generic name rather than brand name. Compare prices in several pharmacies and follow the other suggestions presented in Chapter 19.
- Do not waste money on vitamins and other food supplements. Unless you have a specific medical condition that necessitates supplements prescribed by your physician, a sensible diet will provide all the nutrients you need. If you wish to take supplements regardless, multivitamin and mineral tablets are available for 5¢ a day or less. Do not ingest doses exceeding 100% of the Recommended Dietary Allowances (RDAs) or Daily Values (DVs).
- Read product labels and adhere to any instructions or warnings.
- Learn the names of all medications you use; take them as prescribed.
- Brush and floss your teeth at least once a day. Invest in periodic dental checkups at intervals recommended by your dentist. Support fluoridation of local drinking water, and use other types of fluoride supplementation if recommended by your dentist.
- Be skeptical about the health information you encounter unless you are sure that its source is reliable.
- Purchase health insurance, and make sure that its coverage is adequate to prevent financial catastrophe in case of serious or prolonged illness. An HMO or other managed-care plan may be less expensive and provide appropriate medical services. If you belong to such a plan, be sure to follow its rules regarding preauthorization. Chapter 24 covers these subjects further.
- Maintain a home health library (see Chapter 9). Include at least one book that provides guidance of when to self-treat and when to contact a physician.
- Know the signs of quackery so you can avoid wasting money on senseless products or services.
- Read *How to Cut Your Medical* Bills,[28] by Drs. Art and Val Ulene, which contains many other useful tips.

INSURANCE FRAUD AND ABUSE

Federal officials and insurance company executives believe that insurance fraud and abuse are widespread and very costly to America's health-care system. Fraud involves billing for services that are not rendered. Abuse involves multiple services that are not medically necessary, such as a laboratory test performed on large numbers of patients when only a few should have it. Consumers can detect certain frauds by examining insurance payment reports to see whether they accurately reflect the services rendered.

Although no precise dollar amount can be determined, some authorities contend that insurance fraud constitutes a $100-billion-a-year problem.[29] The United States General Accounting Office estimates that $1 out of every $7 spent on Medicare is lost to fraud and abuse and that in 1998 alone, Medicare lost nearly $12 billion to fraudulent or unnecessary claims.[30] Several large insurance companies have joined forces to develop sophisticated computer systems to detect suspicious billing patterns. The Federal Bureau of Investigation and the Office of the Inspector General (OIG) each have assigned hundreds of special agents to health-fraud projects.[31] These federal agencies have jurisdiction over private insurance plans as well as public ones. The following criminal cases illustrate problems that have been uncovered.

A California nursing home operator filed over 7000 fraudulent Medicare claims, billing for nonexistent medical supplies and submitting false cost reports supported by falsified records and fabricated invoices. He was sentenced to 11 years in prison and ordered to pay fines and restitution of more than $3.5 million.[32]

A Pennsylvania pharmacist was ordered to pay $167,200 and was sentenced to 8 months imprisonment for defrauding Medicaid and Medicare. He had routinely billed Medicaid for brand-name drugs while supplying generic brands. He was also involved in a scheme involving kickbacks, fabricated tests, and forged physician signatures related to the purchase of equipment.[32]

An Illinois durable medical equipment company billed Medicare for female urinary collection devices, which supposedly cost $10 each, when it actually had supplied diapers costing 30¢ each. The case was settled with a civil agreement under which the company and its owner paid $474,730 to the government.[32]

An Arizona osteopath used physical therapy codes to bill for services provided by an acupuncturist who maintained an office next door. They both pleaded guilty and were sentenced to 5 years of probation and restitution of $117,900. The osteopath also had to surrender his license.[33]

A nationwide chain that included more than 60 psychiatric hospitals agreed to pay $379 million in criminal fines and other penalties after pleading guilty to paying kickbacks to physicians and other professionals who referred Medicare and Medicaid patients.[34]

Fresenius Medical Care Holdings, the nation's largest provider of kidney dialysis, agreed to pay $486

What Do You Think?

An insurance company received a hospital bill totaling $1.25 million for a 26-year-old woman who was the first person to receive a new heart, liver, and kidney in the same operation.[35] The operation took 21 hours and involved at least 36 people: 11 surgeons, six anesthesiologists, 15 nurses, one physician assistant, two blood technicians, and one liver technician. During her hospital stay, the woman had seven more operations and spent 113 days in the intensive care unit while doctors struggled unsuccessfully to save her.

When queried by a reporter from *The New York Times*, the hospital refused to release a copy of the bill. But it did provide information on the average payment it receives from Blue Cross-Blue Shield for a $120,000 liver transplantation with no postoperative complications. The main items were:

- $28,000 for hospital and intensive-care rooms
- $20,000 to acquire donor organ
- $20,000 for surgeons, anesthesiologists, a radiologist, an internist, and a neurologist
- $15,000 for radiologic tests, including ultrasound and CT scans
- $8000 to administer blood
- $7000 each for use of the operating room and pharmacy charges
- $4000 each for anesthesia and pulmonary services

The insurance company balked at paying the bill without conducting an audit. The hospital refused to permit an audit until the bill was paid. The reporter noted that a bill this size could have considerable impact on even a large employer's annual health insurance premiums.

The surgeons who operated on the patient acknowledged that even with a single-organ transplant there is a 15% to 25% chance of death within months. Do you think insurance companies should pay for very expensive procedures where the likelihood of prolonging life is small? Do you think the insurance company should pay this bill?

million to resolve civil and criminal charges related to illegal kickback activity, submission of false claims, improper billing for laboratory services, and improper reporting of credit balances.[36]

Two California men received lengthy prison sentences after pleading guilty to multiple felony charges related to a bogus medical testing scheme. After establishing mobile testing laboratories, the men advertised free preventive physical examinations and testing. They and a network of physicians (some unlicensed) then billed insurance companies for a battery of expensive tests. Over a 10-year period the scheme generated more than $1 billion in fraudulent billings that resulted in payment of more than $50 million.[37]

An Illinois physician was sentenced to 25 months in prison and ordered to pay a $25,000 fine and $41,460 in restitution for defrauding Medicare and private insurers. Unable to recruit physicians and sufficient referrals for a multimillion-dollar diagnostic clinic he had built, the physician had billed for $4000 to $6000 for unnecessary tests on every patient who entered the clinic. He also attempted to substantiate the need for testing by entering nonexistent symptoms in patient records.[32]

Consumers who encounter suspicious practices involving Medicare or other federal programs should report them to the OIG Hotline [800-368-5779]. One practice that is easily detectable is the routine waiver of Part B copayments and deductibles. It is legal for providers not to charge Medicare recipients who have a genuine financial hardship, but it is not legal to provide "completely free" care or "discounts" to all patients or to collect only from those who have Medigap insurance. Studies have shown that if patients are required to pay for even a small portion of their care, they will select items or services because they are medically needed rather than because they are free—thus lowering the overall cost of the Medicare program.[38]

NATIONAL HEALTH INSURANCE (NHI)

The United States spends more money and a larger share of its resources for health care than any other country in the world. Yet in 1999, an estimated 44 million Americans had no health insurance and over 30 million more were underinsured.[17,39] (Short and Banthin[40] define the underinsured as people at risk of having out-of-pocket expenses exceed 10% of family income if they incur the large medical bills that they have a 1% chance of experiencing.)

Despite the noble goal of health insurance for all Americans, none of the many NHI proposals have become operational. An ideal system would provide

---

Table 25-5

PROBLEMS IN OUR HEALTH-CARE SYSTEM

In 1993 President Bill Clinton appointed First Lady Hillary Rodham Clinton to preside over a special task force to identify the roots of what has been called America's health-care crisis. After 9 months of intensive investigation the task force released a report identifying seven major problem areas:

1. Americans lack security.
2. Health-care costs are rising faster than other sectors of the economy.
3. Bureaucracy overwhelms consumers and health providers.
4. Quality is uneven.
5. Coverage for long-term care is inadequate.
6. Many Americans cannot obtain quality care.
7. Fraud and abuse cheat everyone.[41]

---

equity, access, efficiency, and quality. There appear to be four general strategies for change:

1. Modify the present private insurance involvement with some increased government support.
2. Combine greater employer-employee participation with government help for the poor and uninsured.
3. Have the federal government set basic rules, but leave it to the states and/or the insurance industry to create and administer the programs.
4. Establish a completely public plan that is controlled, supported, and administered by the government. Canada's system is often mentioned as exemplary.

The Canadian System

Since 1971 the Canadian health-care system has been a partnership between the Canadian federal government and the 10 Canadian provinces (and two territories). The federal government provides some of the funding, but each of the 12 regions administers its own health plan. Christiansen and Christiansen[42] state that the Canadian system rests on five basic principles:

UNIVERSALITY: Each provincial system should cover all of its residents except temporary visitors, transients, people covered by a federal program, and those who have not been in the province for at least 3 months. Each program has the legal authority to raise the necessary funds through taxes or required premiums.

COMPREHENSIVENESS: All medically necessary services must be covered. People who want additional services can pay for them out-of-pocket or through supplemental insurance available from insurance companies or the Canadian government.

Table 25-6

IDEAL CHARACTERISTICS OF A HEALTH CARE FINANCING SYSTEM

- **Universal access:** Every American citizen and legal resident should have access to health care without financial or other barriers.
- **Comprehensive benefits:** Guaranteed benefits should meet the full range of health needs, including primary, preventive and specialized care.
- **Choice:** Every consumer should have the opportunity to exercise effective choice about providers, plans, and treatments. Each consumer should be informed about what is known and not known about the risks and benefits of available treatments and be free to choose among them according to his and her preferences.
- **Equality of care:** The system should avoid the creation of a tiered system; the care provided should be based only on differences of need, not individual or group characteristics.
- **Personal responsibility:** Under health reform, each individual and family should assume responsibility for protecting and promoting health and contributing to the cost of care.
- **Intergenerational justice:** The health-care system should respond to the unique needs of each stage of life, sharing benefits and burdens fairly across generations.
- **Effectiveness:** The new system should deliver care, and innovation that works and that patients want. It should encourage the discovery of better treatments. It should make it possible for the academic community and health-care providers to exercise effectively their responsibility to evaluate and improve health care by providing resources for the systematic study of health-care outcomes.

- **Quality:** The system should deliver high-quality care and provide individuals with the information necessary to make informed health-care choices.
- **Fair distribution of costs:** The health-care system should spread the costs and burdens of care across the entire community, basing the level of contribution required of consumers on ability to pay.
- **Wise allocation of resources:** The nation should balance prudently what it spends on health care against other important national priorities.
- **Effective management:** By encouraging simplification and continuous improvement, as well as making the system easier to use for patients and providers, the health-care system should focus on care rather than administration.
- **Professional integrity and responsibility:** The health-care system should treat the clinical judgments of professionals with respect and protect the integrity of the provider-patient relationship while ensuring that health providers have the resources to fulfill their responsibilities for the effective delivery of quality care.
- **Fair procedures:** To protect these values and principles, fair and open democratic procedures should underlie decisions concerning the operation of the health-care system and the resolution of disputes that arise within it.
- **Local responsibility:** Working within the framework of national reform, the new health-care system should allow states and local communities to design effective, high-quality systems of care that serve each of their citizens.

Source: White House Domestic Policy Council. *The President's Health Security Plan*, 1993.[41]

ACCESSIBILITY: Reasonable access should be available on equal terms and conditions for all, according to need. Access to physicians and hospitals is readily available. Access to services requiring expensive equipment is available, but may not be convenient. Provincial governments will not provide certain expensive equipment (such as MRI machines) to every hospital, so that some patients needing such equipment will have to travel to access it.

PORTABILITY: Canadians are covered when traveling away from their home province or territory, including emergencies that arise when traveling outside of Canada.

PUBLIC ADMINISTRATION: Private insurance companies are excluded from the administration of the system. Before the present system came into effect, overhead costs consumed about 22% of all private health insurance premiums. Under government management the administrative costs have averaged about 5%.

Satisfaction with the Canadian system has fallen sharply during the past 10 years. Budgetary cutbacks have led to restricted access to specialists, longer waiting times for nonemergency surgery, and the closing or merger of many hospitals, resulting in a loss of beds.[43] A 1999 poll found that only 24% of Canadians rated their health-care system as excellent or good, as compared with 61% in 1991.[6]

The Clinton Health Plan
During 1993 a task force appointed by the Clinton administration met with more than 500 experts to enumerate the problems in our health-care system and make detailed proposals for addressing them. Table 25-5 outlines the problems that were identified. Table 25-6 summarizes the principles upon which the task force felt

reform should be based. Clinton's subsequent legislative proposal (the Health Security Act of 1993) spanned 1342 pages and included these provisions:

- Each American citizen and legal resident would receive a health security card.
- Everyone would be enrolled in a health plan through a regional or corporate health alliance, unless they are covered by Medicare or a military, Veteran's Administration, or Indian Health Service plan.
- Employers would pay 80% (or more if they wish) of the premiums, and individuals and families would pay the balance. Additional revenue would be raised by increasing taxes on tobacco products.
- There would be three plan options: fee-for-service, HMO, and PPO. Out-of-pocket costs would be limited.
- Coverage would be comprehensive. It would include: hospital care, emergency care, medical and surgical fees, preventive care, mental health and substance-abuse treatment, pregnancy-related care, hospice care, home health care, extended care, ambulance services, outpatient laboratory and diagnostic services, outpatient drugs and biologicals, outpatient rehabilitation services, durable medical equipment; prosthetic and orthotic devices, vision and hearing care, preventive dental services for children, and health education classes.
- A National Health Board would set standards for quality of care.
- Regional health alliances would negotiate with providers to deliver services within their region and would deal with consumer complaints.
- Claim forms and other paperwork would be standardized and streamlined.
- Residency training programs would have to shift so that half of the physicians-in-training were in primary care and quotas would be established for other specialties.

Consumers Union believes the key issues are universal coverage, comprehensive benefits, cost controls, adequate financing, and public accountability.[44] It prefers a single-payer system[45] and recommends expansion of Medicare to cover prescription drugs and include everyone age 55 and older.[17] It supported most of the Clinton plan but advocates greater standardization of coverage options, more cost controls, additional taxes on alcohol and firearms, federal control over prescription drug prices, and assurance that at least 90% of premium dollars would be used to pay benefits.[46] The AMA supported the provisions that would give more people access to health care, but it opposes any provisions that would limit fee-for-service, set fee schedules, establish a single-payer system, set spending caps, or establish residency training quotas. The AMA also wants substantial malpractice reform.[47] The Health Insurance Association of America attacked the Clinton proposal with television commercials in which "Harry and Louise"

complained that the plan was too restrictive to provide what they really needed.

In addition to making public comments, many organizations promote their views through lobbying activities and campaign contributions. Table 25-7 lists what the 20 largest health-related spenders spent on lobbying activities. Tobacco companies are included because the way they are permitted to market their products will have considerable impact on the nation's ultimate health-care costs. Drug companies were heavily involved because of their concern about prescription drug coverage.

Harvard economist Rashid Fein, Ph.D.,[48] has pointed out that Americans want assurance that they will have access, employers want relief from increasing costs, the federal government wants to reduce its growing deficit, and doctors and hospitals want to replace intrusions into their clinical decisions with more effective ways to control costs. It is not surprising that even though most people want "reform," no plan has been able to satisfy the many competing interests. During the recent election campaign both major parties advocated legislation under which Medicare would help defray the high cost of prescription drugs.[49,50] Aside from that, however, major modification of our health-care system does not appear on our nation's horizon.

Table 25-7
TOP 20 HEALTH-RELATED SPENDERS, 1998*

British American Tobacco	$25,190,000
Philip Morris	23,000,000
American Medical Association	16,820,000
American Hospital Association	10,520,000
Blue Cross/Blue Shield	9,171,572
Pfizer, Inc. (drug company)	6,000,000
RJR Nabisco	5,448,060
Eli Lilly & Co.	5,160,000
Merck (drug company)	5,000,000
Health Insurance Association of America	4,495,000
Schering-Plough (drug company)	4,268,000
Loews Corp (tobacco company)	4,220,000
Biotechnology Industry Organization	3,703,990
Glaxo Wellcome Inc. (drug company)	3,120,000
Pharmacutical Research & Mfrs. of America	3,120,000
Bristol Meyers Squibb (drug company)	2,820,579
SmithKline Beecham	2,680,000
Health Industry Manufacturers Association	2,470,000
American Association of Health Plans	2,040,000
Aetna (insurance company)	1,819,072

*Total 1998 payments to lobbying firms plus in-house expenses for lobbying actibities. It does not include campaign contributions.
Source: Center for Responsive Politics (http://www.opensecrets.org).

It's Your Decision

Assume that you can influence the health-care delivery system for the United States. Rank the following possible characteristics of your system in order of importance.

Rank

1. Everyone should have access to health care without financial or other barriers. _____
2. Guaranteed benefits should meet the full range of health needs, including primary, preventive, and specialized care. _____
3. Each consumer should have the opportunity to exercise effective choice of providers, plans, and treatments. _____
4. The system should provide care based only on differences of need, not financial status or other individual or group characteristics. _____
5. Each individual and family should assume responsibility for protecting and promoting health and contributing to the cost of care. _____
6. The health-care system should spread the costs and burdens of care across the entire community, basing the level of contribution required of consumers on ability to pay. _____
7. Within a national framework, states and local communities should be able to design effective, high-quality systems. _____
8. The system should respond to the unique needs of each stage of life, sharing benefits and burdens fairly across generations. _____
9. The system should provide resources for the systematic evaluation of health-care outcomes so that health care can be improved. _____
10. The amount spent on health care should be balanced against other important national priorities. _____
11. The system should have a democratic way to influence how it works and to resolve any disputes that arise. _____
12. Paperwork and administrative red tape should be minimized. _____
13. The system should deliver high-quality care and provide individuals with the information necessary to make informed choices. _____
14. Treatment policies should be determined with adequate input from clinicians. _____
15. Other (specify) _____ _____

SUMMARY

America is said to be undergoing a "health-care crisis" with skyrocketing costs and inequalities in the distribution of services. This, plus the prospect of greater government intervention, has stimulated rapid and sweeping changes in the way in which the health marketplace is organized. Managed-care enrollment has risen rapidly. Widespread concerns that small organizations will be unable to compete with large ones have been stimulating mergers and other alliances that can achieve economies of scale.

Many of the problems are inherent in the system as it is organized today. Individuals can minimize some of their expenses through prudent consumer strategies.

Insurance fraud is a serious problem. Some frauds can be detected by examining insurance payment reports to see whether they accurately reflect the services rendered.

An ideal national health-care system would provide equity, access, efficiency, and quality. However, even though most people want "reform," no plan has been able to satisfy the many competing interests.

REFERENCES

1. Davies NE and Felder LH: Applying brakes to the runaway American health care system: A proposed agenda. JAMA 263:73-76, 1990.
2. Wunderlich GS and others, editors. Nursing Staff in Hospitals and Nursing Homes: Is It Adequate? Washington, D.C., 1996, National Academy Press.
3. How good is your health plan? Consumer Reports 61:28–42, 1996.
4. National Coalition on Health Care. How Americans perceive the health care system: A report on a national survey. Journal of Health Care Finance 23(4):12–20, 1997.
5. Cromwell J and others. The Nation's Health Care Bill: Who Bears the Burden? Waltham, Mass., 1994, Center for Economics Research.
6. Blendon R and others. Satisfaction with health systems in ten nations. Health Affairs 9(2):185–192, 1990.
7. Donelan K and others. The cost of health system change: Public discontent in five nations. Health Affairs 18:206–216, 1999.
8. Levit KR and others. National health care expenditures, 1990. Health Care Financing Review 13(1)29-54, 1991.

9. National health care expenditures projections. HCFA Web site, Dec 14, 2000.

10. Source Book of Health Insurance Data, 1995. Washington, D.C., 1996, Health Insurance Association of America

11. National health care expenditures. HCFA Web site, accessed Dec 14, 2000.

12. Source Book of Health Insurance Data, 1999–2000. Washington, D.C., 1999, Health Insurance Association of America.

13. Ginzberg E: High-tech medicine and rising health care costs. JAMA 263:1820-1822, 1990.

14. Cooper W, Shulkin D. Can we monitor the monitors of medical costs? Pennsylvania Medicine 93(5):28-29, 1990.

15. Norbeck TB. Telling the truth about rising health-care costs. Private Practice. Feb 1990, pp 11–17.

16. Eastaugh SR. Health Economics: Efficiency, Quality, and Equity. Westport, Conn., 1992, Auburn House.

17. Public opinion and medical technology. Alexandria, Va., 1993, Health Care Technology Institute.

18. Shearer G. The health care divide: Unfair financial burdens. Washington, D.C., 2000, Consumers Union.

19. O'Leary MR. Lexicon: Dictionary of Health Care Terms, Organizations, and Acronyms for the Era of Health Reform. Oakbrook Terrace, Ill., 1994, Joint Commission on Accreditation of Healthcare Organizations.

20. Crane M. Reimbursements: Inching closer to actual charges. Medical Economics 77(22):32–50, 2000.

21. Wenger MF, Shapiro NS. Rethinking utilization review. New England Journal of Medicine 333:1353–1354, 1995.

22. Glasson J and others. Ethical issues in managed care. JAMA 273:330–335, 1995.

23. Azevedo D. Will the states get tough with HMOs? Anti-managed care proposals pile up nationwide. Medical Economics 73(16):172–185, 1996.

24. Managing managed care. American Medical News, Sept 9, 1996.

25. Kletke PR and others. Current trends in physicians' practice arrangements: From owners to employees. JAMA 276:555–560, 1996.

26. Scheier R. Virginia Blues edge closer to for-profit plan. American Medical News, Sept 2, 1996.

27. Pretzer M. The managed-care juggernaut: Explosive growth nationwide. Medical Economics 73(7):64–74, 1996.

28. Ulene A, Ulene V. How to Cut Your Medical Bills. Berkeley, Calif., 1994, Ulysses Press.

29. Borzo G. Smart-bombing fraud: Insurers turn to powerful new computer tools to spot 'aberrant' claims. American Medical News, Oct 10, 1994.

30. Department of Justice Health Care Fraud Report, Fiscal Year 1998. Washington, D.C., 1999, U.S. Department of Justice.

31. Johnson J. Fraud changing with market: Government expands probes, enforcement efforts. American Medical News, Nov 13, 1995.

32. Office of Inspector General. Semiannual Report, October 1, 1995 – March 31, 1996. Washington, D.C., U.S. Department of Health and Human Services.

33. Office of Inspector General. Semiannual Report, April 1, 1995 – September 30, 1995. Washington, D.C., U.S. Department of Health and Human Services.

34. Office of Inspector General. Semiannual Report, April 1, 1994 – September 30, 1994. Washington, D.C., U.S. Department of Health and Human Services.

35. Freudenheim M. Employers balk at high cost of high-tech medical care. The New York Times, April 29, 1990, pp 1, 24.

36. Office of Inspector General. Semiannual Report, October 1, 1999 – March 31, 2000. Washington, D.C., U.S. Department of Health and Human Services.

37. Two men sentenced in one of the largest health insurance fraud cases ever prosecuted. Law Enforcement Report, Winter/Spring 1995, p 6.

38. Kusserow RP. Fraud alert: Routine waiver of copayments or deductible under Medicare Part B. Washington, D.C., 1991, U.S. Departments of Health and Human Services.

39. Second class medicine. Consumer Reports 65(9):42, 2000

40. Short PF, Banthin JS. New estimates of the underinsured younger than 65 years. JAMA 274:1302–1306, 1995.

41. White House Domestic Policy Council. The President's Health Security Plan. New York, 1993, Times Books.

42. Christiansen C, Christiansen P. What is the Canadian system? OT Week, June 30, 1994, pp 16–19.

43. Iglehart JK. Revisiting the Canadian health care system. New England Journal of Medicine 342:2007–2012, 2000.

44. What to watch for in health reform. Consumer Reports 59:396–398, 1994.

45. Can HMOs help solve the health-care crisis? Managed care has become a highly competitive multi–billion–dollar business. But what's good for HMOs may not be good for consumers. Consumer Reports 61:28–35, 1996.

46. The Clinton Health Care Act: What Will It Mean for Consumers? Washington, D.C., 1993, Consumers Union.

47. Painter JT, Bristow LR, Todd JS. AMA's analysis of the Clinton reform plan. In packet distributed to physicians in September 1993 by the American Medical Association.

48. Fein R. Prescription for change. Modern Maturity, July/Aug 1992, pp 22–35.

49. Bush G. Ensuring access to health care. The Bush plan. JAMA 284:2108–2109, 2000.

50. Gore A. Ensuring access to health care. The Gore plan. JAMA 284:2110–2111, 2000.

Chapter Twenty-Six

CONSUMER LAWS, AGENCIES, AND STRATEGIES

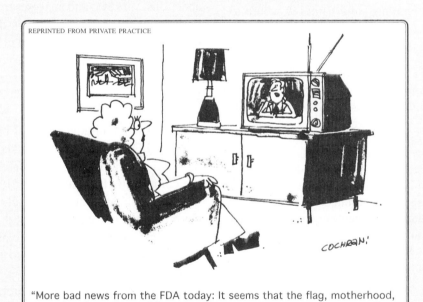

REPRINTED FROM PRIVATE PRACTICE

"More bad news from the FDA today: It seems that the flag, motherhood, and apple pie have all been found to cause cancer-causing agents."

When a situation can be solved with education, we will serve as the instructor. When a sterner approach is called for, we will be the cop.

FRANK E. YOUNG, M.D., PH.D.[1]
FDA COMMISSIONER

The basic principles of consumer protection in health matters were outlined by President John F. Kennedy in a message to Congress in 1962. Although Kennedy's message had little immediate impact, it still provides a framework for future generations: People deserve to be provided with safe and effective foods, drugs, cosmetics, medical devices, and services by health-care practitioners. They must receive accurate information, through advertising and other media, that will enable them to make intelligent and free choices. Individuals have the right to speak out and be heard, to complain, and to know where to complain when they have been misled or exploited.

Implementation of these rights requires five things:

1. Laws ensuring that health products are safe and effective and that health professionals are competent.
2. Government agencies that enforce the laws and keep the public informed.
3. Professional, voluntary, and business organizations that serve as consumer advocates, monitor government agencies that issue safety regulations, and provide reliable information about health products and services.
4. Education of the consumer to permit freedom of choice based on an understanding of scientific data rather than misleading information.
5. Action by individuals to register complaints when they have been deceived, misled, overcharged, or victimized by frauds.

Many agencies help to protect Americans in health matters. This chapter highlights the laws that control the three main federal consumer protection agencies: the Food and Drug Administration (FDA), the Federal Trade Commission (FTC), and the United States Postal Service (USPS). Information is also provided about other government agencies; voluntary, business, and professional groups; consumer education; and actions that intelligent consumers can take to help protect themselves in the health marketplace. Additional sources are listed in the Appendix and on the Consumer Health Sourcebook Web site (http://www.chsourcebook.com). Federal enforcement actions described in other chapters are listed under each agency in the index. State and local actions are listed under "Enforcement actions."

U.S. FOOD AND DRUG ADMINISTRATION

The FDA is part of the U.S. Public Health Service, which is a component of the Department of Health and Human Services. The FDA's main function is to protect the public from health hazards involving foods, drugs, cosmetics, and medical devices. Approximately 25 cents of every consumer dollar in the United States is spent on FDA-regulated products that are made or distributed by about 95,000 companies.[2]

The FDA sets performance standards; conducts inspections, surveys, and analyses to measure compliance with these standards; evaluates drugs, biologics, and devices that require premarket clearance; initiates enforcement actions when necessary; and helps inform and educate industry, health professionals, and the public. In fiscal year 2000 (October 1, 1999, through September 30, 2000), the agency had about 10,000 full-time employees and a budget of $1.2 billion.

The FDA is organized into six regions with 21 district offices and many field offices located throughout the country. Its headquarters offices are located in the Washington, D.C., area and include the Office of the Commissioner, Center for Food Safety and Applied Nutrition, Center for Biologics Evaluation and Research, Center for Drug Evaluation and Research, Center for Veterinary Medicine, and Center for Devices and Radiological Health. Another component, the National Center for Toxicological Research, is in Jefferson, Arkansas. The FDA Commissioner is appointed by the president and confirmed by the U.S. Senate.

Food and Drug Laws

Many federal laws affect the marketing of health-related products. The principal laws are the following, listed in chronologic order.

The original *Pure Food and Drug Act* (1906) was passed in response to public concern about the safety of foods and drugs (see Historical Perspective). The act required that foods be pure and wholesome and that the ingredients of drugs be listed on their label. This law, initially administered by the Agriculture Department's Bureau of Chemistry, did not require that drugs be safe or effective. In 1927 the act's regulatory duties were transferred to the newly created Food, Drug, and Insecticide Administration, which was renamed Food and Drug Administration (FDA) 3 years later. In 1940 the FDA became part of a new Federal Security Agency, which, in 1953, was elevated to cabinet status as the Department of Health, Education, and Welfare (DHEW). In 1979 DHEW became the Department of Health and Human Services (HHS).

The *Sherley Amendment to the Food and Drug Act* (1912) prohibited the labeling of medicines with false therapeutic claims intended to defraud the purchaser.

The *Agriculture Appropriation Act* (1931) gave the Food and Drug Administration its current name.

The *Food, Drug, and Cosmetic (FD&C) Act* (1938) replaced the 1906 law with new and stronger provisions:

- Foods in interstate commerce must be pure and wholesome, safe to eat, and produced under sanitary conditions.
- Drugs and therapeutic devices must be safe.
- New drugs must be approved for safety by the FDA before they can go on the market. (Products marketed before 1938 did not have to meet this requirement.)
- Cosmetics must be safe.
- Labeling must be truthful and not misleading; common names of all ingredients are required; quantities and proportions of potent and habit-forming narcotic and hypnotic substances must be given.
- Drug labeling must include warnings needed for safe use.
- Drugs not safe for self-treatment are restricted to sale by prescription.
- Drug-manufacturing plants must be registered and be inspected by the FDA at least once every 2 years.
- Antibiotics, insulin, and colors used in foods, drugs, and cosmetics must be tested in FDA laboratories before they can go on sale.
- Chemicals added to foods must be proven safe before their use is allowed.
- Pesticide residues on raw crops must not exceed safe tolerances. (The Environmental Protection Agency now establishes the limits, and the FDA enforces them.)
- Penalties are heavier for second offenses and fraud. First offenses might bring up to 1 year in jail.
- The FDA no longer had to prove that defendants intended to defraud their customers. This was important because some promoters were misguided cranks who believed in their products.

The *Public Health Service Act* (1944) contained two sections now enforced by the FDA. Their provisions cover the safety, purity, and potency of biologic products, such as vaccines, sera, and blood for interstate sale and the safety of pasteurized milk and shellfish, as well as the sanitation of food, water, food services, and facilities for travelers on trains, airplanes, and buses.

The *Durham-Humphrey Amendment* (1951) specified that drugs that cannot be safely used without medical supervision must be so labeled and dispensed only by prescription of a licensed health practitioner. Thus a distinction was made between over-the-counter (OTC) and prescription drugs. Before this law took effect, manufacturers decided whether to classify drugs as prescription or OTC drugs. If the FDA disagreed, it could bring the case to court and charge that the product was misbranded.

The *Food Additives Amendment* (1958) prohibited the use of new food additives until the manufacturer had established their safety. Its Delaney Clause gave the FDA additional authority to ban the use of food additives that can cause cancer in humans or animals.

The *Color Additive Amendments* (1960) permitted the FDA to regulate the conditions for the safe use of color additives in foods, drugs, and cosmetics and to require manufacturers to make the necessary scientific investigations to establish safety.

The *Federal Hazardous Substances Labeling Act* (1960) required that labels display prominent warnings regarding household products with hazardous chemicals. This is now enforced by the Consumer Product Safety Commission.

The *Kefauver-Harris Drug Amendments* (1962) overhauled and strengthened the drug provisions of the FD&C Act of 1938. They came about as a result of the foresight of Dr. Frances Kelsey, an FDA medical officer who prevented the release of thalidomide on the U.S. market because of suspected side effects (see Historical Perspective). Strong public support for strengthening the law resulted from news reports about deformed German babies whose mothers had taken thalidomide during their pregnancy. These 1962 amendments included the following provisions:

- Manufacturers must provide substantial evidence that a new drug is effective as well as safe before it can be approved for marketing.
- Previously cleared new drugs may be ordered off the market immediately if new information indicates an imminent hazard to health, and any prior approval may be withdrawn.
- Manufacturers are required to get the patient's consent if experimental drugs are to be used, unless this is not feasible or the investigator believes that obtaining such consent would be contrary to the patient's best interest.
- All drug products must be registered annually with the FDA, and each establishment will be inspected at least once every 2 years.
- The FDA was given broad inspection authority over prescription drugs.

A Brief History of Federal Consumer Protection Laws

The Pure Food and Drug Act (1906) was passed in response to public concerns about the safety of foods and drugs. After the Spanish-American War it was discovered that the army had been supplied with spoiled canned meat and sawdust-adulterated flour. There were also reports that toxic chemicals such as formaldehyde had been used to preserve milk sold in neighborhood grocery stores. Two leaders in the struggle to enact the bill were Dr. Harvey W. Wiley, chief chemist for the Department of Agriculture, and his crusading journalist follower, Samuel Hopkins Adams. Wiley's main concern was the prevalence of fraudulent food products, but he also fought hard for the regulation of patent medicines. Wiley believed that all remedies should have their formula on the label and that none containing alcohol or cocaine should be sold without a doctor's prescription.

In 1905 *Collier's Weekly* magazine began a series of 10 articles by Adams titled "The Great American Fraud." The series attacked nostrum evils and quackery and said that Americans were wasting more than $75 million annually on products containing large quantities of alcohol, opiates, and other questionable ingredients. He noted, for example, that *Dr. King's New Discovery for Consumption*, which had been proclaimed as the world's only sure cure for tuberculosis, contained morphine, chloroform, and 28% alcohol. The chloroform was to allay the cough while the morphine and alcohol drugged the patient into deceptive cheerfulness. The label did not reveal the nature of the ingredients or their possible hazardous effects. Adams explained that patent medicine testimonials were gathered from gullible ignoramuses or secured through various pressures from people in public life.[3] The American Medical Association reprinted his articles as a 172-page booklet and sold nearly 500,000 copies, many of which were distributed by physicians to their patients.

The final impetus to passage of the act was Upton Sinclair's novel *The Jungle*, which was published near the end of 1905. Sinclair was a socialist who railed against American capitalism. His book was aimed at exposing the exploitation of immigrant laborers who were often forced to work long hours at low pay. The setting for his fiction was the meat-packing industry, where, said the book, rats, human fingers, and even whole bodies were processed along with animal parts into sausage and lard. There was no truth in such claims, but the public reacted with outrage—not at the exploitation of immigrants as Sinclair had intended, but at the imaginary conditions he described.[4]

Truth in Labeling

The Pure Food and Drug Act required that medicine labels tell the truth, but not the whole truth. Labels had to indicate the presence and amount of alcohol, opiates, acetanilide, and several other potentially dangerous substances. It was not necessary to identify other ingredients. The label could not provide false or misleading statements about the medicine or its ingredients. The new law did not inhibit self-medication but attempted to make it safer. It was assumed that the average person was intelligent enough to avoid risks when ingredients were known. Products were not required to be effective.

Many product labels changed drastically after 1906. When the law was violated, the government occasionally went to court, where it usually would prevail. However, fines were usually $50 or less, sometimes as low as one cent.

The first court trial under the Pure Food and Drug Act was brought against *Cuforhedake Brane-Fude,* a product that contained acetanilide (an analgesic and antipyretic), antipyrine, caffeine, sodium and potassium bromide, and alcohol. The label stated that the product contained 30% alcohol and 16 grams of acetanilide, but Wiley's analysis revealed only 24% alcohol. The product was claimed to offer "a most wonderful certain and harmless relief" and to contain "no . . . poisonous ingredients of any kind." The government charged that this was misleading. Wiley noted that the product's name appeared to be an evasive spelling for a headache cure and that none of the ingredients was food for the brain. One of Adams's magazine articles had identified 22 headache-remedy users alleged to have had died from acetanilide poisoning.

The manufacturer was found guilty of misbranding, fined $700, and forced to relabel the product. Some two million bottles had been sold for $1 each before the 1908 verdict. This illustrates how the selling of a quack remedy can be extremely profitable despite government enforcement action—a situation that holds true today. Although *Cuforhedake Brane-Fude* is no longer with us, products named after an ailment, body part, or body function are still abundant.

Truth in Advertising

The Pure Food and Drug Act had little effect on misleading advertising. In 1911 the Supreme Court ruled that the Act's prohibition against false labeling did not apply to therapeutic claims, because the misbranding section of the law did not explicitly refer to curative promises. Congressman Swager Sherley of Kentucky sought to correct this problem by obtaining passage in 1912 of an amendment stating that an article would be misbranded "if its package or label shall bear or contain any statement, design, or device regarding the curative or therapeutic effect of such article or any of the ingredients or substances contained therein which is false and fraudulent."[5]

By 1915 the food and drug laws still had not controlled the problem of false and misleading advertising of patent medicines. Observers who claimed that conditions had worsened noted that: the job was too big for a small regulatory staff; fines were small and often unpaid; second offenders could be sent to jail for 1 year, but none had ever been sent; many dangerous drugs were not covered by the law; and newspaper advertisements were still misleading.

Safety Requirements Added

In 1938 the Food, Drug, and Cosmetic Act replaced the 1906 law with new and stronger provisions. As with the original law, public indignation was aroused by a book, *100 Million Guinea Pigs*, by Arthur Kallet and F.J. Schlink. (The book's title referred to the U.S. population at that time.) Several tragedies had occurred, but the most outrageous was the mounting death toll from elixir of sulfanilamide, a product sold over the counter for treating infections, especially gonorrhea.

A Brief History of Federal Consumer Protection Laws - *Cont'd.*

It was the first antibiotic drug and at first was considered a miracle drug. Unfortunately, it contained the toxic substance diethylene glycol and had not been tested for safety. In 1937, 107 people, many of them children, died.

The 1938 law increased public protection but did not clearly distinguish between drugs requiring medical supervision and those suitable for self-medication. New drugs would have to be proven safe before marketing, but proof of effectiveness was still not required. The hazard of permissive refills of prescribed drugs also remained. In the Midwest, a mother of three children was discovered upon admission to a hospital to be a barbiturate addict. She had received a prescription for 30 capsules that had been refilled 16 times within 3 months. Another woman with mild high blood pressure was found dead in her bed. During the preceding 6 months she had received 23 refills of a prescription for 20 barbiturate capsules. Such evidence led to passage in 1951 of the Durham-Humphrey Amendment, which prohibited the refilling of prescriptions without specific authorization of the physician. It also gave the FDA the power to classify drugs as prescription drugs.

Young[5] calls the 25-year period following passage of the 1938 Act "the chemotherapeutic revolution." Its impact on self-medication was enormous. Americans spent less than $200 million per year for nonprescription medications in the 1930s, but by 1957 the sum had reached $2 billion. (Today it is over $30 billion.) This increase was partially due to extensive advertising. Unscrupulous promoters of pseudomedicine were prevalent during this period and their appeals became more sophisticated. Promotions included pamphlets, newspapers, roadside signs, lecturers (some speakers collected $25,000 weekly from fees and sales), and door-to-door salespeople.

Efficacy Requirements Added . . . and Partly Waived

Critics charged in 1961 that the chemotherapeutic revolution had produced a therapeutic nightmare, especially with respect to prescription medications. Although many new drugs could save lives and reduce pain and suffering, many were improperly used, and drug-induced ailments occurred with increasing frequency. Some blame was attributed to physicians because (a) drugs were sometimes prescribed when none was needed, (b) new therapeutic agents were sometimes used without considering their potential dangers, and (c) physicians at times relied too much on the claims of drug manufacturers and salespeople.

Thalidomide, a generic drug, began marketing in 1957 in West Germany as a sleeping tablet, sedative, and antiemetic for pregnant women. In 1960 the manufacturer sought permission to sell it within the United States by submitting a new drug application to the FDA. But Dr. Frances O. Kelsey, an FDA physician, suspected that the drug was hazardous to the unborn child. As a result of her action the application was withdrawn. It soon became clear that babies born to mothers who took thalidomide during pregnancy had a high incidence of similar birth defects. The drug was never marketed in the United States, but some Americans obtained it in Europe.

The thalidomide tragedy led to passage in 1962 of the Kefauver-Harris Amendment to the Food, Drug, and Cosmetic Act. It provided that no new drug could be released to the public unless the manufacturer provided evidence acceptable to the FDA that the drug was effective as well as safe. Drug companies also had to notify the FDA whenever they became aware that an approved drug might have adverse effects. Prior to passage of this law the FDA bore the burden of proving ineffectiveness.

The Dietary Supplement Health and Education Act of 1994, passed in response to an aggressive campaign by the health-food industry, weakened the FDA's ability to protect consumers from misleading promotions for vitamins, minerals, amino acids, herbs, and various other substances marketed as "dietary supplements."

Postal Laws

The Mail Fraud Statute (1872) was enacted to combat a rash of swindles that had erupted after the Civil War. Prior to passage of this law, con artists who used the mail to defraud people were virtually safe from prosecution because local law-enforcement officials were unable to obtain jurisdiction over distant swindlers. By 1895 the Postal Service could stamp letters "fraudulent" and return them to senders, but it was not until 1901 that the Postmaster General, with Dr. Wiley's help, began acting against patent-medicine frauds. Postal authorities assailed the most outrageous quacks who promised sure cures for such problems as cancer, consumption (tuberculosis), epilepsy, blindness, deafness, a drug habit, a tobacco habit, "lost manhood," and "failing womanhood." Proving fraud was easiest against devices said to restore lost manhood or cure all human ills. During the 1920s, frauds involving nostrums for tuberculosis and venereal disease were common. Most current health-related mail frauds involve "miracle" diets and products claimed to enhance beauty, sexual function, or athletic prowess.

The Mail Order Consumer Protection Amendments of 1983 enable the Postal Service to seek large civil penalties for repeat offenders. This law was passed after *Consumer Reports* publicized an investigation by Dr. Stephen Barrett that demonstrated that almost every health-related product sold by mail through magazine advertising was misrepresented.[6] Before that time, swindlers could remain in business indefinitely by modifying products, making new advertising claims, or operating under new company names.

FTC Laws

The Federal Trade Commission Act (1914) was intended to preserve competition in the growing industrial society by providing safeguards against business monopoly. It was designed to prevent unfair methods of competition in commerce by making unfair practices unlawful, thereby protecting consumers as well as other entrepreneurs. The FTC was given authority to investigate, publicize, and prohibit such procedures. The first five commissioners were sworn into office in 1915. The Wheeler-Lea Amendment (1938) provided for regulation of advertising of all health-related products except prescription drugs. The Fair Packaging and Labeling Act (1966) gave the FTC primary jurisdiction over package and label claims in all areas except food, drugs, devices, and cosmetics, which are still delegated to the FDA.

- Prescription drug advertisements must include a summary of side effects, contraindications, and effectiveness.
- All drug labels must bear the established generic name of the drug, and prescription drug labels must list the quantity of each active ingredient.
- Control over the advertising of prescription drugs was passed from the FTC to the FDA.
- Pharmaceutical manufacturers must comply with the Code of Good Manufacturing Practices in testing, processing, packaging, and holding drugs.

The *Drug Abuse Control Amendments* (1965) were enacted to control the manufacture and distribution of depressants, stimulants, and hallucinogens. The amendments required wholesalers and jobbers of these drugs to register annually with the FDA. The agency was also authorized to seize illegal supplies, serve warrants, arrest violators, and require all legal handlers of controlled drugs to keep records of their supplies and sales. A new Bureau of Drug Abuse Control (BDAC) was established for these purposes. In 1968, to consolidate the policing of illegal drug traffic, BDAC was transferred from the FDA to the new Bureau of Narcotics and Dangerous Drugs in the Department of Justice (now called the Drug Enforcement Administration).

The *Fair Packaging and Labeling Act* (1966) provided additional support for the FDA to ensure that food, drugs, medical devices, and cosmetics were honestly and informatively labeled. It required more complete information on labels and packages. The information was to be clearly and prominently stated in terms that would enable consumers to make value comparisons between competing products. Food package labels were required to contain the identity of the food; the name and address of the manufacturer, packer, or distributor; the net quantity of the contents; and an ingredient list. The FTC retained jurisdiction over OTC drug advertising.

The *Radiation Control for Health and Safety Act* (1968) was designed to protect the public from unnecessary exposure to radiation from electronic products such as color television sets, microwave ovens, and x-ray machines. The FDA sets performance standards for these and similar products.

The *Poison Prevention Act* (1970) required special packaging to protect children from accidentally ingesting toxic substances. Poisons identified by the Secretary of Health, Education, and Welfare must be packaged so that most children under the age of 5 would find them difficult to open.

The *Medical Device Amendments* (1976) supplemented the 1938 FD&C Act, which permitted action only if a defect in a product was discovered after the product was in use. The amendments gave new authority over the safety and effectiveness of devices. They enabled the FDA to require premarket approval for some items and performance standards for others.

The *Proxmire Amendment* (1976) prohibited the FDA from limiting the potency of ingredients of vitamin and mineral products that are not inherently dangerous. This bill prevents the FDA from ridding the marketplace of useless "dietary supplement" ingredients and irrational combinations of ingredients. The bill was passed because the health-food industry misled many of its customers into believing that the FDA intended to greatly restrict the sale of supplement products. More than 1 million protest messages poured into Congress as a result.

The *Infant Formula Act* (1980) requires strict controls to ensure the nutritional content and safety of commercial baby foods.

The *Orphan Drug Act* (1983) was passed to facilitate the development of new drugs for more than 5000 rare diseases affecting as many as 20 million Americans. A disease is considered "rare" if it affects fewer than 200,000 people. Drug companies can now claim half of clinical trial costs as a credit against taxes owed. Companies might otherwise be reluctant to develop such drugs and gain FDA approval because the cost is prohibitive. The legislation also authorized grants to fund research to discover useful substances. By 1993, 101 orphan products had been approved, and experts predicted that another 100 would succeed during the next decade.[7] Following approval the manufacturer is entitled to 7 years of marketing exclusivity.

The *Drug Price Competition and Patent Term Restoration Act* (1984) permits the FDA to approve generic versions of previously approved new drugs without requiring their sponsors to duplicate the costly human tests required for the original drugs (see Chapter 19). It allows the term of patents on medicines (17 years) to be extended up to five years to compensate for the time required to get FDA approval.

The *Prescription Drug Marketing Act* (1988) prohibits selling; buying; trading; or offering to sell, buy, or trade prescription drug samples.

The *Safe Medical Devices Act* (1990) gave the FDA the power to (a) obtain earlier knowledge of serious device problems, (b) order recalls to quickly remove defective products from the marketplace, (c) track devices from the manufacturer to the consumer, and (d) apply large civil penalties for violations of the act. The act requires hospitals and other health-care providers to report device-related deaths directly to the FDA instead of to the device manufacturer. Additional provisions are discussed in Chapter 22.

The *Nutrition Labeling and Education Act* (1990) provided for (a) mandatory labeling on most food products; (b) standardization of portion sizes; (c) more appropriate disclosure of fat and cholesterol contents; (d) determination of whether disease-prevention claims can be made for various nutrients; and (e) voluntary guidelines to retailers for nutrition information on raw fruits, vegetables, and fish. Chapter 11 discusses how these provisions have been implemented.

The *Dietary Supplement Health and Education Act* (1994) was passed following a massive lobbying campaign by the health-food industry (see Chapter 12). This law (a) defines the term "supplements," (b) shifted the burden of proof of safety on the FDA, (c) sets standards for the distribution of third-party literature, (d) allows statements of "nutritional support" under certain circumstances, (e) specifies the ingredient and nutritional label information, (f) requires good manufacturing practices, (g) establishes an NIH Office of Dietary Supplements to oversee research and provide advice to other federal agencies, and (h) calls for creation of a commission to make nonbinding recommendations on standards for setting supplement-related health claims. This law has greatly weakened the ability of the FDA to protect consumers against unsubstantiated claims made in product labeling or advertising.[8] Final regulations covering the law's requirements for supplement labeling, health claims, and "statements of nutritional support" took effect in 2000.[9]

The *Food Quality Protection Act* (1996) replaced the Delaney Clause with a more flexible requirement that additives be safe (defined as "reasonable certainty" that no harm will result from their use).

The *FDA Modernization Act* (1997) codified or extended regulations intended to (a) accelerate review of new drugs and devices, (b) increase patient access to experimental drugs and devices, and (c) permit pharmacists to compound certain categories of drug products not commercially available.

Food, Drug, and Cosmetic Act

The Food, Drug, and Cosmetic Act, including amendments, is the primary federal consumer protection law in the United States.[10] It deals with imported products as well as domestic ones. Its purpose is to ensure that foods are safe to eat, drugs and health devices are safe and effective for their intended uses, and cosmetics are safe and are not advertised deceptively. The following are its main provisions.

Food provisions. Food is considered adulterated if it contains (a) poisonous or deleterious substances that are injurious to health; (b) filthy, putrid, or decomposed substances or substances prepared and packed under unsanitary conditions; or (c) unsafe color additives.

Food is said to be misbranded when: (a) the labeling is false and misleading; (b) the food is offered for sale under the name of another food; (c) the food is an imitation of a food and the label does not bear the word "imitation"; (d) the container is so made, formed, or filled as to be misleading about its contents; (e) the food is represented for special dietary use without the label bearing information about the product's vitamin, mineral, and dietary properties; (f) the food contains artificial flavoring, artificial coloring, or chemical preservatives that are not listed on the labels; or (g) the labeling is not conspicuously displayed in terms that consumers are likely to read and understand.

Regulations that took effect in 1994 require manufacturers to provide nutrition information on product labels. The required nutrition panel must state the typical serving size, the amounts per serving of several important nutrients, and Percent Daily Values that indicate how the food fits into the overall diet of people at specified calorie levels. The regulations also permit health claims to be made for certain types of food. Chapter 11 covers the new labeling regulations in detail.

Food additives. Additives must be supported by evidence substantiating their safety before they may be included in a product. The Food Additives Amendment of 1958 authorized the FDA to establish the quantities of certain substances that could be added safely. In addition, the FDA could prevent the use of substances that showed evidence of carcinogenic effect when consumed, not only by humans but also by experimental animals. This was the controversial Delaney Clause.

The Delaney Clause forced the removal of cyclamates (a low-calorie sweetener) from the marketplace and was involved in the debate over removal of saccharin. The food industry, some government regulatory agencies, and the American Council on Science and Health[11] urged that this amendment be repealed or modified because it was rigid and did not attempt to quantify the risk to humans and compare it to a product's possible benefits. Jukes[12] pointed out that (a) the amounts of carcinogens in food and food additives are small, (b) the quantities found naturally in the diet vastly exceed those from human-made sources, and (3) antioxidants protect against low levels of carcinogens. The Council for Agricultural Science and Technology (CAST)[13] noted that substances are now detectable in amounts too small to have a significant effect on health. CAST regarded the Delaney Clause as "hopelessly obsolete" and said a "de minimis" concept should be substituted. (The term comes from a judicial doctrine, *de minimis non curat lex*, which means "the law does not concern itself with trifles.") Various others argued that the Delaney Clause should be retained because it made it easy for the FDA to protect the public from the inclusion of carcinogenic substances in foods. The Food Quality Protection Act of 1996 replaced the Delaney Clause with language calling for a flexible approach based on benefit-risk analysis.[14] The law also required the Environmental Protection Agency to review the risks and benefits of pesticide use and to make suggestions for reducing dietary exposure to pesticides.

The FDA categorizes additives either as regulated food additives or as GRAS (generally recognized as safe) substances. Several thousand compounds can be classified as additives. Regulated food additives are substances that can be added directly to food (such as vitamins to milk or bread) or that get into food from its surroundings, including packaging, manufacturing equipment, and other sources. The GRAS list includes about 700 additives that scientists recognize as safe because of long-established use without evidence of harm to individuals.

Many additives come from food itself. Lecithin, for example, is found in all plants and animals. It is obtained primarily from soybeans and is used mostly as an emulsifier to keep ingredients in processed foods from separating. Calcium and sodium propionate are used in the cheese industry, but propionate also occurs naturally in Swiss cheese. Propionate is used primarily as a mold inhibitor in baked goods. Sodium benzoate prevents mold growth in margarine. Added vitamins and minerals are identical to those found naturally in food.

Food additives are used as (a) nutrient supplements (such as vitamins and minerals), (b) nonnutritive sweeteners (sugar substitutes), (c) preservatives (to prevent microbial spoilage and oxidative chemical change), (d) stabilizers and thickeners (as in ice cream, candy, frozen desserts, jams, jellies, and gelatin), (e) flavors or flavoring agents (such as spices, liquid derivatives of onion and garlic, and the flavor enhancer monosodium glutamate made from corn, beets, or soybeans), (f) bleaching and maturing agents (which speed the aging process of flour), and (g) colors. There are other functional uses, and several additives serve more than one purpose. Ascorbic acid (vitamin C), for example, is a nutrient, an acidifying agent, an antioxidant, and a microbial inhibitor.

Any new substance proposed for addition to food must undergo rigid testing. The FDA also requires information about the chemical composition of the substance, how it is manufactured, and the methods used to detect it and to measure it at the expected levels of use. Data must show that the proposed testing methods are sensitive enough to determine compliance with established regulations. Finally, proof must be provided that the substance is safe for its intended use. This requires tests that administer the additives in various concentrations in the diets of two or more species of animals. The FDA will allow the use of a food additive only if it concludes there is practical certainty that no harm will result from its normal use over a lifetime.

Food irradiation. Irradiation (sometimes called "cold sterilization") can make food safer by killing harmful pathogens, spoilage microorganisms, parasites, and insects and can also extend the shelf-life of fruits, vegetables, and certain other foods by retarding enzymatic spoilage.[15] The FDA regulates food irradiation as an additive, even though it does not "add" anything to food. The process is accomplished by treating foods with ionizing radiation (gamma rays) from radioactive cobalt or cesium or from devices that generate electron beams (beta rays) or electrons. During the 1960s irradiation was approved for use on potatoes to control sprout growth and for insect disinfestation of wheat and wheat flour. Later it was approved for spices and dried herbs (1983), pork (1985), fresh fruits and dry vegetable substances (1986), and meat and poultry products (1990, 1995, 1999).

The American Council on Science and Health[16] believes that irradiation has great potential for use on meats, poultry, fish, fruits, and vegetables. It can kill *Salmonella* bacteria in poultry and trichinosis organisms in pork and can retard spoilage of fruits and vegetables. Extensive studies indicate that foods exposed to low doses of irradiation are safe to eat.[17] The foods do not become radioactive or undergo significant changes in nutrient composition. Some irradiated foods have better flavor and texture than their heat-treated counterparts because, unlike heating, irradiation does not cook the foods. Irradiation is also used to sterilize medical instruments and to prepare special foods for astronauts, military personnel, and cancer patients with impaired immunity. The labels of irradiated foods must carry the internationally used logo of the stylized rose with two petals (Figure 26-1).

Genetically engineered foods. The FDA's policy for genetically engineered foods covers all foods produced by any method of plant breeding.[18] Although GRAS substances are excluded from the requirement for premarket approval, new substances introduced via breeding must be approved as food additives. Genetically engineered food crops that do not contain substances significantly different from those already in the diet do not require approval as food additives, but

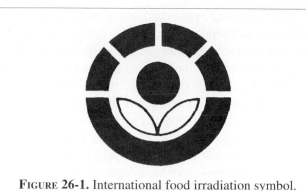

FIGURE 26-1. International food irradiation symbol.

they are required to undergo extensive testing for quality and safety.[19] About 30 companies are developing dozens of products, including tomatoes, melons, potatoes, celery, carrots, cucumbers, a low-cholesterol pig, and cholesterol-free canola oil. These products are also referred to as genetically modified organisms (GMOs).

The FDA has also approved the use of bovine somatotropin (BST), a genetically engineered animal growth hormone that increases milk production in cows. Genetically engineered BST, which supplements the cow's natural supply, does not alter the milk and presents no health risk to consumers.[20] Since there is no detectable difference in milk from treated and untreated cows, the FDA does not require that products from treated cows be labeled. The American Council on Science and Health[21] agrees that genetically engineered foods present no inherent health hazards and will bring substantial benefits to farmers, food processors, and consumers.

Food irradiation and genetic engineering have been unfairly attacked by the health-food industry, the "organic" food lobby, food faddists, and several "consumer" groups (see Figure 26-2). The Foundation

for Economic Trends, for example, which refers to genetically engineered foods as "Frankenfoods," erroneously claims that milk produced with BST will contain "artificial hormones" that "could be hazardous to our health and our children." Food & Water, whose followers bombard potential marketers with boycott threats, falsely asserts that irradiation and BST cause cancer.[22] A few restrictive state laws have been enacted, and boycott threats by radical consumer activists have made many manufacturers and retailers reluctant to market foods produced with these technologies.

Drug provisions for humans. The FD&C Act prohibits misbranding and adulteration of any drug. Drugs are categorized as new, investigational, prescription, or nonprescription:

NEW DRUGS are any drugs that (a) contain a newly developed chemical, (b) contain a chemical or substance not previously used in medicine, (c) have previously been used in medicine but not in the dosages or conditions for which the sponsor now recommends use, or (d) have not been recognized by experts as safe and effective for their intended use. It is illegal to introduce a new drug into interstate commerce without FDA approval. Approval is sought by filing a new drug application (NDA) containing acceptable scientific data that demonstrate safety and efficacy.

INVESTIGATIONAL NEW DRUGS are new drugs intended solely for research use by experts who are qualified by training and experience to investigate the drugs' safety and effectiveness. Their use is permitted under regulations established by the FDA.

PRESCRIPTION DRUGS may be dispensed only when prescribed by a licensed health professional.

NONPRESCRIPTION (OTC) DRUGS are those considered safe for consumer use when label directions and warnings are followed.

Imported drugs must comply with FDA provisions. New drugs approved in other countries must still undergo the FDA's NDA procedure here.

The labeling of a drug must include:

• The name and address of the manufacturer, packer, and shipper
• The strength and quantity
• The active ingredients
• An expiration date
• A warning if a habit-forming substance such as codeine is used
• The quantity of ingredients such as alcohol and ether
• If a prescription drug, a caution that the drug may be dispensed only by prescription
• The established name and trade name clearly identified
• Adequate directions for use, including conditions of use, dosage, frequency, and time of administration
• Adequate warnings, when necessary, to protect the user
• No false or misleading statement

TELL THE FDA
DON'T NUKE MY FRUIT

FIGURE 26-2. Bumper sticker and decal distributed by groups organizing unwarranted boycotts of irradiated and genetically engineered foods.

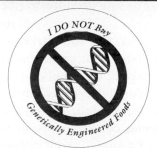

Other drug provisions of the FD&C Act include:

- Drugs must not consist of filthy, putrid, or decomposed substances.
- Drugs must not be dangerous to health when used as directed by the label.
- Nonofficial drugs (those not in any of the official compendia) are considered adulterated if their strength differs from or their purity or quality falls below that which they claim to possess.
- Manufacturers may not ship prescription drugs directly to the public. They may be sent only to firms that are regularly and lawfully engaged in the wholesale or retail distribution of prescription drugs or to hospitals, clinics, physicians, or others who are licensed to prescribe such drugs.
- The official drug compendia are *The United States Pharmacopeia* (USP) (which includes the *National Formulary* [NF]) and the *Homeopathic Pharmacopeia of the United States*. By law, all substances in these references must meet the standards of strength, quality, and purity they set forth.

Clinical testing of drugs. Before a new drug can be approved and marketed, the manufacturer must submit substantial evidence of safety and efficacy. Manufacturers generally must take the following steps:[23,24]

- The drug must be subjected to laboratory and animal tests, which must indicate that it can be safely tested in humans.
- Before the drug is given to people, the sponsor must submit a "Notice of Claimed Investigational Exemption for a New Drug," which is commonly referred to as an "IND." The application must describe the composition of the substance, the results of the animal studies, the design (protocol) of the proposed clinical trial, the measures that will protect the experimental subjects, and the training and experience of the investigators.
- Approved clinical investigations follow three phases: Phase I—About 50 people are exposed to the drug to determine the toxicity, metabolic absorption and elimination, and other pharmacologic reactions; the preferred route of administration; and the safe dosage. Phase II—Initial trials are conducted on a small number of people for treatment or prevention of the specific disease. Additional animal studies to indicate safety may be conducted concurrently. Phase III—Extensive clinical trials take place if Phases I and II demonstrate reasonable assurance of safety and effectiveness, suggesting that the drug's potential value outweighs its possible hazards.
- The manufacturer submits a new drug application (NDA) together with all the data collected plus a sample of the package insert and the proposed label.
- The FDA approves the NDA, asks for further evidence, or rejects the application.
- The FDA can withdraw approval of a drug found to produce unexpected side effects or to be less effective than anticipated.

The FDA drug approval process usually takes several years and has been criticized for delaying the speed with which beneficial new drugs can be marketed. On the other hand, some authorities have expressed concern that speeding up the process may weaken protection against unsafe and ineffective drugs. Sidney Wolfe, M.D., who has criticized the agency for occasional lapses, has stated that "the FDA does a better job of protecting the public from unsafe foods, drugs, medical devices, or other products that it regulates than any other such agency in the world."[25] In response to the AIDS crisis, the FDA has established regulations permitting promising investigational new drugs to be used outside of clinical trials to treat serious or life-threatening conditions when no satisfactory alternative is available.[26]

In 1972 the FDA began the enormous task of reviewing approximately 300,000 OTC products for safety and efficacy (see Chapter 19). Because the number of drugs was so large, the agency decided to investigate the ingredients according to categories rather than each product individually. Each group of drugs was investigated by an expert panel. As the panel reports were issued, many manufacturers reformulated their products by removing ingredients judged unsafe or ineffective and/or adding effective ones. Final rules have been issued for about 80% of the categories,[27,28] but most of the remaining OTC products are safe and effective for their intended purposes.

Device provisions. Before passage of the 1976 Medical Device Amendments, any device could be sold to the public provided it was properly labeled. If the device needed the supervision of a licensed practitioner, the label had to caution that use was restricted. A prescription device could be shipped to a licensed practitioner but not to the patient unless ordered by the practitioner. A device became illegal if it was dangerous to the health of consumers when used as prescribed or suggested on the label. Labels had to contain adequate directions and include warnings to ensure safe use. Despite these rules, many worthless, ineffective, or dangerous products were marketed.

The 1976 amendments enabled the FDA to require that existing devices be safe and effective and that new ones be safe and effective before marketing. The 1990 Safe Medical Devices Act strengthened the FDA's ability to monitor the marketplace, order recalls, and initiate large civil penalties for violations of the act (see Chapter 22 for details).

Cosmetic provisions. Cosmetic preparations distributed in the United States are required to comply with the cosmetic provisions of the FD&C Act and the Fair Packaging and Labeling Act. Cosmetics offered to prevent or cure ailments or to affect the structure and function of the body are subject to the Act's drug provisions. Such products include antibiotic deodorants; hormone creams; and products claimed to remove wrinkles, cure skin diseases, or treat or prevent dandruff. Products must not be injurious to the skin when used as directed on the label. Hair dye preparations that contain skin irritants are an exception. These may be marketed for use as hair dyes if the label bears this statement:

CAUTION: This product contains ingredients which may cause skin irritation on certain individuals, and a preliminary test according to accompanying directions should first be made. The product must not be used for the dyeing of eyelashes or eyebrows, which may cause blindness.

The labeling must contain adequate directions for making the preliminary test.

Color additives used in cosmetics must be approved as safe and certified by the FDA. No coal tar dye is certified for use around the eyes. Containers must not be composed of harmful substances. False and misleading statements are not permitted on labels.

Enforcement Actions

During an average year, FDA investigators inspect about 15,000 companies in the United States and a few hundred abroad. When a food, drug, device, or cosmetic product is defective or hazardous to human health or violates FDA regulations, the FDA can ask the manufacturer to correct the situation. Usually the request will lead to a voluntary recall or correction of faulty labeling. If a manufacturer does not comply, the FDA can seek a court order authorizing seizure of the product. A U.S. marshal will then be directed to take possession of the goods until the matter is resolved.

When products are marketed with improper claims, the FDA may issue a warning letter that specifies the law violations and demands to know how the problem will be corrected. If the letter is ignored or if the FDA decides to begin with more forceful action, the agency can initiate court proceedings for a seizure, injunction, or criminal prosecution. Many warning letters are posted on the FDA's Web site.

If a product is seized, it may be returned to its owner if its labeling can be corrected. If a product is basically unfit to market or if its owner does not contest the seizure, the court will order it destroyed. Injunctions are court orders that tell individuals or companies to discontinue illegal practices (such as marketing drugs that lack FDA approval as safe and effective). If an injunction is violated, the court has considerable discretion in determining the punishment and can order

imprisonment or a large fine. Recalls and seizures are listed in the agency's weekly *Enforcement Report*.

In criminal cases, first-time violators of the Food, Drug, and Cosmetic Act can be imprisoned up to 1 year and repeat offenders can be imprisoned for up to 3 years. The 1984 Criminal Fine Enhancement Act amended all federal criminal laws to allow fines of up to $100,000 (or $250,000 if death results) per offense for up to two offenses.

During fiscal year 1999 there were 1589 warning letters, 3736 product recalls, 25 seizures, 8 injunctions, 41,575 import detentions, and 373 criminal prosecutions.[29] The FDA does not routinely issue statistics indicating how many of its enforcement actions involve health fraud. Table 26-1 summarizes four cases in which FDA-initiated actions stopped products from being marketed with illegal therapeutic claims.

The FDA concentrates its efforts against health fraud on products that are inherently unsafe or are illegally marketed for the treatment of disease. Worthless yet harmless articles promoted to improve health, athletic ability, or appearance—which the agency considers mere "economic frauds"—are considered low priority and are virtually unregulated. Critics of this policy believe that routine use of criminal prosecution would

---

◆ Personal Glimpse ◆

E-mail Quackery Stopped

For several years a New-York-based company called Christian Brothers used unsolicited ("spam") messages to sell apricot seeds with claims that they will completely prevent cancer and can cause cancers to shrink and become harmless. Apricot seeds contain amygdalin, a cyanide-containing compound that has been promoted as a cancer remedy (Laetrile) for many years. (see Chapter 17).

Court documents indicate that the company unlawfully obtained e-mail addresses of America Online (AOL) members and used AOL's computer networks to send more than 20 million messages—at times sending hundreds of thousands of messages per hour. Messages were also distributed through other channels. The messages provided links to several Web sites containing testimonials. AOL sued the company and its president, Jason Vale, and in 1999, was awarded $651,685 award for damages and attorneys' fees. In November 2000, the Justice Department obtained a permanent injunction prohibiting Vale and Christian Brothers from making or distributing amygdalin, Laetrile, or apricot seeds.

Table 26-1

FDA Regulatory Actions

Seller	Product	Disposition
Naturally Good Marietta, Ga. (health-food store)	Gammahydroxybutyrate (GHB), a dangerous product promoted for strength training, muscle-building, weight loss, and sleep induction (see Chapter 1); also known as the "date-rape" drug	Following a criminal search and seizure, owner Joseph Saffar pleaded guilty to introducing a misbranded drug in interstate commerce. He was sentenced to 21 months in prison and fined $30,000.
CTR International New York	Herbal Melange Herbal Drink Formula, falsely claimed to "lower alcohol level," "reduce cholesterol," "create a non-proliferative environment for bacteria and parasites," and cleanse and purify the digestive system	Following receipt of a warning letter and a meeting with FDA officials, product labels and brochures were revised, with all medical and health claims deleted.
Potentials Unlimited Grand Rapids, Mich.	"Hypnotic sleep tapes" on 31 subjects, marketed with false and misleading claims for acne, allergies, bedwetting, facial tic, high blood pressure, tooth and gum problems, and many other ailments	Court ruled that the tapes were "devices" under the law because they were marketed with (illegal) therapeutic claims. The court ordered the tapes constructively destroyed by erasing their contents.
Enzymatic Therapy Green Bay, Wisc.	Raw Thyroid Complex and 55 other products marketed with unsubstantiated claims that they can "support" a large number of organs and bodily functions	A consent decree and permanent injunction prohibit the company from making unsubstantiated health claims for these or similar products.

enable the FDA to deter the marketing of bogus products. As noted by Barrett:

The Internal Revenue Service has made it clear that cheating on income tax can cost people dearly and land them in jail. The FDA should make it clear that cheating on product labels (as well as accompanying literature) can cost just as dearly.[30]

Educational Activities

The FDA distributes many publications about foods, drugs, devices, cosmetics, and hazardous substances. Also, public affairs officers are available to answer questions and to participate in educational programs at schools and elsewhere throughout their districts.[31] *FDA Consumer*, a monthly magazine, provides excellent educational articles and summaries of regulatory actions. "Talk Papers" and "Backgrounders" are available on many subjects. Most of this information is accessible on the agency's Web site at http://www.fda.gov. Details of specific enforcement actions may be obtained by writing to the FDA Freedom of Information Staff, HFI-35, 5600 Fishers Lane, Rockville, MD 20857. Requests should indicate why the information is needed and express willingness to pay a fee if the fee cannot be waived.

Fees are based on the time spent searching for the information and the number of pages copied.

During the mid-1980s the FDA gave high priority to public education about health fraud, which the agency defines as "the promotion, for profit, of a medical remedy known to be false or unproven." In 1984 the FDA and the Council of Better Business Bureaus asked the advertising managers of 19,500 newspapers, magazines, and radio and television stations to check advertising copy more carefully before accepting it for publication. Describing the common characteristics of misleading health ads, both agencies offered to evaluate questionable claims. Between 1985 and 1988 the FDA co-sponsored two national health-fraud conferences and many regional ones. Its current educational outreach is mainly through the Internet.

FEDERAL TRADE COMMISSION

The FTC is an independent federal agency directed by five commissioners nominated by the president and confirmed by the Senate, each serving a 7-year term. The president chooses one commissioner to act as chairman. The FTC's law enforcement work is divided among its Bureaus of Consumer protection, Competition, and Economics. The Bureau of Consumer Protection aims to keep the marketplace free from unfair, deceptive, or fraudulent practices. Its five divisions are credit practices, marketing practices, advertising practices, service industry practices, and enforcement. The Bureau of Competition is the FTC's antitrust arm and seeks to prevent business practices that restrain competition. The Bureau of Economics provides economic analysis and support to the FTC's consumer protection activities.

The FTC's activities are reported in the weekly *FTC News Notes* and an annual report, both of which are available free of charge to interested parties. Annual (fiscal year) reports, news releases, consent agreements, policy statements, consumer advisories, and many other important documents are posted to the agency's Web site (http://www.ftc.gov).

FTC Laws

The *Federal Trade Commission Act* (1914) provides safeguards against business monopoly and makes unfair practices unlawful, thereby protecting consumers as well as other entrepreneurs.

The *Wheeler-Lea Amendment* (1938) enables the FTC to regulate advertising. It states:

It shall be unlawful for any person, partnership, or corporation to disseminate, or cause to be disseminated, any false advertisements—by the United States mails, or in commerce by any means, for the purpose of inducing . . . the purchase of food, drugs, devices, or cosmetics . . . the dissemination . . . of any false advertisement . . . shall be an unfair or deceptive act or practice in commerce.

The *Fair Packaging and Labeling Act* (1966) bans unfair and deceptive packaging and labeling of consumer commodities. It gives the FTC responsibility in all areas except food, drugs, devices, and cosmetics, which are the purview of the FDA.

The *Magnuson-Moss Act* (1975) enables the FTC to adopt trade regulation rules that define unfair or deceptive acts in a particular industry and make it much simpler to stop them.

Enforcement Actions

When the Commission feels that a company is making a false or deceptive advertising claim, it may seek to stop the advertisement or require some other appropriate remedy.[32] FTC actions can be triggered by letters from consumers, businesses, members of Congress, or other interested parties. However, the agency will not usually act unless the matter involves interstate commerce and is believed to involve a significant problem such as a safety hazard or substantial economic harm to the public.

The first step is an investigation. If the FTC concludes that the law has been violated, it may attempt to obtain voluntary compliance by entering into a consent order with the violator. Signers of a consent order need not admit that they have violated the law, but they must agree to stop the practices described in an accompanying complaint. If a consent agreement cannot be reached, the FTC may issue an administrative complaint that leads to an adjudication by an FTC Administrative Law Judge. If a problem is considered serious enough, the FTC can seek a federal court order (injunction) to stop the improper practices. In egregious fraud cases, it can ask the Justice Department to file a criminal action.

When the administrative complaint is disputed, an administrative law judge holds a formal hearing similar to a court trial. Evidence is submitted, testimony is heard, and witnesses are examined and cross-examined. If the judge finds the law has been violated, a cease-and-desist order or other appropriate relief can be issued. Initial decisions by administrative law judges can be appealed to the full Commission, which acts like a court of appeal. Respondents who are dissatisfied with the Commission's decision can appeal their case to the U.S. Court of Appeals and ultimately to the U.S. Supreme Court. The FTC staff may not appeal the Commission's decision.

If a consent agreement is reached or the FTC's complaint is upheld on appeal, a financial penalty may be assessed that can include making restitution available to consumers or donating money for research. Occasionally a company must do "corrective advertising," in which future ads must indicate that previous ads had been false, inaccurate, or misleading. Future violations of consent agreements or cease-and-desist orders can result in fines of up to $11,000 per day for each violation.

Companies going through the administrative or court procedures just described can usually continue the disputed practice(s) if they choose to do so. When the FTC believes that an unfair practice will cause great public harm if allowed to continue, it may ask a federal court to issue an injunction. If a permanent injunction is issued, it may include financial penalties and consumer redress.

When the FTC believes that a problem affects an entire industry, it can promulgate an industry guide or trade regulation rule. Guides are interpretive statements without the force of law. Rules represent the conclusions of the Commission about what it considers unlawful. Before guides and rules are established, interested parties are given the opportunity to comment. Once a rule is established, the Commission can take enforcement action without lengthy explanations about why a particular ad is unfair or deceptive. A reference to the rule is enough. In health matters, problems are almost always handled on a case-by-case basis rather than through rulemaking.

Although FTC actions are powerful, the agency's ability to protect consumers is limited by two factors. The agency does not have sufficient resources to investigate most of the complaints it receives. Its regulatory actions can take years to complete, particularly when contested. Months or even years may go by before an investigation begins or is completed. Unless a consent agreement or injunction is obtained, further delays can occur with each step in the process. This enables some operators to make considerable profits before their improprieties are stopped. Perhaps the most famous case of this type was the FTC's action to remove the word "liver" from *Carter's Little Liver Pills*. Although the pills did nothing for the liver, it took the agency 16 years (1943–1959) to win the case. In another prominent case, the FTC began investigating the J.B. Williams Company's *Geritol* ads in 1959, but the final settlement (a $302,000 fine) did not occur until 1976.

During the 1980s the FTC completed prosecution of about five cases per year involving health-related claims. During the past few years the average has been about 30. The following cases are typical.

In 1985 Joseph Weider and Weider Fitness, Inc., agreed to pay a minimum of $400,000 to settle FTC charges that they had misrepresented two mineral supplements, *Anabolic Mega-Pak* and *Dynamic Life Essence*. Weider and the company agreed not to falsely claim that these products could help build muscles or were effective substitutes for anabolic steroids. They also agreed to make refunds to anyone who had purchased these products and, if the amount refunded was less than $400,000, to donate the difference to fund research on the relationship of nutrition to muscle development. In 2000, Weider Nutritional International agreed to a similar penalty in settling an FTC complaint involving false claims made for two herbal weight-loss products, *PhenCal* and *PhenCal 106*, which it had falsely claimed were as effective as prescription drugs.

In 1986 Meadow Fresh Farms and its president, Roy Brog, agreed to stop claiming that their milk-based dairy substitute could reduce the incidence of cardiovascular disease because it contained less xanthine oxidase (a milk enzyme) than does homogenized milk.

In 1986, after being charged with false advertising, A.H. Robins Company agreed to stop claiming that *Viobin Wheat Germ Oil* could help consumers improve endurance, stamina, vigor, or other aspects of athletic fitness.

In 1987 Phillipe LaFrance USA, Ltd., agreed to pay $600,000 in civil penalties and to make no false claims in the future. The FTC had charged the company with falsely claiming that its "sex nutrient pills" could improve the sexual performance of otherwise healthy men low in "the sex nutrient."

In 1990 Nature's Way and its president, Kenneth Murdock, agreed to stop making unsubstantiated claims that *Cantrol* is helpful against yeast infections caused by *Candida albicans*. The product, which contained acidophilus, evening primrose oil, vitamin E, linseed oil, caprylic acid, pau d'arco, and several other substances, had been promoted with a list of "yes/no" questions asking whether the reader had common symptoms that the manufacturer claimed were associated with yeast problems. The FTC charged that this "self-test" was not valid. The company also agreed to pay $30,000 to the National Institutes of Health to support research on yeast infections.

In 1994 L&S Research and its founder and its chief executive officer agreed to pay $1.45 million to settle charges that they had made numerous false and unsubstantiated claims in the advertising and sale of *Cybergenics Total Body Building System, Cybergenics for Hard Gainers, Cybertrim, Quicktrim,* and *Mega-Fat Burner Tablet* (also called *Super Fat-Loss Tablet*). The FTC had also charged that "before-and-after" photos used in the ads were deceptive because they did not reflect the typical or usual experience of users. The consent agreement prohibits claims that these or similar products can cause a user to gain more muscle or lose more fat than a nonuser of such a product, unless there is reliable scientific evidence to support such an assertion. The agreement also bans unsubstantiated claims that the inclusion of chromium picolinate in a product or program will cause a user to build muscle, lose weight, or lower blood cholesterol.

In 1995 Home Shopping Network and its subsidiaries, Home Shopping Club and HSN Lifeway Health Products, were charged with making unsubstantiated claims that (a) the vitamins in three of its spray products were more fully absorbable than vitamins in pill form, (b) its vitamin C and zinc spray could prevent common colds and heal cold sores, (c) its vitamin B_{12} spray could treat hangover symptoms and increase energy, (d) its antioxidant spray would ensure proper function of the immune system and reduce the risk of contracting infectious diseases, and (e) its *Smokeless Nutrient Spray* would enable users to stop smoking easily. The case was settled with a consent agreement forbidding the challenged claims. In 1999 the company agreed to pay a $1.1 million penalty for making unsubstantiated advertisements for several skin care, weight-loss, and PMS/menopause products in violation of the previous consent agreement.

In 1996 Dr. Atida H. Karr agreed to pay $200,000 to settle charges that she had made unsubstantiated advertising claims that *Acne-Statin* was superior to other acne treatments. The claims also violated a 1979 order prohibiting Karr from making unsubstantiated claims about the effectiveness or superiority of any acne preparation she markets. Infomercials by Karr included endorsements from people who said that the product was effective in treating their severe or cystic acne. An FTC official stated that patients with acne that severe would risk severe facial scarring if they delayed seeking more appropriate treatment. The 1979 settlement had included payment of $175,000 into a consumer refund account.

In 1997, Gerber Products Company settled allegations that the company made false and unsubstantiated "doctor recommended" claims for Gerber baby food. The order bars the company from misinterpreting the results or existence of any survey, test, or research.

In 2000, R-Garden Internationale and its president Donald L. Smyth agreed to pay $375,000 and to stop marketing "Vitamin O" or any other "stabilized" or "aerobic" oxygen product with claims that they can cure disease by increasing oxygen delivery to the cells.

Internet Activities
The FTC has a very agresssive program aimed at frauds promoted through the Internet. Since 1996, it has conducted nine "Surf Days" aimed at providing information to entrepreneurs who may be violating the law. For the first, staff attorneys and investigators were joined by scores of others from federal, state, and local agencies. Over a 3-hour period, this ad hoc task force located over 500 Web sites or newsgroup messages promoting apparent pyramid schemes. The FTC staff e-mailed a warning message to the individuals or companies that had posted these solicitations, explaining that pyramid schemes violate federal and state law and providing a link back to the FTC Web site for more information. A month later, the investigative staff checked and found that a substantial number had disappeared or been improved.

In 1997, the FTC conducted North American Health Claim Surf Day with help from other federal agencies;

18 state attorneys general; and many nonprofit health organizations and consumer protection and information agencies from the United States, Canada, and Mexico. The participants surfed the Internet for questionable claims related to preventing or treating heart disease, cancer, AIDS, diabetes, arthritis, and multiple sclerosis, and sent hundreds of e-mail warnings that claims require adequate substantiation. In November 1998, the process was repeated by an international coalition of 80 government and private agencies and organizations from 25 countries whose participants issued more than 1200 warnings.

Another FTC Internet activity has been the posting of "teaser sites" that mimic pyramid schemes, scholarship scams, false weight-loss claims, and fraudulent vending opportunities—typical frauds that have been practiced on consumers through direct mail, telemarketing, and other means. The teaser sites are registered with major search engines so that they may be encountered by consumers about to become ensnared by plausible but untrue come-ons. Instead of being swindled, the visitors are warned about the deceptive nature of the scams.

U.S. POSTAL SERVICE

The Postal Service has jurisdiction when money is sent through the mail for products or services. Postal inspectors look for misleading advertisements in magazines and newspapers and on radio and television. They also receive complaints from the public and from other government agencies. Postal inspection offices exist in many cities, with about 500 inspectors available to investigate all types of mail frauds. Attorneys in the civil practice section of the agency's law department and postal inspectors with law degrees are available to prosecute cases. The case selection process is decentralized, so that different types of cases are emphasized in different regions of the country.

Postal Laws
Title 39, Section 3005, of the United States Code can be used to block promoters of misleading schemes from receiving money through the mail. If sufficient health hazard or economic detriment exists, an immediate court order to impound mail may be sought under Section 3007 of the code. However, the Postal Service cannot proceed unless the Justice Department approves such action or takes the case itself.

Title 18, Section 1341, provides for criminal prosecution but requires proof of intent to deceive. The maximum penalties are 5 years in prison and a fine for each instance proved. The 1984 Criminal Fine Enhancement Act allows fines of up to $100,000 (or $250,000 if death results) per offense for up to two offenses. However, criminal prosecution is rarely used in cases involving mail-order health products because (a) administrative procedures are simpler and quicker and (b) intent to deceive is difficult to prove when a perpetrator pretends to believe that the product works. The Postal Service does not have jurisdiction when companies take credit card orders by telephone and deliver through private carriers such as United Parcel Service. However, the Justice Department may seek such an injunction under Section 1345, which allows federal district courts to enjoin acts of mail and wire fraud.

When a mail fraud is detected, postal attorneys can file a complaint or seek an agreement with the perpetrator. When a complaint is contested, a hearing is held by an administrative law judge assigned to the Postal Service. If the evidence is sufficient, this judge will recommend that the Postal Service issue a False Representation Order (FRO) blocking money sent through the mail in response to the misleading ads. Although the order can be appealed to the courts, very few companies do this. Each voluntary agreement and FRO is accompanied by a cease-and-desist order that forbids both the challenged acts and similar acts. Under the Mail Order Consumer Protection Amendments of 1983, if this order is violated, the agency can seek a civil penalty in federal court of up to $11,000 per day for each violation. During the past few years, the agency has done very little about misleading ads for mail-order health products. Cases from previous years are archived on its Web site.

In most cases in which health-related products are falsely advertised, the FDA and FTC also have jurisdiction. The FDA can regulate any product intended for use in the cure, mitigation, treatment, or prevention of any ailment, and the FTC has jurisdiction over advertising of all health-related products except prescription drugs. However, the FDA rarely becomes involved with mail-order sales, and the FTC handles relatively few such cases.

Enforcement Actions

Most mail-order health schemes attempt to exploit people's fear of being unattractive. Their promoters are usually "hit-and-run" artists who hope to make a profit before the Postal Service stops their false ads.[33] Common products include "miracle" weight-loss plans, fitness and bodybuilding products, "spot-reducing" devices (claimed to reduce specific parts of the body), antiaging products, and alleged sex aids.[3]

Before the 1983 law was implemented, many unscrupulous mail-order promoters considered legal defense costs and occasional fines as a normal part of their operating overhead. If prosecuted, they would remain in business by changing the wording of an ad, the name of the product, or their company name. The penalty provision of the 1983 law appears to have decreased the number of schemes for mail-order health products. However, in the early 1990s, postal authorities stopped enforcing the law in this area, so the problem has been getting worse. Some examples of previous actions by the U.S. Postal Service follow.

In 1983 Jacob W. Kulp, D.C., a chiropractor from Cheektowaga, New York, entered a plea bargain in which he pleaded guilty to violating a federal food and drug law, and the Postal Service agreed not to prosecute him for mailing out a worthless "nutrient deficiency test." To gather evidence, postal inspectors used an undercover "patient" who took the test and was advised to use wheat fiber tablets to cure "black intestinal plaque."[34]

During 1985 the president of Encore House, Inc., and its advertising director pleaded guilty to criminal mail fraud and received prison sentences for falsely promoting a device called *Figure-Tron II*. Ads for the device had claimed that "tiny micro-electro impulses tone your muscles 500 times a minute," providing the exercise benefit of "3000 sit-ups without moving an inch" or "10 miles of jogging while lying flat on your back." The company also signed a consent agreement with the Postal Service and FTC in which it was assessed $100,000 and a $250,000 restitution fund was set up.[35]

In 1990 postal officials filed a false representation complaint against Nature's Bounty, Inc., of Bohemia, New York (doing business as Puritan's Pride). The complaint charged that at least 19 of the company's nutritional products were falsely advertised in Puritan Pride mail-order catalogs. The products include *Cholesto-Flush, Fatbuster Diet Tea, Kidney Flush, Memory Booster, Prostex*, and *Stress B*. The case was settled with a consent agreement under which the company admitted no wrongdoing but agreed to stop making the challenged claims.

In 1991 postal officials took action against the marketers of *Oncor,* a homeopathic product claimed to alleviate impotence and increase sexual desire in men. An Administrative Law Judge concluded that the product was neither safe nor effective and that the television infomercial used to promote it had been falsely represented as an independent talk show.

In 1993 postal officials charged two men with fraud in connection with the sale of pills guaranteed to cure male impotence. The scheme, which involved several company and product names, generated close to $2 million in sales over a 2-year period. Some victims purchased products from more than one company. In 1995 the perpetrators pleaded guilty and received prison sentences. One agreed to forfeit assets valued at $675,000, while the other agreed to pay $1.6 million in restitution to 25,000 victims who had purchased the pills.[36]

OTHER FEDERAL AGENCIES

The Consumer Information Center stocks and distributes many consumer publications, some available free and some for a modest fee. Its catalog includes many publications on health and nutrition topics.

The Consumer Product Safety Commission (CPSC) distributes information, receives complaints about the safety of products, and can set voluntary guidelines.

The Environmental Protection Agency, among its many duties, sets standards for water quality and pesticide tolerances for foods (which the FDA enforces).

The Federal Bureau of Investigation (FBI) has more than 100 special agents investigating health fraud. Most are cases in which Medicare or private insurance companies have been defrauded.

The Health Care Financing Administration (HCFA) administers Medicare and Medicaid programs, maintains statistics on health-care costs, and oversees federal quality control programs related to health care. Its quarterly journal, *Health Care Financing Review*, reports on the economics of health care.

The National Health Service Corps recruits and places health-care professionals in medically underserved communities.

The National Institutes of Health (NIH) is the federal government's primary agency for supporting and conducting biomedical research and training. Its 306-acre campus in Bethesda, Maryland, houses 14 institutes and a 500-bed hospital. NIH also holds conferences and distributes publications on health matters. The NIH Center for Alternative and Complementary Medicine, which has not been a trustworthy source of information, is discussed in Chapter 8.

The National Health Information Center (NHIC) was established in 1979 as a service of the Office of Disease Prevention and Health promotion of the U.S. Public Health Service. NHIC operates a toll-free hotline through which it refers callers to more than 1000 organizations that can provide health-related information. It also issues reports about information resources. Although NHIC's leads usually are reliable, it may refer people who inquire about nonscientific methods to organizations that espouse them.

The Office of the Inspector General (OIG) of the U.S. Department of Health and Human Services was created in 1976 to help detect and prevent waste, fraud, and abuse. OIG conducts many audits, investigations, and inspections; issues reports; and maintains a hotline for reporting frauds involving Medicare and other government programs. Its activities are summarized each January and July in its *Semiannnual Report*. The most common frauds it investigates involve false claims filed under the Medicare and Medicaid programs.

The U.S. Centers for Disease Control and Prevention (CDC) studies environmental health problems and administers national programs for disease prevention. Its many activities include tracing the source of epidemics, monitoring reportable diseases, and publishing the *Morbidity and Mortality Weekly Report (MMWR)*.

The U.S. Department of Agriculture supports and conducts nutrition research and enforces standards for meat and poultry products. It also publishes periodicals and other reports on nutrition research, food safety, and the food marketplace.

STATE AND LOCAL AGENCIES

State and local agencies that offer information or other help to consumers include health departments, professional licensing boards, consumer protection bureaus, attorneys general, and agriculture departments. Hundreds of counties and cities have offices that deal with consumer affairs, including health matters. Consumers should investigate the resources in their area if they have problems involving health products or services. The *Consumer Protection Report*, published 10 times a year by the National Association of Attorneys General (NAAG), summarizes enforcement actions by state and federal agencies.

During recent years the FTC and state agencies have taken hundreds of joint enforcement actions, most of them against telemarketers.[37] At a 1996 NAAG conference, FTC Chairman Robert Pitofsky noted that cooperation between federal and state consumer protection agencies had never been better, but that all of them were awash in a "sea of fraud."

NONGOVERNMENTAL ORGANIZATIONS

Hundreds of organizations play a role in helping to educate and protect consumers in health matters. These organizations can be broadly classified as voluntary, business, or professional. Their activities include research, publications, advice to consumers, media contacts, testimony to government agencies, lawsuits, and promotion of legislation.

Voluntary Organizations

Voluntary organizations generally are nonprofit corporations formed to assist the public in various ways. Some are supported primarily by dues from their members, some primarily by contributions, and some by both. Consumer groups may address a broad range of consumer issues or focus on limited areas, such as health or health fraud. Many voluntary organizations support research and provide consumer education about a specific disease or diseases. The American Cancer Society and the American Heart Association are two of the most prominent groups of this type. Other organizations, designated "self-help groups," provide information and emotional support for individuals and families affected by particular diseases.

Some voluntary organizations that have had significant impact on the consumer movement in the United States are described below.

Consumers Union (CU), founded in 1936, evaluates products and produces *Consumer Reports, Consumer Reports on Health*, and many books, pamphlets, films, newspaper columns, radio and television programs, and teaching aids. *Consumer Reports* usually covers one or two health topics per month. CU's Washington office monitors government activities and represents consumers through lawsuits and testimony before regulatory agencies.

Consumer Federation of America, founded in 1967, is supported by dues and contributions from about 240 member organizations. It addresses a wide range of issues, most of them economic, and presents its views to Congress and various government agencies. It also publishes a bimonthly newsletter, compiles voting records of congressional representatives on consumer issues, and sponsors an annual assembly on important issues. Its member organizations pay dues and are accorded votes according to the size of their membership; the largest member is Consumers Union.

The National Consumers League, founded in 1899, has a scope of political activity similar to that of Consumer Federation of America. In addition, it develops research and shoppers' guides and helps to resolve grievances. In recent years it has played an important role in combating telemarketing fraud.

The Public Citizen Health Research Group (HRG), founded in 1971 by Ralph Nader and Sidney Wolfe, M.D., is now directed by Dr. Wolfe and staffed by health professionals, attorneys, and researchers. They publish a monthly newsletter; monitor government health agencies; analyze proposed legislation; and take vigorous action—including lawsuits—when they believe that the government is lax in protecting consumers from dangerous foods, drugs, or medical practices. In 1987, for example, HRG forced the FDA to ban interstate sale of unpasteurized milk. HRG also investigates and issues reports on economic and quality-of-care issues. The reports have covered medical fees, hospital evaluation, unnecessary surgery, mental health care, vision care, medical discipline, and many other topics.

The Center for Science in the Public Interest (CSPI) was founded in 1971 by former associates of Ralph Nader and reportedly has 1 million members. It publishes the monthly *Nutrition Action Healthletter*, as well as booklets, posters, computer software, and other materials, most of which concern foods and food choices. It also engages in lawsuits and political activities intended to foster what it believes are better policies toward health and environmental issues by government and industry. CSPI has stimulated many significant government actions to protect consumers. But it also promotes "organic" foods, suggests that everyone should take vitamin supplements, and evinces an alarmist attitude toward the American diet and food supply.

The American Association of Retired Persons (AARP), founded in 1958, provides its 33 million members with guidance on a wide variety of economic and health issues. It publishes the magazine *Modern Maturity* as well as many pamphlets and books. AARP's mail-order pharmacy fills prescriptions and sells many nonprescription products at discount prices. AARP members can participate in social, recreational, educational, and political activities through thousands of local chapters, many of which hold monthly meetings. AARP's health-related publications are usually excellent.

The National Council Against Health Fraud (NCAHF) began in 1977 as the Southern California Council Against Health Fraud, and became national in 1984 see Figure 26-3). It has about 900 members nationwide and chapters in 13 states. Its activities include a bimonthly print newsletter, a weekly electronic newsletter, a media clearinghouse, consumer complaint referral services, legislative action, research on unproven methods of health care, and seminars for professionals and the general public. The Council also appoints task forces to conduct extensive investigations and issue position papers. Its Task Force on Victim Redress helps victims of quackery who want to file suit. Other task forces are concerned with acupuncture, chiropractic, diet and behavior, dubious health-care credentials, broadcast media abuse, dubious credentials, dubious dental

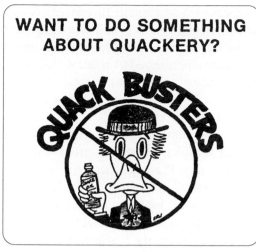

WANT TO DO SOMETHING ABOUT QUACKERY?

FIGURE 26–3. Logo of the National Council Against Health Fraud.

practices, vitamin abuse, ergogenic aids, herbs, questionable addiction treatments, medical neglect of children, cancer quackery, and the quality of information in health periodicals.

Quackwatch is a nonprofit corporation whose purpose is to combat health-related frauds, myths, fads, and fallacies. Its primary focus is on quackery-related information that is difficult or impossible to get elsewhere. Founded by Dr. Stephen Barrett in 1969 as the Lehigh Valley Committee Against Health Fraud, it was incorporated in 1970 and assumed its current name in 1997. Its activities include (a) investigating questionable health claims, (b) distributing reliable publications, (c) reporting illegal marketing, (d) generating consumer-protection lawsuits, (e) attacking misleading advertising, and (f) improving the quality of health information on the Internet. Quackwatch and NCAHF cosponsor *Consumer Health Digest*, a free weekly e-mail newsletter that Barrett edits.

The American Council on Science and Health (ACSH) was founded in 1978 to evaluate issues involving food, drugs, chemicals, the environment, lifestyle, and health. ACSH has more than 300 prominent scientific and policy advisers. It produces peer-reviewed reports, and a quarterly magazine, *Priorities for Health*. It also hosts seminars and press conferences and serves as a clearinghouse for the news media and answers individual inquiries from the public.

The Committee for the Scientific Investigation of Claims of the Paranormal (CSICOP) was founded in 1976 to encourage critical investigation of paranormal and fringe-science claims. It is composed of prominent scientists, educators, and journalists and is assisted by more than 50 scientific and technical consultants. It publishes a bimonthly journal, *Skeptical Inquirer*, and

maintains subcommittees on astrology, education, paranormal health claims, parapsychology, and UFOs. Groups similar to CSICOP exist in many areas of the United States and in several foreign countries.

The Skeptics Society was founded in 1992 to promote science and critical thinking and to disseminate information on pseudoscience, pseudohistory, and fringe claims and groups. It sponsors lectures and telecasts, publishes a quarterly magazine (*Skeptic*), and distributes other educational materials.

Business Organizations

Many business organizations provide information and educational materials to consumers. The Health Insurance Association of America, for example, provides reliable information about the insurance marketplace, and

---

☑ **Consumer Tip**

The Intelligent Health Consumer

- Identifies and uses reliable sources of information. Chapters 2, 9, 16, and 17 and the Appendix list sources that the authors of this textbook consider reliable.
- Is skeptical and investigates the accuracy of health advertising before making purchasing decisions.
- Maintains a healthy lifestyle.
- Understands which types of health problems can be self-treated and which should receive professional care.
- Takes an active role in dealing with health professionals; is assertive but tactful; endeavors to learn the nature of any ailment and the mechanism and potential hazards of treatment; is aware of fees involved.
- Locates and uses a primary physician (or medical group) who provides scientific, considerate, and compassionate care.
- Uses medication properly; carefully reads labels and follows directions for safe use; is aware of common side effects; requests generic drugs when appropriate.
- Is aware of the signs of quackery and health fraud; avoids unsubstantiated products and procedures and any practitioners who recommend them.
- Is familiar with the laws, regulations, and rights that protect consumers.
- Supports, participates in, and seeks help when needed from appropriate consumer organizations.
- Writes letters, makes phone calls, and takes other appropriate action to protest deceptive or fraudulent health practices.

the National Dairy Council provides reliable information about food and nutrition.

The Council of Better Business Bureaus is unique among business groups because it also takes an advocacy role in encouraging truth in advertising and other good business practices through industrial self-regulation. It has published a code for advertising and selling as well as pamphlets to help consumers make wise purchasing decisions.

The Council's National Advertising Division (NAD) receives and adjudicates complaints about nationally circulated advertising and has persuaded a few manufacturers to withdraw health-related ads that have been challenged. However, NAD has exhibited little interest in adjudicating complaints related to vitamin supplements and has even endorsed a fraudulent ad for "nutrition insurance" (see Chapter 4). Local Better Business

Bureau offices can sometimes help consumers with complaints about health products and services provided by local businesses; however, problems with licensed practitioners usually are referred to medical societies or state licensing boards.

Professional Organizations

Health professionals can join a multitude of local, state, and national groups interested in promoting their profession or specialty. The largest such group is the American Medical Association, which evaluates information, publishes books and journals, conducts seminars, engages in lawsuits and legislative activity, offers information to the public and the media, and engages in many other activities. The publications of recognized professional groups are generally reliable and well written; many such groups are listed in the Appendix.

Table 26-2

WHERE TO COMPLAIN OR SEEK HELP*

Problem	Agencies to Contact
False advertising	FTC Bureau of Consumer Protection or regional office National Advertising Division, Council of Better Business Bureaus Editor or manager of media outlet where ad appeared
Product marketed with false or misleading claims	National or regional FDA office State attorney general State health department Local Better Business Bureau Congressional representatives
Bogus mail-order promotion	Chief Postal Inspector, U.S. Postal Service Regional Postal Inspector State attorney general
Dubious telemarketing	State attorney general FTC Bureau of Consumer Protection or regional office National Fraud Information Center hotline
Improper treatment by licensed practitioner	Local or state professional society (if practitioner is a member) Local hospital (if practitioner is a staff member) State professional licensing board National Council Against Health Fraud Task Force on Victim Redress
Improper treatment by unlicensed individual	Local district attorney State attorney general National Council Against Health Fraud Task Force on Victim Redress
Advice needed about questionable product or service	National Council Against Health Fraud Local, state, or national professional or voluntary health groups
Medicare or Medicaid fraud	FBI and HHS Office of the Inspector General hotlines
Junk e-mail, including health-related scams and chain letters	FTC's e-mailbox (uce@ftc.gov)

*See http://www.chsourcebook.com for contact information. When more than one regulatory agency appears to have jurisdiction, contact each of them.
© 2001, Stephen Barrett, M.D.

Consumer Tip

Consumer Protection Insight

The key points of consumer-protection law are: (a) disclosure of ingredients; (b) complete instructions for use, including warnings about potential adverse effects; (c) premarketing proof of safety; (d) a duty to track products to discover any unanticipated adverse effects; (e) premarket proof that a product is effective for its intended purpose; and (f) truthfulness in advertising.

Although some people clamor for "health freedom" (the ability to market whatever they please without government regulation), they cannot demonstrate how any of the above requirements can be set aside without hampering the ability of consumers to make informed decisions. Even though these basic principles are straightforward, it took a great deal of sad experience and political struggle to enact them into law.

CONSUMER ACTION

For society to improve, people must speak out loudly and clearly when they have been misled. Individual consumers as well as agencies and organizations must assume responsibility in this regard. Individuals often feel helpless when cheated, but they must fight back by registering complaints. The system will not change unless people want it to be modified and are willing to take action on their own behalf.

If you encounter a food, drug, device, cosmetic, or other health-related product that appears to be mislabeled or otherwise defective, you can perform a public service by reporting it to the FDA. If you encounter false advertising, you can perform a similar service by reporting it to the FTC or to your state attorney general. When sale through the mail is involved, contact the Postal Service. When services rather than products are involved, a state or local agency is likely to be most helpful.

Table 26-2 summarizes where consumer complaints can be sent. Complaints to federal agencies may receive extra attention when a member of Congress is involved, so it is often a good idea to send a copy of your complaint to your congressional representatives. Where more than one enforcement agency appears to have jurisdiction, it is best to contact all of them.

To make a complaint, record what you have observed and what you think is wrong, and send or deliver this information to the appropriate agency along with any evidence you have collected. If your complaint involves a food or drug, enclose the label or a complete description of the label (including code marks) and indicate where you obtained the product. If your complaint involves a product you have used, check first to be sure you followed the directions. If you have what appears to be an adverse effect to a medication, the problem is most likely an allergy or a side effect known to the FDA rather than poor quality of the medication. Your doctor can be consulted to find this out. If you complain about an advertisement, indicate when and where you observed it.

Information supplied by consumers often leads to detection and correction of a problem. Many people are afraid that making a complaint will subject them to legal action or involve them in a time-consuming process. This is unlikely, however. Complaints made in good faith are privileged—which means the complainant is shielded from liability. Nor is a complainant likely to be needed as a witness in a court proceeding. Regulatory agencies almost always conduct their own investigations and proceed on the evidence gathered by their trained investigators.

SUMMARY

Consumer protection in health matters has two components: education and law enforcement. Intelligent consumers accept personal and public responsibility for the protection of health. They actively pursue the information needed to make wise decisions about health products and services. They are willing to speak out and encourage social and governmental action against misrepresentations and fraudulent practices. Government agencies, in turn, must establish and enforce standards for professional competence and honest marketing of products and services.

REFERENCES

1. Young FE. FDA. The cop on the consumer beat. FDA Consumer 22(3):6–7, 1988.
2. The Food and Drug Administration: Overview. FDA Publication BG99-2, Jan 11, 1999.
3. Young JH. The Toadstool Millionaires: A Social History of Patent Medicines Before Federal Regulation. Princeton, N.J., 1961, Princeton University Press.
4. Reed LW. On Upton Sinclair's *The Jungle:* How a food safety myth became a legend. Consumers' Research 78(8):23–25, 35, 1995.
5. Young JH. The Medical Messiahs. Princeton, N.J., 1992, Princeton University Press.
6. Delusions of vigor: Better health by mail. Consumer Reports 44:50–54, 1979.

7. Henkel J. Orphan products: New hope for people with rare disorders. FDA Consumer 28(5):17–20, 1994.

8. Barrett S. How the Dietary Supplement Health Education Act of 1994 weakened the FDA. Quackwatch Web site, 2000.

9. Food and Drug Administration. Regulations on statements made for dietary supplements concerning the effect of the product on the structure or function of the body; final rule. Federal Register 65:999–1050, 2000.

10. Federal Food, Drug, and Cosmetic Act, As Amended, and Related Laws. Washington, D.C., 1989, U.S. Government Printing Office publication no. 017–012–00347–8. (Obtainable for $7.50 from the Superintendent of Documents, U.S. Government Printing Office, Washington, DC 20402.)

11. Holt T and others. Modernize our food safety laws: Delete the Delaney clause. New York, 1995, American Council on Science and Health.

12. Jukes TH. The Delaney clause: A 1990 appraisal. Priorities, Winter 1991, pp 23–24.

13. Francis FJ. Food safety: Interpretation of risk. Ames, Iowa, 1992, Council for Agricultural Science and Technology.

14. Noah T, Kilman S. New pesticide bill is expected to make foods safer by dumping outdated laws. Wall Street Journal, July 25, 1996.

15. Olson DG. Scientific status summary: Irradiation of food. Chicago, 1998, Institute of Food Technologists.

16. Greenberg RA. Irradiated foods. New York, 1996, American Council on Science and Health.

17. Blumenthal B. Food irradiation toxic to bacteria, safe for humans. FDA Consumer 24(9):11–14, 1990.

18. Maryanski J (interview). Genetically engineered foods: Fears and facts. FDA Consumer 27(1):11–14, 1993.

19. Kessler DA and others. The safety of foods developed by biotechnology. Science 26:1747–1751, 1992.

20. Use of Bovine Somatotropin (BST) in the United States: Its Potential Effects. Washington, D.C., 1994, Executive Branch of the U.S. Government.

21. Huttner SL and others. Biotechnology and Food. New York, 1996, American Council on Science and Health.

22. Katzenstein L. Milking fear to scare up money. Cabot, Vt., 1995, Cabot Creamery.

23. From test tube to patient: New drug development in the United States. HHS publication no. (FDA) 88–3168, Rockville, Md., 1988, U.S. Food and Drug Administration.

24. Basara LR, Montagne M. Searching for Magic Bullets: Orphan Drugs, Consumer Activism, and Pharmaceutical Development. Binghamton, N.Y., 1994, Haworth Press.

25. Clear thinking about regulating medicines: Tidal wave of unfounded attacks on Food and Drug Administration calls for a dispassionate look at agency's record. Public Citizen Health Research Group Health Letter 11(3):1–5, 1995.

26. Young FE. Investigational new drug, antibiotic, and biological drug product regulations; treatment use and sale; final rule. Federal Register 52:19476–19477, 1987.

27. Chelimsky E. Nonprescription drugs: Over the counter and underemphasized. Washington, D.C., 1992, U.S. General Accounting Office.

28. Bradley WW. OTC Review summary. Washington, D.C., Nov 15, 1995, Nonprescription Drug Manufacturers Association.

29. Nordenberg T. FDA takes action to enforce the law. FDA Consumer 34(3):7-8, 2000.

30. Barrett S. Quackery and the FDA: A complicated story. Nutrition Forum 8:41–44, 1991.

31. Adams B, Henkel J. Public affairs specialists: FDA's walking encyclopedias. FDA Consumer 29(4):23–26, 1995.

32. Federal Trade Commission. A guide to the Federal Trade Commission. Washington, DC, 1995, U.S. Government Printing Office.

33. Barrett S. Quackery by mail. New York, 1991, American Council on Science and Health.

34. Postal Inspection Service. Chiropractor causes fiber tablets to become a misbranded drug. Law Enforcement Report, Winter 1983/1984, p 10.

35. Shearing the suckers. Consumer Reports 51:87–94, 1986.

36. Man who sells fake cure for impotency to 25,000 victims gets jail sentence, forfeits home. US Postal Inspection Service Law Enforcement Report, Winter/Spring 1996, pp 3–4.

37. FTC Bureau of Consumer Protection. The Power of Partnerships: FTC-State Cooperative Efforts. Washington, D.C., 1996, Federal Trade Commission.

RELIABLE SOURCES OF INFORMATION

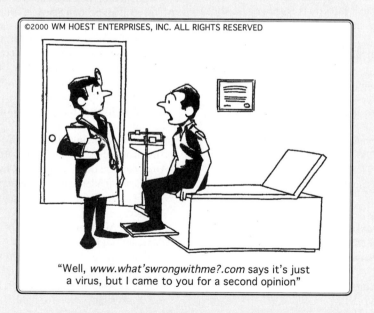

"Well, *www.what'swrongwithme?.com* says it's just a virus, but I came to you for a second opinion"

As you read this, health care consumers are undergoing a radical metamorphosis: They are becoming engaged, empowered, energized e-Health consumers. They represent a vast force that is about to transform the health care world.

DELOITTE CONSULTING, 1999

The organizations and agencies listed in this Appendix offer reliable information. The Consumer Health Sourcebook (http://www.chsourcebook.com) links to their Web pages as well as to other sites that are useful for studying consumer health.

FEDERAL GOVERNMENT AGENCIES

Agency for Health Care Research and Quality (AHRQ)
Center for Food Safety and Applied Nutrition (CFSAN)
Centers for Disease Control and Prevention (CDC)
Consumer Product Safety Commission (CPSC)
Department of Health and Human Services (DHHS)
Environmental Protection Agency (EPA)
Federal Consumer Information Center (FCIC)
Federal Trade Commission (FTC)
Food and Drug Administration (FDA)Health Care Financing
   Administration (HCFA)
National Cholesterol Education Program (NCEP)
National Clearinghouse on Child Abuse and Neglect (NCCAN)
National Guideline Clearinghouse (NGC)
National Health Information Center (NHIC)
National Institutes of Health (NIH)
   National Cancer Institute (NCI)
   National Eye Institute (NEI)
   National Heart, Lung, and Blood Institute (NHLBI)
   National Human Genome Research Institute (NHGRI)
   National Institute of Allergy and Infectious Diseases (NIAID)
   National Institute of Arthritis and Musculoskeletal and Skin
      Diseases (NIAMS)
   National Institute of Child Health and Human Development
      (NICHD)
   National Institute of Dental and Craniofacial Research
      (NIDCR)
   National Institute of Diabetes and Digestive and Kidney
      Diseases (NIDDK)
   National Institute of Environmental Health Sciences (NIEHS)
   National Institute of General Medical Sciences (NIGMS)
   National Institute of Mental Health (NIMH)
   National Institute of Neurological Disorders and Stroke
      (NINDS)
   National Institute of Nursing Research (NINR)
   National Institute on Aging (NIA)
   National Institute on Alcohol Abuse and Alcoholism (NIAAA)
   National Institute on Deafness and Other Communication
      Disorders (NIDCD)
   National Institute on Drug Abuse (NIDA)
   National Library of Medicine (NLM)
   Office of Dietary Supplements (ODS)
National Prevention Information Network (NPIN)
National Maternal and Child Health Clearinghouse (NMCHC)
National SIDS Resource Center (NSRC)
Office of Disease Prevention and Health Promotion (ODPHP)
Office of the Inspector General (OIG)
President's Council on Physical Fitness and Sports (PCPFS)
Substance Abuse and Mental Health Services Administration
   (SAMHSA)
Tobacco Information and Prevention Source (TIPS)
U.S. Department of Agriculture (USDA)
U.S. Postal Service (USPS)

NONGOVERNMENTAL ORGANIZATIONS

Most of the organizations listed below are voluntary groups that draw support and members from the general public as well as professionals. Some have a single national office, while others have chapters in various cities. Most of these organizations provide educational materials on request. Some raise and distribute funds for research. Some conduct educational programs for the public and encourage and develop local support groups. Some offer individual counseling.

Business and professional groups, indicated by an asterisk (*) are composed exclusively or primarily of health professionals or other professionally trained individuals. Most of these groups publish a scientific journal and hold educational meetings for their members. Most of them also help the public by setting professional standards, disseminating information through the news media, and responding to inquiries from individual consumers.

Additional information on most of these organizations can be obtained from the *Encyclopedia of Medical Organizations and Agencies* (Gale Research Company, Detroit), available in the reference department of most public libraries.

Academy for Health Services Research and Health Policy
Action on Smoking and Health (nonsmokers' rights)
Aerobics and Fitness Association of America
Alan Guttmacher Institute (birth control, family planning, and
   women's health issues)
Alexander Graham Bell Association for the Deaf
Alzheimer's Association
*American Academy of Allergy, Asthma, and Immunology
*American Academy of Child & Adolescent Psychiatry
*American Academy of Family Physicians
*American Academy of Ophthalmology
*American Academy of Otolaryngology – Head and Neck
   Surgery
*American Academy of Pediatrics
American Academy of Physician Assistants
American Alliance for Health, Physical Education, Recreation
   and Dance
*American Association for Health Education
*American Association for the History of Medicine
*American Association for Marriage and Family Therapy
*American Association of Blood Banks
*American Association of Endodontists
American Association of Homes and Services for the Aging
American Association of Kidney Patients
*American Association of Pastoral Counselors
*American Association of Plastic Surgeons
American Association of Retired Persons
*American Association of Sex Educators, Counselors, and
   Therapists
*American Association of Suicidology
American Association on Mental Retardation

*American Board of Medical Specialties
*American Burn Association
American Cancer Society
*American Cleft Palate-Craniofacial Association
*American College Health Association
*American College of Cardiology
American Self-Help Clearinghouse
American Society of Clinical Oncology
*American College of Gastroenterology
*American College of Health Care Administrators (nursing homes)
*American College of Healthcare Executives
*American College of Obstetricians and Gynecologists
*American College of Physicians – American Society of Internal Medicine
*American College of Radiology
*American College of Rheumatology
*American College of Sports Medicine
*American College of Surgeons
American Council on Science and Health
*American Counseling Association
*American Dental Association
American Diabetes Association
*American Dietetic Association
*American Epilepsy Society
American Family Foundation (AFF) (cults)
American Federation of HomeCare Providers
American Foundation for AIDS Research
American Foundation for the Blind
*American Geriatrics Society
American Group Psychotherapy Association
*American Headache Society
*American Health Care Association (nursing home standards)
American Heart Association
*American Home Care Association
*American Hospital Association
*American Industrial Hygiene Association
American Kidney Fund
American Liver Foundation
American Lung Association
*American Medical Association
*American Medical Women's Association
*American Medical Writers Association
American Mental Health Counselors Association
*American Nurses Association
*American Occupational Therapy Association
*American Optometric Association
American Pain Foundation
American Parkinson's Disease Association
*American Pharmaceutical Association
*American Physical Therapy Association
*American Podiatric Medical Association
*American Psychiatric Association
*American Psychoanalytic Association
*American Psychological Association
*American Public Health Association
American Red Cross
American Running Association
*American School Health Association
American SIDS Institute
*American Sleep Disorders Association
American Social Health Association (venereal disease)
*American Society for Clinical Nutrition

*American Society for Laser Medicine and Surgery
*American Society for Nutritional Sciences
*American Society for Surgery of the Hand
*American Society of Clinical Hypnosis
*American Society of Clinical Oncology
*American Society of Hematology
*American Society of Law, Medicine, and Ethics
*American Society of Plastic Surgeons
*American Society of Reproductive Medicine
*American Speech-Language-Hearing Association
American Tinnitus Association
*American Urological Association
*American Veterinary Medical Association
Americans for Medical Progress (harm caused by "animal rights" groups)
Americans for Nonsmokers' Rights
Amyotrophic Lateral Sclerosis Association
Anxiety Disorders Association of America
Aplastic Anemia and MDS International Foundation
The Arc of the United States (mental retardation)
*Association for Ambulatory Behavioral Healthcare
*Association for the Advancement of Behavior Therapy
Association for Macular Diseases
Asthma and Allergy Foundation of America
*Better Hearing Institute
Better Vision Institute
*BlueCross BlueShield Association
Cancer Care
Candlelighters Childhood Cancer Foundation
Center for Evidence-Based Medicine
Center for the Study of Services
Children and Adults with Attention Deficit/Hyperactivity Disorder
Children of Aging Parents
Children's Health Care Is a Legal Duty (CHILD)
Children's Leukemia Research Association
Choice in Dying
Committee for the Scientific Investigation of Claims of the Paranormal (CSICOP)
Compassionate Friends
Consumer Federation of America
Consumers Union
Cooley's Anemia Foundation
*Council for Agricultural Science and Technology (CAST)
*Council of Better Business Bureaus
Crohn's and Colitis Foundation of America
Cystic Fibrosis Foundation
*Delta Dental Plans Association (dental insurance)
DOC (tobacco and other preventive health issues)
Drug Policy Foundation
Dysautonomia Foundation
Dystonia Medical Research Foundation
Easter Seals National Headquarters
*ECRI (medical devices, technology, and patient safety)
Endometriosis Association
EngenderHealth (women's health issues)
Epilepsy Foundation
Euthanasia Research and Guidance Organization
Eye Bank Association of America
False Memory Syndrome Foundation
*Federated Ambulatory Surgery Association
*Federation of Societies for Experimental Biology
*Food and Nutrition Board, National Academy of Sciences

Foundation Fighting Blindness
*Gerontological Society of America
Glaucoma Research Foundation
*Health Insurance Association of America
Huntington's Disease Society of America
*Institute of Food Technologists
International AIDS Vaccine Research
International Association for Medical Assistance to Travelers
   (IAMAT)
International Association of Laryngectomees
International Center for Toxicology and Medicine
International Dyslexia Association
International Food Information Council Foundation
*International Hearing Society
*International Life Sciences Institute
Interstitial Cystitis Association
James Randi Educational Foundation (investigation of
   paranormal claims)
*Joint Commission on Accreditation of Healthcare Organizations
Joslin Diabetes Center
Juvenile Diabetes Foundation
La Leche League International (breastfeeding)
Leukemia & Lymphoma Society
Lindesmith – Drug Policy Foundation
Little People of America
Living Bank (organ donor registry)
Lupus Foundation of America
March of Dimes Birth Defects Foundation
Maternity Center Association
Medic Alert Foundation International (emergency medical
   information services)
Muscular Dystrophy Association
Museum of Questionable Medical Devices
Myasthenia Gravis Foundation
National Academy Press
National Alliance for the Mentally Ill
National Alliance of Breast Cancer Organizations
*National Association for Chiropractic Medicine
National Association for Continence
*National Association for Home Care
*National Association of Alcoholism and Drug Abuse Counselors
National Association of Anorexia Nervosa and Associated
   Disorders
National Association of Area Agencies on Aging
National Association of Attorneys General
National Association of the Deaf
*National Association of Social Workers
National Ataxia Foundation (loss of muscle coordination and
   balance)
National Attention Deficit Disorder Association
National Center for Fluoridation Policy and Research
National Center for Nutrition and Dietetics
National Chronic Fatigue Syndrome and Fibromyalgia
   Association
National Committee for Quality Assurance
National Consumers League
National Council Against Health Fraud
National Council on the Aging
National Council on Patient Information and Education

*National Dairy Council
National Depressive and Manic Depressive Association
National Down Syndrome Congress
National Family Caregivers Association
National Family Planning and Reproductive Health Association
National Federation of the Blind
National Foundation for Infectious Diseases
National Fraud Information Center
*National Funeral Directors Association
National Headache Foundation
*National Health Council
National Hemophilia Foundation
*National Hospice and Palliative Care Organization
National Kidney Foundation
National Marfan Foundation
National Mental Health Association
National Multiple Sclerosis Society
National Neurofibromatosis Foundation
National Organization for Rare Disorders (NORD)
National Organization on Disability
National Osteoporosis Foundation
*National Parkinson Foundation
National Psoriasis Foundation
National Safety Council
National Scoliosis Foundation
National Spasmatic Torticollis Association
National Spinal Cord Injury Association
National Stroke Association
National Tay-Sachs and Allied Diseases Association
Obsessive Compulsive Foundation
Oncolink (cancer database)
Oregon Fibromyalgia Foundation
Osteogenesis Imperfecta Foundation
Paget Foundation for Paget's Disease of Bone and Related
   Disorders
Parkinson's Disease Foundation
Planned Parenthood – World Population
Prevent Blindness America
Prevent Child Abuse America
Public Citizen Health Research Group
Quackwatch
Resolve (infertility)
Science & Pseudoscience Review in Mental Health
Scleroderma Foundation
Sickle Cell Disease Association of America
Sjogren's Syndrome Foundation
Skeptics Society
*Society for Clinical and Experimental Hypnosis
Society for Public Health Education
Spina Bifida Association of America
Sudden Infant Death Syndrome Alliance
Tourette Syndrome Association
Tuberous Sclerosis Alliance
United Cerebral Palsy Associations
United Network for Organ Sharing (UNOS)
United Ostomy Association
*United States Pharmacopeial Convention, Inc. (drug
   publications)

GLOSSARY

accreditation: Approval by a recognized accrediting agency that a facility meets its standards. Hospitals and other health-care facilities are accredited by the Joint Commission on Accreditation of Healthcare Organizations. Colleges and professional schools are accredited by agencies approved by the U.S. Secretary of Education or the Council on Recognition of Postsecondary Accreditation (CORPA). The Accreditation Council for Continuing Medical Education (ACCME) manages the accreditation system for continuing education for physicians.

acetaminophen: Nonprescription drug used to relieve pain and reduce fever; the active ingredient in Tylenol and Datril.

acidosis: State in which the blood is more acidic than normal.

activities of daily living (ADLs): Term used to gauge how well people can meet their basic physical needs. The five areas usually considered are bathing, dressing, eating, toileting (includes whether or not the person is incontinent), and transferring (ability to get from place to place).

acupressure (shiatsu): Technique that uses surface stimulation by hand instead of needles at "acupuncture points."

acupuncture: System of treatment purported to balance the body's "life force" by inserting needles (or using other procedures) at points where alleged channels called "meridians" meet on the body's surface.

acute condition: Condition that has rapid onset and follows a short but relatively severe course.

addiction: Persistent, habitual pattern of behavioral excess in which an activity (such as drug taking, eating, or gambling) becomes central to a person's way of life despite its adverse consequences.

administrative complaint: Complaint alleging that a law has been broken, which can lead to a formal hearing before an administrative law judge.

administrative medicine: Occupation that encompasses the operation and management of organizations and institutions such as health departments, hospitals, clinics, and health-care plans.

adrenaline: Hormone, produced and stored by the adrenal glands, which can cause increased heartbeat and other reactions that prepare the body to meet emergency situations.

advance directive: Document in which a person states choices for medical treatment or designates who should make treatment choices if the person should lose decision-making capacity.

aerobic exercise: Exercise that requires large amounts of oxygen and promotes cardiorespiratory fitness.

AIDS (acquired immunodeficiency syndrome): Fatal disease in which the body's immune system breaks down, leaving the body susceptible to certain cancers and serious infections.

alkalosis: State in which the blood is more alkaline (less acidic) than normal.

allergic reaction: Excessive reaction of the body's immune system to a food, drug, or other substance that is ordinarily harmless. In susceptible individuals, exposure to an allergen can cause certain cells to release histamine, which can cause sneezing, wheezing, hives, and other reactions.

allopathy: Term coined by Samuel Hahnemann (founder of homeopathy) to designate medical practices based on the ancient Greek humoral theories that symptoms should be treated with opposites. (Many of his contemporaries, for example, used bloodletting to treat fevers that supposedly represented an excess of "blood humor.") Allopathy has been displaced by medical science, but the term is often used incorrectly to describe modern medical practice.

alopecia: Medical term for baldness.

"alternative" health care: Misleading term used to characterize many types of unscientific methods. Since ineffective methods are not true alternatives to effective ones, the terms "unscientific" or "dubious" are more appropriate.

AMA: Abbreviation for American Medical Association.

ambulatory health care: All types of health services provided to patients who are not confined to an institutional bed during the time the services are rendered; also called outpatient care.

amino acid: Building block of proteins.

anabolism: The phase of metabolism in which simple substances are synthesized into the complex materials of living tissue (e.g., proteins from amino acids).

anaerobic exercise: Exercise, such as sprinting, done without using the oxygen one breathes.

analgesia: Pain relief.

analgesic, external: Topical medicine that can relieve pain.

analgesic, internal: Pain reliever designed to be taken by mouth.

anaphylactic shock: A sudden, life-threatening allergic reaction characterized by a sharp drop in blood pressure, difficulty breathing, and hives.

androgenic steroid: A steroid hormone, such as testosterone or androsterone, that controls the development and maintenance of masculine characteristics.

anecdotal evidence: Reports of personal observations that have not been made under strict experimental conditions.

anesthesia: Loss of sensation, with or without loss of consciousness.

angioplasty: Reconstruction of a blood vessel.

anorexia: Loss of appetite.

anorexia nervosa: Dangerous condition in which victims lose interest in eating and become dangerously thin, usually as a result of false beliefs about being too fat.

antacid: Over-the-counter product used to neutralize hydrochloric acid produced by the stomach.

anthroposophical medicine: Practices based on an occult philosophy said to relate man to his natural environment, with emphasis on color and rhythm.

antihistamine: Drug that counteracts histamine, a substance released during allergic reactions that can cause localized redness, edema, and mucus production.

allergen: Substance that produces an allergic reaction.

antibodies: Protein molecules produced in the blood or tissues in response to a specific antigen, such as a bacterium, virus, or toxin. Antibodies destroy or weaken foreign invaders and neutralize organic poisons, thus forming the basis of immunity.

antigen: Substance that, as a result of coming in contact with appropriate tissues of an animal body, induces antibody formation.

antimicrobial: Any substance that kills germs or inhibits their growth.

antioxidant: Agent that inhibits oxidation and thus prevents rancidity of oils or fats or the deterioration of other substances through oxidative processes. The best-known antioxidants are vitamins A, C, and E; beta carotene; and the food preservatives BHA and BHT.

antipruritic: Any substance that prevents or relieves itching.

antipyretic: Any drug that reduces fever.

aphrodisiac: Any substance claimed to increase sexual stimulation.

aplastic anemia: Life-threatening disorder in which the bone marrow fails to produce adequate numbers of circulating blood cells.

applied kinesiology: Pseudoscience based on the belief that every organ dysfunction is accompanied by a specific muscle weakness.

arrhythmia: Irregular heart rhythm.

arteriosclerosis: Chronic disease characterized by hardening and thickening of artery walls.

aseptic: Devoid of microorganisms.

assisted living: Term used to describe various types of residential facilities that offer help with activities of daily living in a homelike atmosphere.

astigmatism: Uneven curvature of the cornea or surface of the lens of the eye, which distorts vision by preventing proper focus of light rays on the retina.

asymptomatic: Symptom-free.

atherosclerosis: Accumulation of deposits of cholesterol and fibrous tissue within the inner walls of large and medium-sized arteries; extensive buildup can result in blockage of the artery.

autism: a chronic developmental disorder characterized by problems in social interaction, communication, and restrictive and repetitive interests and activities. It is most often identified between the ages of 18 and 30 months.

autointoxication: Unfounded notion that intestinal contents stagnate and putrefy to form toxins that are absorbed by the body and cause chronic poisoning.

autonomic nervous system: Components of the nervous system that regulate many functions of the body that require no conscious effort. Autonomic nerves control the heart, smooth muscles, and glands.

ayurvedic medicine: Practices said to be based on a traditional Indian approach that combines herbs, "purifying" therapies, and "rejuvenation" techniques.

balance billing: Billing a patient for charges exceeding the amount approved by the patient's insurance carrier.

balanced diet: Selection of a wide variety of foods from each of the food groups.

bile: Yellow or greenish fluid secreted by the liver and passed into the small intestine, where it helps in the digestion and absorption of fats.

bioavailability: The ability of a drug or nutrient to participate in metabolic and/or physiologic reactions.

bioequivalent: Term used to describe drug products with equivalent absorption, blood levels, and therapeutic actions.

biofeedback: Relaxation technique using an electronic device that continuously signals pulse rate, muscle tension, or other body function by tone or visual signal.

bioflavonoid: Pigmented substance, not essential in humans, once thought to have vitamin activity. No evidence exists that bioflavonoids are useful for the treatment of any human ailment.

biologic drug product: Preparation, such as a drug, vaccine, or antitoxin, that is synthesized from living organisms or their products and used medically as a diagnostic, preventive, or therapeutic agent.

biopsy: Removal and examination of a sample of tissue from a living patient for diagnosis or prognosis.

biorhythms: Pseudoscientific notion that human performance and susceptibilities can be predicted by charting three biologic rhythms said to begin at the moment of birth.

biotechnology: Use of living organisms or their products to make or modify a substance.

BMI (body mass index): Measure for classifying obesity, calculated by dividing a person's weight in kilograms by the square of the person's height in meters.

board-certified specialist: Health professional who has completed accredited training and passed an examination given by a specialty board.

board-eligible: Person who has the required training and experience to take a certifying examination but has not taken or has not passed the examination. Although the American Board of Medical Specialties has officially abandoned the term, it is still in common use.

bodywork: Umbrella term for practices that include manual massage, manipulation, or exercise of body parts.

bone scan: Diagnostic procedure in which a radioactive substance is injected intravenously and the image of its distribution to the bones is analyzed to detect certain diseases or conditions, most notably cancer.

bran: Outer coat of a cereal grain. Bran contains significant amounts of fiber and several nutrients.

bursa: Sac containing a lubricating fluid (synovial fluid), usually located or formed in areas subject to friction (e.g., where a tendon passes over a bone).

cadaver: Dead body, especially one intended for dissection.

calculus: Hard substance, such as a kidney stone, gallstone, or the hard substance (calcified plaque) that can accumulate on the surface of teeth.

calorie: Unit that expresses the amount of energy the body is able to get from foods. Carbohydrates and proteins provide about four calories per gram, fats provide about nine calories per gram, and alcohol provides about seven calories per gram.

candidiasis hypersensitivity: Fad diagnosis based on the notion that multiple common symptoms are the result of sensitivity to the common yeast *Candida albicans*.

capitation: Method of paying health-care providers according to the number of patients they agree to serve rather than the amount of service rendered per visit.

caplet: Drug tablet shaped like a capsule.

carcinogenic: Cancer-causing.

carcinoma: Malignant tumor of the epithelium. Epithelial cells form the outer layer of the skin and line the gastrointestinal tract, the genitourinary tract, the glands, and other free surfaces within the body.

carcinoma in situ: Cancer that lies within the epithelium and has not invaded adjacent tissues. See *carcinoma*.

cardiovascular: Pertaining to the heart and blood vessels.

cardiorespiratory efficiency: Ability of the heart, blood vessels, and lungs to deliver oxygen to body parts.

caries: Tooth decay.

carotene: Yellow pigment found in various plant and animal tissues that is the precursor of vitamin A. An excessive amount of carotene can cause carotenemia, a condition in which the skin turns yellow.

catabolism: Metabolic breakdown of complex molecules into simpler ones, often resulting in a release of energy.

cataract: Cloudiness of the lens of the eye.

CAT scan: Imaging method in which the density of an area of the body is determined by feeding x-ray data into a computer to create a picture on a screen similar to a cross-sectional photograph; used to study body structures. Also called CT scan.

caveat emptor: Phrase meaning, "Let the buyer beware."

caveat vendor: Phrase meaning, "Let the seller beware."

cease and desist order: Order given by an administrative law judge to stop unlawful activity; if not appealed, the order becomes final.

cellulite: Medically unrecognized term sometimes used to describe dimpled fat commonly found on the thighs of women.

cellulose: Main component of plant cell walls. A component of dietary fiber, celluloses absorb water readily and help make stools bulkier and softer.

cervix: Lower part of the uterus. An opening in the cervix connects the uterus to the vagina.

chakras: Alleged "energy centers" of the body that collect *prana,* the "life force" postulated in yoga (Hindu) philosophy.

CHAMPUS: Abbreviation for Civilian Health and Medical Program of the Uniformed Services, a federal insurance program for military dependents and retirees.

chemosurgery: Use of caustic chemicals to remove diseased or unwanted tissue.

Chinese medicine, traditional (TCM): Collection of practices that includes acupuncture, the use of herbs and dietary procedures, pulse diagnosis, and other procedures.

chiropractic: Conglomeration of practices, most of which are based on the faulty notion that spinal problems are the cause, or an underlying cause, of most health problems (see Chapter 8).

cholesterol level: Concentration of cholesterol in the blood, a factor that can help indicate the risk of heart disease.

chronic condition: Problem that lasts for a long period or recurs frequently.

chronic fatigue syndrome: Illness in which profound fatigue persists or recurs for at least 6 months and is accompanied by several flu-like symptoms, such as throat inflammation, lymph node enlargement, low fever, muscle and joint pains, headache, difficulty in concentrating, and exercise intolerance.

civil procedure: Noncriminal legal action such as an administrative hearing or a civil court action.

clinical: Related to the treatment or examination of patients (e.g., clinical study, clinical practice, clinical psychology).

clinical activities or subjects: Activities or subjects that involve patient care.

clinical ecology: Pseudoscience based on the belief that multiple symptoms are triggered by hypersensitivity to common foods and chemicals.

clinical trial: Investigation into the effects of a drug or vaccine on humans.

closed-panel HMO: Insurance plan that covers services only from specified providers.

coagulate: To change from a liquid to a solid or gel; to clot.

co-insurance: Partial payment beyond the deductible required from the policyholder for services rendered.

colonic irrigation: "High-colonic" enema performed with a rubber tube inserted 20 to 30 inches into the rectum. Warm water is pumped in and out through the tube, typically using 20 or more gallons. The procedure has no medical justification but is used by proponents of "autointoxication."

colonoscope: Instrument passed through the rectum to examine nearly the entire length of the large intestine.

comedo: Plug of dead cells and sebum within a hair follicle; the primary lesion of acne.

"complementary medicine": Approach claimed to combine standard and "alternative" methods, using the best of both; may also be called "integrative medicine."

complete protein: Protein that contains significant levels of all of the essential amino acids.

complex carbohydrates (starches): Compounds composed of long chains of glucose molecules.

comprehensive health insurance: Broad coverage that includes most medical and surgical services in both inpatient and outpatient settings.

conditioner: Hair product intended to restore oils, sheen, elasticity, and manageability after washing.

confidentiality: Ethical principle that information disclosed during the course of treatment may not be revealed without the patient's consent.

confirmatory test: Follow-up test after a positive result from an initial screening test. Confirmatory tests are usually more complex and expensive and often are more invasive than initial screening tests.

congenital: Present at birth.

consent decree (or order): Court-approved agreement (usually to stop behavior that has been challenged by a regulatory agency) that has the force of law.

Consumer Bill of Rights: Principles devised by President Kennedy, who stated that consumers have the right to safety, to be informed, to choose, and to be heard.

consumer health: All aspects of personal enhancement, health maintenance, and consumer protection related to the intelligent purchase and use of health products and services.

continuing medical education (CME): Postgraduate educational activities aimed at maintaining, updating, and extending professional skills. Many professional organizations, state licensing boards, and hospitals require CME participation.

contraceptive: Substance or device used to prevent pregnancy.

contracture: Abnormal (usually permanent) shortening of a muscle or scar tissue. A contracture can cause deformity and loss of joint mobility.

contraindication: Factor that makes it inadvisable to administer a drug or carry out a medical procedure.

coordination of benefits: Insurance policy provision that prohibits collecting benefits from two or more policies for medical care, thereby preventing policy-holders from profiting from being ill. After the primary company pays, other companies will calculate their coverage of the remainder. All group policies contain a coordination clause, but most individual policies do not.

cornea: Transparent, outermost portion of the front of the eyeball.

coronary: Pertaining to the heart.

corrective lenses: Eyeglasses or contact lenses that enable images to be focused on the retina.

cosmetics: Substances intended to be rubbed, poured, sprinkled, or sprayed on the body to cleanse, beautify, increase attractiveness, or alter appearance.

counterirritant: Substance that produces mild irritation of the skin that distracts attention from, and thus relieves, the discomfort of a deeper structure.

CPT codes: A system of code numbers for medical services and procedures. The numbers, which are used for insurance billing, are revised quarterly and are published annually in a book called *Physicians' Current Procedural Terminology*.

crown: Portion of the tooth normally visible above the gum line.

cryosurgery: Destruction of diseased or unwanted tissues by freezing.

cult: Any system that encourages obsessive devotion to a person or an ideal.

cystoscope: Instrument used to look inside the bladder and urinary passageway (urethra).

daily reference values (DRVs): System of food component standards intended to help consumers select food by reading labels wisely (see Chapter 11).

database: Organized compilation of information, usually maintained in a computer system.

decongestant: Drug that constricts blood vessels and membranes of the nose to relieve stuffiness.

deductible: Amount paid out of pocket before insurance coverage takes effect.

defensive medicine: Medically questionable use of procedures (such as x-ray examinations following minor head injuries) to protect the doctor in the event of a malpractice suit.

defibrillator: Device used to administer an electric shock to restart a heart that has stopped beating.

delusion: False belief, not ordinarily accepted by other members of the person's culture, that is firmly held despite obvious proof or evidence to the contrary.

dementia: Chronic mental deterioration characterized by disorientation; confusion; and impaired memory, judgment, and intellect.

dentifrice: Toothpaste, gel, or powder used in brushing teeth.

denturist: Technician who provides dentures directly to the public without supervision or referral from a dentist. Denturism is illegal in most states.

dermabrasion: Process that removes the upper layers of the skin to improve the appearance of scars.

dermatitis: Inflammation of the skin.

diathermy: Generation of heat in tissue by electric currents for medical or surgical purposes.

Dietary Guidelines for Americans (DGA): General guidelines, developed by the U.S. Departments of Agriculture and Health and Human Services, for people who want to decrease their chances of developing certain chronic diseases.

Dietary Reference Intakes (DRIs): Nutrient-based reference values for use in planning and assessing diets and for other purposes (see Chapter 11).

dietary supplement: See *food supplement*.

dilate: Expand or widen.

diopter: Unit of measurement of the refracting power of lenses; the reciprocal of the focal length (in meters). Nearsightedness is designated with negative numbers (e.g., -3.00 D), whereas farsightedness is designated with positive numbers.

diploma mill: Nonaccredited organization that awards degrees without requiring its students to meet educational standards for degrees established and traditionally followed by reputable educational institutions.

diplomate: Person who has passed an examination given by the National Board of Medical Examiners (one route to state licensure) or a specialty board.

disorientation: State of confusion about time, location, or personal identity.

diuretic: Drug that increases the output of urine.

DNR: Abbreviation for "Do Not Resuscitate," a medical order to refrain from cardiopulmonary resuscitation if a patient's heart stops beating.

doctrine of signatures: Principle that the external characteristics (such as shape) of a plant, animal, or other entity signal its magical or healing properties and that relationships exist between the appearance of a source of medicine and the diseases against which it is effective.

dose-response: Gradient response in which exposure to progressively stronger doses produces a progressively greater effect. Two examples are increased sedation with higher doses of sleeping pills, and lung cancer rates that correlate with the number of packs of cigarettes smoked per day.

double-blind test: Experiment in which neither the experimental subjects nor those responsible for the treatment or data collection know which subjects receive the treatment being tested and which receive something else (such as a placebo).

DRGs (diagnosis-related groups): Categories created under Medicare for payment of hospital bills according to the patient's diagnosis rather than the actual length of stay or treatment rendered.

drug (under federal law): Any substance intended to be used for preventing, curing, mitigating, or treating a disease.

durable medical equipment: Long-lasting piece of equipment, such as a cane, wheelchair, respirator, or electric hospital bed.

dysmenorrhea: Menstrual pain.

economies of scale: Cost savings resulting from aggregation of resources or mass production.

edema: Swelling of tissues as a result of the presence of abnormally large amounts of fluid between the cells.

elective procedure: Procedure (usually surgical) that need not be done immediately to prevent death or serious disability.

electroencephalogram (EEG): Record of the electricity of the brain. The encephalography procedure is commonly referred to as a "brain-wave test."

electrolytes: In physiology, various ions, such as sodium, potassium, or chloride, required by cells to regulate the electric charge and flow of water molecules across the cell membrane.

electrosurgery: Use of electricity to destroy benign lesions on skin.

emphysema: Chronic disease in which the ability to move air in and out of the lungs is impaired.

endometriosis: Condition, usually resulting in pain and dysmenorrhea, that is characterized by the abnormal occurrence of functional endometrial tissue outside the uterus.

endometrium: Lining of the uterus.

endorphins: Narcotic-like substances produced by the body that may relieve pain and produce euphoria.

"energy medicine": Term used by practitioners who claim to be able to detect and manipulate "subtle energies," some of which cannot be measured. This category includes the alleged energies involved in psychic healing, prayer, meditation, hope, faith, and the will to live. Energy medicine also is said to encompass acupuncture, electrodiagnosis, homeopathy, and magnet therapy.

enrichment: Addition of specific nutrients to a food to maintain established standards of identity for that food.

enteric coated (tablet): Tablet with a coating that delays release of the medication until the tablet has entered the intestine. This is done to prevent stomach irritation or inactivation of the medication by stomach acids.

"environmental illness": Term clinical ecologists use to describe what they consider "dysregulation" of the immune system. Its proponents claim that multiple symptoms can be triggered by hypersensitivity to common foods and chemicals.

enzymes: Protein substances that trigger and speed up (catalyze) chemical reactions within the body.

epidemiology: Study of the frequency, distribution, and determinants of diseases and disabilities and the impact of interventions in human populations. Epidemiologic evidence can only show associations, not cause-and-effect relationships. However, if additional criteria are met, epidemiologists can infer that an associated factor is causal.

ESADDI: Abbreviation for estimated safe and adequate daily dietary intake. These have been established for certain essential vitamins and minerals for which data are sufficient to estimate a range of requirements but insufficient for developing an RDA.

essential nutrients: Specific nutrients that cannot be synthesized by the body and therefore must be obtained from food.

estrogens: Female sex hormones involved in the development of secondary sexual characteristics and in the maintenance of menstruation; estrogens are contained in birth control pills and may be administered to control menopausal or post-menopausal symptoms.

etiology: The cause or origin of a health problem.

evidence-based medicine (EBM): Medical care based on thorough evaluation of scientific studies.

expectorant: Drug that stimulates the flow of respiratory tract secretions.

extended care: Skilled nursing care.

fallopian tubes: Ducts through which ova can pass from each ovary to the uterus.

false-negative test result: Finding that wrongly indicates normality.

false-positive test result: Finding that wrongly indicates an abnormality.

family practitioner: See *general practitioner.*

fee-for-service care: Professional care for which a fee is earned for each service rendered, as opposed to payment through salary or capitation.

fermentable carbohydrates: Carbohydrates, such as sugars and starches, that can be split into relatively simple substances. In the mouth, saliva and the bacteria in plaque act on these carbohydrates to produce acids that can attack tooth enamel.

fetus: Human developing in the uterus from the end of the eighth week after conception to the moment of birth. (Before that the developing human is called an embryo.)

fiber (dietary): Plant constituents of food that are resistant to digestion by human gastrointestinal secretions; also called roughage. "Crude fiber" is what remains after laboratory breakdown of food with acid and alkali.

flatulence: Excessive intestinal gassiness.

flexibility: Stretching muscles to increase range of movement.

fluoridation: Addition of fluoride to a community's water supply to prevent tooth decay in its users.

food combining: Dietary practice based on the incorrect notion that various food combinations eaten during the same meal can cause or correct ill health.

Food Guide Pyramid: Pictorial representation of U.S. government guidelines for healthy food selection.

food irradiation: Application of ionizing radiation (x-rays, gamma rays, or high-energy electrons) to foods to kill organisms, inhibit sprouting, or delay ripening.

food supplement: Ambiguous term for products used to provide nutrients in addition to those found in one's diet. Most dietary supplements contain vitamins and/or minerals, but the Dietary Supplement Health and Education Act of 1993 includes herbs and many other nonnutritive substances in its definition of "dietary supplement" (see Chapter 12). Various caloric products used for preventing or treating malnutrition are also referred to as supplements.

fortification: Addition of nutrients originally not present (or not present in significant amounts) to make the food more nutritious.

free radical: Atoms or groups of atoms having at least one unpaired electron, which makes them highly reactive.

gangrene: Local death of tissue resulting from loss of blood supply.

gastrointestinal tract: Digestive pathway, including the esophagus, stomach, small intestine, and large intestine.

general anesthesia: Agent, usually given by inhalation or intravenously, that produces unconsciousness and loss of sensation throughout the body.

general practitioner: Physician who provides a wide variety of services for patients of all ages but is not considered a specialist. Family practitioners have the same scope of practice but undergo residency training and are considered specialists.

generic drug: Drug marketed under its simplified chemical name rather than a trade name. Most generic drugs are less expensive but therapeutically equivalent to their brand-name counterparts.

genetic engineering: Techniques of altering plants and animals by modifying their genes. Genetic manipulation has enabled commercial production of insulin, produced several types of hardy crop plants, and shown promise in the treatment of several diseases.

genital: Pertaining to sexual organs.

gingivitis: Inflammation of the gums; the earliest stage of periodontal disease.

glaucoma: Disease in which pressure inside the eye increases; can cause blindness if untreated.

glucose: Simple sugar that is the basic form of food energy for life.

glycogen: Form of glucose that is stored in the body (in the liver and muscles).

grain: In pharmacology, a unit of weight equal to 65 mg.

granola: Common term to describe various mixtures of oats, other grains, fruits, seeds, and nuts. Although granola products are often promoted as "health foods," many of them are high in calories and fat.

gross domestic product (GDP): Total monetary measure of a nation's production of goods and services within the country during 1 year.

hair implantation: Surgical procedure of questionable safety and efficacy in which a hairpiece (or hair that does not take root) is anchored to the scalp with sutures or by other means.

hair transplantation: Surgical grafting of hair-producing tissue from one part of the body to another.

hangover: Unpleasant physical effects that can follow heavy use of alcohol.

HDL (high-density lipoproteins): Substances in the blood that transport cholesterol from various cells to the liver, from which it can be excreted in the bile. Since this helps to protect blood vessels against heart disease, HDL is often referred to as "good cholesterol."

"health freedom": Right to free choice of health practitioners, practices, and products. Although it is desirable for consumers to be free to make informed choices, promoters of quackery promote this slogan to oppose government interference with their ability to mislead consumers.

health maintenance organization (HMO): Managed-care system in which enrollees or their employers pay monthly or quarterly premiums that cover treatment from designated providers.

heart failure: Inability of the heart to pump enough blood to meet the needs of the body.

hemorrhage: Excessive bleeding.

hepatitis: Inflammation of the liver.

herb: Plant or plant part valued for its medicinal, savory, cosmetic, or aromatic qualities.

herniated ("ruptured") disc: Protrusion of a degenerated or fragmented intervertebral disc into the space between the vertebrae through which the spinal nerves exit.

herpes: Family of viruses that can cause acute or periodic skin eruptions, including cold sores (herpes simplex type 1), genital herpes (herpes simplex type 2), "shingles" (herpes zoster), and chickenpox (herpes zoster).

heterosexual transmission (of disease): Transmission from male to female or from female to male.

holistic medicine: Treatment of the "whole person" (physical and psychologic); the term is often used to promote the use of a wide variety of unscientific methods, some of which focus just on specific body parts.

homeopathy: Pseudoscience based on notions that (a) a substance that produces symptoms in a healthy person can cure ill people with similar symptoms and (b) that infinitesimal doses can be highly potent.

homocysteine: Amino acid that, when present in high levels in the blood, can contribute to the development of premature coronary heart disease and stroke (see Chapter 15).

hormone: Substance made in one part of the body that circulates through body fluids to exert its effect on another part of the body.

hospice: Program that enables terminally ill individuals to die as comfortably as possible in a homelike setting.

hypercholesterolemia: Medical term for high blood cholesterol level.

hypertension: Medical term for high blood pressure.

hyperthermia: Treatment method in which the temperature of the body or a body part is raised.

hypoglycemia: Low blood sugar. Physiologic hypoglycemia is normal, moderate lowering of blood sugar in response to the body's insulin and helps make a person feel hungry. Pathologic hypoglycemia is a rare condition in which severe symptoms are accompanied by very low blood sugar.

hysterectomy: Operation to remove the uterus.

iatrogenic: Adverse health problem that results from a diagnostic or treatment procedure.

ibuprofen: Chemical (generic) name for the analgesic/anti-inflammatory drug found in products such as *Motrin* and *Advil*.

ICD-9: Abbreviation for *International Classification of Diseases, Ninth Revision*, a system of diagnostic codes used for submitting insurance claims and for various statistical purposes.

idiopathic disease: Disease having no known cause.

imaging procedures: Examinations that use x-rays, ultrasound, radioactive chemicals, magnetic waves, or other modalities to visualize the structure or function of specified body parts.

impaired physician: Loosely defined term encompassing any form of physical, mental, or behavioral problem that interferes with a doctor's ability to provide appropriate patient care. The problems can include unethical conduct, mental illness, senility, drug abuse, and/or failure to keep up-to-date.

in vitro: Performed in a test tube, tissue culture, or other artificial environment.

in vivo: Performed within a living organism.

incidence: Number of new cases of a disease that develop in a population during a specified period of time, usually 1 year.

indemnity insurance: With respect to health care, an insurance policy that provides benefits specified within a framework of fee schedules, exclusions, and limitations.

infertility: Inability to conceive a child.

inflammation: Local tissue reaction consisting of swelling, redness, and warmth.

informed consent: Permission given by a patient who has been fully apprised of the nature and risks of a proposed treatment.

injunction: Court order forbidding a particular act or acts. When an injunction is violated, the court has great leeway in ordering punishment.

inpatient: Person who is treated at a facility while in residence.

insomnia: Inability to sleep.

Institute of Medicine: Organization chartered in 1970 by the National Academy of Sciences to examine policy matters pertaining to health.

integrated health networks: Corporate linkages of physicians, hospitals, and other health-care facilities into a system that provides comprehensive health care.

interferon: Protein molecule, made in tiny amounts by the body's immune system, that helps the body combat viral diseases and possibly cancer.

intermediate care: Nursing home services that include supervision by a registered nurse for at least one 8-hour shift per day for patients capable of performing some activities of daily living.

international unit (IU): An amount defined by the International Conference for Unification of Formulae—used to express the quantity of certain vitamins, enzymes, and other substances.

interstate commerce: Transactions involving participants or products from two or more states, which means they are subject to federal laws.

intervertebral discs: Structures between the vertebrae that give the spine mechanical strength and cushion the bones. The discs are tough on the outside and jellylike on the inside.

intramuscular injection: Injection into a muscle.

intraocular lens: Plastic lens used to replace an abnormal lens (cataract) of the eye.

intravenous: Administered into a vein.

iridology: Pseudoscience based on the theory that most body abnormalities cause abnormal markings in the eye.

isokinetic exercise: Isotonic activity involving maximum contraction of muscles throughout the full range of motion.

isometric exercise: Contraction of muscles with little or no movement of body parts.

isotonic exercise: Contraction of muscles with movement of body parts.

-itis: Suffix that means inflammation or "disease of."

jaundice: Yellowish pigmentation of the skin, eyes, and other tissues caused by accumulation of bile pigments in the tissues.

JAMA: Abbreviation for the *Journal of the American Medical Association.*

JCAHO: Commonly used abbreviation for the Joint Commission on Accreditation of Healthcare Organizations, formerly called Joint Commission on Accreditation of Hospitals (JCAH). The organization itself never uses "JCAHO" but refers to itself as "the Joint Commission."

joint: Place where bones meet.

ketosis: Abnormal metabolic state brought about by incomplete breakdown of fatty acids into ketone bodies; may result from low-carbohydrate or starvation diet.

kickback: Illegal payment made to someone who refers work to the payer.

kinesiology: Study of the mechanics and anatomy of motion and the functions of muscles; a respectable science, as distinguished from "applied kinesiology," a pseudoscience based on the theory that muscular imbalance is a major factor in most diseases.

labeling (legal definition): Written, printed, or graphic matter displayed on packages or accompanying a food, drug, device, or cosmetic.

laparoscope: Instrument that can be inserted into the abdominal cavity to visualize its contents or perform surgery (such as female sterilization or gallbladder removal).

latent: In a dormant or hidden stage.

LDL (low-density lipoproteins): Substances that contribute to fatty deposits (atherosclerosis) in the major arteries and are associated with increased risk of atherosclerosis. For this reason they are often called "bad cholesterol."

legumes: Group of protein-rich vegetables that includes peas and beans, including black beans, black-eyed peas, broad beans, chick peas, kidney beans, lima beans, pinto beans, soybeans, lentils, split peas, and peanuts.

lesion: Abnormal change in the structure of an organ or body tissue resulting from injury or disease, especially a change that is circumscribed and well defined. Examples are cuts, burns, skin eruptions, and tumors.

leukoplakia: Precancerous condition in which thickened white patches occur on mucous membranes, most commonly those of the tongue, mouth, or female genitalia.

life expectancy: Average number of years that people of a certain age are likely to live.

ligament: Sheet or band of tough, fibrous tissue that connects bones or cartilages at a joint or supports an organ.

lipid: Chemical term for fat.

living will: Document indicating which treatments the signer would or would not want if rendered permanently unconscious or terminally ill and unable to communicate.

long-term care: The continuum of broad-ranged maintenance and health services to chronically ill, disabled, or retarded persons. Services may be provided on an inpatient (rehabilitation facility, nursing home, mental hospital), outpatient, assisted living, or at-home basis.

loss ratio: Percentage of premium dollars an insurance company pays in benefits to policyholders; also called benefit-cost ratio.

macrobiotic diet: Restricted diet, high in whole grains, claimed by its advocates to improve health and prolong life.

macronutrient: Nutrient needed in large amounts.

major medical insurance: Coverage (beyond basic coverage) to offset heavy medical expenses from prolonged illness or serious injury.

malaise: Medical term for general discomfort or uneasiness, which often is an early sign of illness.

malocclusion: Improper alignment of the jaws or teeth.

malpractice: Failure of a professional to provide services that meet prevailing standards of care.

managed care: Health-care system (such as HMO or PPO) that integrates the financing and delivery of services by using selected providers, utilization review, and financial incentives for members who use the providers and procedures authorized by the plan.

mania: Excitement of psychotic proportions manifested by mental and physical hyperactivity, disorganized behavior, and/or elevation of mood.

manic-depressive psychosis: Mental impairment characterized by recurrent periods of mania, depression, or both. Also called manic-depressive illness or bipolar illness.

marker: Substance whose concentration in the blood is monitored to measure the progress of treatment. For example, CD4 counts are used as a marker for AIDS, and other markers are used in managing several types of cancer.

media: Information sources, including radio, television, newspapers, magazines, books, newsletters, pamphlets, and the Internet.

Medicaid: Federally subsidized, state-run program of health care for indigent persons.

medically indigent: Term referring to people who have enough money for most expenses but are unable to pay for sudden high costs of health care. Most medically indigent individuals are employed but cannot afford (or cannot obtain) adequate health insurance.

Medicare: Federal health insurance program for persons 65 years of age or older and for certain disabled younger persons.

megavitamin therapy: Unorthodox treatment using high dosages of vitamins, usually ten times the RDA or more.

menopause: Period of life during which menstruation normally stops—often referred to as "the change of life."

meridian therapy: Term that encompasses acupuncture, acupressure, and other techniques claimed to balance the flow of the body's "life force."

meta-analysis: Review process in which research reports are evaluated by listing desirable attributes, assigning points to each, and scoring each report accordingly. Data from well-designed studies may also be pooled for further statistical analysis.

metabolic therapy: Loosely defined, unorthodox program that may include megadoses of vitamins, oral enzymes, pangamic acid, coffee enemas, and a low-protein diet.

metastasis: Transfer of disease-causing microorganisms or cancerous cells from an original (primary) site to one or more sites elsewhere in the body, usually through blood vessels or lymphatic channels. The secondary cancer is called a metastasis or metastatic tumor.

METs (metabolic equivalents): A measure of the intensity of physical activity. METs are multiples of the resting metabolic rate, which can be expressed in terms of total oxygen consumption or oxygen consumption per unit of body weight. One MET is the amount of oxygen consumed while a person sits quietly at rest: approximately 3.5 milliliters of oxygen per kilogram of body weight per minute.

metabolism: Sum of the physical and chemical processes by which the body is maintained; also, the reactions involved in energy production.

micronutrient: Nutrient needed in only tiny amounts.

misbranding: Misrepresentation, as defined by the Federal Food, Drug, and Cosmetic Act, in the labeling or advertising of a food or drug.

miscarriage: Premature expulsion of a nonviable fetus from the uterus. Also called spontaneous abortion.

MMR: Abbreviation for measles, mumps, and rubella (German measles).

morbidity: Measures of the effects of disease on a population. Incidence and prevalence are both measures of morbidity.

mortality (of a disease or injury): Total number of deaths from a given cause in a population during a specific interval, usually 1 year.

mucous membrane: Mucus-producing tissue that lines the body's air passageways and digestive tract.

naprapathy: Variation of chiropractic based on the philosophy that contractions of the body's soft tissue cause illness by interfering with neurovascular function.

National health insurance (NHI): A federal government-regulated health insurance program for all or nearly all citizens.

National Research Council: Principal operating agency of the National Academy of Sciences and the National Academy of Engineering. It is a private, nonprofit institution that provides science and technology advice under a congressional charter.

natural hygiene: Philosophy of health and "natural living" that emphasizes fasting and food combining; see *food combining*.

naturopathy: Pseudoscientific approach to health care based on the belief that the basic cause of disease is violation of nature's laws.

negative test result: Test result within normal limits.

neurotic reaction: Nervous response, resulting from inner emotional conflict, in which the person generally remains able to distinguish what is real from what is not.

new drug: Drug that is not generally recognized by experts as safe and effective (see *safe and effective*). Drugs cannot be legally marketed in interstate commerce unless they have FDA approval or are generally recognized as safe and effective for their intended use. Intended use can be determined from claims in labeling, advertising, or other promotional channels.

nocebo effect: Unfavorable treatment response that does not result from pharmacologic effect or other direct physical action; opposite of the placebo effect.

nutrient density: Relative concentration of nutrients in the diet, which can be expressed as nutrients per calorie. Foods relatively high in vitamins and minerals and low in calories are said to be nutrient-dense.

nutripathy: Pseudoscience in which urine and saliva tests are used to detect "energy imbalances" that supposedly are correctable with various supplements and special formulas. The data are interpreted using "a mathematical formula for perfect health, based on the biologic frequencies of living matter." The formula was developed by Carey Reams, a self-proclaimed biophysicist who was prosecuted during the 1970s for practicing medicine without a license.

obese: Overweight as a result of excess fat.

obsessive-compulsive disorder: Mental problem in which people have recurrent ideas, thoughts, images, or impulses that they know are irrational but cannot control. They also may engage in repetitive actions, such as excessive handwashing, that they recognize as irrational.

occlusion: Act of closure or state of being closed or obstructed. In dentistry the term refers to the contact between upper and lower teeth (e.g., malocclusion). In medical practice it is used to describe blockage of a body passageway such as a blood vessel or duct.

occult blood: Blood in the feces in amounts too small to be seen but detectable by chemical tests.

off-label use: Prescription of a drug for a purpose that is not FDA-approved.

ombudsman: Someone who investigates complaints, reports findings, and mediates fair settlements, especially between aggrieved parties. In some hospitals patient representatives fill this role.

oncologist: Physician who specializes in the treatment of cancers.

online: Connected to a computer's central processing unit or to a computer network so that databases and/or other stored information are accessible.

open panel: Prepaid insurance plan in which any physician (or other covered type of health professional) can become a provider under the plan.

opportunistic infection: Infection by an organism that normally is harmless but is able to thrive when an individual's immunity is impaired by a serious disease (such as cancer or AIDS) or by treatment with drugs that suppress the immune system.

orthomolecular treatment: Dubious treatment method claimed to treat diseases by administering the "right" nutrient molecules (e.g., vitamins, minerals) at the right time; also called meganutrient therapy.

osteopath: Physician who is a graduate of an osteopathic medical school. Osteopathy was originally based on false beliefs but gradually abandoned them and incorporated the theories and practices of scientific medicine.

osteoporosis: Thinning of the bones, common in post-menopausal women.

otitis: Inflammation of the ear. Otitis media, the most common cause of earaches, is an inflammation of the middle ear.

outcomes research: Studies to determine whether health-care interventions meet predetermined criteria.

outpatient: Person who is treated at a facility without residing there.

over-the-counter (OTC) drugs: Nonprescription drugs.

overweight: Weighing more than the amount listed in a standard height-weight table.

ovulation: Release of a mature egg from an ovary.

palliation: Treatment that lessens symptoms but does not cure.

palpate: To examine by touching with the hands.

palpitation: Noticeably forceful heartbeat.

paradigm: Model or overall understanding of how things work. An example of a faulty paradigm is the claim by "alternative" practitioners that disease is caused by body "weaknesses" that their various methods can correct.

paranormal: Not measurable or explainable by currently accepted scientific methods or theories.

partial hospital: An outpatient psychiatric facility where patients spend 6 to 8 hours a day in a therapeutic atmosphere. Such facilities can avert hospitalizations and help hospitalized patients readjust to community living.

patent medicine: Obsolete term for medicine with a formula that was protected from being copied by a patent from the U.S. Patent Office.

patient package insert (PPI): Leaflet that tells how to use a drug; includes information on the drug's purposes, hazards, and side effects.

Patient's Bill of Rights: Lists of ethical principles that define considerate and ethical treatment in a hospital or nursing home.

pedal: Pertaining to the foot.

peer review: Formal review of clinical work, records, insurance claims, manuscripts, or research by colleagues who are assumed to have equal knowledge. The process is used by insurance companies, managed-care programs, scientific journals, research sponsors, and hospital committees.

percussion: Technique of physical examination in which a body part, usually the chest or abdomen, is tapped with the hand in order to produce a sound that reflects the density of the underlying organ(s).

periodontal disease: General term for inflammatory and degenerative diseases of the gums and other structures that surround the teeth and attach them to their sockets. The word "periodontal" comes from two Greek words meaning "around the tooth."

pharmacognosy: The science of medicines from natural sources.

photochromatic: Term applied to some eyeglass lenses that lighten or darken in response to the amount of ultraviolet light present.

phrenology: Pseudoscience based on the belief that the contours of the skull reflect the person's mental faculties and character.

physical dependence: Physiologic state in which "withdrawal" symptoms are likely to develop when use of a drug is decreased or stopped.

phytochemical: Chemical constituent of a plant.

placebo: Inert substance given with the hope that it will relieve symptoms.

placebo effect: Favorable treatment response that does not result from pharmacologic effect or other direct physical action.

plantar: Pertaining to the sole of the foot.

plaque (atherosclerotic): Deposit that builds up on the inner wall of an artery; see *atherosclerosis*.

plaque (dental): Soft, sticky, colorless, almost invisible film that continuously forms on the teeth and contains bacteria that cause dental decay and periodontal disease.

plasma (blood): The clear, yellowish fluid portion of blood in which the blood cells are suspended.

platelet: Tiny blood cell that promotes clotting.

point of service (POS) plan: Managed care that covers treatment by an HMO physician but permits patients to seek treatment elsewhere with a higher copayment. Patients do not have to choose how to receive services until they need them.

portal of entry: Health-care provider to whom patients have direct access (without referral from another provider).

positive test result: Test result suggesting that something is abnormal.

precertification: Component of managed care in which a plan representative must authorize use of a procedure in order for it to be covered by the plan; also called preauthorization. Precertification is required most often for nonemergency hospital admissions, elective surgery, or psychiatric care.

precursor: Substance from which another substance is derived; commonly used to describe an inactive substance that is converted into an active enzyme, vitamin, or hormone. Beta-carotene, for example, is a precursor of vitamin A.

preferred provider organization (PPO): Prepaid insurance plan in which member hospitals and/or physicians contract with a third-party payer to deliver services for negotiated fees, usually at a reduced rate. Beneficiaries may seek care from nonmember providers, but if they do, the out-of-pocket cost is likely to be higher.

premenstrual syndrome (PMS): Combination of physical and/or emotional symptoms that occur before menstruation and disappear or become minimal during menstrual periods; also called premenstrual tension (PMT).

prenatal care: Care of a pregnant women before birth occurs.

prescription drugs: Drugs that cannot be obtained unless ordered by a physician or other designated health professional.

prevalence: Number of cases of a disease that exist in a population at a specific time.

primary care provider: Health-care professional who provides basic health services, manages routine health-care needs, and is usually the first contact when someone needs care—typically a family practitioner, internist, or pediatrician.

proprietary drug: Drug owned by a private individual or corporation under a trademark or patent.

prosthesis: Artificial device to replace a missing body part, such as an eye or a leg.

protocol (experimental): Written description of the background, objective, design, and intended interpretation of an experiment.

pseudoscience: Theory or methodology that is represented as scientific but has no basis in science. Its proponents typically use scientific terminology and concoct evidence (or distort scientific findings) in support of their beliefs.

psychic healing: Alleged healing through exertion of a paranormal influence without the use of any physical curative agent.

psychic surgery: Sleight-of-hand fakery by individuals who pretend to remove diseased organs during "surgical procedures" that leave the skin intact.

psychomotor retardation: Slowing of the activity of the mind and body, a common finding in severe depression.

psychoneuroimmunology: Hodgepodge of theories and practices based on the idea that brain functioning affects the immune system in ways that positive thinking can modify,

psychosomatic (or psychophysiologic): Pertaining to the effect of emotions on the body.

psychosurgery: Effective but rarely needed method of relieving severe nervous symptoms by severing selected nervous pathways within the brain.

psychosis: Severe form of mental disturbance in which contact with reality is impaired.

psychotherapy: Conversational method used to treat emotional problems.

psychotropic drug: Medication capable of altering someone's mood, perception, or behavior.

puffery: Advertising that uses vague superlatives, exaggerations, or subjective opinions without specific facts.

pyorrhea: Condition in which pus oozes from an infected area, as it may in advanced cases of periodontal disease. The term is sometimes used (mainly by advertisers and laypersons) as a synonym for periodontal disease.

quackery: Promotion of an unproven health product or service, usually for personal gain.

radiograph: Image produced by x-rays passing through the body.

radiopaque: Not allowing the passage of x-rays or other radiation. Radiopaque substances appear white on x-ray films.

RDAs (Recommended Dietary Allowances): Levels of certain nutrients considered adequate to meet the needs of practically all healthy persons.

rebound (from a medication): Situation in which stopping a medication produces a withdrawal reaction opposite to that of the medication. Overuse of nosedrops, for example, can cause rebound congestion, and use of large doses of vitamin C can cause rebound scurvy.

reflexology: Pseudoscience based on beliefs that each body part is represented on the hands and feet and that pressing on the hands and feet can have therapeutic effects in other parts of the body.

regulatory letter: Letter from the FDA warning a seller to stop breaking the law. If corrective action is not taken promptly, the FDA may initiate a seizure or seek an injunction.

remission: Abatement or subsiding of the symptoms of a disease; also, the period during which the signs and symptoms of a disease disappear or are less severe.

renal: Pertaining to the kidney.

respiration: Breathing.

respirator: Device for maintaining artificial respiration.

retina: Light-sensitive membrane at the back of the eye.

risk-benefit analysis: Comparison of the likely benefits and risks of various courses of action (such as undergoing a medical treatment vs doing nothing).

risk factor: Habit, trait, or condition that is associated with increased probability of getting a particular disease, such as atherosclerotic heart disease, cancer, or osteoporosis.

roots (of a tooth): Lower portions of the teeth below the gum.

rubella: German measles.

safe and effective: Legal term used by the FDA to describe drugs that are generally recognized by experts as both safe and effective. Drugs recognized as safe or effective but not both are still considered "not safe and effective."

salt sensitivity: Tendency toward abnormal elevation of blood pressure in response to salt (sodium) intake.

schizophrenia: Any of a group of psychotic disorders typified by disordered thinking, withdrawal from reality, delusions, hallucinations, and/or various other patterns of disturbed emotions or behavior.

scientific method: Principles and procedures for the systematic pursuit of knowledge, involving data collected through observations and experiments; formulation and testing of hypotheses; and peer review.

screening test: Method to identify an unrecognized health problem by sorting out apparently well people who probably have a specific problem from those who probably do not. Abnormal or equivocal findings indicate that further evaluation is needed.

self-help groups: Groups of laypersons who help each other cope with specific problems.

semen: Whitish fluid that carries a male's spermatozoa.

sensitivity (of a test): Likelihood that a test will correctly identify people having the condition that the test is intended to detect. A highly sensitive test will detect all or nearly all with the condition and will have few false-negative results.

serum: Fluid portion of the blood obtained after removal of blood cells and fibrin clot.

"set point" theory: Theory that the body naturally gravitates toward a given weight (largely determined by genes), as if it were set by a thermostat.

sexually transmitted diseases (STDs): Diseases caused by organisms transmitted from one person to another through intimate (usually sexual) contact.

side effect: Effect of a drug that is undesirable or unrelated to the main reason for which it is prescribed.

SIDS: Sudden infant death syndrome.

sigmoidoscope: Hollow tubular instrument that can be passed through the anus into the rectum and part of the large intestine for diagnostic or therapeutic purposes.

simple carbohydrate: Sugar composed of one or two sugar molecules.

single-payer system: Centralized health-care payment system in which one entity, such as the federal government, pays for all health-care services. The best-known example is the Canadian health-care system.

skilled nursing: Rehabilitative inpatient services that include 24-hour nursing coverage.

specificity (of a test): Likelihood that a "positive" test indicates that an individual has the specific condition that the test is intended to detect. A highly specific test will have few false-positive results and often will establish the diagnosis.

speculum: Tubular instrument used to look into an opening of the body, such as the nose, ear, or vagina.

sphygmomanometer: Instrument for measuring blood pressure.

spontaneous remission: Recovery from illness without treatment.

sprain: Stretch or tear of a ligament.

STD: Abbreviation for sexually transmitted disease; formerly called VD (venereal disease).

stenosis: Narrowing of a body passageway such as an artery or duct.

strain: Stretch or tear of a muscle.

stress test: Evaluation in which an electrocardiogram is taken during gradually escalated exercise.

sun protection factor (SPF): Number indicating the degree of protection provided by a sunscreen product against ultraviolet rays. The SPF number is a multiple of the skin's exposure time before burning. SPF 15, for example, means that a person can spend 15 times as much time in the sun before burning than if the person were wearing no sunscreen.

suppository: Drug product administered by insertion into a body opening, usually the rectum or vagina, where it melts to release its active ingredient(s).

synthesis: Formation of compounds by combining simpler compounds or elements.

systemic: Term referring to the body as a whole rather than to a part of the body.

tendon: Band of tough, inelastic fibrous tissue that connects a muscle to a bone or other structure.

TENS device: Battery-powered device that delivers an electric current to an area of the body to relieve certain types of pain.

tertiary care center: Hospital or medical center that offers highly specialized care for severe health problems.

testable hypothesis: Prediction that specific circumstances will produce specific, observable results. Such hypotheses must also be falsifiable (disprovable by negative evidence).

testimonial: Claim by the user that a treatment method has been effective; not a reliable form of evidence.

thermography: Imaging procedure based on the measurement of heat radiating from the body's surface. Scientific practitioners consider thermography unreliable, but it is popular among chiropractors. In 1991 the AMA House of Delegates adopted the position that thermography has not been demonstrated to have any value as a medical diagnostic test.

third-party payer: Payment source other than patient or provider (e.g., insurance company or government program).

TMJ (temporomandibular joint): The jaw joint, which is located in front of the ear near the external ear canal.

tolerance (to a drug): Adaptation to a drug in which higher doses are needed to achieve the effects previously produced by lower doses.

topical use (of a drug): Application to a body surface.

traditional: Mode of thought or behavior that passes from one generation to another. Unscientific practitioners often use this term to describe scientific medicine and to imply that its beliefs (unlike theirs) are rigidly held. This usage is incorrect because medical science evolves in response to valid research.

traditional Chinese medicine (TCM): See *Chinese medicine, traditional*

trans fatty acids: Unsaturated fatty acids that contain one or more double bonds in which the hydrogen ions attached to the carbon atoms at the double bond are on opposite sides of the molecule.

treatment planning: Formal process whereby various staff members of a health-care facility meet regularly to discuss patients, set goals, record the steps necessary to reach the goals, and evaluate the progress of the patients. It is required for the accreditation of psychiatric facilities.

tremor: Abnormal trembling or shaking of a body part.

ultrasound device: Mechanism that transforms electrical energy into sound energy for use in diagnosis, surgery, dental care, or other therapeutic procedures.

unbundling of fees: Billing separately for components of services that should be billed as a single procedure.

United States Pharmacopoeia (USP): Authoritative volume on drugs that contains the official standards for identity, strength, and purity.

unnecessary surgery: Operation performed without a realistic expectation that it will improve the quality or length of a patient's life.

upcoding: Use of a procedure code to falsely represent that a medical service was more extensive than actually rendered.

U.S. RDAs (U.S. Recommended Daily Allowances): Simplified FDA version of the 1968 RDAs used for many years in food and dietary supplement labeling. (See Chapter 11 for current labeling standards.)

USDA: Abbreviation for United States Department of Agriculture.

utilization review: Review, based mainly on medical records, intended to determine the quality and necessity of services provided to the patient.

varicella-zoster virus: Causative agent for chickenpox in children and "shingles" in adults.

varicose: Abnormally swollen or dilated.

vascular: Pertaining to blood vessel(s).

vegan: Strict vegetarian; one who eats no products of animal origin (e.g., red meat, poultry, fish, eggs, milk, cheese, and milk products).

vertebra: Bony segment of the spine that encircles and helps protect the spinal cord and nerves. The plural of vertebra is vertebrae.

vertically integrated system: Health-care system that provides primary care, specialty care, and hospital care under one umbrella.

viscera: The soft internal organs of the body, especially those contained within the abdomen and chest.

vision therapy: Unscientific system of eye exercises claimed to strengthen eyesight and improve learning disabilities.

vitalism: The concept that organisms function because of a "vital principle" or "life force" distinct from the physical forces explainable by the laws of physics and chemistry. Health systems based on this notion (e.g., naturopathy, homeopathy, and traditional chiropractic) maintain that diseases should be treated by "stimulating the body's ability to heal itself" rather than by "treating symptoms."

withdrawal reaction: Symptoms that occur following stoppage or reduced use of a drug upon which someone has become physically dependent.

yo-yo dieting: Repeated weight-loss (through dieting) followed by weight gain; also called weight cycling.

INDEX

A

AARP Pharmacy Service, 438
Abbott Laboratories, 237, 239
Abdominal toners, 318
Abortion, voluntary, 468–469
Abrams, Dr. Albert, 366, 491
Abravanel, Dr. Elliot, 281t, 288
Academy of Certified Social Workers
   (ACSW), 101
Accardo, Pasquale, 15
Accepting assignment, 527
Access to Medical Treatment Act, 173,
   264
Accreditation, 11, 12t, 22, 574
   of acupuncture schools, 22, 143–144
   of ambulatory care centers, 197
   of ambulatory surgical centers, 199
   of chiropractic schools, 22, 147–148
   limitations of, 143
   of managed-care organizations, 524–
      525
   of hospitals, 88, 196, 199–200
   of medical schools, 72
   of naturopathic schools, 22
   of pharmacy schools, 409
Accreditation Association for Ambulatory
   Health Care (AAAHC), 199
Accutane, 447
Acer, Dr. David, 398
Acesulfame K, 288–289
Acetaminophen, 363, 422–423, 422t, 574
Acidophilus, 247t
Acidosis, 574
Acne, 321, 446–447, 466, 561
Acne-Statin, 561
Acquired Immunodeficiency Syndrome;
   see AIDS
ACSM Fitness Book, 307
Activated charcoal, 247t
Activities of daily living (ADLs), 574
Acupressure, 141, 182t, 191, 262, 574
Acupressure earrings, 290
Acupuncture, 141–144, 574
   anesthesia, 142
   and arthritis, 368
   complications, 142–143
   points, 141
   reasons to avoid, 143
   and smoking cessation, 183
Acute condition, 574
Acyclovir, 425–426
Adams, Samuel Hopkins, 550
Addiction, 574
   to smokeless tobacco products, 133
   to *Valium*, 104, 105

Additives
   color, in cosmetics, 442, 557
   food, 110, 251, 371, 377, 553–554
Adequate intake (AI), 217
Administrative complaint, 574
Administrative medicine, 574
Adrenal insufficiency, 166

Adrenaline (epinephrine), 420, 574
Advance medical directives, 107, 496–
   499, 574
Advanced Medical Technology
   Association, 478
Advertising and marketing, 47–67
   AIDS-related, 400–401
   alcohol, 7, 48–49
   antioxidant, 240
   cancer "cures," 378, 381
   chiropractic, 52, 147
   chelation therapy, 170
   cigarette, 7, 48, 59–60
   complaints, where to send, 566t
   corrective, 559
   cosmetic, 48
   costs, 50
   dental, 51, 52
   dietary supplement, 56–58
   ergogenic aids; *see* "Ergogenic aids"
   exercise and fitness products, 63–64,
      319
   food, 7, 56, 58t, 346
   FTC regulation, 51, 56–58, 67, 558–561
   hair analysis, 261–262
   health claims on food labels, 227, 229,
      229t
   hearing aids, 488
   homeopathic products, 58t, 157, 369
   hospital, 53
   influence on magazine contents, 22, 23,
      40, 51, 59
   industry self-regulation, 66–67
   infomercials, 61t, 64, 108
   "low cholesterol" claims, 346
   mail order; *see* Mail-order frauds
   medical ethics and, 51
   misleading nature of, 24, 36–37, 48–50
   misuse of statistics, 18–19
   mouthwash, 126
   multilevel marketing; *see* Multilevel
      marketing
   National Advertising Review Board,
      66–67
   nonprescription drug, 55–56, 237, 416–
      417
   "nutrition insurance," 58t, 238t, 566
   osteopathic, 75
   outlets, 50–51
   patent medicine, 414
   penis enlargement, 455–456
   prescription drug, 53–55
   professional, 51–52
   psychologic manipulation, 48–50, 60
   puffery, 6, 50
   purpose of, 48
   Rodale Press, 63, 265
   sauna devices, 321
   targeting of women, 60
   techniques commonly used, 6–7, 48–50,
      49t
   telemarketing schemes, 66, 151, 489,
      561, 563, 564

   tobacco products, 7, 59–60
   vitamin, 24, 48, 238t
   weasel words, 6, 50
   weight-related claims, 8, 62, 63, 287,
      291, 293
   youth and beauty aids, 62, 63
Aerobic exercise, 304, 574
"Aerobic glasses," 485
"Aerobic oxygen," 561
Aerobics and Fitness Association of
   America, 312t
Ageless Body, Timeless Mind, 167
Agency for Health Care Policy and
   Research (AHCPR), 20, 148
Agency for Health Care Research and
   Quality (AHRQ), 20,
Agranulocytosis, 369
AID (Automated Immunostatus
   Differential) test, 386
AIDS, 395–403, 574
   and cancer, 386, 396
   clinical course, 396–397
   conspiracy theories, 401
   costs, 399–400
   diagnostic criteria, 396–397
   incidence, 396
   prevention, 397–399
   quackery and fraud, 395, 400–403
   testing, 397, 402
   transmission, 397–399, 400
   treatment 399, 556
Aigner, Claire, 258
Alcock, James E., 163
Alcohol
   and cancer, 182, 374, 378
   caloric content, 575
   danger during pregnancy, 182
   dietary guideline, 216t
   and HDL, 349
   and heart disease, 181–182, 349
   "moderate intake," 349
   and NSAIDs, 423
   in OTC drugs, 415
   in patent medicines, 413
   recommended limit, 181–182
   and sleep disturbances, 433
Alexander, Dale, 367
Alexander technique, 167
Alfalfa, 247t
Alfin Fragrances, Inc., 444–445
Alivizatos, Dr. Hariton, 385
Alkalosis, 574
Allergic conditions, 418–420, 574
   desensitization shots, 187, 419
   and electrodermal skin testing, 156
   latex allergy, 490–491
Allied health care personnel, 77t, 120–121
Allopathy, 574
Aloe vera, 247t, 402–403
Alopecia areata, 449, 574
Alpha-fetoprotein screening, 470, 471t
Alpha hydroxy acids, 445
"Alternative agriculture," 245

"Alternative" methods, 7, 22, 137–175, 574; *see also* Quackery and frauds
acupressure, 141, 182t, 191, 262, 574
acupuncture; *see* Acupuncture
and AIDS, 401
anthroposophical medicine, 155–156, 574
applied kinesiology, 262, 575
arthritis and; *see* Arthritis, questionable treatment
astrology, 115, 164
ayurvedic medicine, 166–167, 575
biorhythms, 164–165
cancer and; *see* Cancer treatment, questionable
chelation therapy, 38, 171–172, 355
chiropractic, 144–151; *see also* Chiropractors
classification by NIH, 138
definitions, 36, 138–140, 574
dental; *see* Dentistry, dubious
and drug compounding, 410
fad diagnoses, 38, 132, 168–171
faith healing; *see* Psychic healing
herbal therapy; *see* Herbs and herbal remedies
"holistic medicine," 172–173
homeopathy, 154–158, 583
iridology, 65, 153–154, 580
lack of supporting data, 21, 139
Maharishi Ayur-Ved, 166–167
natural hygiene, 152
naturopathy, 151–152
misleading publicity about, 141
occult practices, 162–164
orthomolecular therapy, 109–110, 581
prevalence of use, 138
psychic healing; *see* Psychic healing
questions for evaluating, 139
reasons for seeking, 141
reflexology, 144, 583
research grants from NIH, 174
satisfaction with, 168
supportive organizations, 172–173
susceptibility to; *see* Quackery, susceptibility to
therapeutic touch, 162
transcendental meditation (TM), 165–167
unscientific medical practices, 168–174
victims of; *see* Quackery, victims of
visual training, 112, 167, 584
yoga, 167
Alternatives to Abortion, 468
Altschul, Dr. Aaron, 297
AMA; *see* American Medical Association
Ambulatory care centers, 197–198
Ambulatory health care, 574
Ambulatory surgery, 88, 198–199
American Academy of Allergy, Asthma, and Immunology, 169, 170, 491
American Academy of Biological Dentistry, 132

American Academy of Dermatology, 452
American Academy of Environmental Medicine, 173
American Academy of Ophthalmology, 112, 483
American Academy of Otolaryngic Allergy, 173
American Academy of Pediatrics, 56, 83, 89, 110, 111, 112, 167, 223, 225, 244, 322
American Advertising Federation, 66
American Association for Accreditation for Ambulatory Surgery Facilities, 199
American Association for Anti-Aging Medicine, 508
American Association for Ayurvedic Medicine, 167
American Association for Marriage and Family Therapy (AAMFT), 101
American Association of Colleges of Pharmacy, 409
American Association of Endodontists, 128
American Association of Naturopathic Physicians, 151, 152
American Association of Nutritional Consultants, 257, 260, 261
American Association of Retired Persons (AARP), 66, 399, 438, 506, 564
American Association of Sex Educators, Counselors, and Therapists (AASECT), 101–102
American Biologics, 391
American Board of Anti-Aging Health Professionals, 508
American Board of Genetic Counseling, 469–470
American Board of Medical Genetics, 469
American Board of Medical Specialties, 52, 72–73, 78–79, 453
American Board of Nutrition, 230
American Board of Opticianry/National Contact Lens Examiners, 481
American Board of Psychiatry and Neurology, 100
American Cancer Society, 161, 374, 377, 381, 392, 473, 502, 564
cancer detection recommendations, 83–84, 185
American Chiropractic Association (ACA), 146
American College of Advancement in Medicine, 173
American College of Gastroenterology, 425
American College of Health Science, 282
American College of Nurse-Midwives, 76
American College of Physicians, 339
Clinical Efficacy Project, 20
American College of Sports Medicine, 305, 306, 312t
American College of Surgeons, 87

American Council on Exercise, 312t
American Council on Pharmaceutical Education, 409
American Council on Science and Health (ACSH), 28, 45, 59, 61, 222, 230, 258, 288, 378, 398, 455, 473, 554, 565
evaluation of nutrition articles, 24t, 25
American Dental Association (ADA), 120, 129, 133, 523
Council on Dental Therapeutics, 125, 128
Council on Scientific Affairs, 125
Seal of Acceptance, 123
American Dietetic Association, 225, 230, 231, 254, 323
American Endodontic Society, 128
American Federation of Home Care Providers, 202
American Health Care Association, 203
American Heart Association, 172, 183, 241, 282, 306, 307, 333, 334, 348
American Holistic Medical Association (AHMA), 173
American Holistic Nurses Association, 173
American Holistic Veterinary Medical Association, 173
American Hospital Association, 72, 201
American Institute of Nutrition, 230
American Lung Association, 183
American Medical Association (AMA), 73, 79, 94, 182, 418, 527, 543, 574
and advertising by physicians, 51
and cigarette advertising, 60
Committee on Allied Health Education and Accreditation, 77
Council on Ethical and Judicial Affairs, 79, 498, 537
Council on Foods and Nutrition, 254, 280
Council on Medical Education, 72
Council on Scientific Affairs, 19, 81, 142, 154, 325–326, 453, 495
Diagnostic and Therapeutic Technology Assessment (DATTA), 19
and health-care reform, 543
and HIV testing, 399
suit against, by chiropractors, 148–149
American Medical Directory, 78
American Mental Health Counselors Association, 101
American Natural Hygiene Society, 152
American Nurses Association, 75, 101
American Nurses Credentialing Center (ANCC), 75
American Optometric Association, 481, 485
American Osteopathic Association, 75
American Pharmaceutical Association, 409
American Podiatric Medical Association, 75
American Preventive Medical Association, 45, 173, 264

American Psychiatric Association, 109–110, 116
American Psychological Association, 101, 111–112
Amercan Public Health Association, 399
American Self-Help Clearinghouse, 192
American Sleep Disorders Association, 433
American Society for AIDS Prevention, 402
American Society for Clinical Nutrition, 230
American Society for Laser Medicine and Surgery, 89
American Society of Plastic and Reconstructive Surgeons, 453, 456
American Speech-Language-Hearing Association, 487
Amino acids, 212, 574
    as "growth hormone releasers," 287, 326
    supplements, unsubstantiated use, 241–242
    L-tryptophan, 259, 434
Aminopyrine, 369
Amniocentesis, 470
Amphetamines, 283
Amway Corporation, 64–65
Amygdalin; see Laetrile
Anabolic steroids, 325–326, 326t
Anabolism, 574
Anaerobic exercise, 304, 574
Analgesics, 574
    acetaminophen; see Acetaminophen
    adverse effects, 422t
    aspirin; see Aspirin
    for arthritis pain, 361–363, 364
    combinations, 421
    comparison of, 422t
    costs, 363, 423
    external, 364, 420–421, 574
    ibuprofen; see Ibuprofen
    internal, 421–423, 574
    ketoprofen, 422t, 423
    for menstrual distress, 461
    naproxen, 422t, 423
    and toothache, 127
Anaphylactic shock, 421, 574
Androgenic steroid, 574
Anderson, Dr. Terence W., 242
Anecdotal evidence, 17, 21, 574
Anemia
    aplastic, 425, 452, 575
    iron-deficiency, 431
    pernicious, 76
Anencephaly, 503
Anesthesia, 574
    dental, 130
Angina pectoris, 17, 335
Angiography, 353
Angioplasty, 355, 574
Animal magnetism, 104, 159
Ankylosing spondylitis, 360
Anorexia nervosa, 278, 574

Antacids, 423–424, 424t, 574
Anthroposophical medicine, 155–156, 574
Antiaging claims
    nutrition-related, 507
    for skin products, 444–445
Antianxiety drugs, 103–104
Antibiotics, 424–426
Antibodies, 574
Antidepressants, 104, 362
    Prozac, 114, 458
Antigen, 418, 574
Antihistamines, 419, 419t, 428, 574
Antimanic agents, 104
Antimicrobials, 426, 574
Antineoplastons, 384
Antioxidants, 23, 240–241, 377, 508, 553, 574
Antiperspirants, 446
Antipruritic, 575
Antipsychotic drugs, 104
Antipyretic drugs, 428, 575
Anxiety attack, 106
"Aphrodisiacs," 426–427, 575
Aplastic anemia, 425, 452, 575
Apocrine glands, 446
Appetite suppressants, 283–284
Applied kinesiology, 262, 575
Aptitude tests, 114
Aquaculture Corporation, 367
Aromatherapy, 167
Aronson, Virginia, 213, 225, 261, 297
Arrhythmia, 575
Arteriosclerosis, 575
Arthritis, 359–371
    common types, 360–361
    guidelines for sufferers, 371
    sources of information, 370–371
    spontaneous remission, 364–365
    treatment, questionable, 365–370
        acupuncture, 368
        aloe vera, 368
        clotrimazole, 368
        devices, dubious, 365–366
        dietary methods, 367
        DMSO, 368, 369, 507
        environmental approaches, 366–377
        medications, dangerous use of, 369, 370
        unethical clinics, 369–370
        venoms, 368
        vitamin/mineral supplements, 367–368
    treatment, scientific, 361–364
        medications, 361–363
        patient's role, 364
        physical treatment measures, 363
        surgery, 363–364
        "weather myth," 367
Arthritis Foundation, 360, 362, 363, 365, 367, 368, 370, 557
Arthritis Today, 370
Artificial sweeteners, 223, 278, 288–289
Asbestos, and cancer, 375
Ascorbic acid; see Vitamin C

Aseptic, 575
Aslan, Dr. Anna, 508
Aspartame, 111, 288
Aspirin, 421–422, 422t
    and arthritis, 361, 362–363
    and cardiovascular disease, 19, 347–348, 422
    in cold remedies, 428
    enteric-coated, 421
    hazards, 412, 421–422, 422t
    and toothache, 127
Assignment of benefits, 515t, 527
Assisted living, 575
Association of American Medical Colleges, 72
Association of National Advertisers, 66
Asthma, bronchial, 187, 418
Astigmatism, 480, 575
Astrology, 115, 164
Astro-Trimmer, 290
Asymptomatic, definition, 575
Atheromas, 334–335
Atherosclerosis, 575
    progression, 334–335
    regression, 345
Athlete's foot, 427
Atkins, Dr. Robert, 265–266, 280
Atkins Diet, 280, 281t
Attention deficit disorder, 105, 110
Audiologists, 77t
Audiometry, 486
Auditing, in Dianetics, 114
Aura, 22
Auriculotherapy, 132
Autism, 575
    questionable treatments, 111–112
Autointoxication theory, 431, 575
Autonomic nervous system, 575
Autopsy, 503
Aversive therapy, 103
Avogadro's number, 155
Avon Products, Inc., 444–445
Ayds, 286
Ayurvedic medicine, 166–167, 575

B
Bach remedies, 108
Back pain, and chiropractors, 148–149
Bad breath, 126
Balance billing, 575
Balanced diet, 575
"Balancing body chemistry," 130, 131
Balch, James and Phyllis, 257
Baldness, 62, 449–450
Barnard, Dr. Christiaan, 445
Barnes, Dr. Carl, 388
Barnum effect, 164
Barrett, Dr. Lisa Feldman, 19
Barrett, Dr. Stephen, v, 7, 22, 23, 25, 42, 43, 123, 137, 139, 155, 213, 217, 225, 240, 244, 258, 260, 267, 297, 364, 367, 410, 558, 565
    investigations by, 25, 64, 67, 188, 262, 551

Basal cell carcinoma, 451
Basic Four Food Groups, 219
Bassler, Dr. Thomas, 303
Bastyr University, 152, 157
Bates method of eye exercise, 480
Battle Creek Sanitarium, 255, 431
Beard Anthrone Test, 386
Beard, H.H., 386
Bee pollen, 247t
Begoun, Paula, 441, 445, 448
Behavioral modification
    and emotional problems, 103
    and weight control, 297
Beltone Electronics Corp., 488
Benecol, 349
Benzocaine, 127, 285, 429
Benzoyl peroxide, 447
Berard, Guy, 111
Berger, Dr. Stuart, 257
Bergman, Dr. Thomas F., 147
Bernadean University, 261
Best, A.M., 523
Beta-carotene, 240–241, 348–349
Beta-glucan, 345
Better Business Bureau, 97, 506; *see also*
    Council of Better Business Bureaus
Beverly Hills Diet, 26, 282
BHT, 508, 574
Bianchini, Magaly, 39
Bias, statistical, 18
Bicycle helmets, 316
Bicycles
    mountain, 316
    stationary, 312, 313t
Bigelow, Charles, 414
Bile, 575
Bill of Rights, 582
    consumer, ix, 548, 576
    hospital, 201, 582
    managed care, 519
    nursing home, 205, 582
Biochemical individuality, 217, 219
Bioequivalence (of drugs), 422, 575
Biofeedback, 103, 575
    questionable gadgets, 108
Bioflavonoids, 236, 247t, 575
Biologic drug product, 575
Biological Homeopathic Industries, 157
Biological response modifiers, 376
Biomagnetic imaging, 87
Biopsy, 575
Biorhythms, 164–165, 575
Biotechnology, definition, 575
Biotin, 214
Birth control; *see* Contraception
Birthright USA, 468
Black Pearls, 369
Blackburn, Dr. George, 271, 279, 289
Blackstrap molasses, 247t
Bland, Dr. Jeffrey S., 291–292
Blood chemistry tests, 82
Blood count, complete, 81
Blood pressure
    high; *see* High blood pressure

measurement, 187–188
    and sodium intake, 225, 229t, 350, 351
Blood sugar tests, 81, 168–169, 187
Blood tests, common, 81–82
Board-certified specialist, 575
Board-eligible, 575
Body mass index (BMI), 272, 273, 274t,
    575
Body odor, 446
"Body types,"
    and ayurveda, 166
    of Dr. Abravanel, 288
Body wrapping, 63, 289
Bodybuilding, questionable products for;
    see "Ergogenic aids"
Bodywork, 575
Bonding, dental, 127
Bone density, 471–472
Bone meal, 247t
Bone scan, 575
Boron, 247t, 327
Bottled water, 489
Bovine albumin, 444t
Bovine somatotropin (BST), 555
Bradford, Robert, 391
"Brain wave synchronizers," 8–9, 108
Bran, 213, 575
    oat, 229, 343, 345
Brandt, Joanna, 382
Brant, Freddie, 92
Braswell, A. Glenn, 61, 63, 451
Breast developers, 25, 62, 63
Breast implants, 453, 454t, 455
Breast self-examination, 83, 375
Breastfeeding, 223, 471
Brewer's yeast, 247t
Brigden, Dr. Malcolm, 379
Brody, Jane, 276
Brog, Roy, 560
Brown, Helene, 373
Brownell, Dr. Kelly, 275
Bulimia, 277t, 278
Bulk producers, 285–286
Bursa, 575
Burton, Dr. Lawrence, 387–388
Burzynski, Dr. Stanislaw R., 384
Buyer's clubs, 400

C
Cabbage soup diet, 282
CABG; *see* Coronary bypass
Cadaver, 575
Caffeine, 105, 186, 249t, 421, 434t, 435
    and insomnia, 433–434
Caisse, Rene M., 381
Cal-Ban 3000, 291
Calcium, and osteoporosis, 225, 229t, 245,
    471–472
Calcium propionate, 554
Calculus, 575
    dental, 124, 129
California Medical Association, 37–38
Callahan Roger J., 113
Callus remedies, 427

Calorie(s)
    definition of, 575
    inaccurate food labeling, 287
    and weight loss, 274–275
Cameron, Dr. Ewan, 242–243
Camphor, as cough suppressant, 428
CanCell, 383
Cancer, 373–393
    and AIDS, 386, 396
    and alcohol use, 182, 374, 378
    and antioxidants, 240–241
    and birth control pills, 466–467
    breast, 83
    causes, 374–375
    and cigarette smoking, 374
    detection, 83–84, 84–85t
        mammography, 84, 85t
        occult blood test, 83–84, 185, 187
        Pap test, 79, 83, 84–85t
        prostate-specific antigen (PSA) test,
            83
        self-examination for, 84
    diagnosis, 375
    and diet, 229t, 374, 375, 376–378
    and hormone-replacement therapy, 473
    immune surveillance theory, 386
    incidence, 374
    insurance coverage for, 518
    and mouthwash, 126
    and "positive attitudes," 386
    and power lines, 375, 493
    prevention, 375, 377–378
        questionable supplements for, 378
    prognosis, 375–376
    prostate, 83–84
    questionable methods, 37, 380, 381–392
        antineoplastons, 384
        CanCell, 383
        corrosive agents, 381
        devices, 385
        diagnostic tests, worthless, 386–387
        diets and dietary supplements, 382–
            383
        Essiac, 381
        fiber-containing pills, 378
        fresh cell therapy, 385
        Gerson diet, 383
        grape cure, 382
        Greek cancer cure, 385
        Hoxsey treatment, 380
        hydrazine sulfate, 383–384
        hyperoxygenation therapies, 383
        Iscador, 383
        immuno-augmentative therapy (IAT),
            387–388
        Krebiozen, 380
        Laetrile, 22–23, 45, 22–23, 388–399,
            557
        Livingston-Wheeler treatment, 385
        "metabolic" therapy, 389
        Mucorhicin, 381
        pau d'arco tea, 382
        promotion of, 22–23, 379, 390–392
        psychologic approaches, 385–386

Cancer—cont'd.
    questionable methods—cont'd.
        Revici Cancer Control, 384–385
        shark cartilage, 382–383
        714X, 384
        vitamin C, 242–243
    reliable information about, 392
    risk factors, 374–375
    skin, 451
    smokeless products and, 133
    spontaneous remission, 376
    testicular, 83
    treatment
        clinical trials, 376
        evidence-based methods, 376
        experimental approaches, 376
        guidelines, 392
        new methods, standards for
            investigation of, 381
        tumor registries, 376
        warning signals, 375
Cancer Control Society, 391
Cancer Treatment Centers of America, 58t,
    392
Candidiasis, 463. 560
"Candidiasis hypersensitivity," 170, 575
CANHELP, 391
Canthaxanthin, 452
Capitation, 515t, 523, 575
Caplet, 575
Caplinger, Gregory Earl, 37
Capsaicin, 364
Carbohydrate loading, 324
Carbohydrates, 212–213
    complex, 212, 576
    fermentable, 578
    food sources, 219t
    simple, 212
Carbon monoxide detectors, 183
Carcinogenic, definition, 575
Carcinoma, 575
    in situ, 575
Cardiac catheterization, 353
Cardiorespiratory efficiency, 305, 575
Cardiovascular disease, 333–356
    and aspirin, 19, 347, 422
    and cholesterol levels; *see* Cholesterol
    and coffee consumption, 335
    coronary heart disease, 334–335, 334t
    and cigarette smoking, 181, 335
    and diet, 229t, 340–346, 344t
    diagnostic tests, 352–354
    and estrogens, 472–473
    heart attacks, 351–352
    high blood pressure; *see* High blood
        pressure
    and homocysteine levels, 337
    prevention advice, 350
    prevalence, 334, 334t, 335
    questionable preventive methods, 348–
        349
    rehabilitation programs, 355
    risk factors, 334–337
    stroke, 334t, 349–350

surgery for, 354–355
in women, 334, 340
Caridex, 127
Caries; *see* Tooth decay
Carnegie Foundation, 73
Carob, 247t
Carotene, 575
Carter's Little Pills, 432t, 560
CAT scan, 86, 576
Cat's claw, 253t
Catabolism, 575
"Catalyst-altered water," 247
Cataracts, 480, 483, 485–486, 576
Caveat emptor doctrine, 48, 576
Caveat vendor doctrine, 576
Cavitational osteopathosis, 132
CD4 cells, 396–397
CDC; *see* U.S. Centers for Disease Control
    and Prevention
Cease-and-desist order, 559, 576
Cell salts, 157
Cellasene, 290
Cellulite, 62, 63, 289–290, 445, 576
Cellulose, 285, 576
Cementum, 124
Center for Advancement for Cancer
    Education, 391
Center for Health Economics Research,
    532
Center for Science in the Public Interest
    (CSPI), 564
Center for the Study of Services, 525
Cephalosporins, 425
Certified milk, 250t
Cervical cap, 465, 465t
Cervix, 576
Cesarean sections, 470
Chakras, 576
Chamlee, C.R., 380, 381
CHAMPUS, 110, 576
Channeling, 163
Chelated minerals, 247-250t
Chelation therapy, 38, 170–171, 355
Chemosurgery, 576
"Chemotherapeutic revolution," 551
Chemotherapy, 376
Chewing tobacco, 133–134
Chi, 140, 141–142
Chicken soup, 17
CHILD, Inc., 160
Child psychiatrists, 100
Childbirth options, 470–471
Chinese medicine, 141–144, 576
Chiropodists; *see* Podiatrists0
Chiropractors, 144–151, 576
    advertising, 52, 147
    antitrust suit by, 149
    avoiding trouble with, 151
    boycott attempt by, 23
    and children, 150
    education, 147–148
    and holistic centers, 172
    and naturopathy, 152
    and nutrition, 150, 260, 262

opposition to immunization, 150
organizations, 146
problems for consumers, 149–151
"preventive maintenance" by, 139, 150
and spinal ultrasound, 87
straights vs. mixers, 146
and "subluxations," 146–147, 150, 151
undercover investigations of, 150
Chitosan, 248t, 286
Chloramphenicol, 425
Chlorhexidine, 126
Chlorophyll, 248t
Cho Lo Tea, 348
Cholecystectomy, 89
Cholecystokinin (CCK), 287
Cholesterol, 214, 335, 576; *see also*
    Lipids, blood
    dietary, 339t, 340
    and CHD death rate, 337
    controversy about screening, 339–340
    and fish oils, 349
    and food advertising, 346
    guidelines, 337–340, 338t
    home testing, 340
    lowering, guidebooks for, 344t
    HDL; *see* HDL
    LDL; *see* LDL
    NCEP classification, 33t
    and obesity, 274, 335
    scam, 348
    testing, 82, 337–338, 340
Choline, 248t
Chondroitin sulfate, 368
Chopra, Dr. Deepak, 27, 166–167
Chorionic villus sampling (CVS), 470
Christian Brothers, 557
Christian Dior Perfumes, Inc., 444–445
Christian Science, 159–160
Christian Science Sentinel, 160
Chromium picolinate, 248t, 286, 292, 327
Chromosome defects, 469
Chronic condition, definition, 576
Chronic fatigue syndrome, 170–171, 576
Chronobiology, 165
Chuifong Toukuwan, 369
Cider vinegar, 248t
Cigarette advertising, 7, 59–60
Cigarette smoking, 181, 335, 374
Circumcision, 89
CITECH, 480
Citizen's Commission on Human Rights,
    114
Citizens for Health, 45, 264, 267
City of Faith, 159
Civil procedure, 576
Clark, Hulda, 381–382
Clark, Dr. Nancy, 325
Clenbuterol, 326, 327
Clinical, definition, 576
Clinical ecology, 169–170, 576
Clinical mental health counselors, 101
Clinical trials, 17, 18, 376, 384, 556, 576
Clinton Health Plan, 542–543
Clinton, Hillary Rodham, 3, 513, 541

Closed-panel HMO, 576
Clostridium difficile, 426
Clotrimazole, 368
Clove oil, 127
Coagulate, 76
Cochrane Collaboration, 20
Cochrane, John D., 96
Codeine, 428
Coenzyme Q$_{10}$, 248t, 349, 507
Coffee enemas, 383, 385, 387, 389
Cognitive therapy, 102–103
Co-insurance, 515t, 576
Cold reading, 164
Cold-pressed oils, 248t
Colds, remedies for, 427–429
Colitis, pseudomembranous, 426
Collagen injections, 447, 454t
Colonic irrigation, 576
Colonoscope, 575, 576
Comedos, 446, 447, 576
Commission E Report, 252
Committee for Freedom of Choice in
    Medicine (CFCM), 45, 391
Committee for the Scientific Investigation
    of Claims of the Paranormal
    (CSICOP), 163, 164, 565
*Compendium of Certified Medical
    Specialists*, 78
"Complementary medicine," 139, 576
Complete protein, 576
Complex carbohydrates, 212, 576
Comprehensive Smokeless Tobacco
    Health Education Act (1986), 133
Computerized axial tomography (CT or
    CAT), 86
Computerized tests for "nutrient
    deficiency," 130, 263
Condoms, 464–465, 465t
Conference of Funeral Service Examining
    Boards, 506
Confidentiality, 576
Confirmatory test, 576
Congenital, definition, 576
Connolly, Dr. Gregory, 133
Conrad, Ruth, 39
Consent decree (or order), 576
Consolidated Omnibus Budget
    Reconciliation Act (1986), 197, 517
Conspiracy claims by quacks, 44, 401
Constipation, 213, 431
Consultations, 95
Consumer Bill of Rights, 576
Consumer Federation of America, 564
Consumer health
    definition of, 4, 576
    "I.Q. test," 4
    questions pertaining to, 5, 13
Consumer Health Digest, 565
Consumer Health Education Council, 405
Consumer Health Sourcebook Web site,
    548
Consumer Healthcare Products
    Association, 416
Consumer Information Center, 563

Consumer Justice Center, 493
Consumer Product Safety Commission,
    312, 479, 563
Consumer protection, 547–567; *see also*
    Enforcement actions; Intelligent
    health consumer; Physicians,
    effective communication with
    analysis of forces, 11–12, 12t
    basic principles, 45, 548, 567
    consumer action, 566t, 567
    federal agencies, 563; *see also* Federal
        Trade Commission; Food and Drug
        Administration; U.S. Postal Service
    laws; *see under* Laws
    need for, 11
    nongovernmental organizations, 563–
        566
        business, 565–566
        professional, 566
        voluntary, 564–565
    state and local agencies, 392, 563
Consumer Protection Report, 563
Consumer Reports, 10, 25, 24t, 50, 81, 106
    122, 125, 132, 151, 158, 171, 187,
    195, 203, 205, 251, 252, 257, 259,
    275, 276, 284, 287, 294, 301, 312,
    316, 318, 325, 351, 412, 428, 430,
    431, 433, 446, 448, 452, 459, 460,
    472, 482, 485, 487, 489, 490, 509,
    521, 524, 525, 531, 551
Consumer Reports Books, 27, 195
Consumer Reports on Health, 26t, 32, 55,
    125, 201, 284, 297, 301, 420, 423,
    432 445, 486, 496
Consumers Digest, 317, 504, 505
Consumers Research, 134
Consumers Union, 173, 398, 534, 543, 564
Contact dermatitis, 418
Contact lenses, 482, 484–485, 484t
Continental Association of Funeral and
    Memorial Societies, 505
Continuing medical education (CME), 576
Continuous passive motion (CPM) tables,
    318
Contraception, 463–468, 464–465t, 576
    barrier methods, 464–466, 465t
    cervical cap, 465, 465t
    condom, female, 464, 465t
    condom, male, 464–465, 465t
    diaphragm, 464, 465t
    emergency, 465t, 467
    fertility awareness (rhythm) methods,
        463–464, 465t
    hormonal methods, 464t, 466–467
    intrauterine devices (IUD), 461, 464t,
        466
    major types, 463, 465t
    spermicides, 465, 465t
    surgical sterilization, 464t, 467–468
    vaginal sponge, 465–466, 465t
    withdrawal, 465t
Contracture, 576
Contraindication, definition, 576
Contreras, Dr. Ernesto, 388

Conversion (of insurance policy), 515t,
    517
Cooper, Dr. Kenneth, 303, 307
Coordination of benefits, 515t, 517, 576
Copayment, 515t
Copeland, Caroline, 39–40
Copeland, Sen. Royal, 155
Copper bracelets, 365
Cornea, 576
Corns, 427
Coronary bypass surgery, 354–355
Corrective advertising, 559
Cosmetic(s)
    for aging skin and wrinkles, 444–445
    camouflage, 456
    categories, 442
    definition, 442, 576
    fade creams, 446
    laws pertaining to, 442, 556–557
    marketing of, 48
    moisturizers, 443–444
    questionable claims, 444–445
    questionable ingredients, 444t
    safety precautions, 443
    shampoos, 447–448
    soaps, 442–443
Cosmetic surgery, 438, 452–456, 454t
    breast enlargement, 453, 454t, 455
    fees, 454t
    liposuction, 290, 292, 454t
    physician selection for, 453
Cough and cold remedies, 415, 427–429
Council for Agricultural Science and
    Technology (CAST), 230, 553
Council for Responsible Nutrition, 263,
    267
Council of Better Business Bureaus, 558,
    566
    National Advertising Division, 66–67,
        239, 566
Council on Chiropractic Education (CCE),
    147
Council on Naturopathic Medical
    Education, 152
Council on Recognition of Postsecondary
    Accreditation (CORPA), 22, 143, 574
Council on Social Work Education, 101
Counterirritants, 421, 577
CPT codes, 527, 528t, 529, 577
Crampton, Lynn and Dale, 243
Cranial osteopathy, 130–131
Creatine, 328
Credentials, dubious, 91, 109, 260–261,
    264, 266, 282, 390
Crelin, Dr. Edmund, 147
Cremation, 504, 505
Criminal Fines Enhancement Act (1984),
    557, 562
Croft, John, 367
Cromolyn, 420
Crook, Dr. William J., 170
Crown, of tooth, 577
Cruzan, Nancy, 499
Cryonics, 509

Cryosurgery, 447, 577
CTR International, 558t
Cuforhedake Brane-Fude, 550
Cult, definition, 577
Curanderas, 140
Curare, 252
Cure for All Cancers, 382
Current Procedural Terminology, 527
Custodial care, 203
Cystoscope, 577

D
Dahlberg, Inc., 488
Daily Reference Values (DRVs), 226, 577
Daily Values (DVs), 226–227, 226t, 553
Dandruff, 448
Dark-field microscopy, 262
DASH diet, 351
Database, 577
Davis, Adelle, 21–22, 265
Davis, Dr. Edward H., 21
Deafness, 486, 487t
Death
    coping with, 495–509
    body disposition methods, 503–506
    certificates, 503
Decibels, 486, 487t
Decongestants, 428, 577
Defensive medicine, 11, 89, 528, 577
Defibrillator, 581
Deficiency diseases, 222
Dehydroepiandrosterone (DHEA), 248t,
    287, 598
Delaney Clause, 549, 553–554
DeLeo, Dr. Vincent, 445
Delusion, 577
Dementia, 577
Densitometry, 472
Dental care, 119–135, 183
    advertisements for, 51, 52
    anesthesia, 130
    auxiliary personnel, 120–121
    bonding of teeth, 127
    dentifrices, 124–125, 577
    dentures, 128–129
    dentists, selection of, 134–135
    denturists, 121, 128–129
    disclosing solutions, 124
    endodontics, 120, 127–128, 131
    fees, 134–135, 535t
    floss and toothpicks, 125–126
    fluoridation; *see* Fluoridation
    implants, 129
    insurance for, 523
    irrigators, 126
    laser drilling, 130
    mouthwashes, 126
    orthodontics, 120, 128
    pain relievers, 127
    periodontal disease, 123–124
    products, 124–127
    quackery, 130–133
    questionable, 130
    restorations, 127

sealants, 122
self-care, 124
specialists, 120
toothbrushes, 125
x-ray procedures, 129–139
Deodorants
    genital, 462
    underarm, 446
Dependence, physical, 582
Depilatories, 449
Depo-Provera, 466, 467
Depression, 100
Derbyshire, Dr. Robert C., 92
Derelian, Dr. Doris, 211
Dermabrasion, 447, 454t, 577
Dermatitis, 577
Desiccated liver, 248t
Desiccated thyroid, 248t
Desirable weights, 273, 273t
Dermatron, 156
"Detergent foods" myth, 124
Detergents, 443, 448
"Detoxification," 43t, 151–152, 255, 387,
    389, 431
Deutsch, Ronald, 245
Devices, health, 477–493
    acupuncture needles, 143
    adverse reports, 478
    for arthritis, 365–366
    Biolator, 165
    blood pressure kits, 187–188
    breast developers, 62, 63
    for cancer, 385
    classification by FDA, 478–479
    E-meter, 114
    EMF protectors, 493
    Electric Ear, 111
    electrodiagnostic devices, 156
    ENS/EMS devices, 64, 313t, 319
    exercise and fitness; *see under* Exercise
        equipment
    hearing aids, 486–489
    humidifiers, 489–490
    intrauterine (IUDs), 461, 464t, 466
    laws regulating, 478–480, 556
    legal definition of, 478
    mastectomy prostheses, 473
    personal emergency response systems,
        206t, 490
    problem reporting system, 478–479
    quack, 8–9, 108, 156, 365–366, 385,
        488, 491–493
    questionable self-help, 182t
    TENS, 363, 584
    ultrasound; *see* Ultrasound
    vision products and services, 480–486
    water purifiers, 489
    weight control gadgets, 290–291
DeVita, Dr. Vincent, 376, 386
DeWys, Dr. William, 242
Dexfenfluramine (*Redux*), 283
Diabetes, self-monitoring, 185
Dial-a-Dietitian, 230
Diamond, Harvey and Marilyn, 152, 282

Dianetics, 113–114
Diaphragm, 464, 465t
Diarrhea remedies, 429
Diathermy, 577
Diet
    and arthritis, 367–368
    assessment, 220–221
    and behavior, 110–111
    and cancer, 229t, 374, 375, 376–378,
        383
    candies, 286
    and cardiovascular disease, 229t, 340–
        346, 344t
    cholesterol-lowering, 340–346
    computer analysis of, 130, 221, 263,
        343
    and constipation, 213
    and heart disease, 229t, 340–346, 344t
    and high blood pressure, 351
    and life-extension claims, 501, 502–503
    sensible, 181, 215–216t
Diet Center, 293, 294, 295
Diet teas, 285
Diet Workshop, 293
Dietary guidelines, 214–215
    Dietary Guidelines for Americans, 215–
        216, 216–217t, 577
    for infants, 222–224
    for cancer prevention, 377–378
    for vegetarians, 225
Dietary Supplement Health and Education
    Act, 45, 62, 235–236, 240, 264, 267,
    551, 553
Dietary supplements, 217, 240–241, 260,
    578; *see also* Vitamin(s), supplements
    amino acid products, 241–242
    antioxidants, 23, 240–241, 377, 508,
        553, 574
    appropriateness of formulations, 260
    appropriate use, 244–245
    consumer confidence in, 236–237
    expenditures for, 236
    fruit and vegetable "concentrates," 241
    legal definition, 235-236
    "meals in a can," 237
    misleading advertisements for, 238t
    multivitamin/mineral combinations,
        236
    "natural" vs. synthetic vitamins, 240
    "nutrition insurance," 237–239, 238t
    phytochemicals, 240, 582
    promotion, 213, 217
    reasons for use, 236
    "stress supplements," 239–240
Diethylstilbestrol (DES), 375
Dietitians, 230–231
Diets; *see also* Weight control
    Atkins, 280, 281t
    Beverly Hills, 282
    cabbage soup, 282
    difficulty with "dieting," 274–276, 278
    fad, shortcomings of, 278–279
    fasting, complete, 279
    fasting, supplemented, 279–280

Feingold, 110–111
Fit for Life, 282
Herbalife system, 282–283
Immune Power, 257
junk, 222–223
low-carbohydrate (high-protein), 280
low-calorie balanced, 295
low-fat (Ornish), 345
macrobiotic, 255, 255, 390–391, 580
Pritikin, 346
questionable, 278–280, 281t, 282–284
Scarsdale Medical, 280
vegetarian, 224–225
very-low-calorie, 279–280
Digitalis, 252
Dimethyl sulfoxide (DMSO), 368–369, 370, 507
Diopter, 577
DiOrio, Father Ralph, 161
Diploma mill, definition of, 577
Diplomates, 577
Dipyrone, 370
Directory of Medical Specialists, 78
Disability insurance, 529–539
Disorientation, 577
Distance Education and Training Council, 261
Diuretics, 577
Diverticulitis, 213
DMARDS, 361–362
DMSO: see Dimethyl sulfoxide (DMSO)
DNA (deoxyribonucleic acid), 469
DNR order, 577
Doctors: see Physicians
Doctrine of signatures, 157, 577
Dodes, Dr. John E., 9, 119, 126, 130, 131, 132, 134, 137
Dolomite, 248t
Doman-Delacato treatment, 111
Donsbach, Kurt W., 260, 264
Donsbach University, 260–261
Don't Go To The Cosmetics Counter Without Me, 445
Dose-response, 577
Doshas, 166
Double-blind study, 17, 577
Doublespeak, 43, 48
Douching, 462
Down syndrome, 469, 503
Doyle, Rodger P., 17
Dr. Atkins' Diet Revolution, 280
Dr. Berger's Immune Power Diet, 257
Dream Away, 287
Drenick, Dr. Ernest, 282
DRGs (diagnosis-related groups), 521–522, 577
Drown, Ruth B., 492
Drug products, 407–438
  acne remedies; see Acne
  advertising, 53–56, 416–417
  allergies to, 418
  allergy products, 418–420, 419t
  analgesics; see Analgesics
  antacids, 423–424, 424t, 574

antianxiety agents, 103–104
antibiotics, 424–426
antidepressants, 104, 362
antihistamines, 419, 419t, 428
antihypertensive, 351
antimicrobials (external), 426
antiperspirants, 446
antipsychotic, 104
"aphrodisiacs," 426–427
arthritis, 361–363, 364
aspirin; see Aspirin
athlete's foot remedies, 427
books about, recommended, 436t
buyer's clubs, 400
cholesterol-lowering, 345, 346–347, 347t
classification of, 408
clinical testing of, 556
compounding, 410
contraceptives; see under Contraception
corn and callus remedies, 427
cost-saving strategies, 437–438
cough and cold remedies, 415, 427–429
definition (under federal law), 577
delivery methods, innovative, 415
deodorants; see Deodorants
diarrhea remedies, 429
estrogens; see Estrogens
expenditures, 410, 416
for the eyes, 429–430
generic; see Generic drugs
hangover products, 430
hemorrhoidals, 430
for home medicine cabinet, 435t, 436
homeopathic; see Homeopathy
imported, 555
interactions with other drugs, 412, 415
Internet pharmacy sales, 415
investigational, 555
iron-containing, 431
labeling requirements, 410, 417
laws pertaining to; see Food, Drug, and Cosmetic (FDC) Act
laxatives, 432–432, 432t
legal definition of, 577
mail-order pharmacies, 437–438
for menstrual distress, 461
motion sickness remedies, 433
"new," 555, 581
off-label use, 581
optometrists, use by, 481
over-the-counter (OTC), 416–418, 555; see also Patent medicines
  banned categories, 416t
  criticism of combination products, 418
  frequency of use, 416
  FDA review of, 417, 556
  limitations, 416
  switch from Rx status, 427
prescription, 408, 410, 555, 582
proprietary, 582
prudent use, 418, 436–438
psychopharmacologic agents, 103–105

rebound from, 583
recalls, 415
safety precautions, 437
sleep aids, 433–434
smoking deterrents, 434
sore-throat products, 429
stimulants for fatigue, 434–435, 434t
suggestions for purchasing, 437–438
sunscreens, 451–452
tolerance to, 584
topical, 584
weight control, 283–284
Drug Topics, 416
Dublin, Louis, 272
Dumping, patient, 197
Durable medical equipment, 577
Durable power of attorney for health care, 496–499
Durovic, Dr. Steven, 380
Dyott, Thomas W., 413
Dyslexia, 112
Dysmenorrhea, 460–461, 577

E
E-Meter, 114
Earl Mindell's Vitamin Bible, 266
Eating disorders, 278
Eccrine glands, 446
Echinacea, 253t
Echo stress testing, 354
Echocardiography, 353–354
Economics, health care, costs; see also Expenditures, health costs; Fees
  AIDS/HIV treatment, 399–400
  ambulatory care centers, 198
  ambulatory surgery, 198
  back-pain treatment, 149
  budgeting for, 535
  cost-control methods, 535–536, 539
  dental care, 120, 535, 536t
  exercise facilities, 319
  eyeglasses, 482
  guidelines for reducing, 437–438, 539
  hearing aids, 487
  home care, 202
  hospice care, 202, 400, 501–502, 579
  hospital care, 534
  insurance, health, 522, 523, 524
  nursing homes, 204, 534
  physician services, 79, 534–535, 535t
  problems with 10–11
Economies of scale, 577
ECT; see Electroconvulsive therapy (ECT)
Eczema, 418
Eddy, Mary Baker, 159
Edema, 577
EDTA, 171
Eggs, fertile, 248–249t
Eisenhower, President Dwight D., 302
Electone, Inc., 488
Elective procedure, 577
Electric muscle/nerve stimulators, 64, 313t, 319
Electroacupuncture devices, 156, 385

Electrocardiogram (ECG), 82, 352
Electroconvulsive therapy (ECT), 105
    opposition to, 114
Electroencephalogram (EEG), 577
Electrolysis, 448, 449
Electrolytes, 214, 577
Electromagnetic fields, 375, 493
Electronic Medical Foundation, 264, 492
Electroshock therapy; see
        Electroconvulsive therapy (ECT)
Electrosurgery, 577
Elkhorn Mining Co., 366–367
Elliptical exercisers, 316
Ellon USA, Inc., 108
Embryo, definition of, 578
EMDR, 111
Emergency care, 79–80
Emergency centers, freestanding; see
        Ambulatory care centers
Emergency medical identification, 80, 420
Emergency medical technicians (EMTs),
        77t
Emergency response systems, 206t, 490
Emery, C. Eugene, Jr., 162
Emollients, 443
Emphysema, 577
Encore House, 562
Encounter groups, 109
Encyclopedia of Medical Organizations
        and Agencies, 192, 570
Encyclopedia of Natural Medicine, 153
Endermologie, 290
Endodontics, 120
Endometriosis, 461, 577
Endometrium, 577
Endorphins, 142, 577
Endorsements
    insurance, 515t
    of products, 6, 20–21
Endurance exercise, 305
Enemas, 432
    coffee, 383, 385, 387, 389
Energy bars, 325
"Energy medicine," 577–578
Enforcement actions, federal, 37, 389; also
        see under Federal Trade Commission;
        Food and Drug Administration; U.S.
        Postal Service
Enforcement actions, state and local, 108,
        113, 239–240, 264, 282, 291, 295,
        384, 399–400, 401–402, 451, 485,
        488, 492–493
Enforma Natural Products, 286
English, Dr. O. Spurgeon, 106
Engrams, 113–114
Enrichment, 251, 578
Ensure, 58t, 237
Entelev; see CanCell
Enteric coating, 578
"Environmental illness," 578
Environmental Protection Agency (EPA),
        374, 489, 543, 554, 563
Environmental tobacco smoke, 181
Enzymatic Therapy, 558

Enzymes, 578
    "deficiency" of, 262
    oral, 248t, 262
Eosinophilia-myalgia syndrome, 259, 434
Ephedra-containing products, 258, 285,
        327
Epidemiology, 17, 578
Epinephrine; see Adrenaline
Epping, Linda, 39
Epstein-Barr virus, 171
Equal; see Aspartame
"Ergogenic aids," 8, 49, 64, 326–327, 560
Erythromycin, 425
Essential nutrients, 577
Essiac, 381
EST; see Electroconvulsive therapy (ECT)
Estee Lauder, Inc., 444–445
Estimated average requirement (EAR),
        217
Estimated Safe and Adequate Daily
        Dietary Intakes (ESADDI), 577
Estraderm, 55
Estrogens, 336, 472–473, 578
    and breast size, 63
    and heart disease, 473
Euthanasia, 502–503
Evans, Gary, 248t
Evening primrose oil, 248t
Evidence-based medicine, 578
"Excedrin headaches," 56
Exclusions (insurance), 515t, 517
Exclusive provider organization (EPO),
        519
Exercise, 301–329
    and anabolic steroids, 325–326, 326t
    and arthritis, 359
    benefits, 181, 303–304
    boredom, prevention of, 307
    calories burned during, 296t, 306t
    and cardiac rehabilitation, 355
    and children, 322
    components of fitness, 304–306
    corporate fitness programs, 323
    equipment and supplies, 66–64, 311–
        312, 310–312t, 316–319, 322, 323
    and ergogenic aids; see "Ergogenic
        aids"
    facilities, 319–322
    guidelines, 306–310, 308t
    historical aspects, 302–303, 327
    in-home, 322
    injuries, 309–310, 310t, 312
    instructors, 312t
    intensity, assessment of, 309
    and longevity, 303–304
    myths, 324t
    and nutrition, 323–325
    power and athletic performance, 309
    programs, 306–310, 311t
    public perceptions, 302–303
    reasons for, 303–304
    sports medicine professionals, 310–311,
        312t
    strength training, 304, 307, 317

    and stress reduction, 304
    stretching, 308–309, 308t
    types, 304
    and vitamin needs, 239, 324
    and weight control, 276, 296t, 297, 323,
        324t
    while traveling, 322–323
Exercise physiologists, 311
Expectorants, 428, 578
Expenditures, health care; see also
        Economics, health care
    chiropractic care, 145
    cold and cough remedies, 428
    drugs, 410, 416
    medical devices, 478
    per capita, 532, 537t
    personal health care, 532, 533t, 537t
    quackery, 3, 35
    skin and beauty aids, 442
    total U.S., 532–533, 533t
    vitamin and mineral supplements, 236
    weight-control products and services,
        278
Extended care, 204, 578
Eyeglasses, 482; see also Sunglasses
Eyes, professional evaluation, 481–482
Eyewashes and decongestants, 429–430

F
Facilitated communication, 111–112
Facts, scientific, how determined, 16–21
Fad diagnoses, 38, 132, 168–171
Faddism, food; see Food faddism
Fade creams, 446
Fair Packaging and Labeling Act (1966),
        551, 552, 559
Faith Assembly Church, 161
Faith healing; see Psychic healing
Fallopian tubes, 578
False memory syndrome, 113
False Representation Order, 562
False-negative tests, 578
False-positive tests, 82, 578
Family therapy, 103
Farsightedness, 480, 481
Fast food, 222
Fasting, 152, 279
Fat(s), 213–214; see also Cholesterol;
        Lipids
    chemical composition, 213, 343
    dietary guideline, 216t
    fatty acid content of fats and oils, 341t
    food sources, 219t, 221t
    infant needs, 223
    percentage in diet, 341, 343
    sterol-enriched margarines, 349
    substitutes for, 289
FDA; see Food and Drug Administration
        (FDA)
FDA Consumer, 32, 558
Feder, Dr. Bernard, 95
Federal Bureau of Investigation (FBI), 66,
        540, 563
Federal Trade Commission (FTC), 11, 12t,

558–561; *see also* Federal Trade Commission Act
and cosmetic claims, 441
and denture adhesives, 129
enforcement actions, 57, 59, 63, 64, 108, 112, 129, 161, 172, 237, 256, 259, 262, 280–281, 287, 291–292, 327, 366–367, 378, 392, 451, 489–490, 493, 559–561, 562
Eyeglass Rule, 482, 484
food advertising rule, 246
functions and responsibilities, 558–559
funeral rule, 505
and hearing aids, 488
industry guides, 559
and infertility services, 469
and infomercials, 64
Internet activities, 561
and personal emergency response systems, 490
and professional advertising, 51
trade regulation rules, 559–560
and telemarketing, 66
and viatical settlements, 499
and water treatment systems, 489
Federal Trade Commission Act (1914), 551, 559
Fair Packaging and Labeling Act (1966), 551, 552, 556–557, 559
Magnuson-Moss Act (1975), 559
procedures and penalties for law violations, 559–560
trade regulation rules, 559–560
Wheeler-Lea Amendment (1938), 551, 559
Federation of American Societies for Experimental Biology, 213, 242
Federation of State Medical Boards, 73, 92
Fee-for-service care, 535–578
Feel Good Again, 188
Fees
at ambulatory care centers, 198
consumer action regarding, 539
cosmetic surgery, 454t
dental, 536t
medical, 534–535, 534t
mental health services, 106
RBRVS, 528t, 529
UCR, 523, 528, 535
Fein, Dr. Rashid, 543
Feingold diet, 110–111
Feldenkrais technique, 167
Fenfluramine (*Pondimin*), 283–284
Fernandez-Madrid, Dr. Felix, 359
Ferrari, Dr. Carl, 112
Fertile eggs, 248–249t
Fertility awareness methods, 463–464
Fetal alcohol syndrome, 182
Fetus, definition, 578
Fiber
dietary, 213, 377, 578
insoluble, 213
and irritable bowel syndrome, 186
label claims permitted, 213, 229t

recommended intake, 213
soluble, 213, 229t, 343, 345
sources, 213
supplements, 213, 285–286, 349
Fibre Trim, 285–286
Fibromyalgia, 360, 362
Figure-Tron II, 562
Finch, Dr. Stuart M., 106
Fish oils, 249t
and arthritis, 368
and cholesterol levels, 349
Fit for Life Diet, 282
Fitness; *see* Exercise and fitness
Fitness Quest, Inc., 64
Fixx, Dr. Jim, 303
Flatulence, 578
Fleiss, Dr. Wilhelm, 164–165
Flexibility, 305, 308–309, 578
Flexner, Dr. Abraham, 73
Florida Department of Citrus, 58t
Florsheim MagneForce shoes, 493
Fluoridation, 122–123, 183, 578
alternatives, 123, 123t
opposition to, 122–123
Fluoride
dentifrices, 125, 442
infant needs, 223
mouth rinses, 123
supplements, 123, 123t, 218, 242
Fluoroquinolones, 425
Fluorosis, 122
Folic acid, 225, 229t, 244, 337
Folk medicine, 140
Food(s); *see also* Diet; Diets; Food faddism; Nutrition
additives, 110, 251, 375, 377, 553–554
adulteration, 553
advertising, 7, 56, 58t, 346
allergies, 418
calories per gram, 220–221
combining, 282, 575
energy, 575
energy bars, 325
enrichment, 251, 578
faddism; *see* Food faddism
faddists, types of, 234t
fast, 222
fat content, 221t
fortification, 225, 251, 578
groups, 219–220
"health," 233, 246, 247–250t
irradiation, 554, 578
junk, 222
labeling; *see* Nutrition, labeling
low-calorie, 287
major components, 212–214
misbranding, 553, 581
myths, 235
"natural," 246, 251
"organic," 245–246, 251
pesticide levels, 245, 251, 554
preservatives, 554
processing, 239, 246
safety, 216t

supplements; *see* Dietary supplements
taste, factors affecting, 245
Food and Drug Administration (FDA), 548–558
and acupuncture needles, 143
and AIDS, 402
and "antiaging" cosmetics, 444–445
and aspirin advertising, 18
definition of health fraud, 36
and device regulation, 478–480, 556
and drug information, 410
drug recalls, 415
and drugs, clinical testing of, 556
educational activities, 558
enforcement actions, 7, 19, 108, 114, 157, 172, 249t, 256, 258–259, 282, 284, 285, 286, 291, 319, 327, 367, 380, 402, 412, 434, 448, 452, 455, 479, 507, 557–558, 558t
enforcement priorities, 557–558
and eyeglass safety, 482
and feminine deodorant sprays, 462
and food additives, 553–554
and food advertising, 342
and gamma hydroxybutyrate (GHB), 7, 558t
and generally recognized as safe (GRAS) list, 554
and generic drugs, 411–412
and hair fibers, implantation of, 479
and HCG, 283
headquarters offices, 548
health-food store investigation, 258
and hearing aids, 488
and homeopathic remedies, 157–158
and irradiation, 554, 578
and *Laetrile*, 388
and latex allergy, 490, 491
laws pertaining to; *see* Food, Drug, and Cosmetic Act
and life-extension products, 507
and low-calorie foods, 282–283
"market basket" studies, 251
and meal-replacement products, 279
Medical Device Surveillance Network, 479
and nutrition labeling; *see* Nutrition, labeling
OTC drug review, 417, 556; *see also* products listed under Drugs and drug products
and phenylpropanolamine (PPA), 284, 428
and prescription drug advertising, 53
procedures and penalties for law violations, 557–558
and *Prozac*, 114
and raw milk, 250t, 564
reporting to, 567
and Scientology, 114
and silicone implants, 453, 455
and "stress supplements," 240
survey of advertisements, 60–61
and tampons, 460

Food and Drug Administration (FDA)—
    cont'd.
    and tanning booths, 452
    and thalidomide, 551
    and thyroid drug labeling, 283
    and tobacco regulation, 60
    and tooth bleaches, 126
    top 10 health frauds, 38
    and vitamin dosage, 236
Food and Nutrition Board, Institute of
    Medicine, 216
Food and Water, 555
Food, Drug, and Cosmetic (FDC) Act,
    478, 549, 550–551, 553–557
    amendments; see under Laws, Food,
        Drug, and Cosmetic Act (1938)
    cosmetic provisions, 442, 556–557
    device provisions, 556–557
    drug (human) provisions, 555
    food provisions, 553
    and homeopathic remedies, 157–158
    procedures and penalties for violations,
        557
Food faddism, 234–235
    definition of, 234
    macrobiotic diets, 255, 390–391, 580
    promoters of questionable nutrition,
        131, 255–256, 263–267
    promotion of questionable nutrition,
        254–263
    roots of, 255–256
    and supplements, 235; see also Dietary
        supplements; Minerals; Vitamin(s)
    and tooth decay, 121, 131
    types of faddists, 234t
    and weight control; see Weight control
Food Guide Pyramid, 215, 218, 219–220,
    578
Forer, Bertram, 164
Fortification, 225, 251, 578
Foundation for Alternative Cancer
    Therapy (FACT), 391
Foundation for the Advancement of
    Innovative Medicine (FAIM), 45,
    173, 266
Foundation for Economic Trends, 555
Foundation for Hospice and Homecare,
    202
Fox, Margaret and Kate, 163
Frauds; see Quackery
Fredericks, Carlton, 265
Free radicals, 240, 578
"Freedom of choice," vii–viii, 43, 44–45,
    173–174, 373, 391
Freedom of Information Act requests
    (FDA), 558
Freireich, Dr. Emil J, 379
Fresh cell therapy, 385
Fresenius Medical Care Holdings, 540–
    541
Fries, Dr. James F., 179, 188, 359, 364
FTC; see Federal Trade Commission
FTC News Notes, 559
Functional intracellular analysis, 262–263

Funerals, 503–506
    profiteering related to, 11, 505

G
Galileo, 21
Gallbladder surgery, 89
Gamma hydroxybutyrate (GHB), 7, 326,
    558t
Gangrene, 578
Garcinia cambogia, 286
Garlic, 252, 253t, 348
Gastric bypass surgery, 292
Gastroesophageal reflux disease (GERD),
    424
Gastrointestinal tract, 578
Gatekeeper, 515t
Gatorade, 325
Genes, 469
General Accounting Office (GAO), 204,
    478
General anesthesia, 578
General Nutrition Inc. (GNC), 258–259,
    287, 378, 451
General practitioner, 578
Generic drugs, 404, 405–407, 407t, 578
Genetic engineering, 578
Genetic testing and counseling, 469–470
Genetically engineered foods, 554–555
Gerber Products Company, 222, 561
Geritol, 57, 560
Germanium, 249t, 383
Gero Vita International, 61
Gerovital H3 (GH3), 508
Gerson, Dr. Max, 383
Gerson diet, 383
Getting Well Again, 386
Gingivitis, 123–124, 578
Ginkgo biloba, 253t
Ginseng, 253t
GlanDiet, 288
"Glandular" products, 157, 249t
Glaucoma, 480, 482, 486, 578
Glucomannan, 285
Glucosamine, 368
Glucose, 212–213, 279, 578
Glucose tolerance test, 168–169
Glycel, 445
Glycogen, 212, 578
Glyoxylide, 374–375
Goldenseal, 253t
Gonzalez, Dr. Nicholas, 387
"Good Health Guides," 257
Goodstein, Dr. David, 20
Gorayeb, Ronald A., 292
Gorski, Dr. Timothy N., 471
Gotu Kola, 256
Gout, 360, 367
Grace period, 515t
Graham, Sylvester, 152, 255
Granfalloons, 39
Granola, 121, 249t, 578
Grant, W.V., 159
Granula, 255
Grape cure for cancer, 382

Grape Nuts, 255
GRAS list, 554
Grave liner, 504
Gravity inversion devices, 318
Great Earth International, 259, 287
Greek cancer cure, 385
Green, Dr. Saul, 384
Green tea, 253t
Green-lipped mussel, 367
Greene, Larry, 402
Greene, Dr. Ralph, 91
Grief, 506–507
Gross domestic product (GDP), 532, 578
Group Health Association of America, 524
Group therapy, 103
Growth hormone, 168, 508
"Growth-hormone releasers," 287, 326
Guaiac test, 185, 187
Guar gum, 284, 285, 291
Guarana, 249t, 327
Guidelines, science-based, 12, 19–20
Gum disease; see Periodontal disease
Gunther, Max, 6, 22, 24
Guthrie, Dr. Helen, 222
Gymnema sylvestre, 286, 327

H
H₂ blockers, 423–424
Hadacol, 414
Haemophilus influenzae, 85
Hahnemann, Samuel, 154, 155, 574
Haidet, Julia, 258
Hair, 447
    analysis, 130, 261–262
    care, 447–451
    conditioner, 579
    dyes, 557
    excess, removal of, 448–449
    hair-growth frauds, 450–451
    implants, 450, 479, 579
    loss of, 449–450
    removal, 448–449
    transplants, 450, 579
Halstead, Dr. Bruce, 391
Handbook of Nonprescription Drugs, 437
Hangover, 579
    alleged remedies, 430
Harkin, Senator Tom, 174
Harper, Dr. Alfred E., 237
Hart, Fred J., 264
Hartman, Samuel Brubaker, 413
Harvard Guide to Women's Health, 469
Harvard Health Letter, 82, 108, 399
Harvard Heart Letter, 349, 350
Hauser, Gayelord, 256
Hay fever, 418
HCG; see Human chorionic gonadotropin
    (HCG)
HDL (high-density lipoproteins), 214,
    337–339, 579
    and alcohol, 349
    and heart attack risk, 336, 337, 579
Healey, John A., 414

Health & Healing, 172
Health care
  attitudes toward, 38, 141, 168
  costs; *see* Economics, health care, costs
  crisis, 532
  dental; *see* Dental care
  emergency, 79–80
  facilities, 195–207
    ambulatory care centers, 197–198
    ambulatory surgery centers, 198–199
    hospices, 202, 400, 501–502, 579
    hospitals; *see* Hospitals
    nursing homes; *see* Nursing homes
    outpatient, 196–199, 198t
    scope and relative cost, 206t
  home care services, 201–202
  medical; *see* Medical care
  mental; *see* Mental health care
  personnel, types and training of
    allied health professionals, 77t, 120–121
    dentists, 120
    medical doctors, 72–73
    medical specialists, 74t
    mental health professionals, 100–102
    nurses, 75–76, 101
    nutrition professionals, 230–231
    optometrists; *see* Optometrists
    osteopathic physicians, 73–75
    pharmacists; *see* Pharmacists
    podiatrists, 75, 311
    scope of practice, 72
  reform
    conflicting attitudes toward, 534, 543
    ideal characteristics of plan, 542t
    need for, 531, 532, 541, 541t
    proposals for, 541–544
  questionable; *see* "Alternative" methods
  science-based, 71–97
  selection of practitioners
    chiropractor, 150
    dentists, 134–135
    infertility specialist, 469
    mental health practitioner, 105–106
    nutrition adviser, 230
    physicians, 76–79
    plastic surgeon, 453
    surgeon, 87
  surgical; *see* Surgery
  system, definition of, 532
Health Care Financing Administration
    (HCFA), 519, 532, 563
Health Care Technology Institute, 533
Health clubs and spas, 319–321
Health devices; *see* Devices, health
Health Employer Data Information
    System, (HEDIS), 524–525
Health-food industry, 256–257
  trade organizations, 267
Health-food stores, 258–259
  advice at, 258, 401
  products sold in, 157, 247–250t
"Health foods," 233, 246, 247–250t
Health Foods Business, 258

"Health freedom," vii–viii, 43, 44–45,
    173–174, 373, 391, 567, 579
Health Freedom News, 264
Health information, 4; *see also*
    Information sources
  for international travel, 80
  problems with, 6–7, 20–30, 174
Health Insurance Association of America,
    522, 523, 543, 565
Health magazine, 25, 27t
Health maintenance organizations
    (HMOs), 518–519, 579
  enrollment, 519t
  "gag clauses," 537
  premiums, 524, 525
  subscriber satisfaction, 521, 524, 525
  types, 518
Health Management Resources, 294
Health on the Net (HON) Foundation, 31
Health Research Group (HRG); *see* Public
    Citizen Health Research Group
Health Science, 152
Healthcare Integrity and Protection Data
    Bank (HIPDB), 93
Healthcare Rights Amendment, 45
HealthComm, Inc., 291
HealthMed, 114
Healthwise, Inc., 27
Healthwise Handbook, 188, 190t
Hearing aids, 486–488
Hearing loss, 486, 487t
Heart attacks, 351–352
Heart failure, 579
Heartburn, 423
Hegsted, Dr. D. Mark, 282
Helicobacter pylori, 425
Helsinki Hair Formula, 451
Hemoglobin test, 81
Hemophilus influenzae type b, 85
Hemorrhage, 579
Hemorrhoidal products, 430
Hendler, Dr. Sheldon Saul, 265
Hennekens, Dr. Charles, 241
Henney, Dr. Jane, 415
Hepatitis, 579
Herbalife International, 282–283
Herbert, Dr. Victor, 7, 23, 137, 139, 155,
    211, 217–218, 233, 240, 244, 258,
    260, 263
Herbs, 8, 251–254, 579
  dangers of, 252–254, 369
  marketing of, 58t, 65, 236
  medicinal use, 251–254
  popular, 253t
Herniated disk, 579
Herpes infections, 54, 425–426, 579
High blood pressure, 349–351
  self-monitoring, 187–188
  sodium and, 225, 229t, 350, 351
High-density lipoproteins (HDL); *see*
    HDL
Hill-Burton Act, 197
Hippocrates, 154, 302
Hirsutism, 448–449

Hives, 418
HMOs; *see* Health maintenance
    organizations
Hoffman, Bob, 327
Hoffman, Cecile, 391
Hoffmann-La Roche, 239
Hohensee, Adolphus, 256
"Holistic dentistry," 130, 131
"Holistic medicine," 172–173, 579
Holmes, Oliver Wendell, 35, 47
Home birth, 471
Home care services, 201–202
Home medicine cabinet, 435t, 436
Home Shopping Network, 560–561
Home Remedies Handbook, 188
Homeopathic Pharmacopeia, 155
Homeopathy, 35, 154–158, 583
  advertising, 58
  attitude of pharmacists toward, 410
  Bach remedies, 108
  dubious products, 9, 157, 172, 290, 562
  and electrodiagnosis, 156
  and FDA regulation, 155, 157–158, 172
  and personality type, 154
  media reports, 141
  "provings," 155
  research studies, 156–157
  use by chiropractors, 150
Homocysteine, 225, 337, 579
Homola, Dr. Samuel, 150
HONcode, 30, 31
Honey, 121
Hoque, F.M. and W. F., 380
Hormone, definition, 579
Hormone replacement therapy, 472–473
Hospices, 202, 400, 501–502, 579
Hospital Bill of Rights, 201, 582
Hospital Santa Monica, 264
Hospitals, 197, 199–200
  accreditation of, 88, 196, 199–200
  characteristics of good, 200
  costs, 534, 540
  emergency departments, 197
  free care at, 197
  infections in, 91
  marketing by, 53
  mental health care in, 107
  number of, 199
  outpatient clinics, 197
  partial, 107, 582
  peer review in, 199, 200
  and physician discipline, 91
  problems for consumers, 201
  selection of, 200–201
  strategies for patients, 91, 200, 201
  types, 199
"Hot flashes," 472
Hot tubs, 321–322
Houdini, Harry, 163
Householder, Michael and Carol, 293
How to Lie with Statistics, 18–19
Hoxsey, Harry, 380, 391
Hoxsey treatment, 380
Hubbard, L. Ron, 113–114

Hudnall, Marsha, 294
Huff, Darrell, 18–19
Huggins, Dr. Hal A., 131, 133
Hughes, Mark, 282
Human chorionic gonadotropin (HCG),
    185, 283, 471
Human immunodeficiency virus (HIV),
    396, 399
Humectants, 443
Humidifiers, 489–490
Humphrey, Derek, 502–503
Hydroquinone, 446
Hydroxycitric acids, 286
Hyman, Dr. Ray, 137, 164
Hyperactivity; *see* Attention deficit
    disorder
Hyperalimentation, 278
Hypercholesterolemia, 579
Hypertension; *see* High blood pressure
Hyperthermia, 579
Hypertrophic cardiomyopathy, 303
Hyperventilation syndrome, 105
Hypnosis, 103, 104, 112–113, 292
Hypoglycemia, 168–169, 579
Hysterectomy, 579

I

Iatrogenic illness, 91, 579
Ibuprofen, 127, 361, 362, 363, 579
ICD-9, 527, 579
Idiopathic disease, 579
Imagery, mental, 22, 386
"Immune boosters," 400, 401–402
Immune milk, 367
Immunizations, 84–86, 85–86t
    bogus, 183
    opposition to, 150, 152
Immuno-augmentative therapy (IAT),
    387–388
Impaired physicians, 90–91, 579
Incidence, of disease, 579
Indemnity insurance, 579
Independent practice association (IPA),
    518
Index Medicus, 19
Infinity², 262
Infertility, 579
    treatment, 469
Inflammation, 579
Infomercials, 64, 108, 291
Information sources, 4, 6–7, 20–32; *see
    also* Advertising
    arthritis, 370–371
    books and pamphlets, 25–27
    cancer, 390–392
    CD-ROMs, 27, 188
    drugs, 409, 416–417, 436t
    educational institutions, 22
    evaluation of, 29–32
    federal agencies, 563, 570
    herbs, 252
    magazines and newsletters, 25, 26t, 27t
    newspapers, 25
    NIH Office of Alternative Medicine, 174

nonprofessionals, 20–21
nutrition, 24t, 26t, 27t, 230–231, 254–
    267
online, 6, 28–30, 193
professionals, 21–22
pseudoscientists, 21
reliable, 230–231, 392, 436t, 570–572
self-help publications, 188–189, 190t
telephone advice, 80
television and radio, 4, 7, 27–28
videotapes, 27
voluntary and professional
    organizations, 564–566, 570–572
Informed consent, 579
Injections, overuse of, 90
Injunction, 579
Inlander, Charles, 191
Inlay, dental, 127
"Innate Intelligence," 140, 145
Inositol, 236, 249t
Inpatient, definition, 515t, 579
Insect stings/bites, 418
"Inside Edition," 384
Insomnia, 105, 433–434, 579
Inspector General; *see* Office of the
    Inspector General
Institute for Aerobics Research, 312t
Institute of Medicine (IOM), 203, 278,
    399, 455, 579
Institutes for Human Potential, 111
Insurance, health, 513–530
    and AIDS, 399–400
    assignment of benefits, 515t, 527
    basic, 514, 516
    benefits, 514, 516
    Canadian plan, 541–542
    claim form, 527
    claim submission, 527, 529
    commonly used terms, 515t
    comprehensive, 516, 576
    contract provisions, 516–517
    cost, 522, 523, 524
    dental, 523
    dependent coverage, 517
    disability, 529–539
    "dread disease," 518
    explanation-of-benefits statement, 528
    fee-for-service plans, 518, 535
    fixed dollar plans, 518
    fraud and abuse, 91, 171, 389, 540–541
    group insurance, 517–518
    health maintenance organizations
        (HMOs); *see* Health maintenance
        organizations
    history of, 514
    hospital indemnity, 518
    indemnity, 515t, 517, 518, 524, 524t,
        525, 579
    long-term care, 522–523
    loss ratios, 523–524, 580
    major medical, 516
    managed care; *see* Managed care
    Medicaid, 92, 522
    medical savings accounts, 525

    Medicare; *see* Medicare
    misleading sales tactics, 521
    national health, 541–543, 541t, 543t,
        581
    portability, 515t, 517
    point-of-service (POS) plans, 519
    preferred provider organizations
        (PPOs), 519, 523
    resource-based relative value scale
        (RBRVS), 528t, 529
    selection, 525, 526t, 527
    single-payer system, 583
    types of plans, 517–519
    uninsured, number of, 10
Integrated health network, 579
"Integrative medicine," 139–140
Intelligence tests, 114
Intelligent health consumer
    and acupuncture, 143
    and advertising, 55, 67
    and arthritis, 371
    and cancer, 392
    and cardiovascular disease, 354
    characteristics of, 12–13, 565
    and chiropractors, 151
    effective communication with
        physicians, 94–97
    evaluation of health information, 28–32
    filing of complaints, 559–561, 566t
    healthy lifestyle, 12–13, 181–183
    and home test kits, 184
    and hospital care, 91, 199–200
    medication use, 55, 418, 436–438
    nutrition decisions, 266
    reducing health care costs, 437–438,
        539
    rights and responsibilities, 79, 538
    and routine periodic interventions, 82–
        85, 84–85t
    self-test, 4
    shopping for eyeglasses, 482
Interferon, 376, 579
Interleukin-2, 376
Intermediate care, 203, 579
International Academy of Nutrition and
    Preventive Medicine, 173
International Academy of Preventive
    Medicine (IAPM), 172–173
International Academy of Somatidian
    Orthobiology, 384
International Association for New Science,
    173
International Association for Medical
    Assistance to Travelers (IAMAT), 80
International Association of Cancer
    Victors and Friends, 391–392
International Association of Clinical
    Nutritionists, 173
International Association of Dentists and
    Physicians, 173
International Chiropractors Association
    (ICA), 146
International College of Applied Nutrition,
    173

International Cosmetic Ingredient Dictionary, 442
International Federation of Bodybuilders, 327
International Health Institute, 387
International Hearing Society, 486
International Journal of Biosocial Research, 264
International Polio Network, 193
International unit (IU), 579
Internet, 28–31
    AIDS fraud, 402
    and cancer quackery, 391
    drug advertising, 53
    extent of health information, 6
    FTC activities, 561
    locating information, 29
    and patient records, 80, 96
    pharmacy sales, 415
    and physician credentials, 78
    prudent use, 28–31
    reliable sites, 29t, 570–572
    signs of a "quacky" Web site, 30
    warning from FTC, 65
Interpersonal psychotherapy, 102
Interro, 156
Interstate commerce, 579
Intervertebral disks, 579
Intraocular lens, 479, 580
Intrauterine devices (IUDs), 461, 464t, 466
Iridology, 65, 153–154, 580
Iron
    deficiency, 57, 462
    infant needs, 223
    overload, 431
    poisoning, 57
    and pregnancy, 244
    products containing, 57, 431
Irradiation, food, 554, 578
Irritable bowel syndrome, 186
Iscador, 383
Isokinetic exercise, 304, 580
Isometric exercise, 304, 580
Isotonic exercise, 304, 580
Ivy, Dr. Andrew C., 22, 380

J
Jackson, James Caleb, 255
Jacob, Dr. Stanley, 368, 369
Jacobs, Dr. Joseph J., 174
Janssen, Wallace, 392
Jarvis, Dr. DeForest C, 255–256
Jarvis, Dr. William T., v, 7, 36, 42, 43, 44, 122, 130, 146, 222, 224, 282, 379, 507, 509
Jaundice, 580
Jaw wiring, 292
JCAHO, 580
Jenny Craig, 292, 295
Jensen, Dr. Bernard, 153
"Joe Camel," 59
Johns Hopkins Medical Letter, 207, 499, 506
Johnson, O.A., 380

Joint Commission on Accreditation of Healthcare Organizations, 88, 196, 197, 502, 574
Joint replacement surgery, 364
Jonas, Dr. Wayne, 174
Journal of Longevity Research, 63
Journal of the American Medical Association (JAMA), 19, 60, 166, 580
Juice Plus+, 65
Jungle, The, 550
"Junk food," 222
Juvenile rheumatoid arthritis, 360

K
Kaiser Permanente, 518
Kallet, Arthur, 550
Kaposi's sarcoma, 397
Karr, Dr. Atida H., 561
Kava, 253t
Keats Publishing, Inc., 257
Keene, M. Lamar, 164
Keeton, Kathy, 384
Kelley, Dr. William, 386–387
Kelley Malignancy Index, 386
Kellogg, Dr. John Harvey, 255, 431
Kelp, 249t
Kelsey, Dr. Frances O., 549, 551
Kennedy, President John F., 298–299, 548
Kent, Saul, 507
Kessler, Dr. David A., 453
Ketosis, 279, 580
Kevorkian, Dr. Jack, 502
Keyes method of gum treatment, 124
Kickapoo Indian Medicine Company, 414
Kickbacks, 540–541, 580
Kilbourne, Jean, 59, 60
Kinesiology, 580
Kinsolving, Rev. Lester, 161
Kiplinger's Personal Financial Magazine, 469, 522
Kirlian photography, 158, 162
Km, 65
Knight, J.Z., 163
Koch, Dr. William, 379
Koch, Robert, 73
Koop, Dr. C. Everett, 59, 222, 395
Kordel, Lelord, 256
Koren Publications, 149
Krebiozen, 22, 380
Krieger, Dr. Dolores, 162
Kuhlman, Kathryn, 158–159
Kroger, Dr. Manfred, v
Kulp, Dr. Jacob W., 562
Kurtz, Dr. Paul, 47
Kushi, Michio, 254

L
L&S Research, 560
Labeling, legal definition, 580
Laboratory tests and procedures, 81–82
    for AIDS, 397
    dubious, 169, 170, 261–263, 384–385, 386–387
    pitfalls of, 82, 91, 340

Lactose intolerance, 186, 247t
Laetrile, 22–23, 45, 22–23, 388–399, 557
Landers, Ann, 271
Lane, Dr. I. William, 382
Lanolin, 443
Lanou, Dr. Amy, 271
Laparoscopic surgery, 580
    gallbladder, 89
    sterilization, 467
Larkin, M., 6, 23
LaRosa, Dr. John, 339
Laser drilling, 130
Laser phototherapy, 456
Laser surgery, 88–89, 449, 456
LASIK, 483
Latex allergy, 490–491
Laws; *also see under* Food, Drug, and Cosmetic Act
    Agricultural Appropriation Act (1931), 549
    and cancer quackery, 392
    Comprehensive Smokeless Tobacco Health Education Act (1986), 133
    Consolidated Omnibus Budget Reconciliation Act (1986), 197, 517
    Criminal Fines Enhancement Act (1984), 557, 562
    Drug Price Competition and Patent Term Restoration Act (1984), 408, 411, 552
    drug substitution, 411
    Fair Packaging and Labeling Act (1966), 551, 552, 559
    Federal Anti-Drug Abuse Act (1988), 325
    Federal Freedom of Access to Clinic Entrances Act (1994), 468
    Federal Hazardous Substances Act (1960), 549
    Federal Trade Commission; *see* Federal Trade Commission Act
    Food, Drug, and Cosmetic Act (1938)
        Color Additive Amendments (1960), 549
        Delaney Clause (1958), 549, 553–554
        Dietary Supplement Health and Education Act, 67, 235–236, 240, 264, 267, 551, 553
        Drug Abuse Control Amendments (1965), 552
        Drug Price Competition and Patent Term Restoration Act (1984), 408, 411, 552
        Durham-Humphrey Amendment (1951), 549, 551
        FDA Modernization Act (1997), 479, 553
        Food Additives Amendment (1958), 549
        Food Quality Protection Act (1996), 547, 554
        Infant Formula Act (1980), 552
        Kefauver-Harris Drug Amendments (1962), 549, 551

Laws—cont'd.
  Food, Drug, and Cosmetic Act (1938)—cont'd.
    Medical Device Reporting Act (1984), 478
    Medical Device Amendments (1976), 478, 552
    Nutrition Labeling and Education Act (1990), 553
    Orphan Drug Amendment (1983), 552
    Poison Prevention Act (1970), 552
    Prescription Drug Marketing Act (1988), 552
    Proxmire Amendment (1976), 236, 552
    Radiation Control for Health and Safety Act (1968), 552
    Safe Medical Devices Act (1990), 478, 552, 550
  General Agreement and Tariff Act (1994), 408
  Health Coverage and Affordability Act (1996), 522
  Health Insurance Portability and Accountability Act (1996), 95, 499, 517
  Health Maintenance Organization Act (1973), 518
  Hospital Survey and Construction Act (1946), 196
  "medical freedom," 173–174
  National Transplant Act (1984), 500
  nutritionist licensing, 231, 261
  Omnibus Budget Reconstruction Act of 1987, 203
  Omnibus Budget Reconciliation Act of 1990, 498
  Organic Foods Production Act (1990), 246
  Physicians Payment Reform Act (1989), 520
  postal; see U.S. Postal Service
  Public Health Service Act (1944), 549
  Pure Food and Drug Act (1906), 548–549, 550
  Saccharin Warning Elimination Employing Science and Technology Act, 288
  Sherley Amendment (1912), 549, 550
  U.S. Organic Foods Production Act (1990), 246
  Uniform Anatomical Gift Act, 500, 501
Laxatives, 432–432, 432t
LDL (Low-density lipoproteins), 214, 335, 337–339, 341, 580
Learning disabilities, questionable treatments, 111–112
Learning Machine, 108
LeBlanc, Dudley J., 414
Lecithin, 249t, 349, 554
Lederer, Dr. Roger, 22
Lederle Laboratories, 239–240
Lee, Dr. Royal S., 264

Lee, Samuel H.P., 413
Lefkowitz, Louis, 245
Legumes, 224, 580
Lesion, 580
Let's Have Healthy Children, 265
Let's Live, 259
Leukoplakia, 580
Levin, Dr. Stephen M., 147
Levitation, 165
Liaison Committee on Medical Education, 72
Libel suits, 23, 26
Licensed practical nurses, 76
Liefcort, 370
Liefmann, Dr. Robert E., 370
Life expectancy, vii, 580
Life Extension: A Practical Scientific Approach, 26–27, 256–257, 287, 507
Life Extension Foundation, 507–508
Life Extension Revolution, The, 507
Lifesavers Guide to Fluoridation, 122
Lifeway Health Products, 560–561
Ligament, 580
Lightsey, David, 328
Lindsey, Ronald, 15
Linoleic acid, 213
Linus Pauling Institute of Medicine, 291
Lipid(s), 580; see also Fat(s)
  analysis (profile), 82, 337–338
  blood, 335, 337
  dietary, 213–214
Lipman, Dr. Marvin, 71
Lipoprotein(a), 333
Liposuction, 290, 292, 454t
Lister, Joseph, 73
Listerine, 126
Lithium products, 104
Live-cell analysis, 262
Live-cell therapy, 385
Living Bank, The, 501
Living wills; see Advance medical directives
Livingston, Dr. Virginia, 385
Lobbying, top health-related spenders, 543t
London, Dr. William M., v, 156
  investigations by, 151, 456
Long-term care, 580
  comparison of facilities, 206t
  insurance, 522–523
Look Younger, Live Longer, 256
Loss ratios, 523–524, 580
Low-calorie products, 287–289
Low-density lipoproteins (LDL); see LDL
L-tryptophan, 259, 434
Lukaski, Frank, 286
Lunelle, 467
Lust, Benedict, 152
Luteinizing hormone, 185
Lutz, William, 48
Lydia E. Pinkham's Vegetable Compound, 413
Lyme disease, 171

M
Ma huang, 258, 285, 327
Macfadden, Bernarr, 152, 255, 303, 327
Macfadden Holdings, 327
MacLaine, Shirley, 163
MacNay, Dr. Donald, 402–403
Macrobiotic diets, 255, 390–391, 580
Macronutrients, 212, 580
Macular degeneration, 241
Magnetherapy, Inc., 492–493
Magnet therapy, 167, 365, 491–493
Magnetic resonance imaging (MRI), 86–87
Magnetic source imaging, 87
Magnetic Therapeutic Technologies, 493
Maharishi Ayur-Ved, 166–167
Maharishi Ayur-Veda Products International, 167
Maharishi Mahesh Yogi, 165, 166
Mail-order frauds
  health products, 8–9, 60–63, 348, 562–563
  laws protecting against, 11, 551, 561–562
Major medical insurance, 516, 580
Malaise, 580
Malocclusion, 580
Malpractice, medical, 37, 90–91, 116, 580
Mammary artery ligation, 17
Mammography, 84, 85
Managed care, 10–11, 517–519, 524–525, 525t, 580
  comparison with indemnity plans, 524–525, 524t
  cost-control strategies, 76, 536–537
  definition, 515t, 517
  effect on pharmacists, 410
  HMO enrollment, 519t
  and Medicare, 521
Mania, 580
Manic-depressive psychosis, 580
Manipulation
  skull, 112, 131–132
  spinal, 143, 148–149, 150–151
Manner, Dr. Harold, 388
Manson, Dr. JoAnn E., 273
Marital and family therapists, 101
Marker, biologic, 580
Marketdata Enterprises, 278
Markle, Dr. George B., 10
Marriage counseling, 103
Martin, Dr. Robert, 318
Mary Kay, 65
Massage, 138
Massage therapists, 311
Mastectomy prostheses, 473
Materia medica, 154
Matol Botanical International, 65
Maximum heart rate, 305
Maximum Life Span, 507
Mayo Clinic Health Letter, 167, 506
Mazel, Judy, 282
McCall, Dr. Timothy B., 82, 179
McCarthy, Dr. Eugene, 88

McCue, Dr. Jack, 498
McGrady, Pat Jr., 391
McKay, Dr. Frederick, 122
McQueen, Steve, 386
MCT oil, 349
Meadow Fresh Farms, 560
Meal-replacement products, 279, 287–288
Media, 580; *see also* Advertising;
    Information sources
  astrology columns, 164
  coverage of "alternative" methods, 141, 174
  effect of libel suits, 23
  functions of, 6, 22
  number of outlets, 4, 6
  as sources of misinformation, 22–28, 38, 40, 254
Medic Alert Foundation, 500–501
Medicaid, 92, 522, 580
  nursing home coverage, 204
Medical assistants, 77t
Medical care; *see also* Health-care
    personnel; Mental health care;
    Physicians; Surgery
  abroad, 80
  basic, 80–87
  choosing a physician, 76, 78–79, 87, 453
  consultations, 95
  lack of continuity, 10–11
  emergency, 79–80
  ethical dilemmas, 93–94
  financial abuse, 91
  "get-acquainted" visit, 79
  iatrogenic illness, 91
  immunizations, 84–86
  impersonal care, 90
  incompetence, 89–90
  laboratory tests and procedures, 81–82
  malpractice, 37, 90–91, 116, 580
  medical imaging; *see under* Medical
    imaging
  patient-physician relationship, 79, 94–97, 115–116
  periodic health examinations, 80–84, 84–85t, 481
  physical examination, 81
  prescientific era, 73, 154
  quality of, 89–91
  reasons for avoiding, 185
  unscientific, 168–173
  when to seek, 185
Medical devices, *see* Devices, health
Medical doctors, training and credentials, 72–73, 74t, 91
Medical imaging, 86–87, 579
  computerized axial tomography (CT or CAT scan), 86
  coronary angiography, 353
  magnetic resonance imaging (MRI), 86–87
  magnetic source imaging, 87
  mammography, 83, 85t
  nuclear magnetic resonance (NMR), 86

positron emission tomography (PET), 86
  radionuclide imaging, 86
  single photon emission computerized tomography (SPECT), 86
  ultrasonography, 87, 353–354
  x-ray films; *see* X-ray films
Medical Information Bureau, 95
Medical Letter, The, 253–254, 284, 347, 422, 450
Medical Overkill, 91
Medical records
  access to, 95
  electronic, 96
  on Web page, 80, 96
Medical savings accounts, 525
Medical societies, 91
Medical specialties and subspecialties, 74t
Medical technologists, 77t
Medical Tribune, 240
Medically indigent, 580
Medicare, 580
  benefits, 520t, 521t
  certification by, 196, 202
  chiropractic coverage, 145
  and Christian Science, 160
  and DRGs, 521–522
  disciplinary action under, 92
  fraud, 540–541
  and HMOs, 521
  hotline, 520
  hospice coverage, 501
  nursing home coverage, 204
  RBRVS fees, 528t, 529
  supplemental (Medigap) insurance, 520–521
Medicine, defensive, 11, 91
Medicine cabinet, products for, 435t, 436
Medicine shows, 414
Medicines from Nature, 58
Medifast, 294
Medigap insurance, 520–521
Meditation, 109, 165
Meditrend International, 157
MEDLINE, 6, 28–29
Megavitamin therapy, 109–110, 242–243, 580
Meinig, Dr. George A., 131
Melanoma, 451
Melatonin, 249t, 508
Memorial societies, 504–505
Meningomyelocele, 503
Menopause, 580
  and heart disease, 334
  hormone-replacement therapy, 472–473
  surgical, 472
Menstrual problems, 460–462
Menstrual products, 460
Mental health care, 99–117
  behavioral therapy, 103
  biofeedback; *see* Biofeedback
  cognitive therapy, 102–103
  cost, 106
  drug therapy, 103–105

electroconvulsive therapy, 105
  group therapy, 103
  hospital care, 107
  hypnosis, 103, 104
  insurance coverage, desirable, 516
  practitioners, 100–102
  psychosomatic disorders, 105
  psychotherapy; *see* Psychotherapy
  questionable practices, 109–117
    auditory integration training, 111
    boundary violations, 115
    Dianetics and "purification," 113–114
    Doman-Delacato treatment, 111
    drugs, overuse of, 104
    electroconvulsive therapy, overuse of, 105
    eye movement desensitization and reprocessing (EMDR), 111–112
    facilitated communication, 111
    false memory stimulation, 113
    Feingold diet, 110–111
    meditation, 109
    megavitamin therapy, 109–110
    Neural Organization Technique (NOT), 112
    Neuro Emotional Technique (NET), 112
    neurolinguistic programming (NLP), 112
    past-life therapy, 112–113
    psychic hotlines, 115
    psychotherapy, mismanagement of, 115–116
    routine personality testing, 114
    sensitivity training, 109
    simplistic advice, 116
    thought field therapy (TFT)
  questionable "self-help" products, 107–108, 182
    Bach remedies, 108
    biofeedback gadgets, 107
    "brain wave synchronizers," 108
    dietary supplements, herbs, and hormones, 108
    Instructional programs, 108
    subliminal self-help, 62, 107–108, 290
  selection of therapist, 105–106
  treatment planning process, 584
  when needed, 100
Menthol, 428
"Mercury amalgam toxicity," 131, 132–133
Meridia, 284
Meridian therapy, 580
Meridians, 141, 142, 156
Mesmer, Franz Anton, 104
Meta-analysis, 580
Metabolic equivalents (METs), 309, 581
Metabolic therapy, 389, 581
Metabolism, definition, 581
Metamucil, 345
Metastasis, 375, 581
Metchnikoff, Elie, 431

Methylsulfonylmethane (MSM), 369
Metropolitan Life Insurance Company, 272, 273t
Mexican clinics, dubious, 264, 369–370, 389, 391, 400
Micro-Dynameter, 366
Micronutrients, 212, 581
Midwives, 76
Mifepristone (RU-486), 468–469
Miles Laboratories, 240
Milk, 225
  certified, 250t
  immune, 367
  raw, 250t, 564
Milk thistle, 253t
Miller, Roger, 47
Mindell, Earl, 266
Minerals, 214
  calcium; *see* Calcium
  chelated, 247-248t
  dangers of excess, 244
  electrolytes, 214
  fluoride; *see* Fluoridation; Fluoride
  food sources, 219t
  and hair analysis, 261–262
  iron; *see* Iron
  sodium; *see* Sodium
  of special concern, 225–226
Minnesota Multiphasic Personality Inventory (MMPI), 114
Minoxidil; *see Rogaine*
Miracle Ear, 488
Mirkin, Dr. Gabe, 15, 273, 280, 282
Misbranding, 553, 581
Miscarriage, 581
Misconceptions
  arthritis and weather, 367
  bowel, 431, 575
  "detergent foods," 124
  about exercise, 324t
  about eyesight, 480
  about generic drugs, 412
  homeopathic products resemble vaccines, 155
  nutrition, 235, 238t
  about placebo effect, 41
  about quackery, 40
  about sugar, 111, 121, 131, 213
  about weight control, 277t
Modern Maturity, 564
Modern Products, 256
Moisturizers, 443–444
Monoclonal antibodies, 376
MORAs, 131
Morbidity, 581
"Morning-after pill," 467
Mortality, 581
Morticians, 503–504
Morowitz, Dr. Harold J., 233
Mourning, 506–507
Mosenkis, Robert, 480
Motion sickness remedies, 433
Motor fitness, 305
Mouthwashes, 126, 429

Moxibustion, 141
MRFIT, 59, 335
MRI, 86–87
MSM, 369
Mucorhicin, 381
Mucous membrane, 581
Multilevel marketing, vii, 9, 22, 36, 64–66, 400
  Amway Corporation, 64–65
  FreeLife International, 267
  Herbalife International, 282–283
  Income from, 64–66
  Infinity², 262
  Juice Plus+, 65
  Mary Kay, 65
  Matol Botanical International, 65
  National Safety Associates, 65
  Nature's Sunshine Products, 65, 288
  Nu Skin International, Inc., 65–66
  Sunrider Corporation, 66
  United Sciences of America, 22
  use of endorsements, 22
Multiple chemical sensitivity, 169–170
Murdock, Kenneth, 560
Muscle & Fitness magazine, 327
Muscle spasms, 309
Muscle testing, 262
Muscular Development magazine, 327
Musgrave, Dr. Katherine, 282
Myocardial infarction, 335, 352
Myths; *see* Misconceptions

N
Nader, Ralph, 564
Naessens, Gaston, 384
Naprapathy, 581
Narcotics, in patent remedies, 413–414
Nasalcrom, 420
National Academy of Sciences, 19
  diet and cancer report, 377, 378
  Food and Nutrition Board, 216
  Institute of Medicine, 203, 278, 399, 455, 579
  National Research Council, 107–108, 109, 167, 182, 226
  Recommended Dietary Allowances; *see* RDAs
National Advertising Review Board (NARB), 66–67
National Alliance for Fraud in Telemarketing, 66
National Association for Chiropractic Medicine, 146
National Association for Home Care, 202
National Association of Alcoholism and Drug Abuse Counselors, 102
National Association of Attorneys General, 563
National Association of Boards of Pharmacy, 415
National Association of Insurance Commissioners, 521
National Association of Social Workers (NASW), 101

National Board for Counselors, 101
National Board of Hearing Instrument Examiners, 481
National Cancer Institute, 124, 392, 502
National Center for Complementary and Alternative Medicine, 174
National Center for Health Statistics, 523
National Center for Homeopathy, 141, 155
National Center for Nutrition and Dietetics, 231
National Cholesterol Education Program, 338, 339, 340, 345
National Coalition on Health Care, 532
National Commission for the Certification of Acupuncturists, 143
National Commission on AIDS, 399
National Committee on Quality Assurance (NCQA), 524–525
National Consumers League, 202, 502, 564
National Council Against Health Fraud, 9, 26, 144, 151, 230, 261, 279, 564–565
National Council for Improved Health, 45
National Council on Patient Information and Education, 410
National Dairy Council, 566
National Enquirer, 327
National Examiner, 25, 371
National Fraud Information Hotline, 66
National Guideline Clearinghouse (NGC), 20
National Health Council, 538
National Health Federation (NHF), 45, 264, 391
National Health Fraud Conference, 402
National Health Information Center, 563
National health insurance, *see* Insurance, health, national
National Health Service Corps, 563
National Hospice Organization, 502
National Institute of Mental Health, 110
National Institute of Nutrition Education (NINE), 261
National Institutes of Health (NIH), 242, 563
  Consensus statements, 19, 144, 225, 292, 306, 433–434
  National Center for Complementary and Alternative Medicine, 174
  Obesity Task Force, 294
  Office of Alternative Medicine, 138, 174
  Office of Dietary Supplements, 553
  Technology Assessment Conference, 276
National Mental Health Consumer Self-Help Clearinghouse, 182
National News Council, 24
National Nutritional Foods Association, 173, 267
National Organic Standards Board, 245, 246
National Physician Data Bank, 93

National Research and Information Center, 506

National Research Council, 107, 109, 167, 182, 375, 398, 493, 581

National Safety Associates, 65

National Safety Council, 426

National STD Hotline, 403

National Survey of Health Insurance, 10

National Task Force on the Prevention and Treatment of Obesity, 275–276

National Testing Laboratories, 489

National Vitamin Gap Test, 263

"Natural" foods, 246, 251

Natural hygiene, 152, 581

Natural Medicines Comprehensive Database, 252

Natural Pharmacist, 410

Naturalife herbal products, 58t

Naturally Good, 558t

Nature's Bounty, 451, 562

Nature's Sunshine Products, 65, 288

Nature's Way, 560

Naturopathy, 140, 151–152, 581

Nearsightedness, 480, 481

Negative ion generators, 385, 488

Negative test result, definition, 581

Nelson, Dr. Merlin, 260

Neonatal intensive care units, 503

Neural Organization Technique (NOT), 112

Neural tube defects, 225, 470, 503

Neuralgia-inducing cavitational osteonecrosis (NICO), 132

Neuro Emotional Technique (NET), 112

Neurolinguistic programming (NLP), 112

Neurotic reaction, 581

Nevyas, Dr. Herbert, 483

New Age Journal, 168

"New Age" movement, 163–164

New drug, 555, 581

New England Journal of Medicine, 19

New York City Department of Consumer Affairs, 295, 327–328, 346, 399–400, 401–402

Newsletters, 25, 26t, 27t

Newsweek, 25, 105, 122–123

Niacin
adverse effects, 347
cholesterol control, 347, 347t
for "purification," 114

Nicotine-replacement therapy, 53, 184, 434

Niehans, Dr. Paul, 385

Nirvana, 165

NMR, 86

Nocebo effects, 42, 581

Nolen, Dr. William A., 159, 387

Nonaccredited schools, 260–261

Nonoxynol-9, 465

Norbeck, Timothy B., 534

NordicTrack, Inc., 292

Norplant, 415, 464t, 466

North American Health Insurance Coordinators, 389

NSAIDs, 361–362, 363, 423, 425, 461

Nu Skin International, Inc., 64–65

Nu-Day Enterprises, 291–292

Nuclear magnetic resonance (NMR), 86

Null, Gary, 265–266, 391

Nurse Healers—Professional Associates International, 162

Nurse's aides, 77t

Nurses
psychiatric, 101
types of, 75–76

Nursing care levels, 201

Nursing homes, 10, 195, 203–205, 206t, 207
alternatives to, 206t, 207
cost of, 522, 534

NutraSweet; *see* Aspartame

Nutri-Books, 254, 256, 257

Nutrient(s)
adequate intake (AI), 217
essential, 578
estimated average requirements (EAR), 217
food sources, 219t
major functions in body, 219t
Recommended Dietary Allowances, 216–217, 237, 583
tolerable upper intake level (UL), 217

"Nutrient deficiency tests," 188, 263, 562

Nutrient density, 222, 581

Nutripathy, 581

Nutri/System, 288, 293, 294, 295

Nutrition, 211–231; *see also* Diets; Food; Food faddism; Vitamins; Weight control
and AIDS, 399
for athletes, 323–325, 324t
Daily Values (DVs), 226–227, 226t, 553
diet and heart disease; *see* Cardiovascular disease, and diet
dietary guidelines, 215–216, 215–216t, 222–224
fads, fallacies, and scams, 233–267
food group systems, 219–221
Food Guide Pyramid, 215, 218, 219–220, 578
human nutrient needs, 214–219
labeling, 226–229, 226t, 287, 346, 553
descriptive terms, 228t, 287
permissible health claims, 229t
sample food label, 227
major food components, 212–214
nutrients of special concern, 225–226
principles of healthful eating, 219
professionals, 230–231
quackery; *see* Food faddism
questionable, promoters of, 131, 255–256, 263–267
questionable, promotion of, 254–263
"roulette," 237
sources of reliable information, 230–231
total parenteral (TPN), 400
vegetarian, 224–225, 367

Nutrition 21, 292

Nutrition Action Healthletter, 564

"Nutrition insurance," 237–239, 238t

Nutrition Labeling and Education Act, 553

Nutrition News, 257

Nutritional Health Alliance, 267

Nutritional Perspectives, 260

Nutritionists
licensing of, 231, 261
reliable, 230–231
sports, 311
unqualified, 9, 261

O

Oat bran, 229, 343, 345–346

Obesity
causes, 272, 275, 277t
clinics, 293–295
definition, 272, 581
health risks, 181, 273–274, 377
incidence, 272
prevention, 274

Obitoriums, 502

Obsessive-compulsive disorder, 581

Occillococcinum, 9

Occlusion, 581

Occult blood test, 83–84, 581

Occult blood, 581

Occult practices, 162–164

Occupational therapists, 77t

Octacosanol, 249t

Office of Dietary Supplements, 553

Office of Technology Assessment, 19–20, 139, 388

Office of the Inspector General, 93, 541, 563
chiropractic reports, 148
and health fraud, 540–541
HMO subscriber surveys, 521, 524

Ohsawa, George, 255

Olestra (*Olean*), 289

Ombudsman, 581

Omega-3 fatty acids; *see* Fish oils

Omni Hearing Systems, 488

Oncologist, 581

Oncor, 157, 562

Online information sources, 6, 28–30, 31, 193

Online Survey Certification and Reporting System (OSCAR), 203

Open enrollment, 515t

Operation Disconnect, 66

Operation Sentinel, 66

Ophthalmologists, 480–481

Opportunistic infection, 581

Opticians, 481

Optifast, 25, 294

Options in Health Care, 191

Optometrists, 9, 481
and visual training, 112, 167, 584

Oral Roberts Evangelistic Association, 159

Orderlies, 77t

Organ donor card, 501

Organ transplants, 499–501, 500t

"Organic" foods, 7, 245–246
Organic Foods Production Act, 246
Orgone Energy Accumulator, 385
Orgotein, 367
Oriental medicine, 141–142
Orlistat, 284
Ornish, Dr. Dean, 345
Orphan drugs, 552
Orthodontics, 120, 128
Orthomolecular Medical Society, 173
Orthomolecular therapy, 109–110, 581
Orthopedists, 311
Oscilloclast, 491
Osler, Sir William, 71
Osteoarthritis, 360, 361, 363
Osteopathic physicians, 73–75, 581
Osteoporosis, 225, 229t, 459, 471–472, 581
Otitis, definition, 581
Outcomes research, 581
Outpatient, definition, 515t, 581
Otolaryngologists, 74, 486
Outcomes research, 17, 585
Over-the-counter (OTC) drugs; *see* Drugs and drug products, over-the-counter
Overeaters Anonymous, 293
Overweight, 272, 582; *see also* Obesity
Ovulation-prediction test, 185
OXYFRESH, 132
Oxygen debt, 304
Oxygen inhalation, by athletes, 326
Oxypathor, 366

P
PABA (para-aminobenzoic acid), 236, 249t, 508
Page, Dr. Melvin, 131
Pain relievers; *see* Analgesics
Pain Stops Here, 493
Palliation, 582
Palmer, Bartlett Joshua, 145
Palmer, Daniel David, 145
Palpitation, 582
Papain, 249t
Papanicolaou (Pap) test, 82, 84–85t
Paracelsus, 154
Paradigm, 582
Paraffin baths, 363
Paranormal, definition, 582
Park, Dr. Robert L., 155
Parker, Wesley, 158
Partial hospitalization, 107, 582
Participating provider, 515t
Passwater, Richard, 261, 266
Past-life therapy, 112
Pasteur, Louis, 73
Patent medicines, 413–414, 582
Patenting requirements, 56
Patient, intelligent; *see* Physicians, communication with, effective
Patient package inserts (PPIs), 582
Patient-physician relationship, 79, 94–97
and psychotherapy, 115–116
Patient representatives, 77t

Patient's Bill of Rights; *see under* Bill of Rights
Pattern for Daily Food Choices, 219
Patterning, 111
Pau d'arco tea, 382
Pauling, Dr. Linus, 242–243
Pavlou, Dr. Konstantin, 271
Pearson, Durk, 257, 287, 507
Pectin, 285
Peer review, 582
by hospital committees, 199, 200, 522
by scientific organizations, 19–20
lack of, among journalists, 23–24
Peet, Dr. Jennifer, 146
Penicillin, 424
Penis enlargement, 455–456
Pennyroyal, 254
People Against Cancer, 45, 391
People's Medical Society, 191
Pepper, Rep. Claude, 3
Percussion, 582
Peridex, 126
Periodontal disease, 123–124, 582
Perkins, Elisha, 491
Personal care facility, 206t
Personal emergency response systems, 206t, 490
Personality tests, 114
Peruna, 413
Pesticides, 245, 543, 554
PET scan, 86
PH, 443
Phacoemulsification, 485
Pharmacists, 409–410
advice from, 259–260, 409–410
compounding, 406
role in promoting food supplements, 36, 259–260, 405–406
and tobacco products, 409
Pharmacognosy, 582
Pharmtech Research, Inc., 378
Phenylbutazone, 370
Phenylketonuria, 288
Phenylpropanolamine (PPA), 284, 428
Philip Morris, 60, 255
Phillipe LaFrance USA, Ltd., 560
Phillips, Marjorie, 402
Phillips, Dr. William P., 380
Phoropter, 482
Photochromatic lenses, 482, 582
PhotoDerm VL, 456
Phrenology, 154, 582
Physical Culture magazine, 327
Physical examinations
by dentists, 134
procedures, 81
recommended frequency, 84–85t
Physical fitness; *see* Exercise and fitness
Physical therapists, 77t, 311
Physician(s); *see also* Medical care
characteristics of good, 76
communication with, effective, 94–95
directories 77, 535
discipline of, 9, 91–93

education of, 72
ethical dilemmas, 93–94
fees, 534–535, 535t
grievance, handling a, 97
impaired, 89–90, 579
medical care, quality of, 89–91
medical doctors, 72–73
meeting prospective, 79
and nutrition advice, 230
osteopathic physicians, 73–75
plastic surgeons, 453
selection of, 76, 78–79, 453
specialties and subspecialties, 74t
sports medicine specialists, 310–311
telephone tips, 95–97
unscientific, 168–173
when to consult, 185
Physician assistants (PAs), 77t
Physician Data Query (PDQ), 392
Physicians' Desk Reference (PDR), 55, 436t
Physicians' Health Study, 18, 349
Physicians Payment Reform Act (1989), 520
Physicians Weight Loss Center, 294, 295
Phytochemicals, 240, 582
Pies, Dr. Ronald, 106
Pinhole glasses, 485
Pitofsky, Robert, 563
Pityrosporum ovale, 448
Pizzorno, Dr. Joseph E, Jr., 152
Placebo, definition, 582
in controlled studies, 17
Placebo effect, 41–42, 41t, 582
Planned Parenthood Federation of America, 463
Plaque
atherosclerotic, 334–335, 337, 346, 353, 582
dental, 123, 124, 125, 126, 129, 582
Plasma, 582
Plastic surgery; *see* Cosmetic surgery
Platelets, 582
Plax, 126
PMS; *see* Premenstrual syndrome
PMS Escape, 461–462
Pneumocystis carinii pneumonia, 396, 399
Podiatrists, 75, 311
Point-of-service (POS) plans, 519, 582
Poison ivy/oak/sumac, 420
Polarity therapy, 167–168
Polaroid lenses, 485
Ponstel, 461
Popoff, Peter, 40, 159
"Poppers," 427
Portability (of insurance), 515t, 517
Portal of entry, 582
Positive test, definition, 582
Positron emission tomography (PET), 86
Post hoc, ergo propter hoc fallacy, 18–19
Post-it advertisements, 61
Post, Charles W., 255
Postal Service; *see* U.S. Postal Service
Potentials Unlimited, 558t

Powwow, 140
Practical nurses, 76
Prana, 140
Pratkanis, Dr. Anthony R., 39
Precertification, 582
Precursor, 582
Pre-existing illness, 515t, 516–517
Preferred Provider Organizations (PPOs),
     519, 523, 582
Pregnancy
     and alcohol, 182
     and aspirin, 421
     and folic acid, 225, 244
     and HIV testing, 398
     iron supplementation, 244–245
     prenatal care, 582
     recommended medical care, 471t
     tests for, 185, 470
Premenstrual dysphoric disorder (PMDD),
     461
Premenstrual syndrome (PMS), 244, 461–
     462, 582
Prenatal care, 470
Presbyopia, 182t, 480, 481
Prescription drugs, 408, 410, 555–556,
     582
     advertising of, 53–55
Prescription for Nutritional Healing, 257
Prescriptions
     how to read, 410t, 411
     obtaining a refill, 96–97
President's Council on Physical Fitness
     and Sports, 327
Prevalence, definition, 582
"Preventative maintenance," by
     chiropractors, 150
Prevention Book Club, 63, 265
Prevention magazine, 24t, 25, 27t, 264–
     265, 509
Preventive Medicine Research Institute,
     345
Price, Dr. Westin A., 131
Price-Pottenger Nutrition Foundation, 131
Primary care, definition, 76, 582
Primrose oil, 248t
Princeton Brain Bio Center, 109
Principia College, 160
Priorities for Health, 24, 32, 565
Pritikin diet, 346
Probe newsletter, 24
Procaine tablets, 508
Procter & Gamble, 289
*Professional's Handbook of
     Complementary & Alternative
     Medicines*, 252
Progesterone, 466, 472
Project Cure, 391
Prometheus Books, 27
Propecia, 450
Propolis, 249t
Prostaglandin, 347, 468
Prostate-specific antigen (PSA) test, 83
Prosthesis, definition, 582
Prosthodontics, 120

Protection, consumer; *see* Consumer
     protection
Proteins, 212
     complete, 576
     sources, 219t
     supplements, 249–251t, 324
Protocol, experimental, 582
Provider, definition, 515t
Provocation-neutralization tests, 169–170
Proxmire Amendment, 236
Prozac, 114, 362, 461
Pseudoscience, 21, 582
Psoriasis, 448
Psychiatric nurses, 101
Psychiatric treatment; *see under* Mental
     health care
Psychiatrists, 100, 101
Psychic healing, 158–162, 582
     Christian Science, 159–160
     evaluation of, 161–162
     evangelical healers, 40, 158–159
     fraud in, 40, 159, 161
     Kirlian photography, 158, 162
     prayer, 160–161
     psychic surgery, 161, 582
     therapeutic touch, 162
Psychic hotlines, 115
Psychoanalysis, 102
Psychoanalysts, 101
Psychologic testing, 100, 114–115
Psychologists, 100–101, 311
Psychomotor retardation, 582
Psychoneuroimmunology, 582
Psychosomatic disorders, 105, 582
Psychosurgery, 583
Psychotherapy, 102–103, 583
     mismanagement of, 115–116
     satisfaction with, 106–107
Psychotic reactions, 100, 104, 583
Psychotropic drug, 583
Psyllium, 345, 432t
Public Citizen Health Research Group, 9,
     93, 521, 564
Puffery, 6, 50, 583
Pulp, of tooth, 127
Pulse, target for aerobic exercise, 305,
     305t
Pulse diagnosis, 142, 166
Pulse monitors, 316–317
Pulse-A-Rhythm, 366
Pumphrey, Jennifer E., 258
Pure Food and Drug Act, 548–549, 550
"Purification program," 114
Puritan's Pride, 562
Pyorrhea, 583
Pyridoxine; *see* Vitamin B$_6$

Q

Qigong, 141–142
Quack(s)
     characteristics, 36, 43t
     definitions, 36
     self-deception, 41
     types, 43

Quackery and frauds, vii–viii, 3, 7–8, 33–
     46; *see also* "Alternative" methods;
     Enforcement actions; Quacks; Mental
     health care, questionable practices
     AIDS, 395, 400–403
     arthritis, 365–370
     breast developers, 62, 63
     cancer; *see* Cancer treatment,
         questionable methods
     congressional investigation of, vii, 38
     cost, 3, 35
     dangers, 3, 39–40, 137, 163, 507
     definitions, 7, 36–37, 583
     dental, 130–132
     device; *see* Devices, health, quack
     fad diagnoses, 38, 132, 168–171
     food faddism; *see* Food faddism
     freedom of choice issue, vii–viii, 43,
         44–45, 373, 391
     hair-growth frauds, 450–451
     health fraud conferences, 398, 558
     insurance fraud, 91, 171, 389, 540–541
     life extension, 507–509
     mail-order products, 8, 60–64, 348
     misconceptions, 40
     nutrition; *see* Food faddism
     promotion of, vii, 7, 22–23, 36, 379,
         390–392
     questionable diagnostic tests, 169, 170,
         261–262, 384–385, 386–387, 455,
         560
     recognizing, 30, 42–44, 43t, 235t, 365,
         390
     telemarketing schemes, 66, 151, 489,
         561, 563, 564
     and terminal illness, 389, 507
     unscientific medical care, 168–173
     Victim Redress Task Force, 565
     victims of, 37, 38, 39–40, 66, 112, 132,
         153, 158, 160, 161, 170, 224, 243,
         254, 265, 293, 369, 387, 388, 390
     vulnerability to, 7–8, 15, 38–39, 364–
         365, 379
     water purifier frauds, 489
     weight control; *see* Weight control,
         questionable products
Quackwatch, 30, 230, 392, 493, 565
Quality assurance, 515t
Questionable health care; *see*
     "Alternative" methods
Quimby, Phineas Parkurst, 159

R

R.J. Reynolds Tobacco Company, 59, 60
Radiance Technique, 168
Radial keratotomy (RK), 483
Radiation, minimizing, 86, 129, 130
Radiation therapy, 376
Radiopaque, 583
Radionics and radiesthesia, 168, 385
Radionuclide imaging, 86
Radon
     and cancer, 183, 374
     mines, and arthritis, 366–377

RAND Corporation, 20, 148
Randi, James, 40, 159, 162, 163
Raso, Jack, 61
Raw milk, 250t, 564
RDAs, 216–217, 237, 583
Reach to Recovery, 473
Rebound (from medication), definition, 583
Rebound scurvy, 244, 583
Recalled By Life, 390
Recommended Dietary Allowances (RDAs); *see* RDAs
Recovery groups, 192–193
Redux, 283–284
Reference Dietary Intakes (DRIs), 214–215, 216–217
References, how to locate, 14
Reflexology, 144, 583
Reflexophone, 491
Refractive surgery, 483
Regulatory letter, 583
Reich, Dr. Wilhelm, 385
Reiki, 168
Relax-A-Cizor, 319
Relman, Dr. Arnold S., 140, 389
Remission, 583
Renewability (of insurance), 517
Renner, Dr. John H., 400
Renova, 445
Rescue factors, 376
Rescue Remedy, 108
Research design, 16–17
Residential care, 203
Resolve, 469
Resource-based relative value scale (RBRVS), 528t, 529
Resperin Corporation, 381
Respiratory therapists, 77t
Resveratrol, 250t
Retin-A, 445
Retina, 583
Revici, Dr. Emmanuel, 384–385
Revlon, 63
Rexall Sundown, Inc., 290
Reye's syndrome, 421
R-Garden Internationale, 561
Rheumatoid arthritis, 360, 361
Risk-benefit analysis, 583
Risk factors, 583
   for cancer, 374–375
   for heart disease, 334–337
   for osteoporosis, 471
   for stroke, 350
Risk markers, 17
Ritalin, 105, 114
RNA/DNA, 250t, 469
Roberts, Oral, 159
Robins, A.H., Co., 560
Rodale Press, 264–265
Rodale, J.I., 264
Rodale, Robert, 245
Rogaine, 449–450
   ads for, 53, 55
Rolfing, 168

Ronsard, Nicole, 289
Root canal therapy, 127–128
   unfair criticism of, 131
Root doctors, 140
Rorschach inkblot test, 114
Rosa, Emily, 162
Rose, Dr. Louis, 161
Rosen, Dr. Gerald, 107
Roughage; *see* Fiber, dietary
Rowing machines, 310, 314t
Royal jelly, 250t
RU-486, 468–469
Rubella, 583
Rutin, 236, 250t
Rx symbol, 410
Rynearson, Dr. Edward H., 265

S
Saccharin, 288
Safe Medical Devices Act of 1990, 478–479, 478, 552, 556
Safety belts, 183
Sagan, Dr. Carl, 15, 16
St. John's wort, 253t
Salaman, Frank, 391, 401
Salt sensitivity, 583
Sampson, Dr. Wallace I., 144, 156, 387, 395, 488
Sargenti method, 128
Sarsaparilla, 251
"Sauna shorts," 321
Saunas, 321
Saw palmetto, 253
Scarsdale Medical Diet, 280
Schafer, Robert, 234
Schauss, Alexander G., 264
Scheel, John, 152
Schering Corporation, 285–286
Schissel, Dr. Marvin J., 137
Schizophrenia, 583
Schlink, F.J., 550
Schuessler, Dr. W.H., 157
Schulte, Fred, 66
Science and Health, 159
Scientific fraud, 20
Scientific method, 16, 583
Scientific research, typical steps in, 18t
Scientology, 113–114
Sclerology, 153
Sclerotherapy, 454t
Screening test, 583
Sea salt, 250t
Sealants, dental, 122
Sebaceous glands, 446, 447
Seborrheic dermatitis, 448
Sebum, 446
Second opinions, 88, 539
Seldane, 53, 415
Self magazine, 23
Self-care, 179–193
   dental, 124–127
   effectiveness of, 181
   health promotion, 181–184, 183t
   home health library, 190t

   home medical tests, 184, 185, 187
   for irritable bowel syndrome, 186
   publications, 188–189
   purposes, 180–181, 181t
   questionable products, 107–108, 182t, 188
   reasons for, 180
   self-diagnosis, 73, 184–185
   self-examination, breasts and testicles, 83, 375
   self-medication, frequency of, 416
   types of, 180
Self-help groups, 189, 191–193, 192t, 583
Self-Help Sourcebook, 192
Self-Test Nutrition Guide, 188
Semen, 583
Sensitivity (of test), 583
Sensitivity training, 109
Serotonin, 461
Serum, 583
"Set point," 583
714X, 384
Seventh-day Adventists, 160, 224
Sex aids, phony, 62, 426–427, 560, 562–563, 575
Sexual therapy, 101–102
Sexually transmitted disease (STD), 466, 583
Shaklee, Forrest C., 303
Shaklee Corporation, 303
Shampoos, 447–448
Shark cartilage, 382–383
Sharks Don't Get Cancer, 382
Shaw, Sandy, 257, 287, 507
Shawnee Mission Medical Center, 90
Shekelle, Dr. Paul M., 146
Shelton, Herbert M., 149
Sherr, Jeremy, 155
Sherley, Rep. Swager, 550
Shiatsu, 574
Shock treatment; *see* Electroconvulsive therapy (ECT)
Shoes, for sports, 317–318
Side effect, 583
Siegel, Dr. Bernie, 386
Siemens Hearing Instruments, 488
Sigmoidoscope, 583
Silicone
   "antibody" tests, 455
   implants, 453, 455
   injections, 455
Simeons, Dr. Alfred T., 283
Simethicone, 423
Simonton, Dr. O. Carl, 386
Simple carbohydrates, 212, 583
Simplesse, 289
Sinclair, Upton, 550
Singer, Dr. Barry, 22
Single photon emission computerized tomography (SPECT), 86
"60 Minutes" (CBS-TV), 28, 132, 368, 382, 387, 502
Skeptical Inquirer, 565
Skeptics Society, 565

607

Ski exercisers, 313t, 316
Skilled nursing care, 203, 583
  insurance for, 516
Skin
  acne care, 446–447
  bleaches, 446
  cancer, 451
  changes with aging, 444
  cross-section, 447
  dry, 443
  testing degree of oiliness, 444
Skin and beauty aids, 441–457; *see also*
  Cosmetics; Cosmetic surgery
Sleep aids, 433–434
Slim-Fast, 287
Slim-Skins, 290
Sloan-Kettering Memorial Cancer Center,
  381
Smith, Dr. Lendon H., 266
Smoke detectors, 183
Smokers' Rights Action Guide, 60
Smokeless tobacco, 133–134
Smoking cessation, 183–184, 375, 434
Smythe, Donald L., 561
Snakeroot, 252
Snuff, dangers of, 133
Soaps, 442–443
Social Security Act, funeral expense
  payment, 504
Social workers, 77t, 101
Society for Cancer Research, 383
Sodium
  Benzoate (food additive), 554
  dietary, 216t, 225–226
  and high blood pressure, 225, 229t, 350,
    351
  infant needs, 223
Solarama Board, 366
"Soldier's sickness," 414
Solomon, Dr. Neil, 290
Sore throat products, 424
Spam e-mail, 30, 557
Spanish fly, 426–427
Specificity (of test), 583
SPECT, 86
SpectraCell Laboratories, 262
Speculum, 583
Speech pathologists, 77t
Sphygmomanometer, 187, 583
Spinal manipulation, complications, 150–
  151
Spiritualism, 163
Spirulina, 250t
Splenda; see Sucralose
Spondylolisthesis, 146
Spondylotherapy, 491
Spontaneous remission, 40–41, 376, 583
Sportelli, Dr. Louis, 144
Sports bras, 318
Sports drinks, 324t, 325
Sports medicine specialists, 310–311
"Spot-reducers," 319
Sprain, 583
Squibb, E.R., and Sons, 239

Stair steppers and climbers, 316
Standard Process Laboratories, 264
Starch blockers, 258, 286
Starches, 212, 576
Starket Laboratories, Inc., 488
Statistics, misuse of, 18–19
Steiner, Dr. Rudolf, 153, 383
Stenosis, 583
Sterilization, surgical, 467–468
Stern, Dr. Judith, 285
Steroid hormones
  and allergies, 420
  "alternatives" to; *see* "Ergogenic aids"
  and arthritis, 363, 369, 370
  use by athletes, 325–326, 326t
Still, Dr. Andrew Taylor, 73–74
Stimulants for fatigue, 434–435, 435t
Stop-loss provisions, 516
Strain, 583
Straus, Charlotte Gerson, 383
Strength training, 304, 307, 317
  equipment for, 317
Streptococcus B screening, 470
"Stress supplements," 239–240
Stress testing, 352–353, 583
  appropriateness, 306–307, 353
Stresstabs, 239–240
Stretching, 308–309, 308t
Stroke, 334t, 350–351
  chiropractic manipulation and, 150–151
  risk factors, 350
Stutz, Dr. David R., 95
Student health services, 197–198, 525
Stye, 430
Subitramine hydrochloride, 284
Subliminal tapes, 62, 107–108, 290
"Subluxations," 146–147, 150, 151
Subscriber (insurance), definition, 515t
Substance abuse counselors, 102
Suburban Water Testing Laboratories, 489
Sucralose, 289
Sucrose, 212, 213
Sugar, 212–213
  infant needs, 223
  myths about, 111, 121, 131, 213
  role in tooth decay, 121, 223
"Sugar blockers," 286
Sugar-free gum, 126
Suicide, assisted, 502–503
Sulfanilamide elixir, 550–551
Sun protection factor (SPF), 451–452, 583
Sunette, 288–289
Sunglasses, 485
Sunlamps, 452
Sunlight, protection from, 451–452
Sunrider Corporation, 66
Superoxide dismutase (SOD), 250t, 367,
  508
Supplements; *see* Dietary supplements
Supportive psychotherapy, 102
Suppositories, 584
Surgery, 87–89
  abortions, voluntary, 468–469
  ambulatory, 88

  arthritis, 363–364
  cancer, 376
  cardiovascular, 354–355
  cataract, 483, 485–486
  cesarean section, 470
  choosing a surgeon, 87
  circumcision, 89
  cosmetic; *see* Cosmetic surgery
  gallbladder, 89
  laser 88–89, 449
  oral, 120
  placebo effect, 41–42, 41t, 582
  plastic; *see* Cosmetic surgery
  and patient responsibility, 88
  and physician responsibility, 88
  preparation for, 87
  psychic, 161, 582
  psychosurgery, 583
  refractive, 483
  second opinions about, 88, 539
  sterilization, 464t, 467–468
  unnecessary, 87–88, 486, 584
  weight control, 292
Swan, Dr. Rita, 160
Sweatshirts, rubber, 319
Systemic, definition, 584
Szasz, Dr. Thomas, 114

T
"T-groups," 109
T-lymphocytes, 396
T-Up, 402–403
Tabloid newspapers, 6, 24, 24t, 371
  advertising in, 61
Take Care of Yourself, 188, 190t
Talcum powder, 318, 430
Tampons, 460
Tanning accelerators, 452
Tanning pills, 452
Tanning salons, 452
Tardive dyskinesia, 104
Tarnower, Dr. Herman, 280
Task Force on Nutrition Support in AIDS,
  399
Teeth, anatomy of, 121
Telemarketing schemes, 66, 151, 489, 561,
  563, 564
Tendon, 584
TENS device, 363, 584
Tension, symptoms of, 105
Tertiary care center, 584
Testable hypothesis, 584
Testimonials, 20–21, 40, 44, 55, 64, 65,
  160, 294, 392, 584
Tetracyclines, 425
Textbook of Natural Medicine, 152
Thalidomide, 549, 551
Theragran Stress Formula, 239
Therapeutic touch, 162
Thermography, 375, 584
Thermometers, mercury in, 133
Third-party payer, 584
Thomas, Adrian, 409
Thomas, Dr. Paul, 237

Thomson, Samuel, 413
Thought field therapy, 113
Thyroid function test, 82
Thyroid hormone, 279
Time magazine, 23, 25, 114, 163
"Tired blood," 57
Tissue salts, 157
TM; *see* Transcendental meditation (TM)
TMJ problems, 128, 131, 132, 584
Tobacco products
    advertising, 7, 59–60
    smokeless, 133–134
Today's Health, 272
Tolerable upper intake level (UL), 217
Tolerance (to drug), 584
Tomatis International, 111
Tonometer, 81
Tooth decay, 121–122
Toothbrushes, 125
Toothpastes, 124–125
Topical use, definition, 584
TOPS (Take Off Pounds Sensibly), 293
Total parenteral nutrition (TPN), 400
Tourette syndrome, 103
Toxic shock syndrome (TSS), 460
Traditional Chinese medicine, 141–144, 576
Trainers
    athletic, 311
    personal, 321
Tranquilizers, 103–104
Trans-fatty acids, 214, 340, 342, 584
Transcendental meditation (TM), 165
Transderm Nitro, 415
Transderm Scop, 433
Transillumination, 375
Traveler's diarrhea, 429
Treadmills, 315t, 316
Treatment planning, 584
Tremor, definition, 584
Tretinoin, 445, 447
Triglycerides, 214
Tubal ligation, 467
Tufts University Health & Nutrition Letter, 27t, 32, 62, 318, 324, 461
Tumor registries, 376
"20/20" (ABC-TV), 150, 505
Twilight sleep, 134
Tye, Joe B., 59
Tylenol; *see* Acetaminophen
Tyler, Dr. Varro E., 286, 382

U
UCR fee, 523, 528, 535
Ulett, Dr. George A., 142
Ultrafast computed tomography, 353
Ultrasound devices, 584
    diagnostic uses, 87, 273, 353–354
    and pregnancy, 470
    therapeutic uses, 363, 485
Ultraviolet light
    and acne, 447
    and cataracts, 485
    and skin cancer, 451

Unbundling, 584
Uniform Anatomical Gift Act, 500
United Network for Organ Sharing (UNOS), 500
United Sciences of America, 22
United States Pharmacopeia, 411, 584
United States Pharmacopeial Convention, 411
University of California at Berkeley Wellness Letter, 446, 489
Unnecessary surgery, 87–88, 584
Upcoding, 584
Urinalysis, 81
Urticaria, 418
U.S. Centers for Disease Control and Prevention (CDC), 85, 170, 180, 225, 305, 326, 338, 360, 396, 397, 398, 563
U.S. Department of Agriculture, 215, 226, 278, 563
U.S. Dietary Guidelines; *see under* Dietary guidelines
U.S. News & World Report, 25, 200, 282, 417, 525
U.S. Office of Education, 143, 147, 574
U.S. Postal Service, 11, 12t, 67, 561–563
    enforcement actions, 157, 259, 287, 291, 366, 402, 562–563
    Mail Order Consumer Protection Amendments Act (1983), 551, 562
U.S. Preventive Services Task Force, 12, 19, 82, 83, 84–85t, 183, 244, 339, 471t, 481
U.S. Recommended Daily Allowances (U.S. RDAs), 584
Utilization review, 88, 515t, 536, 584

V
Vaccination kits, bogus, 183
Vaginal hygiene, 462
Vaginal sponge, 464t, 465–466
Vaginitis, 462–463
Vale, Jason, 557
Valium, 104, 105
Vaporizers, 428
Varicella-zoster virus, 584
Vasectomy, 467–468
Vegan, definition, 224, 584
Vegatest, 156
Vegetarianism, 224–225, 367
Vegetarian Times, 26, 224
Venoms, as arthritis remedy, 364
Vertebra, definition, 584
Vertebral Subluxation Research Institute, 151
Vertically integrated system, 584
Very-low-density lipoproteins (VLDL), 214
Viatical settlements, 499
Vibrators, and arthritis, 365
Vickery, Dr. Donald M., 179, 180, 188
Vinyl chloride, and cancer, 375
Viral infections, and cancer, 375
Viralizer, 489–490

Vis Medicatrix Naturae, 140
Vision Dieter, 290
Vision products and services, 480–486
Visual acuity, 480, 481
Visual training, optometric, 112, 167, 584
"Vital energy," 140
Vital Foods, Inc., 256
Vitalism, 140–141, 584
Vitamin(s), 214; *see also* Dietary supplements; Food faddism
    A, 237, 241
        toxicity, 243
    advertising, 24, 48, 238t
    amounts needed; *see* DRIs
    for arthritis, 367
    B_6
        for premenstrual syndrome, 241, 461
        toxicity, 244
    B_{12}
        injections, 37, 76
        and vegetarian diets, 224
    biotin, 214
    C
        and cancer, 242–243
        and the common cold, 18, 18t, 242, 428
        and false-negative test for occult blood, 187
        and food processing, 239
        and longevity, 509
        and smoking, 239
        and tooth erosion, 122
    D, 214, 471
        dangers of excess, 243–244
    E, 243
        anticoagulant effect, 241,348
        as moisturizer, 444t
        and heart disease, 241, 348
        therapeutic claims, 243
    and exercise, 239, 324
    fat-soluble, 214
    folic acid, 225, 229t, 244, 337
    as food additives, 251, 554
    food sources, 219t
    and hair analysis, 261–262
    K, 214
    and life-extension claims, 507
    losses during food processing, 239, 250t
    megavitamin therapy, 109–110, 580
    niacin; *see* Niacin
    as placebos, 42
    Recommended Dietary Allowances (RDAs); *see* RDAs
    shots, overuse of, 76
    storage in body, 238t
    supplements
        appropriate use, 244–245
        for infants, 223, 244
        and children, 244
        chiropractors and, 260
        expenditures for, 236, 539
        multilevel companies and, 64–66
        "natural vs. synthetic," 240
        needed by vegetarians, 224, 244

pharmacists and, 259–260
and pregnancy, 225, 244
promotion, 56–58
reasons for use, 236
for "special needs," 219
spray products, 560
"stress," 239–240
types of, 236
and weight control, 244
water-soluble, 214
"Vitamin B5," 250t
"Vitamin B15"; see Pangamic acid
"Vitamin B17"; see Laetrile
Vitamin Gap Test, National, 263
"Vitamin O," 561
"Vitamin P"; see Bioflavonoids
Voll, Dr. Reinhold, 156
von Peczely, Ignatz, 153
Voodoo, 140
Vrilium Tube, 366

W
Waist-to-hip ratio (WHR), 273–274
Waiting periods (insurance), 515t, 516
Waiver of premium, 515t
Walford, Dr. Roy, 507
Walker, Dr. Scott, 112
Walsh, Jerry, 38
Warts, 427
Washington Consumers' CHECKBOOK, 76
Water
    bottled, 489
    "catalyst-altered," 247t
    as nutrient, 212, 219t
    purifiers, 489
    testing, 489
Waxman, Rep. Henry, 134
Web sites
    judging credibility, 29–30, 31
    reliable, 29
Weasel words, 6, 50
Weider, Joe, 327
Weider Health and Fitness, Inc., 64, 560
Weight control, 181, 271–298
    basic concepts, 272–276, 277t, 277
    behavior modification, 297

body fat estimations, 273–274
desirable weights, 273, 273t
    dietary guideline, 216t
diets, questionable, 278–283, 281t
difficulty with dieting, 274–277, 279
drugs, 283–284
eating disorders, 278
exercise and, 276, 296t, 297, 323, 324t
gadgets and gimmicks, 290–291
government regulatory actions, 290–292, 294–295
human chorionic gonadotropin (HCG), 283
hypnosis for, 292
low-calorie products, 287–289
marketplace, 278
meal-replacement products, 279, 287–288
myths vs. facts, 277t
"new lifestyle language," 294t
obesity clinics, 293–295
promotions, 62
organizations, 292–295
questionable procedures, 289–290, 292
questionable products, 8, 62, 157, 284–287, 319
risks of obesity, 181, 273–274, 377
suggestions for, 295, 297
surgery, 292
and vitamin supplements, 244
Weight cycling, 275–276
Weight training; see Strength training
Weight Watchers, 293, 294, 294t, 295
Weil, Dr. Andrew, 27, 267
Weiss Rating Guide to HMOs and Health Insurers, 526t, 527
Weiwel, Frank, 391
Weleda, Inc., 155–156
Wennberg, Dr. John E., 88
Wheat germ, 250t
Wheat germ oil, 560
Wheat grass juice, 250t
Whelan, Dr. Elizabeth M., 251
Whirlpool baths, 321–322, 363, 365
Whitaker, Dr. Julian, 60
White, Dr. Philip L., 279

White House Domestic Policy Council, 10, 541t, 542t
Wiley, Dr. Harvey W., 550, 551
Williams, J.B., Company, 57, 560
Winfrey, Oprah, 279
Wisdom tooth extraction, 130
Withdrawal reaction, 584
    caffeine, 105, 435
    nicotine, 434
Wolf, Naomi, 441
Wolfe, Dr. Sidney, 556, 564
Woodrum, Eric, 165
World Chiropractic Alliance, 146
World Health Organization, 402
World Wide Web, 6, 29, 80
    searching, 29
Worrall, Dr. Russell, 153, 485
Wrinkle removers, 444, 445
Wyden, Rep. Ron, 284, 294, 468

X
X-ray examinations
    chiropractic, 150
    dental, 129–130
    medical; see Medical imaging
    osteoporosis screening, 472
Xenical, 284

Y
Yetley, Elizabeth A., 234
Yiamouyiannis, Dr. John, 122
Yo-yo dieting, 274–275, 584
Yoga, 167
Yogurt, 431
York Barbell Co., 327
Young, Dr. James Harvey, 3, 40, 236, 551
Young, Dr. Frank E., 395, 547, 551
Young, Gregory W., 505

Z
Zen macrobiotic diet, 255
Zimmerman, David, 285, 391, 418
Zinc, 223, 250t
Zone therapy; see Reflexology
Zostrix, 364
Zygon International, 108